Ferraro's Fundamentals of Maxillofacial Surgery

Peter J. Taub • Pravin K. Patel • Steven R. Buchman
Mimis N. Cohen
Editors

Ferraro's Fundamentals of Maxillofacial Surgery

Second Edition

Springer

AMERICAN SOCIETY OF MAXILLOFACIAL SURGEONS
ASMS
FOUNDED 1947

Editors
Peter J. Taub, MD
Division of Plastic and Reconstructive Surgery
Mount Sinai Medical Center
New York, NY
USA

Pravin K. Patel, MD, FACS
Pediatric Plastic and Craniofacial Surgery
University of Illinois
Division of Plastic, Reconstructive
and Cosmetic Surgery
Chicago, IL
USA

Steven R. Buchman, MD
Craniofacial Anomalies Program
Division of Plastic and Reconstructive Surgery
University of Michigan Medical School
Ann Arbor, MI
USA

Mimis N. Cohen, MD, FACS, FAAP
Division of Plastic,
Reconstructive and Cosmetic Surgery
University of Illinois
Chicago, IL
USA

ISBN 978-1-4614-8340-3 ISBN 978-1-4614-8341-0 (eBook)
DOI 10.1007/978-1-4614-8341-0
Springer New York Heidelberg Dordrecht London

Library of Congress Control Number: 2014947228

Printed on acid-free paper

Springer is part of Springer Science+Business Media (www.springer.com)

Foreword

This book is designed to give a comprehensive evaluation of maxillofacial surgery, which is the specialty dealing with the diagnosis and treatment of diseases and injuries of the facial craniomaxillofacial skeleton and soft tissues. The fully updated second edition of *Fundamentals of Maxillofacial Surgery* brings together information on a multitude of subjects dealing with this specialty.

This book begins with the embryology and anatomy of the head, neck, and craniofacial regions. It is necessary to understand the normal anatomy of these areas in order to deal with the abnormal shapes and developmental anomalies that can occur. The early chapters also deal with oral anatomy, odontogenesis, and facial aesthetics. Chapters 5, 6, and 7 deal with imaging, regional anesthesia, and fixation techniques necessary to operate in this area. Chapters 8 and 9 discuss the use of bone grafts and newer biomaterials. Chapters 10, 11, 12, 13, 14, 15, 16, 17, 18, 19, and 20 deal with the diagnosis and treatment of fractures of the entire facial skeleton.

Special sections discuss genioplasty, gunshot wounds, microvascular reconstruction, and secondary skeletal and soft tissue reconstruction. The final chapters deal with the evaluation, orthodontic treatment, and surgical treatment of the patient in preparation for orthognathic surgery. Included in this portion of the book is the construction of models with splints and the need for dental prosthetics and extractions to prepare the patient for the impending orthognathic procedures.

It is hoped that with this information, readers will be able to treat most of the cases in the maxillofacial region to which they will be exposed.

Columbus, OH, USA

James W. Ferraro, DDS, MD

Contents

Contributors

Howard Aduss, DDS The Craniofacial Center, Division of Plastic Reconstructive and Cosmetic Surgery, University of Illinois, Chicago, IL, USA

Mairaj K. Ahmed, DDS, MS Department of Dentistry/Oral and Maxillofacial Surgery, Icahn School of Medicine at Mount Sinai, New York, NY, USA

Bassan J. Allan, MD, MBA Department of Surgery, University of Miami, Miami, FL, USA

Anuja K. Antony, MD, MPH, FACS Division of Plastic, Reconstructive and Cosmetic Surgery, University of Illinois, Chicago, IL, USA

Ali Baba Attaie, DDS, MPH Pediatrics and Dentistry, Pediatrics and Dental Medicine, Icahn School of Medicine at Mount Sinai, New York, NY, USA

Stephen Baker, MD, DDS, FACS Department of Plastic Surgery, Georgetown University Hospital, Washington, DC, USA

Thaddeus S. Boucree II, MD, DDS Department of Oral and Maxillofacial Surgery, Larkin Community Hospital, Miami, FL, USA

Sean G. Boutros, MD, FACS Houston Plastic and Craniofacial Surgery, Houston, TX, USA

Emile N. Brown, MD Division of Plastic and Reconstructive Surgery, University of Maryland R Adams Cowley Shock Trauma Center, Baltimore, MD, USA

Karl C. Bruckman, MD, DDS Department of Oral and Maxillofacial Surgery, Thomas Jefferson University Hospital, Philadelphia, PA, USA

Edward P. Buchanan, MD Department of Plastic Surgery, Baylor College of Medicine, Houston, TX, USA

Steven R. Buchman, MD Craniofacial Anomalies Program, Division of Plastic and Reconstructive Surgery, University of Michigan Medical School, Ann Arbor, MI, USA

Stephen A. Chidyllo, MD, DDS Division of Plastic and Reconstructive Surgery, Department of Surgery, Jersey Shore University Medical Center, West Long Branch, NJ, USA

Mimis N. Cohen, MD, FACS, FAAP Division of Plastic, Reconstructive and Cosmetic Surgery, University of Illinois, Chicago, IL, USA

Lisa R. David, MD Department of Plastic and Reconstructive Surgery, Wake Forest University, Winston-Salem, NC, USA

Brent R. DeGeorge Jr., MD, PhD Department of Plastic Surgery, University of Virginia School of Medicine, Charlottesville, VA, USA

Samuel DeMaria Jr., MD Division of Liver Transplantation, Department of Anesthesiology, The Mount Sinai HELPS Center, The Mount Sinai Medical Center, New York, NY, USA

James W. Ferraro, DDS, MD Franklin Park Physical Medicine, Department of Surgery, Columbus, OH, USA

Mark Fisher, BS Division of Plastic and Reconstructive Surgery, University of Maryland R Adams Cowley Shock Trauma Center, Baltimore, MD, USA

Jose I. Garri, MD, DMD Department of Plastic Surgery, University of Miami, Miami, FL, USA

Roop Gill, BM, MRCS (Eng) Department of Plastic Surgery, Vanderbilt University Medical Center, Nashville, TN, USA

Arun K. Gosain, MD Division of Pediatric Plastic Surgery, Lurie Children's Hospital and Northwestern University Feinberg School of Medicine, Chicago, IL, USA

Kevin Han, MD Department of Plastic Surgery, Georgetown University Hospital, Washington, DC, USA

Robert M. Van Haren, MD, MsPH Department of Surgery, University of Miami, Miami, FL, USA

Raymond Harshbarger, MD, FACS, FAAP Craniofacial and Pediatric Plastic Surgery, Dell Children's Medical Center, University Medical Center Brackenridge, UT Austin, Austin, TX, USA

Cathy R. Henry, MD Division of Plastic Surgery, Penn State Hershey Medical Center, Hershey, PA, USA

Joseph L. Hill, MD Division of Plastic Surgery, University of Kentucky College of Medicine, Lexington, KY, USA

Brian Ho, MD Department of Otolaryngology, Georgia Regents University, Augusta, GA, USA

William Hoffman, MD Division of Plastic and Reconstructive Surgery, Department of Surgery, University of California, San Francisco, San Francisco, CA, USA

Larry H. Hollier, MD Department of Plastic Surgery, Baylor College of Medicine, Houston, TX, USA

Department of Plastic Surgery, Texas Children's Hospital, Houston, TX, USA

Reza Jarrahy, FACS, FAAP Division of Plastic and Reconstructive Surgery, David Geffen School of Medicine at UCLA, Los Angeles, CA, USA

Alexandra Junewicz Case Western Reserve University School of Medicine, Cleveland, OH, USA

Patrick Kelley, MD Department of Plastic Surgery, Dell Children's Medical Center, Austin, TX, USA

Kevin J. Kelly, MD, DDS Craniofacial Surgery Center, Department of Plastic Surgery, Vanderbilt University Medical Center, Nashville, TN, USA

David Y. Khechoyan, MD Department of Plastic Surgery, Baylor College of Medicine, Houston, TX, USA

Adam I. Levine, MD Department of Anesthesiology, Icahn School of Medicine at Mount Sinai, New York, NY, USA

Kant Y. Lin, MD Department of Plastic Surgery, University of Virginia Health System, Charlottesville, VA, USA

Lun-Jou Lo, MD Department of Plastic and Reconstructive Surgery, Chang Gung Memorial Hospital and Chang Gung University, Taoyuan, Taiwan

Joseph E. Losee, MD Department of Plastic Surgery, University of Pittsburgh Medical Center, Pittsburgh, PA, USA

Division of Pediatric Plastic Surgery, Children's Hospital of Pittsburgh of UPMC, Pittsburgh, PA, USA

Donald R. Mackay, MD, FACS, FAAP Department of Surgery, Penn State Hershey, College of Medicine, Hershey, PA, USA

Antony Martin Department of Plastic Surgery, Georgia Regents University, Augusta, GA, USA

Carlos A. Martinez, MD Houston Plastic and Craniofacial Surgery, Houston, TX, USA

Mohamad Masoumy, MD Department of Surgery, Georgia Regents University, Augusta, GA, USA

Robert M. Menard, MD, FACS Pediatric Plastic and Craniofacial Surgery, Northern California Kaiser Permanente Craniofacial Clinic, Santa Clara, CA, USA

John M. Mesa, MD Plastic Surgery Center Internationale, Montclair, NJ, USA

Richard Monahan, DDS, MS Pediatric Plastic and Cleft/Craniofacial Surgery, Shriners Hospital for Children, Chicago, IL, USA

Laura A. Monson, MD Division of Plastic Surgery, Michael E. DeBakey Department of Surgery, Baylor College of Medicine, Houston, TX, USA

David E. Morris, MD Division of Plastic Reconstructive and Cosmetic Surgery, University of Illinois, Chicago, IL, USA

Delora L. Mount, MD, FACS, FAAP Division of Plastic Surgery, University of Wisconsin-Madison, Madison, WI, USA

American Family Children's Hospital, Madison, WI, USA

Sanjay Naran, MD Department of Plastic Surgery, University of Pittsburgh, Pittsburgh, PA, USA

Adam J. Oppenheimer, MD Department of Craniofacial Surgery, Seattle Children's Hospital, Seattle, WA, USA

Pravin K. Patel, MD, FACS Pediatric Plastic and Craniofacial Surgery, University of Illinois, Division of Plastic, Reconstructive and Cosmetic Surgery, Chicago, IL, USA

Ivo A. Pestana, MD Department of Plastic and Reconstructive Surgery, Wake Forest University, Winston-Salem, NC, USA

Matthew J. Ranzer, MD Division of Plastic Reconstructive and Cosmetic Surgery, University of Illinois, Chicago, IL, USA

Russell Reid, MD, PhD University of Chicago Medicine Comer Children's Hospital, Chicago, IL, USA

Eduardo D. Rodriguez, MD, DDS Division of Plastic and Reconstructive Surgery, University of Maryland R Adams Cowley Shock Trauma Center, Baltimore, MD, USA

Henry Schupert, DDS The Craniofacial Center, Division of Plastic Reconstructive and Cosmetic Surgery, University of Illinois, Chicago, IL, USA

Darren M. Smith, MD Department of Plastic Surgery, University of Pittsburgh Medical Center, Pittsburgh, PA, USA

Magdalena Soldanska, MD Division of Plastic and Reconstructive Surgery, Mount Sinai Medical Center, Icahn School of Medicine at Mount Sinai, New York, NY, USA

Jordan P. Steinberg, MD, PhD Northwestern University Feinberg School of Medicine, Chicago, IL, USA

Mitchell A. Stotland, MD, MS Section of Plastic Surgery, Dartmouth-Hitchcock Medical Center, Geisel School of Medicine at Dartmouth, Lebanon, NH, USA

Kristoffer B. Sugg, MD Division of Plastic and Reconstructive Surgery, University of Michigan Medical School, Ann Arbor, MI, USA

Peter J. Taub, MD Division of Plastic and Reconstructive Surgery, Mount Sinai Medical Center, New York, NY, USA

Seth Thaller, MD, DMD Division of Plastic and Reconstructive Surgery, Department of Surgery, University of Miami, Miami, FL, USA

Henry C. Vasconez, MD, FACS Division of Plastic Surgery, University of Kentucky College of Medicine, Lexington, KY, USA

Derrick C. Wan, MD Division of Plastic and Reconstructive Surgery, Stanford University Medical Center, Palo Alto, CA, USA

Bo Wang, MD Department of Surgery, University of Miami, Miami, FL, USA

Neil Warshawsky, DDS The Craniofacial Center, Division of Plastic Reconstructive and Cosmetic Surgery, University of Illinois, Chicago, IL, USA

William M. Weathers, MD Department of Plastic Surgery, Baylor College of Medicine, Houston, TX, USA

Andrew M. Wexler, MD, MA Department of Plastic Surgery, Craniofacial Services Southern California, Kaiser Permanente, U.S.C., Los Angeles, CA, USA

S. Anthony Wolfe, MD Department of Plastic and Reconstructive Surgery, Miami Children's Hospital, Miami, FL, USA

Erik M. Wolfswinkel, MD Department of Plastic Surgery, Baylor College of Medicine, Houston, TX, USA

Jeffrey Y. Wu Section of Plastic Surgery, Dartmouth-Hitchcock Medical Center, Geisel School of Medicine at Dartmouth, Lebanon, NH, USA

Jack C. Yu, MD, DMD, MS Ed, FACS Department of Plastic Surgery, Georgia Regents University, Augusta, GA, USA

Linping Zhao, PhD Division of Plastic, Reconstructive and Cosmetic Surgery, Department of Surgery, University of Illinois, Chicago, IL, USA

Part I

The Basics

Embryology of the Head and Neck

1

Peter J. Taub and John M. Mesa

Prenatal Development

Following fertilization, the fusion of two haploid germ cells, a diploid zygote with 46 chromosomes is produced. Mitotic division produces two daughter cells, each half the size of the original cell but containing the full complement of genetic information. Subsequent divisions produce a solid mass of cells by the fourth day ("morula"). As fluid accumulates within the morula, one group of cells accumulates on one side ("embryoblast") while the remaining group of cells surrounds the periphery ("trophoblast"). This new cystic structure is named a "blastocyst" (see Fig. 1.1). The outer trophoblast layer, from "tropho-" meaning nutrition, will become the placenta following implantation in the uterus by day 6. The inner embryoblast layer will become the embryo.

During the second week of gestation, the inner embryoblast differentiates into two germ cell layers to form a bilaminar embryo ("germ disk") that is surrounded by two fluid-filled cavities: the amniotic cavity and the primary yolk sack. The cell layer close to the trophoblast is named "epiblast" and the layer bellow is named "hypoblast" (see Fig. 1.2).

A localized thickening of the bilaminar embryo them forms, called the "prechordal plate," which gives polarity to the bilaminar disk. It will ultimately give origin to the mouth opening at the cephalad region of the embryo. Caudal to the prechordal plate, a cleft in the epiblast called the "primitive streak" will allow the migration of epiblast cells (neural crestal cells and other differentiating cells) into the space between the epiblast and hypoblast to create the mesoderm, endoderm, and notochord. The epiblast will become the ectoderm as part of a trilaminar embryo (see Fig. 1.3).

The Embryonic Period (Fourth to Eighth Weeks)

At approximately 22 days (third week), the neural tube begins to form, which will develop into the brain and spinal cord. The trilaminar embryo folds itself along the axis of the primitive streak/notochord to form a trilayer cylindrical structure that fuses ventrally and ultimately gives rise to the fetus (see Fig. 1.4). The head begins to form also around the fourth week, followed by the eyes, ears, nose, and mouth of the face. The cardiovascular system develops as a single blood vessel that goes on to form the heart. A heartbeat can be detected for the first time. During the fifth week, the arms and legs appear as buds off the sides of the embryo. At this stage, the embryo weighs just one gram and is about one inch in length.

The Fetal Period (Ninth Week to Birth)

The period of fetal development begins during the ninth week of gestation, when cell differentiation is mostly complete. This stage of prenatal development lasts the longest. By the end of the third month, all parts of the body will be present. Previously formed organ systems continue to develop and the genital system appears as the last to develop. The neural tube develops into the brain and spinal cord and neurons form. At this point, the fetus weighs around three ounces. During the fourth through sixth months, the brain and central nervous system become responsive and the heartbeat grows stronger. The fetus increases quite dramatically in size, increasing about six times in size. From 7 months until birth, the lungs begin to expand and contract.

P.J. Taub, MD (✉)
Division of Plastic and Reconstructive Surgery, Mount Sinai Medical Center, 5 East 98th Street, 15th Floor, New York, NY 10029, USA
e-mail: peter.taub@mountsinai.org

J.M. Mesa, MD
Plastic Surgery Center Internationale, Montclair, NJ, USA

P.J. Taub et al. (eds.), *Ferraro's Fundamentals of Maxillofacial Surgery*,
DOI 10.1007/978-1-4614-8341-0_1, © Springer Science+Business Media New York 2015

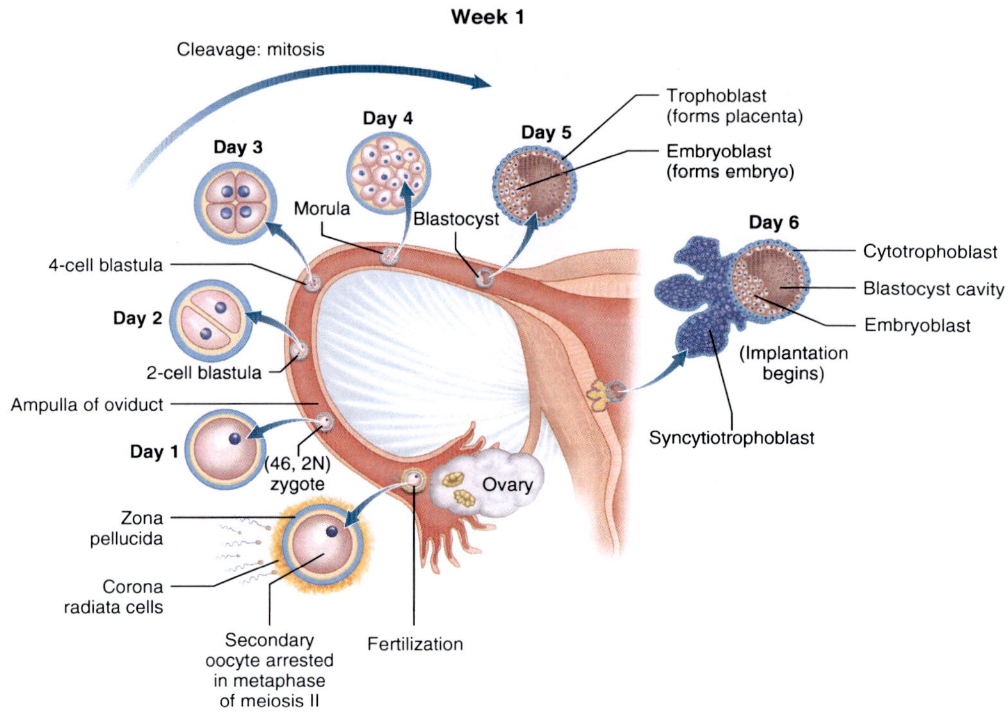

Fig. 1.1 Fertilization, embryogenesis, and implantation

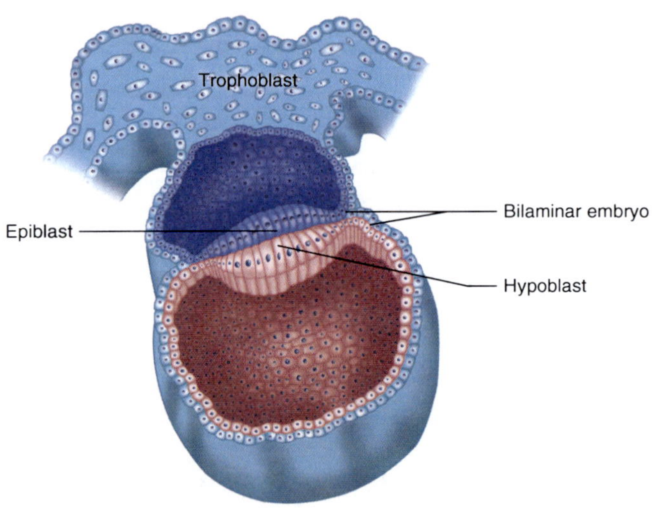

Fig. 1.2 Bilaminar embryo

Development of the Skull

The bones of the craniofacial skeleton originate from one of two sources. They form either from mesoderm that first transforms into cartilage and then into bone ("endochondral ossification") or from direct ossification of mesenchyme ("membranous ossification"). The majority of the cranial vault bones (frontal, temporal, parietal, and part of the occipital bone) originate from membranous ossification. The bones of the cranial base (the sphenoid, ethmoid, mastoid, and petrous portions of the temporal bone and the base of the occipital bone) originate by endochondral ossification. The facial bones (maxilla, mandible, zygomatic bone, squamosal portion of the temporal bone, and the primary hard palate) are also formed through by membranous ossification (see Fig. 1.5). Although the first pharyngeal arch (that will form the mandible) forms cartilage rod known as Meckel cartilage, this cartilage does not give origin to the mandible. The Meckel cartilage serves as a template for the mandible formation (that originates from membranous ossification of the mesenchyme). The Meckel cartilage then disappears.

The individual bones in the infant skull are held together by strong, fibrous, elastic cranial sutures that converge at fontanelles (see Fig. 1.6). The sutures and fontanelles are needed for brain growth and development. During childbirth, the sutures allow the bones to overlap so the head can pass through the birth canal. The fontanelles gradually close in infancy while the sutures remain open often into early adulthood. The posterior fontanelle usually closes by 1–2 months of age. The anterior fontanelle remains open longer, usually closing between 9 and 18 months of age. Except for the metopic suture, cranial sutures do not normally close until adulthood. The metopic suture is the earliest to close, usually by 2 years of age. The sagittal, coronal, and lambdoidal sutures close in the third decade of life, while the squamosal suture closes between 35 and 39 years of age.

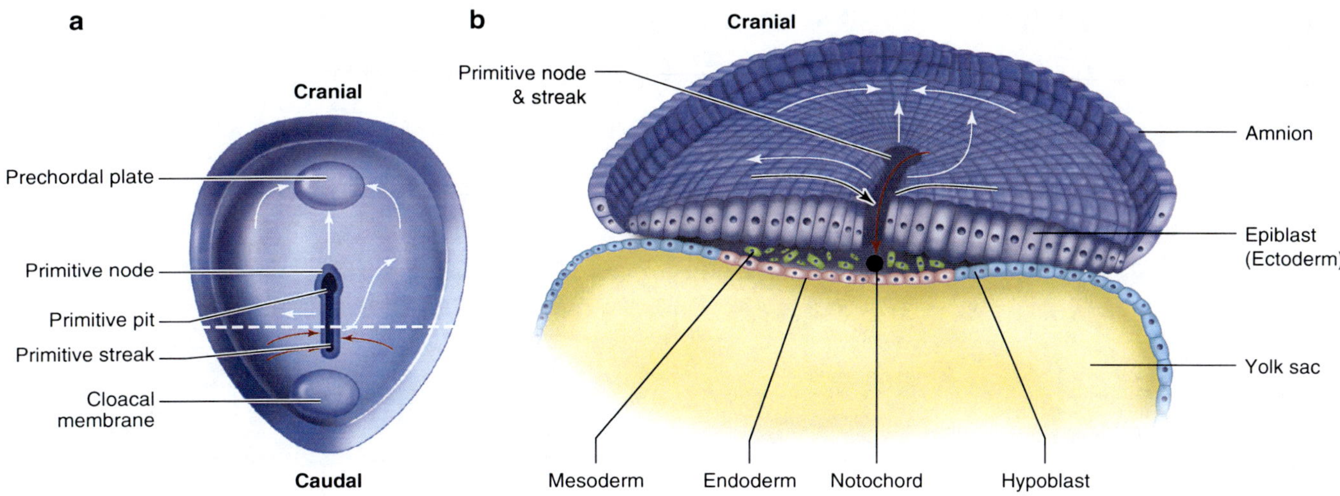

Fig. 1.3 Formation of the trilaminar embryo: endoderm, mesoderm, and ectoderm

Fig. 1.4 Folding of the trilaminar embryo

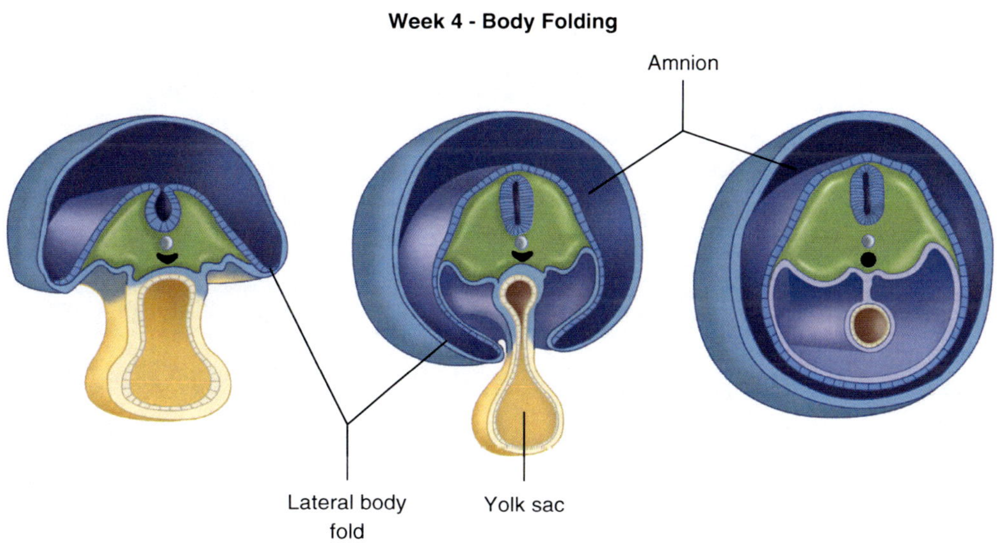

Clinical Correlate

With the exception of the metopic suture, the cranial sutures remain patent until the third decade of life. The sagittal suture starts fusing on the average at age 22 years. The coronal suture starts fusing at age 24 years. The lambdoid suture starts fusing at age 26 years. Although early studies placed the onset of metopic suture fusion at 2 years of age, recent evidence has indicated that fusion begins as early as 3 months and is complete by 8 months of age. Premature closure of the bones of the skull results in craniosynostosis. It occurs in 0.04–0.1 % of live births. Specific suture fusion produces characteristic deformations of the calvarial vault. Sagittal synostosis – the most common type (50–60 %) – produces an elongated skull in the anterior-posterior plane with narrowing of the bitemporal width. Coronal synostosis (20–30 %) produces anterior asymmetry most notable in the unequal appearance of the orbits (see Fig. 1.7). Metopic synostosis (5–10 %) produces a triangular shaped forehead with hypotelorbitism and retrusion of the lateral orbital bar. Lambdoid synostosis – the least common (2–4 %) – produces posterior asymmetric with elongation of the ipsilateral mastoid area.

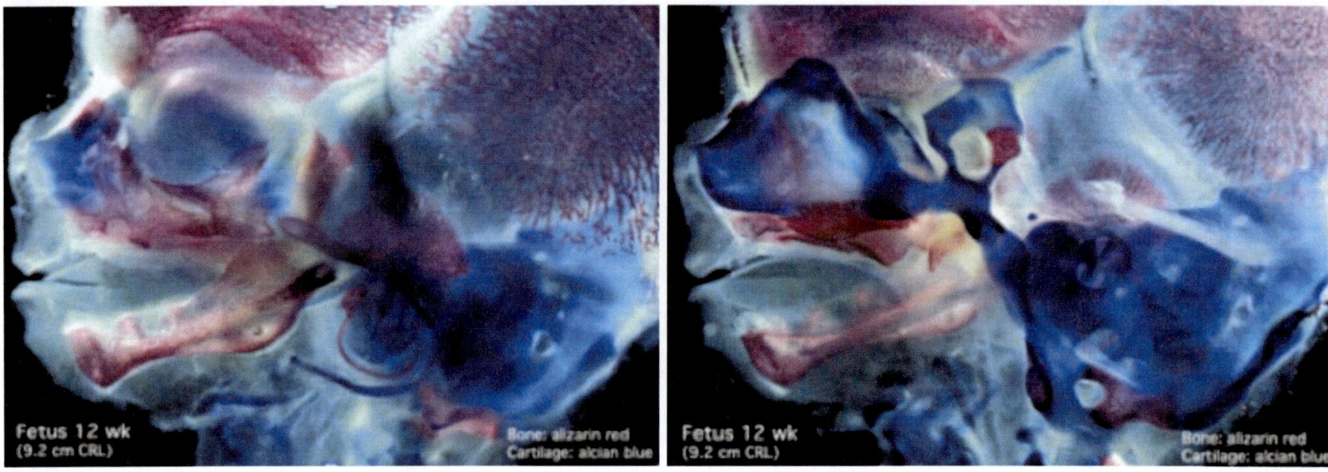

Fig. 1.5 (**a**, **b**) Development of the facial bones

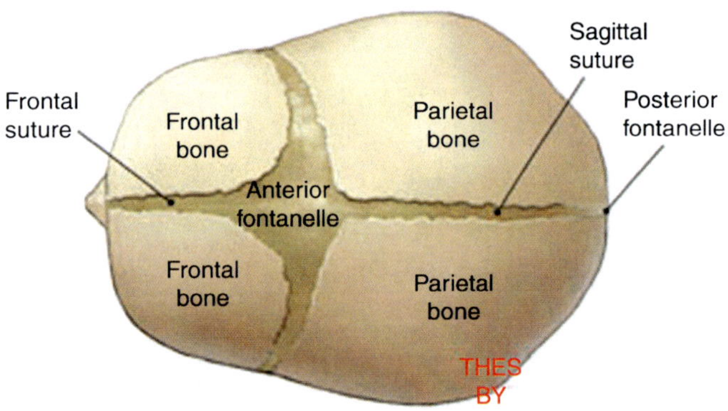

Fig. 1.6 Calvarial bones of the infant skull

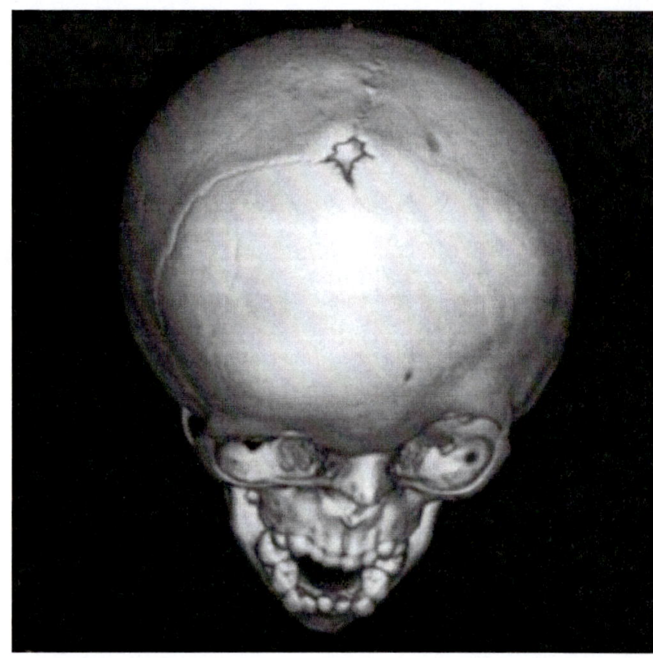

Fig. 1.7 Three-dimensional CT scan of a patient with coronal synostosis

Clinical Correlate
Encephaloceles represent herniation of neural tissue through defects in the calvarial bones. They may contain meninges (meningocele) or brain matter and meninges (encephalomeningocele), or they may communicate with a ventricle (encephalomeningocystocele).

Development of the Face

Facial development largely occurs between the fourth and eighth weeks of gestation, and takes on a clearly human appearance by age 10 weeks. The cephalic portion of the cylindrical embryo will give rise to the skull and the face. Near the prechordal plate, the future site of the oral cavity, a series of swellings limited by indentations appear. These "pharyngeal arches" (or "branchial arches") will give origin to most of the facial structures (see Fig. 1.8a). The pharyngeal arches consist of a series of swellings of mesoderm covered by ectoderm externally and endoderm internally. Each pharyngeal arch is separated by an external indentation ("pharyngeal groove") and an internal indentation ("pharyngeal pouch") (see Fig. 1.8b). The human embryo develops five pharyngeal arches numbered 1, 2, 3, 4, and 6 (the fifth one, present in most of inferior vertebrate species, does not form in the human embryo). Both the pharyngeal arches and pouches are also numbered accordingly to the immediately cephalic pharyngeal arch.

Development of the face and neck structures derives from the pharyngeal arches, groves, and pouches. The mesoderm

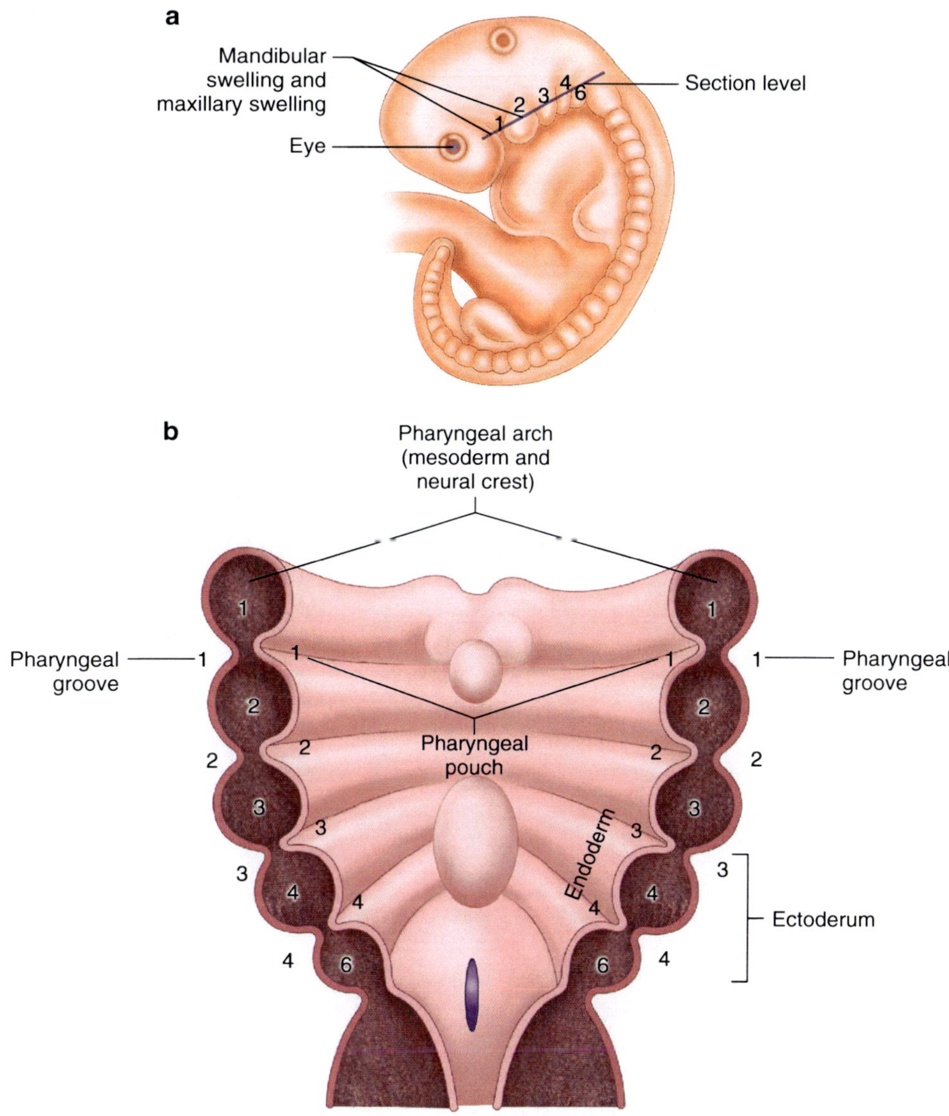

Fig. 1.8 (**a**) Development of the branchial arches. (**b**) Infant cranial skeleton, including bones and sutures

of each pharyngeal arch gives origin to the nerves, soft tissue, blood vessels, and bony structures. The ectoderm and endoderm give rise to skin, membranes, and glandular structures. Each pharyngeal arch is associated with a cranial nerve, and therefore, the muscles originated from a specific arch have a distinct cranial nerve innervation pattern (see Table 1.1).

The first arch divides into two paired swellings or prominences, two maxillary and two mandibular, that will give rise to the maxilla (and secondary palate) and mandible, respectively. A cranial, midline swelling not associated with the pharyngeal arches, the frontonasal process, also forms and fuses with the two maxillary swellings to give origin to the upper portion of the human face: dorsum of the nose, philtral column, and primary palate (see Fig. 1.9).

The first pharyngeal grove and pharyngeal pouch deepen toward each other to form the external auditory canal (pharyngeal groove), middle ear, and Eustachian tube (pharyngeal pouch). The cells that separate them form the tympanic membrane. The second arch grows caudally and covers the surface of both the reminder pharyngeal arches and pharyngeal grooves. The overgrowth of the second pharyngeal arch gives origin to the structures of the neck, including the platysma muscle. The second pharyngeal pouch will give origin to the tonsillar fossa and tonsils. The third pharyngeal pouch invaginates and migrates caudally to give origin to the inferior parathyroid glands and thymus. The fourth pharyngeal pouches also invaginate and migrate caudally, but not as far as the third, to give rise to the superior parathyroid gland (see Fig. 1.10).

Table 1.1 Neural, skeletal, and muscular elements derived from the pharyngeal arches

Arch	Nerve (neural ectoderm)	Skeletal/cartilage (neural crest)	Muscle (mesoderm)	Artery (aortic arch mesoderm)
1	V (trigeminal CN)	Maxilla Mandible *Middle ear bones*: Incus Malleolus	*Muscles of mastication* Masseter Temporalis Lateral pterygoid Medial pterygoid *Plus*: Anterior digastric Mylohyoid Tensor tympani Tensor veli palatini	
2	VII (facial CN)	*Middle ear bones*: Stapes Styloid process Lesser horn and upper body of hyoid bone	*Muscles of facial expression* Plus: Posterior digastric Stylohyoid Stapedius	
3	IX (glossopharyngeal CN)	Grater horn and lower body of hyoid bone	Stylopharyngeus	Right and left common carotid arteries Right and left internal carotid arteries
4	X (vagus CN) Superior laryngeal Pharyngeal branches	Thyroid cartilage	Cricothyroid muscle Soft palate Pharynx (five muscles)	Right subclavian artery (right arch)
6	X (vagus CN) Recurrent laryngeal	All other laryngeal cartilages	Intrinsic muscles of larynx (except cricothyroid muscle)	Right and left pulmonary arteries Ductus arteriosus (left arch)

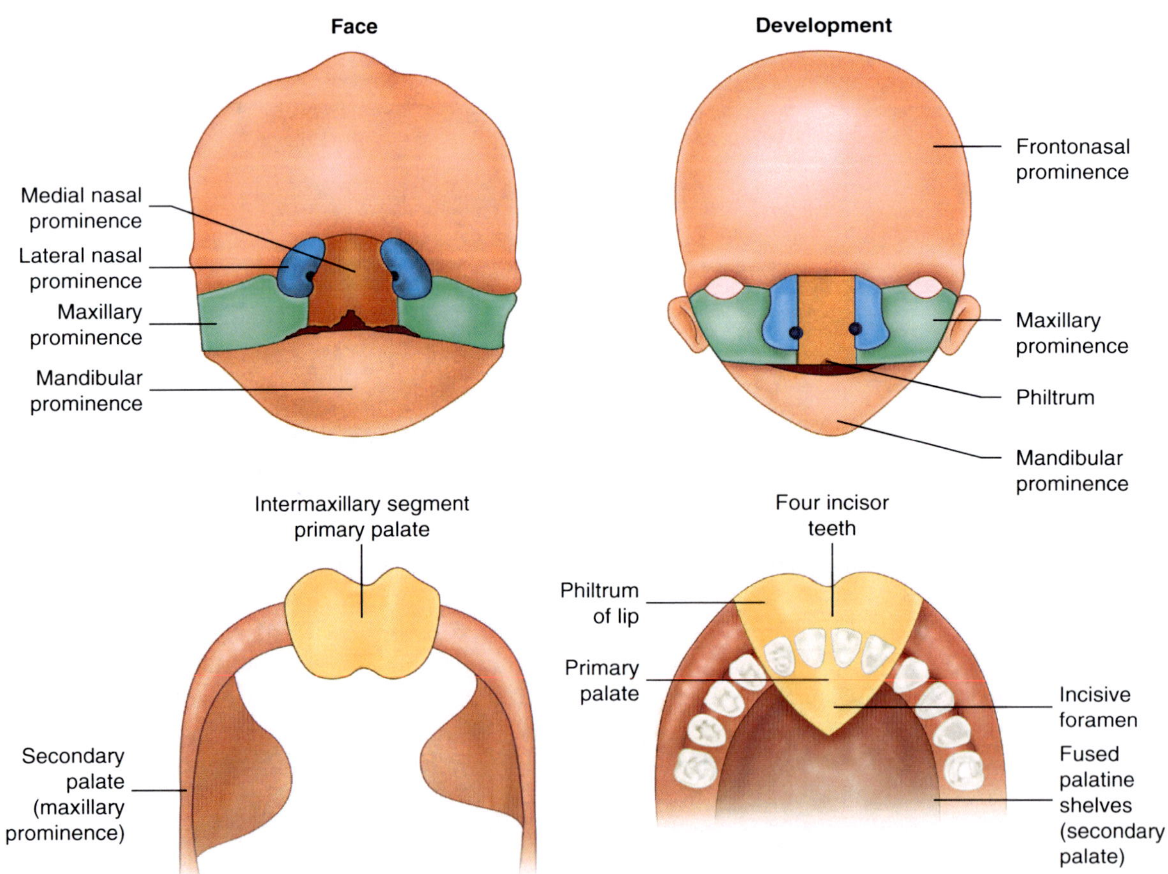

Fig. 1.9 Development of the midface

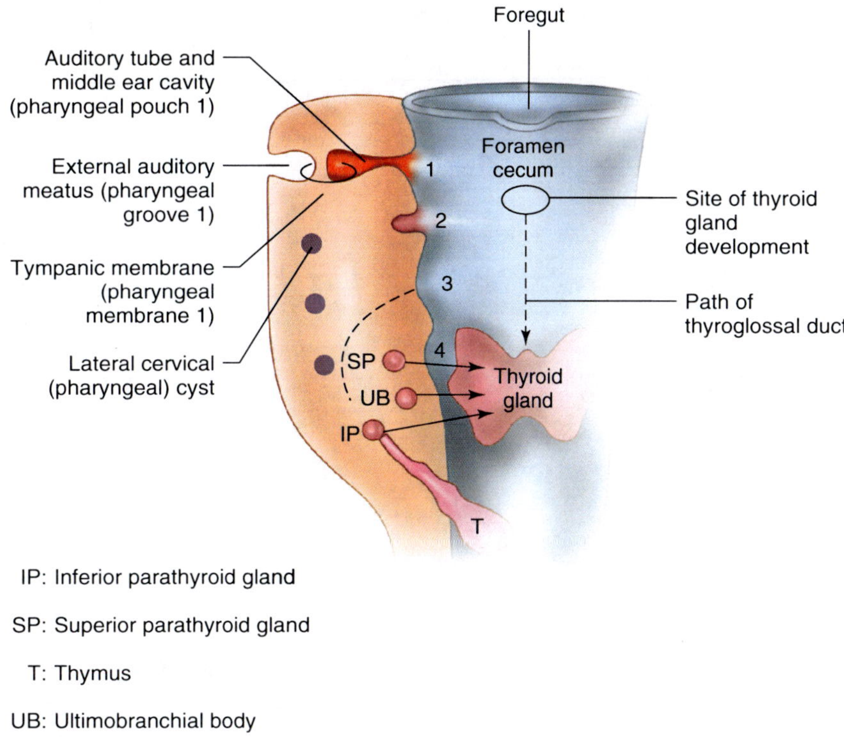

Fig. 1.10 Development of the external auditory canal, tympanic membrane, middle ear, and Eustachian tube

Clinical Correlate
Inadequate or incomplete obliteration of the pharyngeal groves 3, 4, and 6 results in formation of the lateral cervical cysts or sinuses that are usually located along the anterior border of the sternocleidomastoid muscle.

Development of the Nose

The nose starts forming by the fourth week when bilateral thickenings of the surface ectoderm, called nasal placodes, located at the inferior, lateral aspect of the frontonasal prominence appear. With further elevation of the margins of the nasal placodes, the sides develop into the medial and lateral nasal prominences, while the depressed central region of the placodes develops into the nasal pit (see Fig. 1.11a–c). The nasal pits, initially in contact with the stomodeum, are precursors of the nares. The paired maxillary prominences continue to migrate medially, also affecting medial migration of the medial and lateral nasal prominences. Fusion of the medial nasal, lateral nasal, and maxillary prominences produces continuity between the nose, the upper lip, and the palate. Fusion of the medial nasal and maxillary prominences results in separation of the nasal pits from the stomodeum and subsequent separation of the oral and nasal cavities. Merging of the medial nasal prominences forms the philtrum and Cupid's bow region of the upper lip, the nasal tip, the premaxilla and primary palate, and the nasal septum. The lateral nasal prominences form the nasal alae. The nasolacrimal groove develops as a furrow separating the lateral nasal prominence from the maxillary prominence.

Clinical Correlate
Nasal *dermoids* are the most common congenital nasal anomalies. They represent epithelial-lined cavities or sinus tracts with variable numbers of skin appendages. They arise from trapped epithelial cells or from failure of ectodermal extensions into the fetal nasal septum to disappear as the septum fuses and ossifies. *Arhinia* is an extremely rare anomaly which describes absence of the external nasal structures and nasal passages.

Development of the Eyes

Each eye develops from an outpouching of the central nervous system and an outpouching of the surface ectoderm. The eye is first noticeable at 22 days of gestation as two optic groves, which appear along the neural tube. These grooves then further deeper into vesicles off the developing forebrain. The adjacent surface ectoderm invaginates to form a lens placode then a rounder lens pit. As the distal vesicle further invaginates, it forms a double-walled cup around the lens pit. The retina develops from the two walls of the proximal optic cup. The proximal vesicle collapses to form an optic stalk

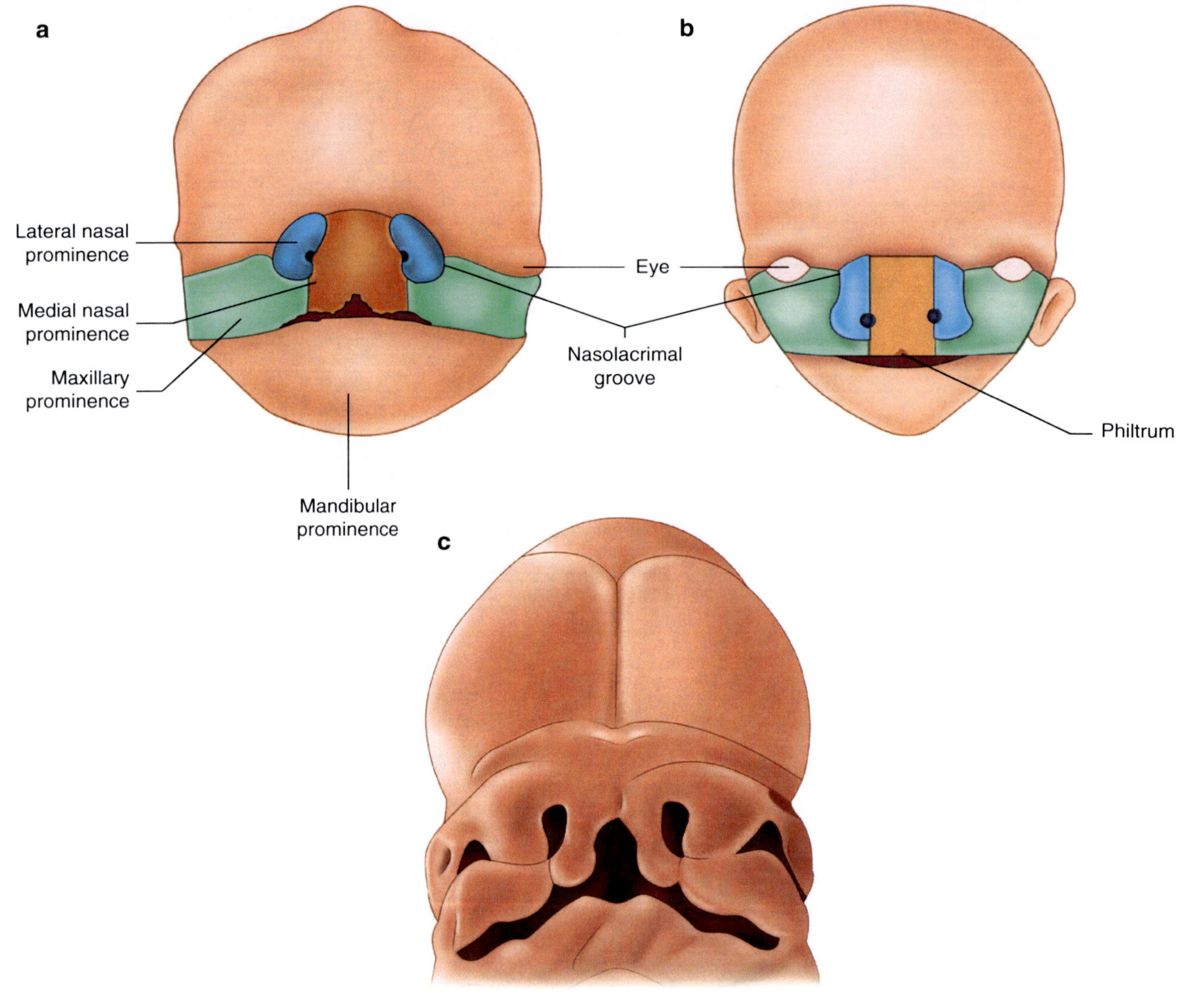

Fig. 1.11 Development of the anterior face

but retains an opening on the ventral aspect to allow passage of vasculature elements. This fissure closes around 6–7 weeks of gestation. The central portion becomes populated with axons of the optic nerve.

Development of ciliary body and iris arises from anterior portions of the optic cup and surrounding mesenchyme. The ciliary muscle, which functions in the accommodation reflex, is derived from mesenchyme near the margin of the optic cup. The iridial muscles, the dilator, and sphincter pupillae muscles are smooth muscles derived from neuroectoderm of the optic cup. These control the size of pupillary aperture.

The extraocular muscles develop from somitomeres I–IV, which are paraxial mesoderm cranial to the occipital somites. They are innervated by cranial nerves III, IV, and VI, which function to coordinate movements between the two eyes. The pupillary light reflex appears at 30 weeks gestation. Accommodation of the eyes and constriction of the pupil remain under parasympathetic control, while dilation is under sympathetic control. Pupillary constriction occurs as oculomotor efferent axons from the Edinger-Westphal nucleus signal ciliary muscle to contract. This reduces tension on suspensory ligaments of lens causing the curvature of lens to increase. In addition, the oculomotor nucleus signals both medial recti muscles to contract. The smaller pupil sharpens the image on retina and reduces light intensity. Pupillary dilation (a sympathetic activity) results from activity of a chain of three neurons: axons in the hypothalamus travel to the T1–T2 roots of the spinal cord, where preganglionic axons from the spinal cord travel to the superior cervical ganglion, and finally postganglionic axons from the superior cervical ganglion to the dilator pupillae muscle.

Clinical Correlate

Numerous congenital anomalies occur from abnormal development of the eye and/or ocular adnexa. Microphthalmia (small globe) may result from interference with the process of eye growth after birth, while anophthalmia (complete absence of the globe) originates earlier during fetal development. Microphthalmia in newborns is sometimes associated with fetal alcohol syndrome or infections during pregnancy. *Aphakia* (absence of the lens) and *aniridia* (absence of the iris muscle) are both extremely rare. Congenital *cataracts* may occur as a result of with infection with rubella virus. They form within 2–3 weeks of birth as a result of galactose accumulation in the lens. Congenital *glaucoma* is characterized by abnormal development of the drainage channels of the eye that normally drain aqueous humor from inside the globe.

Colobomas are defects in closure of optic (choroid) fissure.

Agenesis of the extraocular muscles usually occurs with a single muscle rather than multiple muscles. Failure to align visual axes results in *strabismus*, which potentially may result in diplopia (double vision). *Amblyopia* refers to reduced or absent visual ability in one eye.

In most cases of *congenital ptosis*, the lower eyelid position results from a localized myogenic dysgenesis of the levator muscle. Rather than normal muscle fibers, fibrous and adipose tissues occupy much of the substance, diminishing its ability to contract and relax. The overall incidence is unknown, but in 70 % of cases, it is unilateral. Most cases are sporadic; however, an autosomal dominant pattern of inheritance may be seen.

Development of the Ears

The ears are composed of three distinct portions: the inner ear, the middle ear, and the outer ear. In the third week of gestation, surface ectoderm ("otic placode") invaginates to form a depression ("otic pit"). In the fourth week, the edges of the pit fuse to become an otocyst. The dorsal portion of this cyst develops three diverticula, which go on to become the semicircular canals. The ventral saccular portion forms a tubular diverticulum, the "cochlear duct," which lengthens in a spiral fashion to become the membranous cochlea. The organ of Corti, containing the auditory hair cells, differentiates from cells along the wall of the cochlear duct. Vibrations in the fluid of the cochlea produce a shearing force in the superficial hairs of these cells each of which contains its own auditory nerve receptor. In the sixth week of gestation, neuroectoderm develops into the spinal and vestibular ganglia and corresponding sensory nerves. The mesodermal elements around the otocyst then form a cartilaginous otic capsule, which ossifies by 25 weeks. Vacuoles containing the perilymph develop within the otic capsule. The vacuoles enlarge and unite to form the perilymphatic space, which divides into the scala tympani and the scala vestibuli. The cartilaginous otic capsule ossifies to form the bony labyrinth of the inner ear.

The middle ear develops from the endoderm of the first pharyngeal pouch. The lining cells of the middle ear form the tympanic cavity. The connection to the pharynx elongates to form the Eustachian tube. The cartilage of the first and second pharyngeal arch derived from mesoderm forms the ossicles. Cartilage from the first arch – "Meckel's cartilage" – forms the head of the malleus and the body and short process of incus. Cartilage from the second arch – "Reichert's cartilage" – forms the long process of the malleus, the long process incus, and the stapes. The footplate of the stapes forms from the otic capsule. The ossicles are full-sized by 15 weeks gestation and ossify by 25 weeks.

The external ear develops from the surface ectoderm covering the dorsal end of the first pharyngeal groove. A solid epithelial plate develops at the bottom of the funnel-shaped pharyngeal groove. The tympanic membrane is composed of an inner layer endoderm, a middle layer mesoderm, and an outer layer ectoderm. There are six hillocks composed of mesoderm. The first pharyngeal arch develops into the tragus, the helical root, and the helix itself. The second pharyngeal arch develops into the antihelix and antitragus (see Fig. 1.12).

Clinical Correlate

Congenital deafness occurs in 1 out of every 1,000–2,000 births, roughly half the incidence of acquired deafness from aging or trauma. It may be inherited or non-inherited. Of the inherited causes, an autosomal recessive pattern is most common, accounting for more than 75 % of all congenital cases. Specific syndromes associated with congenital deafness include Alport syndrome, branchio-oto-renal syndrome, Charcot-Marie-Tooth, Oculoauriculovertebral dysplasia (OAVD) or Goldenhar syndrome, Stickler syndrome, Treacher Collins syndrome, and Waardenburg syndrome. Non-inherited causes of congenital deafness account for roughly 20 % of congenital cases.

In a *Stahl's ear deformity*, there is an abnormal third antihelical crus that extends from the normal antihelix, through the scapha (scaphoid fossa), and up through the rim of the helix (see Fig. 1.13). The normally hollow cartilage of the scapha is bent forward. This is different from *cryptotia*, in which the cartilage of the upper ear is hidden but palpable beneath the skin of the temporal scalp. *Microtia* (see Fig. 1.14) and *anotia* refer to incomplete and absent development of the ear, respectively.

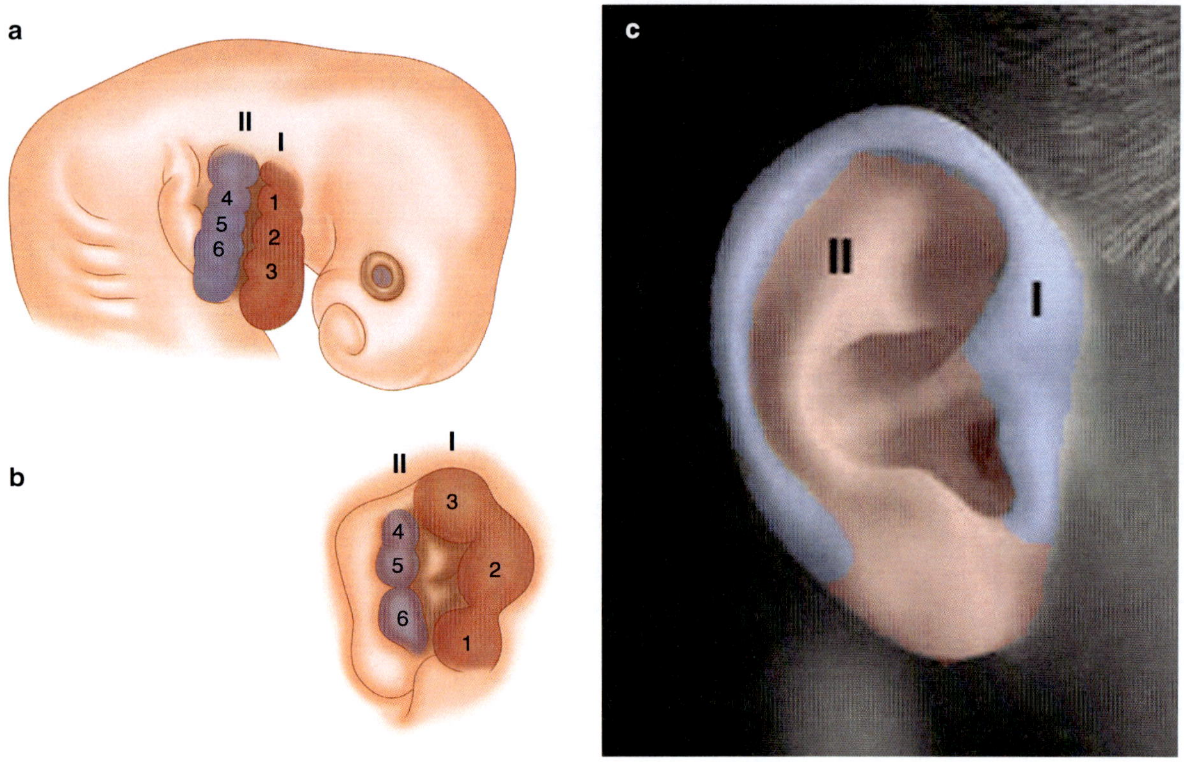

Fig. 1.12 (**a–c**) Development of the external ear

Microtia occurs one in every 6,000–12,000 births. It usually occurs in conjunction with an absence of the ear canal and patients usually have severe hearing loss on the affected ear. Although there is a hearing loss in children with microtia, the inner ears on both sides are usually normal. Microtia may be caused by local ischemia during development. Since the kidneys develop about the same time as the ears, an ultrasound of the kidneys is recommended as part of the work-up.

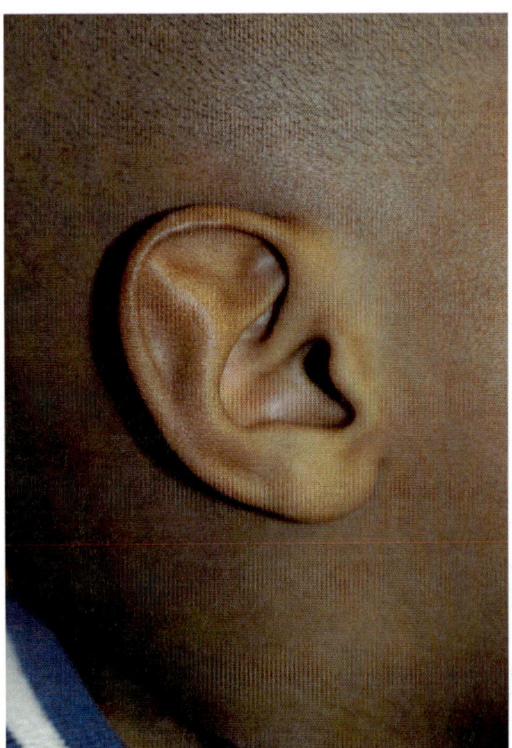

Fig. 1.13 Stahl's ear deformity

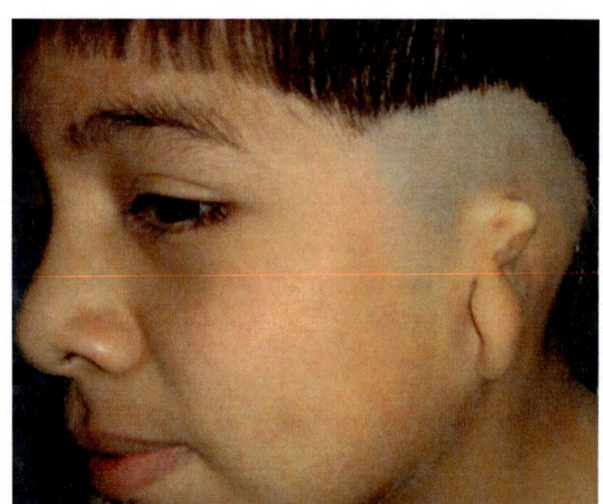

Fig. 1.14 Congenital microtia

Development of the Mouth and Palate

Development of the mouth derives from structures that arise from the first pharyngeal arch. The actual opening forms from a gap between the frontonasal process, the maxillary prominences, and the mandibular prominences. The palate develops in two key stages from outgrowths from the maxillary segments. It is formed during the embryonic period and during the early fetal period, involving the fusion of maxillary components of the first pharyngeal arch (lateral) and the frontonasal prominence (midline) as well as transition from epithelial to mesenchymal elements.

The median nasal process gives rise to the primary palate. The secondary palate is a structure that helps to separate the nasal passage from the pharynx and arises from the lateral palatine processes that derive from the maxillary prominences. Initially the medial primary palate and bilateral lateral palatine processes (secondary palatal shelves) are separated and located around the tongue. The secondary palatal shelves have initially a vertical position (see Fig. 1.15). During the eighth week, as the mandible grows and the tongue displaces anteriorly, the orientation of the lateral palatal shelves alters from vertical to horizontal to initiate their fusion in the midline. Fusion also then occurs between the lateral palatine processes and the median palatine process. The junction of the medial and lateral palatine processes is known as incisive foramen. The median palatine process and anterior potion of the lateral palatine processes undergo intramembranous ossification to form the hard palate. The posterior portion of the lateral palatine processes becomes the soft palate. Errors of development caused by genetic, mechanical, or teratogenic factors can occur at any of these steps and frequently result in a cleft of the primary, second-

Clinical Correlate

Absent or partial fusion of the medial nasal processes and the maxillary processes results in the common form of a cleft lip (see Fig. 1.16). The less common median cleft lip occurs when the two medial nasal processes fail to fuse. *A median cleft of the lower lip* results from failure of fusion of the two mandibular arches. A cleft palate results from failure of the palatine shelves to fuse with each other and/or with the primary palate.

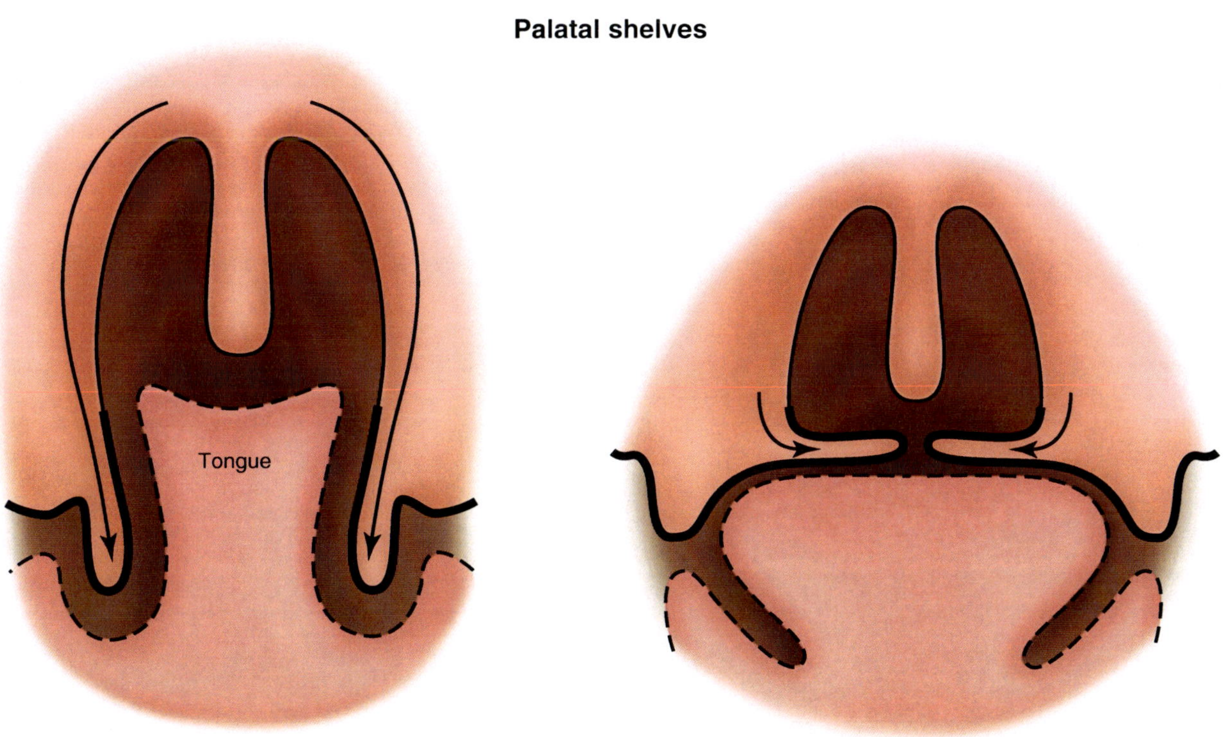

Fig. 1.15 Development of the palate

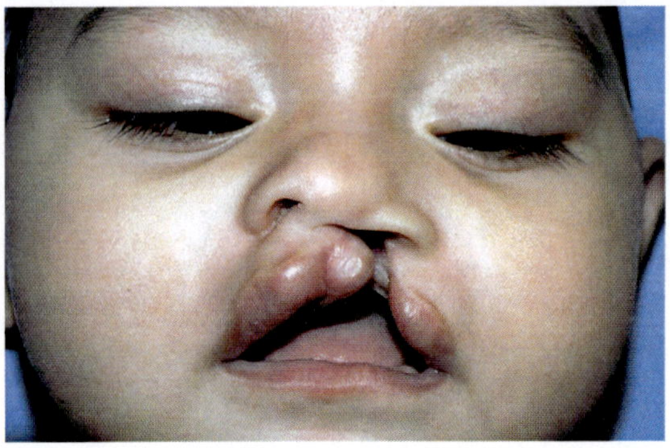

Fig. 1.16 Right unilateral cleft lip deformity

ary, and for primary and secondary palate unilaterally and/or bilaterally.

Development of the Tongue

Development of the musculature of the tongue arises from somites in the occipital region. This tissue, originally posterior to the pharyngeal arches, is supplied by the hypoglossal nerve (CN XII). Development of the tongue mucosa from the pharyngeal arches is more complex. Mesoderm from the first arch forms the anterior two-thirds of the tongue to the foramen cecum. Mesoderm from the third and fourth arches forms the mucosa in the posterior one-third.

The tongue starts developing during the fourth week. A median bud elevates from the floor of the primitive pharynx to form part of the tongue. Two additional lateral buds (lingual swellings) grow over the tuberculum to form the anterior two-thirds of the tongue. These median and lateral swellings originate from the mesenchyme of the first branchial arch and are supplied by the lingual nerve (CN XII), a branch of the mandibular division of the trigeminal nerve (CN V). The second, third, and fourth pharyngeal arches contribute to the development of the posterior one-third (pharyngeal part) of the tongue. The glossopharyngeal nerve (CN IX) and the superior laryngeal branch of the vagus nerve (CN V) supply the sensory innervation to this part of the tongue. The facial nerve (CN VII from the second pharyngeal arch) does not provide sensory innervation to the posterior one-third of the tongue. The anterior two-thirds of the tongue is separated from the posterior one-third of the tongue by a V-shaped groove known as the terminal sulcus. The hypoglossal nerve innervates all muscles of the tongue except for the palatoglossus. The latter muscle is innervated by the vagus nerve (CN X).

Bibliography

Cohen MM. Sutural biology and the correlates of craniosynostosis. Am J Med Genet. 1993;47:681–716.

Francis-West PH. Craniofacial development: the tissue and molecular interactions that control development of the head. Berlin/New York: Springer; 2003.

Kokich VG. The biology of sutures. In: Cohen MMG, editor. Craniosynostosis: diagnosis, evaluation and management. New York: Raven; 1986. p. 81–103.

Larsen WJ. Human embryology. 3rd ed. New York: Churchill Livingstone; 2001.

Moore KL. The developing human: clinically oriented embryology. 9th ed. Philadelphia: Saunders; 2011.

Saint-Jeannet J. Neural crest induction and differentiation. New York: Springer; 2006.

Serafin D. Pediatric plastic surgery. St. Louis: Mosby; 1984.

Sperber GH. Craniofacial embryology. 4th ed. London: Wright; 1989.

Thorne CH. Grabb and Smith's plastic surgery. 6th ed. Philadelphia: Wolters Kluwer Health/Lippincott Williams & Wilkins; 2007.

Todd TW, Lyon DW. Cranial suture closure. Am J Phys Anthropol. 1925;8:23–31.

Weinzweig J, Kirschner RE, Farley A, et al. Metopic synostosis: defining the temporal sequence of normal suture fusion and differentiating it from synostosis on the basis of computed tomography images. Plast Reconstr Surg. 2003;112:1211–8.

Anatomy of the Head and Neck

2

Andrew M. Wexler

Successful maxillofacial surgery requires an intimate knowledge of static and functional anatomy of the head and neck. This chapter will provide a brief review of these areas that are of greatest importance to the maxillofacial surgeon. The present chapter is organized by what is encountered operatively, beginning with the most superficial areas and proceeding inward to the deeper structures. For each plane, the important structures are addressed. Areas of particular interest, such as the orbit and submandibular region, will be highlighted separately.

Facial Innervation: The Trigeminal Nerve

The skin of the face and scalp derives its sensation from the terminal branches of cranial nerve V, the trigeminal nerve. The trigeminal nerve has three sensory roots that arise from the gasserian ganglion (see Figs. 2.1 and 2.2).

Ophthalmic (V_1): The ophthalmic division of the nerve exits through the superior orbital fissure and divides into three major branches—the frontal, the lacrimal, and the nasal ciliary:

1. The *frontal* branch exits at the superior rim of the orbit as the *supratrochlear nerve*, which gives sensation to the conjunctiva and the skin of the upper lid and the forehead, and the *supraorbital nerve*, which gives sensation to the upper lid, the forehead, and the scalp.

> **Operating Notes**
> The supratrochlear nerve lies roughly 1.7 cm off the midline at the supraorbital rim. The supraorbital nerve lies roughly 2.7 cm off the midline. The latter may exit within a notch or through a foramen. When turning down a coronal flap, the foramen may need to be opened with a small osteotome to release the neurovascular structures.

2. The *lacrimal nerve* provides sensation to the conjunctiva and skin of the upper eyelid and also carries postganglionic parasympathetic fibers from the pterygopalatine ganglion to the lacrimal gland (see Fig. 2.2).
3. The *nasociliary nerve* carries sensation to the nose, to the sclera, and to the cornea of the eye. Its nasal branches provide sensation to the nasal septum in the lateral wall of the nasal cavity as well as to the skin of the ala, the apex, and the vestibule of the nose. The anterior and posterior ethmoidal branches provide sensation to the ethmoidal and frontal sinuses.

Maxillary (V_2): The maxillary division exits the cranium through the foramen rotundum and passes through the pterygopalatine fossa, where it gains postganglionic parasympathetic fibers that are carried with the nerve to the nasal and palatine glands. The nerve then branches to form the greater palatine nerve, the lesser palatine nerve, and the nasopalatine nerve:

1. The *zygomaticotemporal* nerve.
2. The *zygomaticofacial* nerve.
3. The nerves off the sphenopalatine ganglion include the *greater palatine nerve*, which supplies sensation to the hard palate to the incisor teeth; the *lesser palatine nerve*, which supplies sensation to the soft palate, uvula, and tonsils; and the *nasopalatine nerve*, which runs across the roof of the nose, traverses the nasal septum, and exits through the incisive foramen where it innervates the anterior hard palate and the alveolar margins of the incisors.
4. Of particular interest to the maxillofacial surgeon are the posterior, middle, and anterior superior alveolar nerves. The *posterior superior alveolar nerve* supplies sensation to the first, second, and third molars.
5. The *middle superior alveolar nerve* supplies sensation to the upper molars, and the anterior superior alveolar nerve supplies sensation to the upper incisors and canine teeth.
6. The *anterior superior alveolar nerve*.
7. The maxillary branch then courses along the floor of the orbit, exiting the maxilla below the infraorbital rim, exiting as the *infraorbital nerve* to provide sensation to the

A.M. Wexler, MD, MA
Department of Plastic Surgery, Craniofacial Services Southern California, Kaiser Permanente, U.S.C., Los Angeles, CA, USA
e-mail: surgiwex@gmail.com

P.J. Taub et al. (eds.), *Ferraro's Fundamentals of Maxillofacial Surgery*,
DOI 10.1007/978-1-4614-8341-0_2, © Springer Science+Business Media New York 2015

Fig. 2.1 Sensory innervation of the face

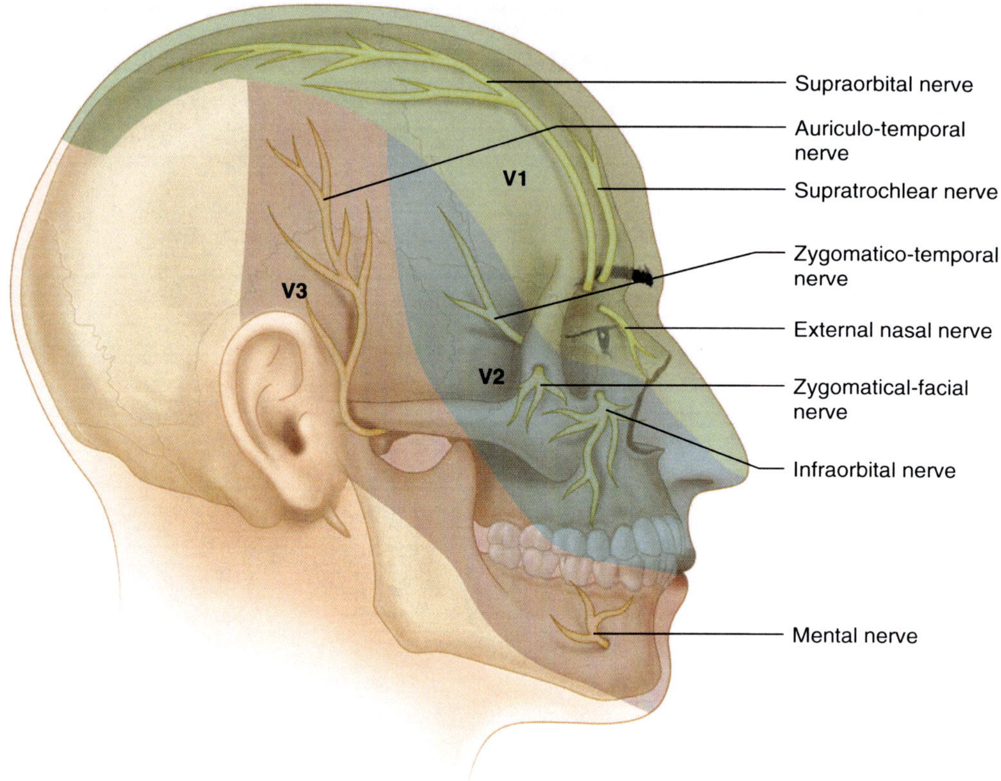

skin of the lower eyelid, the anterior part of the cheek, the malar prominence, the upper lip, and the anterior part of the temple.

Operating Notes
Fractures of the inferior floor of the orbit frequently transverse the infraorbital canal, which results in hypoesthesia along the infraorbital nerve distribution. Accordingly, patients who present after trauma with decreased sensation of the upper lip and anterior cheek should be suspected of having a fracture of the floor of the orbit.

Mandibular (V_3): The mandibular division exits the cranium through the foramen ovale, passing deep to the lateral pterygoid muscle and lateral to the eustachian tube and otic ganglion. Its sensory branches then pass through the semilunar ganglion. These sensory branches are then joined by a motor branch, and together they form the main trunk of the mandibular nerve. The main trunk gives off three motor branches to the medial pterygoid, the tensor tympani, and the tensor palatini muscles. The nerve then divides into an anterior and a posterior division:

1. The anterior division provides motor innervation to the muscles of mastication as well as one sensory branch, the long buccal nerve, which is responsible for sensation to the buccal mucosa and lower gums. Its motor fibers innervate the pterygoid, masseter, temporalis, and tensor palatini muscles. The buccal nerve passes often with the anterior deep temporal branch between the two heads of the lateral pterygoid. It then runs downward along the medial insertion of the temporalis muscle, pierces the buccal fat pad, and is then distributed to provide sensation to the inner cheek and gingiva.
2. The posterior division, as it passes inferiorly in line with the ramus of the mandible, gives off an *auriculotemporal nerve* that provides sensation to the temporomandibular joint, the skin over the temporal region of the ear, the lateral aspect of the scalp, and the tympanic membrane. Prior to entering the inferior alveolar canal on the medial side of the mandible, the posterior division of the mandibular nerve gives off the *lingual nerve*, which courses posterior to the retromolar trigone and enters the tongue to provide general sensation to the anterior two-thirds of the tongue, the floor of the mouth, and the gums. Prior to entering the tongue, the lingual nerve receives the *chorda tympani* from the facial nerve, a branch of the seventh cranial nerve that carries taste fibers from the anterior two-thirds of the tongue. The chorda tympani also carries autonomic parasympathetic nerves to the submandibular and sublingual glands. After giving off the lingual nerve, the mandibular nerve then enters the inferior alveolar foramen and is now designated the *inferior alveolar nerve*. The inferior alveolar nerve runs within the inferior alveolar canal to the substance of the body of the mandible. The inferior alveolar nerve gives off motor branches to

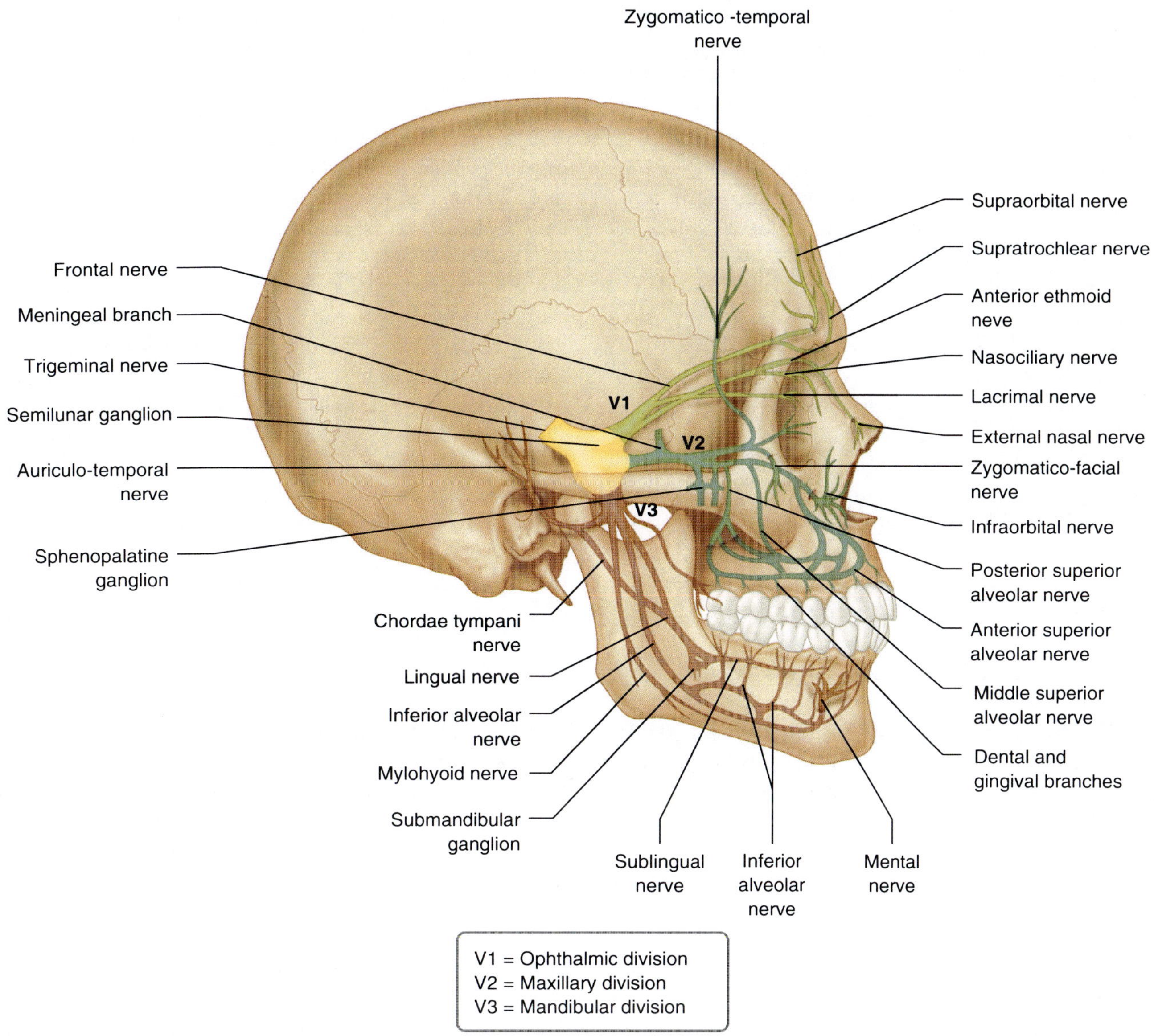

Fig. 2.2 Anatomy of the trigeminal nerve

the mylohyoid muscle and the anterior belly of the digastric muscle, as well as sensory branches to the premolar and molar teeth of the mandible. The terminal sensory branch of the nerve exits the mandible as the *mental nerve* where it provides sensation to the lower lip and chin.

The posterior trunk of the nerve runs lateral to the tensor and levator palatini. The auriculotemporal nerve, in close proximity to the medial meningeal artery, is the first branch given off from the posterior trunk. The posterior trunk then passes in the preauricular region posteriorly and medial to the temporomandibular joint, and anteriorly to the external acoustic meatus, where it accompanies the superficial temporal artery to supply sensation to the anterior ear, the auditory meatus, and the skin of the temple. The posterior trunk of the mandibular nerve then divides into the inferior alveolar and lingual nerves prior to leaving the infratemporal fossa.

Operating Notes

The diverse interconnections of the trigeminal nerve throughout its facial distribution are responsible for a multitude of referred pain syndromes. A common example of these would be a sinusitis of the maxillary sinus being referred through the maxillary sensory branches to the pharyngeal nerve and being perceived as a pain in the back of the throat. Similarly, pain from dental caries of the mandible perceived through the inferior alveolar nerve, or a carcinoma of the tongue, perceived through the lingual nerve, might be referred through the mandibular branch of the trigeminal nerve to the auriculotemporal nerve and be perceived as pain in the tympanic membrane.

The mental nerve exits the anterior surface of the mandible below the second bicuspid, where it may lie within a fracture line. Fractures of the mandible that transverse the inferior alveolar canal are frequently associated with decreased sensation in the chin and lip on the involved side. Within the bone, the nerve may run several millimeters lower than the foramen where it is vulnerable to injury from bicortical screws. Plating a parasymphyseal fracture requires placement of the plate along the lower border of the mandible well below the foramen of the nerve.

The inferior alveolar nerve is also vulnerable during a sagittal split of the mandible. Care must be taken to orient osteotomes along the inner surface of the outer cortex to keep the nerve surrounded by cancellous bone within the proximal segment of bone.

The Musculofascial Collars of the Neck

Directly beneath the skin and subcutaneous tissue of the neck lies the platysma, a broad flat muscle that originates from the superficial fascia of the thorax, just inferior to the clavicle, and inserts into the outer body of the mandible at its inferior border. The platysma is considered a muscle of facial expression and accordingly is innervated by a branch of the facial nerve, the cervical branch. The muscle fibers of the platysma have been noted to blend with the orbicularis oris, enhancing the depressor function of the lower lip. The anterior jugular veins lie beneath the platysma anteriorly, while the external jugular veins lie more laterally. Dissections in the subplatysmal plane, frequently performed in rhytidectomy procedures, should avoid these vessels so as to avoid a hematoma.

Deep to the level of the platysma, the outer muscle collar encircles the neck (see Fig. 2.3). This musculofascial collar is composed of the sternomastoid muscle and the trapezius muscle, along with the dense fascia, which both covers and runs between them. The sternomastoid muscle is composed of two separate heads: the round sternal head originating from the superior portion of the front of the manubrium, and a flat clavicular head, originating from the upper surface of the medial third of the clavicle. The two heads of the muscle insert into the outer surface of the mastoid process of the temporal bone and the lateral part of the superior nuchal line. The muscle is innervated by the eleventh cranial nerve, the accessory nerve, along with branches from cervical nerves 2 and 3. The normal function of the sternomastoid muscle is to flex the head and the neck and assist in the rotation of the skull. Traumatic injury of the sternomastoid muscle at birth is not uncommon, with resultant scar tissue formation shortening the muscle. This results in congenital torticollis, which may result in development of an asymmetrical skull, plagiocephaly, from the pull of the shortening. The sternomastoid muscle anatomically divides the posterior triangle of the neck from the anterior triangle of the neck.

The posterior triangle is covered by a dense fascia that originates in the prevertebral area and sweeps forward, splitting anteriorly and posteriorly to enclose both the trapezius and the sternomastoid muscle. The fascia, known as the roofing fascia of the posterior triangle, is renamed the investing layer of the deep cervical fascia when it splits to surround the sternomastoid. Anterior to the sternomastoid, the fascia provides separate investments for the strap muscles, the trachea, and the thyroid glands as the pretracheal fascia. The superficial portion of the deep cervical fascia, which passes as the superficial investing layer of the sternomastoid, extends inferiorly from the scapula, clavicle, first rib, and manubrium to the superior nuchal line, mastoid process, and lower border of the body of the mandible. This fascia then becomes contiguous with the superficial musculoaponeurotic system (SMAS), which extends upward from the border of the mandible to the zygomatic arch. In doing so, it creates separate fascia pockets for the parotid and submandibular glands. Accordingly, the parotid gland cannot be said to have a capsule, as it is only the superficial portion of the gland that is covered by this fascia. This same layer of fascia that is briefly broken by the zygomatic arch is seen to continue superior to the arch as the superficial layer of the temporal fascia, also known as the temporal parietal fascia. We may therefore consider the SMAS and in fact the superficial temporal fascia as being extensions of the superficial portion of the deep cervical fascia (see Fig. 2.4). It has been noted that this fascia is pierced anteriorly by the anterior jugular vein and laterally by the external jugular vein. In addition, four sets of nerves pierce the fascia on the lateral aspect of the neck: the lesser occipital nerve, running to the scalp, behind the ear, along the posterior border of the sternomastoid; the greater auricular nerve, running vertically on the sternomastoid muscle toward the ear; the anterior cutaneous nerve, which courses horizontally forward across the sternomastoid muscle to the anterior triangle; and multiple supraclavicular nerves, providing sensation to the anterior neck. All of these nerves are derived from the anterior rami running through the cervical plexus.

The Muscles of the Facial Expression

The muscles of facial expression (see Fig. 2.5) are all innervated by the facial nerve (CN VII). These muscles, which are all interconnected, may be divided into four major groups: the scalp and ear, the orbits, the nose, and the mouth. All of these muscles insert into the skin and most have a bony origin, except the orbicularis oris, whose multiple interconnected fibers encircle the mouth. Table 2.1 gives an outline of these muscles.

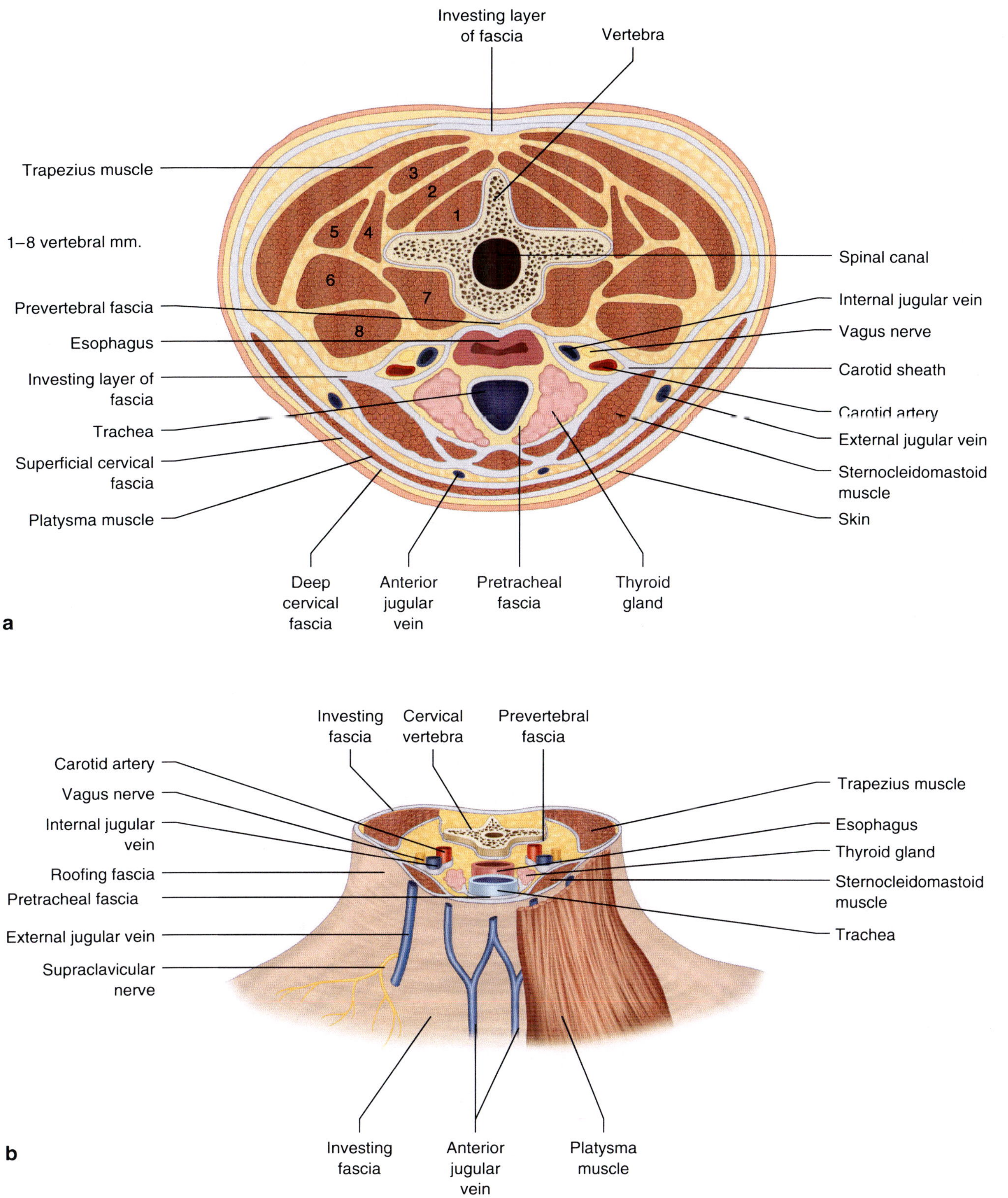

Fig. 2.3 Anatomy of the neck

Fig. 2.4 Fascial layers of the head and neck

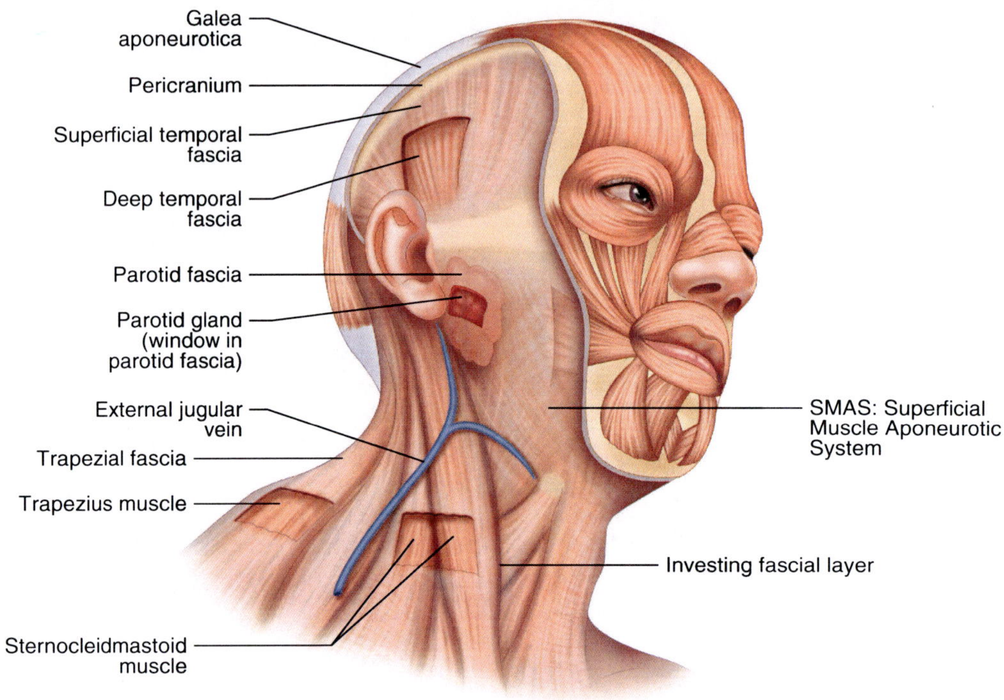

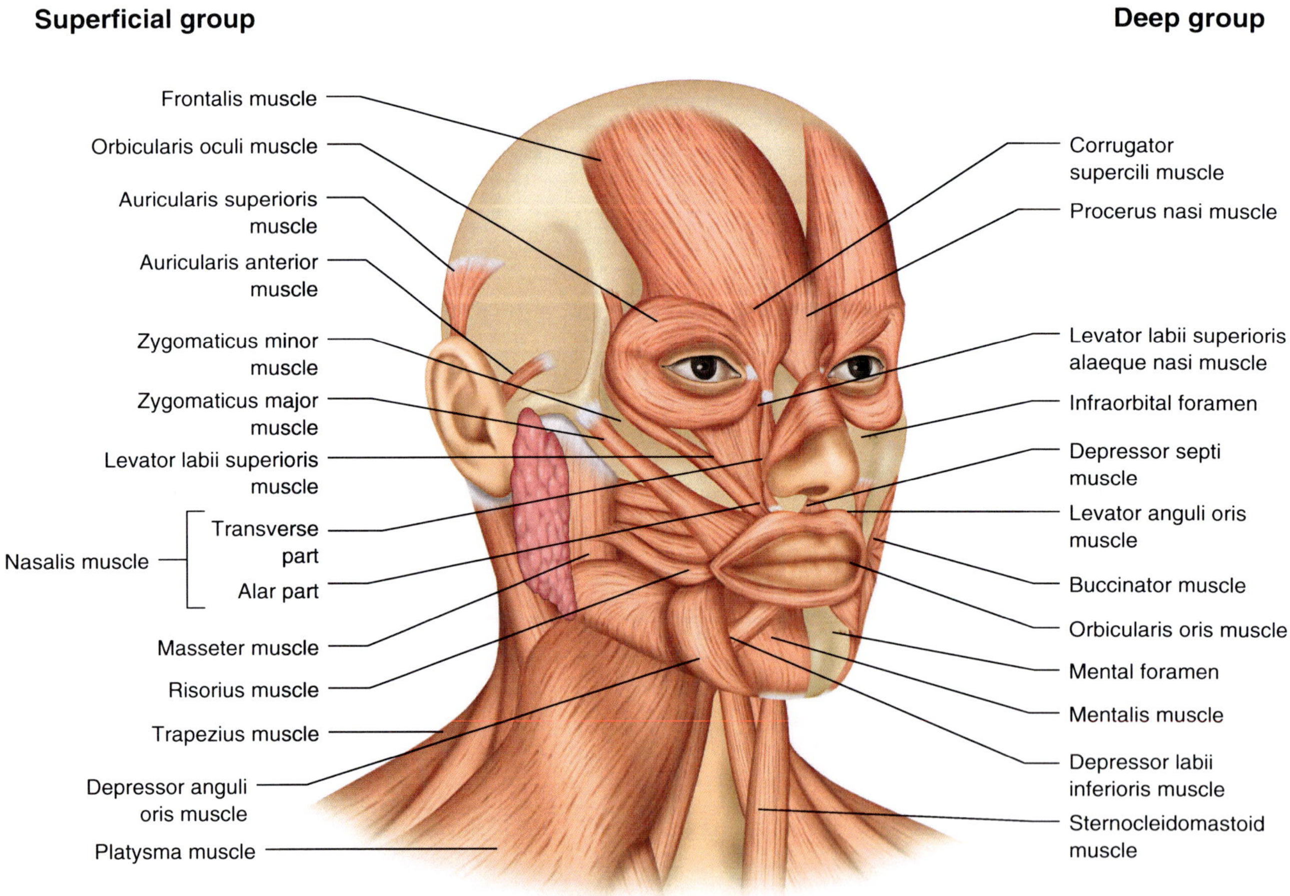

Fig. 2.5 Superficial (**a**) and deep (**b**) muscles of the head and neck

Table 2.1 Muscles of facial expression

Muscle	Origin	Insertion	Innervation	Function
Muscles of the scalp and ears				
Frontalis	Tendonous galea	Skin of forehead	Temporal	Moves scalp and forehead
Occipitalis	Mastoid portion of temporal bone	Skin of scalp	Posterior auricular	
Superior auricularis	Galea	Auricle	Posterior auricular	Elevation of the ear
Anterior auricularis	Galea	Helix	Temporal	Draws ear forward
Posterior auricular	Base of mastoid	Concha	Posterior auricular	Retracts and elevates ear
Muscles surrounding the orbit				
Orbicularis oculi, orbital portion	Medial palpebral ligament, nasal portion of frontal bone, frontal process of maxilla	Skin surrounding the eyes	Zygomatic and temporal	Closes eye, depresses forehead, elevates cheek
Orbicularis oculi, palpebral portion	Medial palpebral ligament, posterior lacrimal crest	Loose connective tissue below skin	Zygomatic and temporal	Closes eye, depresses forehead, elevates cheek
Procerus	Nasal bone	Skin root of nose	Zygomatic and temporal	Transverse wrinkling of the root of the nose
Corregator supercili	Frontal bone	Medial eyebrow	Zygomatic and temporal	Draws eyebrows medially. Vertical wrinkling above the root of the nose
Muscles of the nose				
Transverse	Maxilla	Nasolabial fold	Zygomatic and buccal	Dilates nares
Alar	Maxilla over lateral incisor	Greater alar cartilage	Zygomatic and buccal	Depresses nares
Depressor septi	Incisive foramen of maxilla	Septum and posterior ala	Zygomatic and buccal	Narrows nares
Muscles around the mouth				
Orbicularis oris	Skin of lips and fibers of surrounding muscle	Skin of lips and mouth	Buccal	Sphincteric action
Depressor anguli oris	Body of mandible below premolar and first molar teeth	Corner of mouth skin and orbicularis	Marginal mandibular	Depresses angle of mouth
Depressor labii inferioris	Anterior mandible	Skin and mucosa of lower lip	Marginal mandibular	Depresses central lip
Mentalis	Root of lower incisors	Downward into skin of chin	Marginal mandibular	Draws skin of lip upward, forces lower lip against lower teeth and gums
Platysma	Clavicle and upper portions of thorax	Border of jaw superficial to facial muscles and depressor angular oris	Cervical	Contracts skin of neck, depresses lower lip at corners
Risorius	Subcutaneous tissue over parotid	Mucosa and skin of lateral corner of mouth	Buccal	Draws corner of mouth laterally and somewhat upward
Zygomaticus major	Posterior lateral zygoma	Skin and mucosa corner of mouth	Buccal and zygomatic	Draws corner of mouth laterally and upward
Zygomaticus minor	Zygoma medial to z-major	Skin and mucosa corner of mouth	Buccal and zygomatic	Draws corner of mouth laterally and upward
Levator labii superioris	Infraorbital margin of maxilla	Skin and lateral half of lip	Buccal and zygomatic	Raises upper lip
Levator labii superioris alacque nasi	Frontal process of maxilla along the nose	Skin of and nasal ala of nose and skin of upper lip	Buccal and zygomatic	Lifts the lip and widens the naris
Buccinator	Pterygomandibular raphe, upper medial mandibular at the ramus body junction and posterior alveolar process of maxilla	Orbicularis and mucosa and skin of lips	Buccal branches of facial	Flattens cheek against teeth, moves food from buccal sulcus onto teeth

The Scalp and Paracranium

The soft tissue covering of the skull is composed of hair-bearing skin, subcutaneous tissue, and epicranial aponeurosis, all firmly bound together. Below this lies the periosteum of the skull. The vessels of the scalp are contained in the subcutaneous layer and are adherent to the noncompliant aponeurosis.

Operating Notes

The aponeurosis of the scalp prevents effective constriction of the blood vessels when they are cut. This fact allows even minor scalp wounds to bleed more profusely than wounds in other locations. Although bleeding under the aponeurosis can spread over the skull dome, bleeding between the periosteum and the skull is restricted to the individual skull bone to which the periosteum is attached.

Lymphatics

The lymphatic drainage of the head and neck runs to five major groups of nodes, which encircle the head from the occiput to the submental region. Proceeding from posterior to anterior, these major groups are the occipital group, a posterior auricular group overlying the mastoid area, a preauricular group lying both superficially and deep to the parotid, a submandibular group lying inferior and posterior to the mandible, and a submental group anterior and inferior to the mandible.

The relationship of the parotid gland to the preauricular nodal group may make parotidectomy a necessary adjuvant in the resection of certain facial and scalp carcinomas. The occipital and posterior auricular lymph node groups drain primarily into the superficial cervical glands surrounding the external jugular vein lying on the sternomastoid muscle. The superficial cervical glands, in turn, drain to the external jugular glands or deep to the anterior group of the cervical nodes that surround the internal jugular veins. A superior deep cervical group of nodes drains the preauricular, submandibular, and submental lymph nodes although they may also drain directly into the inferior deep cervical group. The inferior deep cervical group also receives drainage from the axilla and pectoral regions, as well as the pharynx, the upper part of the thyroid gland, and the larynx.

The Facial Blood Supply

The blood supply to the face is provided by the facial artery, which arises from the external carotid artery coursing close to the pharynx (see Fig. 2.6). It then runs upward, deep to the posterior digastric muscle, giving off tonsillar branches. The artery loops around the posterior part of the submandibular gland and appears at the inferior border of the mandible where it can be palpated just anterior to the border of the masseter muscle.

Operating Notes

Palpation of the facial artery and identification of the location of the marginal mandibular nerve are important landmarks when making a Risdon incision to access the ramus of the mandible.

From the border of the mandible, the artery runs superiorly and medially deep to the platysma, risoris, and zygomaticus. The vessel then courses along the side of the nose toward the medial angle of the eye, where it terminates in the angular artery. Along the way, the facial artery gives off a superior and inferior labial artery, which runs deep to the orbicularis and superficial to the submucosa of the inner lip.

Operating Notes

The inferior labial artery serves as the axial blood supply for the Abbe flap. The artery's submucosal position allows for division of a majority of the lip, the creation of a thin pedicle, and subsequent ease of flap rotation.

The anterior facial vein runs parallel and posterior to the artery. The vein begins as the angular vein at the angle of the nose and eye. The angular vein communicates with the orbital vein and consequently with the cavernous sinus. Infections of the face, especially around the upper lip and nose, have the potential for intercranial extension and cavernous sinus thrombosis.

The anterior facial vein empties into the common facial vein and then into the internal jugular vein. The common facial vein also receives the anterior division of the posterior facial vein. The posterior facial vein is formed opposite the temporomandibular joint, where it receives drainage from the scalp, the temple, and the pterygoid plexus. The vein divides into an anterior division, which drains the common facial vein, and a posterior division, which joins with the posterior auricular vein, to drain into the external jugular.

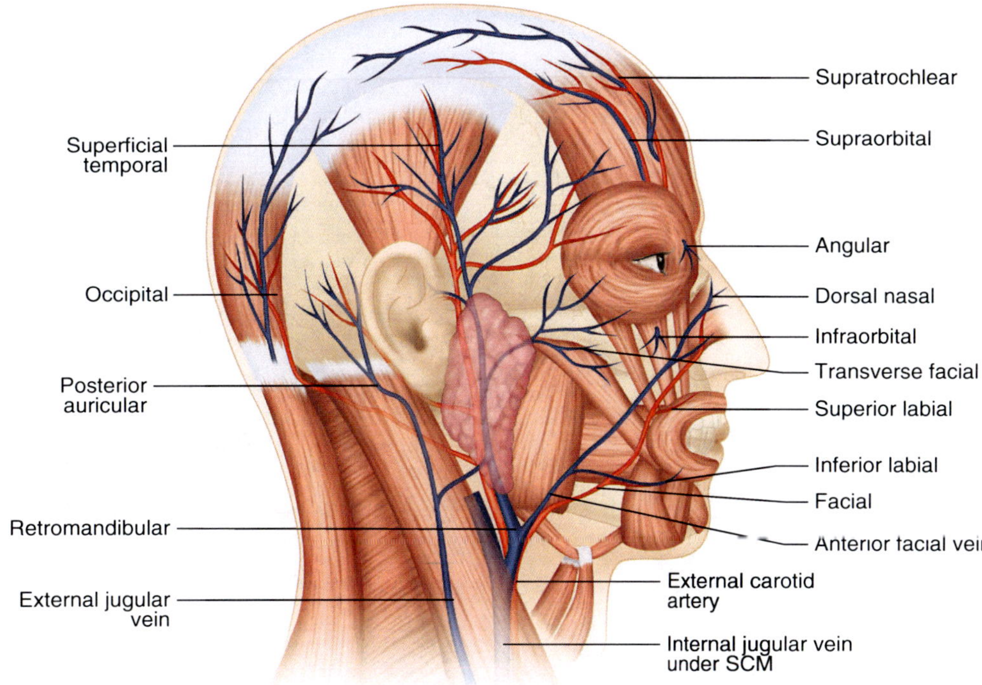

Fig. 2.6 Vascular supply of the head and neck

The Parotid Gland

The parotid is the largest of the salivary glands. It wraps itself in a horseshoe-shaped manner around the posterior ramus of the mandible. The deep segment of the gland lies medial to the medial pterygoid along the medial surface of the ramus, while the superficial segment lies lateral to the masseter muscle, along the lateral surface of the ramus. Note that although the parotid has a deep and a superficial segment, it is not divided into two separate lobes, nor does it possess its own fascial capsule. Instead, it is covered superficially by an extension of the superficial layer of the deep cervical fascia. At the most inferior portion of the gland, this fascia joins with the fascia running deep to the parotid gland to form the stylomandibular ligament, which separates the parotid from the underlying submandibular gland (see Fig. 2.7).

At the anterior edge of the superficial portion of the gland, the parotid (Stensen's) duct may be found exiting the gland and coursing anteriorly across the masseter muscle on a line running roughly between the lobule of the ear and the base of the nasal ala. At the anterior border of the masseter muscle, which lies along a vertical line extending downward from the lateral canthus, the duct turns medially, piercing the buccinator, and enters the mouth through the buccal mucosa at the parotid papilla. The papilla can be found at the level of the junction of the crown and root of the second maxillary molar.

Piercing the parotid's substance posteriorly is the main branch of the facial nerve (CN VII). The facial nerve trunk exits from the stylomastoid foramen, passes under the protection of the mastoid process, and then divides within the gland's substance into its five major branches. Arborization of the nerve branches takes place within the gland's substance (Fig. 2.7).

Operating Notes

Facial lacerations encountered anterior to a vertical line drawn between the lateral canthus and the lateral oral commissure need not be explored for either parotid duct damage or facial nerve damage, as the duct will have already pierced the buccinator muscle and the facial nerve will have sufficiently arborized to an extent that makes repair both difficult and unnecessary (see Fig. 2.8). The surgeon should be aware that in a child under the age of 4, the main trunk of the facial nerve runs very superficially in the preauricular region and is not afforded the protection of the mastoid process, which at this stage is not fully developed. Accordingly, lacerations or surgical incisions made in this area risk transecting the facial nerve trunk.

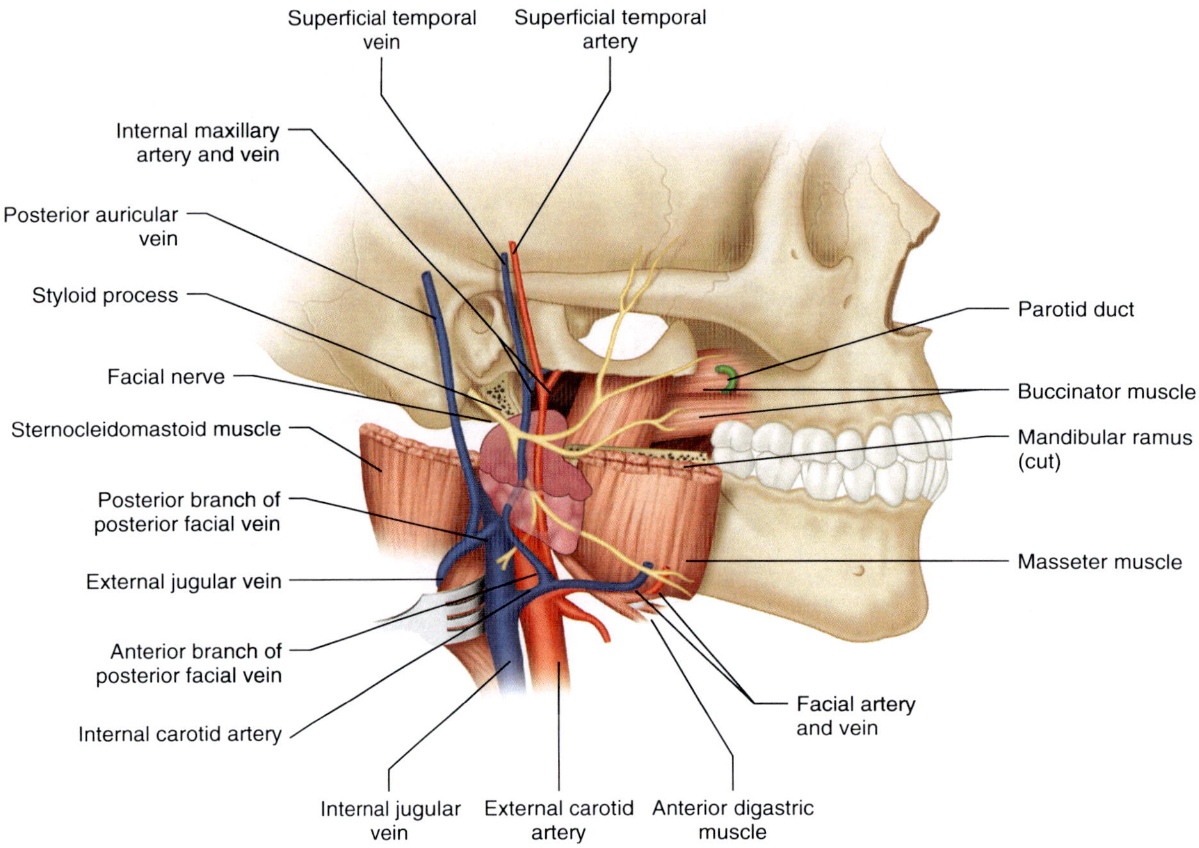

Fig. 2.7 Relationship of the facial nerve to surrounding structures

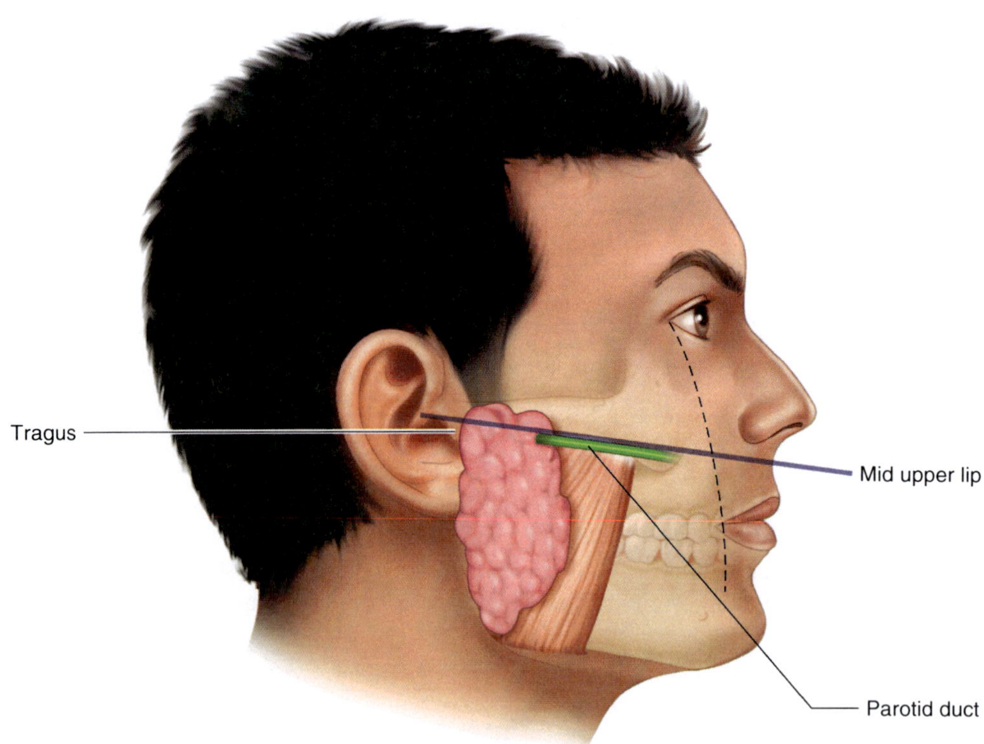

Fig. 2.8 Anatomic landmarks for the course of the parotid duct

The parotid's parasympathetic innervation is primarily derived from the glossopharyngeal nerve (CN IX) via the auriculotemporal nerve, a branch of the trigeminal nerve (CN V). Sympathetic innervation of the gland is via the fibers carried along the adjacent arteries.

The Infratemporal Region

The infratemporal region lies below and medial to the zygomatic arch. The infratemporal fossa is superiorly bordered by the infratemporal crest of the greater wing of the sphenoid. The medial limit is the lateral pterygoid plate. The lateral borders are the ramus and coronoid process of the mandible. Anteriorly, the fossa is bound by the infratemporal surface of the mandible and posteriorly by the posterior border of the mandible. Within the infratemporal region lie most of the muscles of mastication as well as the major blood vessels and nerves to the mouth region.

The mandibular division of the trigeminal nerve (CN V) is the main nerve of the infratemporal region, and the maxillary artery (internal maxillary) is the major vessel. The maxillary artery takes its origin from the external carotid artery, which ascends deep to the posterior belly of the digastric and stylohyoid muscles, running approximately parallel to the posterior border of the ramus of the mandible.

After giving off the facial artery at the level of the angle of the mandible, the external carotid continues superiorly to give off the maxillary artery and the superficial temporal artery as well as additional smaller branches to the face and neck (see Fig. 2.9). The maxillary artery usually passes

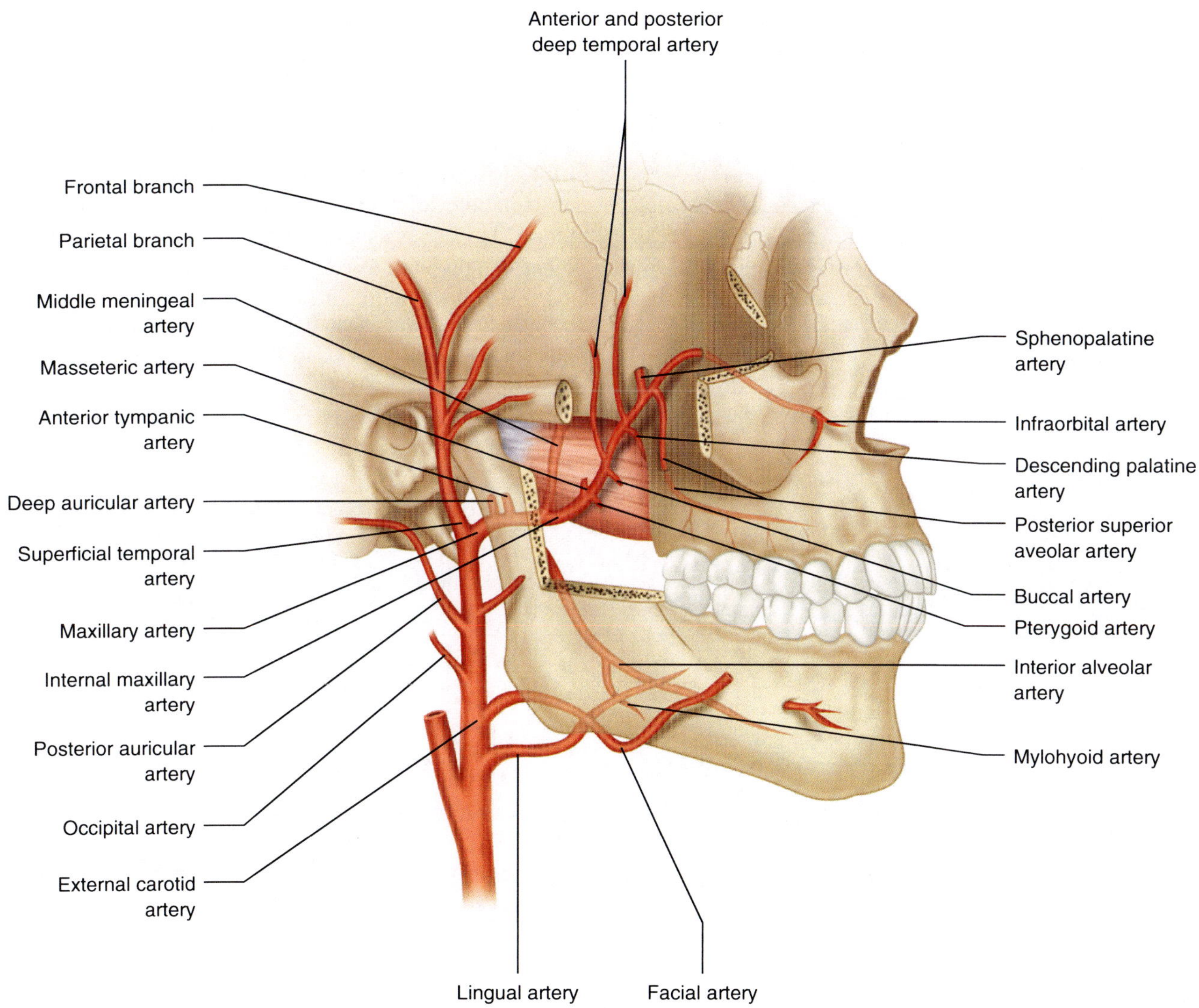

Fig. 2.9 Branches of the external carotid artery

across the lateral surface of the lateral pterygoid muscle, though it may run deep to the muscle for a short distance and then surface further forward between its two heads. The course of the maxillary artery is anatomically considered in three portions as it traverses the infratemporal region. The first portion is medial to the mandible and posterior to the lateral pterygoid. Four branches arise from this first part of the artery. The deep auricular and anterior tympanic arteries pass upward to supply the external acoustic meatus and the middle ear cavity. The middle meningeal artery, the most important branch clinically, runs upward to enter the skull through the foramen spinosum. The inferior alveolar (dental) artery descends, accompanied by the inferior alveolar nerve, into the mandibular canal where it supplies the lower teeth.

The second part of the artery lies in contact with the lateral pterygoid muscle. The branches of this portion of the artery accompany nerves of the same name to the surrounding musculature. The arterial branches are the masseteric, the buccal, two deep temporals, and branches to both pterygoids. The third portion of the artery is that which enters the pterygopalatine fossa in the posterior lateral aspect of the maxilla. The branches of this portion of the artery are the posterior superior alveolar artery to the upper teeth; the infraorbital artery, which enters the infraorbital canal and gives off orbital and superior alveolar branches; the descending palatine artery with its greater and lesser palatine branches; and, last, the sphenopalatine artery, which supplies the nose. Surrounding the lateral pterygoid muscle is a plexus of veins draining the areas supplied by the maxillary artery. The pterygoid plexus drains into the alveolar and posterior facial vein.

Operating Notes

In maxillofacial trauma, the sphenopalatine vessel is often a source of profuse bleeding. Inability to control bleeding through reduction of the fracture or nasal packing may require either intraluminal occlusion of the vessel (by interventional radiology) or direct exposure of and ligation of the artery.

The Muscles of Mastication

The four muscles of mastication all pass through the infratemporal fossa. Their functional anatomy is of primary importance to the maxillofacial surgeon. The masseter muscle originates from two heads. The superficial portion arises from the lower border and the anterior two-thirds of the zygomatic arch. The muscle fibers slant downward and backward, overlying the deep head of the muscle to insert into the lateral and inferior portion of the ramus of the mandible. The deep head of the muscle originates from the inner surface of the posterior one-third of the zygomatic arch, where it then runs vertically downward to join the insertion of the superficial head at the ramus. The masseter muscles are strong elevators of the mandible. The deep head of the muscle also serves as a mandibular retractor.

The temporalis muscle originates in the temporal fossa, passes lateral to the maxillary artery and lateral to the pterygoid, and beneath the zygomatic arch, to insert into the coracoid process and the medial side of the ramus of the mandible. The temporalis muscle is covered by two layers of fascia, the tem-

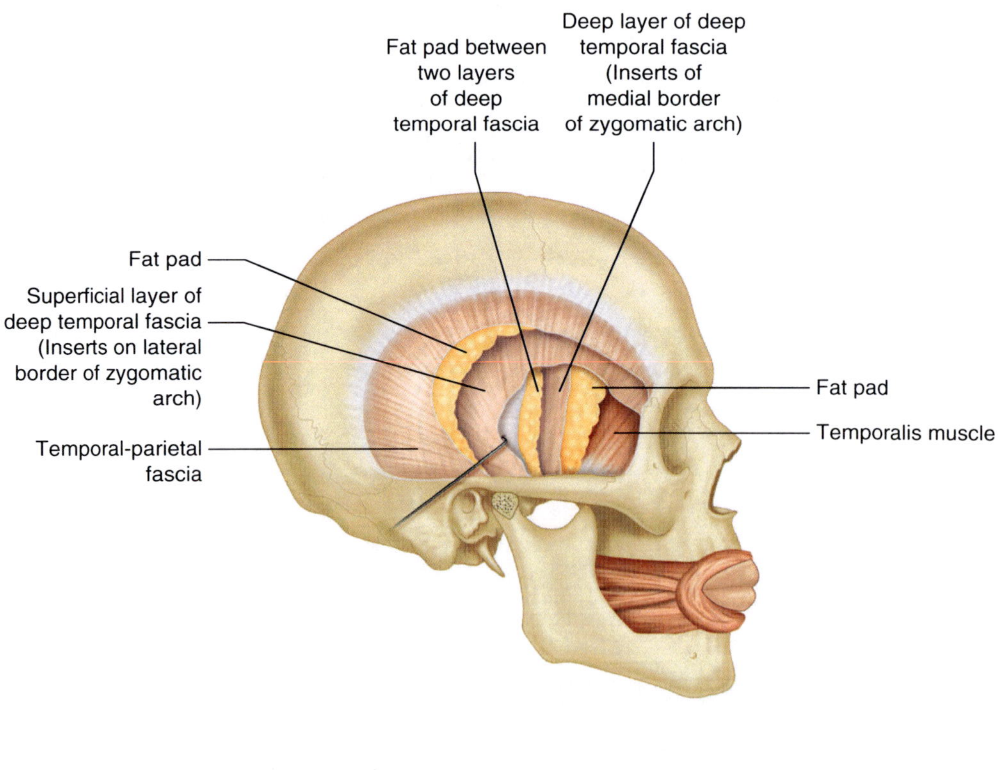

Fig. 2.10 Soft tissue layers of the temporal scalp

poral parietal (most superficial layer of the fascial layers) and the deep temporal fascia (see Fig. 2.10). The deep temporal fascia is further subdivided into a superficial and a deep layer. The temporal parietal fascia and deep temporal fascia are separated by a layer of loose areolar tissue. As one approaches the zygomatic arch, the superficial and deep layers of the deep temporal fascia are separated by the superficial temporal fat pad.

The frontal branch of the facial nerve is encompassed by the temporal parietal fascia at two fingerbreadths lateral to the lateral orbital rim and two fingerbreadths above the zygomatic. The temporal branch of the facial nerve is also encompassed by the temporal parietal fascia at the level of the arch (see Fig. 2.11). When performing a coronal approach to the upper facial skeleton, the operating surgeon should separate the superficial and deep layers of the deep temporal fascia, reflecting the superficial deep layer and the temporal parietal fascia with the frontal nerve enclosed.

The superficial layer of deep temporal fascia inserts into the lateral border of the zygomatic arch, while deep layer inserts into the medial border of the arch. To elevate and reduce a malar complex fracture through a Gillies approach, posterior to the temporal hairline, the surgeon must pass the elevator to the deep layer of the deep temporal fascia and follow the muscle toward its insertion on the coronoid. In this way the elevator is certain to be posterior to the zygomatic arch and malar complex. The temporalis muscle elevates and retracts the mandible.

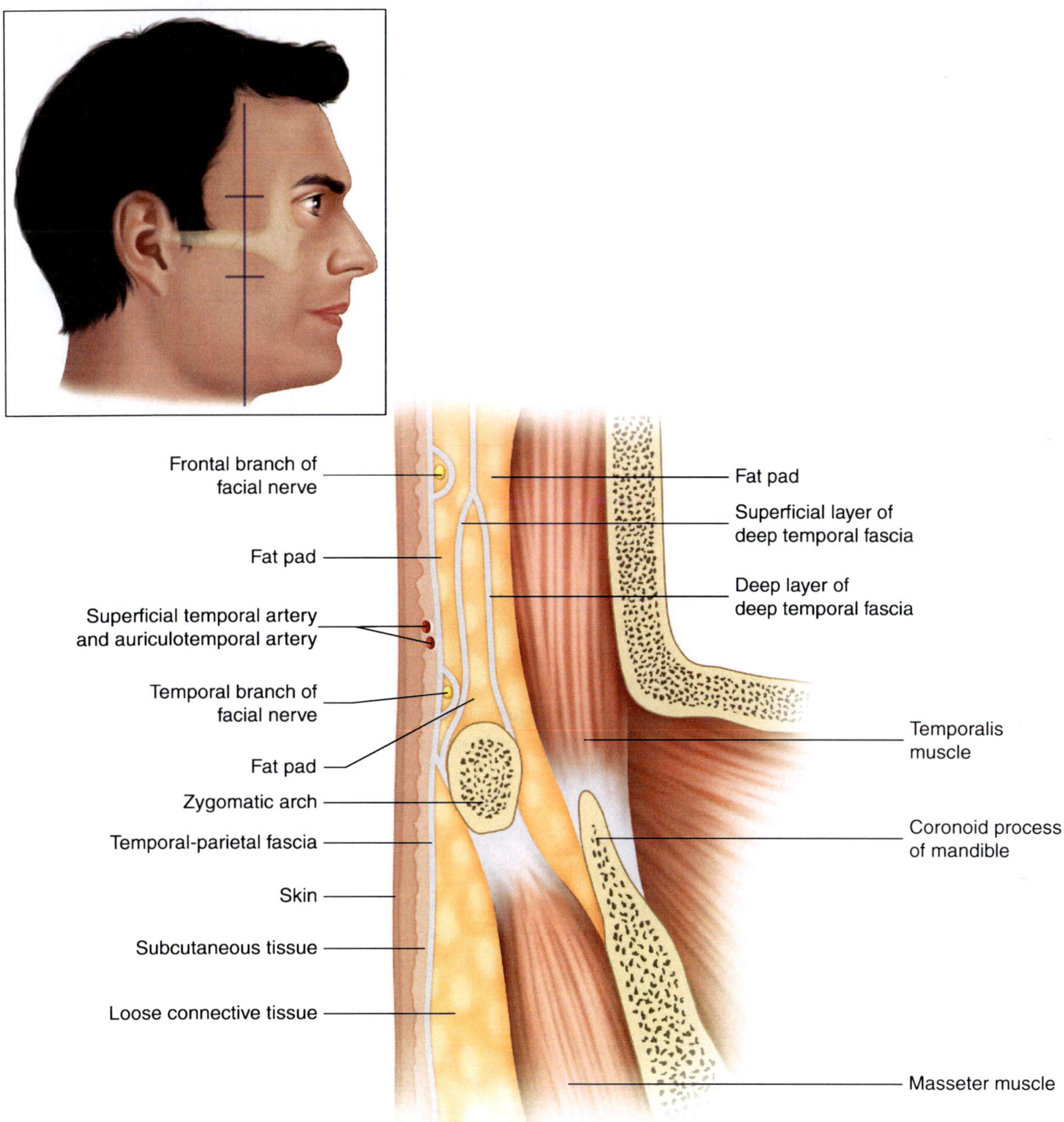

Fig. 2.11 Cross-section of the temporal scalp and zygomatic arch

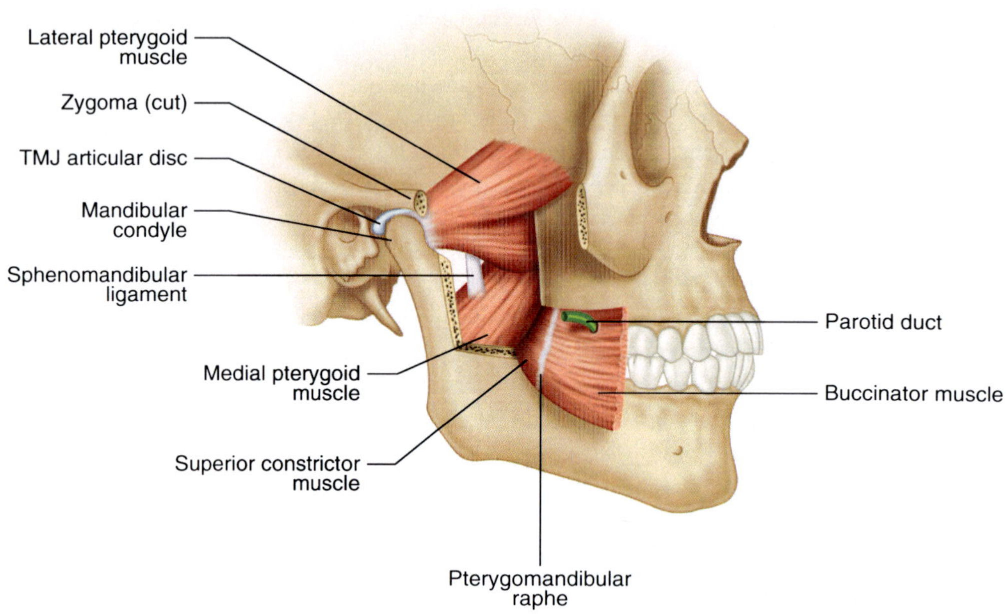

Fig. 2.12 Muscles of mastication

Though there are two pterygoid plates, a medial and a lateral, the pterygoid muscles both take their origin from the lateral pterygoid plate (see Fig. 2.12). The lateral (external) pterygoid muscle arises from two heads. The superior head originates from the infratemporal surface of the greater wing of the sphenoid and sweeps downward to its insertion into the articular surface and disk of the temporomandibular joint. The inferior head arises from the lateral surface of the lateral pterygoid plate and runs slightly upward and straight back to insert into the pterygoid fovea on the neck of the mandible. The pull of the muscle exerted on the mandible is primarily forward and medial. The lateral pterygoid is primarily a protruder of the mandible. In fractures or resections of the mandible, this segment is pulled upward and lingually. Understanding this action is essential for the intraoperative alignment of occlusion.

Operating Notes

In a LeFort-type fracture, the action of the lateral pterygoid pulls the maxillary segment inferior and posterior, resulting in premature contact of the molar teeth. This molar blocking produces an anterior apertognathia (open bite deformity), a frequent presenting sign of the maxillofacial trauma patient.

The medial (internal) pterygoid muscle has its origins from the medial surface of the lateral pterygoid plate. The fibers of this muscle run downward laterally and posteriorly, inserting into the medial and inferior border of the ramus of the mandible, forming a sling with the masseter muscle around the mandibular ramus. The pull of the medial pterygoid is inward and upward, elevating and medially directing the mandible. This pull results in a superior and medial pull of proximal mandibular fracture fragments (see Fig. 2.13).

Other Muscles of the Mandibular Region

The geniohyoid muscles are paired muscles whose origin is the mental spine of the inner aspect of the symphysis of the mandible. They insert on the body of the hyoid bone. The muscle is innervated by the hypoglossal nerve (CN XII) as well as fibers from cervical nerve 1 (C-1). The muscles act as depressors and retractors of the mandible.

The digastric muscle is composed of a posterior and an anterior belly connected by a long tendon. The posterior belly originates on the medial mastoid process, passes forward and inferiorly, and becomes tendonous as it passes through a fascial sling at the level of the hyoid bone. The tendon then courses abruptly upward and forward, becoming the anterior belly of the digastric and inserting into the digastric fossa on the lower medial surface of the mandible. The digastric muscle has two innervations. The posterior muscle is innervated by the facial nerve (CN VII), while the anterior belly is innervated by the trigeminal nerve (CN V) by way of the mandibular segment of the nerve, whose inferior alveolar branch gives off the mylohyoid nerve, which further branches to supply the digastrics. The digastric muscle similarly acts as a depressor and retractor of the mandible (see Fig. 2.14).

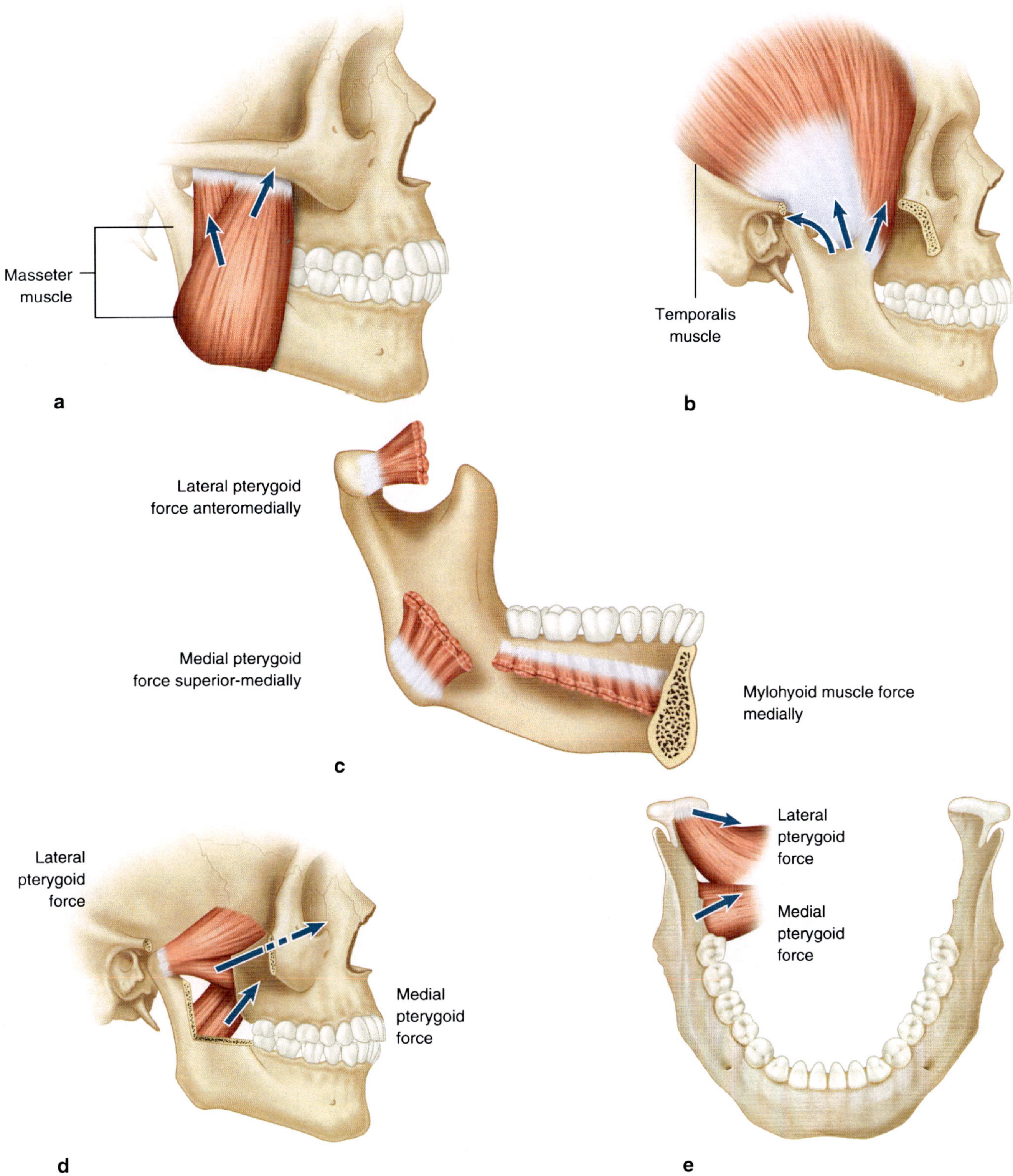

Fig. 2.13 Isolated muscles of mastication

Fig. 2.14 Muscles of the neck

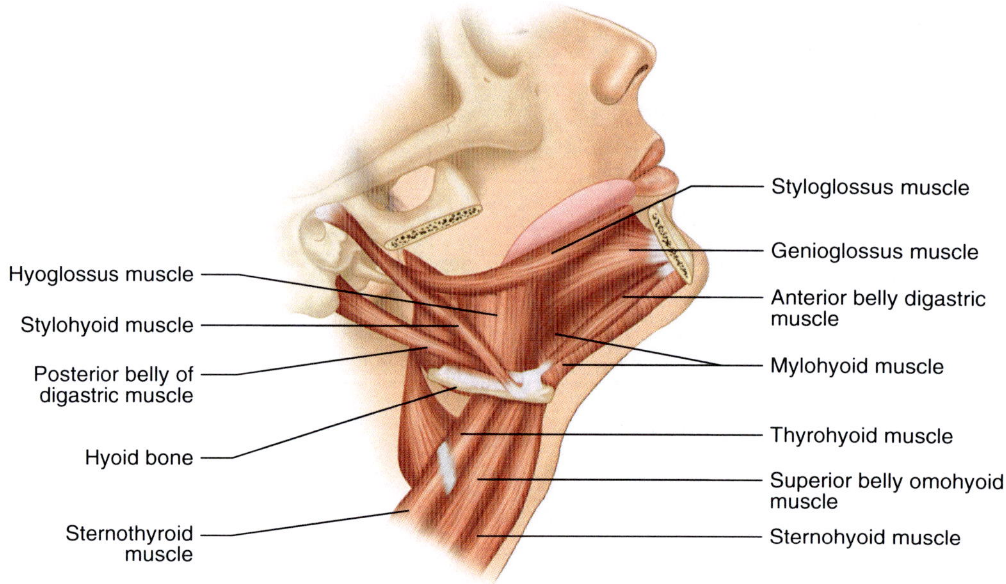

The mylohyoid muscles form a muscular diaphragm, extending across the inner surface of the mandible as well as posteriorly to the body of the hyoid bone. Superior to the muscle lie the geniohyoid and the muscles of the tongue. Inferiorly lie the digastric muscle and the paired submandibular glands. The muscle is supplied by the mylohyoid branch of the mandibular nerve. The mylohyoid functions to elevate the tongue during swallowing.

Operative Notes

With a parasymphyseal fracture, the muscle pulls on the bone producing a lingual inversion of the fractured segment. Placement of a simple inferior border wire on the mandible would be insufficient alone to maintain the proper occlusion in a fractured body segment. The resultant action of the geniohyoid and digastric muscles is to pull anterior fractured segments inferior and posterior (see Fig. 2.15). Overcoming these forces is required to properly reduce bilateral anterior or parasymphyseal fractures. The degree of displacement of mandibular fractures is dependent upon the pull of the musculature with regard to the line of fracture (see Fig. 2.16).

The Submandibular Region

The submandibular region is considered anterior to the border of the sternocleidomastoid muscle, inferior to the floor of the mouth, and superior to the line of the hyoid.

Operative Notes

The surgical approach to this area might involve an incision approximately one fingerbreadth below the border of the mandible, extending from the ramus forward to the chin. Directly below the border of the platysma, which overlies the mandible, the facial vein and artery are encountered about halfway between the ramus of the mandible and the chin. The vessels can be palpated at the border of the mandible. Running in the subplatysmal plane is the marginal mandibular branch of the facial nerve. The nerve runs along the border of the mandible, sometimes above and sometimes below. The nerve crosses superficial to the facial artery and vein. The use of a nerve stimulator in the surgical approach to this area is highly recommended to avoid damaging this nerve.

The submandibular gland forms a U shape around the free posterior lateral border of the mylohyoid. Just as the posterior ramus of the mandible delineates the parotid into a deep and a superficial segment, so too does the mylohyoid separate the submandibular gland into a deep and a superficial segment. The deep segment of the gland lies on the hyoglossus muscle, which arises from the length of the greater horn of the hyoid and extends superiorly to insert at the side of the tongue. The hyoglossus pulls the sides of the tongue downward. It is innervated by the hypoglossal nerve (CN XII), which runs in the space between the deep

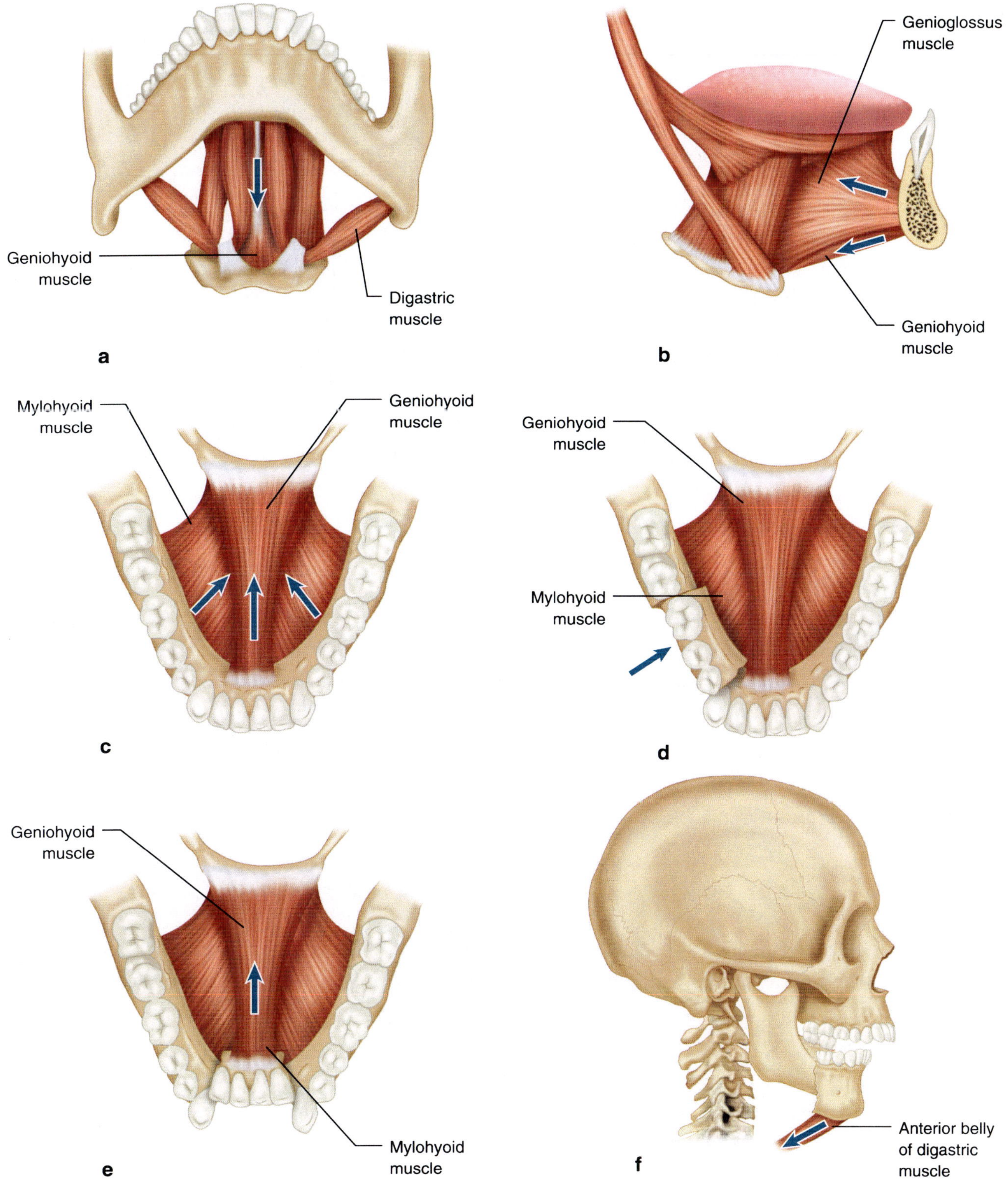

Fig. 2.15 Muscles surrounding the mandible

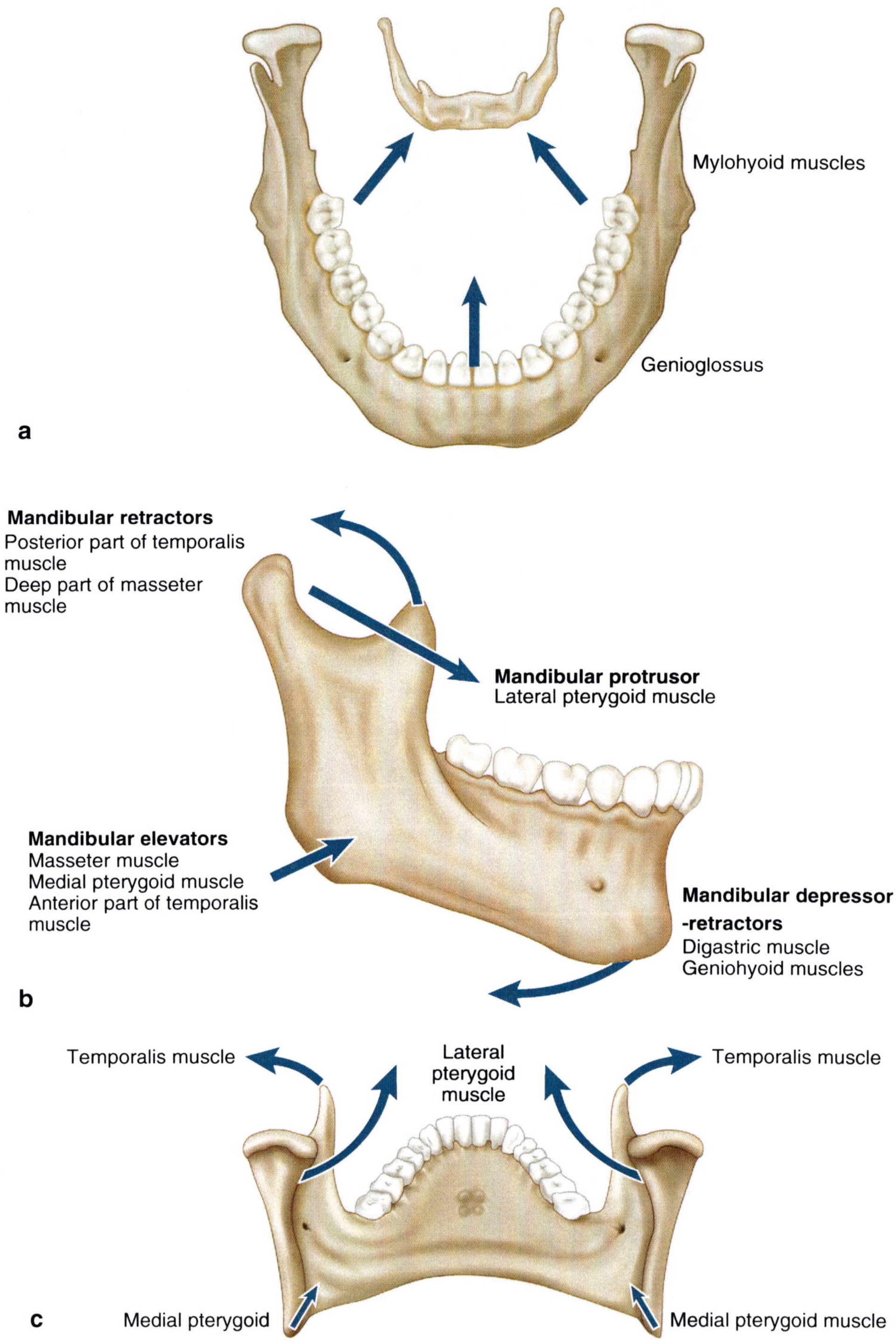

Fig. 2.16 Specific function of the muscles of mastication

portion of the submandibular gland and the hyoglossus. Within this space is also found the submandibular ganglion, from which postganglionic fibers pass to the submandibular and sublingual glands. The submandibular duct (Wharton's) exits from the deep part of the gland, running forward first on the hyoglossus and then on the genioglossus to open through the floor of the mouth into the mouth cavity by a small raised papilla close to midline. The lingual nerve, on its way to supply the tongue, runs first above the deep portion of the submandibular gland and then encircles the duct by first lying lateral to, then below, and then medial to the duct.

The sublingual gland lies anterior to the deep portion of the submandibular gland and just lateral to the lingual nerve and submandibular duct as they course along the lateral side of the genioglossus. The anterior portion of the gland lies in contact with the anterior portion of the contralateral gland, directly below the mucous membrane of the anterior floor of the mouth. The gland is drained by multiple small ducts, some of which drain into the submandibular duct and others that empty directly into the floor of the mouth.

Operative Notes
An incision through the mucous membrane just lateral to the tongue passes into the area on the lateral side of the hyoglossus, giving a clear view of the sublingual gland and lingual nerve. The submandibular gland is, however, best operatively approached from below the mandible.

The Tongue

The tongue lies on the floor of the mouth posteriorly attached by its root, through which its nerves and vessels pass. The upper surface of the tongue is covered with mucosa in which reside several different types of papillae. At the apex to a "V" formed by the large circumvallate papillae lies the foramen cecum, a small area indicating the embryologic origin of the thyroid gland. A mass presenting in this area of the tongue first discovered at puberty may represent a lingual thyroid gland. In some 70–80 % of patients, this may be the only thyroid gland present.

The sensory innervation of the tongue is derived from the first, second, and third branchial arches from which it takes its embryologic origin. The anterior two-thirds of the tongue is supplied with general sensation from the lingual nerve branches of the trigeminal nerve. The lingual nerve also carries the taste fibers from the chorda tympani, a branch of the facial nerve. The posterior one-third of the tongue is supplied with both taste and general sensation by the glossopharyngeal nerve (CN IX). A small area on the lateral posterior lingual tonsil is supplied by the vagus nerve (CN X).

The tongue is a muscle divided into extrinsic and intrinsic muscle fibers. The extrinsic muscles of the tongue are the genioglossus, the styloglossus, the hyoglossus, and the palatoglossus. The genioglossus muscle extends from the mental spine posteriorly in a fan-shaped manner along the entire area of the tongue from apex to base. The genioglossus acts as a protruder and depressor of the tongue.

The styloglossus originates at the styloid process and stylomandibular ligament. It extends downward and anteriorly to the lateral side of the tongue. The lower fibers of the muscle are related laterally to a portion of the sublingual gland. The styloglossus acts primarily as a retractor of the tongue.

The hyoglossus arises from the lateral body and greater cornu of the hyoid. It then passes upward and forward laterally to the posterior genioglossus, where it then interlaces with the styloglossus and intrinsic muscles of the tongue. Its action is that of a tongue depressor.

The palatoglossus (more a muscle of the palate than the tongue) extends from the palatine aponeurosis at the side of the tongue to form the anterior tonsillar pillar. The palatoglossus elevates the root of the tongue. Unlike the other extrinsic and intrinsic muscles of the tongue, which are all supplied by the hypoglossal nerve (CN XII), the palatoglossus, being more related to the palatal musculature, is supplied by the vagus nerve (CN X).

The intrinsic muscles of the tongue are oriented longitudinally, vertically, and horizontally, with extensive interdigitation of fibers. The intrinsic musculature functions to shape the tongue for swallowing and speech. The main arteries supplying the tongue are the paired lingual arteries off the external carotid. They are accompanied by the lingual veins. The deep lingual vein (or ranine vein) can be seen in the floor of the mouth at the side of the frenulum. The various veins of the tongue drain ultimately into the internal jugular.

Operative Notes
Coverage of intraoral defects may utilize a flap of tongue based on the lateral blood supply. In most cases, the donor site may be closed primarily without significant deformity.

The Pharynx

The pharynx may best be considered as a mucosal-covered muscular tube open anteriorly through its entire length until it becomes the closed esophagus at its most inferior aspect. The upper portion of the tube, the nasopharynx, opens to the nasal chambers. The middle portion of the tube, the oropharynx, opens into the mouth. The lower portion of the tube, the laryngeal pharynx, opens to the larynx at the level of the hyoid bone and upper hyoid cartilages. The muscles that form the pharyngeal tube include the superior, middle, and inferior constrictors. Each of these muscles sweeps posteriorly from its anterior origins to join with the corresponding muscle from the opposite side at the pharyngeal raphe of the posterior midline.

The superior constrictor has a broad origin: superiorly from the posterior border of the medial pterygoid plate and its hamulus, inferiorly from the pterygomandibular raphe along the posterior border of the buccinator, and most inferiorly from the posterior part of the hyoid bone over the mandible and the side of the root of the tongue. The connection of the superior constrictor to the buccinator and through the buccinator to the orbicularis oris provides for a continuous ring of musculature from the neck through the lower face.

Operative Notes
Clefts of the lip break the dynamic balance of this ring, and it may be hypothesized that the muscular forces exerted through the broken ring now contribute to the gradual distraction of the cleft segments with every swallow. Repair requires reorientation and reapproximation of the muscle to itself.

The middle constrictor arises from both the lesser and greater cornua of the hyoid bone. Superiorly, it overlaps the superior constrictor and is in turn overlapped at its inferior border by the inferior constrictor.

The inferior constrictor arises from the oblique line of the thyroid cartilage, along the tendonous line to the cricoid cartilage. This tendonous line also gives attachment to the thyrohyoid and sternothyroid muscles. The cricopharyngeal portion of the inferior constrictor is also known as the cricopharyngeal muscle (see Fig. 2.17).

An additional muscle of the pharynx of note is the stylopharyngeus, which originates from the medial aspect of the styloid process and passes downward and medially to pass into the pharyngeal wall in the gap between the superior and middle constrictors. The muscle functions to elevate the pharynx to the esophagus. Like most of the palatal musculature, the constrictors are innervated by the vagus nerve (CN X), while the stylopharyngeus is innervated by the glossopharyngeal nerve (CN IX).

Filling the gap between the upper border of the superior constrictor and the base of the skull are two small muscles, the tensor veli palatini and levator veli palatini. These muscles reinforce the pharyngeal wall in this area, though they are primarily concerned with the soft palate.

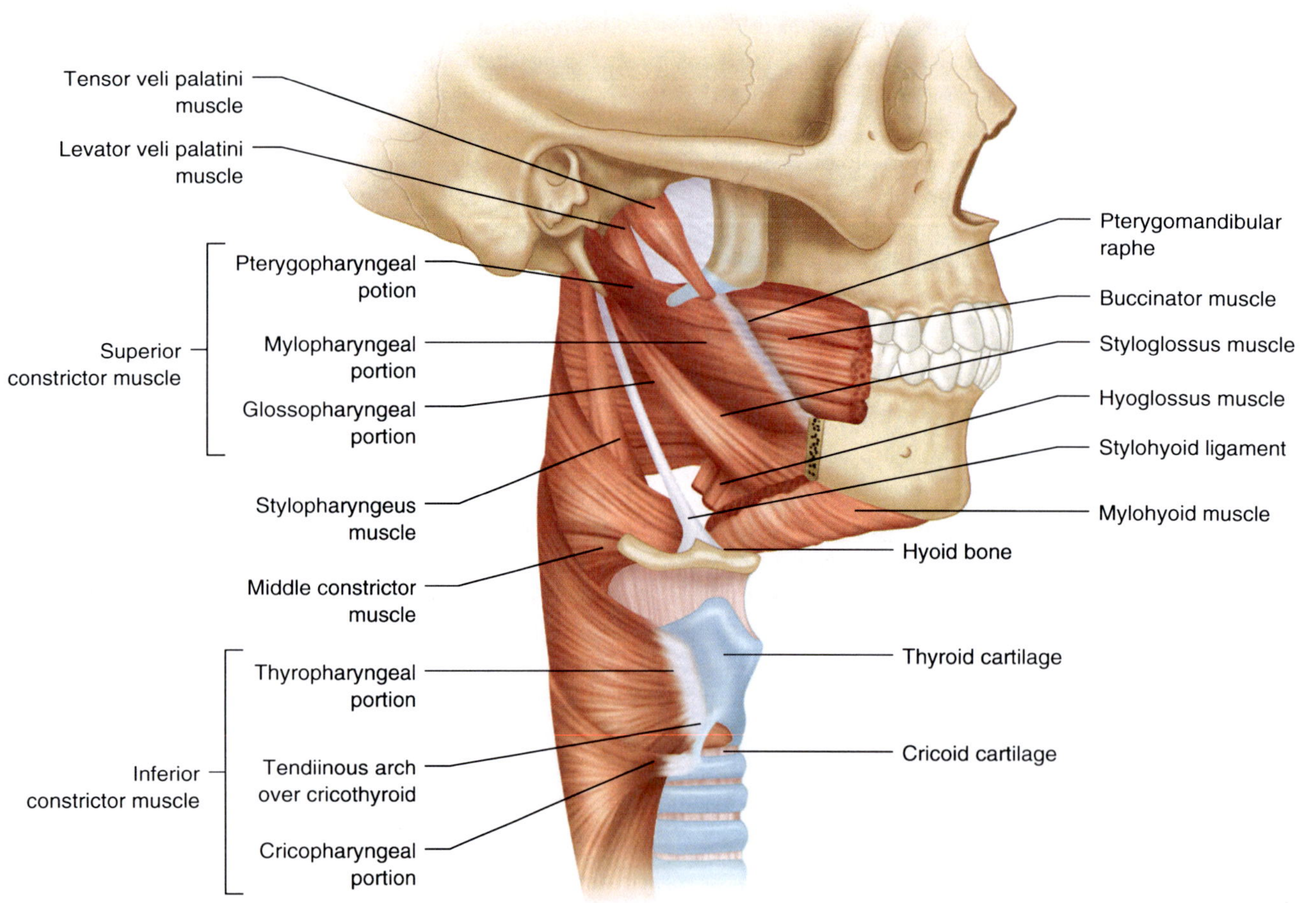

Fig. 2.17 Muscles of the pharynx and hypopharynx

Operative Notes
As with the lip, reorientation and reapproximation of the levator muscle to itself across the midline of the soft palate is important in the creation of normal velopharyngeal function and resonance.

The Palate

The palate separates the nasopharynx from the oropharynx. Proper speech and swallowing functions are directly dependent on the ability of the palate to completely separate these two areas. The palate is composed of a bony hard palate and a muscular soft palate.

The hard palate is formed by the palatine process of the maxilla and the horizontal process of the palatine bones. The maxillary portion is continuous with the alveolar process of the maxilla anteriorly and laterally. The hard palate is divided into a primary portion anterior to the incisive foramen and derived from the premaxilla and a secondary portion posterior to the incisive foramen derived from the palatine process of each maxilla. The hard palate is covered by mucosa firmly attached to the underlying bone by a tough connective tissue known as the mucoperiosteum. Numerous minor salivary glands are contained in the mucoperiosteum. The blood supply to the hard palate comes anteriorly via the sphenopalatine branch of the maxillary artery, which exits through the incisive canal, and posteriorly via the paired greater palatine branches of the maxillary artery. These branches descend in the greater palatine foramina just medial to the third maxillary molars. More posteriorly there are also the lesser palatine foramina, through which emerge minor palatine vessels. The nerve supply to the hard palate comes from the sphenopalatine and greater palatine branches of the maxillary division of the trigeminal nerve (CN V). These branches exit with their respective arteries.

Operative Notes
With LeFort osteotomy, the down-fractured maxillary segment remains supplied by the paired greater palatine arteries posterior to the maxillary sinus. Care should be taken to protect these vessels by not running a saw or osteotome across the posterior wall of the sinus but rather performing a controlled fracture of this area to mobilize the inferior segment. If posterior impaction of the maxilla is required, careful freeing of the vessel and direct removal of the bone with a rongeur is recommended.

The soft palate, or velum, is composed of a muscular structure bound together by the palatine aponeurosis of connective tissue and covered by mucosa on both its nasal and oral side. The uvula projects downward from the posterior midline of the soft palate. The soft palate musculature is composed of five muscles: the tensor veli palatine, the levator veli palatini, the palatoglossus, the palatopharyngeus, and the muscularis uvulae (see Fig. 2.18).

The palatoglossus is the most superficial palatal muscle on the oral side of the soft palate. Its fibers sweep transversely from the midline of the palate, laterally and inferiorly downward to the lateral margin of the tongue, forming the anterior tonsillar pillar on its way.

The palatopharyngeus is the most superficial of the palatal muscles on the pharyngeal side of the soft palate. This muscle, more a pharyngeal muscle than a palatal one, forms the palatal pharyngeal arch along the posterior tonsillar pillar. The muscle sweeps upward into the soft palate, where its anterior and posterior fibers separate to surround the musculari uvulae. The normal action of the palatoglossus and the palatopharyngeus muscle is to draw the soft palate downward and help provide inward lateral pharyngeal wall motion.

Operative Notes
It is the tonsillar portion of the palatopharyngeus muscle that is elevated on a superior base and used to perform a sphincter pharyngioplasty.

The muscularis uvulae lies deep to the palatopharyngeus, and its fibers run longitudinally down the midline of the soft palate and posteriorly into the uvula. The action of the muscularis uvulae is to draw the uvula forward and upward.

The levator veli palatini, the largest muscle of the soft palate, originates at the apex of the petrous bone at the base of the skull and along the medial cartilage of the eustachian tube. It sweeps forward, downward, and medially into the soft palate lying between the muscularis uvulae and the anterior layer of the palatopharyngeus. Constriction of this muscle elevates the palate and pulls open the eustachian tube.

The tensor veli palatini originates broadly from the scaphoid fossa of the medial pterygoid plate and the lateral eustachian tube cartilage. The muscle passes downward between the medial pterygoid muscle and the medial pterygoid plate to the hamulus. The fibers of the muscle are adherent to the hamulus, at which point they continue to sweep medially at a right angle across the palate, attaching themselves to the posterior hard palatal shelf and joining with the

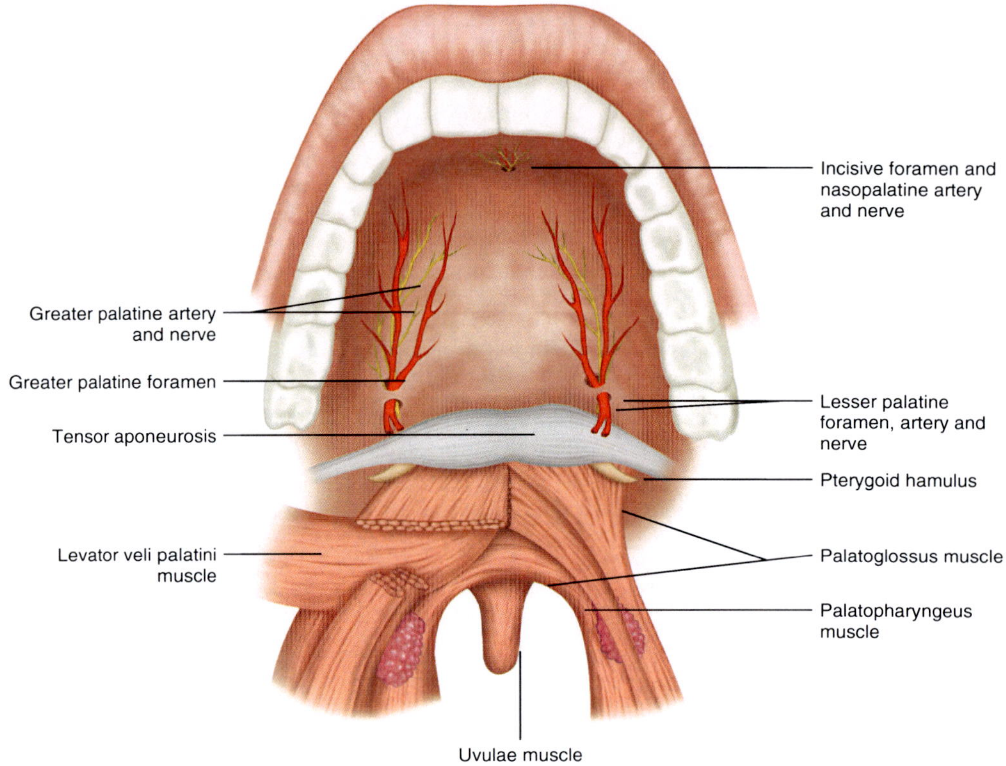

Fig. 2.18 Muscles of the soft palate

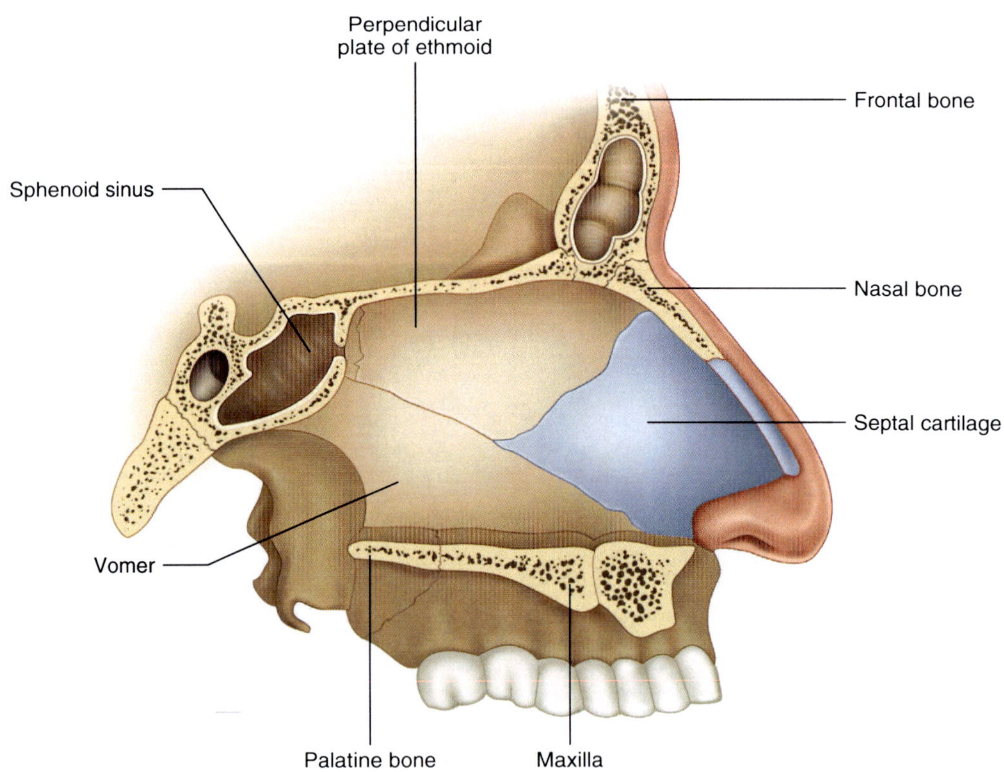

Fig. 2.19 Nasal septum

Operating Notes

In palatal repair, the tightening action of the tensor may inhibit the medial transposition of the palatal tensor muscle. Stripping the attachment of the muscle from the hamulus at the time of palatal repair may ameliorate this tension.

contralateral muscle at the soft palate midline. The tensor, as the name implies, tenses the soft palate and depresses it somewhat in the midline. It also serves as the primary opener of the eustachian tube. Unlike the other muscles of the soft palate, which receive their innervation by the vagus nerve (CN X), the tensor is innervated by a branch of the mandibular division of the trigeminal nerve (CN V).

The Nose

The pyramidal shape of the nose and its gently curving nasal ala is determined by its underlying bony and cartilaginous structure. The upper third of the nose is supported by the paired nasal bones, which are considered separate facial bones. The middle third is supported by the upper lateral cartilages, which extend, tentlike, from their junction with the nasal septum at the dorsum toward the maxilla. The lower lateral cartilages support the lower third, including the ala and nasal tip.

The nasal septum divides the nasal chamber into right and left nasal cavities (see Fig. 2.19). The septum extends from the hard palate below, arising from the vomer and perpendicular plate of the ethmoid, to the undersurface of the anterior cranial fossa. The cartilaginous quadrilateral septal cartilage forms a large portion of the septum. A septum deviated to one or both sides may obstruct the airway.

The roof of the nasal cavity is formed by the frontal bone, the cribriform plate of the ethmoid, and the body of the sphenoid. Special smell receptors, located in the mucous membrane of the upper nasal cavity, transmit their information via rootlets of the olfactory nerve, which pierce the roof of the cribriform plate beneath the crista galli. Sensory innervation of the nose is carried by the sphenopalatine nerve, which innervates the majority of the nasal septum and the anterior third of the hard palate. The anterior ethmoidal nerve supplies sensation to the anterior part of the nasal septum.

The lateral wall of the nose is formed principally by the maxilla and ethmoid. The lateral wall of the nasal cavity separates the nose from the air cells of the paranasal sinuses. Drainage from these sinuses takes place through openings in the lateral nasal wall. The upper part of the lateral nasal wall is formed by the ethmoid, whose air cells form a prominent bulge into the nasal cavity, referred to as the ethmoidal bulla. More anteriorly, a thin spur of ethmoid, known as the uncinate process, is present and is separated from the ethmoidal bulla by a shallow groove known as the hiatus semilunaris. The maxillary sinus drains into this groove (see Fig. 2.20).

Overlying the bulla and air cells are delicate scrolls of bone covered by mucus membrane. These scrolls are known as the conchae. There are four conchae, separated from one another by grooves, known as meatae. Each meatus is named after the concha to which it is related: "supreme," "superior," "middle," and "inferior" concha. All but the inferior concha are outgrowths of the ethmoidal bone. The inferior concha is considered a separate facial bone. The space between the superior concha in front and the sphenoid behind is the sphenoethmoidal recess.

The sphenoid sinus drains into the sphenoethmoidal recess. The posterior ethmoidal sinus drains into the superior meatus. The anterior and middle ethmoidal sinuses drain through the bulla, while the maxillary antrum and the frontal sinus open into the hiatus semilunaris. The drainage from these areas appears below the middle concha. The nasolacrimal duct opens into the inferior meatus.

The Orbit

The Bony Orbit

The bony orbit is pyramidal in shape, with its apex lying posteromedially. There are four walls: a medial wall, a lateral wall, a roof, and a floor. The medial wall of the orbit lies almost directly within the sagittal plane, while the lateral wall diverges laterally outward from apex to base. The optic nerve enters posteriorly through the optic foramen at the apex, approximately 43 mm posterior to the orbital rim. The orbit also communicates intracranially via the superior orbital fissure, through which runs the oculomotor, trochlear, and abducens nerves (see Fig. 2.21). The orbital rim forms the base, although the widest portion is actually found approximately 1.5 cm behind the orbital rim, where the circumference of the globe is widest.

There are eight separate bones that contribute to different portions of the orbit. The roof is composed of the frontal bone and lesser wing of the sphenoid. The lateral wall is composed of the greater wing of the sphenoid and the zygomatic bone. The medial wall is composed of the ethmoid bone posteriorly and the lacrimal bone anteriorly, while the floor is made up of the maxilla, comprising the roof of the maxillary sinus and a small posterior segment of the palatine bone. The floor of the orbit, after initially dropping inferiorly, posterior to the inferior rim, starts a gentle upward slope. The continuity of the floor is broken by the inferior

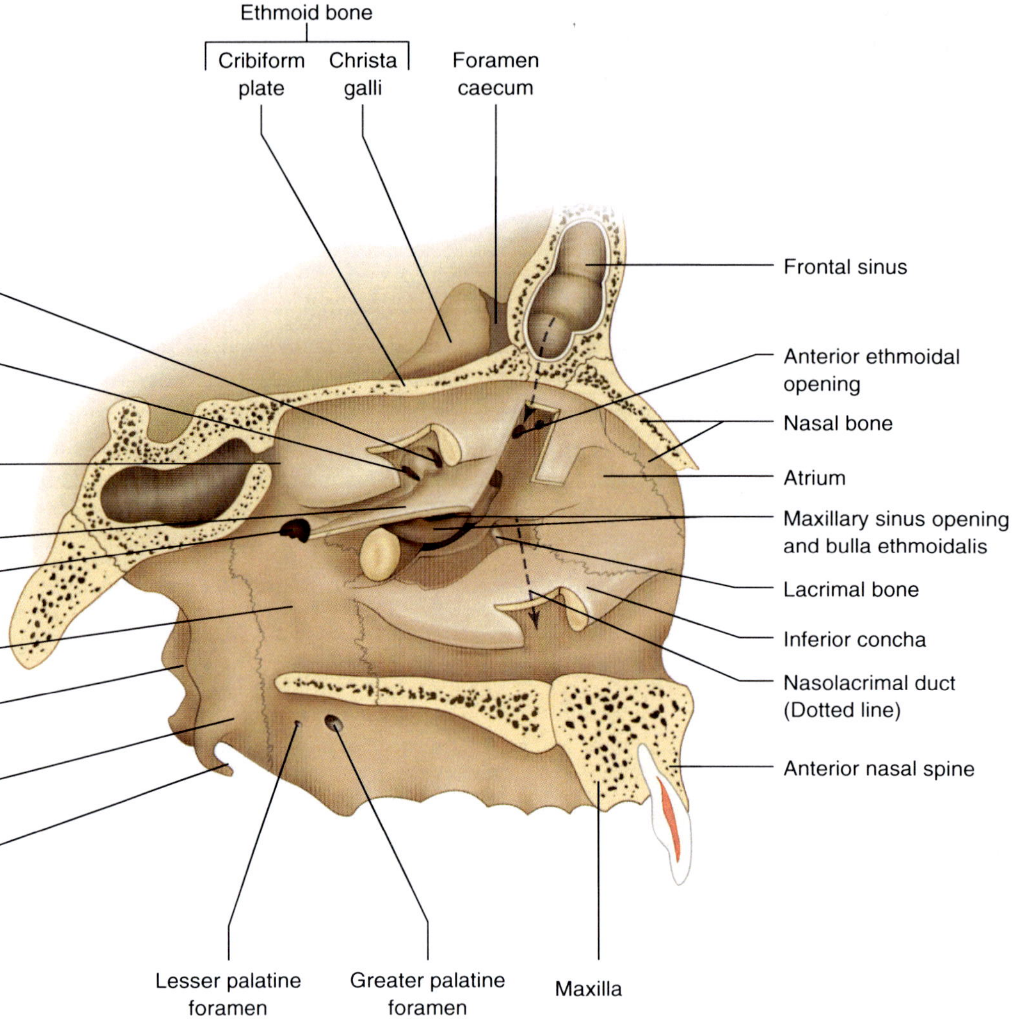

Fig. 2.20 Drainage of the craniofacial sinuses

orbital fissure, which communicates with the infratemporal space, and the infraorbital canal, which accommodates the infraorbital nerve.

Operating Notes

A lower eyelid incision is frequently used in maxillofacial surgery to gain access to the bony orbit, most often for repair of orbital blowout fractures. Dissection within the subperiosteal plane elevates the orbital contents from the bony orbit. The optic nerve lies approximately 44 mm posterior to the orbital rim. A helpful landmark to gauge the depth of one's dissection is the posterior wall of the maxillary sinus, which is found at approximately 38 mm from the orbital rim and is easily palpated with an instrument through a floor fracture. The medial wall of the orbit is pierced by the anterior and posterior ethmoidal arteries at approximately 24 mm and 34 mm, respectively, from the orbital rim. Identification of these arteries will provide a more bloodless dissection for the surgeon.

The inferior orbital fissure serves as an important landmark for osteotomies in the orbit. It is from here that an osteotomy in the lateral wall begins and moves superiorly and an osteotomy of the floor proceeds medially.

The orbital floor is weakest along the canal, and accordingly, orbital floor and malar complex fractures frequently occur along this line, resulting in compression of the infraorbital nerve with resultant hypoesthesia.

A second area of structural weakness is along the medial orbital wall separating the orbit from the ethmoidal air cells. This area is referred to as the lamina papyracea (paper wall) and is frequently blown out in orbital fractures.

Fig. 2.21 Bones of the orbit

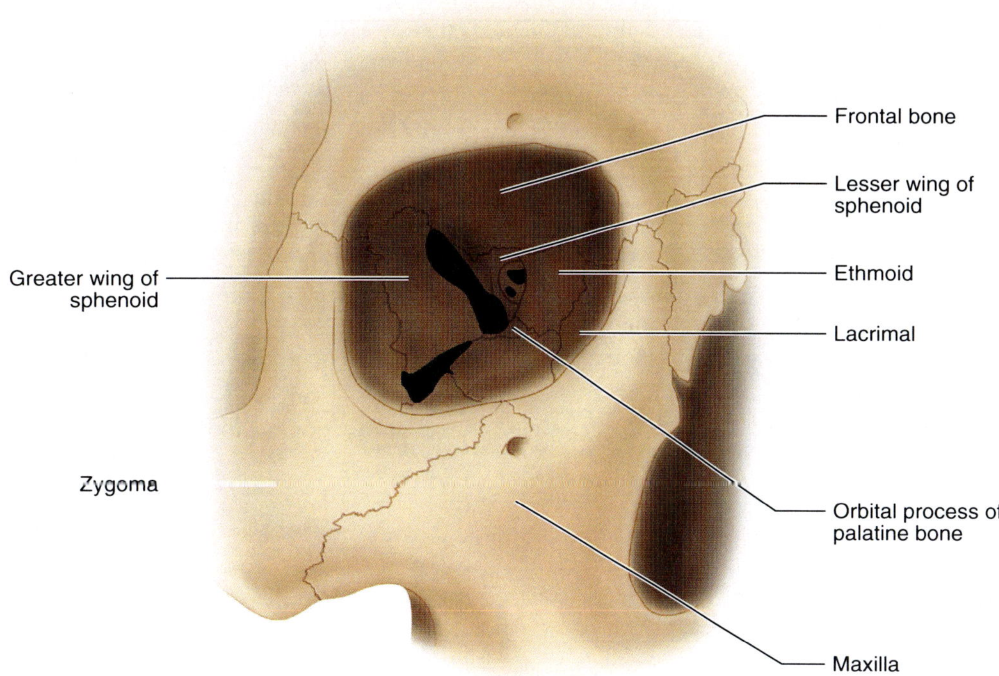

The Periorbita and Rectus Muscles

The bony orbit is lined by a loosely connected periosteum referred to as the periorbita. The periorbita sweeps backward to become continuous with the dural sheath at the optic foramen. Surrounding the area of the optic foramen and superior orbital fissure, the periorbita thickens into a circular structure from which arise the tendonous origins of the four rectus muscles. As the four recti pass anteriorly from the tendonous annular ring to their respective attachments on the globe, they form a cone of muscle that anatomically separates the retrobulbar area into intraconal and extraconal spaces.

The Extraconal Space

Removal of the orbital roof will reveal the superior portion of the extraconal space. Immediately apparent from this approach is the superior orbital fissure. The ophthalmic division of cranial nerve V is easily identified within the canal. This sensory nerve divides into three branches. The nasociliary branch of the nerve passes into the muscular cone, while the lacrimal and frontal branches continue extraconally.

The lacrimal nerve passes laterally in the orbit to the lacrimal gland and surrounding conjunctiva. The frontal nerve passes anteriorly between the roof of the orbit and the superior levator. Before crossing the superior orbital rim, the nerve divides into the supraorbital and supratrochlear nerves, which carry sensation from the skin, the conjunctiva of the medial canthus, the forehead, and the scalp, from as far posterior as the lambdoidal suture. The trochlear nerve (CN IV) also passes into the orbit via the superior orbital fissure, but unlike the other nerves to the ocular muscles, the trochlear nerve runs outside the muscular cone, passing medially across the superior levator to innervate the superior oblique muscle. As described earlier, the superior levator runs along the undersurface of the superior orbit into the tarsal plate. Medial and inferior to the superior levator is the superior oblique muscle. The superior oblique muscle arises outside of the annulus, superior and medial to the optic canal. It runs superior and medial to the medial rectus, becoming tendonous prior to passing through the trochlea, a U-shaped cartilage lined by synovial tendon sheath and attached to the spine of the frontal bone. The superior oblique muscle, on passing through the trochlea, turns sharply posteriorly, laterally, and inferiorly to where it then makes a fan-shaped attachment to the posterior superior quadrant of the globe. The action of this muscle is to pull the pupil into a downward-looking position. When unopposed by the inferior rectus secondary to oculomotor nerve palsy, the pupil is deflected nasally.

Outside the muscular cone, in the inferior orbit, lies the inferior oblique muscle, which takes its origin just posterior to the medial orbital rim, lateral to the nasal lacrimal canal. The inferior oblique passes laterally, superiorly, and posteriorly, between the periorbita and the inferior rectus muscle, to attach to the posterior lateral aspect of the globe, beneath the lateral rectus muscle. The inferior oblique is innervated by a branch of the oculomotor nerve, which passes through the muscular annulus. The action of the inferior oblique is to rotate the globe into an upward gaze and, when unopposed by the superior oblique, into a lateral gaze as well.

Operating Notes
The inferior oblique muscle may be injured during lower blepharoplasty as fat is dissected between the medial and middle compartments or during exposure of the orbital floor for fracture repair. Patients with this injury will complain of difficulty walking upstairs.

The Intraconal Space

The structures within the intraconal space are best appreciated with regard to their anatomic relationship to the optic nerve. The nerve is accompanied by the ophthalmic artery, which runs directly beneath it. The nerve passes through the common tendonous ring to enter the eyeball medial to its posterior pole. The optic nerve is accompanied by an extension of the meninges as far as its entry into the eyeball.

The nasociliary branch of the ophthalmic division of the trigeminal nerve enters the orbit via the optic foramen, passes through the muscular cone lateral to the optic nerve, and then passes superior and medial to the optic nerve, where it then divides into the anterior ethmoidal and infratrochlear nerves. Prior to this division the nerve gives off a sensory root, passing directly into the eyeball. It also branches the two long ciliary nerves, which carry sympathetic fibers from the internal carotid artery directly into the eyeball. Sympathetic stimulation of these nerves functions to dilate the pupil. The anterior ethmoidal nerve carries sensation from the ethmoidal air cells and the tip of the nose. The infratrochlear nerve carries sensation from the bridge and the side of the nose.

The oculomotor nerve (CN III) enters the orbit via the superior orbital fissure and immediately passes within the muscular cone. The nerve then divides into the motor branches for all the ocular muscles except the lateral rectus and superior oblique. A convenient formula to remember for the ocular muscle innervation is LR_6SO_4, indicating the lateral rectus muscle innervation by CN VI and the superior oblique by CN IV. The remainder of the orbital muscles are all innervated by CN III.

The ophthalmic artery enters the orbit through the optic foramen inferior to the optic nerve. The artery passes through the tendonous ring into the muscular cone. The artery first branches into the central artery of the retina and numerous ciliary branches that supply the eyeball. The artery then spirals laterally, sending a branch to the lateral orbital wall. The artery then crosses over the optic nerve to the medial wall of the orbit. There are numerous branches of the artery that supply all the ocular structures, including the conjunctiva and the skin of the lids. The ophthalmic veins run along with the arteries and coalesce to form the superior and inferior ophthalmic veins. The superior ophthalmic vein passes back through the superior orbital fissure and into the cavernous sinus. The inferior ophthalmic vein passes back through the inferior orbital fissure to communicate with the plexus and cavernous sinus. It is this arrangement of venous drainage that makes orbital and upper facial infections potentially so dangerous, as bacteria can travel from an extra- to intracranial location with resultant meningitis.

The Lacrimal Apparatus

The lacrimal apparatus is composed of the lacrimal gland, the lacrimal ducts, the lacrimal sacs, and the nasolacrimal duct. The lacrimal gland lies in the superior lateral orbit, between the eyeball and the roof of the orbit. The gland is folded about the posterior border of the levator aponeurosis, which separates the gland into an orbital and a palpebral portion. The orbital portion lies directly behind the orbital septum.

Operating Notes
During an upper blepharoplasty, an inferiorly displaced or "herniated" lacrimal gland may be mistaken for resectable orbital fat. Accordingly, care should be taken to preserve the gland, which can be pexied into its proper position.

Tears produced by the lacrimal gland flow inferiorly and medially across the globe of the eye to accumulate in the lacrimal lake at the medial lower lid. The tears then drain into two small ducts, the lacrimal canaliculi, which lie on the medial end of each eyelid. The visible openings of each of these ducts, the lacrimal punctum, lie on the medial end of each eyelid. Initially, the canaliculi pass perpendicular to the lid margin, but after about 2 mm they turn sharply medially to converge on the lacrimal sac. The canaliculi are each approximately 8 mm in length from the punctum to the lacrimal sac. The lacrimal sac, about 12 mm in length, lies in a groove at the anterior end of the medial orbital wall. As described earlier, its upper end is immediately posterior to the medial canthal ligament. From the lacrimal sac, the tears pass through the nasolacrimal duct, entering the nose beneath the inferior meatus. The lacrimal gland receives its parasympathetic fibers from cranial nerve VII, through the sphenopalatine ganglion.

Operating Notes
Procedures or disruptions of the lacrimal drainage system via trauma or infection will cause tears to accumulate and spill over the lower lid, which is referred to as epiphora. This may require placement of a tube from the punctum to the nose or creation of a new pathway for drainage directly through the lateral wall of the nose (dacryocystorhinotomy).

Eyelids

The eyelids consist of several layers. Approached from a skin incision, one encounters skin, subcutaneous tissue, orbicularis oculi muscle, orbital septum, tarsus, and conjunctiva. Additionally, behind the orbital septum of the upper lid, one encounters first the levator palpebrae superioris muscle and, beneath it, the superior tarsal or Muller's muscle. The levator arises from the bone at the apex of the orbit just above the common tendonous ring and passes forward, lying on the superior rectus to insert into the upper border of the tarsal plate. Muller's muscle is a thin sheet of smooth muscle, sympathetically innervated, which is firmly attached to the posterior surface of the levator and inserts into the upper border of the tarsus. The loss of sympathetic innervation to Muller's muscle, as in Horner's syndrome, leads to a ptosis of the upper lid.

The tarsi are anchored medially and laterally by the medial and lateral canthal ligaments, which connect each plate to the adjacent orbital margin. The medial ligament originates at the medial angles of the two tarsi and extends medially. The majority of the ligamentous fibers pass directly in front of the lacrimal sac to attach to the frontal processes of the maxilla at the anterior lacrimal crest. A few ligamentous fibers will pass behind the sac to attach to the posterior crest.

Operative Notes
Operative detachment of the canthus from its bony insertion is to be avoided if possible, as the medial angle of the palpebral fissure is difficult to reestablish. A transnasal canthopexy is generally required to reestablish an adequate reattachment.

The lateral canthus originates from the lateral borders of the tarsi and makes its bony attachment to the zygoma at the lateral orbital tubercle.

The Cranial Facial Skeleton

As discussed in the chapter on embryology, the cranial facial skeleton has its origins in both membranous and cartilaginous bone. There are ten cranial bones (see Figs. 2.22 and 2.23): one frontal (Fig. 2.24), two ethmoid, two sphenoid (Fig. 2.25), one occipital, two parietal, and two temporal bones (Fig. 2.26). The facial bones are 15 in number and are all paired except for the solitary vomer (Fig. 2.27). The rest are listed as follows: two nasal, two lacrimal, two inferior nasal conchae, two maxillae (Fig. 2.28), two zygomatic (Fig. 2.29), two palatine (Fig. 2.30), and two hemi-mandibles (Fig. 2.31).

It is of interest to note that the superior and middle nasal concha are part of the ethmoid and are hence classified as cranial bones, while the inferior nasal conchae are independent facial bones. The cranial bones are composed of inner and outer cortical tables separated by vascular cancellous bone, making up the diplopic space.

Operating Notes
As the inner table of cranial bone is thin, care must be taken when harvesting bone grafts not to lever the osteotome against the inner table, as this may lead to a depressed skull fracture.

The cranial bones are joined along their respective suture lines. The coronal suture joins the frontal bone to the parietal bones. The lambdoidal suture joins the occiput to the parietal bones. Running anterior to posterior at the midline, the sagittal suture extends between the frontal and lambdoidal suture lines. The point of intersection of the coronal and sagittal sutures is the bregma. The point of intersection between the lambdoidal and sagittal sutures is the lambda. Directly below the sagittal suture runs the sagittal sinus, the major venous drainage of the brain. The dome of the cranium extends from the superciliary arches, posteriorly to the external protuberance and superior nuchal line.

Operating Notes
The cranial bone should not be harvested from the sagittal midline, to avoid disruption of the sagittal sinus. If the midsagittal portion of bone is to be removed, all lateral osteotomies should be completed first, leaving only the osteotomies that cross the midline until last. In this way the bone flap may be removed as quickly as possible if excessive bleeding is noted from the sagittal sinus.

The temporal fossa includes portions of the frontal and parietal bones, as well as the squamous portion of the temporal bone, and greater wing of the sphenoid. The temporal bone itself may be divided into a squamous portion and an inferior petrous portion, as well as the mastoid, styloid, and zygomatic processes (see Fig. 2.32).

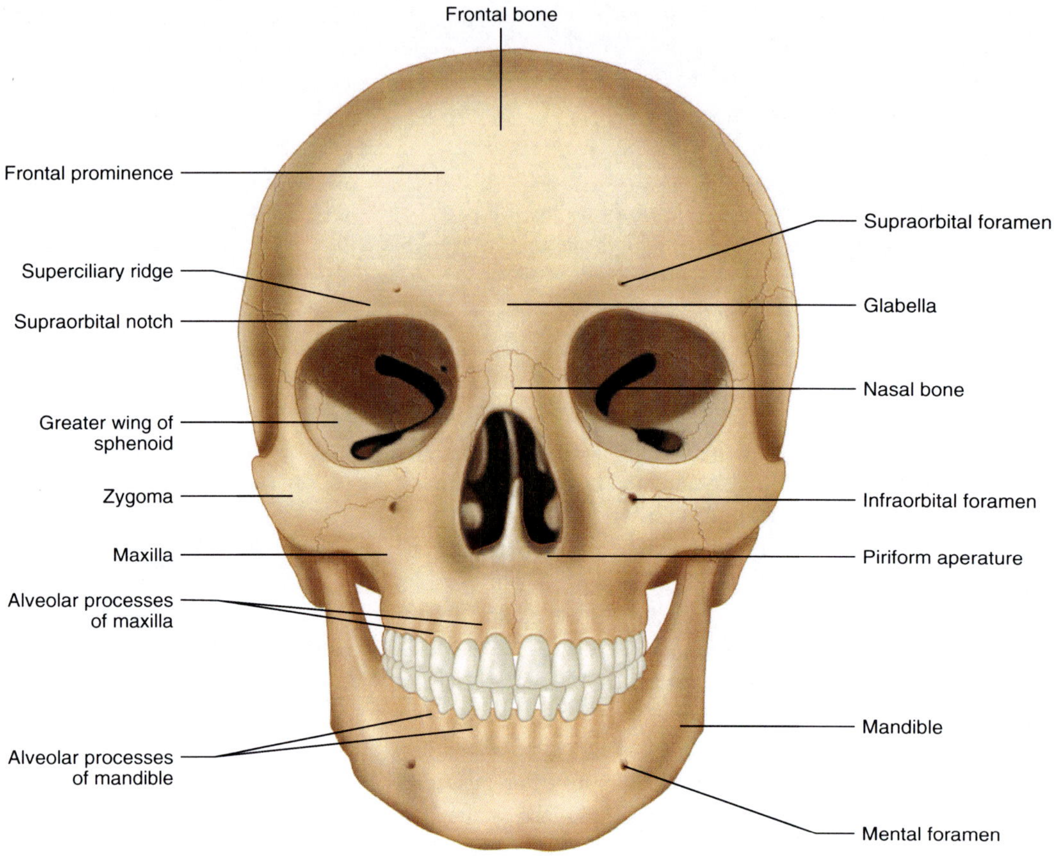

Fig. 2.22 Anterior view of the crainofacial skeleton

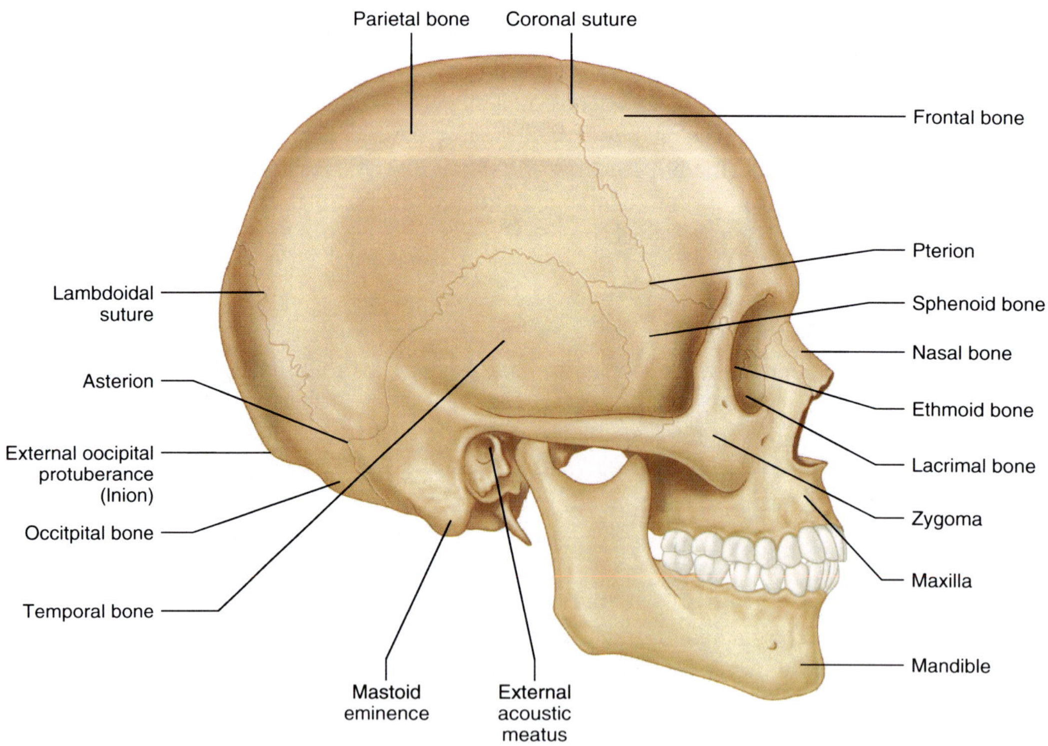

Fig. 2.23 Lateral view of the craniofacial skeleton

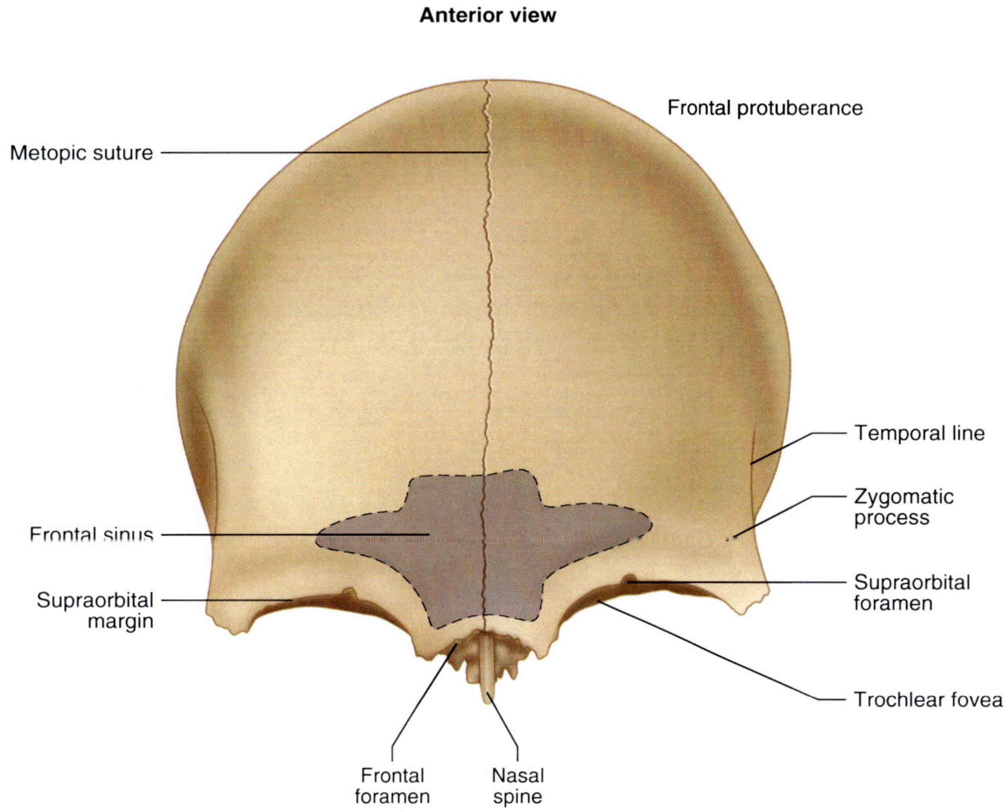

Fig. 2.24 Anatomy of the frontal bone

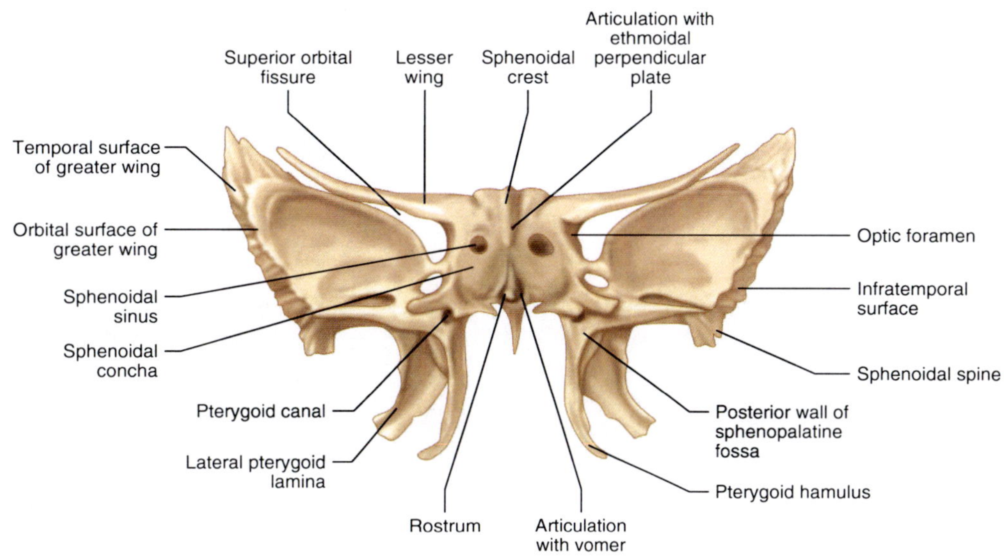

Fig. 2.25 Anatomy of the sphenoid bone

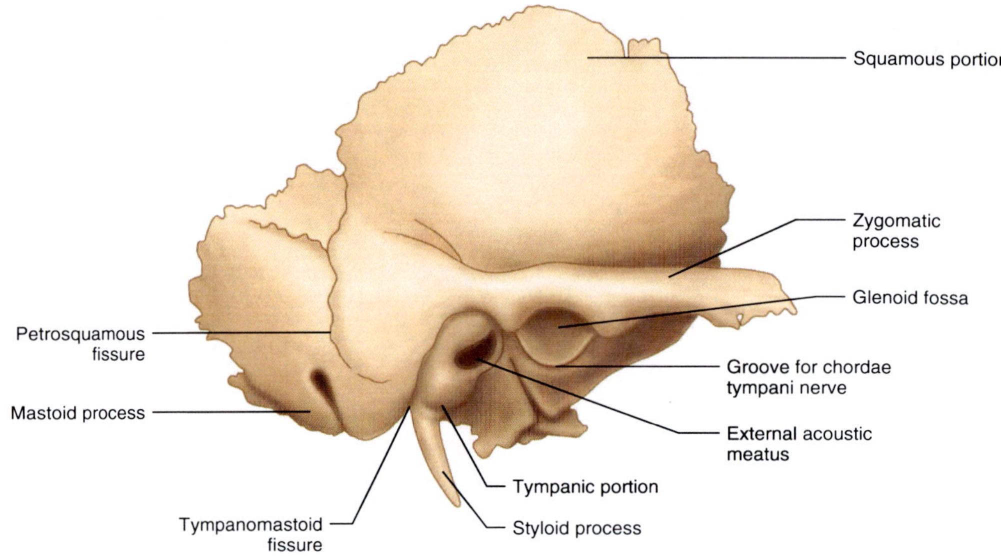

Fig. 2.26 Anatomy of the temporal bone

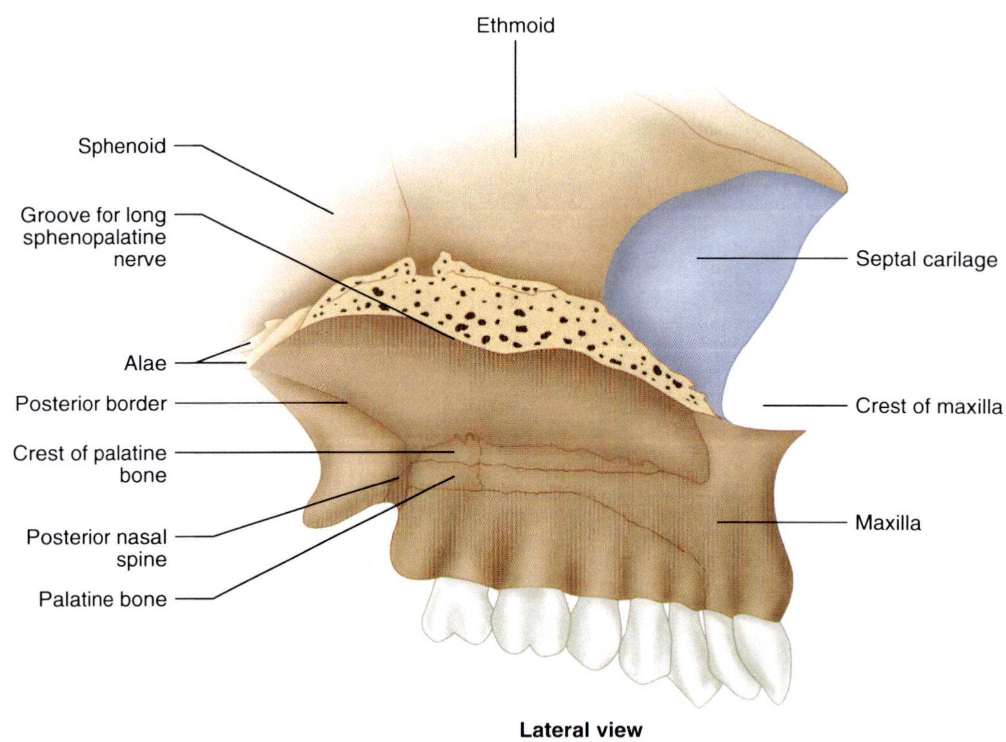

Fig. 2.27 Anatomy of the vomer

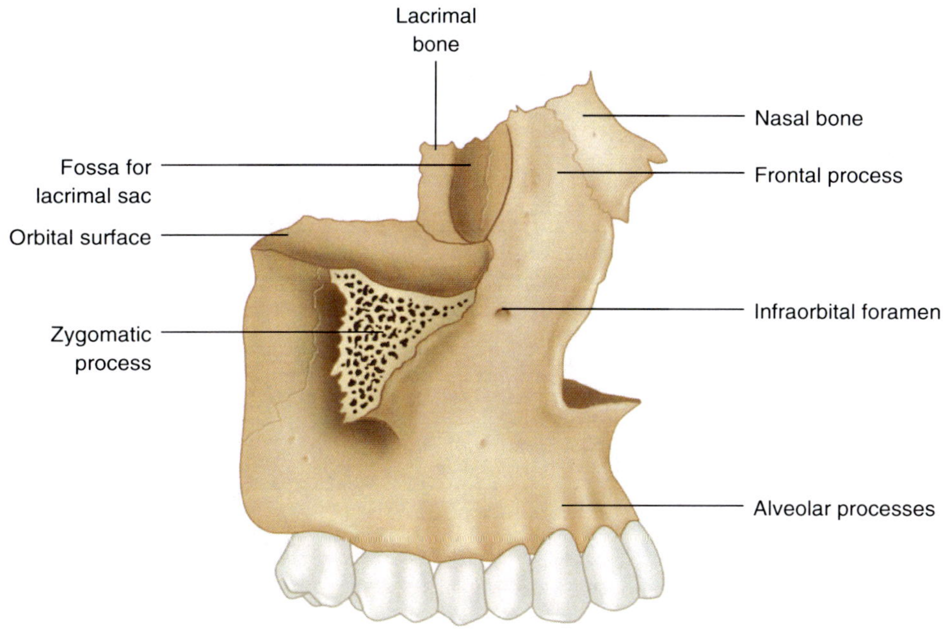

Fig. 2.28 Anatomy of the maxilla

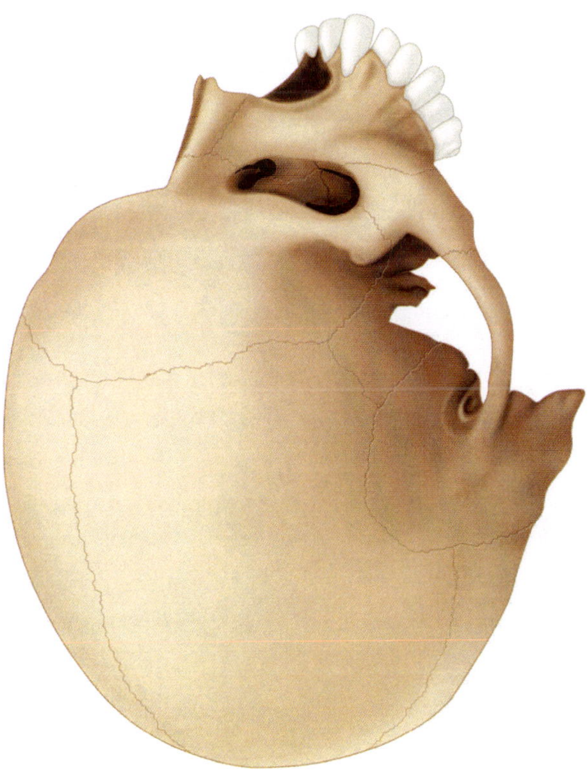

Fig. 2.29 Anatomy of the zygomatic arch

The basal aspect of the skull may be considered from anterior to posterior. The alveolar process of the maxilla is first encountered along with the teeth of the upper jaw. Proceeding posteriorly from the alveolar process, one encounters the palatine process of the maxilla, fused at the midline to make up the anterior two-thirds of the hard palate. The posterior one-third of the hard palate is formed by the horizontal plate of the palatine bone, which lies between the medial pterygoid plates of the sphenoid bone. The lesser palatine nerves pierce the palatine bone on the way to the soft palate. The sphenoid bone fills the cranial base between the occipital bone and the palatine bone. Centrally the paired choanae join with the vomer midline. Extending laterally, one encounters the pterygoid process, which includes the medial and lateral pterygoid plates, as well as the hamulus. More laterally, the greater wing of the sphenoid joins with the temporal bone laterally and posteriorly. Piercing the sphenoid bone are the foramen ovale, through which passes the mandibular nerve, and the foramen spinosum, through which passes the middle meningeal artery.

Posteriorly, at midline, the sphenoid joins with the basilar part of the occipital bone, anterior to the foramen magnum. Laterally, the sphenoid is separated from the occipital bone by the petrous portion of the temporal bone. At the junction of the posterior sphenoid and the petrous portion is the foramen lacerum, through which runs the internal carotid artery (see Fig. 2.33).

The petrous portion of the temporal bone includes the stylomastoid foramen, through which exits the facial nerve, and the jugular foramen, through which exit the internal jugular vein and CNs IX, X, and XI. Posterior to the petrous portion of the temporal bone, the remainder of the skull base is composed of the occipital bone.

Fig. 2.30 Anatomy of the palate

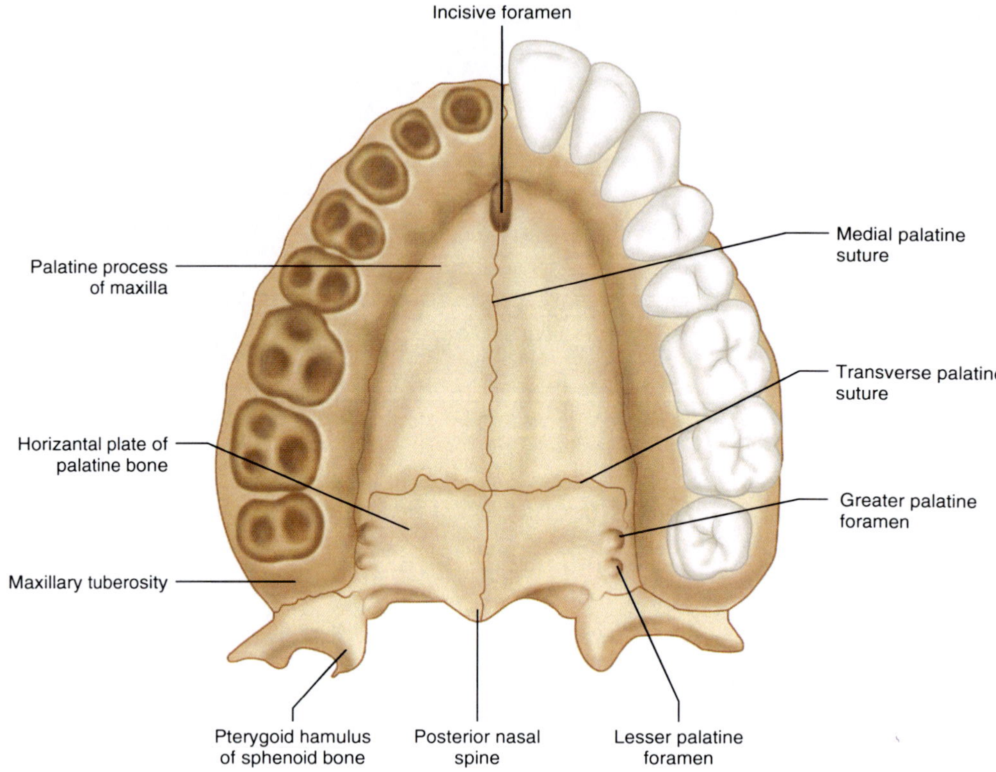

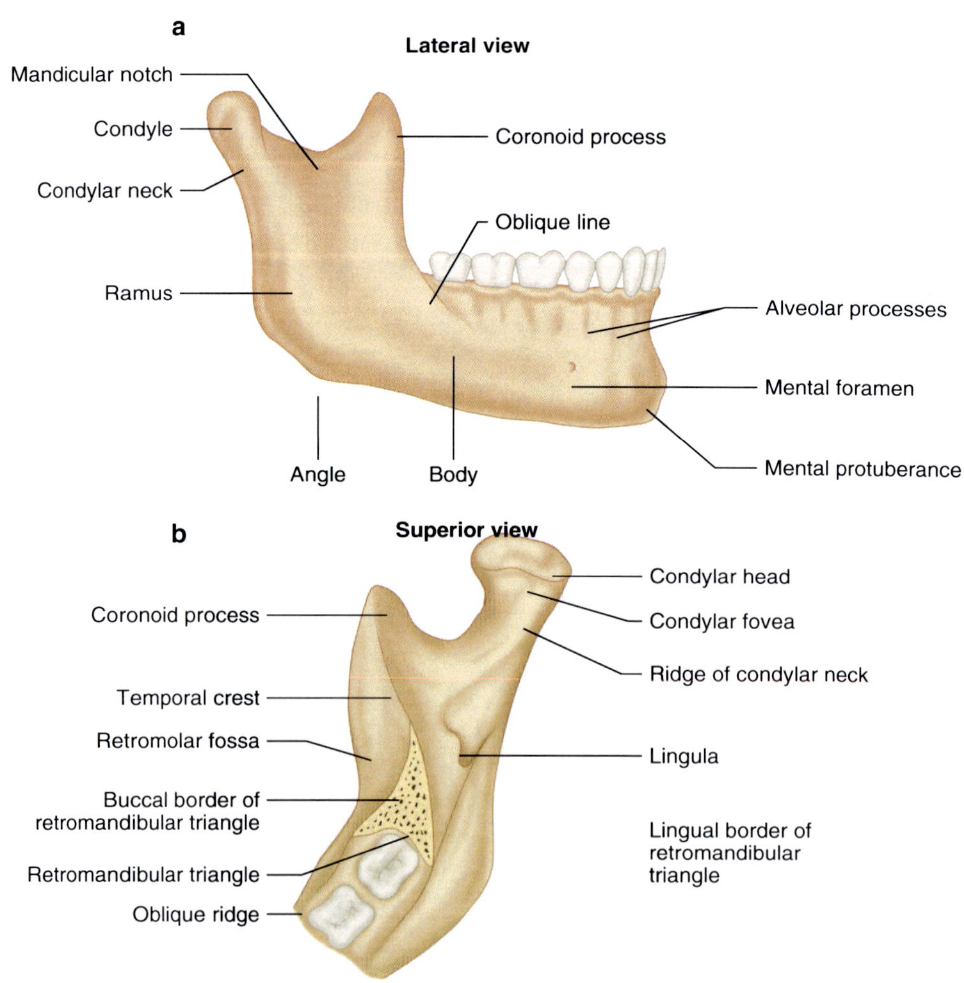

Fig. 2.31 Anatomy of the mandible

Fig. 2.31 continued

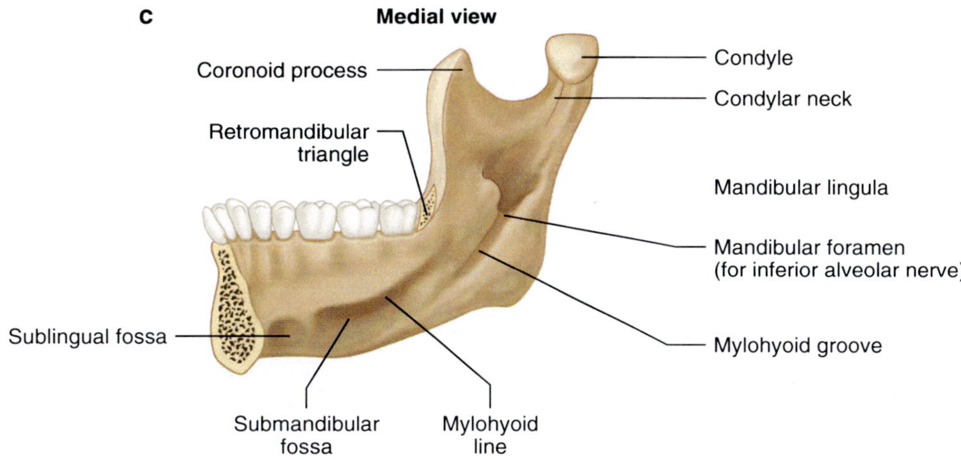

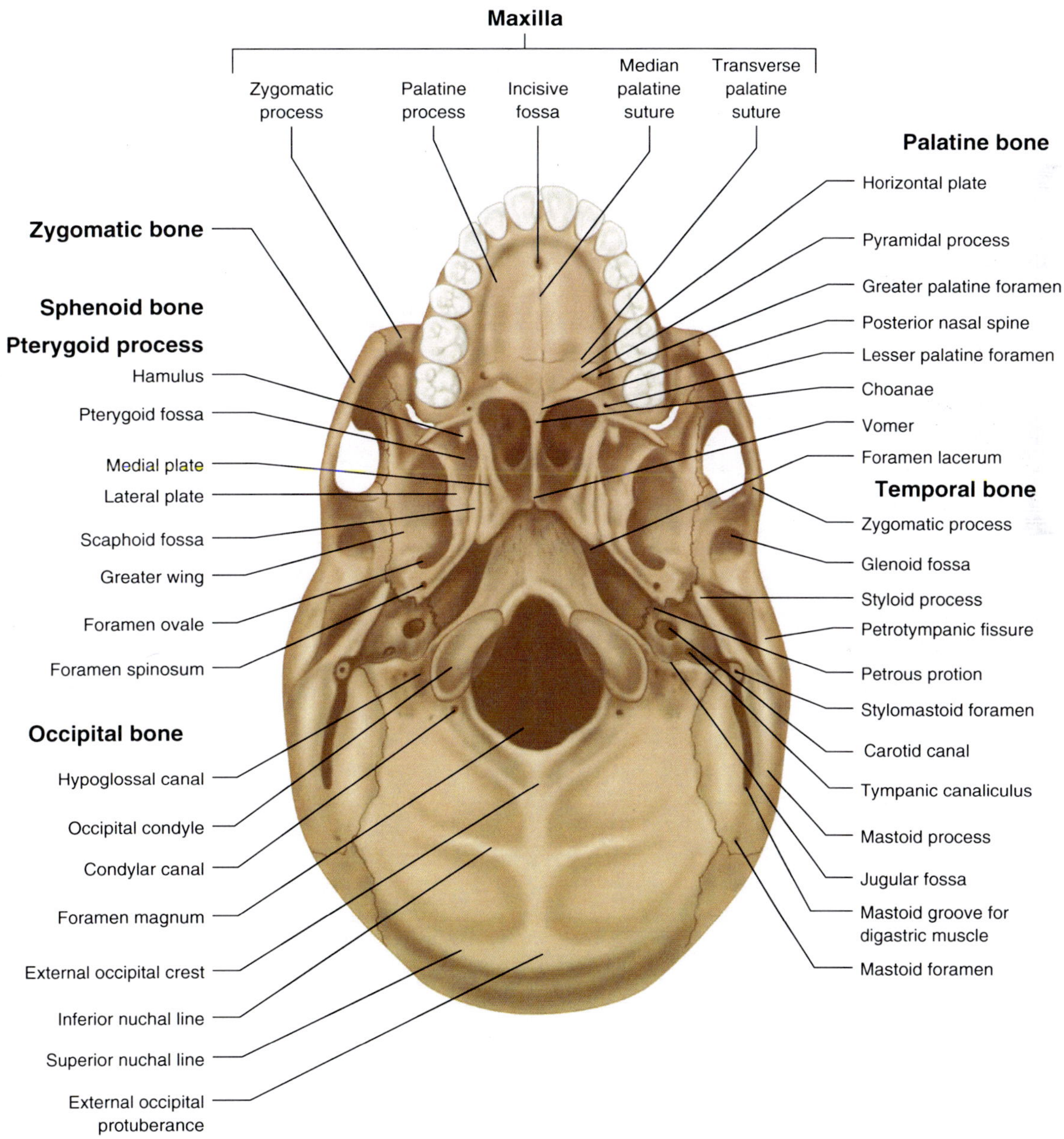

Fig. 2.32 Inferior aspect of the skull

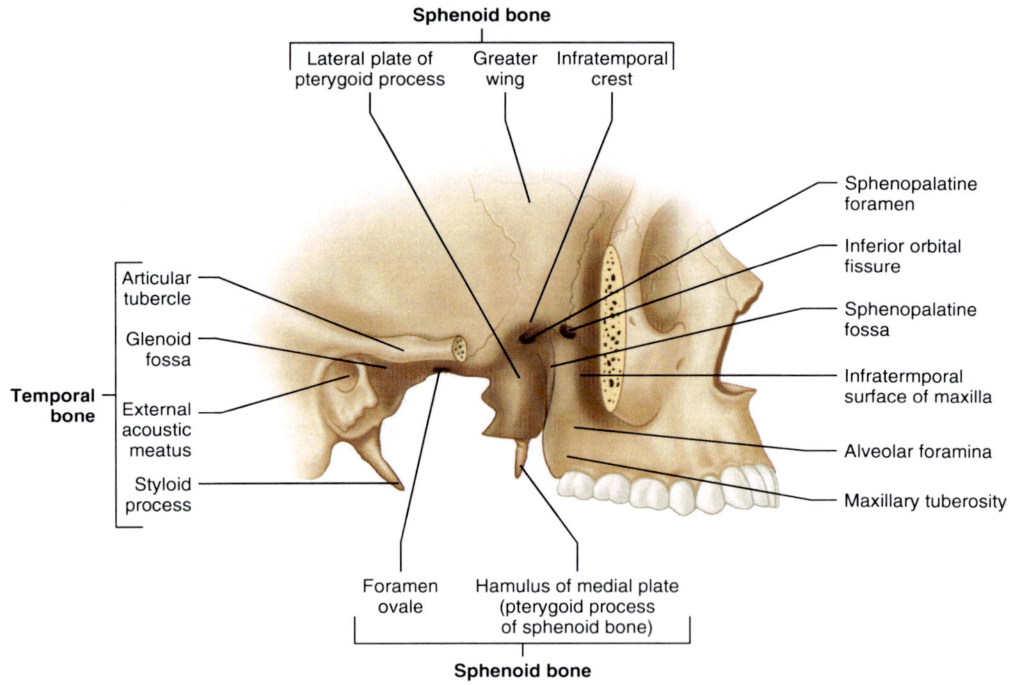

Fig. 2.33 Junction of the sphenoid and temporal bones

3 Oral Anatomy

Ali Baba Attaie and Mairaj K. Ahmed

The oral cavity consists of an outer vestibule and an inner oral cavity proper. It is bound anteriorly by the lips, laterally by the cheek mucosa, inferiorly by the floor of the mouth, posteriorly by the oropharynx, and superiorly by the hard and soft palate. In addition to being a site for mastication and propulsion of bolus, enzyme release and salivation concurrently occur in order to initiate the digestive process. Additional roles of the oral cavity include tissue mobility and lubrication for speech and swallowing, vital chemosensory functioning, and an alternative respiratory passage.

The oral cavity is lined by a mucous membrane consisting of a stratified squamous epithelium, which may or may not be keratinized. In areas of functional, chemical, and mechanical challenge, the mucous membrane is keratinized and tightly attached to the underlying bone. Conversely, in areas requiring mobility of tissue and elasticity, the mucosa is nonkeratinized and loosely attached to the underlying periosteum.

The mucous membrane is composed of two layers: the surface epithelium and an underlying connective tissue layer, the lamina propria. The submucosa underlying the lamina propria is highly variable. As a result of the variability in the type of epithelium present, as well as the characteristics of the connective tissue, several regions can be distinguished: lining mucosa, masticatory mucosa (mucoperiosteum), specialized mucosa, and a transitional zone (vermillion zone).

The true mucous membrane of the lips and cheeks is characterized by a relatively thin, nonkeratinized epithelium with a thin lamina propria. In these areas, where the lining mucosa covers muscles (lips, cheeks, and ventral surface of the tongue), the submucosa is fixed to the underlying fascia of the muscles. The mucosa here is smooth and very elastic and acts as a safeguard in functional mastication. If it were not elastic it would fold and produce creases that could be traumatized when chewing if it protruded between the teeth.

The mucosa of the soft palate is a transition zone between the mucosa of the lips and cheeks and that of the vestibule and floor of the mouth. The vestibular mucosa and that of the floor of the mouth are loosely attached and allow for the movement of labial and lingual frenum attachments, which are critical for speech, mastication, and swallowing. The mucosa of the vestibule (alveolar mucosa) is quite pink and red in color and very flexible when compared to the attached mucosa over the gingiva.

The attached mucosa is specialized depending on its position within the oral cavity. It is subjected to the forces and friction of mastication (hence the term masticatory mucosa) and thus is thick and keratinized with a dense, firm lamina propria. It is tightly adherent to the teeth and bone due to its dense bands of fibrous connecting tissue that join the mucous membrane directly to the underlying periosteum and bone. The submucous space in the mucosa of the hard palate is subdivided into irregular and intercommunicating compartments of various sizes that are filled with fat in the anterior palate and glands in the posterior palate. The submucous space of the gingiva does not exist, and instead the lamina propria continues into the depth of the tissues and fuses directly with the periosteum of the alveolar process or the cervical region of the teeth.

Dentition

In humans, the teeth are composed of a core, the dental pulp, which is rich in nerves and blood vessels. The bulk of the tooth is formed from dentin, with that portion exposed to the oral cavity called the crown, which is covered with an ectodermal derivative (enamel) (Fig. 3.1). The portion of the tooth embedded in the bony socket is covered by a mesodermal derivative (cementum) that is by its nature almost exactly like bone (Fig. 3.2). The junction of the root and the crown is the cementoenamel junction.

A.B. Attaie, DDS, MPH (✉)
Pediatrics and Dentistry, Pediatrics and Dental Medicine,
Icahn School of Medicine at Mount Sinai, New York, NY, USA
e-mail: alibaba@hellosmile.com

M.K. Ahmed, DDS, MS
Department of Dentistry/Oral and Maxillofacial Surgery,
Icahn School of Medicine at Mount Sinai, New York, NY, USA

P.J. Taub et al. (eds.), *Ferraro's Fundamentals of Maxillofacial Surgery*,
DOI 10.1007/978-1-4614-8341-0_3, © Springer Science+Business Media New York 2015

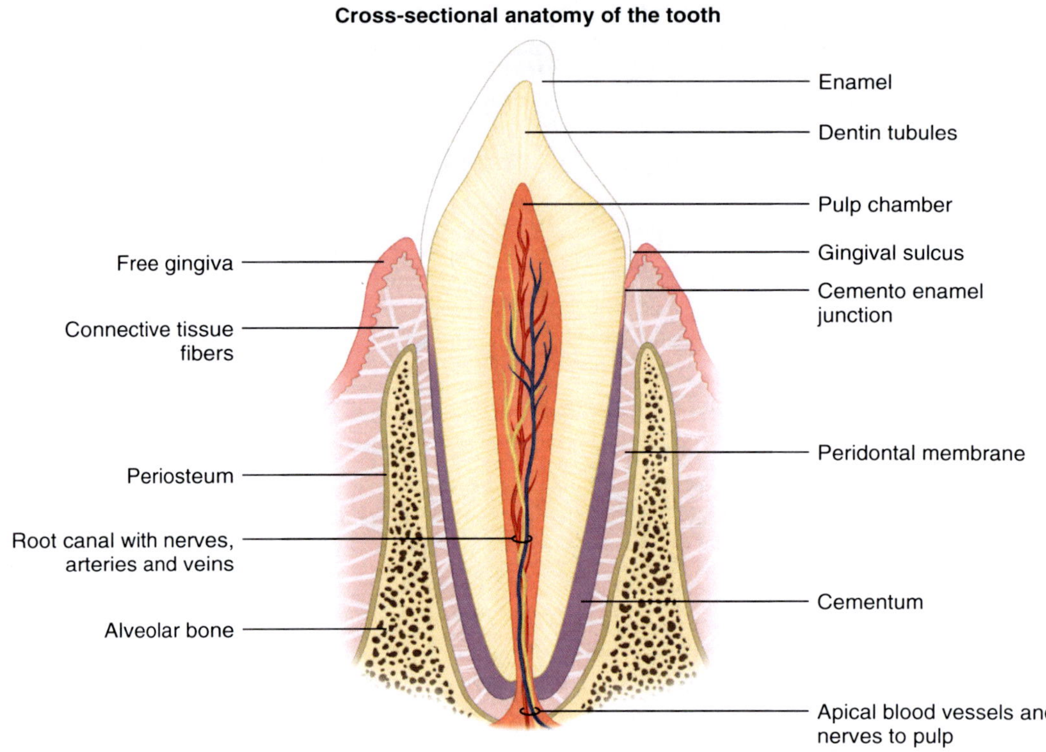

Fig. 3.1 Cross section of a canine tooth

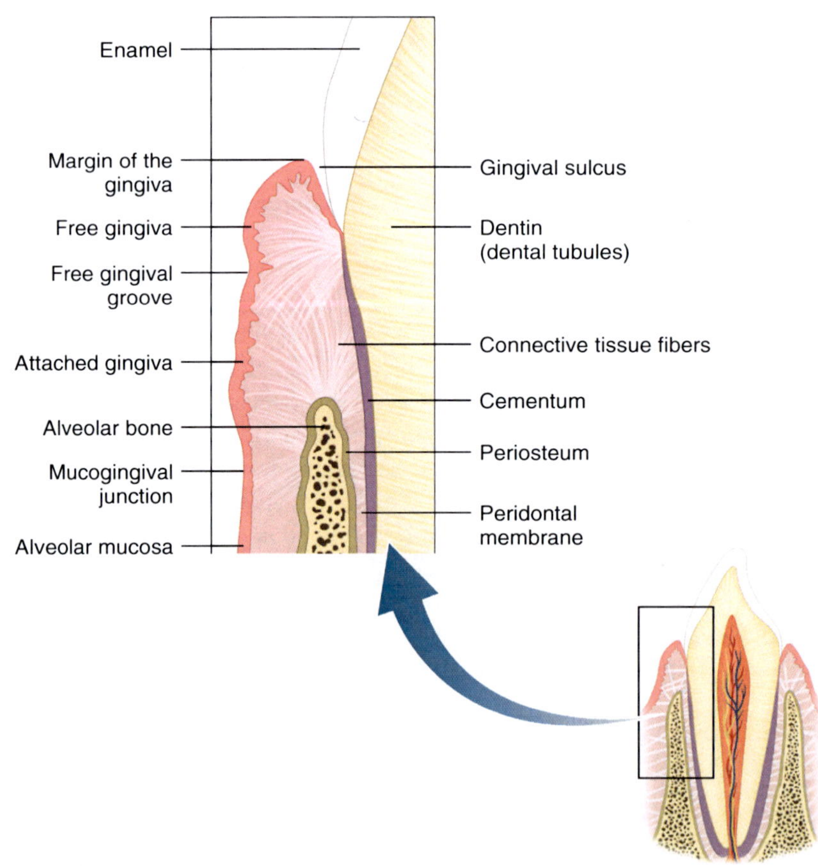

Fig. 3.2 Close-up of dental attachment to the gingiva

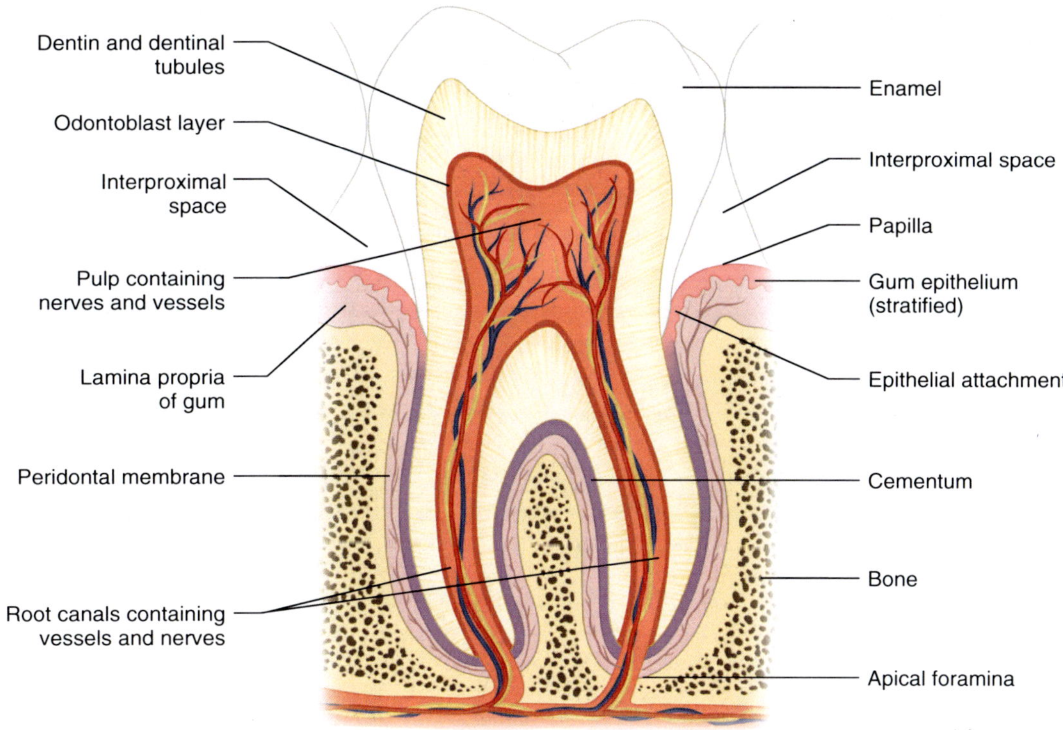

Fig. 3.3 Neurovascular supply to a molar tooth

Once the tooth is developed and it erupts through the gingival surface, a gingival margin and cuff forms at the junction of the dentoenamel junction. The gingival surface is not attached to the crown of the tooth but rather is attached below the cementoenamel junction by collagenous nonelastic fibers called Sharpey's fibers of the alveolar crest fibers of the periodontal membrane. It is these Sharpey's fibers that attach the bone to the cementum, acting as a "shock absorber" and thereby protecting the tooth and the adjacent bone from the constant trauma of chewing. These fibers make up the bulk of the periodontal membrane. The periodontal membrane or periodontium is attached from the junction of the crown and the root and extends all the way down around the apex of the fully developed root as well as around the gingiva at the cementoenamel junction. It is divided into three segments:

1. The gingival segment where the free gingival fibers attach to the cementum near the neck of the tooth.
2. The transeptal or interdental ligament. These fibers in a strict sense are not contained in the periodontal space but run across the interdental space from one tooth to the next and serve to unite all the teeth of one arch into a functional unit.
3. The alveolar ligament, which is horizontal and oblique fibers running from the alveolar bone to the cementum of the root.

If there is any breakdown of the periodontium from inflammation, there will be a destruction or degeneration of the periodontal membrane. Associated with this is the inflammatory destruction of the adjacent alveolar bone. This results in progressive weakening of the tooth in the socket because of its lack of bony support. A relationship between periodontal disease and systemic disease (such as diabetes, preterm, low birth weight, cardiovascular) has been demonstrated.

In a multirooted tooth, the same structures are present and the attachment of the tooth itself is exactly the same as a single-rooted tooth, except that there are more roots, meaning that there are more areas of attachment of that tooth. Also in the periodontal membrane are remnants of the epithelial root sheath of the developing tooth (as mentioned earlier in this chapter) called the epithelial rests of Malassez. They are elliptical segments that can appear as round islands of epithelial cells near the root of a tooth especially at the apex. They are of no consequence except they may proliferate in association with inflammation and have been implicated as forming the epithelial lining of a radicular cyst at the apex of the tooth.

The pulp canal in the roots and the main pulp chamber in the crown, with its arterial, venous, lymphatic, and neural structures, are seen as they pass from the pulp chamber through the apex of the fully formed root (Fig. 3.3). Nerves and vessels are plentiful as they exit through the apex of each tooth and have a wide communication with the blood supply coming from the adjacent bone through the periodontal membrane and the adjacent mucosa. If we consider the presence of a wide plexus, we can easily understand how a tooth's pulp can be removed and yet the viability of the tooth structures can be maintained. Fig. 3.4 shows the mean lengths of teeth. Cleft lip/palate has been associated with significantly different mean lengths.

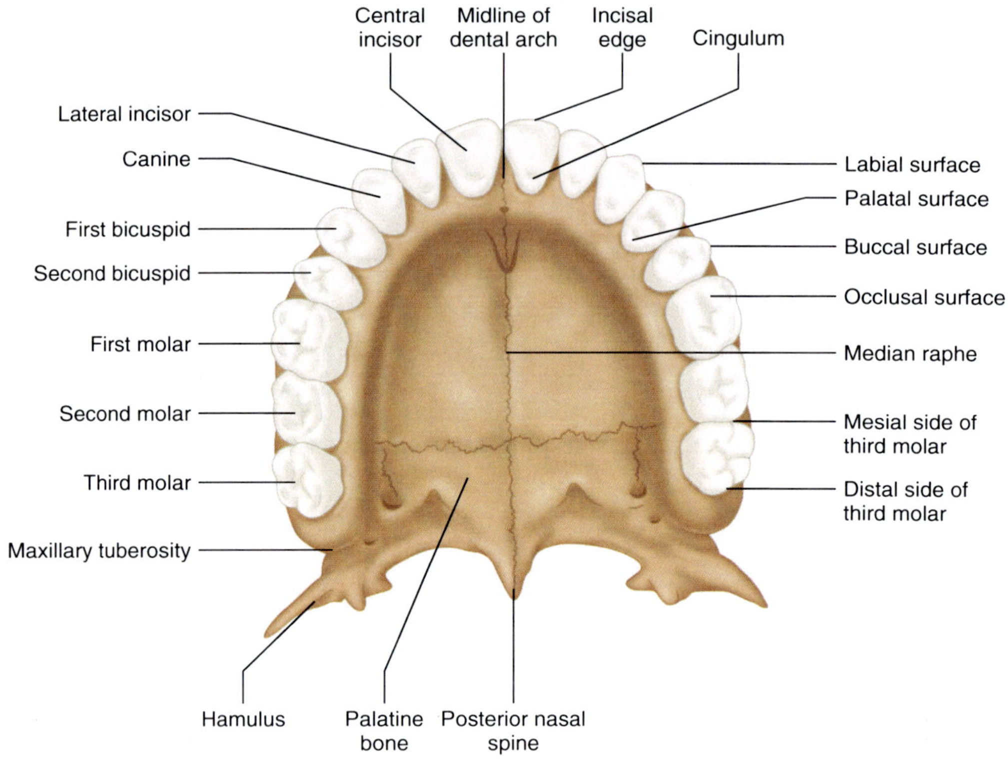

Fig. 3.4 Palatal surface of the maxilla demonstrating 16 teeth

Sensibility and Viability

The term viable tooth tissue refers to a tooth with an intact blood supply either from the pulp or the adjacent tooth tissue. The term sensate refers to the ability of that tooth to emit the sensation of pain when the tooth's pulp is stimulated with an electric or cold stimulus. The two terms, sensate and viable, are not mutually exclusive. A tooth without a pulp (pulp chamber being removed by endodontics) still will be viable because of the blood supply coming in from the adjacent periodontal membrane, but that same tooth, however, will not emit a painful stimulus from a pulp tester and is therefore viable but nonsensate. The same principal occurs when we cut the maxilla in a Le Fort I osteotomy. All the teeth have lost their nerve supply because of the osteotomy and the transection of the posterior, middle, and anterior superior alveolar nerves. Yet if the blood supply is maintained via the palatal vessels, the teeth will remain viable and be maintained in the alveolar process of the maxilla. If, however, the blood supply is cut and the segment becomes avascular and the viability is destroyed, then the tooth and the adjacent bone will be sloughed from the arch. If the labial or palatal blood supply is maintained, segmental bony structures can be mobilized and moved into various positions.

Description and Nomenclature of the Dentition

If a line is drawn between the central incisors down the medial raphe of the maxilla, it divides the arch into right and left components (Fig. 3.5). Terms such as mesial and distal are used to denote teeth position in the arch and surfaces on the tooth itself. For example, the central incisor is mesial to the lateral incisor, which is mesial to the cuspid. The first bicuspid is distal to the cuspid and the second molar is distal to the bicuspids and first molar. Similarly the central incisor has a mesial surface (towards the midline) and a distal surface (away from the midline). The lateral incisor and all the other teeth also have a mesial and distal surface depending on the surface and its relationship to the midline.

The lingual surface of all the teeth is that surface next to the tongue. The outer surface, however, is different. The anterior six teeth (central through cuspid on each side), because they are next to the lips, have a labial surface. The anterior teeth (bicuspids and molars), because they are next to the cheek, have a buccal surface.

The anterior six teeth have a sharp edge called the incisal surface, whereas the bicuspids and molars, because their surface is flatter and are used to grind food, have an occlusal surface. Thus, the surfaces of molars are mesial, distal, lingual, buccal, and occlusal. The surfaces of the anterior incisors are mesial, distal, labial, lingual, and incisal. The mandibular teeth surfaces are named exactly the same.

The anterior teeth have one more peculiar anatomical segment. Each of these teeth has a cingulum. The cingulum is a small area and is adjacent to the lingual surface of the anterior teeth. The bicuspids erupt in the adult dentition where the deciduous molars are present in the primary dentition. Each of these teeth has two cusps, a buccal and a lingual cusp. These teeth are chewing and grinding teeth and can also tear food, but not as effectively as the incisors and canines. The molars are multicusped teeth (four or more) that also have multiple roots (Fig. 3.6). The shape of the dental arches varies considerably. However, in the

	Deciduous	Permanent
Upper central incisor	18 mm	24 mm
Upper lateral incisor	16 mm	22.5 mm
Upper cuspid	20 mm	27 mm
Upper first bicuspid	—	21.7 mm
Upper second bicuspid	—	21.5 mm
Upper first molar	16 mm	21.3 mm
Upper second molar	18 mm	21.2 mm
Upper third molar	—	Too variable
Lower central incisor	17 mm	21.4 mm
Lower lateral incisor	17 mm	23.2 mm
Lower cuspid	19 mm	25.4 mm
Lower first bicuspid	—	22.7 mm
Lower second bicuspid	—	23.2 mm
Lower first molar	15.5 mm	22.8 mm
Lower second molar	18 mm	22.8 mm
Lower third molar	—	Too variable

Fig. 3.5 Lengths of the deciduous and permanent teeth

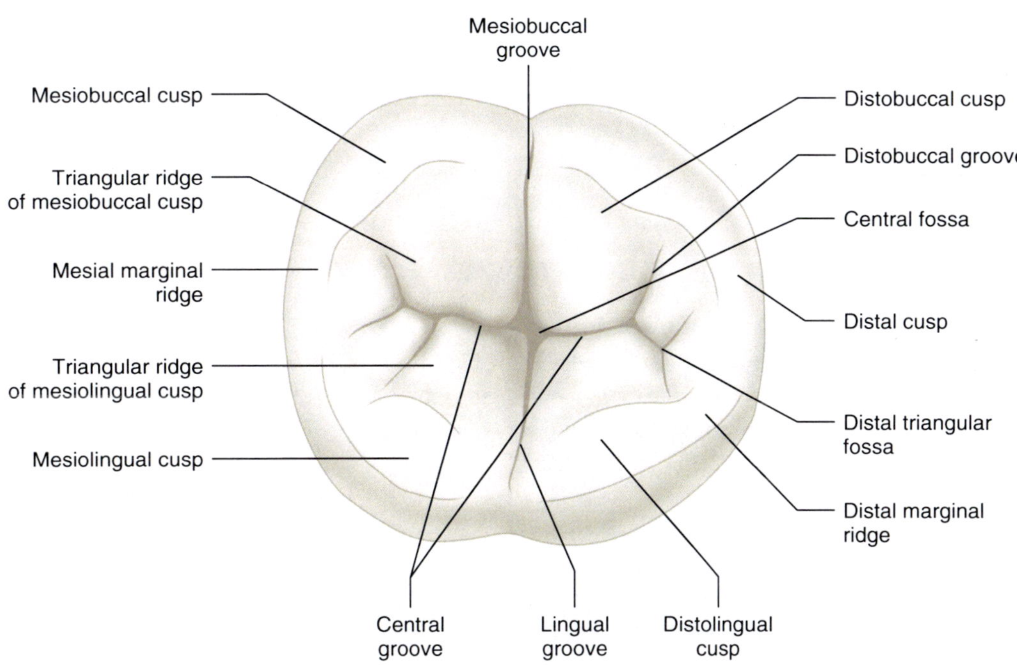

Fig. 3.6 Occlusal surface of a molar tooth

average individual, the arch has two curves in space. In the horizontal plane, the arch form is somewhat U-shaped with the labial surfaces of the six anterior teeth. As we progress to the bicuspids, this plane is continued. It is not until we reach the distal cusps of the first molar that the curve begins to bend towards the lingual. This curve of the arch is important because it prevents the teeth from biting the cheek and gives clearance for the coronoid process of the mandible to move within the zygomatic arch.

Deciduous Dentition

The deciduous dentition closely resembles their permanent successor; however, they have smaller crowns and shorter root lengths (Fig. 3.7). The anterior incisors have more curvature on their labial surface when compared to the adult version. The height of contour of the molars is closer to the gingiva than the permanent molars, thus making it much harder to get wires below the height of contour so that they will hold tight to the teeth when applying arch bars. As a result, acrylic splints, circumandibular and transmaxillary wires, drop wires from the piriform apertures, or zygomatic buttresses are frequently used to hold the arch bars in young patients.

The permanent dentition, in contrast, has contact points at the upper third of the clinical crown above the interproximal papillae. Fixation of arch bars in the permanent dentition can be easily secured with interdental wires if the dentition is intact. The deciduous teeth in the anterior are replaced in kind by the permanent teeth. However, in the case of the deciduous molars they are

Deciduous dental erupt ion schedule				
	Calcification of crown begins (fetal months)	Tooth erupts (months)	Calcification of root ends (years)	Tooth sheds (years)
Central incisors	4	6–7 1/2	1 1/2	7
Cateral incisors	4 1/2	7–9	1 3/4	8
Canines	5	16–18	3 1/4	12
First molars	5	12–14	2 1/2	10
Second molars	6	20–24	3	11

Permanent dental eruption schedule

	Calcification of crown begins	Calcification of crown ends (years)	Tooth erupts (years)	Calcification of root ends (years)
Central incisors	3–4 months	4–5	6–8	9–10
Lateral Incisors	3–12 months	4–5	7–9	10–11
Canines	4–5 months	6–7	9–12	12–15
First premolars	1 1/2–2 years	5–6	10–12	12–13
Second premolars	2–21/2 months	6–7	10–12	12–14
First molars	At birth	2 1/2–3	6–7	9–10
Second molars	2 1/2–3 years	7–8	11–13	14–16
Third molars	7–10 years	12–16	17–21	18–25

Fig. 3.7 Dental eruption schedule

replaced by permanent bicuspids. Because there are no bicuspids in the deciduous dentition, there are only 20 teeth in the arch. In comparison, the three permanent molars erupt de novo and as a result, there are 32 permanent teeth in the adult arch.

Dental Formula

There are many formulas one can use to indicate the position of a permanent or deciduous tooth in the arch. In this text, two basic methods are discussed. One method frequently used is where a cross was made and the vertical line would separate the right side from the left, while the horizontal line would separate the upper from the lower jaws. Looking at that cross, it would be as though the patient were looking at you.

The deciduous dentition is marked in Roman numerals or letters (A through E), while Arabic numbers are used to represent any erupted permanent teeth (Fig. 3.8). Another method to denote the dentition in the arch is to use a formula where the teeth are numbered starting in the right upper quadrant and going forward all the way around the arch (1–18). The lower left third molar is now 19 and then around to the full complement of teeth in the lower arch to the right third molar, which is 32. Here, for example, the lower left central would be 24 and the lower right cuspid would be 27.

It must be mentioned that the eruption schedule is only a guide because eruption patterns of human teeth vary considerably. It is only those eruption times that are significantly outside the ranges that are considered as pathologic. The eruption of the deciduous teeth generally follows front to back with the upper centrals and laterals erupting first and the cuspids next and on back to the molars erupting at age 3 years. The sequence in the permanent teeth is quite different. Here, the upper and lower first molars are the first teeth to erupt into the arch. They position themselves just behind the deciduous second molars and are usually fully erupted by age 6 or 7. This is an important concept, for these teeth act as pillars, so that if the loss occurs before the dentin is completely erupted, a disturbance in the occlusion is likely to occur. As stated by Angle, "all teeth are essential yet in function and influence some are of greater importance than others, the most important of all being the first permanent molars." These teeth act to maintain the dynamic balance of the occlusion between the forces of the anterior arch with the forces of the molars on the posterior portion of the arch. Early loss of these teeth results in tilting of adjacent teeth, overeruption of the opposing teeth, and migration of the adjacent teeth into the first mandibular space, creating marked dental disharmony.

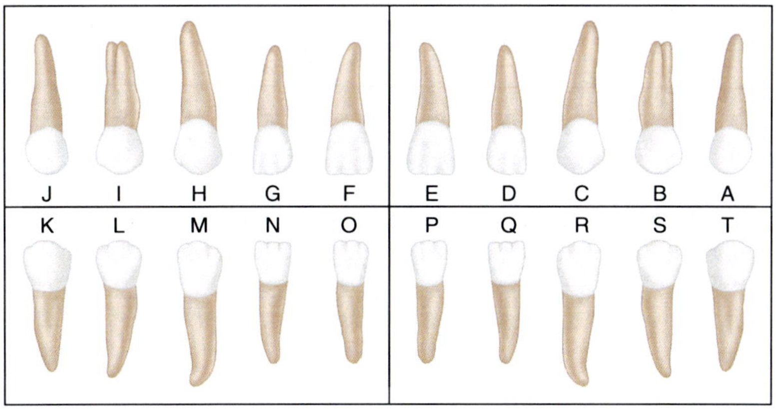

Fig. 3.8 Pediatric dental nomenclature

- Maxillary Central Incisor: This tooth has a broad crown and a shovel shape. When the tooth first erupts, it (as well as the lateral incisors in both the maxillary and mandibular arches) has three rounded cusps called mamelons. These are quickly worn away with occlusal abrasion. It is important to note that if in an adult you still see mamelons present on the centrals and laterals, you can assume that very little contact has been made between these teeth, as is frequently seen in class III malocclusions or open bite deformities. The root of the fully formed central incisor is relatively short (about 12 mm) and cone shaped and as a result can be pulled easily inferiorly with a wire or elastic traction. As a result, interproximal wires should not be placed around this tooth and attached to an arch bar. This could easily result in partial extrusion of the tooth below the upper incisal plane. The same is true of the maxillary laterals and the mandibular central and lateral incisors.
- Maxillary Lateral Incisor: This tooth is similar to the central but has a slightly narrower crown width mesially to distal. The root frequently has a slight distal bend at its apex. The root length is also about 12 mm. This tooth has a higher rate of being congenitally missing or malformed.
- Maxillary Cuspid: Here, the incisal edge has a sharp point. It has a short blunted lingual cusp or cingulum. The root is longest and strongest in the dental arch (16 mm) with an overall tooth length of 27 mm. The apex of the root curves distally. This root structure is why this tooth should be included when placing arch bars. However, because of the low lingual crown anatomy, it is necessary to loop the arch wire around the arch bar to hold the wire as close to the neck of the tooth as possible.
- Maxillary First Bicuspid: These teeth are the first to have a true occlusal surface. The buccal cusp is similar to the cuspid but here the cingulum is now a fully developed lingual cusp. The root of the maxillary first bicuspid can have either one or two roots. Sicher states that over 50 % of these teeth had two roots with two root canals.
- Maxillary Second Bicuspid: This tooth is somewhat smaller than the first bicuspid. It has a lingual and buccal cusp of equal height. The root is rarely divided. It frequently has a deep groove and its root canals may be totally separate or may fuse at variable distances from the apex of the roof.
- Maxillary First Molar: Here the occlusal surface is rhomboid shaped. It frequently has an extra cusp on the mesial lingual surface called the cusp of Carabelli. Sicher states it is present in 10–15 % of upper first molars as a well-developed cusp, but a remnant such as a pit or groove may be present in the mesial lingual cusp in up to 40 % of upper first molars. The roots are three, with the lingual (or palatal) and a distal and mesial root.
- Maxillary Second Molar: The overall shape in this tooth is similar to the upper first molar except there is no cusp of Carabelli. The roots are also similar, except they do not diverge as much and are more frequently fused into one mass but still maintain the three separate root canals.
- Mandibular Central Incisor: The crown of this tooth is narrow with a sharp mucosal edge. As with the upper central incisors, there are mammelons present in the newly erupted lower central incisors that quickly are worn away with incisal function. The root is straight and the overall tooth size is quite small, and therefore it too should not be attached to an arch bar because it could easily be avulsed from its socket.
- Mandibular Lateral Incisor: This tooth is very similar to the central incisor, only it is a little longer.
- Mandibular Cuspid: This tooth is smaller and shorter than the maxillary cuspid (overall length 25 mm vs. 27–28 mm for the upper cuspid). Because of its similar shape to the upper cuspid, it must also be wired to the arch bar with a loop wire. The root is shorter than the maxillary cuspid and not as strong, but it should be used to help retain the lower arch bar because it does have good retentive strength.
- Mandibular First Bicuspid: Here, there are two cusps, a buccal and lingual, but when compared with the upper first bicuspid, the lingual cusp is smaller and shorter. The root here is singular with one root canal.

- Mandibular Second Bicuspid: The crown of the mandibular second bicuspid is larger than the first with a larger, more developed, lingual cusp. Its root is also singular with a root canal but is longer and stronger than the lower first bicuspid.
- Mandibular First Molar: This tooth has five cusps, three on the buccal and two on the lingual. It is rectangular shaped. The lingual cusps are slightly higher than the buccal ones because they fit into the central fossa of the upper first molar. There are two roots, a distal and mesial root with two canals, and these roots frequently deviate distally in the arch
- Mandibular Second Molar: The crown has two lingual and two buccal cusps. Both are of equal height. The roots also are two, a mesial and distal root with two root canals.

Eruption of a Tooth

When there is pressure exerted in living bone, it responds either by osteoblastic proliferation (bone formation) or osteoclastic activity (bone resorption). As the tooth develops in its dental sac, there is a resorptive surface at the periphery of the dental sac that permits the growth and development of the crown of the tooth. This is called the preeruptive phase of eruption. With the development of the root, the active phase of eruption begins. As the root grows down into the alveolar bone, the resultant force is upward in the mandible and downward in the maxilla. This process of eruption proceeds as the tooth emerges through the mucosa and continues until the erupting tooth comes in contact with the tooth of the opposite arch. Eruption also occurs in a rotational axis or in a transverse labiolingual or buccolingual axis (tilting or tipping of teeth). Finally, a tooth may move parallel to its long axis or drift, as can occur when an adjacent tooth is absent and the tooth migrates into the adjacent tooth space. Once the tooth is fully developed, it still can erupt if, for example, it has no opposing tooth. It is believed that the negative force created by the unopposed tooth results in bone apposition at the apex of the tooth and facilitates the eruption until opposite contact is made.

In the mandible of a child, the larger size of the developing teeth results in crowding. The follicles of these permanent teeth may be rotated or staggered in the arch and frequently are just above the inferior border of the mandible or just below the orbital floor in the maxilla. The permanent bicuspid crowns are smaller than the overlying deciduous molars and develop immediately below the bifurcation of these molar roots.

The position and growth of the permanent molar teeth is dependent on the forward growth of the mandible. When the permanent molars begin to develop, they lie in the base of the ascending ramus of the mandible. The developing upper molars lie in the expanded maxillary tuberosity. If horizontal growth of the mandible fails to occur or the maxilla is hypoplastic, these molar teeth may be unable to erupt because they become "blocked out" by the erupted adjacent teeth and remain in the bone in an oblique or horizontal position.

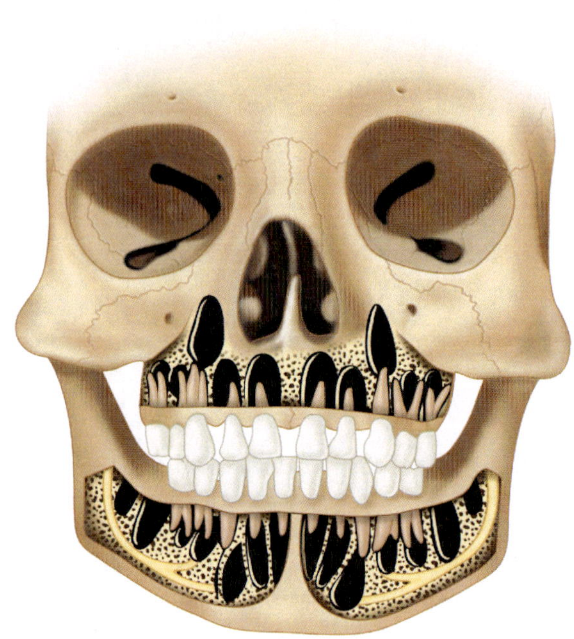

Fig. 3.9 Location of the permanent dentition within the pediatric maxilla

The position of the developing and erupting teeth also demonstrates how difficult reduction of fractures of the maxilla and mandible are in the young child (Fig. 3.9). There is little or no room to place plates and screws without risking injury to these teeth. An osteotomy of the maxilla would also be extremely difficult because of the absence of the maxillary sinus and the high position of the developing cuspid and bicuspids in relation to the orbital floor.

Maxillary Sinus

The maxillary sinus at the time of birth is very small - about the size of a pea (Fig. 3.10). As the face grows and the teeth erupt, the sinus enlarges in an inferior direction. This may explain why the maxillary sinus ostium is at the upper end of the adult maxillary sinus cavity. In most individuals, Sicher states the maxillary sinus continues to expand throughout life. This expansion penetrates deeper into the alveolar process and thus we frequently see the apices of the molar teeth sticking up into the sinus floor. The maxillary sinus may even invade into the body of the zygomatic bone. The enlargement of the maxillary sinus explains in part why

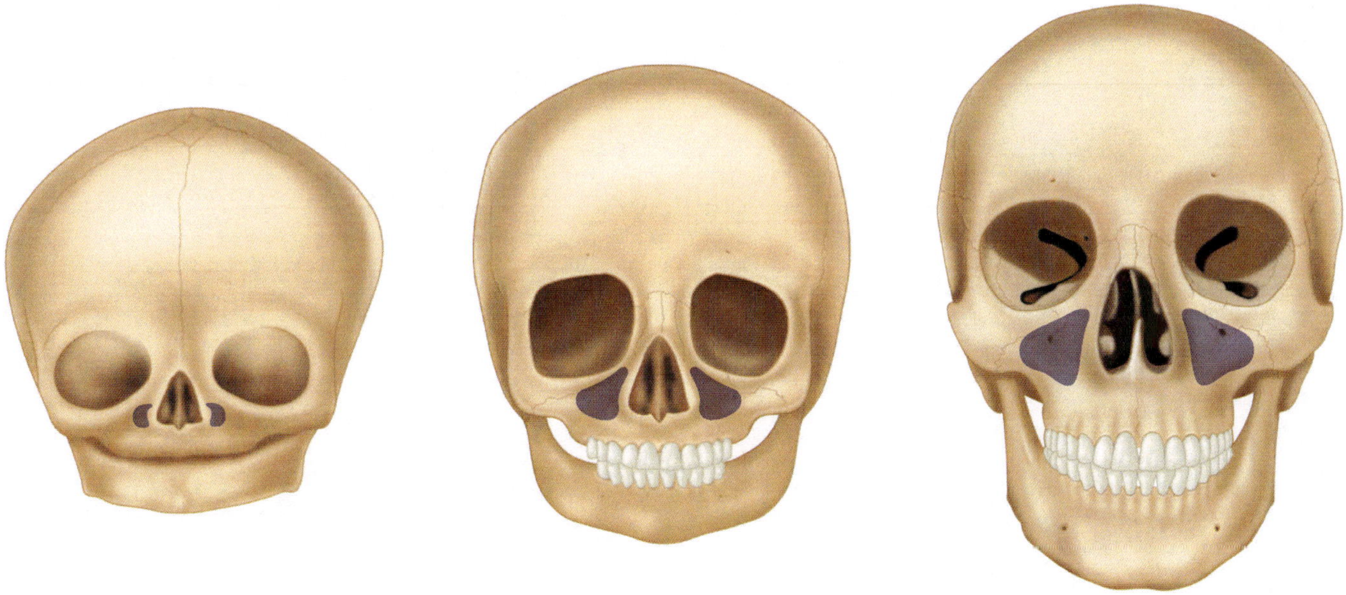

Fig. 3.10 Growth and aeration of the maxillary sinus with age

maxillary fractures are less often seen in children than in adult patients. Also, the intimate relationship of the sinus to the roots of the bicuspid and molar teeth explains why with maxillary sinusitis one can have a feeling of pressure or pain referred to these teeth.

Curve of Spee

When looking at the maxillomandibular occlusion from the buccal surface, an anterior position curve is noted. This curve is called the curve of Spee. It extends from the tip of the mandibular cuspid and follows along the buccal cusps of the mandibular posterior teeth (Fig. 3.11). This curve is usually slight and only in a few patients does it have a pronounced arc. It is believed to be an adaptation of the teeth to a balanced occlusion and it is caused by the tendency of a single tooth to assume a position in the jaw where its long axis is best suited to the forces of mastication. The long axis of the upper and lower arches form reciprocal curves, which are convex in the maxilla concave in the mandible. This position gives each tooth the optimal resistance under maximal force from the muscles of mastication. The obliquity of the resultant force produces an angular position of the teeth in the arch and is affected by the arc of rotation and angulation of the condyle in the glenoid fossa and by the forces of the muscles of mastication. This curve permits the maximum utilization of tooth contacts during function that would not be possible if there was a flat occlusal plane.

The teeth are not in continual contact in normal individuals. Instead there is a position the mandible assumes when the patient is erect and the muscles of mastication are relaxed. This is called the mandibular rest position. Here the teeth are not in contact but have a space of 2–3 mm between them, the freeway space. When the patient is in rest position, even though the muscles are relaxed, there is still some muscle activity present, the muscle tonus, which is present throughout the body unless the patient is paralyzed under general anesthesia. This freeway space is important and must be maintained. If the bite is artificially "opened" and exceeds the freeway space distance, the muscles of mastication, especially the external pterygoid, become chronically stretched with an increase in tone. This can result in fatigue and increased muscle irritation, with muscle spasm and pain.

Centric Relation and Centric Occlusion

Centric relation refers to the most retruded unstrained position of the mandibular condyle in the glenoid fossa. This is also called the terminal hinge position. Centric relation does not in itself indicate occlusion of the teeth. It is simply a condylar glenoid fossa relationship. Centric occlusion, on the other hand, refers to the maximal contact of the incline planes of the opposing cusps of the mandibular and maxillary arches. In this relationship of maximal contact, there must be bilateral symmetrical contact and a balanced and unstrained relationship of the condyle in the glenoid fossa. With premature contact of the cusps (due to loss of teeth and overeruption of the opposing teeth, restorations with too high an occlusal contact, malpositioned teeth, and/or skeletal discrepancy), the centric occlusion can be compromised. Orthodontics and orthognathic surgery serve to reestablish a normal jaw relationship so that when there is centric relation

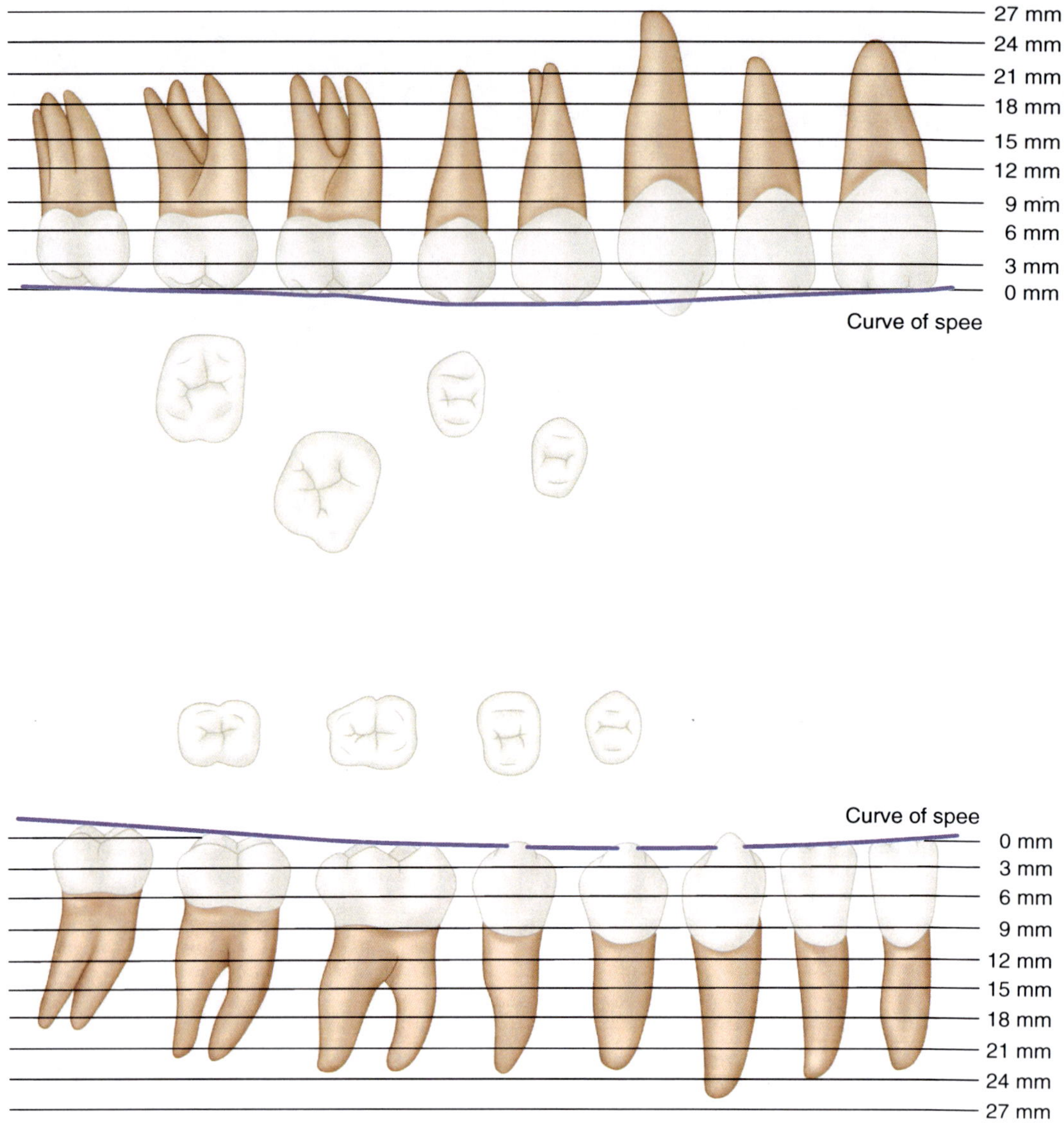

Fig. 3.11 Curve of Spee

of the condyle in the glenoid fossa, there is also centric occlusion of the dentition.

One other term must also be discussed, and that is habitual occlusal relationship. This is the occlusion a patient goes into when they occlude their teeth several hundred times a day while swallowing, talking, and so forth. It is imperative for dental and temporomandibular joint health that the habitual occlusion and centric occlusion position be the same so that there is harmony between the occluding teeth and the condyle in the glenoid fossa.

Overbite, Overjet, and Crossbite

The normal interarch relationships of the anterior teeth show two different types of overlap: a vertical and a horizontal overlap. The horizontal distance from the labial incisal edge of the lower central incisor to the labial incisal edge of the upper central incisor when the jaws are in centric occlusion is called overjet (Fig. 3.12). In a class II malocclusion, there is frequently an increased amount of overjet (This may not be the case in class II, division 2, and cases with deep bites). In the vertical plane, the vertical overlap is called overbite and is represented by the distance from the incisal edge of the upper central incisor to the incisal edge of the lower central incisor while the teeth are in centric occlusion. A class II, division 2 case with a deep bite will have an increased overbite whereas an end-to-end bite (class III) will have no overbite whatsoever. Some patients may even have a distinct gap between the incisal edges of the central incisors when the molars are in centric occlusion. This is referred to as an anterior open bite deformity and is more likely to be seen in patients with vertical maxillary excess and/or steep mandibular plane angles.

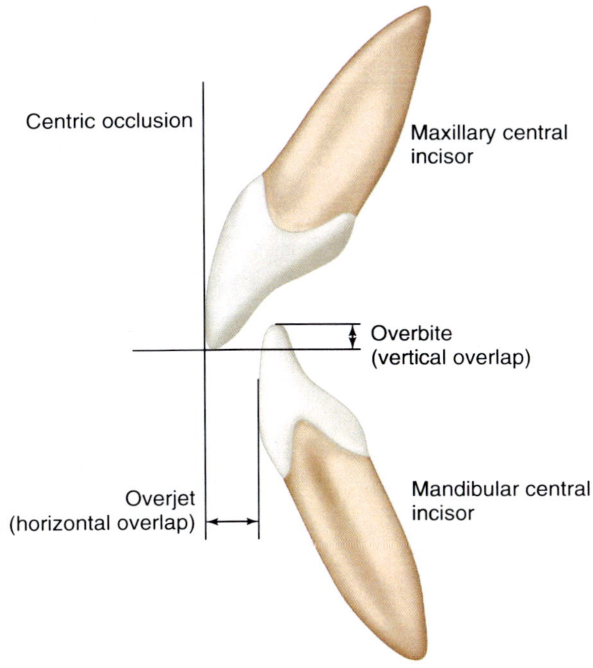

Fig. 3.12 Representation of "overjet" and "overbite"

The occlusion of the posterior teeth can also demonstrate overjet, overbite, open bite, and crossbite. In the normal buccolingual arch relationship of the mandibular and maxillary molar teeth, the mandibular buccal cusps occlude in the central fossae of the maxillary molars and the maxillary lingual cusps articulate in the central fossae of the mandibular teeth. This is explained because in the normal individual the total length of the maxillary arch is 128 mm, whereas the mandibular arch is only 126 mm. This produces some degree of overjet and overbite in this molar region. If there were a gap between the maxillary and mandibular occlusion, then a lateral posterior open bite could exist as well. The overlap of the maxillary molars prevents the cheek from being entrapped when the molar teeth occlude.

When the position of the maxillary teeth versus the mandibular teeth is excessive in the buccal dimension, a "buccal crossbite" or "Brodie bite" can result. When this situation is reversed, then a posterior crossbite can exist. It may be bilateral or unilateral. In this type of malocclusion, the mandibular lingual cusp articulates in the central fossa of the maxillary teeth and the maxillary buccal cusp articulates on the central fossa of the mandibular teeth.

Classification of Malocclusion

The differences in the mesiodistal diameters of the upper and lower incisors cause a distal position of the upper cuspids, bicuspids, and molars to their counterpart in the lower arch. Thus, the upper cuspid occludes distal to the lower cuspid, between it and the lower first bicuspid. In the molar region, this distal position of the upper dentition results in the mesial buccal cusp of the upper first molar to articulate with the buccal groove of the lower first molar, which is the basis for Angle's classification of occlusion. He divided malocclusions into three broad classes dependent on the relationship of the maxillary and mandibular first molars: class I neutroclusion, class II distoclusion, and class III mesioclusion.

Malocclusion can be divided into dental dysplasia, skeletal dysplasias, and skeletal soft tissue dysplasias. Angle's classification serves as a tool to describe the anterior-posterior relationships of the maxillary and mandibular dental arches. Using it makes it possible to scientifically categorize malocclusions and gives us "common ground" to communicate information to our colleagues. It has more recently been expanded to include skeletal and soft tissue relationships of the upper and lower jaws.

There are a variety of environmental effects on malocclusion. These include respiratory patterns (mouth breathing causing a high-arched palate and transverse constriction of the palate and maxillary teeth) and habits such as thumb sucking and tongue thrusting. Possible equilibrium influences, whether from masticatory forces, periodontal fibers, and swallowing posture, can have a role in tooth alignment and are dependent on magnitude and duration of force against teeth.

The patient's basic hereditary or ethnic pattern, which can result in discrepancy in the size and number of the teeth in relation to the size and shape of the skeletal support of the jaws, also has a role on occlusion. In a large study of 21,328 children, 6–18 years of age, by Dr. Woeffel in the USA, 71.7 % had dental malocclusions, whereas 28.3 % had an acceptable occlusion. When classified according to Angle's classification, 28.3 % had class I occlusions, 22 % had class II occlusions, and 5.7 % had class III occlusions.

Class I (Neutroclusion)

With class I occlusion, the anterior-posterior relationship of the maxillary and mandibular molars is in neutral position. The mesiobuccal cusp of the maxillary first molar articulates with the buccal groove of the mandibular first molar (Fig. 3.13). The anterior occlusion may display dental abnormality, such as flaring, crowding, or excessive lingual tilt. It is also possible to see a class I molar and cuspid relationship but have the entire upper and lower dentition positioned forward on their alveolar bases (called bimaxillary protrusion). Another possibility is having the posterior molar relationship class I, but the anterior teeth and bicuspids out of contact, producing an anterior open bite. It is important to remember that an open bite may also occur in class II and III malocclusions as well. The effects of these malpositioned teeth on the soft tissues may produce excessive eversion of the vermilion, protruding lips in the bimaxillary protrusive case, or the lip incompetence that is frequently seen in anterior open bite or severe overjet cases.

Fig. 3.13 Class I ("neutral") occlusion

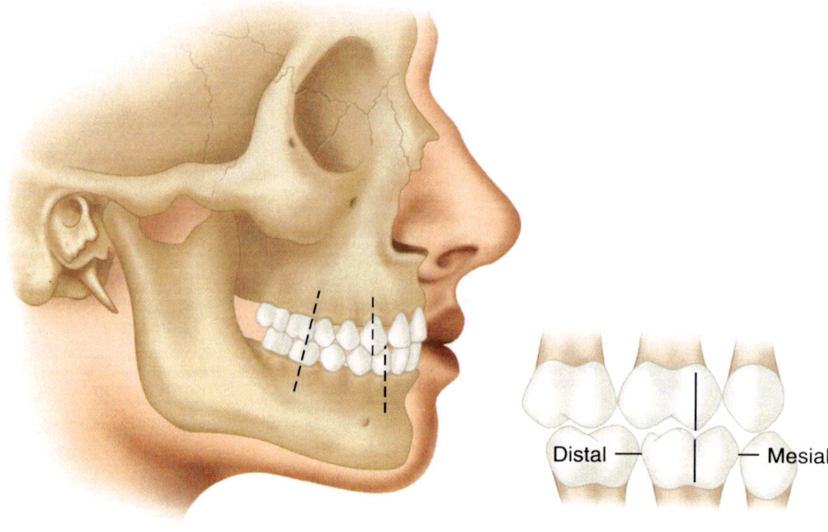

Class II (Distoclusion)

With class II malocclusion, the mandibular arch is in a distal or posterior position in relation to the maxillary arch. The mesial buccal cusp of the maxillary first molar articulates with the distal portion of the mandibular second bicuspid and the mesial cusp of the first molar (Fig. 3.14). The remaining teeth reflect this distal position of the mandible. Angle subdivided this class II into division 1 and division 2, depending on the relationship of the anterior teeth to each other.

In division 1, the molar relationship is as described above but the anterior teeth are proclined, producing a significant overjet. This results in muscle imbalance with loss of upper and lower lip competence. Here, the lower lip frequently becomes everted because of its contact with the proclined maxillary central and lateral incisors. The arch form is frequently V shaped, rather than U shaped, due to narrowing in the cuspid and bicuspid regions. This narrowed maxillary arch tends to constrict the tongue, which then puts pressure on the anterior teeth with swallowing and thereby accentuates the labial proclination and excessive protrusion of the anterior maxillary teeth.

In division 2, the mandibular molar relationship is class II or in a distal position when compared to the maxillary dentition. The anterior dental relationship, however, is quite different than in division 1. The maxillary dental arch is not narrow but instead may be quite wide. There is an excessive curve of Spee with super eruption and lingual retroclination of the mandibular anterior incisors. This produces a deep bite that can result in trauma to the maxillary palatal gingiva in excessive cases. The maxillary lateral incisors are either flared or in lingual version also. Because this is a deep bite, the forced lingual retroclination of the lower anterior incisors may cause their apices to protrude through the labial plate of bone. The mandibular incisors may occlude on the anterior portion of the hard palate, including the incisive papilla, and cause severe tissue damage and, in certain cases, damage to the roots of the maxillary incisors. This tight locked bite can also force the mandible and its condyle into a retruded position in the glenoid fossa, which may lead to symptoms of temporomandibular joint pain, frequently associated with deep bite patients. These malocclusions can present with strong labial musculature.

Class III (Mesioclusion)

With class IIII malocclusion, the mandibular dentition is mesially positioned when compared to the maxillary dentition. The mandibular first molar articulates with the maxillary first and second bicuspid teeth (Fig. 3.15). In the anterior teeth, there is either an end-to-end bite or a crossbite relationship. In cases of true prognathism, the mandibular incisors are usually lingually displaced because of the increased mandibular length and forward mandibular position. This results in an increased lingual pull by the muscles of the lips on these anterior mandibular incisors, resulting in their lingual retroclination. At the same time, there is a decreased force by the tongue labially because it lies easily in the floor of the mouth, which is larger because of the increased mandibular length. The lingual retroclination of the lower incisors and the labial proclination of the maxillary incisors seen in this class of malocclusion are called dental compensations. These dental compensations must be overcome orthodontically and be placed correctly over basal bone before surgery is performed to correct this malocclusion. A class III relationship can be due to midface hypoplasia, mandibular prognathism, or a combination of both. In addition to the anterior-posterior relationship, the vertical growth pattern and transverse relationship of the maxilla and

Fig. 3.14 (**a**, **b**) Class II malocclusion, including divisions 1 and 2

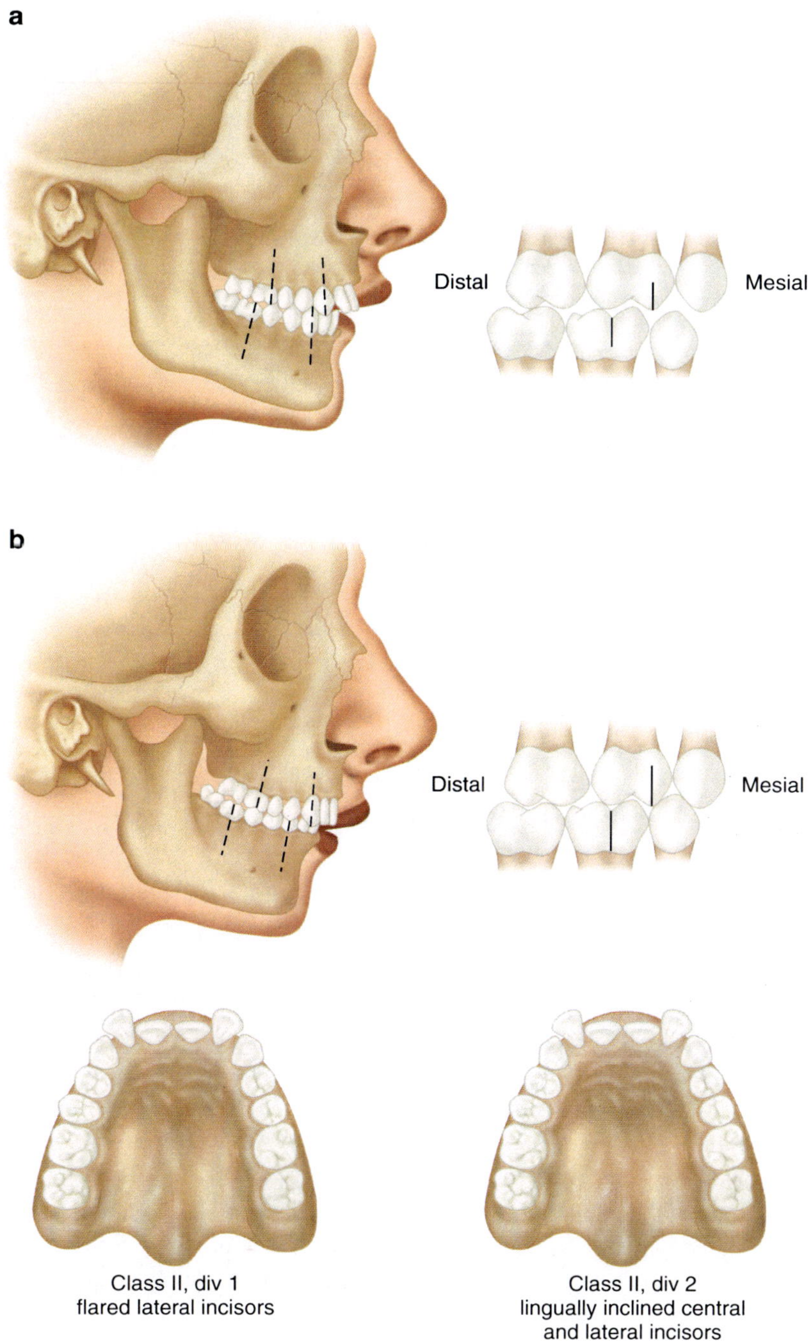

mandible have significant effects on the treatment plan. A proper diagnosis of must be completed prior to orthodontic and surgical correction in order to ensure an ideal result.

Gingiva

The mucous membrane surrounding the teeth, the gingiva, is subjected to forces of friction and pressure in the process of mastication. The gingiva is sharply limited on its outer surface of both jaws by a scalloped line (mucogingival junction), which separates it from the alveolar mucosa. The gingiva is normally pink, sometimes with a grayish tinge, a variable partly caused by differences in the thickness of the stratum corneum. The alveolar mucosa, on the other hand, is red, showing numerous small vessels close to the surface. A similar line of demarcation is found on the inner surface of the lower jaw between the gingiva and the mucosa on the floor of the mouth. In the palate, there is no sharp dividing line because of the dense structure and firm attachment of the entire palatal mucosa.

Fig. 3.15 Class III malocclusion

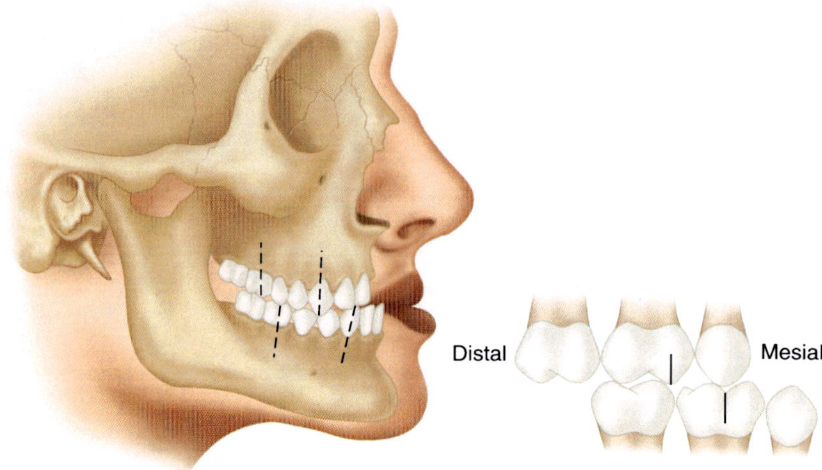

Fig. 3.16 Schematic diagram of gingiva

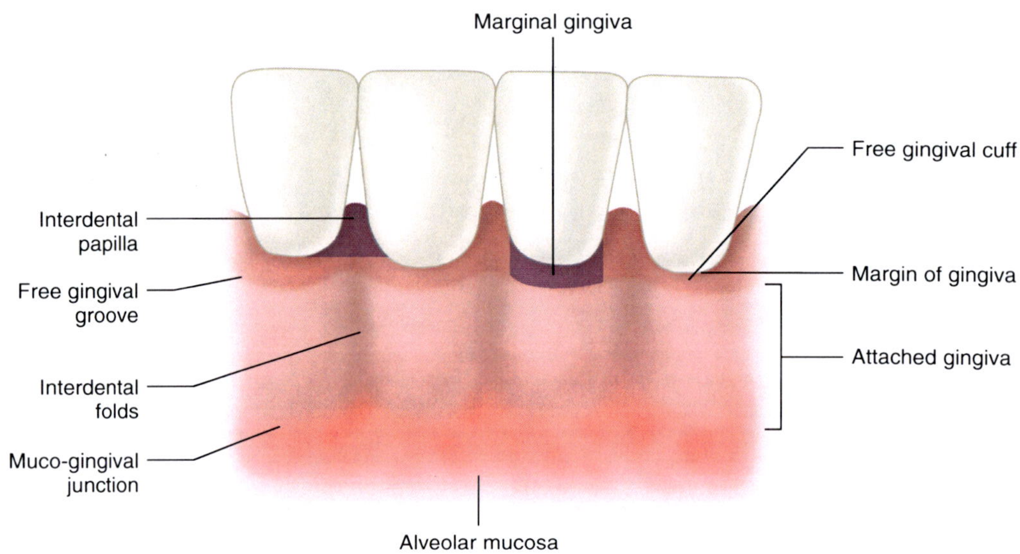

Normally the epithelium of the gingiva is cornifed on its surface and contains a granular layer. In the absence of cornification, there is no granular layer and the flat surface cells contain nuclei that are frequently pyknotic. The epithelium that covers the margin of the gingiva also continues into the epithelial lining of the gingival sulcus. The cells of the basal layer here may contain pigment granules (melanin). While pigmentation is a normal occurrence in blacks, it may also be found in Caucasians, especially those with a dark complexion. When found, it is most abundant in the basal areas of the interdental papillae. If, however, there is increased pigmentation of the interdental papillae, especially when associated with increase in pigmentation of the skin, Addison's disease can be suspected.

The lamina propria of the gingiva consists of dense connective tissues that are not highly vascular. The papillae of the attached gingiva are characteristically long, slender, and numerous. The presence of these numerous papillae permits a sharp demarcation of the gingiva with that of the alveolar mucosa, which usually has fewer and flatter papillae. The tissues of the lamina propria contain only a few elastic fibers that are, for the most part, confined to the walls of the blood vessels. The gingival fibers of the periodontal membrane enter into the lamina propria, attaching the gingiva firmly to the cementum. The gingiva is immovable and firmly attached to the periosteum of the alveolar bone because of the presence of large, coarse collagen bundles that extend from the lamina propria into the bone.

The gingiva may be divided into the free gingiva and attached gingiva (Fig. 3.16). The dividing line between these two parts of the gingiva is the free gingival groove, which runs parallel to the margin of the gingiva at a distance of 0.5–1.5 mm. The free gingival groove is, on histologic section, a shallow, V-shaped groove corresponding to the heavy epithelial ridge that divides the free and attached gingiva. The free gingival groove develops at the level of, or somewhat apical to, the bottom of the gingival sulcus.

The attached gingiva is characterized by high connective tissue papillae elevating the epithelium the surface of which appears striped. The stippling is most probably an expression of functional adaptation to mechanical impacts. The degree of stippling varies with different individuals. The disappearance of stippling is an indication of edema, secondary to chronic inflammation such as gingivitis. It is important to distinguish between attached gingiva and alveolar mucosa. This is because teeth will not erupt through alveolar mucosa but will most assuredly erupt through attached gingiva. This is especially important in patients in which bone grafting is being performed in the region of the alveolar clefts. If the erupting cuspid is covered by alveolar mucosa, it will not properly erupt into the oral cavity, whereas if attached gingiva is brought over the area of the bone graft, the erupting cuspid can easily erupt into the oral cavity in its normal dental position. It is also important not to bring alveolar mucosa down around the necks of erupted teeth because the alveolar mucosa will not attach to the adjacent tooth structure with a normal architectural pattern. Periodontal pockets can easily develop, the mucosa appears red and beefy, and it will not withstand the forces and friction of mastication as attached gingiva will.

Attached gingiva appears slightly depressed between each tooth, corresponding to the depression of the alveolar bone process between eminences of the sockets. In these depressions, the attached gingiva often forms slight vertical folds. The interdental papilla is that part of the gingiva that fills the space between two adjoining teeth and is limited at its base by a line connecting the margin of the gingiva at the center of one tooth to the center of the other. The interdental papilla is composed of free gingiva and attached gingiva in various relations, depending largely upon the relationship of the neighboring teeth.

Bibliography

Akcam MO, Toygar TU, Ozer L, Ozdemir B. Evaluation of 3-dimensional tooth crown size in cleft lip and palate patients. Am J Orthod Dentofacial Orthop. 2008;134(1):85–92.

Angle EH. Classification of malocclusion. Dent Cosmos. 1899;41:248.

Graber TM. Orthodontics; principles and practice. 3rd ed. Philadelphia: W B Saunders Co; 1972.

Nance HN. The limitations of orthodontic treatment; part I. Am J Orthod Oral Surg. 1947;33:177–223.

Newman Dorland WA. Dorland's Illustrated medical dictionary. 27th ed. Philadelphia: WB Saunders Co.; 1988.

Okeson JP. Fundamentals of occlusion and temporomandibular disorders. St. Louis: CV Mosby Co.; 1985.

Orban B. Oral histology and embryology. 4th ed. St Louis: CV Mosby Co.; 1957.

Proffit WR, Fields Jr HW, Sarver DM. Contemporary orthodontics. 4th ed. St. Louis: Elsevier Science Health Science Division; 2006.

Seymour GJ, Ford PJ, Cullinan MP, Leishman S, Yamazaki K. Relationship between periodontal infections and systemic disease. Clin Microbiol Infect. 2007;13 Suppl 4:3–10.

Sicher MD, Harry DSC. Oral anatomy. 7th ed. Saint Louis: CV Mosby Co.; 1980.

Sicher H, Tandler J. Oral anatomy. 4th ed. Saint Louis: CV Mosby Co.; 1965.

Spee FG. Prosthetic dentistry. 4th ed. Chicago: Medico-Dental Publishing Co.; 1928.

Facial Aesthetics

4

Sean G. Boutros and Carlos A. Martinez

The primary aim of facial aesthetic surgery is to enhance the natural attractiveness of the face by restoring or maintaining youthful features while preserving functionality and dynamics. Beauty can be defined as a combination of qualities that are pleasing to the senses or the mind. As a philosophical concept, Alexander Baumgarten, the eighteenth-century philosopher who established aesthetics as a separate field of philosophy, created the term derived from the Greek word for perception (aesthesis). Therefore, the study of aesthetics will comprise the evaluation and comprehension of the beautiful and, its counterpart, the unpleasant or ugly.

Various cultural, social, genetic, and even environmental factors contribute to the definition of an aesthetically beautiful face, and despite the historical era, youth has always been considered the cornerstone of beauty. Romm acknowledged that individuals bestowed with balanced and well-defined skeletal features would best preserve a younger facial profile through the ravages of time than others with insufficient or poorly defined facial features. Furthermore, an abundance of facial soft tissue can be found in the teenage population, providing the underlying structure essential for the harmonious appearance of a youthful face.

The long-standing perspective of beauty in the mid- to late nineteenth century, preceding the introduction of detailed and complex guidelines, was that average facial features contributed as the main factor of the aesthetic and attractive face. The advent of technology to the field of plastic surgery in the form of digital imaging confirmed this perception; digital composites of faces created from different facial features were rated the most attractive when compared to their individual components among infant population, and digital composites could gain higher attractiveness ratings by increasing the number of components. This demonstrated not only the instinctive predisposition of infants to recognize facial beauty but also that facial features closer to the average can increase the attractiveness of an individual. Despite the appraisal of contemporary literature for facial averageness as aesthetically pleasing or that commonly observed facial features are considered particularly appealing, the most beautiful faces will also show extreme features. The complexity of a beautiful face might go beyond averageness as depicted by Perrett et al. after comparing facial features among a group of female individuals. He found that a facial composite that was the average of a total of 60 female faces was considered to be less appealing than composite faces of the top 15 most attractive females from the same sample, where features were exaggerated, thus making the images more appealing. Thus, we can conclude that a beautiful face will always include average features, but unique and distinguishing qualities will have a higher rating in aesthetic standards and will lend to above-the-average beauty.

Caucasian women, especially models and mainstream media personalities, are considered the main reference when depicting ideal beauty. Few studies address the qualities of the aesthetic male profile. Mature features such as a square-shaped jaw with a projecting chin, prominent cheekbones, or thick eyebrows rank among the predominant features that a population of female observers finds attractive. Michiels et al. found that the chin, upper lip, and nose are considered the most important factors that contribute to female attractiveness. Other authors determined that the oral region, with marked attention to the fullness and shape of the lips, is the major determinant of a beautiful face. In further studies, men have shown an increased attraction to female faces with central baby-like features, as revealed by Baudouin and Tiberghien where women with large eyes, prominent malar eminences, thin eyebrows, and a small or finely contoured nose and chin ranked among the particularly beautiful profiles. Questions regarding how pronounced these features should be, in order to increase the attractiveness rather than diminishing it, remain vague; hence, the surgeon's opinion should meet the expectations of the patient in order to obtain ideal results.

S.G. Boutros, MD, FACS (✉) • C.A. Martinez, MD
Houston Plastic and Craniofacial Surgery, Houston, TX, USA
e-mail: drseanboutros@drseanboutros.com

P.J. Taub et al. (eds.), *Ferraro's Fundamentals of Maxillofacial Surgery*,
DOI 10.1007/978-1-4614-8341-0_4, © Springer Science+Business Media New York 2015

Photography

Photography is essential in the evaluation of patient's facial features. Because of its affordability and versatility, two-dimensional images remain the gold standard for preoperative planning or intraoperative decision-making, as well as a method for evaluating postoperative results. The surgeon should take procedure-specific photographs in standard views, including frontal, right and left lateral, and right and left oblique, as well as detailed close-ups of the areas that may require special attention in order to obtain an efficient surgical evaluation. The position of the head must remain unchanged during the different photographic angles. The patient can assume a natural head position (NPH) or one that places the Frankfort horizontal parallel to the floor (the infraorbital rim will be level with the supratragal notch).

Preoperatively, photography will assist during consultation with the patient, as some may be surprised by their look in pictures taken straight ahead. Uniqueness of the face is something to be discussed with the patient in full detail, and the aim of the surgeon is to find individualized and optimal results for each facial procedure. Further use of photographic imaging includes medicolegal documentation and learning purposes.

Computerized Analysis

The use of computer imaging represents a vast, yet underused, instrument in the field of plastic surgery. By increasing the level of detail for a complete evaluation and the information available to be discussed with the patient, the use of the computer should be considered a first-tier tool. The surgeon will be able to visualize the potential end results of the procedure to be performed while allowing the patients to express their own considerations and possible modifications. Discrepancies between the self-image of the patient and the surgeon's professional expectations are a possibility. Furthermore, differences in aesthetic interpretations can occur, and computerized imaging in the preoperative consultation will allow the patients to view themselves with another perspective, one that they usually don't see or otherwise is difficult to perceive with more rudimentary techniques of evaluation. Also, these state-of-the-art devices can manipulate different structures of the face, thus yielding various results and setting realistic patient expectations.

Proportions

In order to achieve a well-balanced face, some relative proportions must exist between the numerous visualized structures. When evaluating the patient prior to any surgical procedure, the relationship between these structures must be taken into consideration. Moreover, isolated or individual assessment of a part can be counterproductive, as modification of one portion can produce an undesired effect on the others. Evidence in the form of quantifiable data, derived from studies with groups of subjects, did not become available for clinical use until the 1970s. Until that time, clinicians interested in the enhancement of facial appearance had to rely on guidelines based on the opinion of artists. Ancient Egyptians were among the first to try to describe the facial and bodily proportions using mathematical methods, followed by ancient Greeks. Sculptures of the human form were widely reproduced during that time, where methods as simple as comparing the size of the hand with the length of the head were thoroughly used. The so-called golden or *divine* proportion was recognized early by the Greeks as a mathematical phenomenon, a ratio with a numerical value of 1.61803 and represented by the Greek letter *phi* (ϕ). Believed to have originated with the sculptor Phidias, hence the representation with the letter *phi*, it has been used as an aesthetically pleasing relationship of horizontal and/or vertical structures, where a line consisting of two uneven segments so that the ratio of the shorter segment to the longer segment is the same as the ratio of the longer segment to the line (Fig. 4.1).

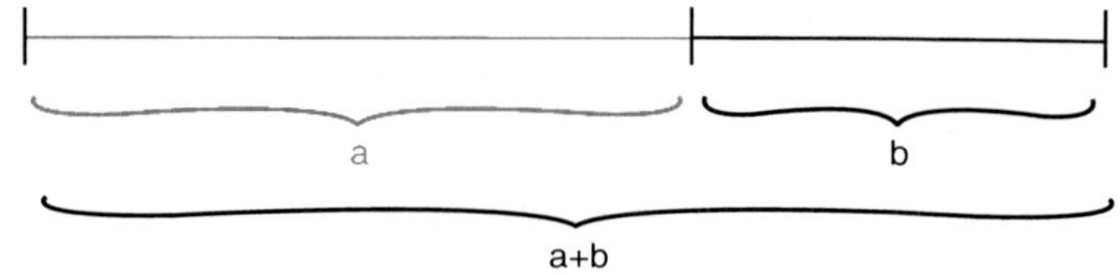

$$\frac{a}{b} = \frac{a+b}{a} = 1.618... = \phi$$

Fig. 4.1 Classical depiction of the *divine proportion* and its *phi* (ϕ) representation

Hellenist Greeks found several proportions between different structures of the body that corresponded with the golden ratio. Such knowledge was later adopted by the Romans, where prominent minds like physician and philosopher Galen or the architect Vitruvius made significant contributions, as in the trisection of the face in equidistant and balanced portions (Fig. 4.2). Furthermore, the golden ratio, along with the Greek and Roman description of facial proportions, is present in Leonardo da Vinci's paintings, masterpieces with an intrinsic harmony or beauty particularly appealing to the human eye. The most common example today is the credit card, whose size ratio is based on the divine proportion.

Following the introduction of cephalometric and anthropometric studies, several criteria and canons were created in order to fulfill the absence of "evidence-based" standards for the evaluation of the aesthetically beautiful face.

Cephalometric analysis was initially used in the field of maxillofacial surgery, mostly because of the enormous impact in the representation of facial proportions. The information however was two-dimensional at the level of the bones, with no soft tissue-based measurements rendering it incomplete. This leads to the advent of anthropometry and the direct measurement of living subjects. Advantages of this approach included its noninvasive nature and its incorporation of a comprehensive database of age- and sex-matched standards (although limited to Caucasian population). These key anthropometric measurements summarized neoclassical "cannons" of beauty.

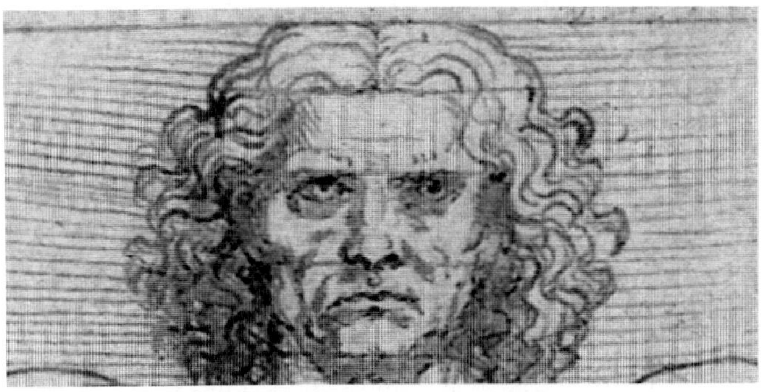

Fig. 4.2 Vitruvius trisection of the face as depicted by Leonardo da Vinci

Initial Assessment

As a plastic surgeon, knowing what to look for is a key aspect of the initial evaluation. Every face will present with asymmetries and disproportions that might be not evident at first glance, and many of these may be unknown to the patient. Patients are evaluated in *natural head position* (NPH). The Frankfort horizontal (Fig. 4.3b) can be deviant due to biological alterations. Frontal and lateral views are used to examine facial proportions and symmetry (Fig. 4.4).

Analysis of the Frontal Face

To assess the length of the face, the patient must be in a standing position. The ratio of facial height to facial width ("facial index") is used to assess the different facial outlines (Fig. 4.5a). A height to width ratio of 1.3:1 for females and 1.35:1 males on a frontal view is considered aesthetically

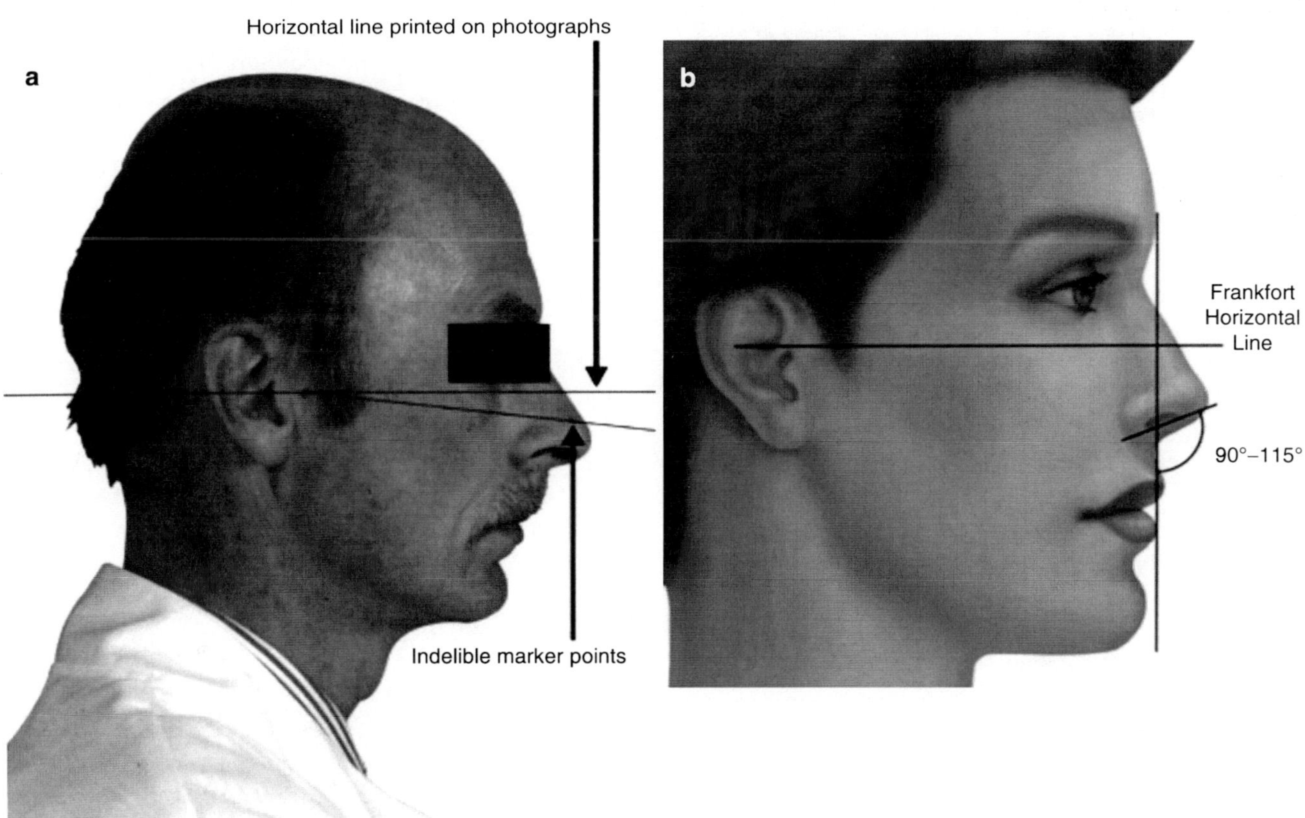

Fig. 4.3 (**a**) The horizontal axis in NPH. (**b**) The Frankfort horizontal: A plane passing through the inferior margin of the orbit and the upper margin of the external auditory meatus (**a**: is an example proposed from Walker F, Ayoub AF, Moos KF, Barbanel J. Face bow and articulator for planning orthognathic surgery: 1 face bow. Br J Oral Maxillofac Surg. 2008;46(7):567–72, and **b**: is an example proposed from Ira D. Papel. Principles of facial plastic and reconstructive surgery. 2008;9:365)

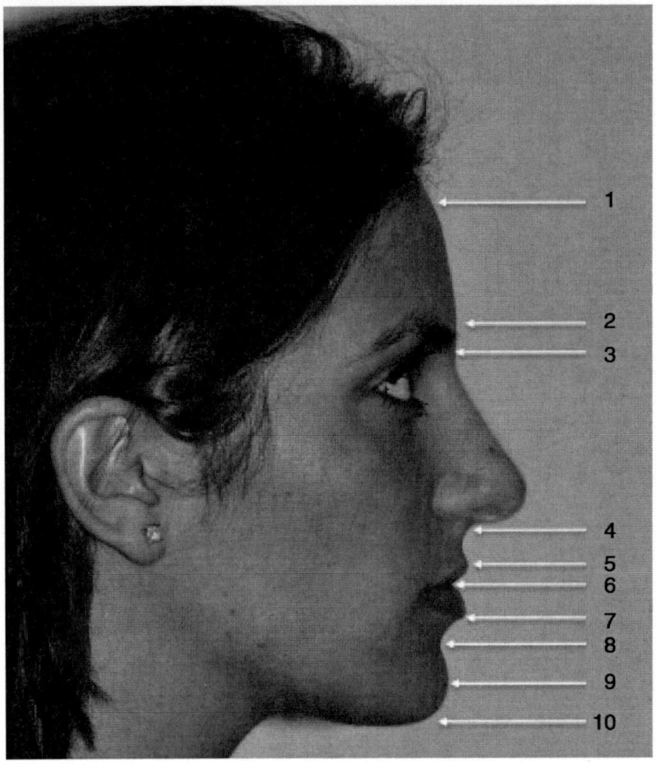

Fig. 4.4 Facial soft tissue landmarks in the profile view: Facial soft tissue landmarks in the midsagittal plane (profile view). *1* Trichion (hairline). *2* Glabella (most prominent point of the forehead soft tissue). *3* Soft tissue nasion (deepest point of the concavity between the forehead and the nose). *4* Subnasale (point where the base of the nasal columella intersects the upper lip). *5* Labrale superioris (point denoting vermilion border of the upper lip). *6* Stomion (midpoint of interlabial fissure). *7* Labrale inferioris (point indicating vermilion border of the lower lip). *8* Labiomental fold (point of highest concavity on the contour of the lower lip between the labrale inferioris and the soft tissue portion of the menton). *9* Soft tissue pogonion (the protruding point on the soft tissue chin), and *10* Soft tissue menton (the inferior point on the soft tissue chin)

proportionate and allows categorizing an individual's face as "square" or "long," among others. A line traced between each zygion (the most lateral point of the zygomatic arch), the bizygomatic facial width, will have an ideal value of approximately 70 % of the vertical facial weight. The bitemporal width, drawn between the most lateral points of the forehead, ideally will measure 80–85 % of the bizygomatic width, whereas the bigonial width, measured from each soft tissue gonion (the most inferior, posterior, and lateral point on the angle of the mandible), should be 70–75 % proportion to the bizygomatic width.

The transverse face is evaluated using the "rule of fifths" (Fig. 4.5b), where each fifth roughly equals the width of the palpebral fissure. Vertical lines dropped from the lateral canthi should approximate with the width of the neck. The outer fifths on the frontal view will extend from the lateral canthus to the most lateral point of the helical rims. The width of the oral commissure should equal the distance between the medial aspects of both irises. Also, the intercanthal space should be equal to the nasal alar base width.

The vertical face is evaluated by dividing the face into thirds: trichion to the glabella, glabella to subnasale, and subnasale to the pogonion. Ideally, these *facial thirds* should be equal (Fig. 4.5c), although in males, the lower third can be slightly greater than the middle third. The lower third can be further subdivided into thirds: the upper lip (subnasale to stomion) makes up one-third, while the lower lip and chin (stomion to pogonion) make up the inferior two-thirds.

Analysis of the Profile Face

A convex profile can be indicative of an underlying Class II skeletal pattern, where maxillary prognathism or mandibular retrognathism are the likely causes. On the other hand, facial concavity is an indication of an underlying Class III skeletal pattern due to maxillary retrognathism or mandibular prognathism. The anteroposterior position of the maxilla can be evaluated by dropping a vertical from the nasion (point where the nasal and frontal bones of the skull meet) that is perpendicular to the Frankfort line while the patient is in NHP. Ideally, the subnasale must be located within this line. Signs of maxillary hypoplasia can include paranasal hollowing or flatness. The facial vertical (Gonzalez-Ulloa and Stevens line or SG line) is a line drawn from the nasion that is perpendicular to the Frankfort plane and is used to evaluate the anteroposterior position of the chin. Ideally the soft tissue pogonion should be 0–2 mm posterior to this line. It is important to assess the overlying soft tissue thickness located anteriorly to the bony chin, as it may be the cause of an overprojected chin. Evaluating the anteroposterior position of the lip is also done primarily using the Steiner line (S-line). Ideally the lips should touch this line, which is drawn between the pogonion and the midpoint between the nasal tip and the subnasale (Fig. 4.6).

Forehead/Eyebrows

The forehead comprises the upper third of the face. Ideally, it should have a gentle convexity on a lateral view, with its most anterior point located above the nasion, at the level of the supraorbital ridge. The nasofrontal angle is formed between the nose and the forehead. A tangent that passes through the

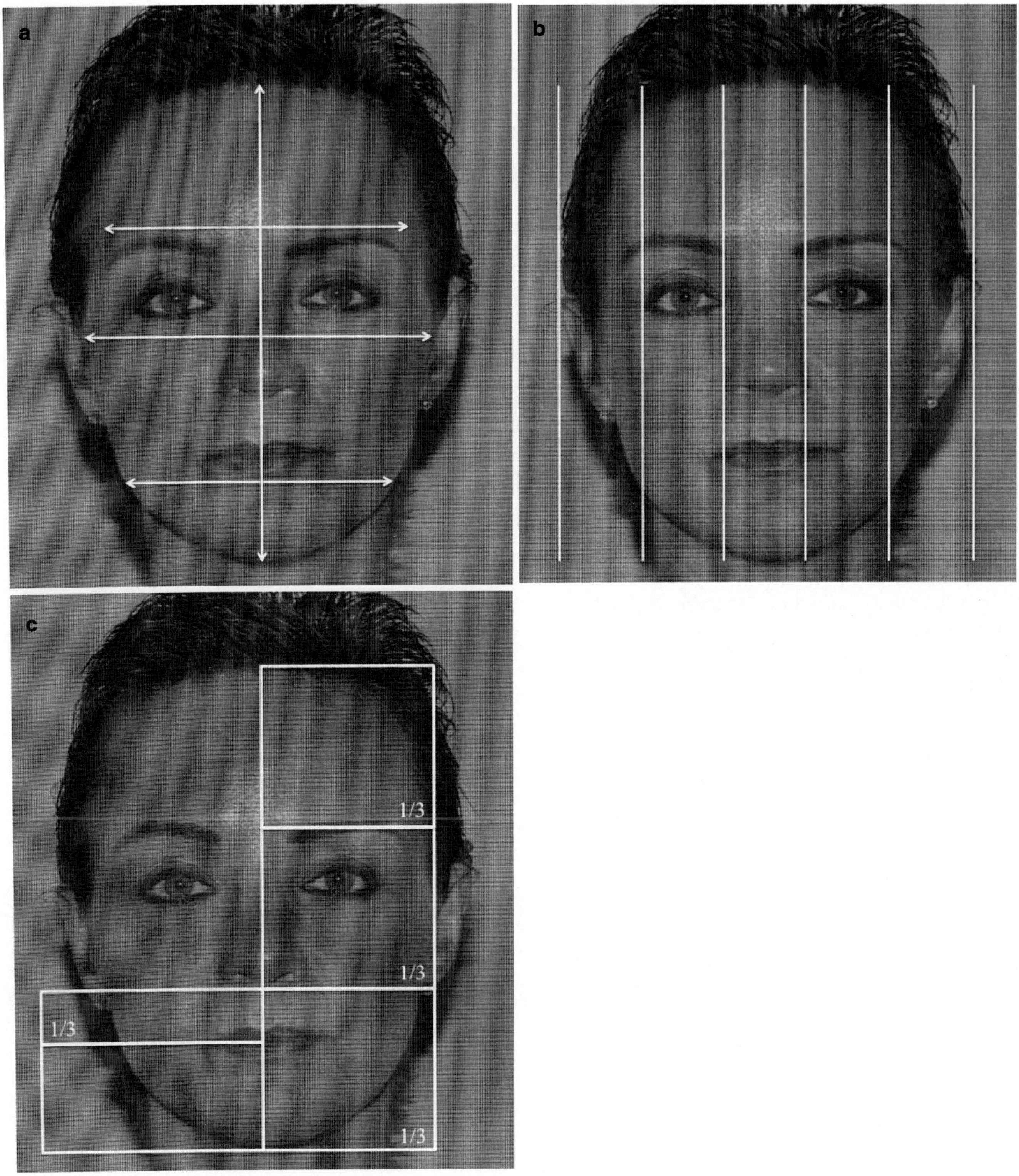

Fig. 4.5 (**a**) Facial index (facial height to width ratio). (**b**) Transverse facial proportions (rule of fifths), each with the width of an eye. (**c**) Vertical facial trisection, with lower facial third proportions

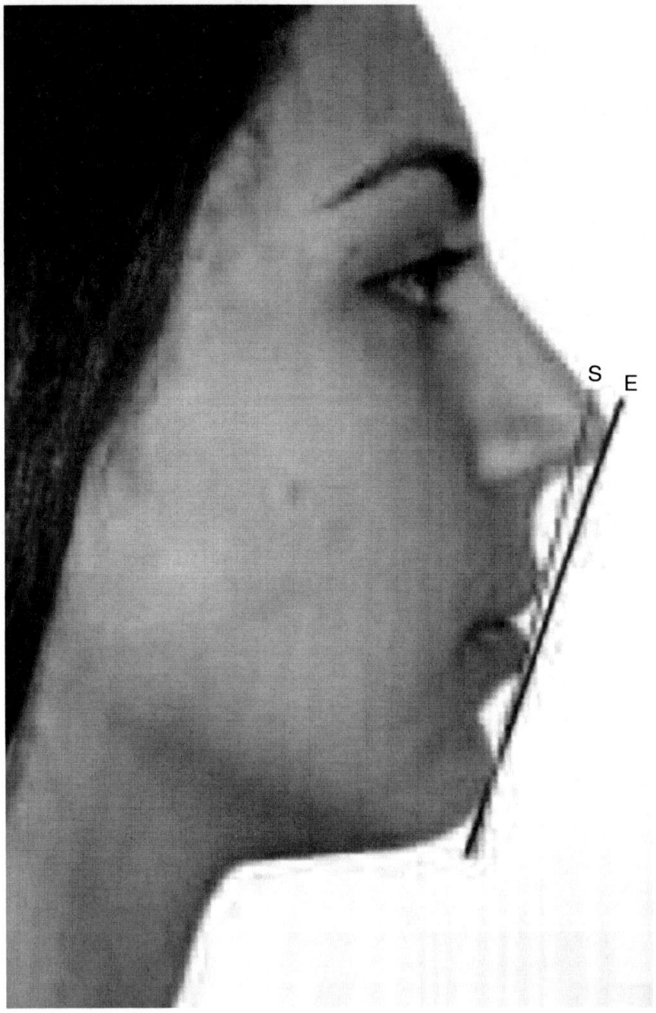

Fig. 4.6 The anterior portion of the lips should touch the *S-line* (Attached is an example proposed from Dent Update. 2008;35:166)

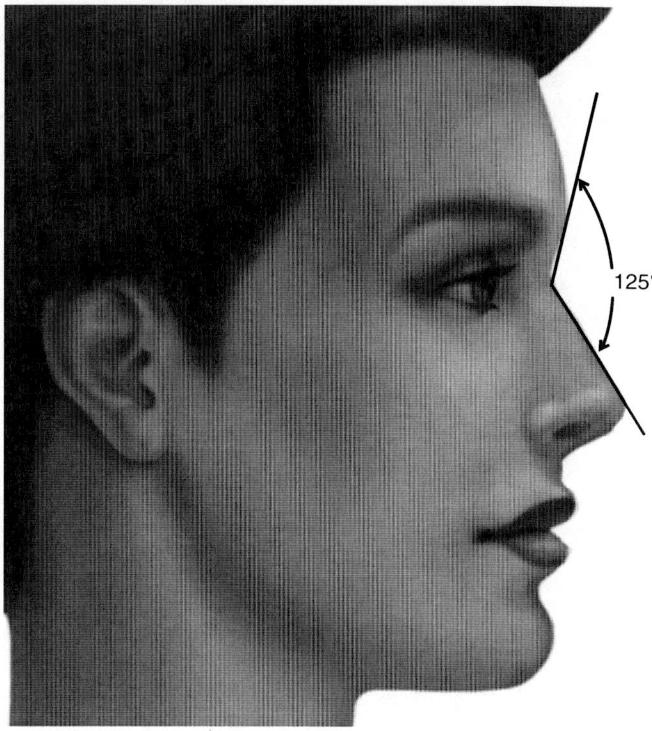

Fig. 4.7 The nasofrontal angle should lie between 115° and 130°. A more obtuse angle is favorable in females, whereas an acute angle is favorable in males (Example proposed from Ira D. Papel. Principles of facial plastic and reconstructive surgery 2008;9:102)

glabella and nasion and meets a line located along the nasal dorsum determines this angle (Fig. 4.7).

There are three fundamental forehead contours: sloping, flat, and protruding. The shape of the forehead influences the perception and appearance of the nose due to its proximity. An exaggerated look of the nose will be seen in patients with a forehead that slopes posteriorly from the brow to the hairline. On the other hand, a vertical and flat forehead, or even protruding, will result in a diminished appearance of the nasal length.

The brow separates the upper and middle portions of the face while framing the eyes. Aesthetically, the brow begins medially at the level of a vertical line drawn from the alar base to the medial canthus. The medial edge passes through the lateral portion of the nasal ala and approximately 1 cm above the medial canthus of the eye. The central portion should have a club-shaped configuration, fashioning a smooth climb of 10–20° until the lateral end, without giving the appearance of a "surprised" face. From the eyebrow to the crease of the eyelid, it should measure 1.6 cm, and from the eyebrow to the middle portion of the pupil, it is 2.5 cm. The distance from the eyebrow to the supraorbital rim is 1 cm and finally to the hairline is 5–6 cm. Ideally, an arch-shaped eyebrow is desirable in women, with its highest point at the level of the lateral canthus or lateral limbus. Some feel that this high point of the brow should preferably be in a more lateral position, specifically the apex positioned along a vertical line located through the lateral canthus, as opposed to the lateral limbus. In men, the arch can be less noticeable and lie slightly lower, close to the level of the supraorbital rim.

Soft tissue laxity and increased skin associated with aging and persistent gravitational forces pulling the structures downward can generate brow ptosis. This can be easily misdiagnosed as upper-eyelid ptosis or dermatochalasis; thus, it is important that the assessment of the resting eyebrow position is performed after the patient closes his eyes for 10–15 s.

Eyes

Asymmetries seen in the eyes are of special concern, as they are arguably the most expressive parts of the face. Aging effects are prematurely noticeable in comparison with other parts of the face, mainly related to skin laxity of the eyelids and pseudoherniation of fat through the orbital septum.

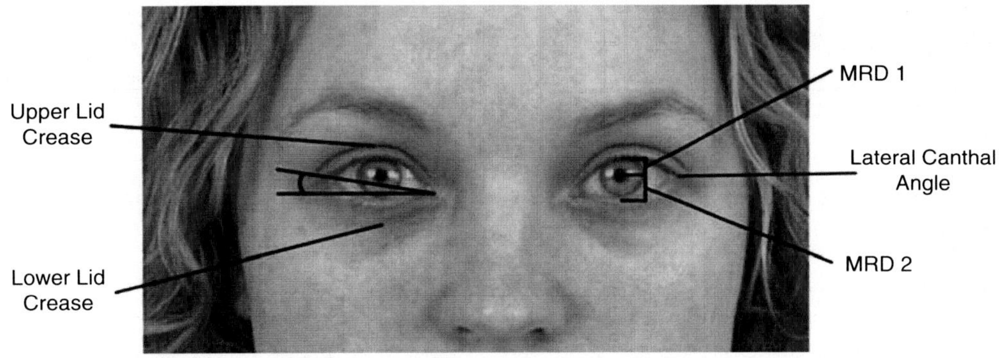

Fig. 4.8 MRD1 and MRD2 measurements evaluate the position of the *upper* and *lower* lids (Example proposed from Maria Z. Siemionov. Plastic and reconstructive surgery 2010;22:304)

Neoclassical standards divide the face vertically into fifths, where the width of each eye, intercanthal space, and nasal width all measure one-fifth. Variations in these proportions were found between Caucasian and Asian populations, where the width of the eyes and nose was often either greater or lesser than the width of the intercanthal space.

On a well-proportionated face, the distance between the central portions of the pupils should be equal to the distance between the nasion and the superior border of the upper lip. Aesthetic eyes are often described as almond-shaped, where the position of the medial canthus, one of the few landmarks that remain unchanged during aging, should be at least 5–10° lower than the lateral canthus. When the head is in a neutral position, the supraorbital rim should lie slightly anterior to the infraorbital rim.

A subtle yet distinctive upper-lid crease is essential. The distance between the upper-lid margin and the lowest part of the brow should be 12–15 mm. The fold lies approximately 7–12 mm above the upper-lid margin, and a variation from 7 to 15 mm in the distance from the lash line to the lid crease is considered ideal and is closely related to body weight, ethnicity, and thickness of underlying skin. The upper lid should cover a small portion of the iris and should not be in touch with the pupil. There should be minimal visualization of the sclera below the iris with the lower lid showing a slight concavity and shaped in a tapered-scroll fashion. An upward projection of 5–10° should be noted on the lateral half of the lower lid while presenting a smooth transition with the zygomatic portion of the midface.

The margin reflex distance-1 (MRD1) is measured between the central border of the upper eyelid and the central portion of the pupil, and the margin reflex distance-2 (MRD2) is the distance between the central border of the lower eyelid and the central portion of the pupil. A palpebral distance of less than 10 mm with an MRD1 of less than 4 mm is typically due to ptosis of the upper eyelid (Fig. 4.8).

Cheek

A prominent cheek is often a hallmark of facial beauty as strong malar prominences can masquerade the otherwise noticeable aging effects. The aesthetic and attractive cheek should resemble a well-defined and ovoid-shaped structure, where fullness and a distinctive projection of the malar region are often considered the most attractive configuration. The malar eminence is formed by the zygomatic and the maxillary bones along with the overlying soft tissues and can be easily located with a method described by Wilkinson, where a line is dropped from the lateral canthus to the inferior mandibular border, and then dividing it into thirds; it should lie just lateral to the point situated one-third from the canthus. Ideally the fullest portion of the cheek should be in a center and high position over the zygoma. A gradual inward sloping of the malar cheek is seen inferior to this point, where a flat, or even slightly concave, submalar cheek is formed.

The optimum height of the malar eminence should be between 25 and 27 mm from the lateral canthus, with an ideal angle of 40°, and approximately 1 cm above the Frankfort line and 1 cm posterior to the lateral orbital rim. A deepening of the nasolabial crease and accentuation of the nasolabial fold are changes associated with aging. In fact, the nasolabial fold should be subtle, with a jowl area flat or even slightly concave.

Nose

The nose, due to its position in the midline of the facial central third and prominence in the sagittal plane, is probably the most significant aesthetic feature of the face. Analysis of the patient and the relationships between the nose and surrounding structures is always assessed prior to a nasal procedure, where harmony between these structures is essential for ideal aesthetic results. Powell and Humphreys detailed guidelines regarding the proportions of the aesthetic and attractive nasal-facial structures, in terms of its length, projection, rotation, and width, providing further assessment and planning in facial rejuvenation.

Symmetrical dimensions of the nose can be evaluated from a *frontal view*. Any deviation of the nose can be easily noted by bisecting the nasal bridge and the tip with a line from the glabella to the chin point. The alar base can also be assessed via this view, where the width should be equal to

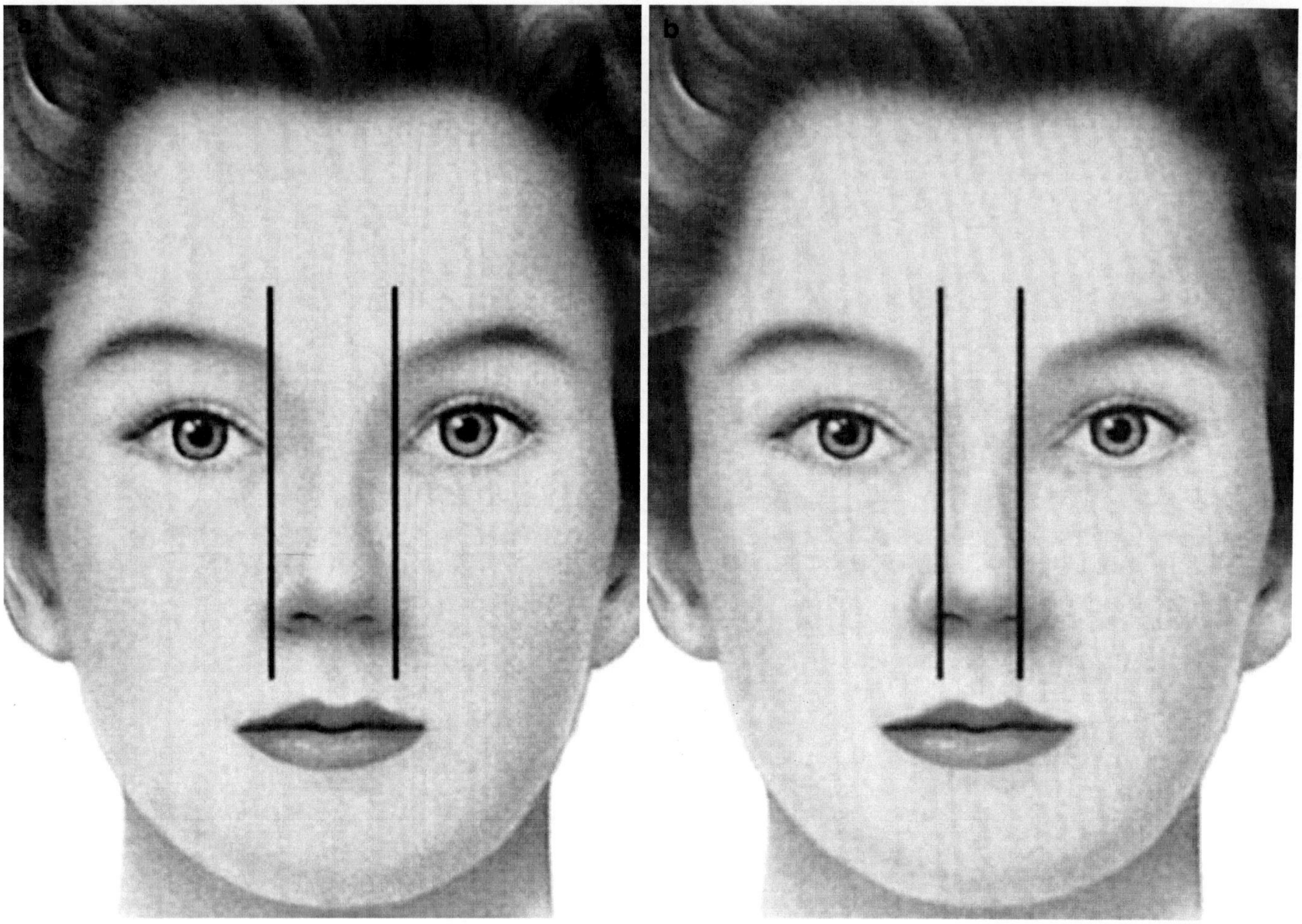

Fig. 4.9 (**a**) Alar base should equal the intercanthal space. (**b**) The bony portion should approximate 80 % of the alar base width (Example proposed from Ira D. Papel. Principles of facial plastic and reconstructive surgery. 2008;9:363)

the intercanthal space. The measured width of the osseous portion of the lateral walls should be 70–80 % of the normal alar base (Fig. 4.9). Frontal visualization of the tip can evaluate asymmetries in the domes of the lower lateral cartilage. Also, the tip may appear wide if the lower lateral cartilages are not united. Excessive visualization of the nostrils may indicate an overly rotated nasal tip or asymmetries of the alar rims. Ideally, the columella is seen just inferior to the alar rims and should be scarcely visualized on frontal view.

The *lateral view* can be used to assess the nasofrontal angle, which connects the nasal dorsum with the glabellar domain. It is measured at 115–130°, although no well-established parameters have been described; therefore, the surgeon must use judgment to determine the ideal depth. The nasion, the deepest point of the nasofrontal angle, should lie at the level of the supratarsal crease. As described by Crumley and Lancer, nasal projection is determined from the profile and can be measured by a triangle. Nasal projection and length proportion are represented by a 3:5 ratio, thus making nasal projection 60 % of nasal length; measurements are made from the alar-facial crease perpendicular to the Frankfort horizontal plane to the nasal tip. Another method for the evaluation was described based on its relation with the upper lip. Adequate nasal projection is represented when 50–60 % of the horizontal projection of the nose lies anterior to the superior labial border (Fig. 4.10a–b). Dimensions over 60 % are considered overprojected, while less than 50 % are considered underprojected.

The nasolabial angle can be evaluated by drawing a line between the nasal columella and the upper-lip slope. The ideal angle for men ranges from 90 to 95°, while in women is from 95 to 115°. It is important to remember that this angle is dependent of the anteroposterior position of the maxillary incisors and the maxilla, the vertical position of the tip of the nose, and the morphology and underlying tissue of the upper lip. Two to four millimeter of the alar-columellar relationship should be visible from the profile view. Retraction of the alar lobule may result from excessive projection of this area.

Finally, orientation, size, and shape of the base of the nose are carefully assessed, along with the symmetry of the nostrils and the length of the columella and lobule. A teardrop-shaped nostril with a 45° angle on the long axis in relation to

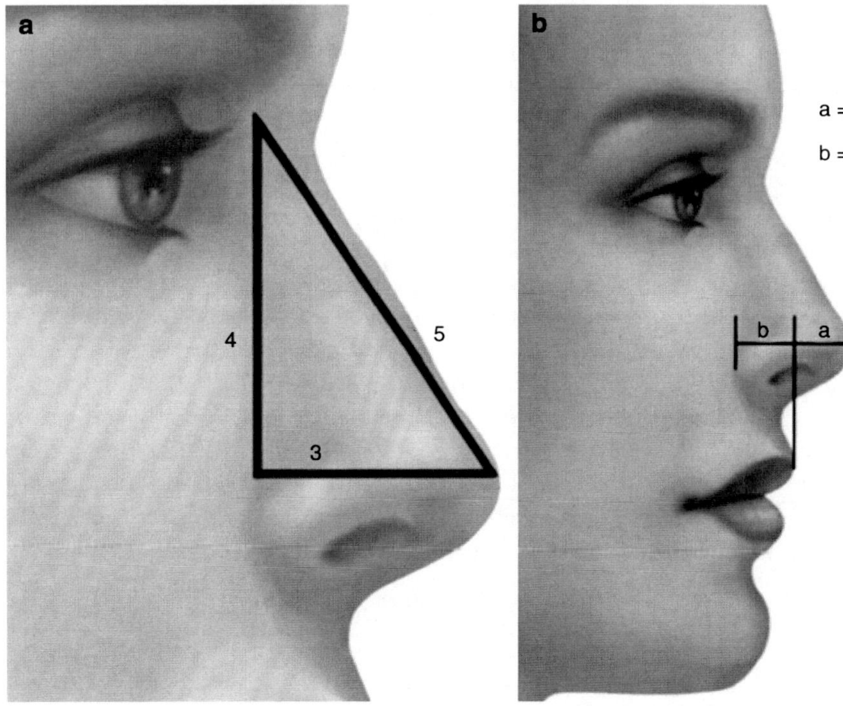

Fig. 4.10 (**a**) Crumley's and (**b**) Simons' methods for tip projection (Example proposed from Ira D. Papel. Principles of facial plastic and reconstructive surgery 2008;9:362–5)

the columella is ideal; width of the nostrils should be similar as the width of the columella.

With age, the cartilaginous structures of the nose weaken, causing tip ptosis, lengthening, broadening, and even airway obstruction. Furthermore, widening of the nostrils and a sharper visualization of the columellar-labial angle may also develop.

Lips

The lips are an expressive and active part of the facial anatomy. The upper lip should have a more prominent anterior projection than the lower lip, although the latter should be fuller in volume. A strong definition of the philtrum along with fullness of the lips is associated with youth, while aging process of the lips include flatness, loss of highlights and a thin vermillion. The underlying dental structures will define the posture of the lips, designated as recumbent or procumbent. The commissures should be vertically aligned with the medial limbus. Constructing a line between the subnasale and the soft tissue pogonion can assess the horizontal lip position. The upper and lower lips should rest 3.5 and 2.2 mm anterior to this line, respectively. Another method used to assess the position of the lips is to draw a line between the nasal tip and the pogonion. Both lips should lie posterior to this line, called nasomental or aesthetic line (E-line). Ideally, the upper lip will be situated 4 mm behind this line, and the lower lip 2 mm behind this line. Both lips should be 57–62 mm in width, with a vertical height of 8.5–9 mm for the upper lip and 9.5–10 mm for the lower lip. The philtrum, at the junction with the vermilion, should measure 10–11 mm. A distinctive feature of the upper lip, the "Cupid's bow," should be upward tilted 10–20° from the commissure. The labial ledge, the distance between the base of the columella and the Cupid's bow, should be equal to or shorter than the distance between the supratarsal crease and the lower-lid lash line. A *competent* posture of the lips is seen when the lips are held together at rest, whereas an *incompetent* posture is seen when lips are help apart at rest by more than 3–4 mm. Finally, the gingiva should be exposed 0–2 mm when smiling. Increased muscular activity of the upper lip or a long bony midface ("vertical maxillary excess") can lead to a *gummy smile*.

Mandible

The mandible is included in the evaluation of the lower portion of the face and also as part of the length of the lower lip. The jawline must be smooth and well defined from lateral and frontal views, with a relative absence of ptotic fat, in order to have a pleasant form. A subtle yet sharply defined menton is associated with a more feminine aesthetic, while a highlighted masseter region, representation of the underlying fat and muscle, is a more attractive feature in the masculine face. The anterior limit of the chin is determined by a vertical line (SG line) from the brow. The tip should slightly touch a line drawn from the nasion down to the nasal spine, perpendicular to the Frankfort plane. A definite yet gentle mentolabial sulcus separating the cutaneous lower lip from the chin is essential. The deepest point should lie approximately 4 mm behind a line drawn in between the inferior border of the lower lip and the pogonion. The nasomental line is measured from the pogonion to the nasal tip and ideally ranges from 120 to 132° (Fig. 4.11).

The dorsal line, which constitutes the upper line of the angle, depends on nasal projection, as previously described. The line located in the inferior portion, the nasomental line, is modified by the position of the mandible. The labiomental angle is formed between the inferior point of the lower lip and the chin. A value range of 100–130° is considered aesthetically ideal, although it depends on the inclination of the lower incisor and the height of the anterior lower face. It is important to recognize that many conditions may lead to an acute labiomental angle, such as a prominent chin, an excess in lower incisor proclination, or a reduced lower anterior facial height.

The mentocervical angle should also be assessed. It evaluates the neckline and its relationship with the inferior portion of the face. It is determined by drawing a line between the cervical point and the lowermost point on the chin, the menton, and the angle will be obtuse if there is evidence of mandibular retrognathia, retrogenia, or excessive submental fat. The ideal measurement ranges from 80 to 95°.

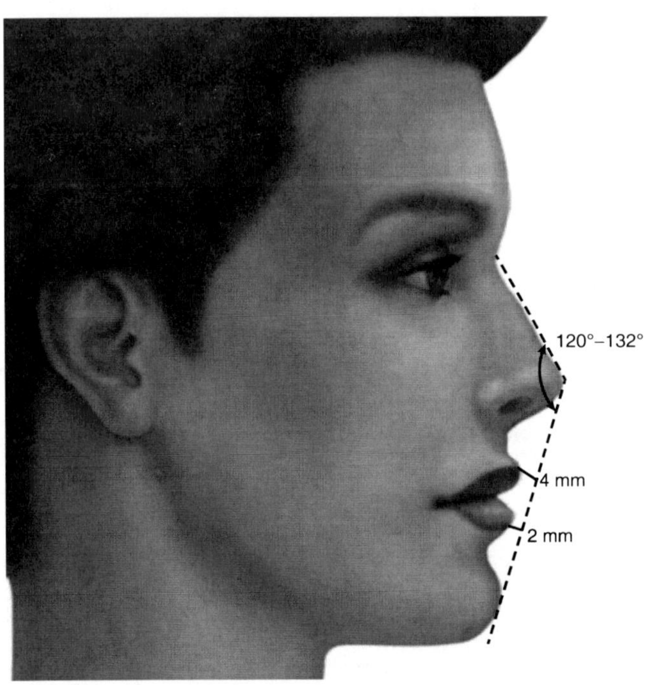

Fig. 4.11 The nasomental angle is defined by a line from the nasion to tip intersecting the tip-to-pogonion line (Example proposed from Ira D. Papel. Principles of facial plastic and reconstructive surgery. 2008;9:106)

Symmetry

Perception of attractiveness can be enhanced by high facial symmetry or low fluctuating asymmetries (FA), which are single variations between the left and right hemispheres of the face, in traits that are usually symmetrical. The correlation between facial (and bodily) symmetry and the healthy individual, which provides "quality" genetic material, has been a historical dogma. Many authors are convinced that a perfectly symmetrical face has a definitive influence in the perception of beauty.

Absolute symmetry is impossible; slight unevenness of the commissures, eyelids, or eyebrows, even unmatched nostrils, will be present in every face. Differentiating "normal" facial asymmetries from "abnormal" can be challenging, and the surgeon's sense of imbalance combined with the patient's perception is the most valuable tool to be used during evaluation. Furthermore, during the evaluation, an extensive discussion regarding this matter is indispensable, mostly because the majority of patients are often not aware of the quantitative or qualitative presence of their own asymmetry. Facial symmetry can be evaluated by tracing a line through the midsagittal plane of the face and comparing both sides; the axis should lie within the forehead, nose, lips, and chin. As previously mentioned, the face can be divided into fifths, and comparison between the balances of each fifth can be done. The simplest method of evaluating asymmetry is a non-reversing mirror. This reverses the typical side and highlights subtle differences. Also, computerized reconstruction can be performed, where a composite image of the patient's hemisphere is mirrored to the contralateral side, thus creating a symmetrical image that will contribute to a more efficient evaluation. This will also help illustrate that facial asymmetries are essentially normal and, in most cases, can remain unnoticed.

Contour

The forehead (along with the supraorbital region) and the pyriform-maxillary territory are also considered promontories, although they remain of lesser importance to the overall aesthetic appearance. Reduction or enhancement of these promontories can create or restore facial harmony and beauty as desired by the patient. Such modification in the shape or size of any of these promontories will directly and inversely affect the aesthetic appearance of the others. The skin should be assessed for quality and thickness and the subdermal and deep fat for its adequacy. Soft tissue evaluation must include the muscle tone or the presence of ptosis.

Augmentation of the mandible and the malar eminence will result in a reduced magnitude of the nasal appearance. An accentuated malar eminence will diminish the importance of the nose and the chin. Finally, if the nasal prominence is reduced, relative sizes of the midface and the jawline will assume a more visual significance. Therefore, the visual appearance of one element can be easily affected by a poorly assessed alteration of the other, resulting in an unbalanced relationship between the major promontories.

Nose

On a frontal view, the ideal nose resembles an hourglass, formed by two divergent and concave lines that extend from the tip to the medial portion of the eyebrow (*brow-tip aesthetic line*). They should narrow at the middle nasal vault and widen slightly along the alar margins. The transition between the middle nasal vault and the tip should be subtle, with a slight divergence as it approaches the alar margins. A bulbous appearance of the tip can result from excessive fullness in the supratip region, thus an undesirable shadowing might be seen. This fullness may be due to excessive vertical height or a cephalic position of the lateral crura. Fullness in the supratip area should be eliminated in order to create an ideal supratip shadow, resulting in an attractive nasal tip.

Malar Eminence

During the assessment of the malar eminence, the position should be evaluated in the context of other skeletal relationships and facial features: the deepness of the nasolabial folds, the shape of the nose, the prominence of the chin, and the overall facial outline. As previously noted by Mladick, seven groups might benefit after alteration of the malar eminence, including the aged face, the flat or "dish face," the round and full face, post-traumatic depressions, congenital deformities, and patients with an unbalanced aesthetic triangle. Aesthetic modifications to the contour of the malar eminence can be achieved by fashioning volumetric changes of the malar space, providing support for ptotic soft tissues and promoting harmony between the promontories.

Mandible

Although the nose is the most prominent structure of the facial mosaic, the chin remains as an important portion to the overall appearance, where dissonant bony and skin features can become a challenge for the surgeon in the search for an attractive mandibular line. The mandible is the major component that provides structure to the lower third of the face. Changes in the position of the chin therefore play an important role in altering the appearance of the face. Notable differences in aesthetic standards between men and women have been described, where a marked anterior projection of the chin is more acceptable in men. The displacement of the origins of the mentalis muscle can create a "drooping chin" deformity, allowing a downward dislocation of the soft tissue and musculature overlying the area. This is a special concern in patients with an inherited globular, round, and prominent central soft tissue chin mound or aging patients that develop an adjacent lateral soft tissue sulcus between the central chin mound and the ptotic, lateral jowl elements. This sulcus is commonly referred as the anterior mandibular sulcus or "marionette groove."

Conclusion

Analysis of the facial aesthetics is an important aspect of any cosmetic evaluation. Understanding the canons of beauty along with the facial proportions helps the surgeon to identify deviations from these canons and proportions. It is this understanding of both the standards and deviations which aids the surgeon in identifying what is beautiful and what is lacking in a face. This, together with the patient desires, allows the surgeon to formulate a plan, which will enhance the patients' facial aesthetics.

Bibliography

Auger TA, Turley PK. The female soft tissue profile as presented in fashion magazines during the 1900s: a photographic analysis. Int J Adult Orthodon Orthognath Surg. 1999;14:7–18.

Baudouin JY, Tiberghien G. Symmetry, averageness, and feature size in the facial attractiveness of women. Acta Psychol (Amst). 2004;117:313–32.

Bishara SE, Burkey PS, Kharouf JG. Dental and facial asymmetries: a review. Angle Orthod. 1994;64:89–98.

Broadbent Sr BH, Broadbent Jr BH, Golden WH. Bolton standards of dento-facial developmental growth. St. Louis: Mosby; 1975.

Burnstone CJ. Lip posture and its significance in treatment planning. Am J Orthop. 1967;53:262.

Cellerino A. Psychobiology of facial attractiveness. J Endocrinol Invest. 2003;26:45–8.

Cook TA, Brownrigg PJ, Wang TD. The versatile midforehead browlift. Arch Otolaryngol Head Neck Surg. 1983;115:163–8.

Crumley RL, Lancer R. Quantitative analysis of nasal tip projection. Laryngoscope. 1988;98:202–8.

Edler RJ. Background considerations to facial aesthetics. J Orthod. 2001;28:159–68.

Ellenbogen R. Transcoronal eyebrow lift with concomitant upper blepharoplasty. Plast Reconstr Surg. 1983;71:490–9.

Farkas LG. Anthropometry of the head and face. New York: Elsevier; 1981.

Farkas LG, Munro IR. Anthropometric facial proportions in medicine. Springfield: Charles C. Thomas Pub Ltd; 1987.

Farkas LG, Hreczko TA, Kolar JC. Vertical and horizontal proportions of the race in young adult North American Caucasians: revision of neoclassical canons. Plast Reconstr Surg. 1985;75(3):328–38.

Faure JC, Rieffe C, Maltha JC. The influence of different facial components on facial aesthetics. Eur J Orthod. 2002;24:1–7.

Grammer K, Thornhill R. Human [Homo sapiens] facial attractiveness and sexual selection the role of symmetry and averageness. J Comp Psychol. 1994;108:233–42.

Hume D. "Of Tragedy" in essays, literary, moral and political. London: Oxford University Press; 1963.

Hutchenson F. An inquiry into the original of our ideas of beauty and virtue. Indianapolis: Liberty Fund; 2004.

Johnston VS, Franklin M. Is beauty in the eye of the beholder? Ethol Sociobiol. 1993;14:183–99.

Kant I. The critique of judgement. London: Oxford University Press; 1973.

Kerr WJ, O'Donnell JM. Panel perception of facial attractiveness. Br J Orthod. 1995;17:299–304.

Langlois JH, Roggman LA, Casey RJ. Infant preferences for attractive faces: rudiments of stereotype? Dev Psychol. 1987;23:363–9.

Langlois JH, Kalanakis LE, Rubenstein AJ. Maxims or myths of beauty: a meta-analytic and theoretical overview. Psychol Bull. 2000;126:390–423.

Larrabee WF, Makielski KH, Herderson JL. Variations in facial anatomy with race, sex, and age. Surgical anatomy of the face. Philadelphia: Lippincott Williams & Wilkins; 2004. p. 22–8.

Michiels G, Sather AH. Validity and reliability of facial profile evaluation in vertical and horizontal dimensions from lateral cephalogram and lateral photographs. Int J Adult Orthodon Orthognath Surg. 1994;9:43–54.

Mladick RA. Alloplastic cheek augmentation. Clin Plast Surg. 1991;18:29–38.

Moorrees CFA, Kean MR. Natural head position: a basic consideration in the interpretation of cephalometric radiographs. Am J Phys Anthropol. 1958;16:213–34.

Peerlings RH, Kuijpers-Jagtman AM, Hoeksma JB. A photographic scale to measure facial aesthetics. Eur J Orthod. 1995;17:101–9.

Perrett DI, May KA, Yoshikawa S. Facial shape and judgments of female attractiveness. Nature. 1994;368:884–7.

Pogrel MA. What are normal esthetic values? J Oral Maxillofac Surg. 1991;49:963–9.

Popovich E, Thompson GW. Craniofacial templates for orthodontic case analysis. Am J Orthod. 1977;71:406–20.

Powell N, Humphreys B. Proportions of the aesthetic face. New York: Thieme-Stratton; 1984.

Rhodes G, Sumich A, Byatt G. Are average facial configurations attractive only because of their symmetry? Psychol Sci. 1999;10:52–8.

Rickets RM. A foundation for cephalometric communication. Am J Orthod. 1953;39:729–55.

Romm S. Art, love and facial beauty. Clin Plast Surg. 1987;14:579.

Scheib JE, Gangestad SW, Thornhill R. Facial attractiveness, symmetry and cues of good genes. Proc Biol Sci. 1999;266:1913–7.

Shackelford TK, Larsen RJ. Facial asymmetry as an indicator of psychological, emotional, and physiological distress. J Pers Soc Psychol. 1997;72:456–66.

Steiner CC. Cephalometrics for you and me. Am J Orthod. 1953;39:729–55.

Tardy ME. Rhinoplasty: the art and the science. Philadelphia: WB Saunders Co; 1996.

Tardy ME, Becker OJ. Surgical correction of facial deformities. Diseases of the nose, throat and ear. Philadelphia: Lea & Febiger; 1977.

Tatarunaite E, Playle R, Hood K. Facial attractiveness: a longitudinal study. Am J Orthod Dentofacial Orthop. 2005;127:676–82.

Tessier P. The definitive plastic surgical treatment of the severe facial deformities of craniofacial deformities of craniofacial dysostosis: Crouzon's and Apert's diseases. Plast Reconstr Surg. 1971;48:419–42.

Thornhill R, Gangestad SW. Facial attractiveness. Trends Cogn Sci. 1999;3:452–60.

Tolleth H. Concepts for the plastic surgeon from art and sculpture. Clin Plast Surg. 1987;14:585.

Valen LV. A study of fluctuating asymmetry. Evolution. 1962;16(2):125–42.

Wilkinson TS. Complications in aesthetic malar augmentation. Plast Reconstr Surg. 1983;71:643–7.

Wolfe SA, Vitenas P. Malar augmentation using autogenous materials. Clin Plast Surg. 1991;18:39–54.

Regional Anesthesia

5

Adam I. Levine and Samuel DeMaria Jr.

The use of regional anesthesia for head and neck, and more specifically, maxillofacial procedures has a long history in anesthesiology. Indeed, the introduction of local anesthetics such as cocaine and procaine revolutionized much of these procedures as early as the late 1800s, when Koller began using cocaine as an anesthetic. Today, a working knowledge of the pharmacology of local anesthetics and of head and neck anatomy is all that one needs to safely and effectively utilize regional anesthetic techniques for intraoperative maxillofacial surgery and for acute postoperative pain management strategies.

Essentials of Regional Anesthesia

Regional anesthesia can be described as either central or neuraxial regional anesthesia including spinal and epidural anesthesia and peripheral nerve anesthesia. The use of regional anesthetic techniques has evolved from their use as a sole anesthetic, under which a surgical procedure could be performed, to a way of providing intraoperative anesthesia as one component of a balanced anesthetic and as but one strategy for postoperative analgesia. An evolution has occurred from relying on surface landmarks to the increased use of nerve stimulation and direct visualization with ultrasound technology that has certainly improved patient comfort and perhaps safety and efficacy of peripheral nerve block techniques. The role of these newer technologies in OMFS procedures is less well defined, however.

A.I. Levine, MD (✉)
Department of Anesthesiology, Icahn School of Medicine at Mount Sinai, New York, NY, USA
e-mail: adam.levine@mssm.edu

S. DeMaria Jr., MD
Division of Liver Transplantation, Department of Anesthesiology, Icahn School of Medicine at Mount Sinai, New York, NY, USA

Indications

Instituting regional anesthesia is dependent on a number of conditions: the patient's considerations including comorbities, anatomy, and procedural consent, and the surgical considerations including the planned surgical procedure and technique, the surgeon's request, and lastly the availability of necessary resources. Although the use of regional anesthetic techniques is not without risk, it offers a very viable alternative to general anesthesia or "deep" monitored anesthetic care (MAC) that risks aspiration and apnea/hypoxemia. The disadvantages of peripheral nerve blocks include local anesthetic toxicity, permanent nerve damage and paresthesias, and potential damage of surrounding structures (depending on the block performed, this may include the eye, other nerves, or even brain injury).

When planning to perform head and neck procedures under regional anesthesia, it is critical that the anesthetic and surgical teams have a clear understanding of surgical and anesthetic expectations. Due to the proximity of the surgical site to the airway, patients must remain cooperative, breathe spontaneously, and, because of the risk of fire in oxygen-enriched areas, require minimal supplemental oxygen and airway support. Therefore, the surgical team must be aware that heavy sedation will not be considered a safe option since a major goal for anesthesiologists in these cases is to limit oxygen supplementation. If the surgical team is not confident that they will be able to accomplish the planned surgery given these conditions, then general anesthesia with a protected airway should be employed to reduce the risk of fire and respiratory compromise.

Patient Education and Selection

As with all cases preformed under regional anesthesia as the primary technique, patient education, motivation, and selection are critical. This is especially important in

P.J. Taub et al. (eds.), *Ferraro's Fundamentals of Maxillofacial Surgery*,
DOI 10.1007/978-1-4614-8341-0_5, © Springer Science+Business Media New York 2015

maxillofacial surgery given the proximity of the surgical site to the face and airway. Preoperatively, patients must be educated and have a clear understanding of the surgical procedure and a clear understanding of the anesthetic expectations. Patients presenting for and requesting regional anesthesia for their surgery must understand that minimal sedation will be employed to assure their cooperation, airway maintenance, and oxygenation. With this knowledge, many patients may opt for general anesthesia. Patients should be mature and generally free of anxiety disorders or claustrophobia to cooperate. The ability to communicate with the patient intraoperatively is also critical. There should be no language barrier between providers and patients undergoing head and neck surgery under regional anesthesia. If these conditions do not exist, the option to perform the procedure exclusively under a regional anesthetic must be questioned. It should be kept in mind that in such a situation use of both a general anesthetic supplemented with a regional block is a viable alternative and affords the benefit to reduce intraoperative anesthetic exposure will be providing postoperative analgesia.

Contraindications

Most contraindications to peripheral nerve blockade using local anesthetics are relative. Local infections or tumors at the sight of the injection are absolute contraindications and although extremely rare hypersensitivity to local anesthetics would preclude their use. Bleeding disorders, bloodstream infections, and preexisting neuropathy are relative contraindications. Patient refusal is of course an absolute contraindication.

In adult patients, neuraxial or peripheral regional anesthesia is generally not instituted after the induction of general anesthesia for fear of undetected neuronal injury. However, most procedural regional anesthesia for maxillofacial surgery is essentially a “field block” and can be performed safely even after the induction of general anesthesia.

Premedication

Premedication with small doses of a benzodiazepine and/or opioid helps reduce anxiety and raise the pain and seizure (in the case of benzodiazepines) thresholds. Intravenous midazolam 1–2 mg for most adults is a safe and effective dose. Fentanyl 25–50 mcg IV is similarly effective. In general, only light sedation is desirable so the patient can report paresthesias during the performance of regional nerve blockade. While placing the block supplemental oxygen should generally be administered to all patients via nasal cannula or facemask to reduce the incidence of hypoxemia following even light sedation.

Local Anesthetics

Overview

Local anesthetic agents are a group of heterogeneous drugs that reversibly block transmission of nerve conduction to diminish or abolish sympathetic, sensory, and or motor function. The injection of local anesthetics near nerves is most often used in regional anesthesia either as a stand-alone technique or in conjunction with monitored anesthesia care or general anesthesia. Local anesthetics can also be infiltrated and applied topically to mucous membranes and skin to provide anesthesia. Local anesthetics have wide-ranging application in maxillofacial surgery, from minor office procedures to more invasive open surgeries. Application of local anesthetic appears to decrease postoperative pain in common head and neck procedures. Of course, local anesthesia is also used successfully for regional anesthesia of the head and neck whereby entire surgeries may be performed without general anesthesia and postoperative pain relief may be effectively achieved.

Pharmacology

Local anesthetics are sodium channel blocking drugs that decrease neural transmission of nociceptive signals. Normally, following activation by excitatory signals, activation of voltage-gated sodium channels leads to an action potential that travels down the axon. Impulses are then expedited down the axon by hopping from successive nodes of Ranvier (saltatory conduction). Local anesthetics function by binding to the inner aspect of neuronal sodium channels in order to inhibit this impulse propagation. Local anesthetics preferentially block small, myelinated, and high-frequency firing nerves. In general, blockade of sympathetic nerve fibers occurs first, sequentially followed by pain and temperature, touch, and then motor fibers. Due to the presence of sodium channels, the central nervous and cardiovascular systems are the sites where local anesthetic toxicity will predominate.

Structurally, local anesthetics are composed of an aromatic ring and an amine group, linked centrally by either an ester or amide bond (Table 5.1). This central portion is used to classify the two groups, either esters or amides. Esters are generally metabolized to p-aminobenzoic acid (PABA) by plasma cholinesterase, have a short half-life in the plasma (<1 min), and are more likely to elicit (rare) allergic reactions (due to PABA). Cocaine is a unique ester local that undergoes extensive liver metabolism. Amides are degraded in the liver and have a half-life of 2–3 h. All local anesthetics are weak bases with a pKa of 7–9, existing mainly in the cationic form at physiologic pH.

Table 5.1 Physiochemical and pharmacological properties of commonly used local anesthetic agents for subcutaneous infiltration

Local anesthetic	Pka	Onset	Duration	Maximum dose[a] (mg/kg)
Esters				
Procaine	8.9	Slow	Short	11 (13)
Chlorprocaine	8.5	Fast	Short	10 (12)
Tetracaine	8.4	Slow	Long	1.5 (2)
Amides				
Prilocaine	7.9	Fast	Moderate	5 (7)
Lidocaine	7.9	Fast	Moderate	5 (7)
Mepivacaine	7.6	Fast	Moderate	3 (5)
Bupivacaine	8.1	Moderate	Long	2 (2.5)
Ropivacaine	8.1	Fast	Long	2 (2.5)
Etidocaine	7.7	Slow	Long	4

[a]Dose in parenthesis is the maximum dose in mg/kg with the addition of epinephrine

Local anesthetics must first cross the cell membrane in the uncharged state before binding to the inner pore of the sodium channel (Fig. 5.1). With the exception of chloroprocaine, local anesthetics with a pKa closer to physiologic pH are more likely to exist in the unprotonated, more hydrophobic form and therefore have a faster onset of action. In general the speed of onset of local anesthetics is therefore inversely related to the pKa. Adding sodium bicarbonate to a local anesthetic solution in order to increase the unprotonated fraction may speed the rate of onset.

Potency of local anesthetics is related to their lipid solubility. Protein binding (to α-1 acid glycoprotein), peripheral vascular effects, and lipid solubility determine duration of action. Epinephrine (1:200,000) can be added to local anesthetic solutions to prolong the duration of action by causing local vasoconstriction and decreasing systemic absorption. Use of epinephrine is best avoided in very peripheral nerve blocks, patients with heart disease, and uncontrolled hypertension. Refer to for pharmacological properties of individual local anesthetic agents.

Toxicity

Central Nervous System

When two different local anesthetics are used, the maximum safe dose should be assumed to be additive and not independent. The most likely adverse effects of local anesthetics are due to their initial excitatory (seizures) and ultimately depressive (coma) effects on the central nervous system. Patients generally will first complain of lightheadedness or dizziness, followed by tinnitus and/or perioral numbness. They may then become agitated which could progress to tonic-clonic seizures. If left untreated reversible coma (general anesthesia) will follow. It is essential to have immediate access to resuscitation and intubation equipment in addition to anticonvulsant medications (midazolam 0.03–0.06 mg/kg or propofol 0.5–1 mg/kg) when performing nerve blocks. This is especially true in head and neck blocks where delivery of local anesthetics directly to the central nervous system can be incredibly efficient. Hyperventilation may help lessen this toxicity by avoiding acidosis and hypercarbia, which increases cerebral blood flow and decreases local anesthetic binding to serum proteins.

Cardiovascular System

Local anesthetics are class 1 antiarrhythmic agents that have depressant effects on cardiac conduction, hence the use of lidocaine to treat excitatory arrhythmias. Excessive inhibition of these channels, however, can lead to prolonged conduction and decreased inotropy. Local anesthetic overdose also leads to arteriolar dilation and hypotension. The exception to this trend is cocaine, which inhibits reuptake of norepinephrine and dopamine, leading to hypertension, increased inotropy, tachyarrhythmias, and coronary spasm. Therefore, cocaine should be used cautiously in patients with cardiac disease as it can precipitate myocardial ischemia and even cerebrovascular accidents.

Bupivacaine has increased affinity for sodium channels and is more likely to produce severe cardiotoxic effects. Refractory ventricular tachycardia or fibrillation from bupivacaine is particularly resistant to treatment and is often fatal. The use of 20 % intralipid solution has been found to be effective as a rescue agent in malignant dysrhythmias and cardiovascular collapse from bupivacaine that is unresponsive to traditional resuscitation protocols. Ropivacaine is a stereoisomer of bupivacaine that has reduced affinity for cardiac sodium channels and is accordingly less cardiotoxic (although still more cardiotoxic than lidocaine). With all local anesthetics, aspiration prior to injection decreases the risk of intravascular injection. Figure 5.2 below outlines the American Society of Regional Anesthesia and Pain Medicine Guidelines for the treatment of local anesthetic toxicity (LAST).

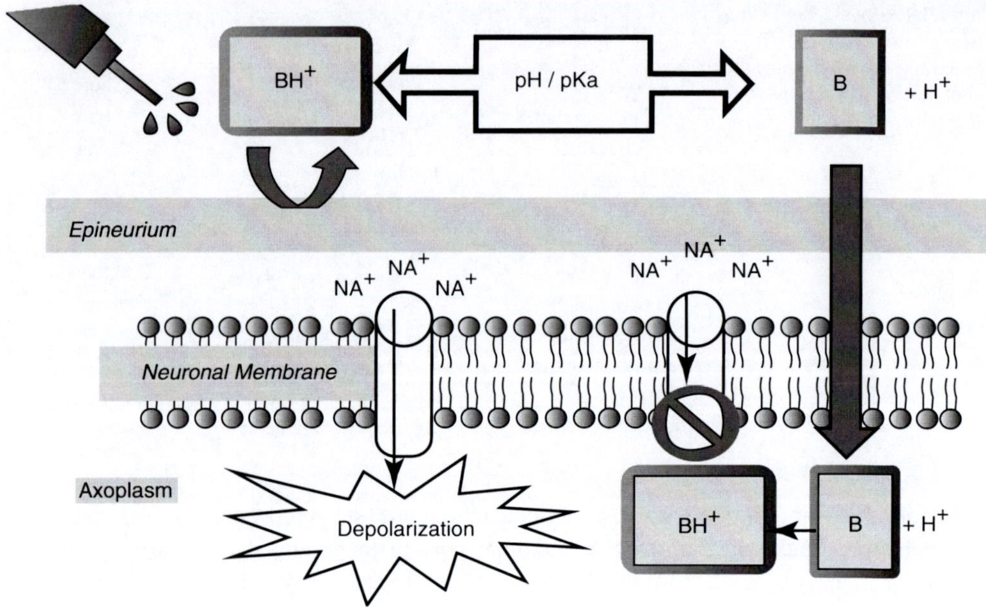

Fig. 5.1 Diagram of mechanism of local anesthetic action. Local anesthetic exists as both a charged (*BH*+) and uncharged (*B*) basic structure. The proportion of each is determined by the pKa of the anesthetic and the pH of the environment. Once the uncharged form reaches the intracellular environment, it is protonated and is able to block the sodium channel

- ☐ Get Help
- ☐ Initial Focus
  - ☐ Airway management: ventilate with 100% oxygen
  - ☐ Selzure suppression: benzodiazepines are preferred; AVOID propofol in patients having signs of cardiovascular instability
  - ☐ Alert the nearest facility having cardiopulmonary bypass capability
- ☐ Management of Cardiac Arrhythmias
  - ☐ Basic and Advanced Cardiac Life Support (ACLS) will require adjustment of medications and perhaps prolonged effort
  - ☐ AVOID vasopressin, calcium channel blockers, beta blockers,or local anesthetic
  - ☐ REDUCE individual epinephrine doses to <1 mcg/kg
- ☐ Lipid Emulsion (20%) Therapy (values in parenthesis are for 70kg patient)
  - ☐ Bolus 1.5 mL/kg (lean body mass) intravenously over I minute (~100mL)
  - ☐ Continuous infusion 0.25 mL/kg/min (~18 mL/min: adjust by roller clamp)
  - ☐ Repeat bolus once or twice for persistent cardiovascular collapse
  - ☐ Double the infusion rate to 0.5 mL/kg min if blood pressure remains low
  - ☐ Continue infusion for at least 10 minutes after attaining circulatory stability
  - ☐ Recommended upper limit: Approximately 10 mL/kg lipid emulsion over the first 30 minutes
- ☐ Post LAST events at www.lipidrescue.org and report use of lipid to www.lipidregistry.org

Fig. 5.2 American Society of Regional Anesthesia and Pain Medicine Guidelines for the treatment of local anesthetic toxicity

Hematologic System

Some local anesthetics can cause the development of methemoglobinemia, a condition characterized by excessive methemoglobin. The iron moiety of methemoglobin is oxidized (ferric [Fe^{3+}] rather than ferrous [Fe^{2+}]). Oxygen delivery is compromised resulting in tissue hypoxia. Patients report feeling short of breath, appear cyanotic, and have a pulse oximeter reading that approaches 85 %. Their blood will classically look "chocolate brown." Intravenous methylene blue (a reducing agent) 1–1.5 mg/kg intravenous is the treatment.

Local Anesthetic Selection

Although regional anesthesia of the head and neck generally does not require the use of large volumes of local anesthesia, toxicity must be considered in light of the agents' individual characteristics such as onset duration and their use in close proximity to major blood vessels. Good surgical anesthesia is obtained only when local anesthetic is injected close to the nerve(s) to be blocked. Common local anesthetic solutions that are used for surgical anesthesia include lidocaine 1.5–2 %, mepivacaine 2 %, bupivacaine 0.5 %, levobupivacaine 0.5 %, or ropivacaine 0.5 %. In general more dilute solutions are recommended for postoperative analgesia due to the decreased motor blockade; since motor blockade may be less of a concern with head and neck surgery, the authors recommend using more concentrated solutions for improved efficacy and duration of action.

Utility as Topical Anesthetics

Besides use by injection in regional nerve blocks and tissue infiltration, local anesthetic agents can also be used topically. Local anesthetic sprays are available for application to the esophagus and larynx for endoscopic procedures. Several agents can be sprayed into the larynx and trachea prior to intubation to reduce the incidence of coughing during emergence from anesthesia (i.e., laryngotracheal anesthesia) and decrease the sympathetic response to tracheal intubation. The cricothyroid membrane may also be punctured with a small needle for the direct application of local anesthetic to the larynx and trachea. Local anesthetics can be delivered via nebulizer for endoscopy or awake intubation.

Eutectic mixture of local anesthetics (EMLA) is a cream composed of 2.5 % lidocaine and 2.5 % prilocaine that may be applied to intact skin as a local anesthetic. Use is limited by onset time (requires at least 30 min) and the risk of methemoglobinemia.

Applications in Maxillofacial Surgery

Anatomy

Understanding the sensory innervation of the head and neck is critical in planning and conducting regional anesthesia for the head and neck (Table 5.2).

The majority of the sensory input of the face, head, and neck is supplied by the trigeminal nerve (CN V) and the cervical plexus (C2, C3, and C4). Whereas the sensory innervation of the nasal cavity is predominately from the V1 and V2 branches of CN V, the sensory innervation of the tongue is complex and comes from both trigeminal (anterior 2/3) and the glossopharyngeal (CN IX) (posterior 1/3). In general, the use of regional anesthesia (and analgesia) for maxillofacial procedures can be divided by anatomical distribution of the trigeminal nerve and the cervical plexus. After originating at the gasserian ganglion, the trigeminal nerve branches into the ophthalmic (V1), maxillary (V2), and mandibular (V3) nerves – each providing targets for regional anesthetics. For maxillofacial procedures, V2 and V3 nerves will be targeted more commonly. The superficial portions of the cervical plexus (C2–C4) provide sensation to the posterior region of the head and neck (Figs. 5.3 and 5.4) (see Chap. 2).

Ophthalmic Branch (V1)

The ophthalmic division of the trigeminal nerve divides into the supraorbital, supratrochlear, and nasociliary nerves. The nasociliary branch innervates the sinuses and mucous membrane of the nasal cavity. Regional anesthesia of the ophthalmic division of the trigeminal nerve can be utilized in ophthalmologic, neurologic, and frontal sinus surgery. Ocular injury is a significant risk during blocks of these nerves. For maxillofacial procedures, these nerves will generally not be targeted as commonly as blocks of V2 and V3.

Table 5.2 Sensory innervation of the head and neck

Trigeminal nerve (CN5-V1 V2 V3)	Face, head, tongue
Glossopharyngeal nerve (CN9)	Tongue
Cervical plexus (C2 C3 C4)	Head, mandible, neck

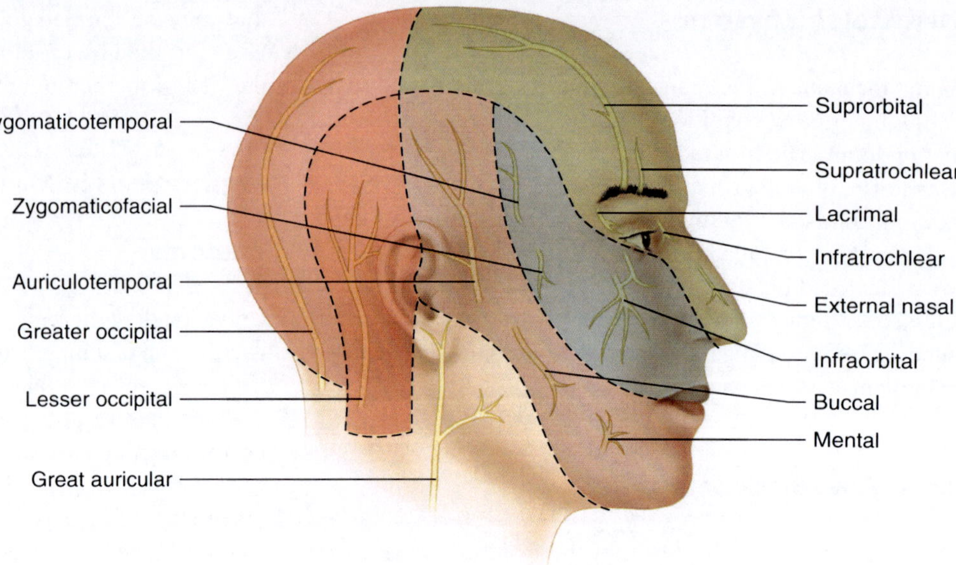

Fig. 5.3 Terminal branches of the trigeminal nerve

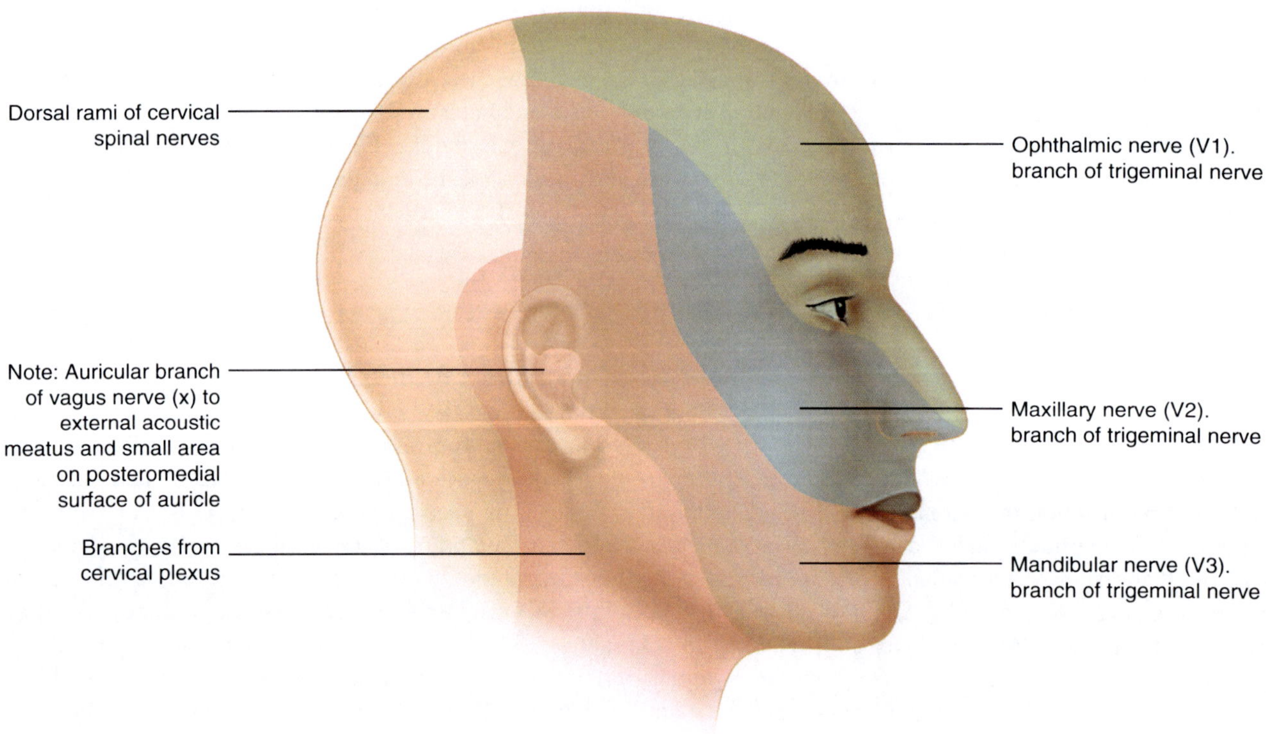

Fig. 5.4 Supraorbital and supratrochlear nerve block distribution

The Frontal Nerve Block

The so-called frontal nerve block can be used to block both the supraorbital and supratrochlear nerves as well as the infratrochlear nerve, which exits a foramen below the trochlea and provides sensation to the medial upper eyelid, canthus, medial nasal skin, conjunctiva, and lacrimal apparatus (Figs. 5.5 and 5.6). When injecting this area, use the free hand to palpate the orbit and prevent inadvertent injection into the globe. One can block all three nerves by injecting 2–4 ml of local anesthetic solution from the central brow proceeding to the medial brow.

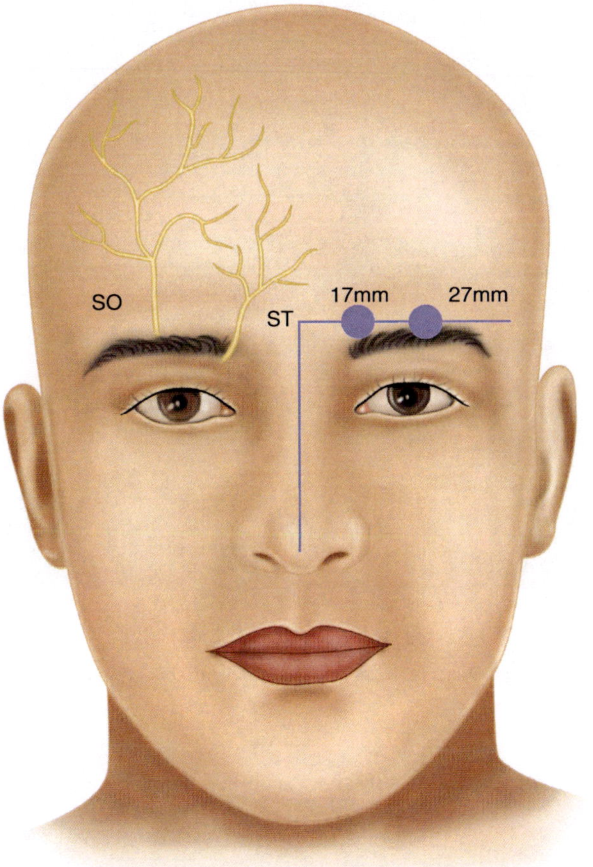

Fig. 5.5 Frontal nerve block. The frontal nerve exits at the superior orbital rim approximately 27 mm lateral to the glabellar midline. This supraorbital notch is readily palpable in most patients. The supratrochlear nerve exits approximately 17 mm from the glabellar midline and supplies sensation to the middle portion of the forehead. *SO* supraorbital nerve, *ST* supratrochlear nerve

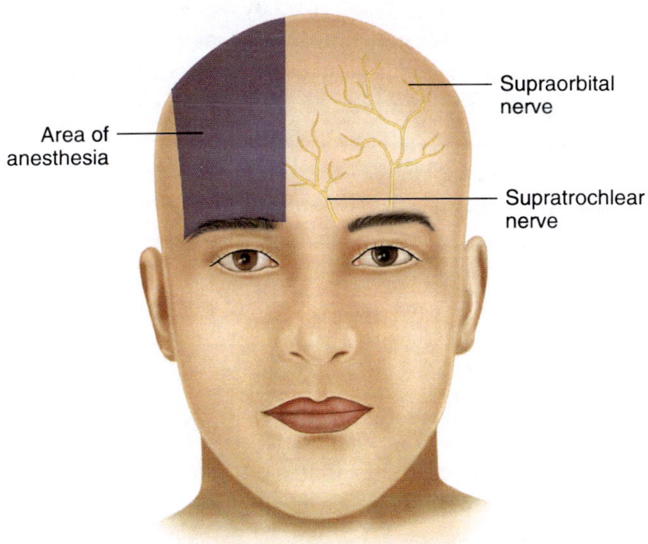

Fig. 5.6 Sensory innervation of the forehead

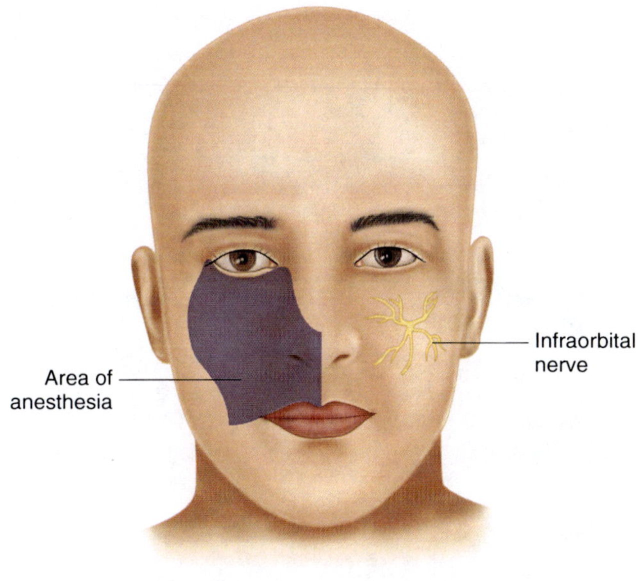

Fig. 5.7 Infraorbital nerve block distribution

Maxillary Branch (V2)

The maxillary division (V2) becomes the infraorbital nerve (IFON) and pterygopalatine branches from V2 travel to the pterygopalatine ganglion or sphenopalatine ganglion (SPG) and the postganglionic fibers form the greater and lesser palatine nerves. The IFON provides innervation to the palate, teeth (5–8 from the right and 9–12 from the left), gums, nasal mucosa, lower eyelid, and upper lip. In combination with the nasociliary branch of the ophthalmic division, the infraorbital nerve also provides sensation to the sinuses and nasal mucosa. The SPG supplies the lacrimal gland, paranasal sinuses, the mucosa of the nasal cavity and pharynx, the gingiva, and the mucous membrane of the hard palate.

The Infraorbital Nerve Block

The infraorbital nerve is a relatively simple nerve to locate and block using regional anesthesia techniques. The infraorbital nerve provides sensation to the cheek, upper lip, eyelid, and lateral aspect of the nose (Fig. 5.7) and has been used successfully for a variety of these structures procedures. Bilateral or unilateral blocks may be used for surgery of the upper lip, nasal fracture reductions, and dental work on maxillary teeth. The infraorbital nerve exits the infraorbital foramen approximately 1 cm below the inferior orbital ridge, palpable with a finger, along a vertical line from the medial limbus of the eye. Three approaches are possible in order to block the infraorbital nerves: a transcutaneous (direct), intra- or transoral, or an intra- or trans-nasal approach.

To locate the nerve, the infraorbital foramen is first palpated approximately 2–3 cm from the midline of the face and

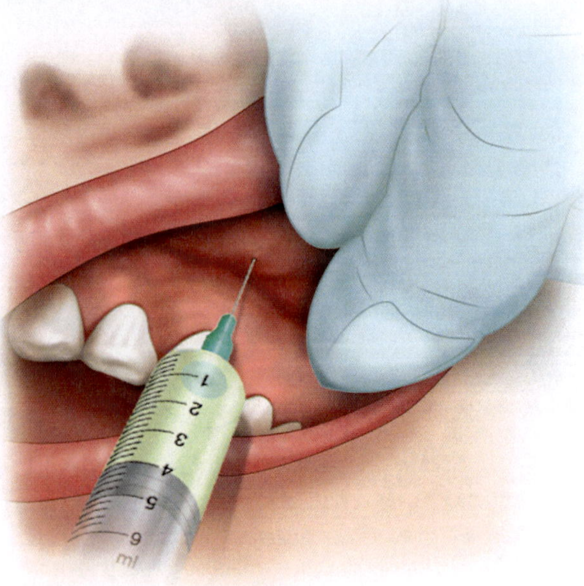

Fig. 5.8 Transoral approach to the infraorbital nerve block

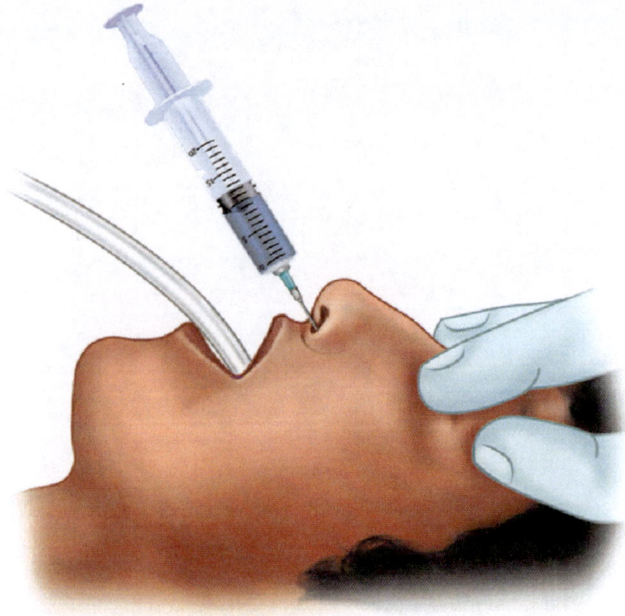

Fig. 5.9 Trans-nasal approach to the infraorbital nerve block

inferior to the orbit. The infraorbital notch can be palpated with a fingertip rolled over the inferior orbital rim. In the direct approach, the needle is placed 0.5–1 cm inferior to the foramen and directed toward the nerve in order to prevent direct passage of the needle through the foramen and into the orbit and globe of the eye. Indeed, ocular injury has been reported and is a potential and severe complication of these blocks.

One to three milliliters of local anesthetic is injected after a negative aspiration for blood or vitreous humor. In the transoral approach, the needle is inserted into the superior buccal groove (between the gums and lip) and directed superolaterally until the tip of the needle is positioned midway between the nasal labial fold and the infraorbital foramen (Fig. 5.8) (We recommend leaving the finger over the foramen for the reasons mentioned previously.)

The trans-nasal approach may be used to block the infraorbital nerve. For the trans-nasal technique, the index finger of the nondominant hand is placed over the infraorbital foramen. During the trans-nasal approach, a 1.5-in. 25-gauge needle is inserted through the nares and tunneled under the skin toward the foramen (Fig. 5.9). After negative aspiration, injection occurs when the tip of the needle is located midway between the nasal labial fold and the infraorbital foramen delineated by the procedures finger. The fingertip is maintained over the foramen throughout the procedure to identify the nerve origin and to prevent the needle from entering the foramen and potentially causing ocular injury. A total of 2 ml of 0.5 % bupivacaine or 0.75 % ropivacaine is injected. This technique should not be performed in patients with pathology such as neoplasms or AV malformations involving the nasal cavity such as the septum and nasal vestibule. In such cases we perform the procedure using the transoral approach.

The Sphenopalatine Ganglion (Greater Palatine Nerve) Block

Located within the pterygopalatine fossa under a thin layer of connective tissue and mucous membrane, the SPG is traditionally accessed either trans-nasally or transorally. The sphenopalatine ganglion (SPG) originates from the maxillary branch of the trigeminal nerve (V2) and provides sensory innervation to the lateral wall of the nasal cavity and inferoposterior portions of the nasal septum. The greater palatine nerve gives off branches to innervate the inferior nasal cavity mucosa and then exits through the greater palatine foramen to provide sensation to the hard palate. The lesser palatine nerve also provides branches to the nasal cavity mucosa and then travels through the lesser palatine foramen to innervate the soft palate and tonsils.

The sphenopalatine ganglion or pterygopalatine ganglion supplies the lacrimal gland, paranasal sinuses, the mucosa of the nasal cavity and pharynx, the gingiva, and the mucous membranes of the hard palate. The ganglion may be blocked via the greater palatine foramen approach. SPG blockade is currently indicated in the treatment of a variety of painful conditions including cluster headaches, acute migraines, atypical facial pain, and trigeminal neuralgia as well as an analgesic adjunct for major sinonasal and palatal surgeries.

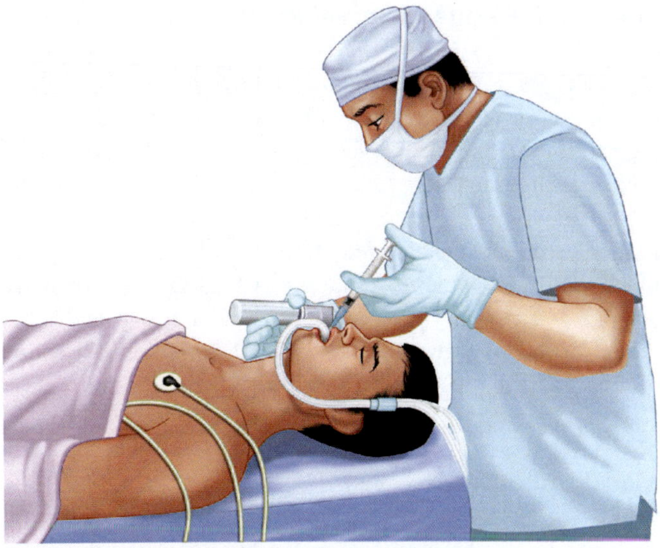

Fig. 5.10 Mac 3-assisted SPG blockade. The SPG block is performed with the practitioner at the head of the bed using gentle anterior pressure to displace the tongue and visualize the hard palate

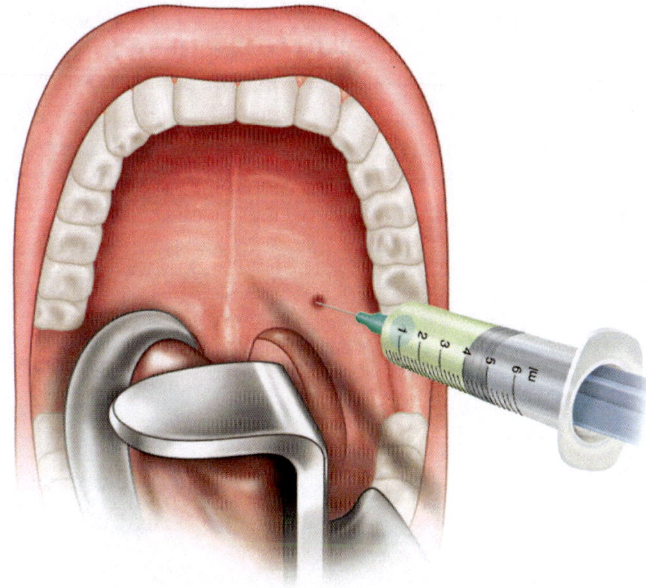

Fig. 5.11 Sphenopalatine ganglion blockade with blanching of hard palate from epinephrine-containing local solution. Correct placement of the SPG block is confirmed by resistance to local anesthetic injection and by blanching of the hard palate due to maxillary artery vasoconstriction with epinephrine

The trans-nasal approach to the SPG involves use of a cotton-tipped applicator soaked in local anesthetic that is then topically applied through the nasal cavity into the posterior pharynx. This approach is difficult, however, when dealing with inflamed and enlarged nasal mucosa, as is the case with many patients undergoing ESS. The transoral approach requires identification of the greater palatine foramen with subsequent injection of a local anesthetic into the pterygopalatine canal and is considered to be more technically challenging due to difficulty in identification of the appropriate anatomy within the hard palate. The approach involves use of finger palpation to identify the greater palatine foramen, which is located posteromedial to the second or third maxillary molar and anteromedial to the maxillary tuberosity and pterygoid hamulus. Identification simply by finger palpation, however, is not always consistent and varies greatly depending on individual anatomy. A transoral approach using direct visualization with the help of a Macintosh 3 blade or a headlamp with "loops" may also be used as a technique for SPG blockade.

When used in conjunction with a general anesthetic, the block is performed after anesthetic induction and placement of the endotracheal tube (ETT) but prior to surgical incision. With the patient supine, and with neck extension, a Macintosh 3 blade is used in similar fashion as in direct laryngoscopy but without advancing to the vallecula in order to displace the tongue anteriorly (Figs. 5.10 and 5.11). This provides direct exposure to a well-lit hard palate without disrupting the ETT.

The greater palatine foramen is then visualized by identifying a shallow groove located approximately 0.5–1 cm medial to the space between the second and third maxillary molars. A 25-gauge, 1.5-in. needle bent at a 90° angle 1.5 cm from the tip is used to limit the depth of entrance into the pterygopalatine canal and avoid the theoretical risk of intraorbital penetration. The needle tip, once in the foramen, should feel as though it has "fallen into a space." The needle should then be advanced no further than the length of the bent portion. If the foramen is not easily visualized and accessed in this manner, the tip of the needle is used to probe through the mucosa in the expected anatomic location until the needle slips easily into the canal, located approximately where the hard palate adjoins the mucosa. We use 1–1.5 ml of 1 % lidocaine with epinephrine 1:100,000 bilaterally for a total of 2–3 ml injected with aspiration throughout needle insertion to avoid intravascular injection. Resistance met during injection of the local anesthetic verifies correct placement of the block within the shallow pterygopalatine canal rather than the nasopharynx. Appropriate placement is further confirmed by blanching of the hard palate on the side that is blocked. The vasoconstriction is due to the spread of the local anesthetic into the pterygopalatine fossa, where the vasoconstricting agent in the anesthetic (i.e., epinephrine) acts on the internal maxillary artery and its terminal branches. This region is highly vascular and significant systemic absorption is minimized by use of epinephrine. In addition, the added vasoconstriction will be helpful in creating a "bloodless" surgical field. Used in combination with general anesthesia, this nerve block helps to provide both local anesthesia and vasoconstriction for the endoscopic sinus surgeon.

It should be noted that this technique has been associated with complications such as intravascular injection, infraorbital nerve injury, and transient diplopia. It should be avoided in cases where pathology may involve the pterygopalatine fossa since inadvertent trauma to the tumor may occur. An alternative option is to infiltrate the region overlying the foramen and not inject into the foramen itself.

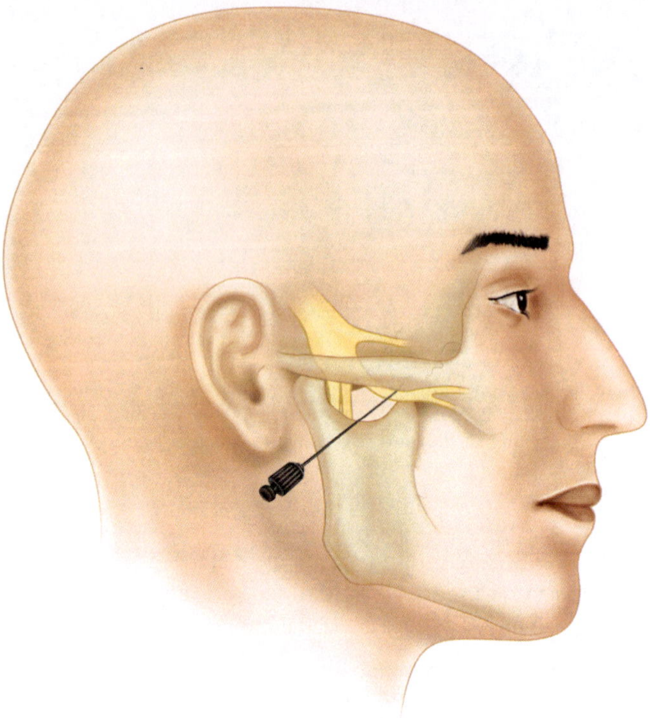

Fig. 5.12 Maxillary nerve block

The Total Maxillary Nerve Block

It is sometimes necessary to block all the divisions of maxillary nerve for extensive surgical procedures. In these cases, the extraoral maxillary nerve block can be used. Under strict aseptic technique, the zygomatic process is located and the depression in its inferior surface is marked. A 1.25-in., 25-gauge needle is inserted perpendicular to the sagittal plane until it touches the lateral pterygoid plate (usually around 3–4 cm deep). The needle is withdrawn and redirected cephalad and anteriorly. After aspiration, 2–3 ml of the local anesthetic solution is injected slowly (Fig. 5.12).

Mandibular Branch (V3)

The mandibular branch (V3) is the largest of the three trigeminal branches and supplies both motor and sensation to the face. V3 exits the scull from the foramen ovale and enters the infratemporal fossa. There it divides into anterior (predominately motor; mastication) and posterior divisions (predominately sensory) (Fig. 5.13). The posterior division divides into three branches: the auriculotemporal nerve, lingual nerve, and inferior alveolar nerve. The auriculotemporal nerve provides sensation from the preauricular area, the lingual nerve provides sensation from the anterior two-thirds of the tongue, and the inferior alveolar nerve provides sensation of the mandibular teeth, buccal mucosa, gingiva, and mandible. The mental nerve, a terminal branch of the inferior alveolar nerve, emerges from the mental foramen and together with input from the facial nerve provides sensory input from the skin of the chin and the mucous membrane of the lower lip. Blockade of the mandibular nerves prior to bilateral man-

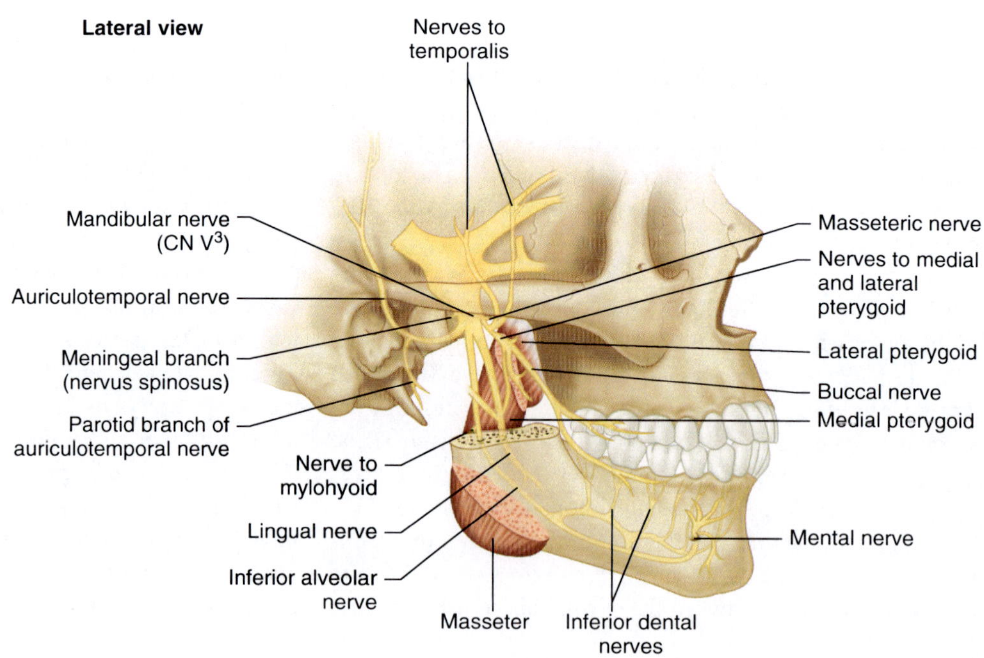

Fig. 5.13 Sensory braches of V3

dibular osteotomy has been shown to effectively decrease total perioperative opioid consumption. A computed tomography (CT)-guided approach to the foramen ovale to block the mandibular nerve in a patient with mandibular deformity caused by segmental mandibulectomy has been successfully performed as an approach to chronic pain therapy.

The Auriculotemporal Nerve Block

The auriculotemporal nerve (ATN) crosses the superior portion of the parotid gland and ascends behind the temporomandibular joint (TMJ), supplying sensation to the skin of the auricle, external auditory meatus, tympanic membrane, temporal region, and temporomandibular joint. Although the sensory innervation of the external ear and surrounding structures is complex and procedures on the ear would require anesthesia of branches from the trigeminal nerve, the vagus, and the cervical plexus, surgery on the TMJ can general be accomplished under ATN block.

To perform the ATN block, the patient is supine with the head turned to the contralateral side. The periauricular area is sterilized. To identify the location of the ATN, the temporal artery is palpated as it crosses the zygomatic arch. Using a 25–27 gauge needle 2–4 ml of 0.5 % bupivacaine is infiltrated in this area (Fig. 5.14).

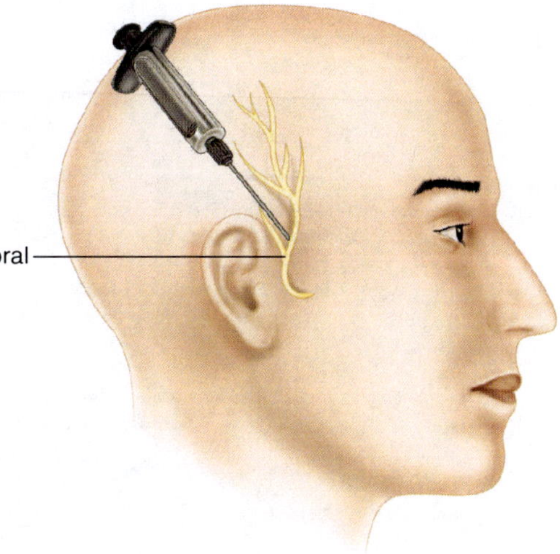

Fig. 5.14 Auriculotemporal nerve blockade

The Inferior Alveolar Nerve Block

The inferior alveolar branch of the mandibular nerve descends in the region between the lateral aspect of the sphenomandibular ligament and the medial aspect of the ramus of the mandible. It travels along with, but lateral and posterior to, the lingual nerve. The nerve travels along with the inferior alveolar artery and vein within the mandibular canal and divides into the mental and incisive nerve branches at the mental foramen. The lingual nerve occupies the pterygomandibular space between the medial aspect of the mandible and the lateral aspect of the pterygoid muscle. It then travels deep to the pterygomandibular raphae and terminates deep to the sublingual gland. The lingual nerve provides sensory innervation to the anterior two-thirds of the tongue, mucosa of the floor of the mouth, and lingual gingiva. Due to the proximity of the lingual and inferior alveolar nerves (IAN), both nerves can and will be blocked simultaneously during an IAN block.

The inferior alveolar nerve block is one of the most common nerve blocks for maxillofacial and dental procedures and is routinely used for surgical procedures involving the mandible, all mandibular teeth, the floor of the mouth, the anterior two-thirds of the tongue, the gingivae on the lingual and labial surface of the mandible, and the mucosa and skin of the lower lip and chin. IAN blocks are the most common blocks for maxillofacial procedures, yet they carry a high failure rate (10–15 %) compared to maxillary blocks due to nerve root inaccessibility. This block may not provide complete anesthesia and may require supplemental nerve blocks (e.g., the buccal nerve) to increase success. The limited success rate of the standard inferior alveolar nerve block (IANB) has led to the development of alternative approaches to mandibular anesthesia. Although a detailed description of these procedures exceeds the scope of this chapter, the Gow-Gates technique requires that the patient be able to open their mouth widely, while the Akinosi-Vazirani closed-mouth technique (as the name implies) can be used with patients with limited mouth opening, TMJ disorders, or trismus. Both techniques are considered reliable alternatives to the traditional IAN block. Nerve stimulation techniques have also been attempted to decrease the failure rate of these blocks without considerable success. If successful, the IAN block simultaneously blocks the mental, incisive, and lingual nerves.

The target for the IAN block is the mandibular nerve as it travels on the medial aspect of the ramus, prior to its entry into the mandibular foramen. A 25-gauge long needle (1.5–2 in.) in length is used for this technique. The patient is positioned supine and with the mouth open maximally, the coronoid notch and the pterygomandibular raphe are identified. Retracting the cheek, the needle is placed at the injection site from the contralateral premolar region (Fig. 5.15a, b). Local anesthesia can be deposited at the injection site. The needle is advanced until the mandible contacted at approximately 25–35 mm of depth. Once the mandible is contacted, withdraw the needle one millimeter and redirect the needle slightly posterior. After confirming a negative aspirate for blood (a positive aspiration is encountered in approximately 10–15 %), 4 ml of 0.5 % bupivacaine is injected. While withdrawing the needle, an additional 1 ml of bupivacaine should be injected to assure that the lingual nerve is blocked.

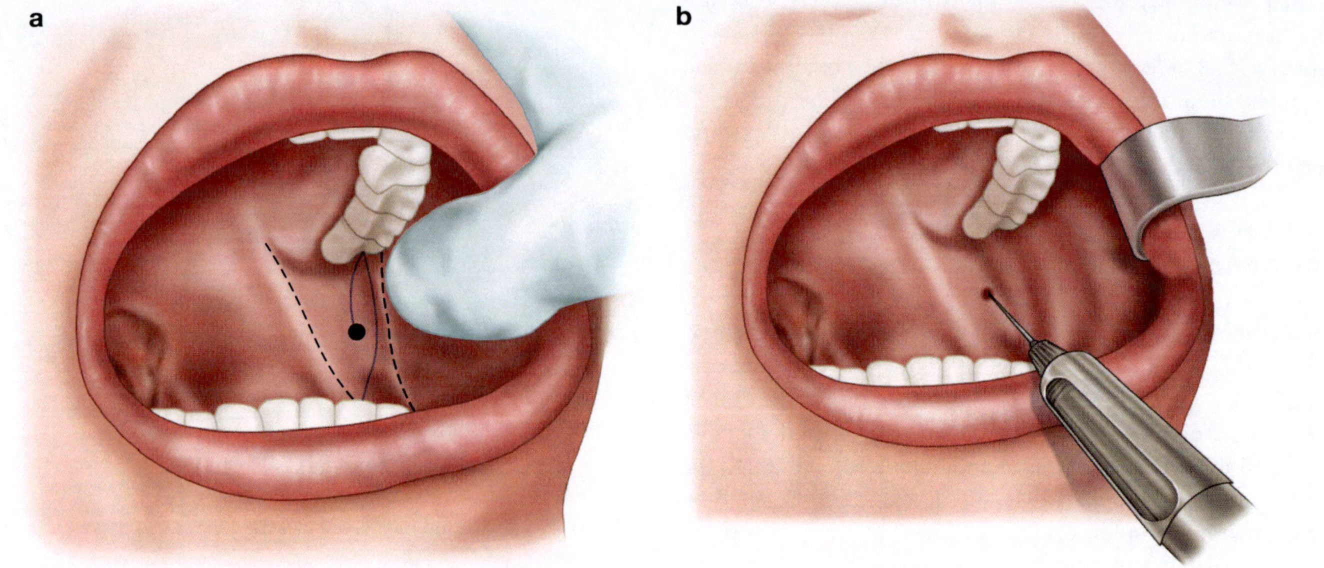

Fig. 5.15 Inferior alveolar nerve blockade. (**a**) The cheek is retracted to reveal the appropriate injection site. (**b**) Injection of local anesthesia using a long 25 g needle and retractor

The Incisive and Mental Nerve Blocks

Both the mental and incisive nerves are terminal branches of the inferior alveolar nerve and will be blocked with a successful IAN block. One can however block these nerves individually. The incisive nerve provides sensory innervation to the mandibular anterior teeth. The mental nerve emerges from the mental foramen and provides sensory innervation to the skin of the chin and lower lip.

The mental nerve can be blocked either from the external skin or intraorally. To perform the block externally, the mental foramen can be palpated midway between the upper and lower borders of the mandible directly below a vertical line from the pupils (Fig. 5.16a, b). Since the canal of the mental foramen angles medially and inferiorly, a 25-gauge needle is inserted 0.5 cm in depth and placed lateral and superior to the foramen. 2 ml of 0.5 % bupivacaine is injected after a negative aspiration. The intraoral approach is accomplished by placing a 25-gauge needle between the two premolar teeth immediately below the tooth root. 2–3 ml of anesthetic is injected after a negative aspiration.

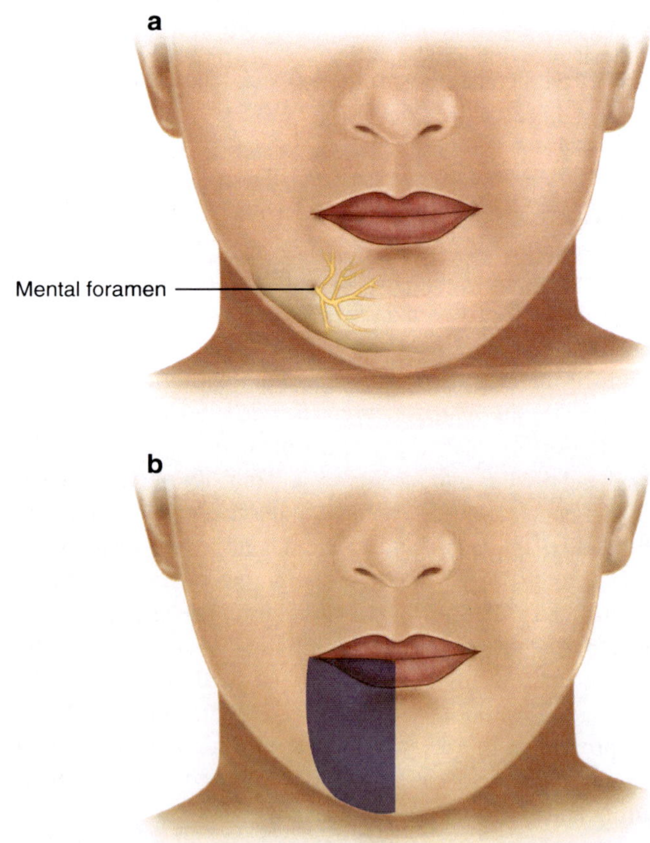

Fig. 5.16 Site for direct mental nerve block (**a**) and accompanying distribution of anesthesia (**b**)

Cervical Plexus

The cervical plexus is comprised of the ventral rami of spinal nerves C1 through C4. Although the plexus is deep to the sternocleidomastoid (SCM), nerves formed from the plexus emerge at the midway point of the sternocleidomastoid and supply sensory input from the back of the head and neck. Anesthetizing the nerves as they emerge from behind the (SCM) is known as a superficial cervical plexus block (SCPB). The plexus can also be blocked as the rami exit the vertebral column. This is known as a deep cervical plexus block (DCPB), which is in essentially a cervical paravertebral block. Regional blockade of the plexus can provide surgical anesthesia for procedures of the anterior (bilateral block will be required) and lateral neck, jawline, posterior auricular region, and the back of the head including otoplasty, cochlear implant, thyroidectomy, parathyroidectomy, tympanomastoid surgery, and carotid endarterectomy. The use of SCPB and DCPB for postoperative analgesia has also been demonstrated in several studies, while others have dismissed its usefulness. Although many clinicians employ the use of both the deep and superficial block in their practice, bilateral DCPB is contraindicated since bilateral phrenic nerve blockade will result. Care should also be used in patients with significant pulmonary disease who might not tolerate even a unilateral phrenic nerve block. In a review of 69 papers that included nearly 10,000 patients undergoing cervical plexus block for CEA, it was determined that the anesthetic quality was no different when superficial block was used alone compared to a combination of deep and superficial. More importantly the group that had the combined technique required a conversion to general anesthesia and had more complications than those patients where only the superficial block was employed. This might be explained by the increased incidents of phrenic nerve block and the increased potential of intravascular and intrathecal injections. Some no longer employ the use of deep cervical plexus block for either intraoperative anesthesia or postoperative analgesia. For completeness we will describe both blocks below.

The Deep Cervical Block (Cervical Paravertebral Block)

Although our group no longer advocates the use of the deep block because the literature suggests the risks outweigh the benefits, the block, if performed, must only be done unilaterally and used with caution with patients with significant pulmonary disease. The patient is positioned supine with their head turned to the contralateral side at approximately 45–60°. After confirming the surgical site, the following landmarks are identified: the mastoid process and Chassaignac's tubercle (CT) of cervical vertebrae C6 (at the level of the cricoid cartilage). Using a marker, a line is drawn from the mastoid to CT. With a ruler, 2, 4, and 6 cm distances from the mastoid are marked along this line; they represent the position of the transverse processes of C2, C3, and C4 respectively. Once the landmarks are identified and demarcated, the skin is prepped and draped sterilely. The DCB can be accomplished using three individual injections of 5 ml of local anesthesia (0.5 % bupivacaine, .75 % ropivacaine, or 2 % lidocaine) or a single injection at C4 with 10–15 ml of local anesthesia. Regardless of technique, the needle position and injection technique are the same. A 21-gauge needle with flexible tubing attached to a syringe is employed. The needle is advanced perpendicular to the skin at the injection points. The transverse process should be contacted at approximately 1.5–2 cm in depth. After contact the needle should be withdrawn 1–2 mm, a negative aspiration confirmed and the local injected. This is repeated at each transverse process. If the transverse process is not contacted, the needle should be withdrawn to the skin, redirected 10–15° caudad, and advanced. If failure to make contact still occurs, the reconfirmation of landmarks must be considered. The needle should never be redirected cephalad as this may increase the risk of an intrathecal or intravascular (vertebral artery) injection.

The Superficial Cervical Plexus Block

Superficial cervical blocks can be accomplished bilaterally, unilaterally, while the patient is awake or under general anesthesia. Because the block is accomplished with the deposit of very superficial local anesthesia, the change of traumatizing a major structure (i.e., pneumothorax intraneural injection) or an inadvertent intrathecal or carotid injecting is rare. The patient positioning, landmarks, and site preparation are the same as for the DCB describe above. For this block, it is critical to identify the posterior boarder of the sternocleidomastoid. This is done with the patient awake regardless if the plan is to place the block after the induction of anesthesia. Having the patient lift their head against the practitioner's opposing hand positioned on the patient's fore head easily identifies the contracted muscle. A marker is used to demarcate this border. The mastoid and the level of Chassaignac's tubercle (CT) are also identified. The midway point between the mastoid and CT is marked along the muscle boarder and is where the nerves of the cervical plexus emerge. Ten to 15 ml of local anesthesia placed superficially along this boarder establishes the block (Fig. 5.17).

Although some describe inserting the needle at the midway point and fanning the needle caudad toward the level of CT and cephalad toward the mastoid process, maintaining a superficial needle is important because brachial plexus injury can occur at this level. We recommend alternatively placing the needle at the level of CT and staying very superficial,

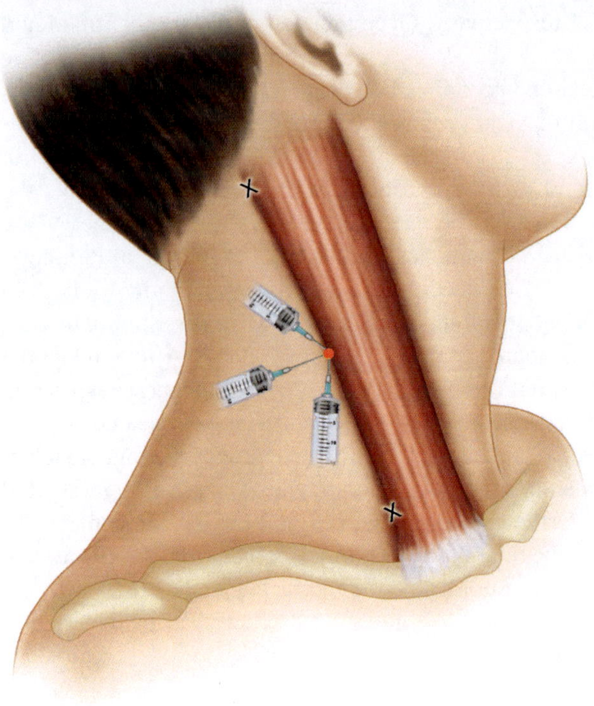

Fig. 5.17 Landmarks and needle fanning for superficial cervical plexus blockade

injecting local anesthesia creating a skin wheal as the needle is advanced toward the mastoid process.

Conclusions

Regional anesthesia for patients undergoing maxillofacial surgery and procedures provides excellent intraoperative surgical conditions as a sole technique or as a component of a balanced anesthetic. Additionally patients benefit from the use of regional anesthetic techniques for acute postoperative pain management. To employ regional techniques for maxillofacial procedures requires a working knowledge of the pharmacodynamics and kinetics of local anesthetics and in depth knowledge of head and neck anatomy.

Bibliography

Akinosi JO. A new approach to the mandibular nerve block. Br J Oral Surg. 1977;15:83–7.

ASRA – Publications – Consensus Statements – Practice Advisories – Local Anesthetic Systemic Toxicity. 2010. At http://www.asra.com/publications-local-anesthetic-systemic-toxicity-2010.php.

Becker DE, Reed KL. Local anesthetics: review of pharmacological considerations. Anesth Prog. 2012;59:90–101; quiz 102–3.

Chan BJ, Koushan K, Liszauer A, Martin J. Iatrogenic globe penetration in a case of infraorbital nerve block. Can J Ophthalmol. 2011; 46:290–1.

Cho D-Y, Drover DR, Nekhendzy V, Butwick AJ, Collins J, Hwang PH. The effectiveness of preemptive sphenopalatine ganglion block on postoperative pain and functional outcomes after functional endoscopic sinus surgery. Int Forum Allergy Rhinol. 2011;1:212–8.

de Sousa AA, Filho MAD, Faglione W, Carvalho GTC. Superficial vs combined cervical plexus block for carotid endarterectomy: a prospective, randomized study. Surg Neurol. 2005;63 Suppl 1: S22–5.

DeMaria S, Govindaraj S, Chinosorvatana N, Kang S, Levine AI. Bilateral sphenopalatine ganglion blockade improves postoperative analgesia after endoscopic sinus surgery. Am J Rhinol Allergy. 2012;26:e23–7.

Donlon WC, Truta MP, Eversole LR. A modified auriculotemporal nerve block for regional anesthesia of the temporomandibular joint. J Oral Maxillofac Surg. 1984;42:544–5.

Goerig M, Bacon D, van Zundert A. Carl Koller, cocaine, and local anesthesia: some less known and forgotten facts. Reg Anesth Pain Med. 2012;37:318–24.

Gow-Gates GA. Mandibular anaesthesia. Aust Dent J. 1978;23:117.

Gow-Gates GA. The Gow-Gates mandibular block: regional anatomy and analgesia. Aust Endod J. 1998;24:18–9.

Haas DA. Alternative mandibular nerve block techniques: a review of the Gow-Gates and Akinosi-Vazirani closed-mouth mandibular nerve block techniques. J Am Dent Assoc. 2011;142(Suppl): 8S–12.

Kanakaraj M, Shanmugasundaram N, Chandramohan M, Kannan R, Perumal SM, Nagendran J. Regional anesthesia in faciomaxillary and oral surgery. J Pharm Bioallied Sci. 2012;4:S264–9.

Kodama Y, Seo K, Tanaka R, Arashiyama T, Ajima H, Takagi R. Placement of mandibular nerve block using computed tomography to locate the foramen ovale in a patient with severe dislocation after segmental mandiblectomy. Br J Oral Maxillofac Surg. 2009;47:407–8.

Van Lancker P, Abeloos JV, De Clercq CA, Mommaerts MY. The effect of mandibular nerve block on opioid consumption, nausea and vomiting in bilateral mandibular osteotomies. Acta Anaesthesiol Belg. 2003;54:223–6.

Levin M. Nerve blocks in the treatment of headache. Neurotherapeutics. 2010;7:197–203.

Manavi MV. Lipid infusion as a treatment for local anesthetic toxicity: a literature review. AANA J. 2010;78:69–78.

Masters RD, Castresana EJ, Castresana MR. Superficial and deep cervical plexus block: technical considerations. AANA J. 1995;63:235–43.

McAdam D, Muro K, Suresh S. The use of infraorbital nerve block for postoperative pain control after transsphenoidal hypophysectomy. Reg Anesth Pain Med. 2005;30:572–3.

Pandit JJ, Satya-Krishna R, Gration P. Superficial or deep cervical plexus block for carotid endarterectomy: a systematic review of complications. Br J Anaesth. 2007;99:159–69.

Pipolo C, Bussone G, Leone M, Lozza P, Felisati G. Sphenopalatine endoscopic ganglion block in cluster headache: a reevaluation of the procedure after 5 years. Neurol Sci. 2010;31 Suppl 1:S197–9.

Salam GA. Regional anesthesia for office procedures: part I. Head and neck surgeries. Am Fam Physician. 2004;69:585–90.

Sved AM, Wong JD, Donkor P, Horan J, Rix L, Curtin J, Vickers R. Complications associated with maxillary nerve block anaesthesia via the greater palatine canal. Aust Dent J. 1992;37:340–5.

Maxillofacial Imaging

6

Richard Monahan and Linping Zhao

Introduction

The information gained from an imaging study is called the "diagnostic yield." The higher the diagnostic yield, the more information the clinician receives about his/her patient. However, the information gained must be of clinical relevance to the surgeon. It must provide answers to diagnostic questions that allow the surgeon to better understand the anatomic or pathologic condition under consideration.

For legal, insurance, and documentation purposes, an imaging study always requires a diagnostic report. Along with appropriate patient information, the report must state the type of study completed, the radiographic findings, and a diagnostic impression.

Select anatomic conditions and pathologic entities will be used in this chapter to illustrate the presentation of each imaging modality. The bibliography at the end of the chapter guides the clinician to resources that cover the broad spectrum of diagnostic challenges relevant to the maxillofacial region.

Clinically Relevant Radiation Biology

Traditional projection imaging (lateral cephalometric, skull and panoramic studies done on film or in digital format) as well as computed tomography and cone beam computed tomography utilize ionizing radiation to create an image. Magnetic resonance imaging (MRI) does not. MRI utilizes a combination of radiofrequency waves and magnetism to manipulate hydrogen protons within the body and generate an image. To date, there are no scientifically documented harmful effects from the clinical utilization of MRI.

Ionizing radiation, also called X-rays, is a form of electromagnetic energy that has a wavelength of approximately a millionth of a millimeter. By comparison, television waves, also a form of electromagnetic radiation, have a wavelength of approximately 2 m and radio waves have a wavelength of 100 m. The smaller the wavelength, the more powerful the radiation. The small wavelength of X-rays makes them powerful enough to harm living tissue.

Two distinct reactions caused by X-rays contribute to the damage/risk they inflict on our patients. One reaction, called the direct effect of ionizing radiation, takes place when an X-ray collides directly with a macromolecule and breaks one of the bonds within the molecule. Altered structure and function can result. Additionally, when the molecular damage involves reproductive tissue, the deleterious effects can be passed on to future generations. The second reaction, called the indirect effect of ionizing radiation, occurs when an X-ray collides with a molecule of water and splits the water into two reactive ions: H* and OH*. These ions may result in the formation of H_2O_2 (hydrogen peroxide) which can cause damage to the intracellular environment.

While the body may possess the power to repair some of the damage caused by ionizing radiation, current theory states that complete healing never occurs and the residual effects of ionizing radiation are cumulative. Therefore, limiting the patient's lifetime exposure to X-rays is essential.

Prescribing an Imaging Study, ALARA, and the American College of Radiology

Based on the clinical examination, medical history, and treatment objectives, the surgeon decides what, if any, imaging study is essential for a given patent. This is a professional judgment based on prevailing evidenced-based best practices. Once the decision to image has been made, strict adherence to the concept of ALARA is essential. ALARA (as low as rea-

R. Monahan, DDS, MS (✉)
Pediatric Plastic and Cleft/Craniofacial Surgery, Shriners Hospital for Children, Chicago, IL, USA
e-mail: monahan@shrinenet.org

L. Zhao, PhD
Division of Plastic, Reconstructive and Cosmetic Surgery, Department of Surgery, University of Illinois, Chicago, IL, USA

P.J. Taub et al. (eds.), *Ferraro's Fundamentals of Maxillofacial Surgery*,
DOI 10.1007/978-1-4614-8341-0_6, © Springer Science+Business Media New York 2015

sonably achievable) is often misinterpreted to be a guideline on *when* a patient should be imaged. As stated above, the decision on when a patient should be imaged lies within the professional judgment of the surgeon. What ALARA dictates is that once the decision is made that imaging is necessary, the clinician prescribes an imaging study that will provide the required diagnostic yield and, at the same time, subject the patient to the lowest amount of ionizing radiation as possible. Inherent in the concept of ALARA is that the doctor limits the field of view to the anatomic area under consideration. Another concept embraced by ALARA is that the patient has adequate shielding during the imaging procedure. Having X-ray machines properly calibrated, avoiding repeat examinations when possible, and utilizing imaging equipment with the lowest possible dose to the patient are all encompassed in ALARA.

The American College of Radiology states:

The ACR advises that no imaging exam should be performed unless there is a clear medical benefit that outweighs any associated risk. The ACR supports the as low as reasonably achievable (ALARA) concept which urges providers to use the minimum level of radiation needed in imaging exams to achieve the necessary results.

http://www.acr.org/Search?q=ALARA

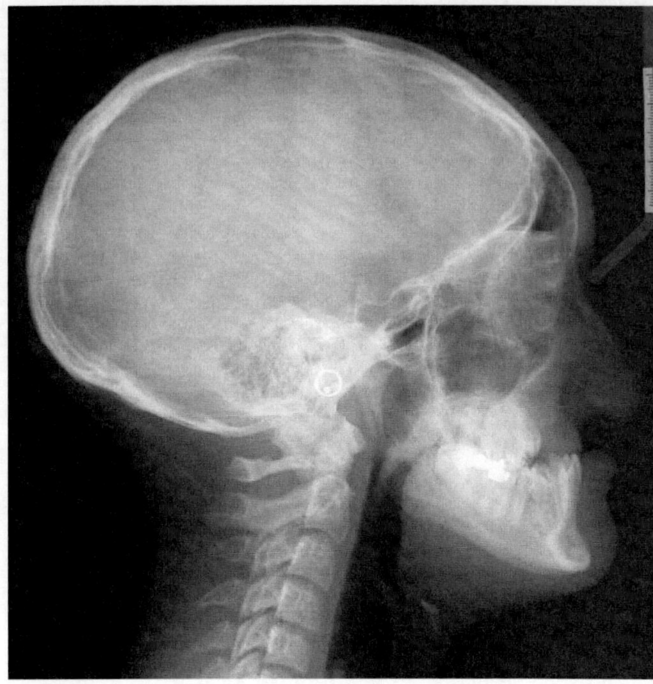

Fig. 6.1 The lateral cephalometric projection illustrates the relative osseous relationship of the mandible to the maxilla and the maxilla to the craniofacial base. The resultant image is compromised due to inherent magnification, distortion, and overlap of adjacent structures

Two-Dimensional Images: Advantages, Limitations, and Alternatives

Projection radiology (*PR*) has been used for a century to provide relatively reliable diagnostic information. In PR the patient is placed between the X-ray source and the imaging receptor. Selective absorption (attenuation) of the X-ray beam as it passes through the patient creates a pattern that reflects the various anatomic structures being imaged. In general, the thicker and denser the anatomic structure being imaged, the more X-rays it will attenuate. Areas of high attenuation (bone) result in a relatively white (radiopaque) impression within the final image. Areas of low attenuation (air, soft tissue) result in a radiolucent presentation.

The lateral cephalometric projection (see Fig. 6.1) illustrates the relative osseous relationship of the mandible to the maxilla and the maxilla to the craniofacial base. The resultant image, like all PR images, is compromised due to inherent magnification, distortion, and overlap of adjacent structures. It does however provide baseline osseous relationships relevant to treatment planning craniofacial surgery and related orthodontic/orthognathic procedures. Image filtering allows portrayal of the soft-tissue profile. With its ease of acquisition, relatively low radiation dose and its long history of clinical utilization, the lateral cephalometric image is one of the most prescribed images for initial patient evaluation and follow-up. The frontal cephalometric image (see Fig. 6.2) can be utilized to display relative osseous symmetry from the coronal perspective.

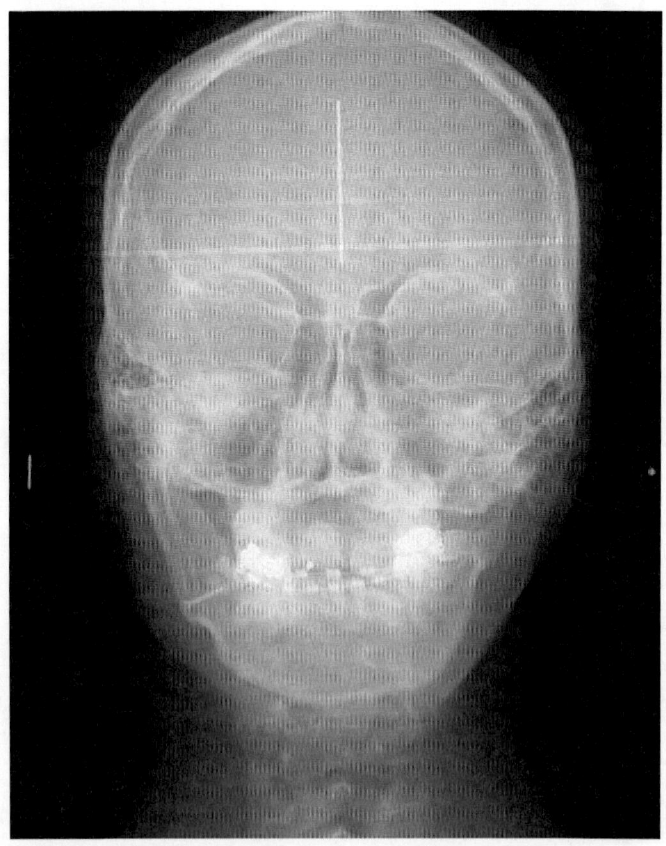

Fig. 6.2 The frontal cephalometric image can be utilized to display relative osseous symmetry from the coronal perspective. The resultant image is compromised due to inherent magnification, distortion, and overlap of adjacent structures

Several previously used skull projections have been replaced by modern cross-sectional imaging. These include

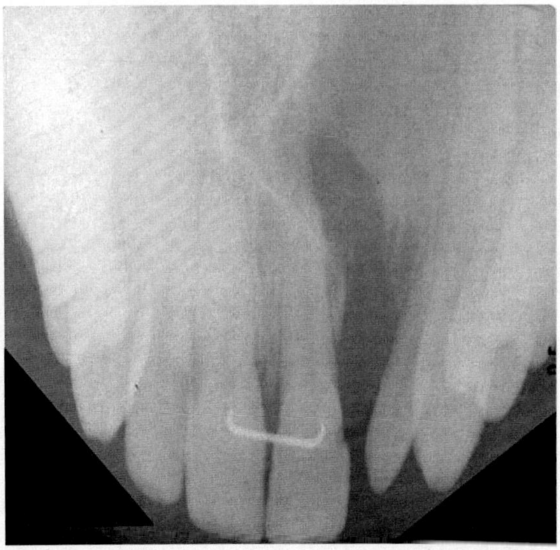

Fig. 6.3 An occlusal projection can offer essential diagnostic information when evaluating the dimensions of a cleft palate and the adjacent maxillary dentition to regional anatomic structures

the Waters projection for portrayal of the maxillary sinus, the Caldwell projection for evaluation of the orbits, the lateral jaw projection for imaging the body of the mandible, the anterior-posterior projection for imaging the occipital bone, and the reverse Towne projection for evaluating the TMJ complex. The diagnostic yield of a tomographic study (computed tomography/cone beam computer tomography) is sufficiently higher then these traditional skull images and the additional radiation dose may be warranted when evaluating the complex anatomy under consideration.

Dental intraoral images provide exceptional resolution and contrast but have a field of view limited to the teeth and adjacent anatomy. One related form of intraoral imaging called an occlusal projection can offer essential diagnostic information when evaluating the mesial-distal dimension of a cleft palate, pathology of the hard palate, or the relationship of adjacent maxillary dentition to regional anatomic structures. This imaging technique should have the central X-ray beam projecting directly through the area of interest and strike a 60° angle with the image receptor. Although the image suffers from the distortion and overlap inherent in all projection geometry images, anatomic relationships are portrayed with minimal radiation dose to the patient. The occlusal image in (see Fig. 6.3) demonstrates a cleft palate.

Panoramic radiology is a maxillofacial imaging system that utilizes a coordinated movement of the radiation source and an image receptor to create a relatively clear zone or layer of anatomy that includes the jaws and surrounding structures. The panoramic image suffers from distortion and structural overlap, but its ease of acquisition, low dose, and relative clarity make it an invaluable addition to the maxillofacial imaging armamentarium. Its anatomic coverage includes portions of the osseous structures of the mandible,

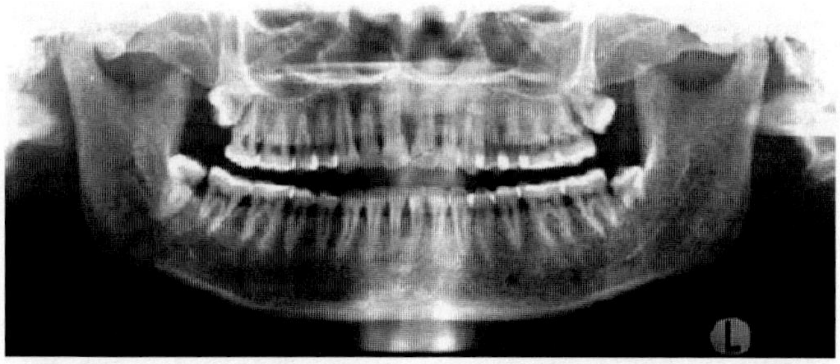

Fig. 6.4 The panoramic image provides an osseous overview of the lower face. While panoramic radiology has diagnostic strengths in the tooth-bearing areas, it can be inherently nondiagnostic in the mid-maxilla and temporomandibular joint

the maxilla inferior to the orbit, the external auditory meatus, and the zygomatic process of the temporal bone. It provides an osseous overview of the lower face (see Fig. 6.4). While panoramic radiology has diagnostic strengths in the tooth-bearing areas, it can be inherently misleading in the mid-maxilla and temporomandibular joint.

Projection radiology, in both analog and digital formats, continues to provide a relatively low radiation dose, technically straightforward, patient-friendly, and financially attractive means of acquiring structural anatomic relationships. When a higher diagnostic yield is necessary, a tomographic (cross-sectional) imaging system can provide undistorted images without the drawback of anatomic superimposition. The radiation dose to the patient (the radiation burden) is increased so a heightened risk-benefit analysis is mandatory before a tomographic study is prescribed. Often termed "advanced imaging," these cross-sectional systems include computed tomography and the more recently developed cone beam computed tomography. The clinical applications, advantages, and disadvantages of each of these modalities will now be considered.

Computed Tomography

Invented in 1972 by Georges Hounsfield at EMI Institute in London, CT (also called CAT scan for computed axial tomography) has become the gold standard for maxillofacial imaging. Like projection images, CT uses ionizing radiation that is selectively absorbed as it traverses the body. The pattern formed by the X-ray beam after it exits the patient is captured by a detector. How CT differs from projection radiology is that as the X-ray source turns or revolves around the patient, the detectors capture snapshots or profiles of the attenuated X-ray beam. The profiles are fed to a computer that uses algorithms to generate slices of the internal anatomy captured in the area of interest (also called the field of view). Early clinical CT machines would generate a thin, fan-shaped X-ray beam that would revolve around a movable patient bed (the gantry). The gantry would incrementally move the patient as the X-ray beam would slice or knife its way through the anatomic area of interest. A set of

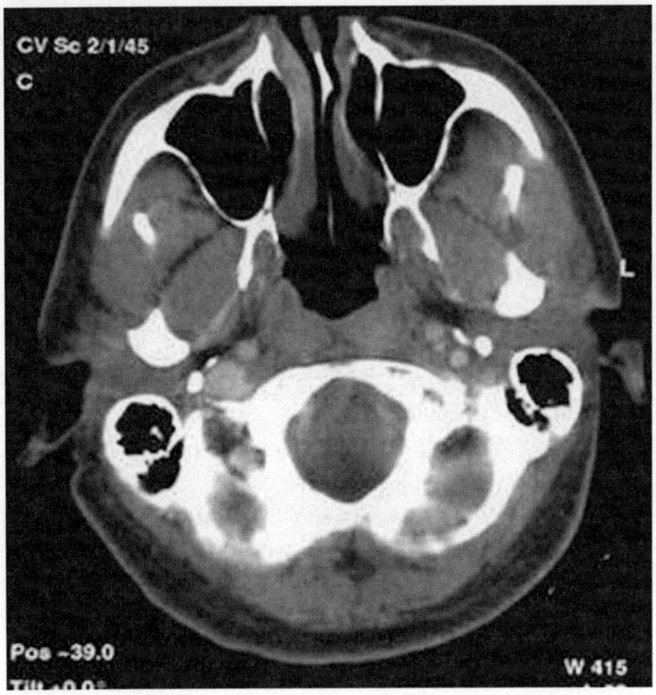

Fig. 6.5 CT image set to optimize soft tissue. The pterygoid muscle is easily identified

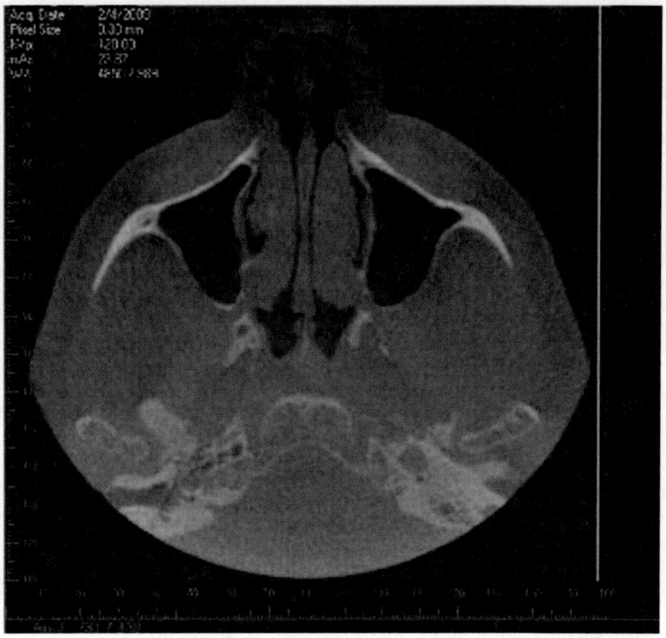

Fig. 6.6 CT image set to a "hard tissue" window. A clear outline of the osseous boundaries of the maxillary sinus is visible, but the image lacks any soft-tissue detail

ring-like detectors synchronized with the X-ray beam captured the attenuated radiation pattern as it leaves the patient and feed the data to a computer for image reconstruction and display.

Contemporary CT scanners utilize multiple arrays of X-ray detectors and sophisticated helical-shaped radiation emission patterns that allows for faster scans, more robust data collection, and undistorted image display in all anatomic orientations (called MPR for multiplanar image reconstruction).

All clinical CT data sets allow for several standard viewing options termed "windows." A soft-tissue window will present the clinician with a view of the patient's anatomy that accentuates or focuses on those attenuation densities that provide optimal viewing of soft tissues (versus bone). (see Fig. 6.5) is an example of a CT image set to optimize soft tissue. The pterygoid muscle is easily identified. Osseous structures are viewable when the computer displays anatomy in the soft-tissue window setting but with suboptimal resolution and contrast. The reverse is true when a clinician selects the "bone window" alternative. (see Fig. 6.6) shows a clear image of the osseous boundaries of the maxillary sinus but lacks any soft-tissue detail. Other window display combinations can be tailored to specific diagnostic evaluations (e.g., knee, brain).

CT data manipulation can generate three-dimensional images, volumetric display, transparency of select anatomic structures, surgical models, and surgical stents and provide simulated outcome predications based on individualized treatment plans. (see Figs. 6.7, 6.8, 6.9, 6.10, 6.11, 6.12, and 6.13) illustrate the vast amount of diagnostic information available utilizing state-of-the-art digital image processing software.

The tremendous diagnostic yield of a CAT scan comes with a risk in terms of radiation dose to the patient. Although advances in technology strive to reduce the X-ray exposure needed to obtain a scan, CT uses far more X-rays than traditional projection radiology.

While the American College of Radiology acknowledges that ionizing radiation poses risks to the patient, it makes the following policy statement in regards to CT:

> There is significant debate and uncertainty regarding the cancer risks associated with the X-rays used for diagnostic imaging. However, some studies of large populations exposed to radiation have demonstrated slight increases in cancer risks even at low levels of radiation exposure, particularly in children.
> The conclusions of (these studies) rely largely on data which equates radiation exposure and effects experienced by atomic bomb survivors to present day patients who receive CT scans. Atomic bomb survivors experienced instantaneous exposure to the whole body… and were exposed to X-rays, particulate radiation, neutrons, and other radioactive material. The known biological effects are very different in these two scenarios.
> http://www.acr.org/About-Us/Media-Center/Position-Startements

Cone Beam Computed Tomography

Relatively new to maxillofacial radiology, cone beam computed tomography possesses a set of strengths that makes it a welcome addition to the spectrum of diagnostic imaging options. Utilizing a relatively low dose of ionizing radiation, CBCT allows for image capture that displays excellent

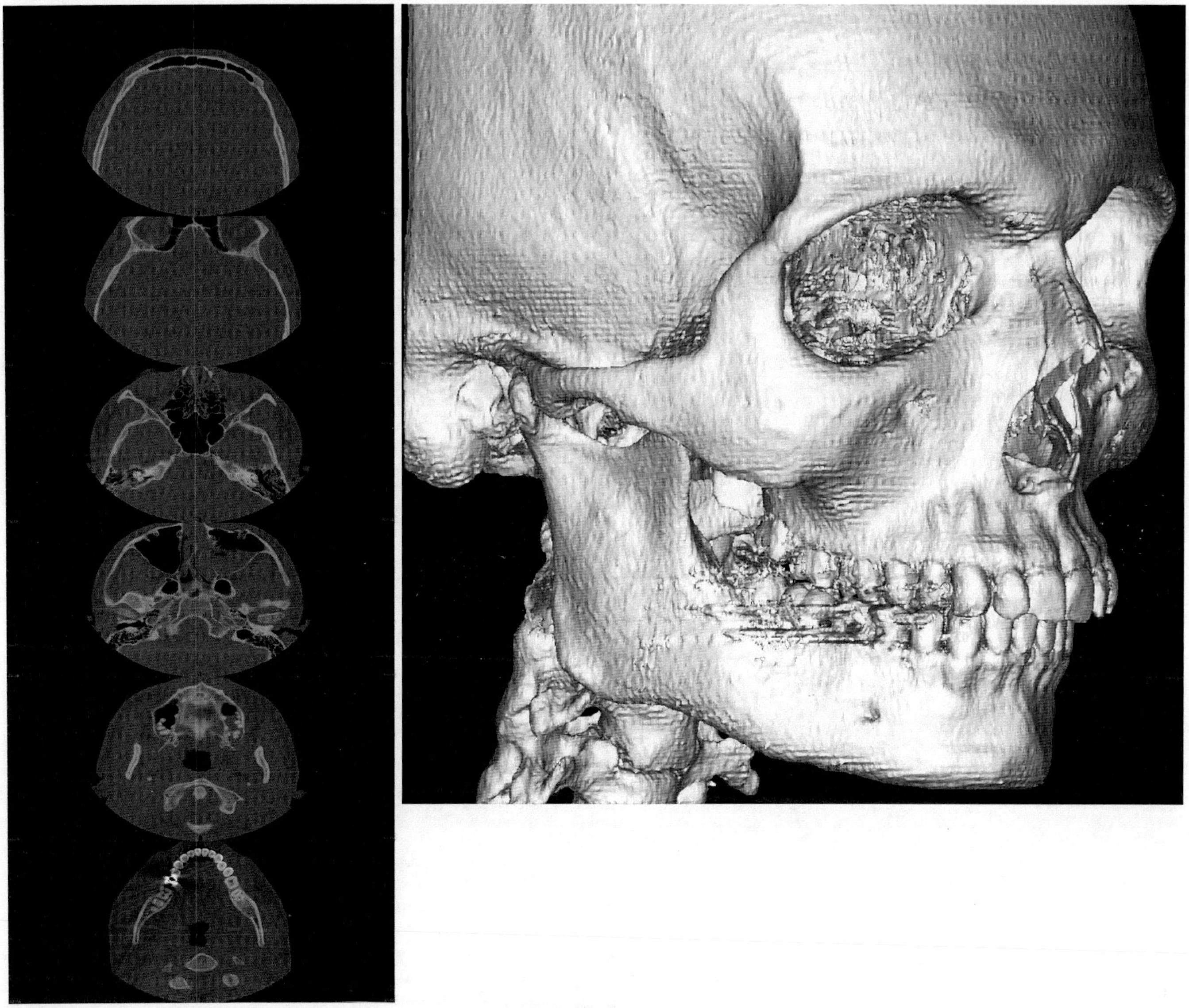

Fig. 6.7 A stack of 2D image slices from CT scan (*left*) is utilized to build a 3D volumetric object (*right*)

spatial resolution (image detail) of hard tissue in a patient-friendly imaging system that is both technically easy to operate and carries a relatively light economic burden.

Traditional CAT scanners can be thought of as using multiple slices or ribbons of X-rays that cut through the patient creating an attenuation pattern that is collected by arrays of detectors. In contrast, a CBCT scan uses a cone-shaped X-ray beam that turns around the patient one time and covers the entire anatomic area of interest. Profiles or snapshots of the attenuated radiation beam are captured on a single flat-panel detector which feeds into a local computer for instantaneous display and manipulation. Like a traditional CT scan, CBCT data sets can be integrated with diagnostic software programs.

A standard cephalometric projection (see Fig. 6.14) can be generated from the CBCT data set. As depicted in (see Fig. 6.15), anatomic areas of interest such as the osseous component of the temporomandibular joint can be evaluated in successive cross sections. (see Figs. 6.16, 6.17, and 6.18) illustrate multiple views of a tumor that occupies the left body and ascending ramus of the mandible. Volumetric analysis of the airway can be obtained using task-specific software applications (see Fig. 6.19).

While these qualities are comparable with traditional CT units, an important advantage of CBCT is the relatively low radiation dose needed to capture the data set. Although imaging parameters affect the actual radiation dose of each tomographic imaging system, a radiation reduction approaching 90 % can be achieved with CBCT.

When compared with a CAT scan, a CBCT study can demonstrate excellent anatomic detail. Unfortunately, all CTBT studies exhibit relatively poor contrast resolution. Therefore, while the viewing parameters can be adjusted in a CBCT study to display the optimal inherent diagnostic yield,

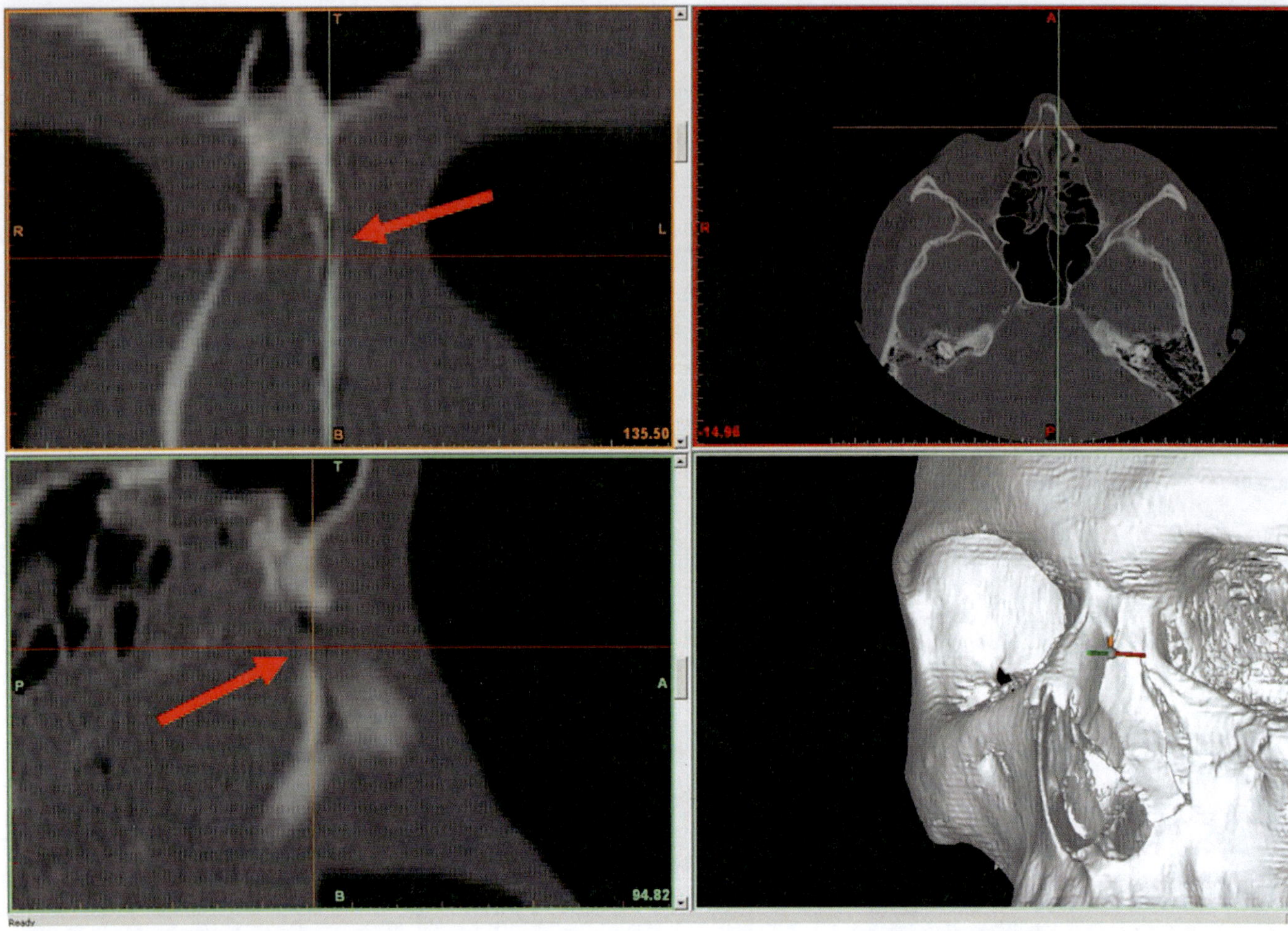

Fig. 6.8 Identification of skeletal fracture is facilitated by both 2D images and 3D objects: (*top left*) coronal view, (*top right*) axial view, (*bottom left*) sagittal view, and (*bottom right*) 3D view. *Red arrows* in coronal and sagittal views are corresponding to the 3D locator in 3D view

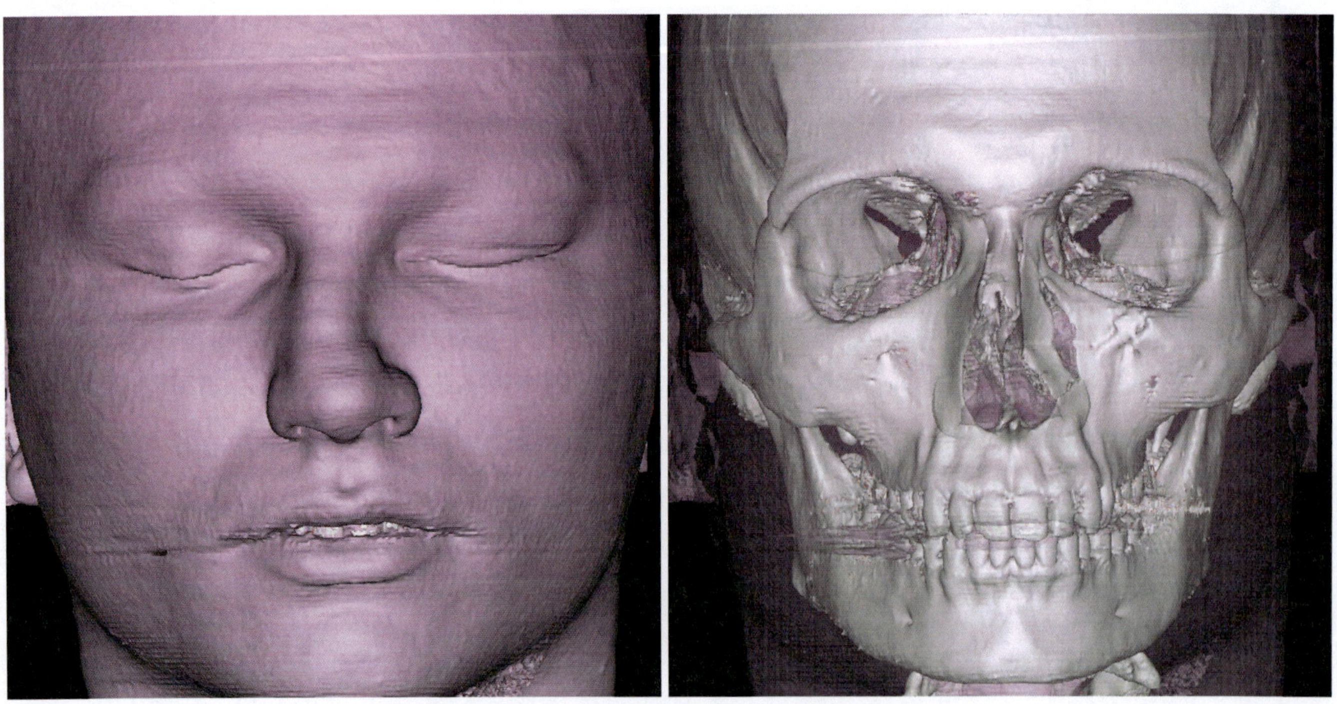

Fig. 6.9 Transparency of soft tissue reveals the nasal deformity in soft tissue (*left*) and associated with skeletal facture (*right*)

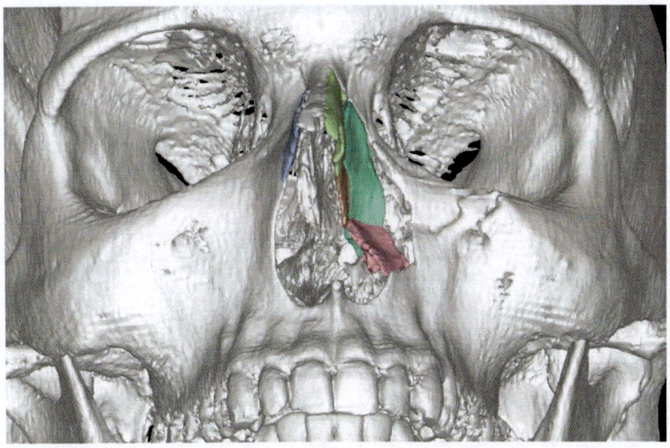

Fig. 6.10 Segmentation of fractured skeletal components is highlighted via various colors

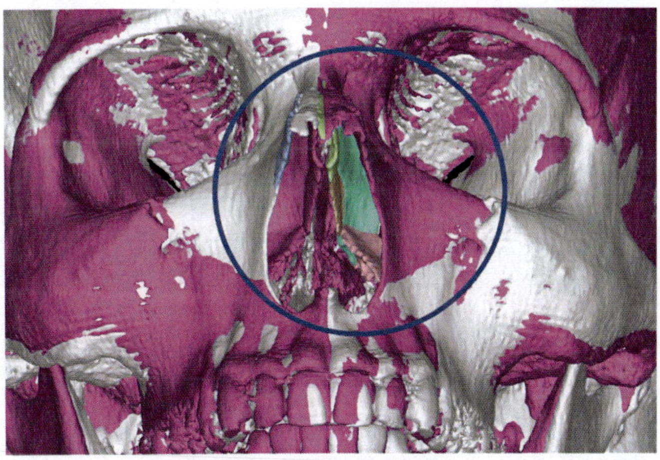

Fig. 6.11 Mirrored skeletal structure (*pink*) is superimposed on the skull (*white*) and reveals the skeletal deformity including the deviation of the septum (within the *blue circle*). It provides reference for both diagnosis and treatment planning

there is no true window that allows the clinician to distinguish soft-tissue anatomic structures of similar tissue density. When the radiographic work-up calls for differentiation of internal soft-tissue structures, CT should be considered superior to CBCT. In addition, the use of injectable contrast media to highlight vascular tissue, enhance lymph node visibility, or outline anatomic boundaries is not clinically feasible with CBCT at this time. It is estimated that 40 % of the CT examinations performed in the USA are done with contrast injections. CBCT would be inappropriate for this subset of imaging studies.

The USFDA endorses the principle of ALARA and makes the following statement regarding the use of CBCT:

> CBCT provide a fast, non-invasive way of answering a number of clinical questions. CBCT images provide 3D information, rather than the 2D information provided by a conventional X-ray image. This may help with the diagnosis, treatment planning and evaluation of certain conditions.

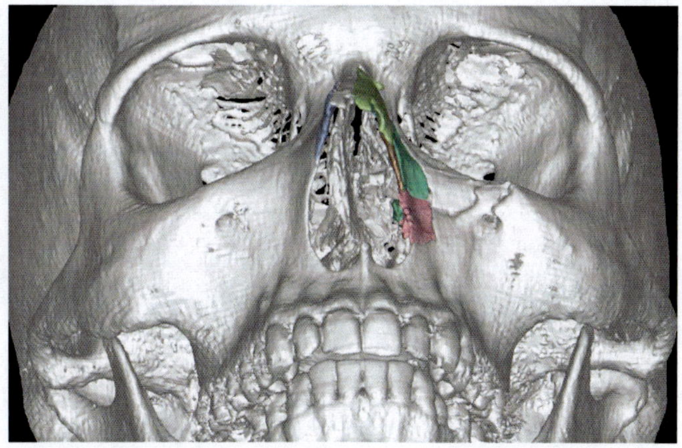

Fig. 6.12 One of many predictions of the skeletal reconstruction outcome

http://www.fda.gov/RadiationEmittingProducts/RadiationEmittingProductsandProcedures/MedicalImaging/MedicalX-Rays/ucm315011.htm

Magnetic Resonance Imaging

MRI imaging is unique in that it does not use ionizing radiation. Instead of X-rays, MRI utilizes a combination of magnetic energy and radiofrequency waves to generate an image. During the examination, the patient is placed in a large magnet and electromagnetic energy temporarily changes the alignment and orientation of the hydrogen protons within the body. The area being examined is then subjected to radiofrequency waves. The energy of the radiofrequency waves is transferred to the hydrogen protons which causes a momentary shift in their orientation and alignment. When the RF waves cease, the absorbed energy is released and detected by an antenna. This signal is then processed into a measurable density that is reflective of the imaged anatomy.

The abundance of hydrogen in the water and fat of soft tissue provides an excellent source of protons which can be used to generate a detailed MRI image. Differences between adjacent soft tissue, such as fat and muscle, can be easily distinguished. MRI can also distinguish blood vessels and nerves from surrounding soft tissue. This type of anatomic differentiation is far superior to other imaging modalities and constitutes the principal benefit of an MRI study. (see Fig. 6.20) illustrates an MRI image of the temporomandibular joint complex. Note arrow "b" identifies the TMJ disk. Diagnostic imaging systems that utilize ionizing radiation rather than magnetic energy are unable to produce this level of soft-tissue visualization.

Hard tissue, such as bone, contains less water and consequently less available hydrogen protons than soft tissue. Since protons are used to generate an MRI image, bony structures are not well defined in MRI. CT/CBCT remains the state of the art when evaluating osseous contours, defin-

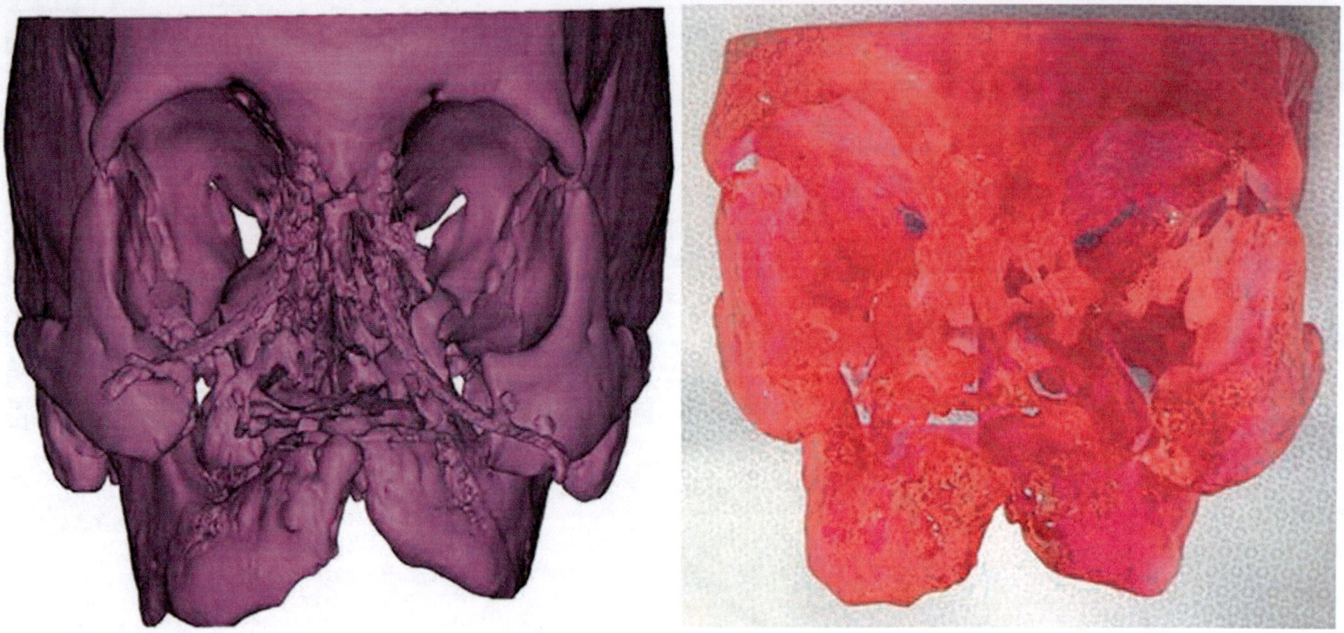

Fig. 6.13 An acrylic model (*right*, *white*) fabricated via additive manufacturing technology, based upon 3D reconstruction (*left*, *yellow*) of CT scan data

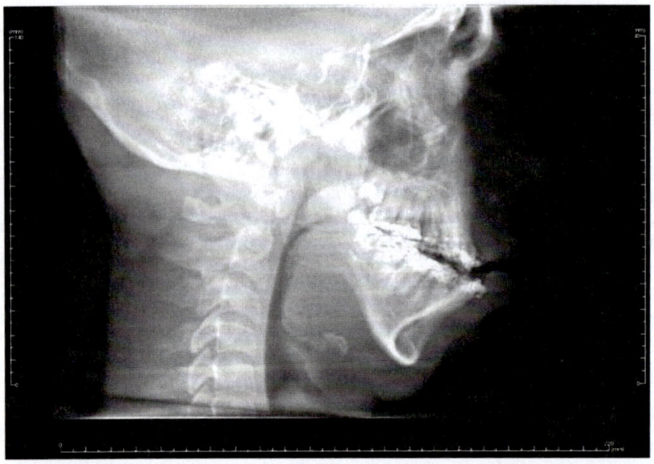

Fig. 6.14 Traditional lateral cephalometric skull image extracted from a CBCT scan

ing clefts, diagnosing fractures, or detecting subtle changes in cortical bone.

According to the ACR:

> Possible contraindications (to MRI) include, but are not limited to, the presence of cardiac pacemakers, ferromagnetic intracranial aneurysm clips, certain neurostimulators, certain cochlear implants, and certain other ferromagnetic foreign bodies or electronic devices. Possible contraindications should be listed on a screening questionnaire. All patients should be screened for possible contraindications prior to MRI scanning. Published test results and/or on-site testing of an identical device or foreign body may be helpful to determine whether a patient with a particular medical device or foreign body may be safely scanned. There is no known adverse effect of MRI on the fetus. The decision to scan during pregnancy should be made on an individual basis.
> http://www.acr.org/~/media/ACR/Documents/PGTS/guidelines/MRI.pdf

Conclusion

This chapter presents an overview of the major imaging systems applicable to the maxillofacial/craniofacial complex. Each system has its strengths and weaknesses, its advantages and limitations. The key to taking advantage of each imaging modality is to frame the clinical question in terms of diagnostic yield: "What information will the imaging study provide that will affect how I manage this case?" The answer to that question is then balanced with the principle of ALARA. When the radiology report is integrated with the clinical examination and patient dialogue, the surgeon can then provide optimal treatment.

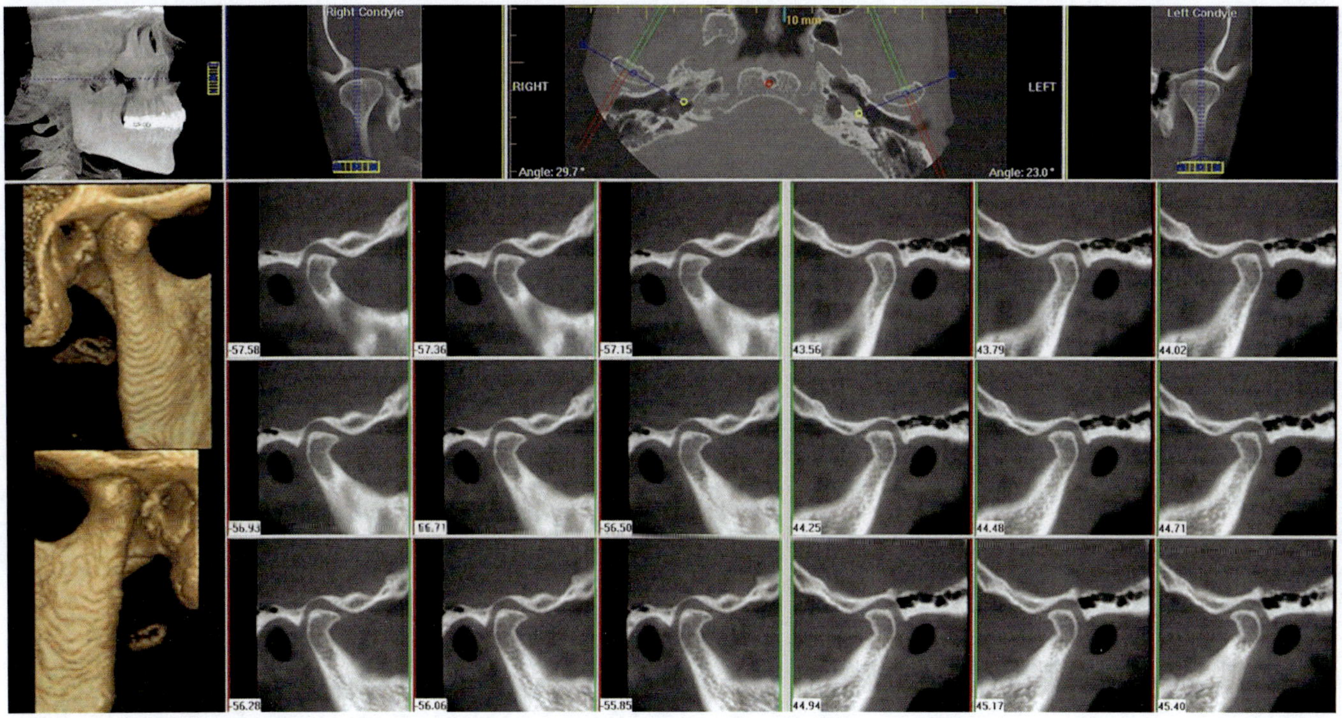

Fig. 6.15 Cross-sectional depiction of the osseous components of the TMJ as generated from a CBCT scan

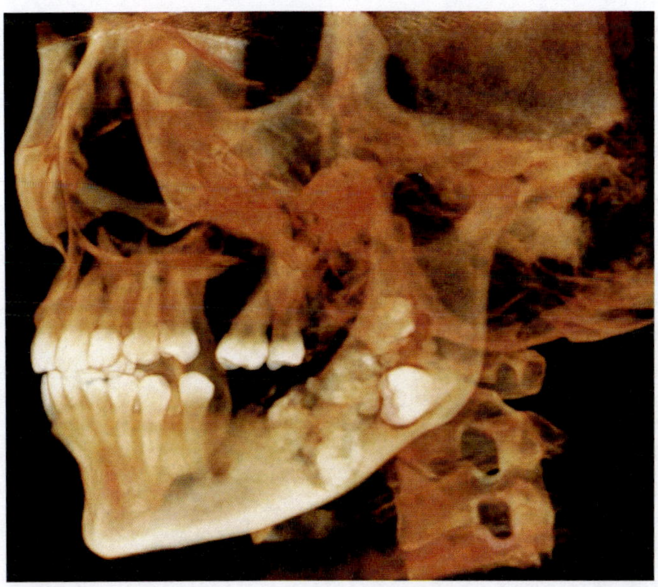

Fig. 6.16 Three-dimensionally rendered skull image generated from a CBCT scan. Note the pathology occupying the left body/ascending ramus of the mandible. Additional views of this tumor are seen in Figs. 6.17 and 6.18

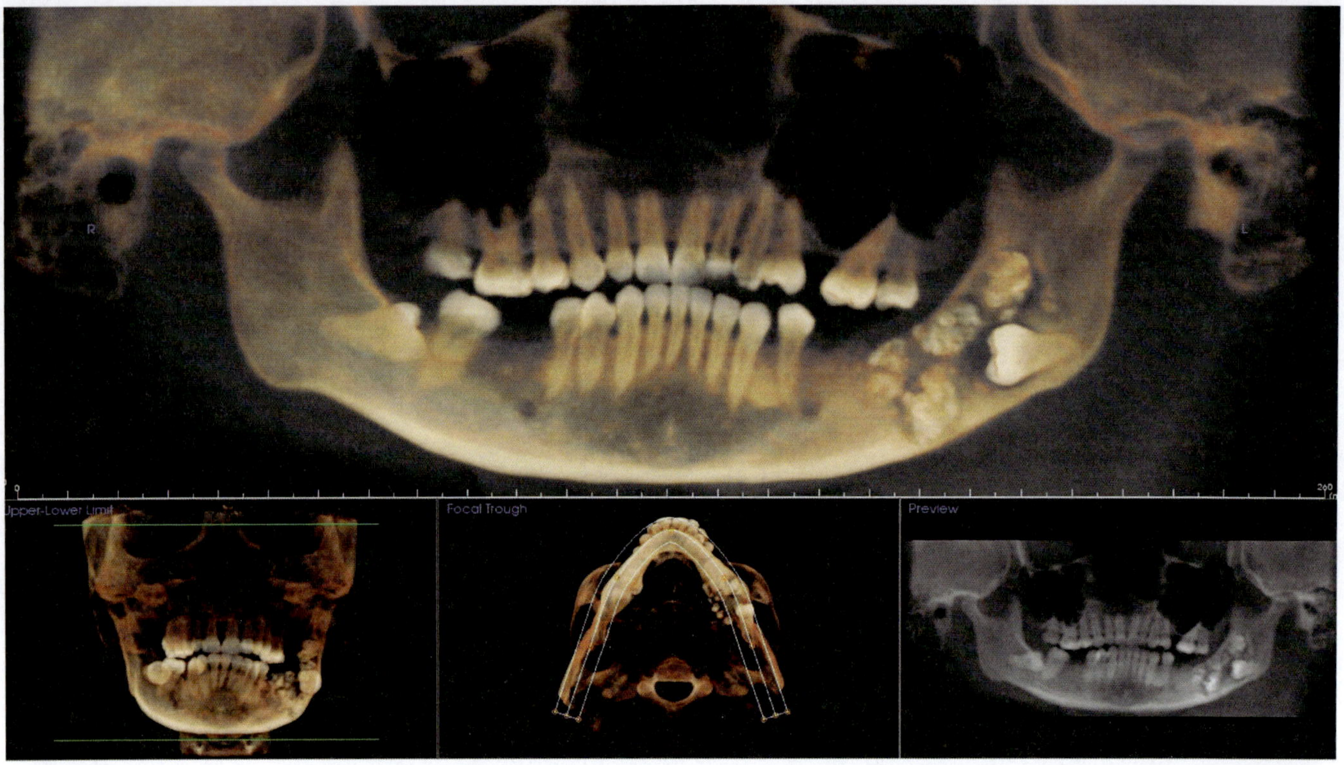

Fig. 6.17 Tumor occupying the left body/ascending ramus of the mandible demonstrated in CBCT three-dimensionally rendered format

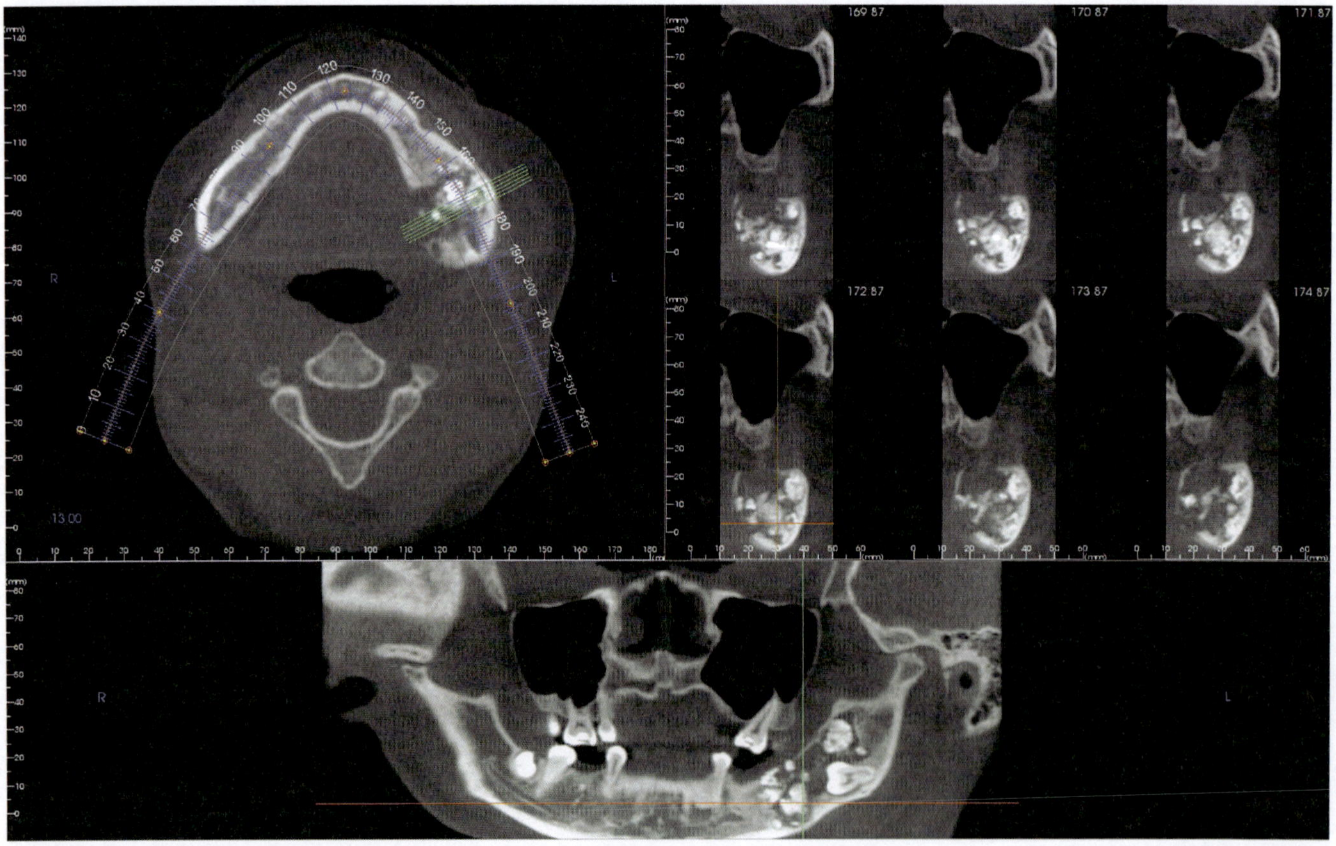

Fig. 6.18 Standard CBCT cross-sectional images of the tumor shown in Figs. 6.16 and 6.17

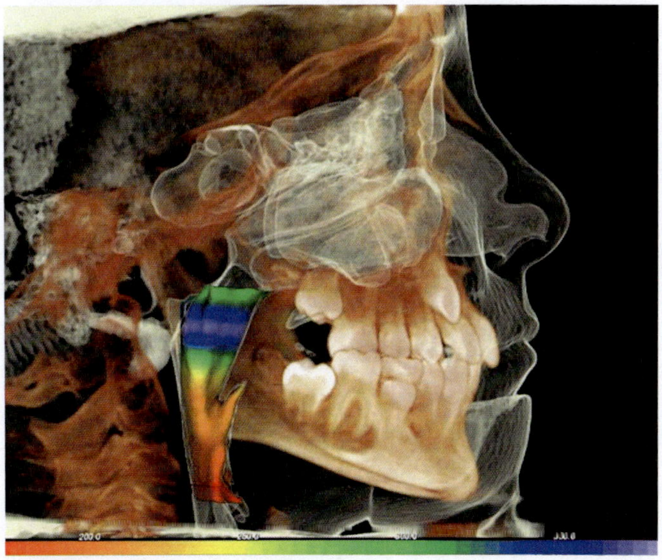

Fig. 6.19 Volumetric analysis of the airway can be obtained using task-specific CBCT software applications

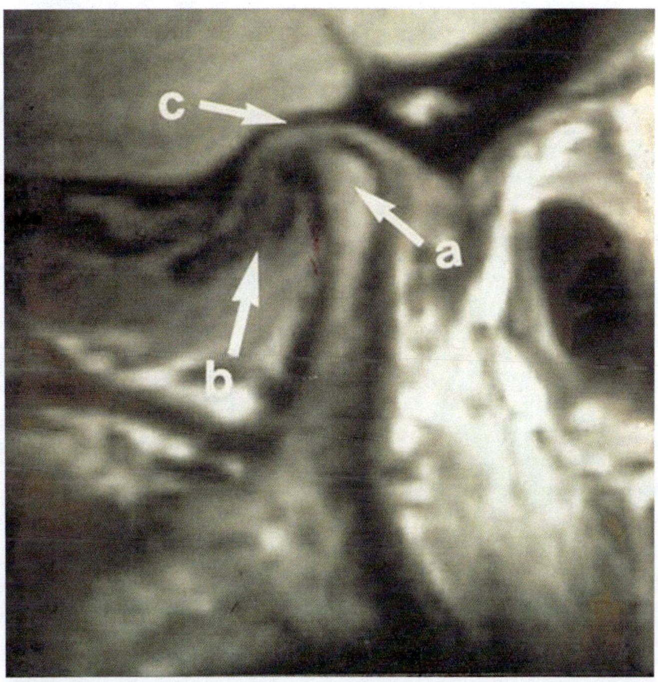

Fig. 6.20 MRI image of the temporomandibular joint complex. Note *arrow* "*b*" identifies the TMJ disk. Hard tissue, such as the head of the condyle (*a*) and the roof of the glenoid fossa (*c*), contains less water and therefore cannot generate the signal strength necessary for diagnostic detail

Bibliography

Harnsberger HR, Glastonbury CM, Michel MA, Koch BL, Phillips CD, Mosier KM, et al. EXPERTddx. Head and neck. Salt Lake City: Amirsys Press; 2009.

Kennedy DW, Bolger WE, Ziinreich SJ. Diseases of the sinuses. London: BC Decker; 2001.

Koenig LJ. Diagnostic imaging oral and maxillofacial. Salt Lake City: Amirsys Press; 2012.

MacDonald D. Oral & maxillofacial radiology. Chichester: Wiley-Blackwell; 2011.

Robb RA. Biomedical imaging, visualization, and analysis. New York: Wiley-Liss, Inc.; 2000.

Zhao L, Patel PK, Cohen M. Application of virtual surgical planning with computer assisted design and manufacturing technology to cranio-maxillofacial surgery. Arch Plast Surg. 2012;39(4):309–16.

Fixation Techniques

7

Jack C. Yu, Antony Martin, Brian Ho, and Mohamad Masoumy

Introduction

Reduction and fixation are two principal components of fracture treatment. Without proper reduction, the correct anatomic form is not restored, and without the proper form, the functional restoration may be incomplete. Fixation is to hold the bony fragments in the desired position until healing can occur. Even properly reduced fragments can undergo secondary displacements, if the forces producing displacements exceed those that resist them. However, once healing has progressed to the point that the bone fragments are sufficiently united and that they now can withstand the average deforming forces, it would be important for the fixation system used to permit the transfer of load-bearing function back to the bone. This chapter will review basic biomechanics pertinent to fracture fixation, the fixation devices and techniques, and important underpinning biological principles. The learning objectives are as follows:

1. Be able to explain fixation using biomechanical concepts and terms such as force, load, stress, strain, yield stress and yield strain, ultimate stress and ultimate strain, interfragmentary strain, tension, compression, shear, rigid, load bearing, load sharing, cyclic loading, fatigue, endurance limit, modulus of elasticity, and viscoelastic deformation.
2. Be able to articulate why fractures are fixated the way they are when treated by open reduction and internal fixation.
3. Be able to compare and contrast between the following fixation methods used in craniofacial skeleton: maxilla-mandibular fixation, Ivy loops, inter-fragmentary wiring, mono-cortical plates, non-locking plates and screws, locking plates and locking screws, self-drilling and self-tapping screws, and lagging and lag screws.
4. Be able to formulate a workable treatment plan to fixate maxillary and mandibular fractures and measures to reduce complications.

Basic Biomechanical Principles

The bone is a living, rigid, porous viscoelastic composite. It is the only living tissue that is perpetually hard. Rigidity, or hardness, is that materials property which resists deformation when subjected to external forces. Force is measured in newtons, N for short; it is 1 kg mass accelerating at 1 m/s/s, or 1 kgm/s^2. When this force is normalized (divided) by the cross-sectional area on which it is acting, the resulting N/m^2 is the stress. 1 N/m^2 is 1 Pa. Load is not a very precise term; some authors use it to refer to force, while others used it to mean stress. The better terms to use are force and stress. When the object's deformation, either elongation or foreshortening, is measured and expressed as a fraction original length, it is called the strain, tensile if larger than 0 and compressive if less than 0. As the force increases, the stress and strain will go up, to a certain point, called the yield point; above that, the deformation becomes permanent. If the force continues to increase, the object will break. That point is the failure point and the corresponding stress and strain are the ultimate stress and ultimate strain. The bone has an ultimate strain of only 1–2 % which means when stretched more than 2 % of its length, it will break. The ultimate tensile stress for human cortical bone is about 135 million Pa, or 135 MPa. Its compressive ultimate stress is better, 205 MPa. What the bone does not tolerate well is shear stress; it has ultimate shear stress of 67 MPa. After fracture, the gap has certain

J.C. Yu, MD, DMD, MS Ed, FACS (✉) • A. Martin
Department of Plastic Surgery, Georgia Regents University, Augusta, GA, USA
e-mail: jyu@georgiahealth.edu

B. Ho, MD
Department of Otolaryngology, Georgia Regents University, Augusta, GA, USA

M. Masoumy, MD Department of Surgery, Georgia Regents University, Augusta, GA, USA

P.J. Taub et al. (eds.), *Ferraro's Fundamentals of Maxillofacial Surgery*,
DOI 10.1007/978-1-4614-8341-0_7, © Springer Science+Business Media New York 2015

finite length; this length is called the gap length and when bone fragments move, the gap length will change; this change when expressed as a fraction of the original gap length is the all-important inter-fragmentary strain. No bone can form if this is above the ultimate tensile strain. Simply stated, the goal of fixation is to reduce inter-fragmentary strain.

The rate at which stress is applied and thus the rate at which strain is developed are known as the stress rate and strain rate, respectively. They are important. Sudden fast strain rate is not as well tolerated. The pattern of force application, one time or multiple repeated applications, also produce different responses. The latter is called cyclic stress and produces cyclic strain. The slope of the straight portion of stress–strain curve is Young's modulus, a quantitative measure of material's stiffness. The material's property will deteriorate under cyclic stress because of the development of microscopic cracks. Human bone is very good at repairing such, and they can stand decades of cyclic stress and strain, because the remodeling mechanism can repair these microscopic cracks. No man-made materials, to date, can do that. Titanium or stainless steel, after high enough cycle numbers at sufficient stress level, even though well below the ultimate stress, will demonstrate deterioration of the elastic modulus. This is known as fatigue damage—the reason why the bone must take over the function of resisting deformational forces from the plates and screws. Without bone healing and restoration of the continuity, plates and screws will have to undergo repeated cycles of stress and strain; eventually, when endurance limit is reached, they will break. That inability to transfer the stress-bearing function back to the bone due to excessively strong plates and screws is stress shielding and must be avoided. The proper way is to start out with plates and screws bearing the stress but gradually split the stress, i.e., load sharing, and eventually the bone, once healed, becomes the load-bearing part.

Means to Reduce Inter-fragmentary Strains

Inter-fragmentary strain naturally decreases as fracture site is occupied by tissues of progressively higher tensile modulus and lower ultimate tensile strain. The pain, edema, and muscle spasm associated with acute fracture immediately reduce movements of the bone ends, creating in essence a splint around the fracture. The replacement of hematoma by granulation tissue increases the cellularity, vascularity, and strength of the fracture gap. Eventually, when motion has been reduced to produce inter-fragmentary strain in the range less than 1 %, ossification starts. Surgeons use many means to hasten the inter-fragmentary strain reduction by using stainless steel inter-fragmentary wires, or maxilla-mandibular fixations, external fixators, or plates and screws. Plates and screws are the most standard way internal fixation is achieved today, though inter-fragmentary wiring still has its place, either as the sole fixation or as a temporary measure to allow plate osteosynthesis. Unlike fractures of the appendicular skeleton, the maxilla and mandible house numerous teeth with precise indexing called intercuspations. This position of maximum intercuspation is used to reduce the fractures. If the maxilla is intact, it is used to reduce mandible and vice versa. Even when both jaws are fractured, the intact portion of one arch serves as a template for the fracture reduction of the other. In some fractures, maxilla-mandibular fixation, MMF, is sufficient and gives very nice long-term results. The requirement for such treatment method is, of course, good premorbid dentition, with sufficient firm teeth for MMF. External fixators are reserved, in today's management strategies, to secondary treatment when internal infections have occurred. Pins are driven into the fragments and fastened to rigid metal rods to maintain stability.

Screws are the workhorse in rigid fixation, and until very recently, it was impossible to achieve any form of rigid fixation, internal or external, without screws. Screws belong to a general group of fasteners like nails, bolts, and rivets. Figure 7.1 shows the various parts of a standard, non-locking, self-tapping screw. These devices connect two or more loose parts together into a single rigid structure. Nails work like K-wires and achieve fixation by friction; they are long cylinders with a pointed end. When a slotted head and threads are added to that cylinder, a screw is born, one of the six simple machines. The head has a larger diameter than the cylinder (core) and therefore a large moment arm when turned, applying the principle of wheel and axel. The threads are wrapped

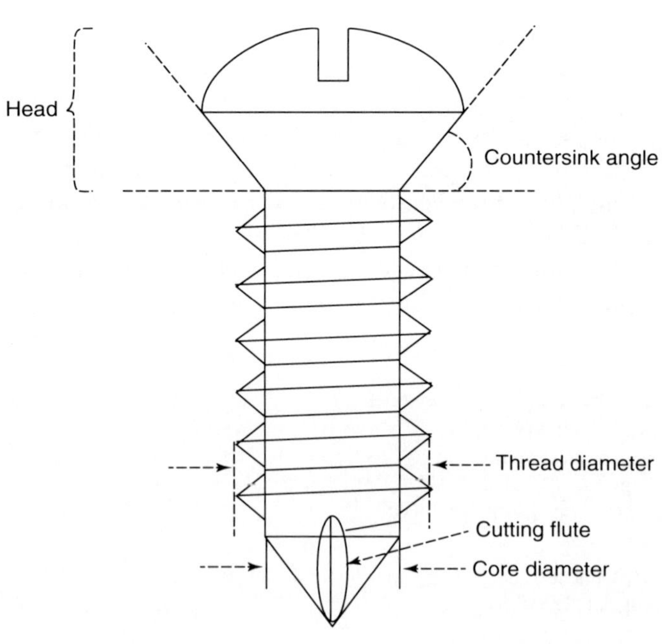

Fig. 7.1 The anatomy of a standard non-locking, self-tapping, screw

around at an angle, like rolling an inclined plane onto a post. The slope of this incline dictates the distance between the threads and is called pitch. The threads add to the core diameter and 2× thread with + core diameter = the thread diameter.

The thread diameter is what is used to identify the various sizes of the screw: a 2.0 mm screw has a core diameter smaller than 2.0 mm, and if a 2.0 mm bit is used to drill the hole, the 2.0 screw will simply spin freely in the 2.0 mm hole. The pilot hole must be drilled using the bit having the same diameter as the core. Some screws cannot tap by themselves, due to softness of the material they are made of or the lack of cutting flutes, and require tapping, a process of cutting the precise threaded hole by using a separate instrument called a tap. If the cutting flute is designed such that the screw can be advanced without first drilling the pilot hole, it is a self-drilling screw. Self-drilling screws cannot be made too long or too large because the resistance builds up and force required to turn becomes too high or too damaging to the bone. Drilling produces heat and debris. Heat must be dissipated by cooling using continuous saline irrigation so that the temperature in the surrounding bone does not rise. It took only 45 °C for a few seconds to coagulate the cytoplasm within the cells such as endothelial cells, osteocytes, and osteoblasts, denaturing the proteins and killing the cells. Necrosis caused by overheating is a major reason for delayed screw loosening and increase in inter-fragmentary strain and infected nonunion.

Plates and screws are the most common fixation devices used. There are two major types of plates: locking and non-locking. In non-locking plates, the compression of the plate to bone surface when screws are tightened produces a great deal of friction, resisting any movements between bone segments and the plate, thus reducing the inter-fragmentary strain. Crucial in their deployment is good adaptation of the plates. If the plates are not conforming to the bone contour, the bone fragments will be displaced as the screws tighten, dictated by the plates. The principle advantages of the locking plates and locking screws are that the screws will firmly "lock" into the plate—without the need for intimate contact between the bone surface and the plate, thus permitting better periosteal blood flow and accepting a plate that is not as well adapted.

Lag screws are special screws with differential advancement along its length achieved by varying pitch so that each rotation of the screw advances more at the point closer to the screw head (near cortex) than at the tip (far cortex). Any regular screws with uniform thread pitch can be deployed in a lagging fashion by making the hole larger in the near cortex (closer to the screw head) so as to prevent the engagement of the thread while keeping the hole closer to the tip (in the far cortex) small to permit the thread engagement when turned. The larger hole is the gliding hole, and the smaller one is the threaded hole. The gliding hole is placed in the near, or proximal, cortex and the threaded hole is in the far, or distal, cortex. When the screw is turned, the distance between the screw head and the far cortex will decrease, resulting in compression of the fracture. The prerequisites for this elegant and efficient technique are perfect coaxial alignment of the gliding and threaded holes and perpendicular orientation of the screw to the fracture if all possible. If there is excessive deviation from orthogonal placement, shear stress builds up at the fracture and can cause slippage of one fragment relative to the other. When properly placed, the compressive force generated is in the range of 2,500 N. The elastic modulus of the titanium, the material making up the screw, is 100 GPa, more than 5× that of the cortical bone (15–20 GPa), and contributes to the stability of the fixation.

Key Steps in Fracture Fixation

After proper exposure and reduction, the surgeon must hold the bone fragments in their reduced, anatomic positions and deploy the definitive fixation to keep them reduced until healing can occur. This temporary fixation and final hardware placement represent the bulk of the hardest tasks in fracture treatment. Some may say that they are the *sine qua non* of ORIF and require planning and practice.

Temporary fixation can be achieved by the following means:

1. Bone clamps
2. Border wires
3. K-wires
4. Arch bars
5. Ivy loops (See Figs. 7.2 and 7.3.)

Bone clamps can deliver very high compressive forces to hold the bone fragments in very close coaptation. For fractures with large fracture surface areas, such as oblique or spiral fractures, clamp is placed perpendicular to the long axis of the bone. This is not possible when the fracture itself is more transverse, perpendicular to the long axis. In such cases, small holes are drilled at appropriate distance (3–4 mm from the fracture on each side, depending on the configuration of the clamp) as close to the neutral axis as possible, crossing the fracture at 90°. The neutral axis is where compression zone changes to tension zone, and as such it experiences the least amount of both. Think about the mandibular body as a beam; compression in the inferior border has the tendency to cause tensile forces to be exerted on the occlusal border. To overcome that, arch bars or Ivy loops should be used whenever there is inferior compression. Similarly, unopposed compression at the occlusal border by Ivy loops or arch bars tends to distract the inferior border. Compression at the external (buccal) border can distract the internal (lingual) border. 1° of deviation at anterior mandible produces about 8 mm of lateral displacement at the condyles. It is thus important to visualize all borders.

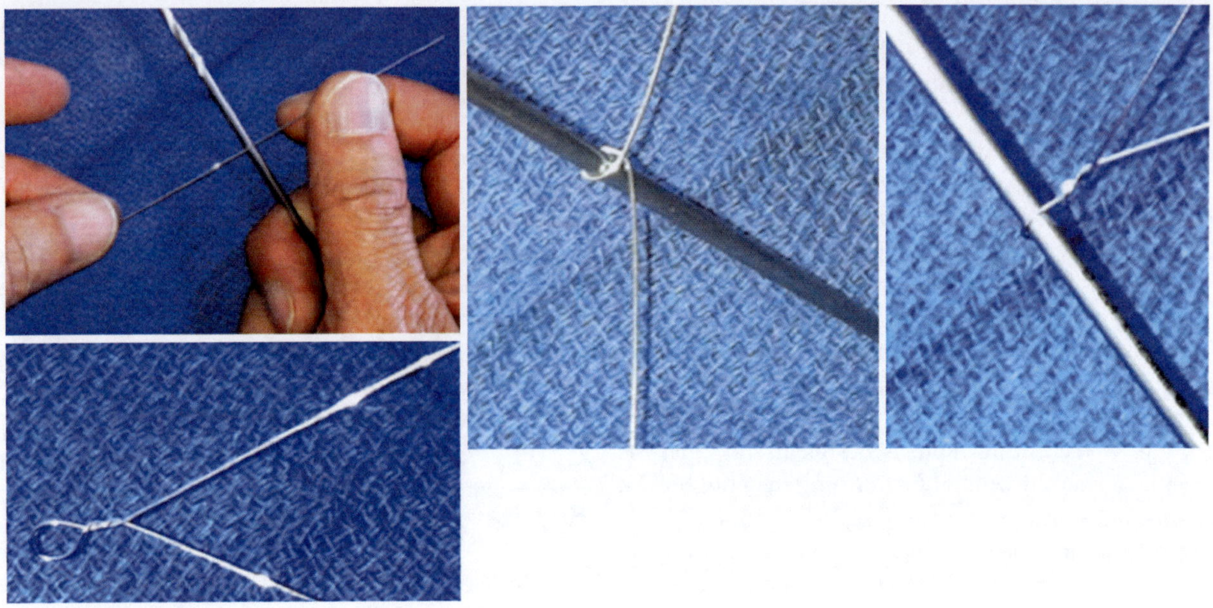

Fig. 7.2 Making Ivy loops. Ivy loops can be easily constructed from 24G wires over any rigid cylindrical instruments of 3–4 mm diameter, such as a suction cannula or drill bit. The twists are clockwise and should correspond to interdental widths (4–6 mm)

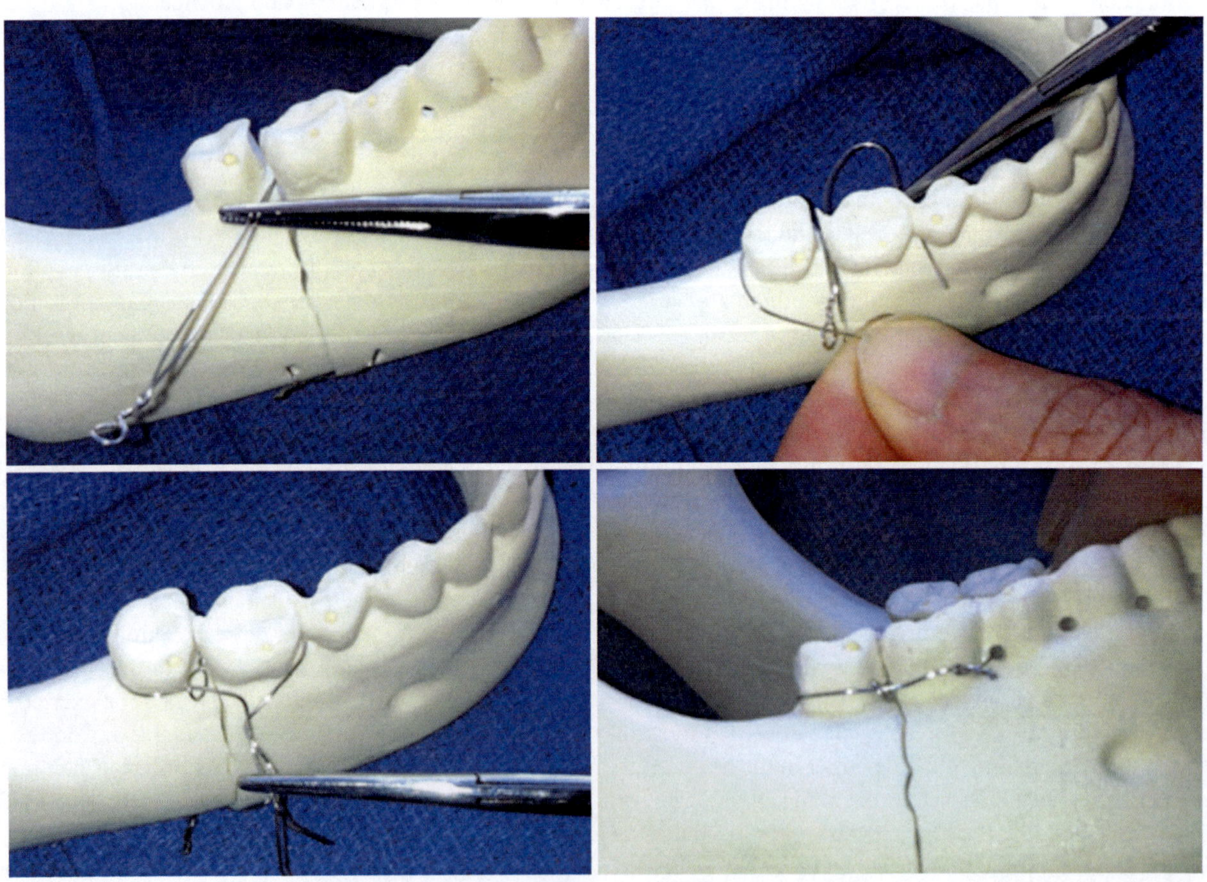

Fig. 7.3 Placement of Ivy loops. Both tails are first passed through selected interdental space from buccal to lingual. The tails are turned and passed from lingual to buccal through the interdental space mesial (anterior) and distal (posterior) to the initial interdental space. The distal end is passed anteriorly through the eyelet and twisted to the anterior tail end, after each tail end has been seated and pulled tight individually

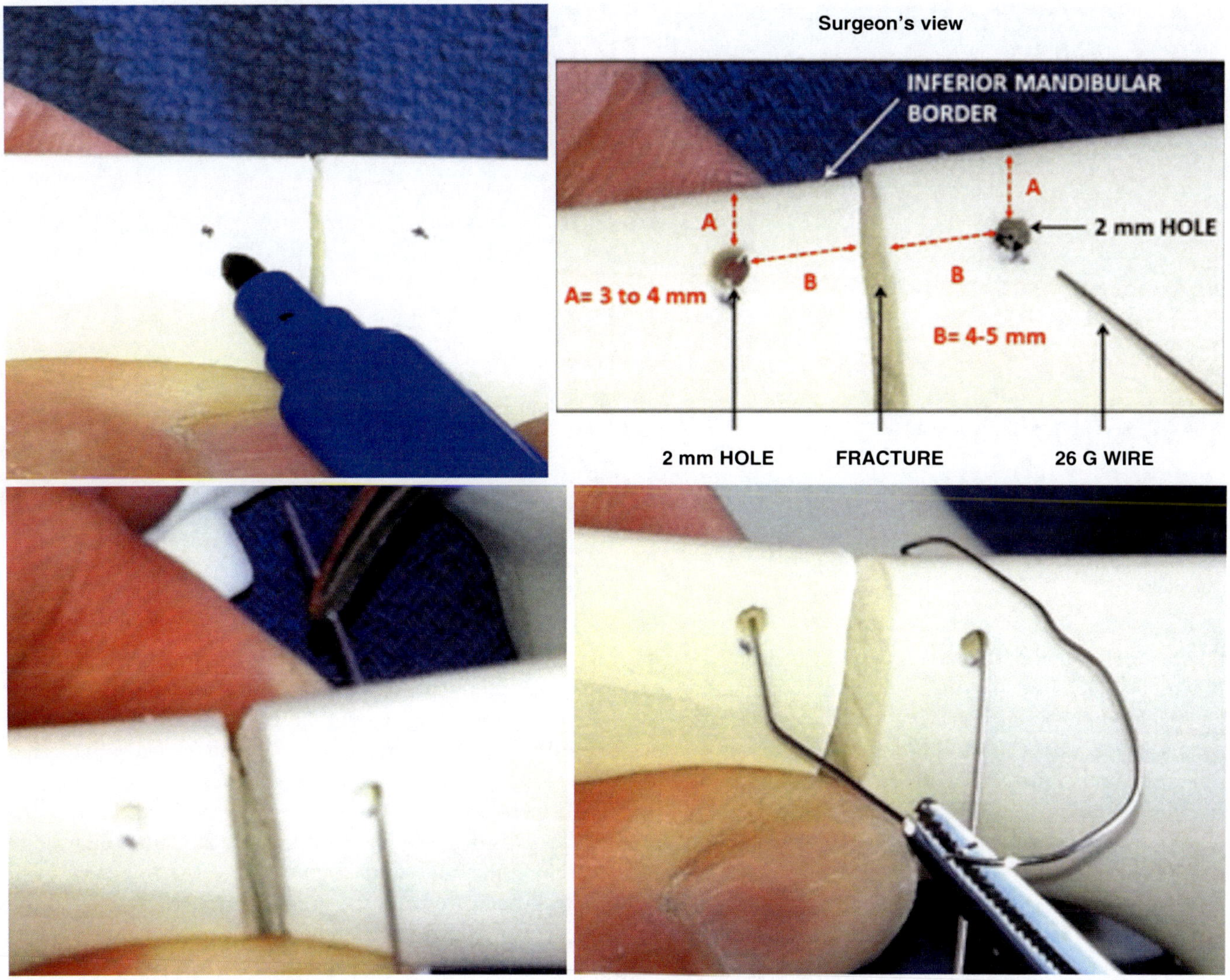

Fig. 7.4 The placement of inferior border figure-of-eight wire, for right mandibular angle transverse fracture by a right-handed surgeon standing at the 12 o'clock position. The 2 mm holes must be drilled precisely as ultimately they determine the position of bone fragments. The 26G, or 24G, wire is passed from "outside-in" in both passes, avoiding the more difficult "inside-out" passes

Inferior border figure-of-eight wiring is very versatile and easy to do; importantly, it can be done without an assistant surgeon. (See Figs. 7.4 and 7.5.) On both sides of the fracture, at a point 3 mm back from the inferior border and 4 mm back from the fracture, two 2 mm holes are drilled with constant irrigation, through both cortices. A 26G stainless steel wire is passed from outside in and retrieved. That inside end is then passed again in an outside-in fashion though the hole on the opposite and retrieved.

The two ends are twisted clockwise till tight. The positions of the holes are very important and must be equidistant from the inferior border; otherwise, the tightening of the wire will cause the bone fragments to move out of alignment. It also must be sufficiently away from the fracture to allow the wires not to "fall" into the fracture.

Technical Considerations

Angle of Mandible

MMF is always established first. Exposure is through a lower buccal sulcus for simple fractures or Risdon incision for more complex ones. After the fracture site is cleansed of any soft tissue interposition, temporary fixation is used to hold the reduction. The fracture line is inspected and the proper occlusion rechecked. The reduction can be maintained with bone holding forceps placed across the mandible for oblique fractures. For fractures crossing closer to 90° to the long axis of the bone, bone clamp is harder, if not impossible, to place. Inter-fragmentary wiring can be used instead. (See Figs. 7.4 and 7.5.) Using direct visualization and with CT imaging of

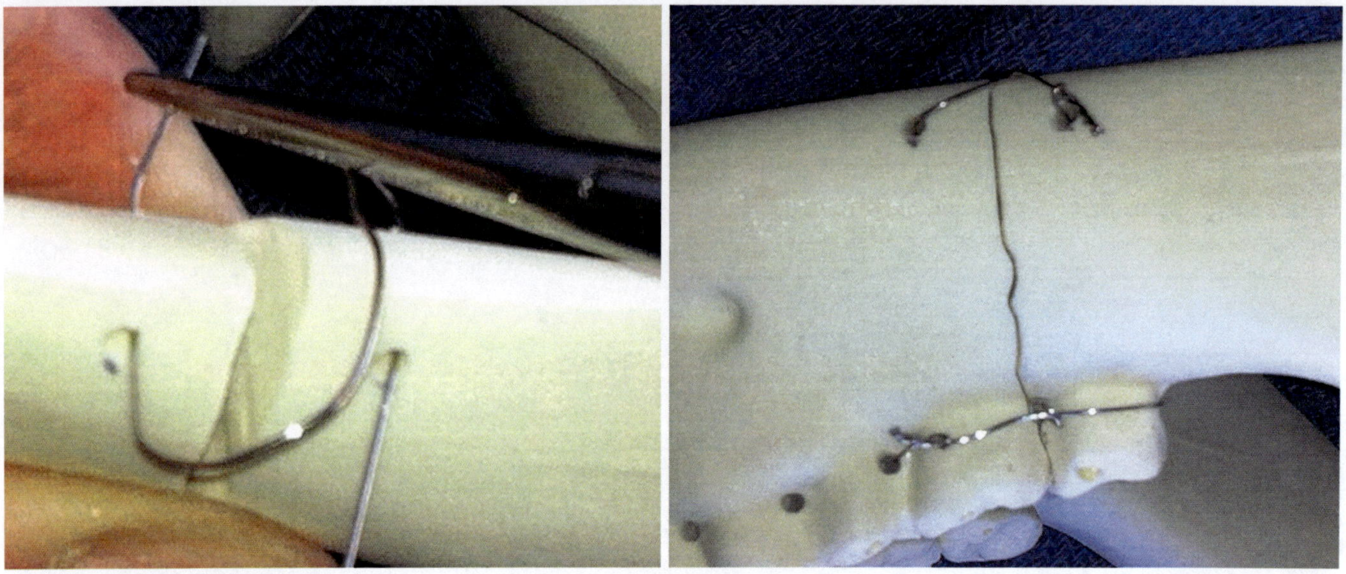

Fig. 7.5 Tightening the inferior border figure-of-eight wire. Each end of the wire is pulled tight and then twisted clockwise, providing compression inferiorly

the fracture, an optimal site of entry is selected, and a 0.035″ K-wire is driven bisecting the angle formed from a line perpendicular to the fracture and the long axis of the bone. For a right-handed surgeon treating left mandibular angle fracture, the path is from caudal posterior lateral to cranial anterior lingual, and usually the inferior alveolar nerve will be missed. The oblique fractures can also be temporarily fixated using K-wire, passing perpendicular to the surface of the external cortex. A stab incision is then made on the skin for the drill guide. To avoid slippage of the drill bit, an indentation on the cortex at the site of entry point is made using a 2 mm burr. Another option is directing the drill bit perpendicular to the bone just enough to gain purchase of drill bit and changing it to parallel the K-wire. When using this technique, it is essential to avoid over-drilling the near cortex which may preclude the surgeon from changing the angle of drill bit. If bone clamp is used, it may be relaxed just enough to allow visualization of burr entering the fracture gap and that it is heading towards the far cortex, avoiding the problem of missing it. The forceps are re-clamped and the far cortex is drilled.

For average-size adults, 2.4 or 2.7 mm cortical screws provide sufficient strength for lagging the fracture of angle of mandible. The near cortex is drilled using a bit of the same diameter as the screw (2.4 mm bit for 2.4 mm screw and 2.7 mm bit for 2.7 mm screw), creating a gliding hole. A concentric drill guide with appropriate outer diameter is then used to drill the far cortex, creating the pilot hole using 1.7 mm bit for the 2.4 mm screw and 1.9 mm bit for the 2.7 mm screw. The length is measured using a depth gage, and near cortex is countersunk and a self-tapping screw of the correct length is placed. A second screw can be placed in the similar fashion, at the 0.035 in. K-wire site if one was used. MMF is removed at the end of operation in unilateral fractures and kept for a week for bilateral fractures. Some authors remove lag screw routinely 6 months after surgery. Third molar is also removed at this time if it is indicated. (See Figs. 7.5, 7.6, 7.7, and 7.8.)

If there is comminution, plate osteosynthesis is the workhorse. This begins with precise plate adaptation followed by attaching the plate to the appropriate bone fragment, using plate holding forceps or screw. The plate must be strong enough to reduce inter-fragmentary strain to less than 1 % during healing but not so strong as to cause stress shielding. In-plane bending is done before out-of-plane bending. Locking plates and screws have more tolerance by providing dual fixations: from bone to screw and from screw to plate. Once the major fragments have been fixated, reestablishing mandibular continuity, the comminuted fracture becomes a simple transverse or oblique fracture and can be managed as such. While lag screw is contraindicated by itself in treating comminuted fractures, it can certainly be used in addition to plate osteosynthesis (Fig. 7.9).

Symphyseal Fractures

Plate osteosynthesis of symphyseal fractures needs considerably more extensive periosteal stripping and more devascularization of bone and may cause dysfunction of lower lip muscles and neuropraxia of mental nerve. Lag screw is ideally suited in short oblique or vertical fracture in the symphyseal or parasymphyseal regions. Comminuted fractures are not suitable for this mode of fixation. Patients with poor dentition may not be suitable candidates as this method requires the use of arch bars as tension band at the superior border.

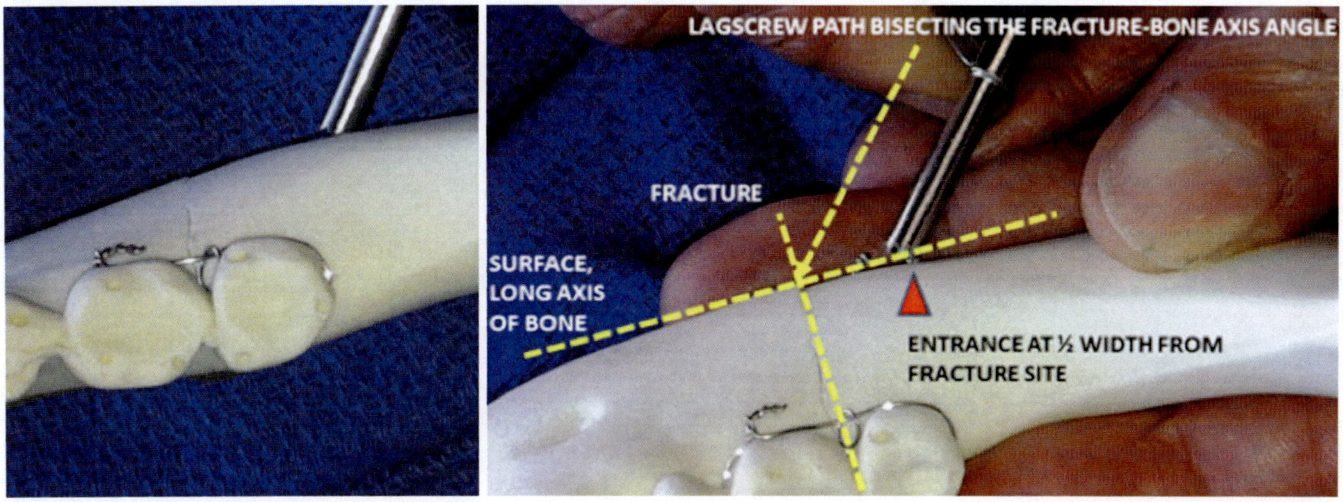

Fig. 7.6 Lag screw fixation of transverse fracture of posterior mandible after initial, temporary stabilization with figure-of-eight wiring at inferior border and tension band at superior border by interdental Ivy loop. The near cortex is drilled using a burr corresponding to the thread diameter of the screw. The entrance is at a point ½ the width of the mandible posterior to the fracture and directed at an angle bisecting the fracture plane and the surface (or long axis) of the bone. The path is from lateral inferior posterior to medial anterior superior

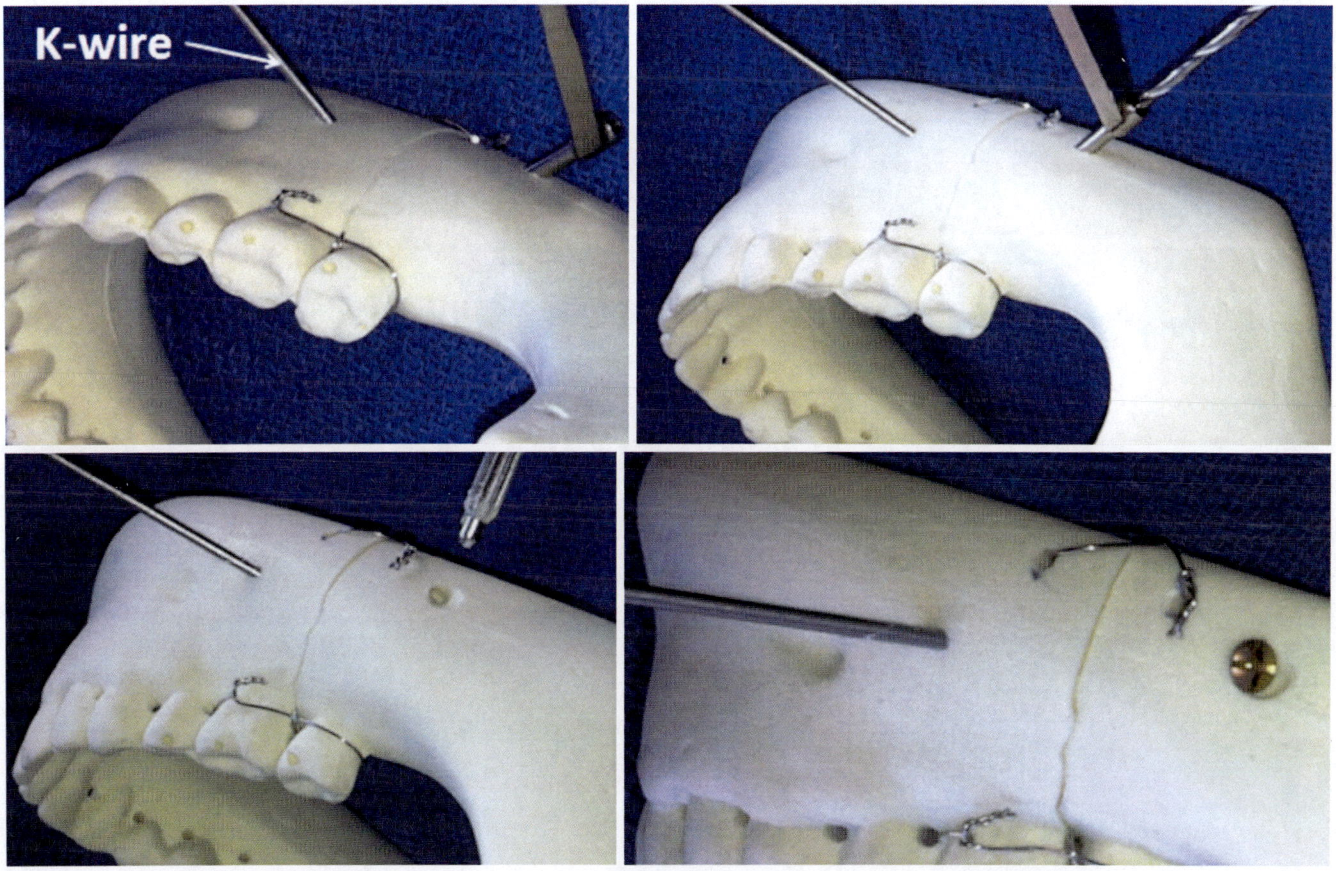

Fig. 7.7 A concentric drill guide is placed into the gliding hole for drilling the pilot hole in the far cortex. The K-wire provides additional stability and is optional. The hole is depth-gaged, countersunk and screw deployed

For symphyseal fractures arch bars are applied first, either segmentally or loosely first, and only tightened once in proper occlusion using 24G wires. After establishing MMF, lower labial sulcus incision is made. Fracture site is exposed and cleared of any soft tissue. A reduction clamp is used to keep the fracture site reduced. A drill guide through reduction clamp itself if available can obviate the need for a separate hole. Otherwise, a separate stab incision may be needed for the drill guide. Lag screw is done using technique described above. While tightening the screw, it is important to prevent opening of fracture on the inner cortex or the occlusal border of mandible. This is achieved either by holding the two rami of mandible together while tightening lag screw or by placing the screw exactly in the neutral axis of the mandible. The arch bar, serving as a tension band, reduces splaying of fracture site on the superior border. Postoperatively MMF is released in a week and arch bars are removed at 5–6 weeks. (See Fig. 7.10.)

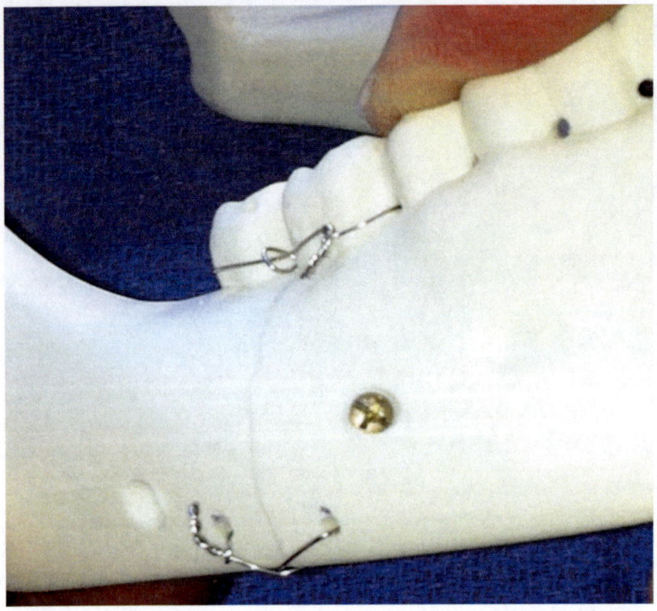

Fig. 7.8 The alternative lag screw placement: from anterior inferior lateral to posterior superior medial. If a K-wire was used, it may be removed when tightening the first screw and then the space used for the placement of the second lag screw. When correctly deployed, the fracture is compressed to a barely perceptible thin line

How to Avoid Complication

The oral cavity is normally colonized with aerobic and anaerobic bacteria, communicating directly to the external environment. This coupled with poor dental hygiene, malnutrition, and trauma, severe infections can occur when hardware is deployed in the maxillofacial skeleton for fixation. Most surgeons would use antibiotics perioperatively. Zallen et al. noted four decades ago that the infection rate was nearly 50 % with compound mandibular fractures in those who did not receive antibiotics. Another study divided patients into a

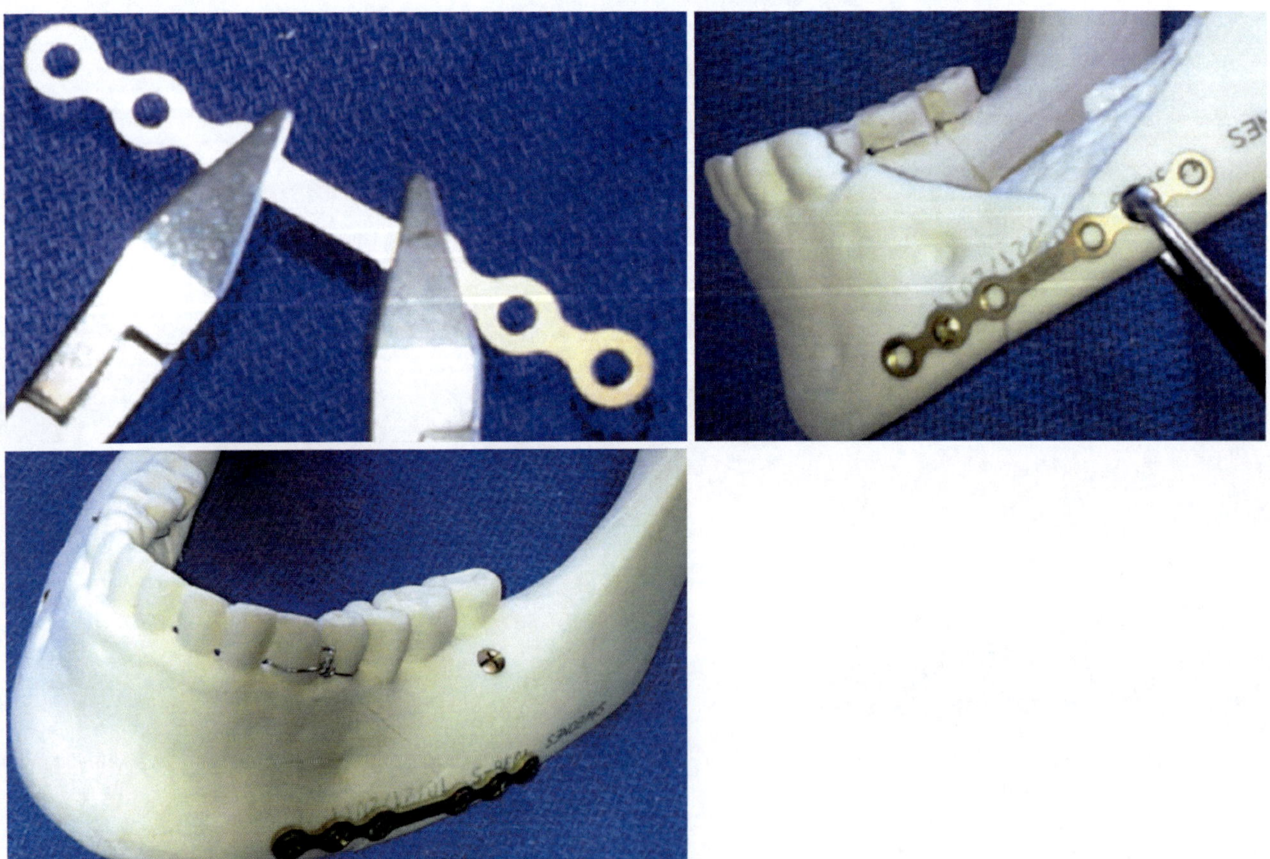

Fig. 7.9 Plate osteosynthesis of comminuted left posterior mandibular fracture. The plate is adapted using plate benders. It is then attached to the appropriate major fragment and screws placed. The plate can then be clamped in place, temporarily holding the major distal segment, reconstituting mandibular continuity. Once the plate is securely fixated near the inferior border, the additional fragments can be fixated using lag screws. Notice the compression provided by the lag screw can reduce the additional fracture to a very thin line, permitting primary bone repair

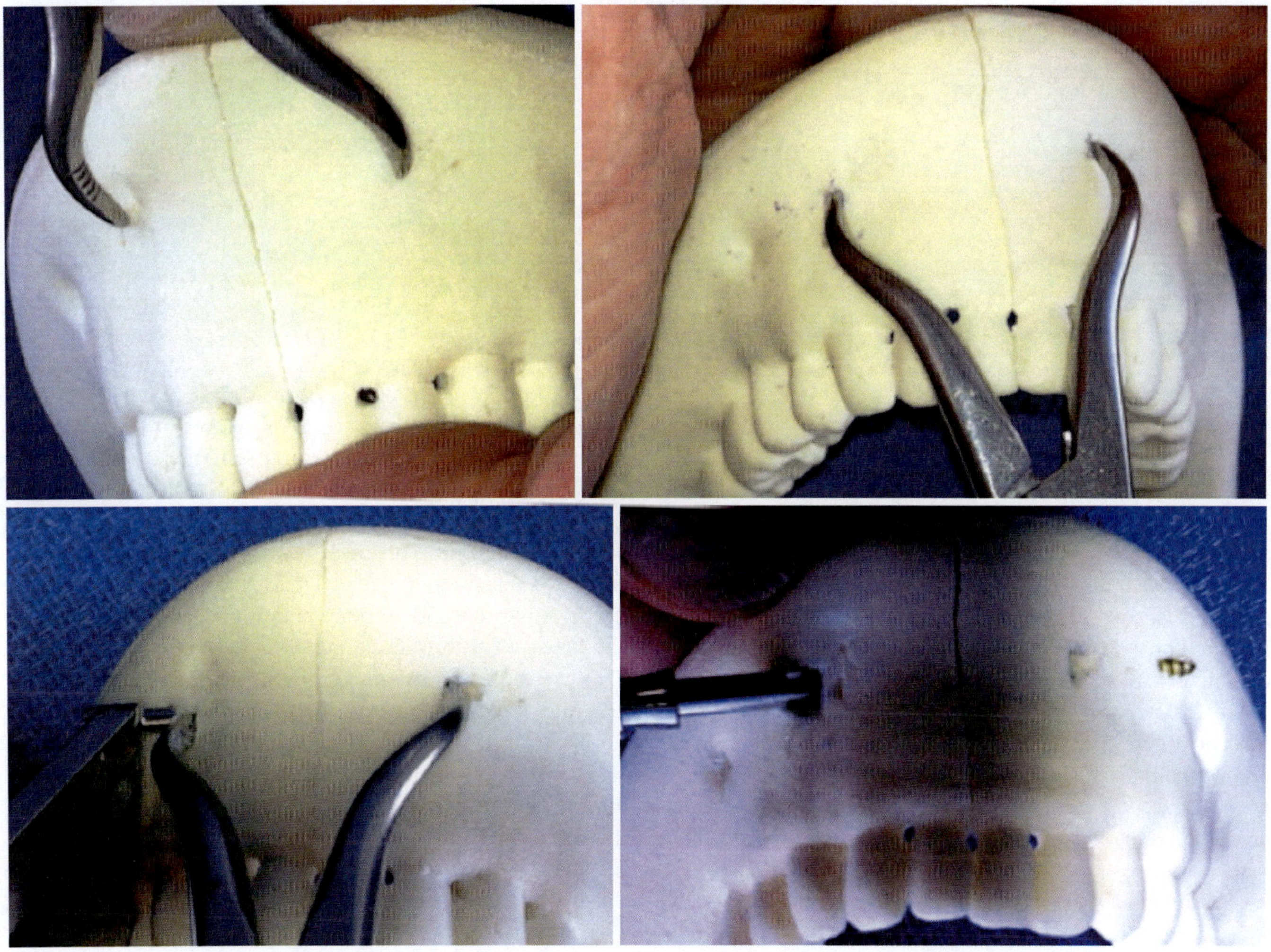

Fig. 7.10 Lag screw fixation of mandibular symphyseal fracture. The position of the purchasing holes for the reduction forceps is marked by placing reduction forceps across the fracture, low enough to avoid tooth roots but high enough to reduce splaying of the superior border. They also must be sufficiently apart to allow compression by the forceps. Once the temporary fixation is achieved, the lag screw placement is fairly straightforward

"prophylactic antibiotic group" and a "non-therapy" group with 50 % of the "non-therapy" group developing wound infections at the operative site, as opposed to only 6 % in the antibiotic group. The antibiotic used in this study was penicillin. There have been multiple studies since then, and the general consensus is that there is increased infection if antibiotics are not used within 72 h of the fracture. Most of these infections are due to normal resident oral flora, such as facultative and obligate anaerobes. Traditionally, clindamycin was used extensively for trans-oral procedures, including oncologic resections and basic lacerations. Schaefer and Caterson reported the rate of infection using clindamycin in ORIF of the mandible was 19.35 %. This infection rate was significantly over the 7.59 % in the ampicillin/sulbactam (Unasyn) group. Chole and Yee postulate that the typical 5-day course of antibiotics was equivalent to short-term prophylaxis. Antibiotic prophylaxis should, therefore, be stopped at 24 h post procedure, as there is little evidence to support longer use. The head and neck area has rich blood supply and is thus more resistant to infection, but the oral cavity is laden with microbes, and any mandibular fractures involving teeth are by definition compound fractures. Because of this, the complication rate is high. Infection can lead to osteomyelitis, ischemia, and bone and soft tissue necrosis. These ischemia and necrosis impede the delivery of antibiotics, making the osteomyelitis difficult to treat. Osteomyelitis may lead to the loss of further bone stock at the fracture site. A multistep treatment process is needed, including debridement, irrigation, antibiotics, and possible bone grafting. Many infective postoperative complications have preventable intraoperative root causes.

Intraosseous blood supply to the mandible is inferior alveolar vessels which can be compromised from the original, traumatic event; the healing process will then depend on the soft tissue envelope, especially the periosteum. Excessive stripping to expose the bone will reduce the blood supply and is to be avoided. Comminution with damage to the periosteum, muscle, and mucosa poses particularly difficult challenges. One way to avoid periosteal stripping or to allow infection to clear after hardware removal is external fixation which can be applied effectively and quickly. (See Fig. 7.11.)

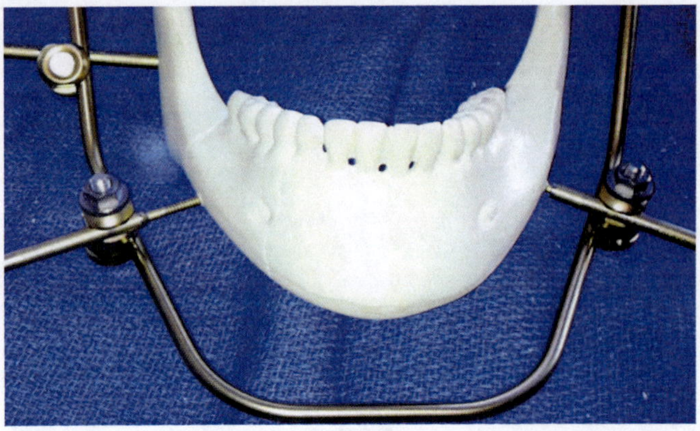

Fig. 7.11 External fixation. This is used after infected hardware removal, or when there is excessive amount of comminution and preservation of periosteal blood supply becomes paramount

Delayed union occurs when the normal healing is prolonged and can result from excessive inter-fragmentary strain due to inadequate fixation or supraphysiological loading. Impaired host healing due to advanced age, malnutrition, and chronic diseases contributes to this as well. Nonunion is failure to achieve osseous healing. This is uncommon in the maxilla but occurs occasionally in the mandible. Delayed union and nonunion occur in about 3 % of fractures, with technical error as the most common etiology. Excessive inter-fragmentary strain due to poor immobilization can be associated with lack of stable teeth and difficulty in obtaining MMF. Overheating during drilling can cause bone to die back resulting in hardware loosening. Fracture lines should be meticulously inspected for dental root fractures. Devitalized teeth can lead to periapical abscesses that can potentially spread to the marrow space, causing osteomyelitis. Poor vasculature impairs healing and patients are strongly encouraged to not smoke. Cannel et al. demonstrated a higher incidence of both delayed and nonunion in patients who consumed ethanol. This is possibly due to poor nutrition and mineral deficiencies associated with alcoholism. The treatment of these two groups (delayed and nonunion) is best addressed by treating the source. If the process is due to poor plate adaptation or inadequate fixation, the hardware should be removed and wounds cleansed and properly re-fixated. Constant irrigation is a must and arch bars must be applied properly in fractures involving tooth-bearing segments of the mandible as malocclusion and malunion can result if arch bar is wired tight prior to proper reduction.

Malunion is described as osseous union with displacement still present. It should be noted that there are instances of subclinical malunion because they are asymptomatic. Subclinical malunion can occur in edentulous patients or fractures that involve the ramus or condyle. Malunion becomes symptomatic when there is malocclusion. Malocclusion is prevented with proper MMF. Malocclusion can be corrected and treated with continued MMF at the beginning stages of healing or with orthodontics, osteotomies, or occlusal equilibration by selective grinding after the patient is taken out of MMF. These procedures should not be performed at a minimum of 6–12 months to allow for possible self-resolution and osseous remodeling.

Nerve Injury

Similar to orbital fractures and the inferior orbital nerve, comminuted or displaced mandible fractures can lead to inferior alveolar/mental nerve injury. At the initial evaluation, thorough medical documentation should be made of preoperative nerve function. Clinical symptoms of nerve injury may be due to neuropraxia (edema) or true neurotmesis (nerve and axon severing).

The inferior alveolar nerve can also be damaged intraoperatively at the time of lower buccal sulcus dissection. The nerve is subject to a degree of manipulation and edema during traction and plate manipulation. Surgical technique should be used to free the nerve to prevent excess traction. This can be performed with proper identification of the nerve and then tracing the nerve using a small curved clamp into the soft tissue superficially. The extra length can greatly reduce injury to the nerve while operating. Obvious intraoperative nerve injuries or transections should be repaired at the level of the epineurium with nurolon sutures. Most instances of neural symptoms are transient and regenerative distally or centrally reorganize.

If an inferior approach is to be utilized for debridement and fixation, meticulous surgical technique should be instilled to identify the marginal mandibular branch of the facial nerve. The marginal mandibular nerve is located roughly 3 cm (2 fingerbreadths) inferior to the mandibular border and in the investing fascia of the submandibular gland. If the fascia is reflected superiorly, this will then protect the nerve, and then dissection can proceed to the mandibular border. Patients may develop postoperative House-Brackmann scale deficiencies of the marginal mandibular nerve. Most of these are self-limited but if severe nerve injury persists may require dynamic slings.

Ankylosis is a rare yet feared complication after reduction and fixation. This process occurs more frequently in the pediatric population and is thought to occur due to intracapsular fractures leading to intra-articular hemorrhage and fibrotic ankylosis. This can also lead to severe growth disturbance and developmental derangement of the affected joint. Ankylosis is more common with intracapsular fractures and prolonged MMF, especially in pediatric patients younger than the age of 10 years. As with many processes, the best treatment is that of prevention. Prevention of TMJ ankylosis is achieved with shorter periods of MMF, which early motion of the joint. Length of MMF is a difficult clinical decision in younger children or unreliable adults. Taking patients out of fixation and allowing them to their own devices can lead to malunion (as described above). Rubber bands can be used over arch bars to assist with occlusion and fixation while still allowing some mobility to prevent joint fixation. No rule can be made for this and physicians should use their best judgment based on physical examination. In general, once the fracture is no longer tender to palpation, MMF release should be contemplated. Once ankylosis develops, its treatment may require temporomandibular joint arthroplasty, possible coronoidectomy, cartilage disc reconstruction, condylectomies, and joint replacements.

Bibliography

Cannell H, Boyd R. The management of maxillofacial injuries in vagrant alcoholics. J Maxillofac Surg. 1985;13:121–4.

Chole RA, Yee J. Antibiotic prophylaxis for facial fractures. A prospective, randomized clinical trial. Arch Otolaryngol Head Neck Surg. 1987;113:1055–7.

Chuong R, Donoff RB, Guralnick WC. A retrospective analysis of 327 mandibular fractures. J Oral Maxillofac Surg. 1983;41:305–9.

Dodson TB, Perrott DH, Kaban LB, Gordon NC. Fixation of mandibular fractures: a comparative analysis of rigid internal fixation and standard fixation techniques. J Oral Maxillofac Surg. 1990;48:362–6.

Ellis 3rd E. Use of lag screws for fractures of the mandibular body. J Oral Maxillofac Surg. 1996;54:1314–6.

Forrest CR. Application of minimal-access techniques in lag screw fixation of fractures of the anterior mandible. Plast Reconstr Surg. 1999;104:2127–34.

Hindawi YH, Oakley GM, Kinsella Jr CR, et al. Antibiotic duration and postoperative infection rates in mandibular fractures. J Craniofac Surg. 2011;22:1375–7.

Mathog RH, Rosenberg Z. Complications in the treatment of facial fractures. Otolaryngol Clin North Am. 1976;9:533–52.

Munro IR, Chen YR, Park BY. Simultaneous total correction of temporomandibular ankylosis and facial asymmetry. Plast Reconstr Surg. 1986;77:517–29.

Niederdellmann H, Shetty V. Solitary lag screw osteosynthesis in the treatment of fractures of the angle of the mandible: a retrospective study. Plast Reconstr Surg. 1987;80:68–74.

Perren SM. Evolution of the internal fixation of long bone fractures. The scientific basis of biological internal fixation: choosing a new balance between stability and biology. J Bone Joint Surg Br. 2002;84:1093–110.

Schaefer EH1, Caterson EJ. Antibiotic selection for open reduction internal fixation of mandible fractures. J Craniofac Surg. 2013;24:85–8.

Topazian RG. Etiology of ankylosis of temporomandibular joint: analysis of 44 cases. J Oral Surg Anesth Hosp Dent Serv. 1964;22:227–33.

Zallen RD, Curry JT. A study of antibiotic usage in compound mandibular fractures. J Oral Surg. 1975;33:431–4.

Bone Grafting: Physiology and Techniques

8

Sanjay Naran and Robert M. Menard

Craniofacial anatomy represents one of the few places in the body where bony anatomy is truly married to that of soft tissue. As well as providing structural support and protecting sensory anatomy, the skeletal component of craniofacial anatomy is essential in fulfilling perhaps the face's most important role: to look like a face. Given this unique marriage of form and function, the goal of this chapter is to review the principles of bone anatomy, physiology, histochemistry, repair and regeneration, and reconstruction and grafting techniques, as they pertain specifically to craniofacial surgery.

Bone Anatomy

The craniofacial skeleton is made up of a total of 29 bones; 8 comprise the cranium, 14 the facial area, 6 form the auricular ossicles, and finally there is the hyoid. As well as providing protection of vital sensory organs, bone provides structural support and serves as an attachment point to facilitate movement of the facial soft tissues. Bone also serves as a reservoir for growth factors and minerals, although to a lesser degree in the craniofacial skeleton than elsewhere in the body. Bones are often described as either flat or tubular; the craniofacial skeleton is composed primarily of flat bones. These differ from tubular bones in that they do not contain the three distinct regions seen in tubular bones (diaphysis, metaphysis, and epiphysis) and are primarily cancellous with a thin cortical shell.

Bone may be classified either as cortical or cancellous. These differ greatly in terms of density, structure, and metabolic activity. Cortical bone makes up the majority of all bony tissues (~80 %) and forms the outer layer of the skeleton. A dense, fibrous, bilayered membrane known as periosteum covers this shell. A thin layer of connective tissue that lines the surface of the bony tissue that fashions the medullary cavity of long bones forms what is known as the endosteum. Cortical bone is resistant to torsional and bending stresses and is 5–10 % porous, which is what provides it with its compressive strength. Cortical bone is composed of osteons, or haversian units, each of which consist of concentric layers or cortical tissues, or lamellar, of compact bone tissue surrounding a central, or haversian, canal (Fig. 8.1). Perforating holes, known as Volkmann's canals, run perpendicular to the haversian canals within the osteons and interconnect the haversian canals with each other and the periosteum. It is within the haversian and Volkmann's canals that nutrient vessels and nervous tissue tract. Conversely, cancellous bone is 50–90 % porous, which allows it to be compressible, and also has a higher rate of metabolic activity owing to its greater surface area.

Composition

While an understanding of bone composition and function of those components is important for the craniofacial surgeon, detailed histology and discussion of the intricate signaling pathways of the cellular components is beyond the scope of this text.

Bone is made up of inorganic matter, organic matter, and water. The inorganic component, which comprises 60 % of bone, is primarily made up of hydroxyapatite, which is a naturally occurring mineral form of calcium apatite. The inorganic bone matrix therefore sequesters 99 % of the body's storage of calcium. The hydroxyl component may be replaced by minerals such as phosphate, which allows for bone to function as a reservoir. The organic phase, which makes up 30 %, is primarily composed of type I collagen. Other components include proteoglycans, growth factors, and glycoproteins.

S. Naran, MD
Department of Plastic Surgery, University of Pittsburgh, Pittsburgh, PA, USA

R.M. Menard, MD, FACS (✉)
Pediatric Plastic and Craniofacial Surgery, Northern California Kaiser Permanente Craniofacial Clinic, Santa Clara, CA, USA
e-mail: rmmenard@stanford.edu

P.J. Taub et al. (eds.), *Ferraro's Fundamentals of Maxillofacial Surgery*,
DOI 10.1007/978-1-4614-8341-0_8, © Springer Science+Business Media New York 2015

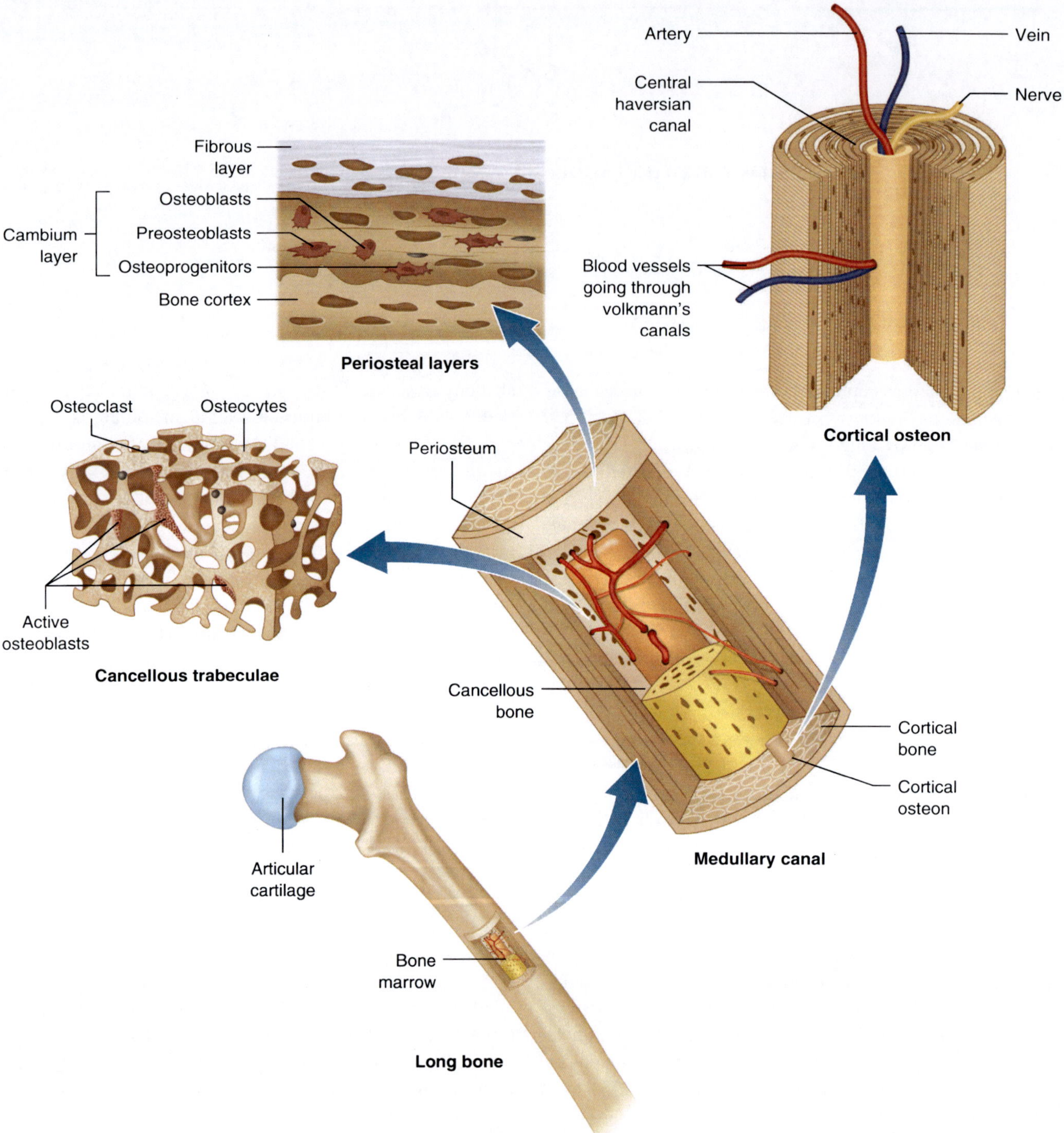

Fig. 8.1 Bone microanatomy. Most bones are comprised of a hard cortical component and a "spongy" cancellous component. Cancellous trabecular packets are arranged to maximize surface area for nutrient diffusion and exposure to circulating cytokines and hormones important in bone and mineral homeostasis. The external surface of bone is covered by a periosteum, which provides additional vascular supply, and osteoprogenitor cells important in the initial stabilization of fracture callus

Cells within bone may be divided into two groups: osteoprogenitor cells and osteoclasts. Osteoprogenitor cells arise from pluripotent mesenchymal stem cells and differentiate to form osteoblasts and osteocytes, whereas osteoclasts arise from hematopoietic cells. Osteoblasts are located on the surface of the bone and form a dense, active, remodeling surface. Osteoblasts are rounded, basophilic cells. When active, they produce bone matrix and in doing so release alkaline phosphatase, which serves as a marker of osteogenesis. Upon activation, they either remain as osteoblasts, terminally differentiate into osteocytes, or revert back to an osteoprogenitor cell.

Osteocytes are embedded within the lacunae, which is akin to a bone corpuscle. These lacunae are connected to one another by canaliculi, which are thin cytoplasmic projections that extend from the osteocyte upon activation. Osteocytes are therefore stellate cells. Osteocytes are essential for mineral homeostasis, particularly calcium, and bone resorption when stimulated by parathyroid hormone.

Osteoclasts are large, multinucleated cells with a ruffled border that are located within Howship lacunae, shallow grooves/pits of endosteal and periosteal that form over the surface of bone. In areas of active remodeling, they form deeper cavities known as cutting cones. Osteoclasts resorb bone, adhering to bone matrix and dissolving it through acidification. This process is of particular importance clinically in instances of pathologic and dysfunctional resorption.

The extracellular matrix is formed primarily by osteoblasts. It is primarily composed of type I collagen, but also contains myriad other collagens, noncollagenous phospho- and glycoproteins, and growth factors. It is this matrix from which bone derives the majority of its strength.

Bone Regeneration

Differing from collagen deposition in the process of scar formation, bone is unique in its ability to heal through cellular regeneration via mineral matrix production and constant remodeling. Much like any other molecular process, there exists an intricate milieu that governs migration, proliferation, and differentiation. Identification of key factors within these cascades, as well as the ability to spatially control their effects, continues to be the basis for much of today's research. The following serves as an introduction to the more prolific of these key factors, with specific craniofacial clinical applications discussed here and in subsequent sections.

Bone Morphogenetic Protein

Bone morphogenetic proteins (BMPs) are members of the transforming growth factor-β superfamily and are essential in the regulation of cellular growth and differentiation. They also serve to attract osteoblasts and mesenchymal cells. With 20 unique isoforms identified, BMPs play different roles at various stages of development. They are critical to skeletogenesis, epidermal induction, and neural crest cell development. BMP is expressed during fracture repair by mesenchymal cells, as well as by osteoblasts and osteoclasts. Many studies have elucidated the role of BMP with regard to the specific aspects of the craniofacial skeleton, including its role in accelerating bone deposition in the mandible during distraction, as well as in the regeneration of cranial defects. Furthermore, BMP is the only signaling molecule capable of singly inducing de novo bone formation. Clinically, rhBMP-2 and rhBMP-7 are the only two isoforms that are currently Food and Drug Administration approved for human application and are most often utilized for spinal and orthopedic procedures. Most notably in the field of craniofacial surgery, BMP has been shown to accelerate mandibular regeneration and therefore may be utilized to augment distraction osteogenesis within the craniofacial skeleton. Its use in alveolar cleft bone grafting has also been documented.

Transforming Growth Factor-B

Transforming growth factor-β (TGF-β) is also a member of the transforming growth factor-β superfamily and controls proliferation, cellular differentiation, motility, as well as many other functions in a wide variety of cell types. It plays a role in many human diseases, including cancer, heart disease, diabetes, and acquired immunodeficiency disorder. TGF-β is released in three isoforms, with TGF-β1 having been shown to play an important role in bone physiology. TGF-β1 is the primary isoform secreted by bone, and in addition to being critical in inducing mesenchymal cell differentiation to chondrocytes or osteoblasts, it has been implicated in osteogenesis, osteoclastogenesis, and bone resorption and repair.

Fibroblast Growth Factor

Fibroblast growth factors (FGFs) play important roles in all stages of human life. Involved in angiogenesis, wound healing, and embryonic development, they are a heparin-binding glycoprotein and are key in a wide range of aspects of cellular developmental biology. With regard to bone, FGFs regulate prenatal and postnatal bone formation, controlling osteoprogenitor cell replication and osteoblast differentiation and function. While TGF-β and BMP are indirect regulators of angiogenesis, FGF, specifically FGF-2, is a direct regulator and therefore increases this process during fracture repair. Furthermore, dysfunction of FGF signaling has been implicated in human skeletal dysplasias and cranial suture disorders and therefore may provide a molecular basis for developing clinical therapeutic strategies.

Platelet-Derived Growth Factor

Platelet-derived growth factor (PDGF) is a polypeptide chain, made up of disulfide-bonded dimers, which promotes organogenesis, skeletal development, angiogenesis, and wound healing. PDGF increases chemotaxis of osteoblasts and is secreted by osteoblasts and macrophages during fracture repair, promoting matrix deposition and turnover. PDGF has also been shown to increase the production of osteoprotegerin, an inhibitor of osteoclastogenesis and bone resorption. With specific regard to craniofacial biology, PDGF directly and indirectly increases bone turnover in periodontal tissue in humans.

Bone Healing

Craniofacial bones develop, grow, and heal by direct ossification of mesenchyme rather than preformed cartilage. As such, unlike bones of the appendicular skeleton, cartilage within craniofacial bone only acts as a scaffold and does not act as a bone precursor. This is important for a number of reasons, but in regard to craniofacial reconstruction, one must be cognizant that therapeutics designed for long bone healing may not directly translate to that of the craniofacial skeleton.

As is the case elsewhere in the body, bone repair following fracture repeats the process undergone during skeletogenesis for that particular anatomy. For the majority of bones within the body, this may be either primary healing (direct cortical healing without a cartilaginous intermediate through the deposition of bone by osteoblasts) or secondary healing (callus bone repair whereby a cartilaginous intermediate is formed within the periosteum, soft tissues, and bone marrow). However, similar to its development, bones of the craniofacial skeleton do not heal via a callus model as described above, but rather through a process akin to secondary endochondral bone union whereby preexisting cartilaginous matrix is replaced with osseous precursors which in turn lead to new woven bone formation.

Variables Influencing Craniofacial Bone Repair

Key elements in fracture healing closely resemble elements critical in wound healing, with the exception of the addition of fracture fixation. Adequate blood supply is essential for bony healing. Revascularization may occur through a process known as haversian remodeling. Vascular endothelial growth factor (VEGF) is the prototypical molecule described in the direct regulation of angiogenesis. A dimeric glycoprotein expressed by osteoblasts, osteoclasts, and mesenchymal cells, VEGF increases vascular sprouting, endothelial cell migration, and proliferation adhesion. The therapeutic promise of VEGF continues to be elucidated. The persistence of devitalized bone even in the setting of a well-vascularized environment remains possible. In such cases, devascularized bone is unable to activate remodeling and, over a period of 6–12 months, will transition to become necrotic bone and predispose itself to repeat fracture. An important variable that is often encountered during craniofacial reconstruction is the effect of radiation following the treatment of head and neck cancers. Radiation-induced changes limit options for primary salvage and impair secondary reconstruction by inhibiting bone healing and growth, choking microvascular supply, and decreasing the integrity of surrounding soft tissue.

Fracture fixation, while pervasive today, has a relatively short history in craniofacial surgery. Over the past several decades, there has been a constant evolution and refinement of the principles of craniofacial fixation, resulting in enhanced understanding of its benefits. While the scale of fixation systems has decreased with time, the principles of application remain the same. Critical to the stability and success of bony healing is the reduction in the degree of motion of fracture fragments. At the same time, micromotion at fracture sites has been shown to increase the degree of bone healing through the enhancement of chondrogenesis and osteogenesis. In the setting of insufficient fixation, fibrous tissue is subsequently deposited within the fracture gap, creating a callus that may be visualized radiographically. In some instances, the fibrous tissue provides sufficient stabilization of the bony fragments to result in differentiation of the callus into bone. If this is not the case, which is occasionally the outcome in the craniofacial skeleton where bones are subject to the forces of muscular movement during expression and mastication, cartilage forms within this gap, resulting in nonunion. These same principles hold true for stabilization and survival of bone grafts.

Age brings with it a number of physiologic changes that affect multiple factors ranging from angiogenesis and stem cell function to signaling cascades and periosteal structure, each of which are essential to bone healing and repair. This is evidenced by the observation that pediatric bone heals at a faster rate than adult bone, likely secondary to increased angiogenic potential of younger bone.

Bone Remodeling

Bone and bone grafts regenerate through three mechanisms: direct spontaneous formation (direct osteogenesis), osteoinduction, or osteoconduction. Combinations of varying degrees of each can occur in a single setting. When implant materials are utilized, a process of osseointegration also occurs, with osteoinduction or osteoconduction occurring in the context of the architecture and composition of the implant.

Osteoinduction

Osteoinduction is the process whereby undifferentiated pluripotent cells are stimulated to transform into bone-producing cells through the release of active factors and thereby form bone in an area previously devoid of it. BMP is the most studied and the most prolific bone-inducing agent, occurring naturally during the genesis of bone or following fracture repair, or via exogenous stimulation. For bone grafts, the architecture of the graft (cancellous versus cortical) dictates the success of incorporation. Cancellous bone graft incorporation tends to be more favorable compared to cortical bone, owing to its open architecture which allows for more rapid revascularization and differentiation of osteoprogenitor cells into bone-forming osteoblasts.

Osteoconduction

Osteoconduction describes bone formation from either adjacent bone or periosteum via the ingrowth of capillaries and osteoprogenitor cells from the recipient bed into, around, and through a bone graft or bioimplant. Therefore, the graft or bioimplant acts as a scaffold for new bone formation. Unlike osteoinduction, this process occurs in an environment already containing bone. Osteoconduction can be more broadly described as the facilitation of bone growth along a scaffold of autogenous, allogenic, or alloplastic materials. In the case of nonvascularized bone grafts, partial necrosis initially occurs, followed by an inflammatory phase where the majority of grafted bone is replaced with new bone, a process described as creeping substitution.

Osseointegration

Osseointegration refers to the direct structural and functional connection between living bone and the surface of a load-bearing artificial implant. Osseointegration of implants results in union without a cartilaginous intermediate. Therefore, the composition and architecture of the implant is integral to its ability to osseointegrate. Implant materials may be classified as either inert or bioactive. Inert materials may generally be used in areas where adjacent soft tissue quality is satisfactory, whereas reconstruction of load-bearing architecture as well as tooth-bearing areas generally requires bioactive materials.

Distraction Osteogenesis

Distraction osteogenesis (DO) is the surgical process of lengthening bones of the body, whereby new bone is formed between two vascularized bone surfaces as those surfaces are slowly mechanically separated. Alessandro Codivilla, an Italian surgeon, introduced surgical practices for lengthening of the lower limbs in 1905. However, like many medical endeavors, early techniques were plagued with high complication rates often resulting in subsequent therapeutic failure. It was not until after the contributions of Gavril Ilizarov, a Russian orthopedic surgeon, that the technique was popularized. Ilizarov's technique was based upon the biology of bone and founded upon the fact that soft tissues regenerate under tension.

Reconstruction of both congenital and acquired craniofacial defects often requires the elongation of facial bones. As such, it was not long before Ilizarov's principles were explored within the craniofacial skeleton. Unique challenges were appreciated with respect to the three-dimensional movement of bone within the face, as well as lower thresholds for cutaneous scarring. Clinical reality was not achieved until 1992, when McCarthy et al. published the first report of gradual mandibular elongation in humans. The same basic principles are adhered to (1) a cut around the perimeter of the bone to be elongated; (2) application of a rigid fixator/distractor; (3) following a short latency period, gradual separation/distraction of the opposing bone surfaces; and (4) consolidation of the newly formed bone. Mechanisms have evolved from external devices with a single vector to both external and internal devices that may move bone in multiple vectors. Most devices are still dependent upon manual turning and are not yet capable of continuous distraction. However, spring-mediated distraction, capable of gradual continuous distraction, has shown promise in craniofacial applications. More so than with long bones, movement of bones within the craniofacial skeleton must be carefully planned. Three-dimensional planning tools are currently available to simulate the entire process of distraction osteogenesis and in doing so calculate the necessary trajectory needed.

Clinical Applications of Bone Grafts

Bone grafting materials may be classified according to origin or architecture. Autografts are taken from the host and are the "gold standard." They are the only grafts that are truly osteogenic, i.e., osteoblasts originating from the bone graft contribute to new bone formation, in addition to bone formation via osteoinductive and osteoconductive processes. Allografts are taken from the same species and are usually cadaveric; incorporation is via osteoconduction, and possibly osteoinduction if osteoinductive cell mediators are still present in the graft. Xenografts are taken from different species and are usually of bovine or porcine origin. Synthetic grafts are not taken from living donors and have no cellular or protein products; calcium phosphate derivatives such as hydroxyapatite are among the most common.

Indications for Bone Grafting

Bone grafts can be used for (1) the filling of acquired bone defects, such as following tumor extirpation or continuity defects following trauma; (2) surface augmentation, such as placement of bone graft for zygomatic or chin augmentation; and (3) reconstruction of congenital defects, such as bone grafting for alveolar cleft defects or for mandibular ramus reconstruction.

Bone Graft Healing and Graft Survival

Bone graft healing parallels that of fracture repair, as outlined earlier, and as such differs in the craniofacial skeleton versus elsewhere in the body. Osteocyte activity is primarily at the recipient site, as osteocytes of the donor seldom survive following transplantation. Bone viability should be maintained during the harvest. The duration of exposure to air should be minimized. Grafts should be covered in a blood-soaked sponge with a moist saline gauze over top. Graft should be kept below 42 °C, and antibiotic washes used with caution owing to their cellucidal properties. The graft recipient site should be well vascularized, and if it is the case, cancellous grafts should be abutted to a cancellous bed.

Decreased viability secondary to poor technique may result in decreased healing capacity, as well as poorer biomechanical properties of the grafted bone and resulting bone regenerate. Viability is dependent upon the size and thickness of the graft, as well as its application to the recipient site. Onlay bone grafts tend to resorb, whereas inlay bone grafts have more favorable survival, with osteogenesis being favored over resportion.

Techniques of Harvest and Sources of Autologous Bone Graft

Sources of autologous bone run the entire topography of the human body. The choice depends upon quantity of bone desired, as well as desired architecture and shape. Traditionally, the ilium, tibia, calvarium, rib, and mandible have served as the preferred donor sites for craniofacial applications. The importance of using the correct instruments, and for those instruments or be in optimum condition, cannot be stressed highly enough.

Iliac

The ilium is a workhouse donor site for the majority of craniofacial applications. Iliac bone graft harvest may be divided into anterior iliac (AI) and posterior iliac (PI) harvest. Iliac harvest allows for a dual surgical team approach and may provide free bone as well as vascularized bone grafts. Given that most craniofacial procedures require the patient to be supine, the anterior ilium is the site of choice in most cases. Bone may be harvested in a variety of states: cancellous, thin cortical, corticocancellous, and bicorticocancellous (Fig. 8.2). The ilium, therefore, serves all indications for bone grafts for craniofacial procedures. The ilium is also the primary donor site for alveolar bone grafting.

The primary goal, in addition to the harvest of quality bone graft, is preservation of the shape and regenerative ability of the iliac crest and the avoidance of postoperative pain. The approach for AI graft harvest is made by first appropriately positioning the patient either supine or with the hip slightly raised. A skin incision 3 cm lateral to the iliac crest, 5 cm below the lateral femoral cutaneous nerve, is made (Fig. 8.3). The skin and subcutaneous tissue is pulled medially to allow for an incision straight down through the superficial fascia and muscular aponeurosis to the periosteum at the top of the iliac crest. There is no need to elevate the periosteum on the crest ridge. Care should be taken to avoid unnecessary superior dissection, which places the lateral cutaneous branch of the T12 subcostal nerve at risk of being stretched or cut (Fig. 8.4). In adults, the fascia overlying the bone must be separated. In the pediatric population, the crest is padded with a cartilaginous growth area that should be preserved in order to avoid growth disturbances.

With a saw or a chisel, the iliac crest is split into two segments. The medial segment remains attached to the insertion of the abdominal muscles, and lateral segment to the insertion of the gluteal muscles. This split is extended ~10 mm anteriorly and posteriorly through the crest, down to the anticipated graft harvest zone. The marrow may be harvested with a sharp curette from this exposure. For corticocancellous harvest, the dissection continues deeper, with careful subperiosteal elevation of the medial iliac and lateral gluteal muscles; care should be taken to avoid laceration of these muscles. The medial iliac crest segment, having been split in an inferomedial direction, is reflected medially with the abdominal muscles attached, and the lateral part of the crest, having been split posterolaterally, is reflected

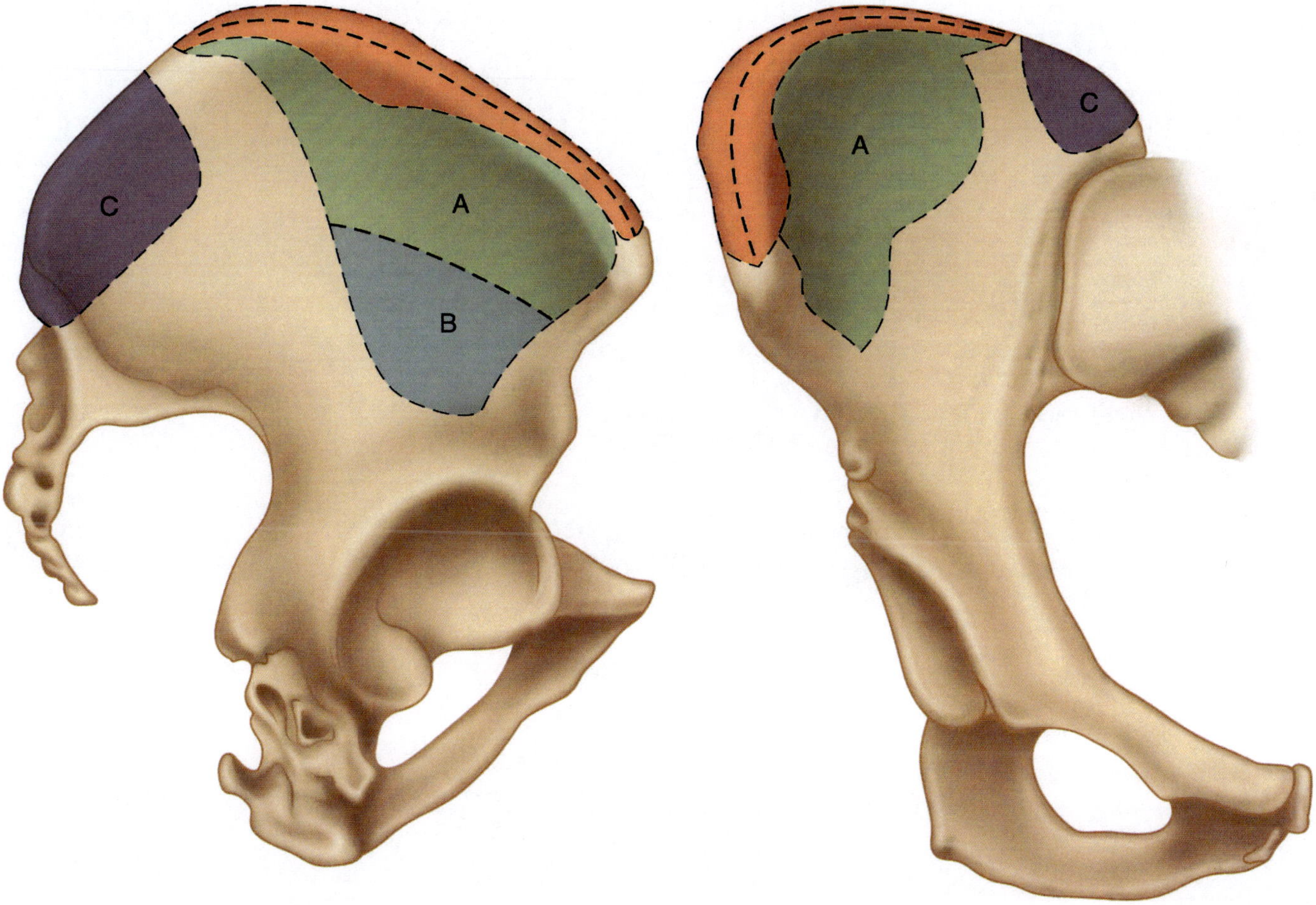

Fig. 8.2 (*Left*) The outer aspect of the anterior and posterior iliac crests, showing (*A*) the large subcrest 5 × 8 cm corticocancellous graft that can be harvested, (*B*) cancellous bone harvest area down to the cotyloid ridge, and (*C*) the posterior corticocancellous graft donor site. (*Right*) The inner aspect of the anterior and posterior iliac crests, with (*A*) the large 6 × 10 cm innercorticocancellous donor site and (*C*) the smaller inner table posterior iliac crest donor site

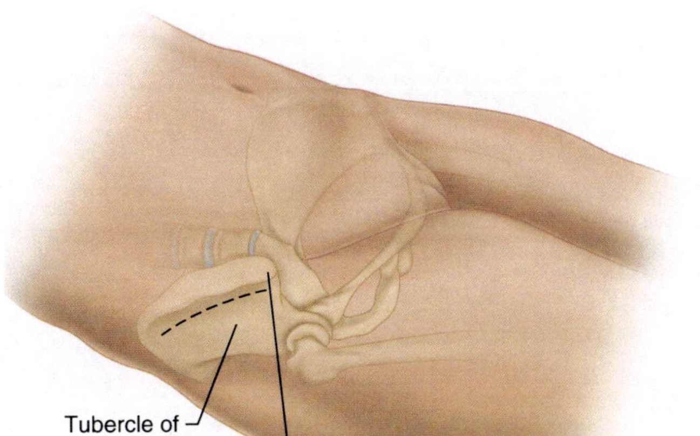

Fig. 8.3 Location of the skin incision 3 cm lateral to the iliac crest. The incision is drawn after marking the locations of (1) the anterior iliac spine and (2) the tubercle of the iliac crest

laterally with the gluteal muscles attached (Fig. 8.5). The lateral dissection can be avoided in the harvest of a medial monocortical graft. Mono- or bicortical grafts can then be harvested using straight or curved thin osteotomes or with a reciprocating saw (Figs. 8.6 and 8.7). Gelfoam is then used to preserve the periosteal pocket of the donor site, and the medial and lateral segments of the split crest are then repositioned and secured with either a sturdy resorbable suture or 26 gauge wires (Fig. 8.8). Harvest from the posterior iliac follows the same tenets. While classically the patient is positioned prone, the patient may be positioned supine following the technique of Tessier et al. The posterior pelvis is raised on a sandbag, with the legs turned to the contralateral side. The skin incision is made on the medial third of the crest, and the exposure is then achieved as previously described (Fig. 8.9). The complication rate for iliac bone graft harvest is reported to be as low as 0.5 %, with postoperative pain being most predominant. This

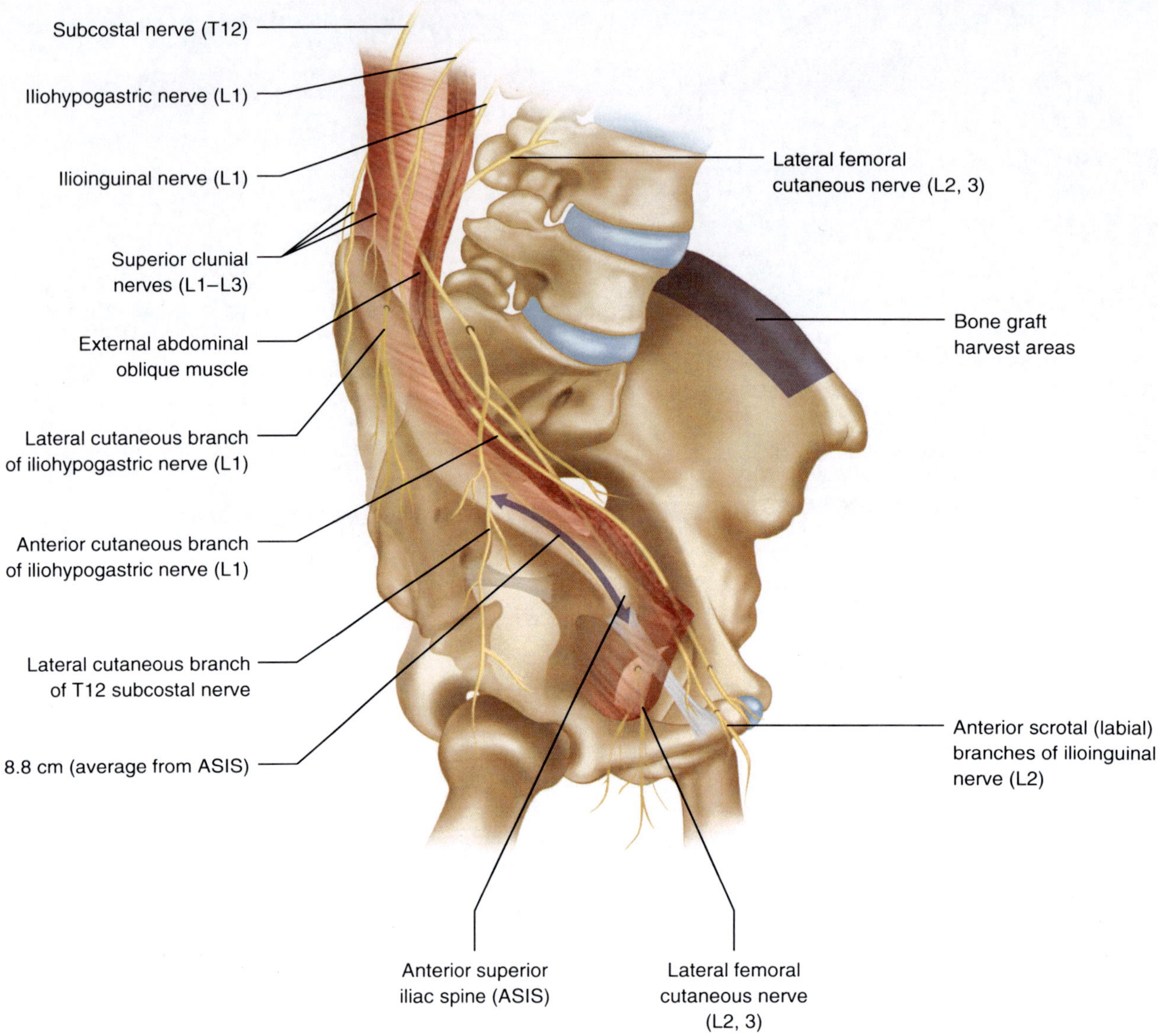

Fig. 8.4 Planned line of osteotomy to split iliac crest, with lateral cutaneous branch of the T12 subcostal nerve at risk for injury at the superior margin and the lateral femoral cutaneous nerve at risk for injury on the lateral and inferior margins

may be reduced utilizing a minimally invasive approach. Percutaneous hollow needle technique has been described to reduce blood loss as well as postoperative pain versus conventional open harvest (Fig. 8.10). Similarly, in comparing a minimally invasive technique utilizing a trephine system versus conventional open harvesting of cancellous bone, the minimally invasive technique was found to be a superior alternative, with shorter operative time, decreased requirement for pain medications, less pain on discharge, and a shorter hospital stay. Placement of continuous release analgesic systems has also been shown to be safe as well as reduce pain scores and time to first narcotic compared to traditional open techniques. Fractures of the leaves of the split crest, hematomas (0.1 %), infection (0.02 %), hernia (0.02 %), parasthesia (0.18 %), and hardware failure (0.14 %) have also been reported among the complications associated with iliac harvest.

Tibia

The proximal tibia has long been used as an excellent source of cancellous bone with minimal morbidity. Cancellous bone volumes equaling or exceeding that of the iliac crest can be harvested. Volumetric analyses of the proximal tibia using three-dimensional imaging reconstruction have shown an average of 77 cm^2 of cancellous bone available for harvest in the proximal tibia, two to three times the accepted

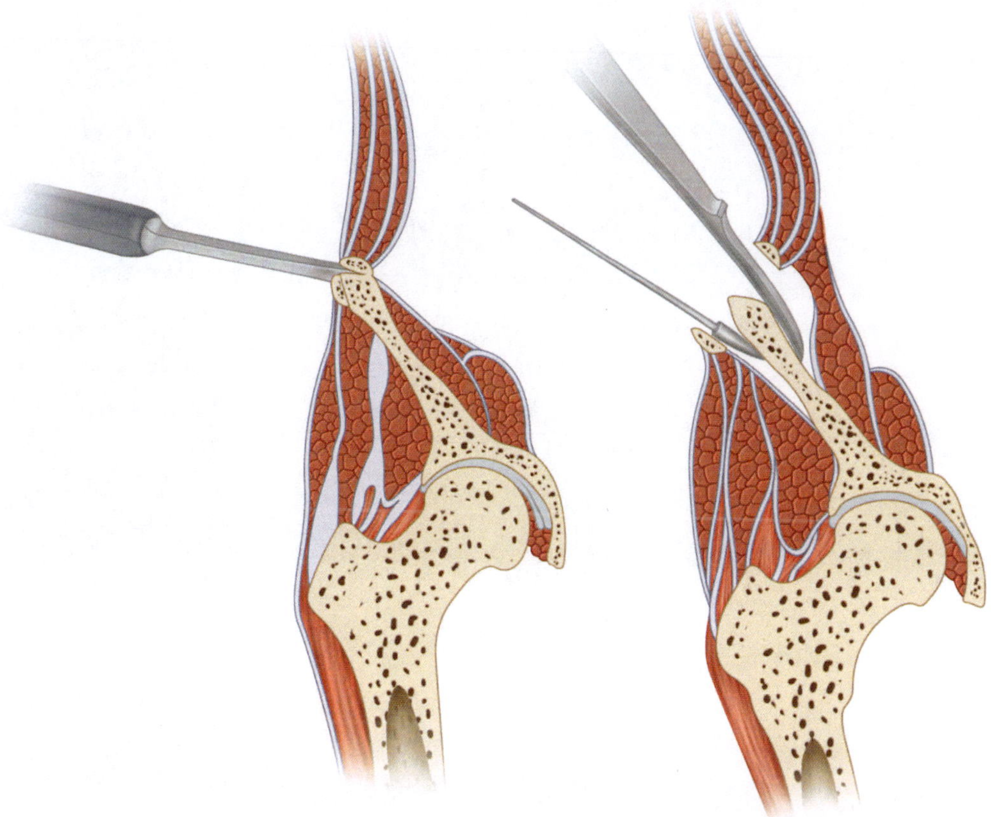

Fig. 8.5 (*Left*) The iliac crest is split medially and laterally, leaving the abdominal muscles attached medially, and the gluteal muscles attached laterally. (*Right*) Subperiosteal dissection can then be performed medially and laterally to allow for the harvest of corticocancellous grafts

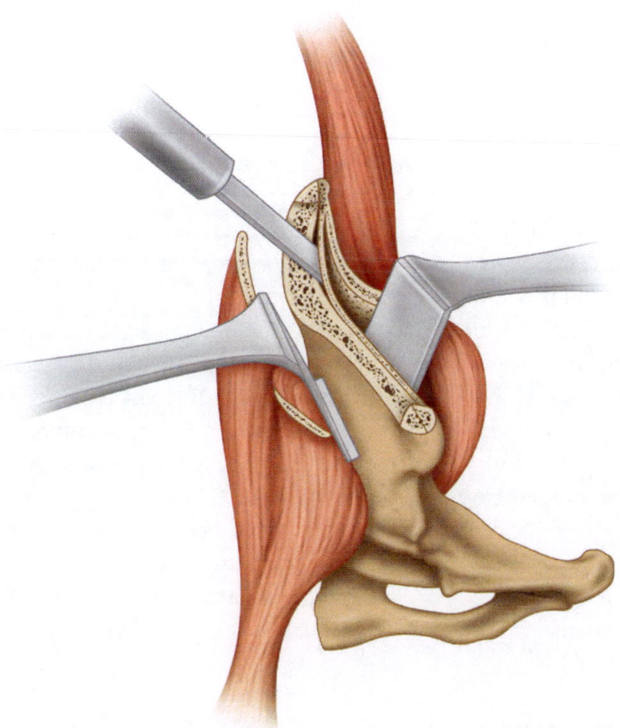

Fig. 8.6 Following splitting of the crest and medial subperiosteal elevation, corticocancellous bone graft can be harvested with osteotomes

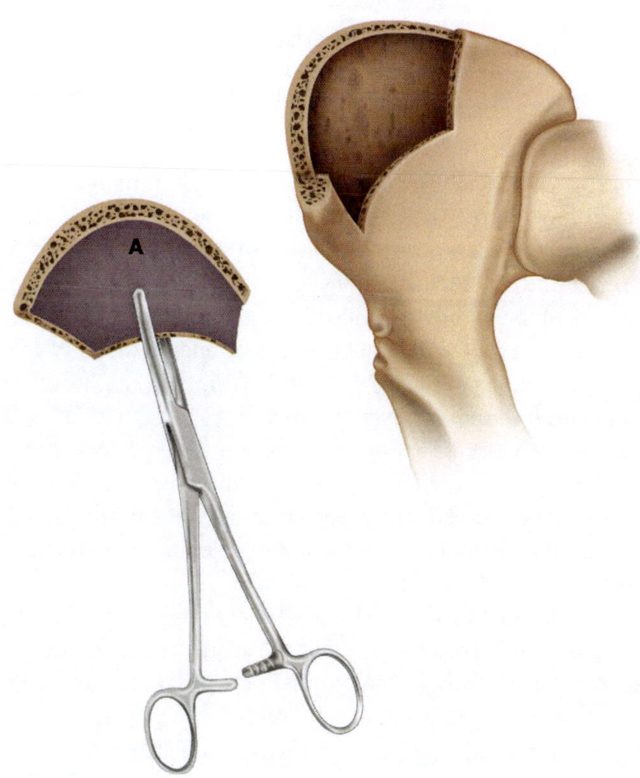

Fig. 8.7 Harvest of a large corticocancellous graft, up to 6 × 10 cm, can be achieved

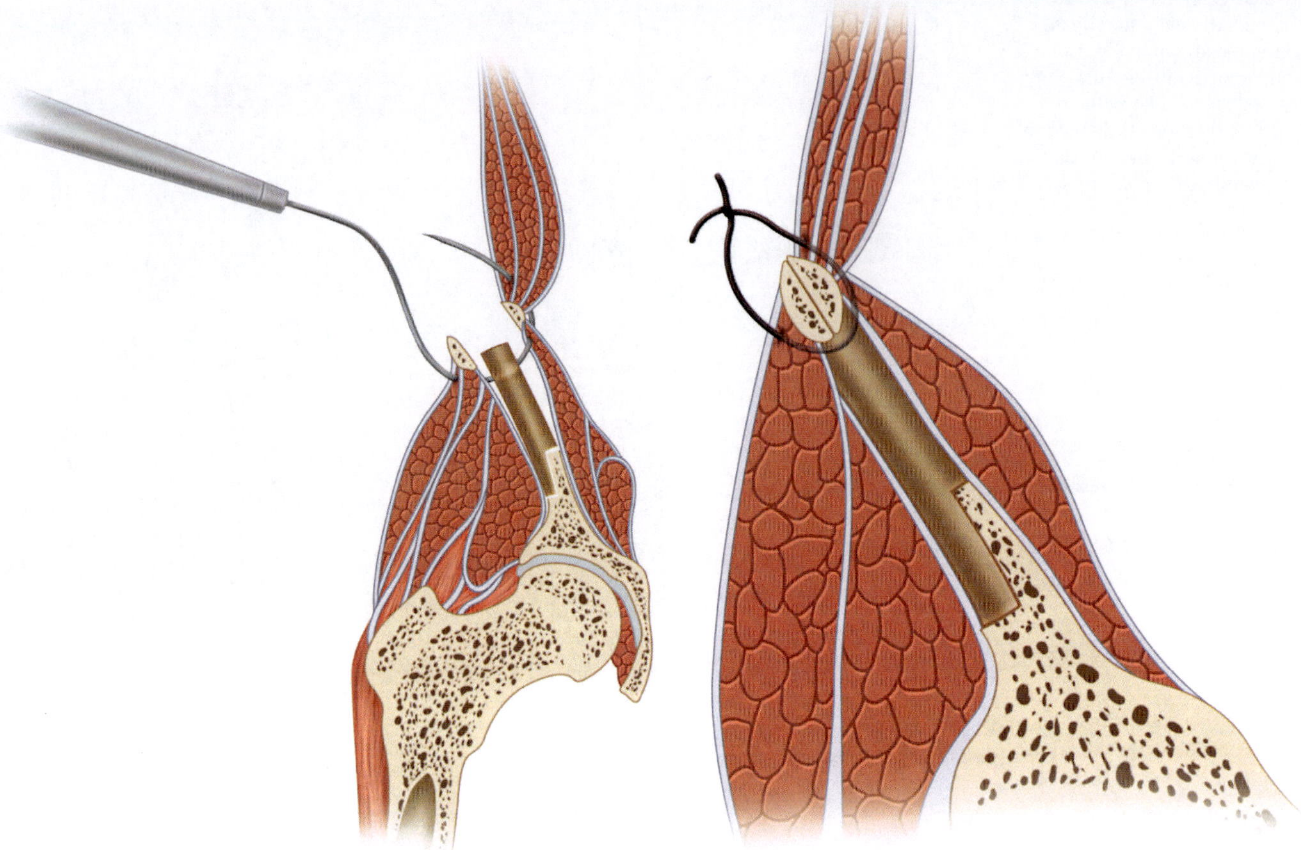

Fig. 8.8 Closure of the donor site is achieved by passing four 26 gauge wires or sturdy resorbable sutures to reapproximate the medial and lateral leafs of the split iliac crest. The reapproximated leaves should rest on the anterior superior iliac spine to provide stability and can be fixed to the ASIS with wire or suture

average. Due to their rigidity, tibial cortical grafts are more difficult to contour than calvarial grafts, but remain a potential source of strong cortical bone graft. With regard to graft harvest, the procedure begins by palpating and marking Gerdy's tubercle. Gerdy's tubercle is the bony protuberance between the patellar ligament (midline) and the head of the fibula, which is palpable 90° laterally (Fig. 8.11). A tourniquet is used for hemostasis, and local anesthetic with adrenaline is also used for vasoconstriction and postoperative pain control. A 3 cm incision is made directly over Gerdy's tubercle, and dissection proceeds through the thin soft tissue layer and periosteum down to the tubercle. A 1 cm^2 cortical window is made using osteotomes, or a circular window using a surgical drill; a circular window has the theoretical advantage of less stress than at the angles of a square or rectangular window in the cortical bone. Curettes are then used to harvest the cancellous bone from the tibial plateau and down the tibial shaft, with great care taken to avoid entering the joint space superiorly (Figs. 8.12 and 8.13). If a 1–2 cm wide strip of cortical bone is required, the approach is modified, utilizing a skin incision that begins under the tibial tuberosity and arcs medially as it courses down the leg, and through the superficial fascia. The fascial edges are reflected to expose the tibia. The periosteum is incised in a slightly larger area than the planned donor site, maintaining a connected edge. A sharp osteotome is then driven into the cortex and used to mark the donor site, and a corticoperiosteal flap pedicled superiorly at the tuberosity is preserved for later closure. Cancellous bone is then extracted from the upper epiphysis using curettes (Fig. 8.14). The donor site may be packed with Gelfoam, and the corticoperiosteal strap unfolded to cover the donor site. Closure is completed in layers, with closed suction drainage and a pressure dressing applied from the toes to the knee.

Complications are few and have been reported as low as 0.3 %. They include transient postoperative pain, hematoma requiring drianage, infection, and fracture of the tibial eminence.

Calvarium

Calvarial bone is extensively utilized in craniofacial reconstruction, with Tessier outlining the use of autologous calvarial bone grafts for facial and cranial reconstruction. Its rich diploic vascular system allows for rapid revascularization

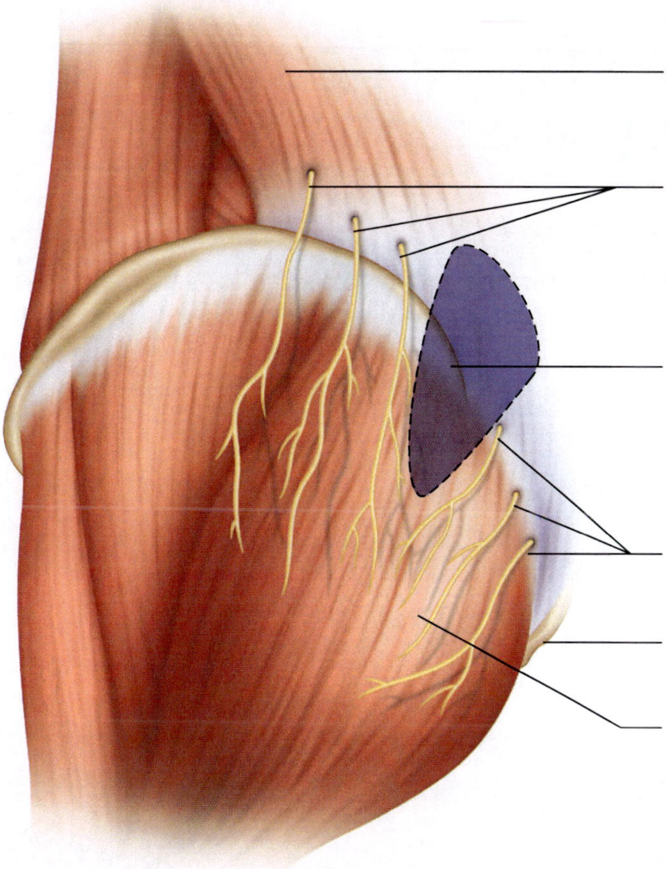

Fig. 8.9 Posterior iliac crest harvest. In order to avoid injury to the superior and middle cluneal nerves during harvesting of a posterior iliac bone graft, a linear incision approximately 2.5 cm anterior to the PSIS and perpendicular to the long axis of the posterior iliac crest is recommended. Subperiosteal dissection over the PSIS on each side of the axis of the incision (2.5 cm on each side) will most likely avoid injury to the superior and middle cluneal nerves

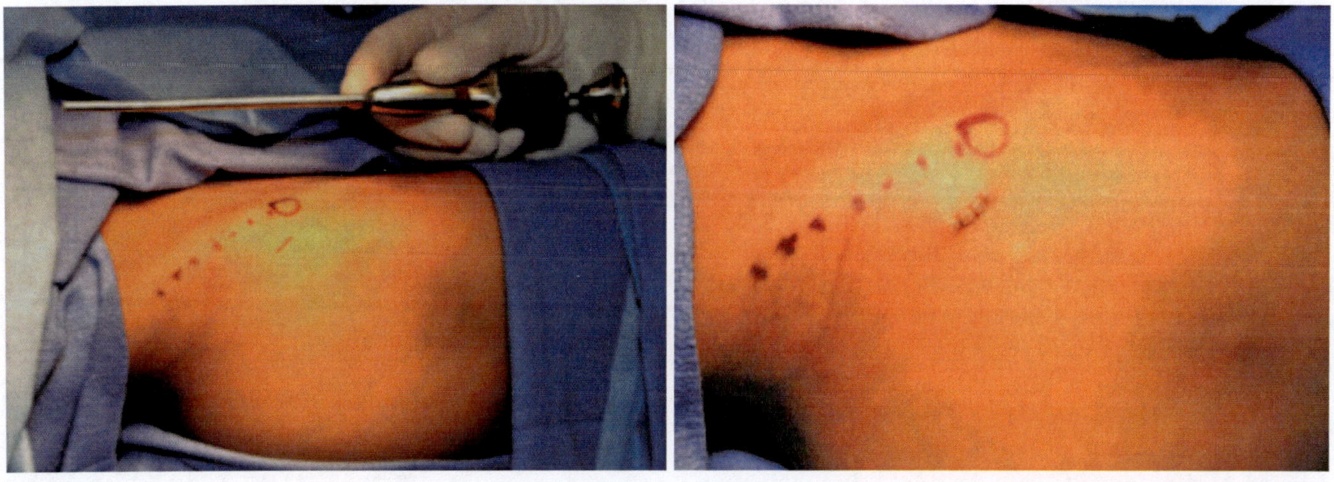

Fig. 8.10 Percutaneous harvest of iliac bone graft. The skin incision is made 3 cm posterior and inferior to the ASIS (marked with a *circle*)

and decreased resorption compared to other corticocancellous grafts. Furthermore, the calvarium is an intramembranous bone, which is thought to undergo less resorption than endochondral bone. Proximity to the recipient site, as well as minimal donor site morbidity, makes these grafts ideal for calvarial, orbital, nasal, and midfacial applications. Calvarial grafts can be selected based upon natural shape, but contour may be improved with bone benders. Attention must be paid to the location of the coronal and sagittal sutures (Fig. 8.15), as well as the posterior perforating vessels, the anterior temporal crest, and the intraosseous lateral vein. A preoperative coronal CT scan is of use in assessing the thickness of the parietal bones for harvesting grafts and of any potential midline abnormalities.

Harvest of calvarial grafts may be achieved through a variety of techniques. A coronal incision is made through the

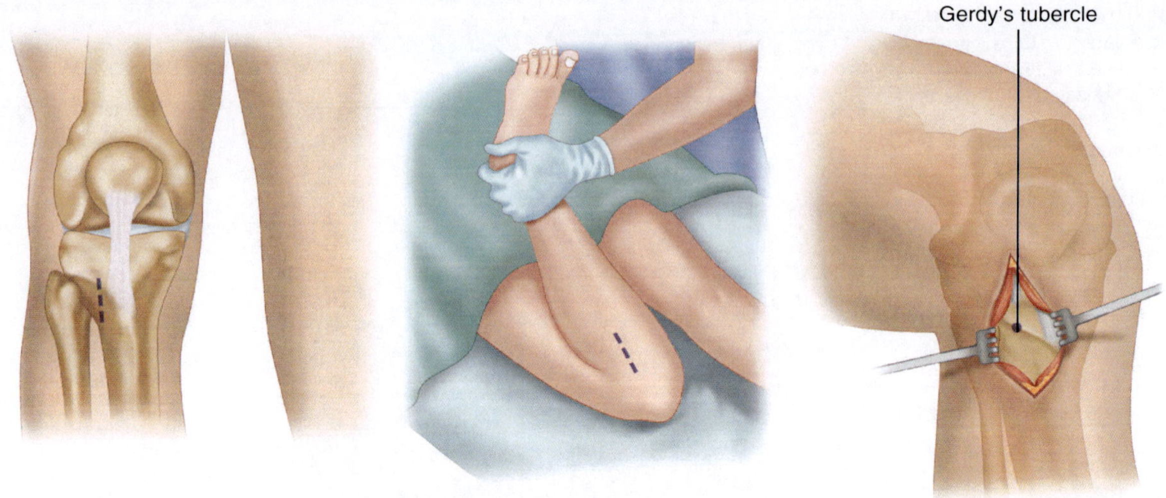

Fig. 8.11 Gerdy's tubercle is the tuberosity on the anterolateral side of the upper end of the tibia giving attachment to the iliotibial tract; it is located between the tibial tuberosity in the midline and the fibular head laterally. As there are no vital structures overlying Gerdy's tubercle, an approach centered over it is safe and effective

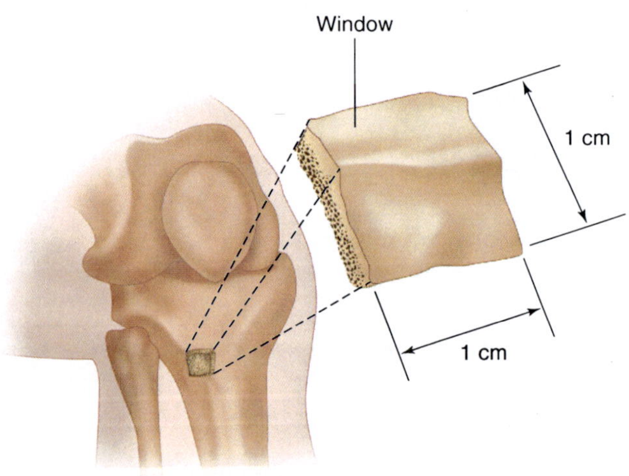

Fig. 8.12 A square or circular 1 × 1 cm ostetomy is made through Gerdy's tubercle, exposing the cancellous bone

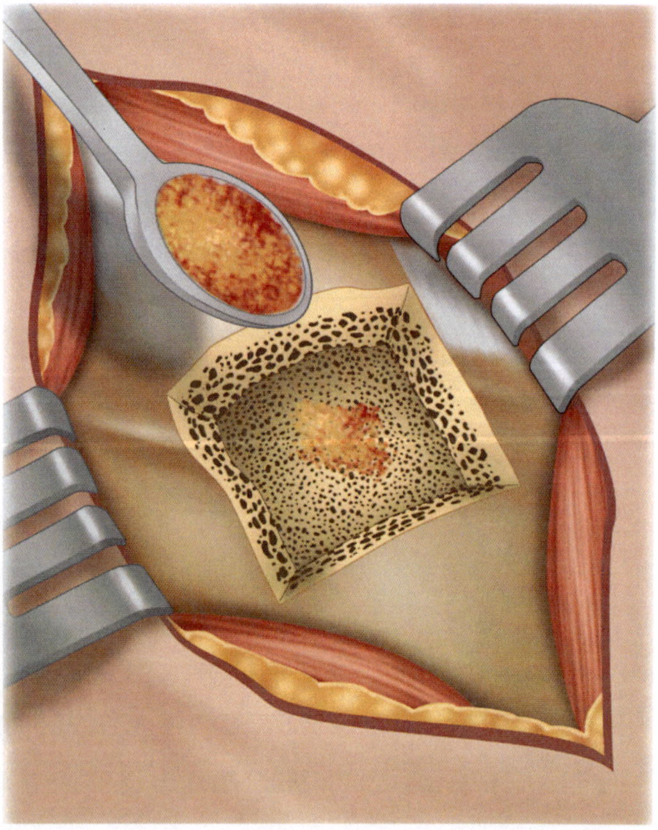

Fig. 8.13 Around 70 cm^2 of cancellous graft can be harvested from the proximal tibia; care must be taken during superior graft harvest to avoid injury to the tibial plateau and entering the joint space

scalp and galea. The pericranium is then incised and elevated with wide Obwegesers, with Gelfoam and bone wax used to help achieve hemostasis. For split in situ grafts, the outline of the donor site is first scribed with a saw or chisel. An oval 6 mm, side-cutting bur is then used to delineate the bone grafts. A narrow anterior strip is scribed and removed in order to allow room to keep the calvarial splitting osteotomes tangential. Alternating straight and curved osteotomes of varying widths are then used to split the bone. Following removal of the cortical segments, the diploe may be removed in sheets with a straight osteotome. This harvest may extend as far back as the lambdoid suture. The donor site may be covered with a large sheet of Surgicel. Closure is completed in layers, with the pericranium sutured over the donor site, the galea approximated, and a closed suction drain placed before final closure of the scalp with sutures or staples (Fig. 8.16).

An intracranial approach may be a better option, especially in the pediatric patient where in situ splitting may not be feasible secondary to a thin or irregular skull. A team approach with a neurosurgeon is recommended in these instances.

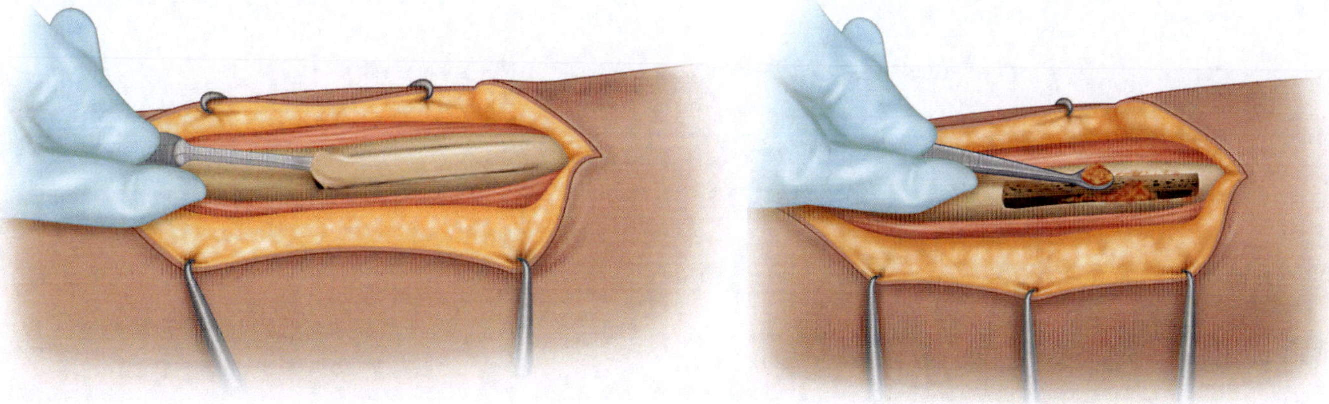

Fig. 8.14 (*Left*) Elevation of the superiorly based corticoperiosteal flap, used for closure, prior to removal of the outer tibial cortex. (*Right*) Following removal of the cortex, cancellous bone can be easily harvested from the upper epiphysis

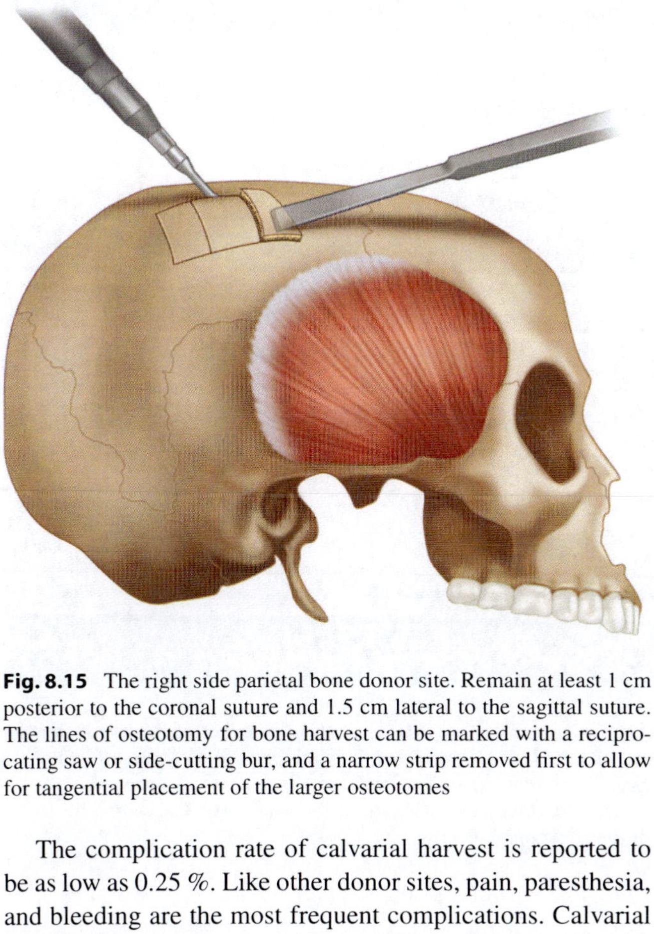

Fig. 8.15 The right side parietal bone donor site. Remain at least 1 cm posterior to the coronal suture and 1.5 cm lateral to the sagittal suture. The lines of osteotomy for bone harvest can be marked with a reciprocating saw or side-cutting bur, and a narrow strip removed first to allow for tangential placement of the larger osteotomes

The complication rate of calvarial harvest is reported to be as low as 0.25 %. Like other donor sites, pain, paresthesia, and bleeding are the most frequent complications. Calvarial irregularities may also occur; however, these are often camouflaged by hair. Alopecia along the scalp incision line may be avoided by minimizing thermal injury along this area.

Rib

Free rib grafts can be harvested in a variety of ways: full thickness, split thickness, and as composite costochondral grafts. They are suitable for reconstruction of the mandible, as well as defects of the zygoma, orbits, and calvarium. They contain little cancellous bone with a thin cortex and are best fixed using wires. Careful microplate fixation, such as in cantilever rib grafts for salvage rhinoplasty, is also a possibility.

Preoperative markings and landmarks are dependent upon the amount of harvest required. Regardless of the extent of harvest, the technique follows the same principles. In the case of single rib harvests, an incision is made directly over the rib to be harvested; if two ribs are being harvested, an incision is made over the rib between those that will be harvested. Skipping ribs when harvesting multiple ribs will help maintain chest wall stability and avoid contour deformities. Incisions are usually made over the fifth, sixth, or seventh rib on the right side of the chest (Fig. 8.17).

These are often hidden within the breast fold of female patients. Costal cartilage graft harvest occurs more medially. Taking advantage of short incisions and appropriate retractors will help avoid unnecessary subcutaneous dissection and will decrease the risk of pneumothorax. Skin and superficial thoracic fascia is first incised, followed by the deep thoracic fascia directly over the targeted rib. The periosteum is incised longitudinally over the lateral surface and an angled elevator used to elevate tissues subperiosteally along the edges of the rib. Ribs should be divided close to the costochondral junction. Once the rib is divided, Semb elevators are used to continue the subperiosteal dissection posteriorly. The use of Semb elevators will reduce the risk of pneumothorax. Retractors should be repositioned as the dissection progresses deeper (Fig. 8.18).

The wound should be irrigated and checked for any air leak. Closure is achieved in a layered fashion: edges of the periosteum, followed by approximation of the deep fascia and muscles, followed by closure of the superficial fascia and skin (Fig. 8.19). A costal cartilage graft, such as those used in microtia repair, requires partial division of the rectus, which must be repaired during the final closure.

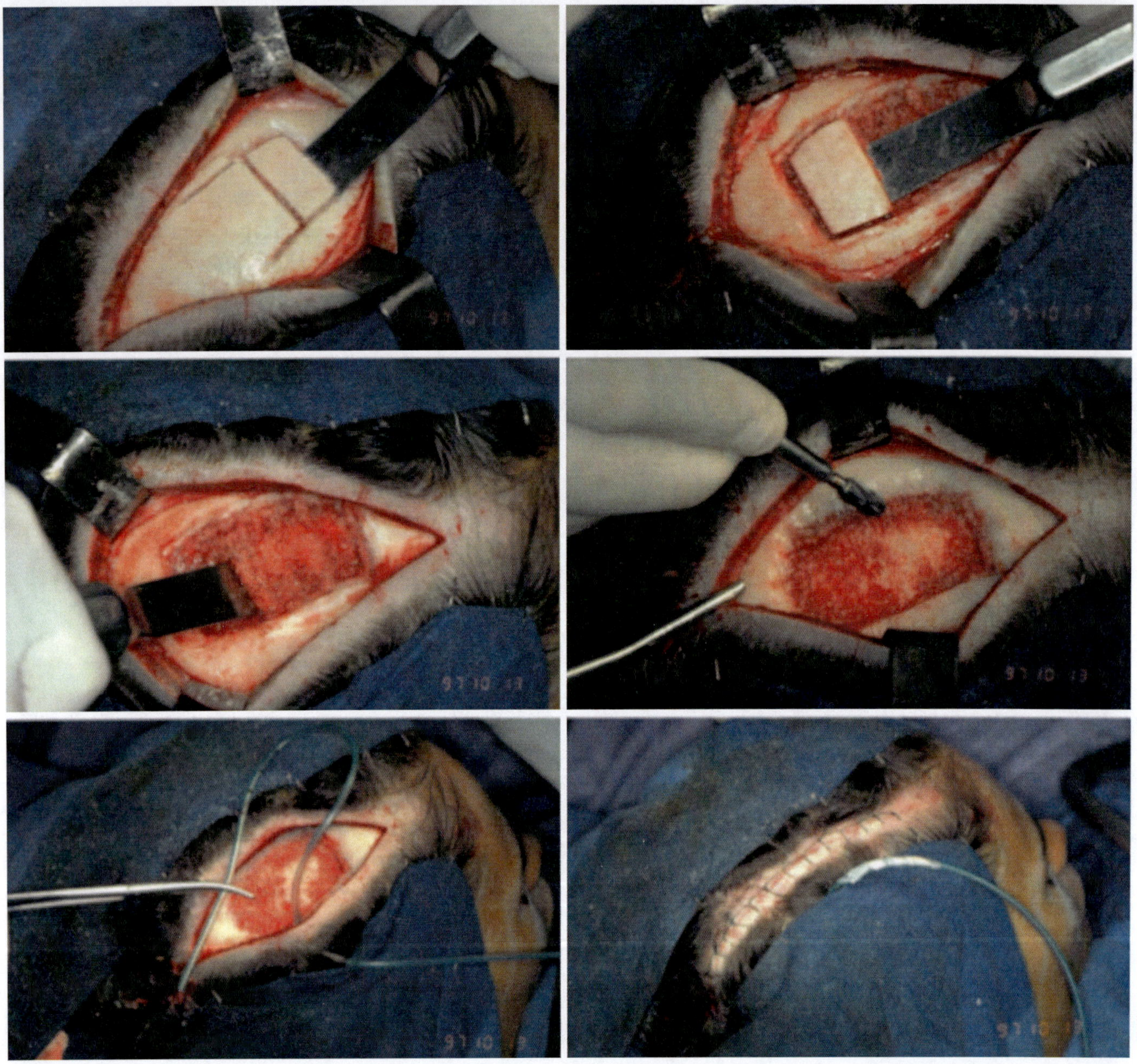

Fig. 8.16 (*Top left*) Following scalp incision, periosteal elevation, and osteotomy line scoring, grafts can be removed with a sharp osteotome. (*Top right*) Removal of the final graft. Grafts can be harvested to within 1 cm of the lambdoid suture. (*Middle left*) Following removal of the corticocancellous graft, diploic cancellous graft can be harvested with curettes or osteotomes. (*Middle right*) The edges of the donor site can be smoothed with a pineapple burr to decrease any step-offs palpable through the scalp. (*Bottom left*) Drain placement to help avoid fluid collection. (*Bottom right*) Closure of the scalp over Gelfoam with either sutures or staples

The overall complication rate for ribs harvested using the above technique is 0.9 %. One of the primary concerns regarding harvest of rib grafts is the risk of pneumothorax. This is a relatively low risk (1 %) when proper technique and tools are utilized. Also, when harvesting multiple rib grafts, skipping ribs will help avoid chest wall contour deformities as well as maintain chest wall stability.

Mandible

The mandible provides a local source of membranous (body and ramus) and endochondral (condyle) bone. As well as the advantage of proximity to the recipient site, bone may be harvested intraorally, which eliminates the morbidity of cutaneous scarring.

Harvest approach and technique is dependent upon the specific mandible donor site. For a mandibular symphysis harvest, one may approach with a vestibular or a sulcular incision, the latter being used in cases of healthy dentition without any crowns (Fig. 8.20).

The vestibular incision is made 1.5 cm from the gingival sulcus and continues through the mentalis muscle while preserving the gingival, periosteal, and mentalis insertion attachments superiorly, similar to an osseous genioplasty approach. For the sulcular approach, an incision is made along the gingiva from second bicuspid to second bicuspid, with oblique relaxing incisions made at the distal buccal line. A full thickness mucoperiosteal flap is then elevated, enabling complete visualization of the symphysis and bilateral mental neurovascular bundles. In either approach, the superior osteotomy should be at least 5 mm below the root apices, as well as 5 mm from the mental foramina, and should penetrate the labial cortex. Depth is dependent upon graft thickness (Fig. 8.21). Closure is achieved in a layered fashion, with care to avoid the complication of mentalis or chin ptosis in the case of the vestibular approach.

When harvesting from the ramus and body, an incision is made distal to the most posterior tooth and continues to the retromolar pad and up the ascending ramus (Fig. 8.22).

Oblique incisions may be made at the posterior extent of the incision. The incision extends along the buccal sulcus opposite the first bicuspid. The temporalis is stripped from the bone with an elevator superiorly, and a full thickness mucoperiosteal flap reflected inferiorly. Three complete osteotomies are made: one superior and two vertical. Another horizontal bone groove is made at the inferior border. The superior osteotomy is created with a small fissure

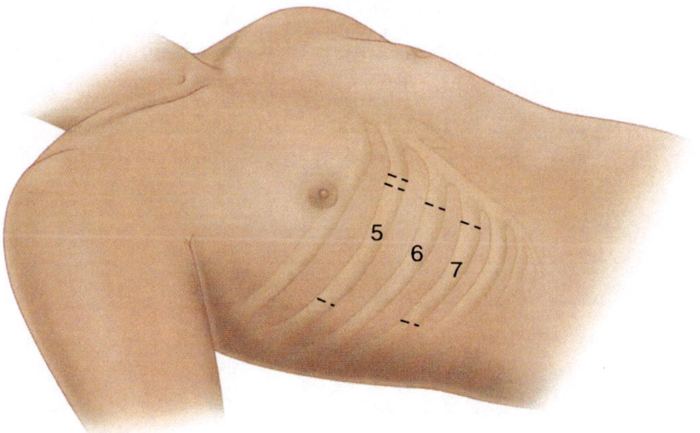

Fig. 8.17 The fifth, sixth, or seventh ribs are most commonly used for either costal or costochondral grafts

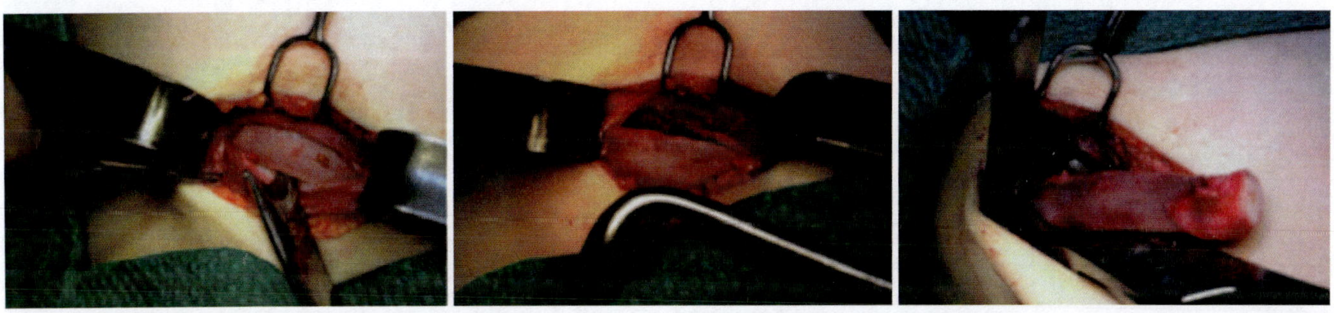

Fig. 8.18 (*Left*) Following dissection straight down to the rib, the perisosteum is incised and elevated from the superior and inferior (pictured) surface of the rib. (*Center*) A Doyen elevator can then be passed from inferiorly to superiorly in the subperiosteal plane and used to free the periosteum from the rib posteriorly. (*Right*) A cartilagenous cap can be left on the medial surface of the rib, as in ascending ramus reconstruction in hemifacial microsomia, and the rib can be divided laterally using a costotome

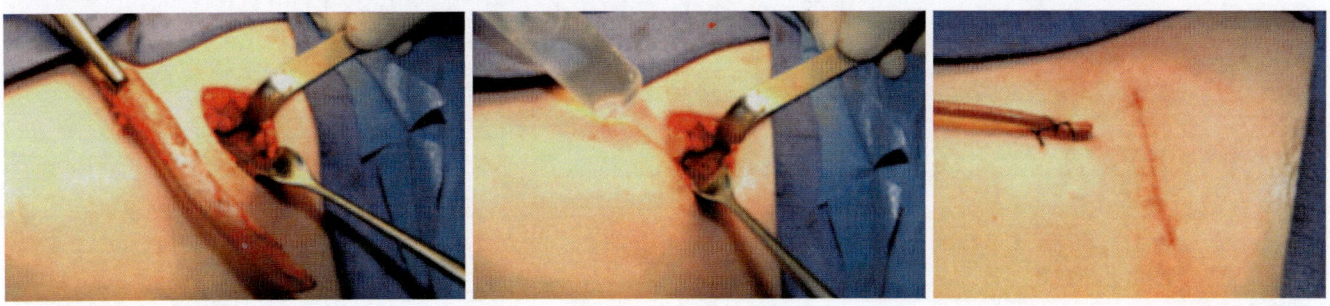

Fig. 8.19 (*Left*) A long section of rib (15 cm) can be harvested through a smaller incision. (*Center*) Prior to closure, the wound should be filled with normal saline and positive pressure breaths given to look for bubbles, which would be indicative of a pleural tear. (*Left*) Closure of the incision (with drain optional placement)

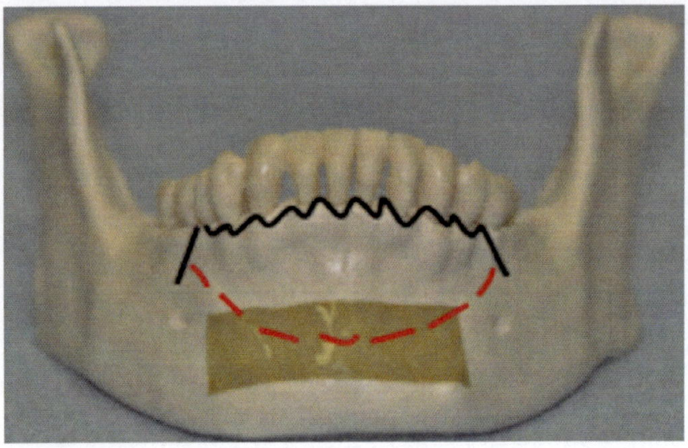

Fig. 8.20 Mandibular symphysis bone grafts can be harvested via vestibular (*dotted red line*) or sulcular (*curvilinear black line*) incisions. The sulcular incision should be reserved for those patients with healthy dentition without anterior crowns

bur 4–5 mm medial to the external oblique ridge. The superior osteotomy begins at the mandibular first or second molar and continues posteriorly along the ascending ramus depending on the required size. Anterior and posterior vertical osteotomies begin at each end of the superior cut and are made 10–12 mm in length in the superoinferior direction. Finally, a groove connecting the inferior aspect of each vertical osteotomy is made using a round bur. The graft is then split at the osteotomies using sharp chisels and is fractured along the inferior groove (Fig. 8.23). Care is taken to avoid injury to the inferior alveolar neurovascular bundle, which is visible 10–12 % of the time. Sharp edges may be smoothed with a large round fissure bur. Following adequate hemostasis, closure is achieved in layered fashion.

Harvest of mandibular bone may be complicated by temporary mental nerve hypersthesia, parasthesia, and altered sensation, with each of these being higher in cases of symphysis

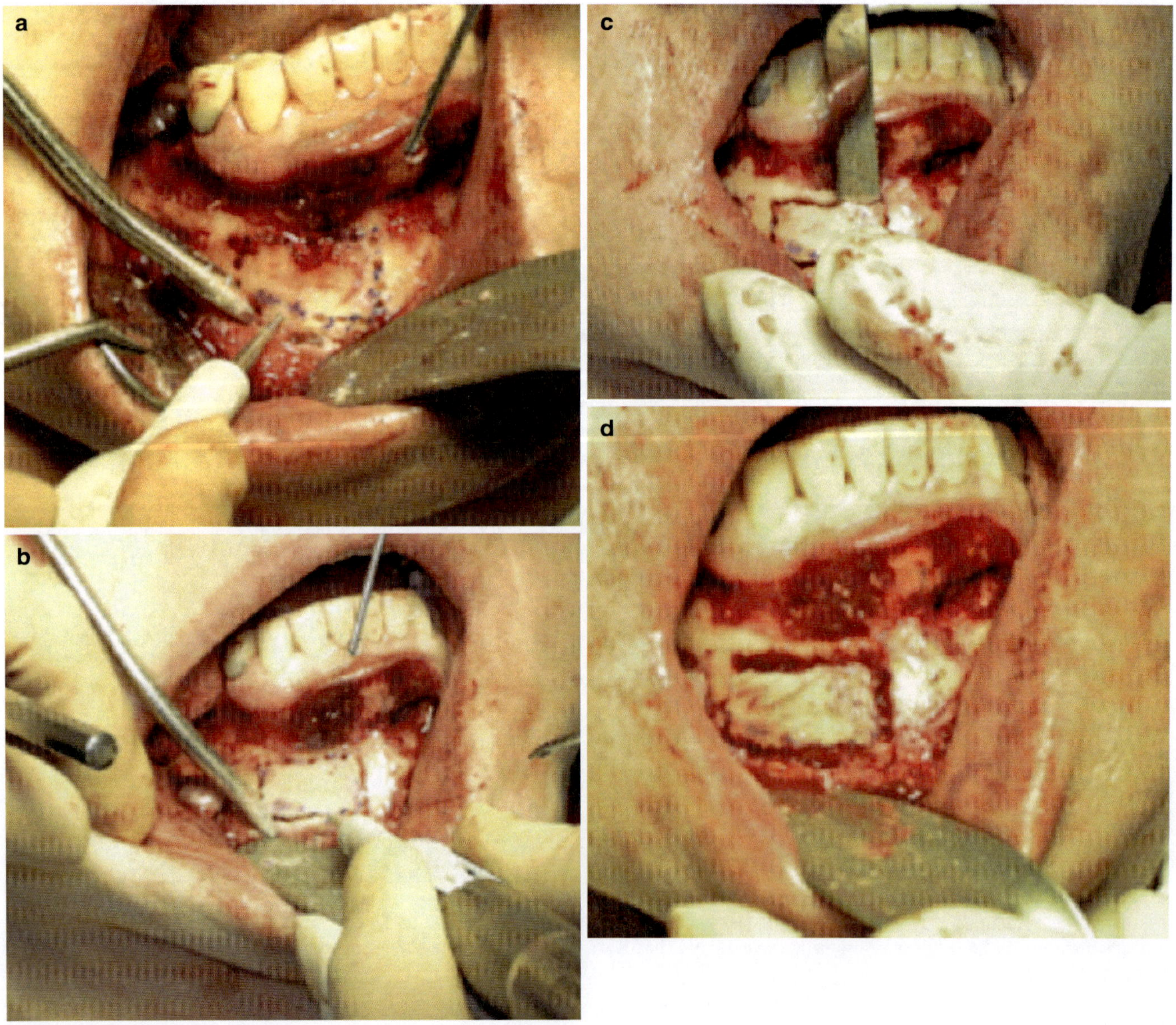

Fig. 8.21 (**a**) Marking the osteotomy of the mandibular symphysis with a marking pen. (**b**) Using a small round bur to incise the labial cortex. (**c**) Harvesting the labial cortex using a small osteotome. (**d**) The freed corticocancellous block harvested from the right mandibular symphysis

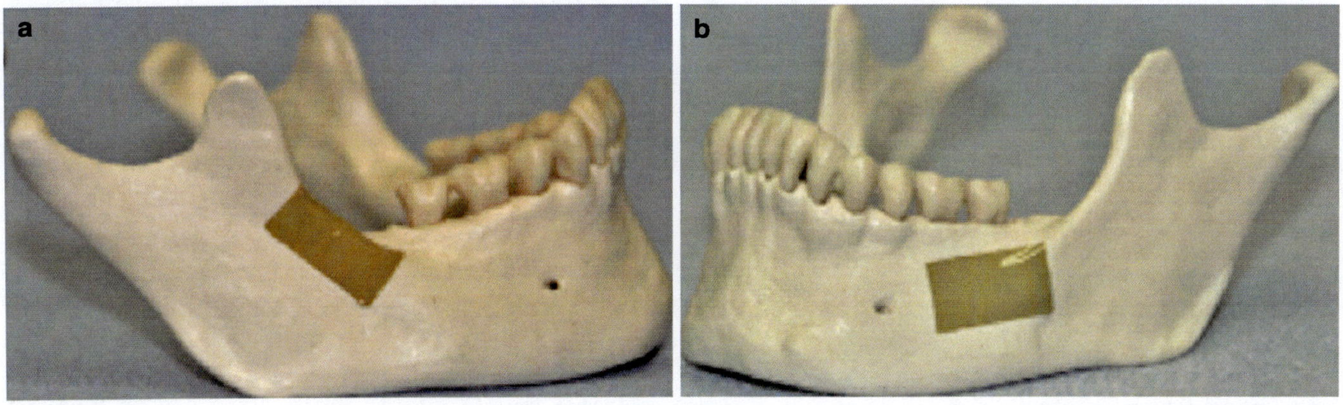

Fig. 8.22 Bone grafts can be harvested from the ascending mandibular ramus (**a**) or mandibular body (**b**)

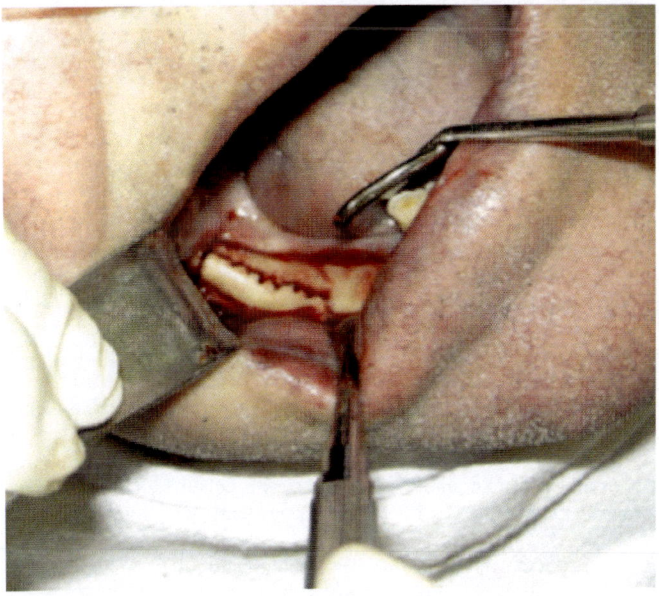

Fig. 8.23 Bone graft harvest from the right ascending mandibular ramus. Care must be taken to avoid injury to the inferior alveolar neurovascular bundle

harvest. Infection rates and permanent neurosensory deficits are reported to be less than 1 %. The vestibular approach for symphysis harvest may also result in chin ptosis, scar band formation, as well as postoperative pain. The ramus/body approach therefore offers the advantages of similar bone stock with decreased risk of neurosensory disruption.

Allogenic Bone Grafts

Allografts are taken from the same species and are usually cadaveric. They may also be harvested from living donors. The ideal allograft would provide a combination of space maintenance, osteoconductive structural guidance for bone regeneration, acceleration of bone remodeling, and may act as a carrier for antibiotics, growth factors, or other tissue-engineering approaches. Allografts retain osteoinductive (they release BMPs) and osteoconductive properties, but lack osteogenic properties because of the absence of viable cells. While these constructs are acellular, there remains concern regarding the association of allogenic material and the risk of transmission of viral diseases, malignancies, systemic disorders, or toxins. The use of allografts has increased recently given improvements in processing and preservation, but this has resulted in a decrease of the osteoinductive properties. Allografts come in a variety of shapes and sizes: complete bone segments, corticocancellous or cortical grafts, cancellous chips, and most commonly, demineralized bone matrix (DBM). Allografts are also not without additional cost. The benefits, however, include abundant supply, potential addition of growth factors, and decreased donor site morbidity.

Specifically for craniofacial reconstruction, allogenic DBM has been used to supplement cancellous autograft. DBM is prepared by pulverizing allogenic bone to a consistent size, followed by extraction of the mineralized phase of bone. This results in a composite of noncollagenous proteins, growth factors, and collagen, which lacks any structural stability. DBM is usually available in a variety of constitutes including putty block form, moldable paste with bone chips, gel form, and an injectable bone paste. DBM application is therefore limited to structurally stable environments. The addition of supplemental DBM allograft and cancellous allograft to iliac autograft in cleft alveolar defects has been shown to be safe and effective, resulting in low morbidity, shorter operative times, and higher rates of bone graft survival when compared to autograft alone. Similarly, a randomized controlled clinical trial comparison of the utility of synthetic biomaterials, bovine-derived bone substitutes, and human-derived allografts to autograft in maxillary sinus augmentation resulted in human-derived allograft providing the second highest rate of de novo bone formation, behind that of autograft. For most all other craniofacial reconstruction applications, however, autograft remains preferred over allograft.

Vascularized Bone Grafts

Vascularized bone flaps are superior to nonvascularized grafts, owing to a lack of dependency on recipient bed vascularity. Indications include irradiated and chronic defects as well as those whose vascularity is compromised by extensive scarring. By bringing with it a robust blood supply, free bone flaps in turn increase blood flow to the recipient site and may be tailored to include skin, muscle, and nerves in addition to bone. Vascularized bone grafts are covered in detail elsewhere.

Xenogenic Bone Grafts

Xenografts are taken from different species and are usually of bovine or porcine origin. These are rarely used in the setting of craniofacial surgery as they are void of growth factors and proteins and therefore are inferior in their utility to autografts and allografts.

Bibliography

Andrew JG, Hoyland JA, Freemont AJ, Marsh DR. Platelet-derived growth factor expression in normally healing human fractures. Bone. 1995;16(4):455–60.

Ang E, Black C, Irish J, Brown DH, Gullane P, O'Sullivan B, Neligan PC. Reconstructive options in the treatment of osteoradionecrosis of the craniomaxillofacial skeleton. Br J Plast Surg. 2003;56(2):92–9.

Ashinoff RL, Cetrulo CL, Galiano RD, Dobryansky M, Bhatt KA, Ceradini DJ, Michaels J, McCarthy JG, Gurtner GC. Bone morphogenic protein-2 gene therapy for mandibular distraction osteogenesis. Ann Plast Surg. 2004;52:585–90.

Boyle WJ, Simonet WS, Lacey DL. Osteoclast differentiation and activation. Nature. 2003;423:337–42.

Buck DW, Dumanian GA. Bone biology and physiology: part I. The fundamentals. Plast Reconstr Surg. 2012;126(6):1314–20.

Buckwater JA, Glimcher MJ, Cooper RR, Recker R. Bone biology. J Bone Joint Surg Am. 1995;77:1256–75.

Chou D, Storm P, Campbell J. Vulnerability of the subcostal nerve to injury during bone graft harvesting from the iliac crest. J Neurosurg. 2004;1:87–9.

Ehrenfeld M, Hagenmaier C. Autogenous bone grafts in maxillofacial reconstruction. Craniomaxillofacial reconstructive and corrective bone surgery. New York: Springer; 2002.

Englestad M, Morse T. Anterior iliac crest, posterior iliac crest, and proximal tibia donor sites: a comparison of cancellous bone volumes in fresh cadavers. J Oral Maxillofac Surg. 2010;68:3015–21.

Engstand T. Biomaterails and biologics in craniofacial reconstruction. J Craniofac Surg. 2012;23(1):239–42.

Fallucco MA, Carstens MH. Primary reconstruction of alveolar clefts using recombinant human bone morphogenetic protein-2: clinical and radiographic outcomes. J Craniofac Surg. 2009;20(2):1759–64.

Feldmeier JJ. Hyperbaric oxygen and wound healing in the head and neck, in essential tissue healing of the face and neck. Shelton: People's Medical Publishing House; 2009.

Fisher C, MacIsaac ZM, Grunwaldt LJ, Boretsky K, Kumar AR. Examining the effects of regional anesthesia on iliac crest bone graft harvest during alveolar cleft repair. Presented at The Ohio Valley Society of Plastic Surgeons 55th annual meeting, Cleveland, May 2012.

Gateno J, Teichgraeber JF, Aguillar E. Computer planning for distraction osteogenesis. Plast Reconstr Surg. 2000;105(3):873–82.

Graham S, Leonidou A, Lester M, Heliotis M, Mantalaris A, Tsiridis E. Investigating the role of PDGF as a potential drug therapy in bone formation and fracture healing. Expert Opin Investig Drugs. 2009;18(11):1633–54.

Hardy SP, Wilke RC, Doyle JF. Advantages of percutaneous hollow needle technique for iliac bone harvest in alveolar cleft grafting. Cleft Palate Craniofac J. 1999;36(3):252–5.

Havlik RJ. Rigid fixation and bone healing in craniofacial surgery, in craniofacial surgery. Philadelphia: W.B. Saunders Company; 2002.

Howell TH, Fiorellini JP, Paquette DW, et al. A phase I/II clinical trial to evaluate a combination of recombinant human platelet-derived growth factor-BB and recombinant human insulin-like growth factor-I in patients with periodontal disease. J Periodontol. 1997;68(12):1186–93.

Kanaan RA, Kanaan LA. Transforming growth factor beta1, bone connection. Med Sci Monit. 2006;12(8):164–9.

Karsenty G. The genetic transformation of bone biology. Genes Dev. 1999;13:3037–51.

Kolk A, Handschek J, Drescher W, Rothamel D, Kloss F, Blessmann M, Heiland M, Wolff KD, Smeets R. Current trends and future perspective on bone substitute material – from space holder to innovative biomaterials. J Craniomaxillofac Surg. 2012;40:706–18.

Lauritzen C, Davis C, Ivarsson A, Sanger C, Hewitt T. The evolving role of springs in craniofacial surgery: the first 100 clinical cases. Plast Reconstr Surg. 2008;121:545.

MacIsaac ZM, Rottgers SA, Davit III AJ, Ford M, Losee JE, Kimar AR. Alveolar reconstruction in cleft patients: decreased morbidity and improved outcomes with supplemental demineralized bone matrix and cancellous allograft. Plast Reconstr Surg. 2012;130(3):625–32.

Maeda M, Bryant MH, Yamagata M. Effects of irradiation on cortical bone and their time-related changes. A biomechanical and histomorphological study. J Bone Joint Surg Am. 1998;70:392–9.

Marie PJ. Fibroblast growth factor signaling controlling bone formation: an update. Gene. 2012;498(1):1–4.

Marie PJ, Coffin JD, Hurley MM. FGF and FGFR signaling in chondrodysplasias and craniosynostosis. J Cell Biochem. 2005;96:888–96.

Marx RE. Bone and bone graft healing. Oral Maxillofac Surg Clin North Am. 2007;19(4):455–66.

McCarthy JG, Schreiber J, Karp N. Lengthening the human mandible by gradual distraction. Plast Reconstr Surg. 1992;89:1–8.

McCarthy HS, Williams JH, Davie MW, Marshall MJ. Platelet-derived growth factor stimulates osteoprotegerin production in osteoblastic cells. J Cell Physiol. 2009;218(2):350–4.

McKibbin B. The biology of fracture healing in long bones. J Bone Joint Surg. 1978;60-B:150–62.

O'Keeffe Jr RM, Riemer BL, Butterfield SL. Harvesting of autogenous cancellous bone graft from the proximal tibial metaphysis. J Orthop Trauma. 1991;5(4):469–74.

Oppenheimer AJ, Tong L, Buchman SR. Craniofacial bone grafting: Wolff's law revisited. Craniomaxillofac Trauma Reconstr. 2008;1:49–61.

Ouaki J, Dadure C, Bringuier S, Raux O, Rochette A, Captier G, Capdevilla X. Continuous infusion of ropivacaine: an optimal postoperative analgesia regimen for iliac crest bone graft in children. Paediatr Anaesth. 2009;19(9):887–91.

Pikos MA. Mandibular block autografts for alveolar ridge augmentation. Atlas Oral Maxillofac Surg Clin North Am. 2005;13:91–107.

Polley JW, Figueroa AA, Kidd M. Principles of distraction osteogenesis in craniofacial surgery, in craniofacial surgery. Philadelphia: W.B. Saunders Company; 2002.

Rever LJ, Manson PN, Randolph MA, Yaremchuk MJ, Weiland A, Siegel JH. The healing of facial bone fracture by the process of secondary union. Plast Reconstr Surg. 1991;87(3):451–8.

Ripamonti U, Heliotis M, Ferretti C. Bone morphagenetic protein and the induction of bone formation: from laboratory to patients. Oral Maxillofac Surg Clin North Am. 2007;19(4):575–89.

Roden Jr RD. Principles of bone grafting. Oral Maxillofac Surg Clin North Am. 2010;22:295–300.

Rogers GF, Greene AK. Autogenous bone graft: basic science and clinical implications. J Craniofac Surg. 2012;23:323–7.

Salisbury Palomares KT, Gleason RE, Mason ZD, et al. Mechanical stimulation alters tissue differentiation and molecular expression during bone healing. J Orthop Res. 2009;27:1123–32.

Schmitt CM, Doering H, Schmidt T, Lutz R, Neukam FW, Schlegel KA. Histological results after maxillary sinus augmentation with Straumann® BoneCeramic, Bio-Oss®, Puros®, and autologous bone. A randomized controlled clinical trial. Clin Oral Implants Res. 2013;24(5):576–85.

Seitz IA, Teven CM, Reid RR. Repair and grafting of bone, in plastic surgery, vol. 1. 3rd ed. New York: Elsevier/Saunders; 2013.

Sharma S, Scheinder LF, Barr J, Sarabi S, Chibbaro P, Grayson B, Cutting CB. Comparison of minimally invasive versus conventional open harvesting techniques for iliac bone graft in secondary alveolar cleft patients. Plast Reconstr Surg. 2011;128(2):485–91.

Shubailat GF. Rib grafting in salvage rhinoplasty. Aesthetic Plast Surg. 2003;27:281–5.

Sittitavornwong S, Gutta R. Bone graft harvesting form regional sites. Oral Maxillofac Surg Clin North Am. 2010;22:317–30.

Snyder CC, Levine GA, Swanson HM, Browne Jr EX. Mandibular lengthening by gradual distraction: preliminary report. Plast Reconstr Surg. 1973;51:506–8.

Tessier P. Autogenous bone grafts taken from the calvarium for facial and cranial applications. Clin Plast Surg. 1982;9:531–8.

Tessier P, Kawamoto H, Matthews D, Posnick J, Raulo Y, Tulasne JF, Wolfe SA. Taking bone grafts from the anterior and posterior ilium-tools and techniques: II. A 6800-case experience in maxillofacial and craniofacial surgery. Plast Reconstr Surg. 2005a;116(5):25S–37.

Tessier P, Kawamoto H, Matthews D, Posnick J, Raulo Y, Tulasne JF, Wolfe SA. Complications of harvesting autogenous bone grafts: a group experience of 20,000 cases. Plast Reconstr Surg. 2005b;116(5):72S–3.

Tessier P, Kawamoto H, Matthews D, Posnick J, Raulo Y, Tulasne JF, Wolfe SA. Taking calvarial grafts, either split in situ or splitting of the parietal bone flap ex vivo-tools and techniques: V. A 9650-case experience in craniofacial and maxillofacial surgery. Plast Reconstr Surg. 2005c;116(5):54S–71.

Tessier P, Kawamoto H, Matthews D, Posnick J, Raulo Y, Tulasne JF, Wolfe SA. Taking long rib grafts for facial reconstruction-tools and techniques: III. A 2900-case experience in maxillofacial and craniofacial surgery. Plast Reconstr Surg. 2005d;116(5): 38S–46.

Tubbs R, Levin M, Loukas M, Potts E, Cohen-Gadol A. Anatomy and landmarks for the superior and middle cluneal nerves: application to posterior iliac crest harvest and entrapment syndromes. J Neurosurg Spine. 2010;13:356–9.

Wan DC, Nacamuli RP, Longaker MT. Craniofacial bone tissue engineering. Dent Clin N Am. 2006;50:175–90.

Wang K, Almeida L, Olsson A. Volume analysis of the proximal tibial metaphysis. J Oral Maxillofac Surg. 2007;65:2425–9.

Wolfe SA. On the maintenance and sharpening of instruments. Plast Reconstr Surg. 2005;16(5):89S–91.

Zouhary KJ. Bone graft harvesting from distant sites: concepts and techniques. Oral Maxillofac Surg Clin North Am. 2010;22:301–16.

Biomaterials

9

Russell Reid

Alloplastic cranioplasty is an ancient concept. From the Incan use of precious metals, to the first documented use of a synthetic material to repair a cranial defect (Fallopius, sixteenth century), to Meekeren's use of canine bone in a human subject, the quest for a suitable nonautologous material has been almost epic. In this quest, the characteristics of the ideal bone substitute have been established. The ideal bone substitute should be (1) chemically inert, (2) hypoallergenic or incapable of inducing a foreign-body reaction, (3) easily contoured, (4) stable and durable shape retention, (5) noncarcinogenic, and (6) capable of incorporation into or replacement with living tissue from the recipient. Although this ideal has not been reached, several products are available. The following discussion is based upon the three broad categories of substitutes used in clinical practice: (1) cement pastes, (2) biomaterials replaced by bone, and (3) prefabricated polymers.

Cement Pastes

Calcium Phosphates

Resembling the inorganic phase of bone, hydroxyapatite and related composites have been FDA approved for clinical use since 1994. Calcium phosphate substitutes have emerged as a more superior form of substitute compared to calcium sulfate variants due to their closer resemblance to bone, higher biocompatibility, and their tendency to undergo less resorption. Two main forms are available for use: ceramic pastes and cement pastes. Ceramic hydroxyapatite substitutes (e.g., Interpore, Interpore International, Irvine, CA) are difficult to mold. However, they demonstrate less resorption and better osteoconduction than their cement counterparts, as demonstrated in a series of animal experimentation. It has been shown that the higher the pore size, the greater degree of osteoconduction and osteoinduction, as substitutes composed of pure ceramic hydroxyapatite, or cement forms of higher tricalcium phosphate (80 % tricalcium phosphate/20 % hydroxyapatite) exhibited greater replacement by lamellar bone histologically. In turn, the higher tricalcium phosphate content, which yields to resorption and replacement by macropores, is typically more osteoinductive. The cement form of this material has been quite popular, due to its biocompatibility, malleability, and relative ease of handling.

Bone Source

The first commercially available calcium phosphate cement, BoneSource (Stryker Leibinger, Inc.) is composed of tetracalcium phosphate and dicalcium phosphate dehydrated and activated with water at a 4:1 ratio prior to use. After an isothermic reaction, the resulting paste can be contoured on the field, setting into pure hydroxyapatite within 20–25 min. Final set time is 4–6 h. A dry operative field is mandatory for this biomaterial to reach its final cured state. In this state, BoneSource achieves a compressive strength of 50 MPa and a diametral strength of 8 MPa. Several formulations exist to decrease the set time and make the substitute easier to handle in a wet field.

BoneSource has been used in numerous applications on the craniofacial skeleton. In one of the largest series to date, Burstein and colleagues reviewed their experience with this product in 61 patients, retrospectively (20-month mean follow-up). Inlay and onlay grafting were performed over a 3-year period. Postoperative complications were present in 11 % of patients, mainly seromas. Interestingly, the authors used slow-release antibiotic therapy (1 g cephalosporin mixed with 10 g of cement prior to use). In another large trial in cranioplasty patients ($n = 103$), 446 an overall infection rate of 5.8 % was achieved.

R. Reid, MD, PhD
Department of Surgery, Division of Pediatric Plastic Surgery, University of Chicago Medicine Comer Children's Hospital, Chicago, IL, USA
e-mail: rcube91298@yahoo.com

P.J. Taub et al. (eds.), *Ferraro's Fundamentals of Maxillofacial Surgery*,
DOI 10.1007/978-1-4614-8341-0_9, © Springer Science+Business Media New York 2015

Norian SRS/CRS

Norian (Synthes, Inc.) was a unique carbonated calcium phosphate that mimicked the inorganic phase of bone. Conferring solubility at a low pH, Norian had the theoretical advantage of resorption and replacement by true bone. This calcium phosphate cement was produced intraoperatively by mixing a base powder (monocalcium sulfate, monohydrate, a-tricalcium phosphate, calcium carbonate) and a solvent-containing sodium phosphate at room temperature. After a 5-min interval, the material was ready for use, and continued to cure for approximately 24 h to become a microporous polycrystalline apatite with a maximum compressive strength of 50 MPa and tensile strength of 2.1 MPa. For comparison, the compressive and tensile properties of cancellous bone are 1.9 and 2.42 MPa, respectively.

FDA-approved in 1998, Norian CRS was subjected to long-term clinical outcome analysis. Providing the largest series specific to this bone cement in the context of craniofacial surgery, Gilardino and colleagues reported a rather substantial complication rate (26 % overall), when using this product regardless of the type of cranioplasty (onlay, full-thickness inlay). The majority of complications were infectious, attributable to the sheer amount of material used, or its use in a contaminated field. Stratifying according to type of cranioplasty (inlay vs. onlay), the authors reported the following limitations with Norian: (1) increased trending complication rate when >25 cm^2 inlay defects were reconstructed with this bone cement; (2) statistically significant increased complication rate when onlay constructs were placed in areas of high bacterial contamination (paranasal sinuses). Such results indicated that this bone cement, not dissimilar to others, failed to osteoconduct. Due to these findings and clinical experience, Norian was taken off of the market in 2011.

Osteoactive Materials

Osteoactive materials include bioactive glass (Nova Bone, Porex Surgical Inc.) and demineralized bone matrix (DBM). Composed of silica dioxide, sodium dioxide, calcium dioxide, and phosphate, bioactive glass confers its osteogenic properties when these components are mixed together to form an apatite surface layer. This layer recruits and stimulates osteoprogenitor cells to produce cytokines that have an autocrine and paracrine effect. Osteoblasts proliferate and differentiate on this surface, leading to new bone formation. In turn, the particulate glass undergoes resorption via osteoclastic activity.

The formulation that comprises demineralized bone matrix is based upon the landmark work of Urist and Strates, as well as Reddi and Huggins. This bone substitute is produced with a standard methodology: human cadaver long diaphyses are morselized to 250–600-mm particle sizes, demineralized in 0.6 N hydrochloric acid, and washed with deionized water, ethanol, and ethyl ether. In contrast to bioactive glass, DBM contains trace amounts of bone morphogenic protein (BMP), which makes this biomaterial both osteoconductive and osteoinductive. DBM alone, however, is hard to handle. In order to improve handling characteristics, various types of carriers have been added (e.g., glycerol, gelatin, calcium sulfate). It follows that not all preparations of DBM are the same. Acarturk and Hollinger have performed comparative analysis of all commercially available DBMs. In an athymic rat critical-sized calvarial defect model, they found that there was indeed a differential bone regenerative effect among the different types. One unifying principle was that those formulations which provided better handling [DBM + glycerol (Grafton, Osteotech, Inc.), DBM + hyaluronan (DBX, Synthes USA)] demonstrated statistically significantly higher bone formation than other groups as assessed by histomorphometry. Overall, however, the bone regenerative capacity was not as robust as the authors predicted.

Prefabricated Polymers

Methyl Methacrylate

An acrylic-based construct, methyl methacrylate forms from a powdered mixture of methyl methacrylate polymer, methyl methacrylate-styrene copolymer, and benzoyl peroxide monomer. The reaction is caustic, leading to an exothermia that approaches 85 °C and pungent fumes that are carcinogenic. The premixing recommendations of methyl methacrylate therefore demand use in an approved fume hood. After mixing 8–10 min, the polymerization process yields a rigid, durable material that can be contoured, and can be fixed rigidly to the cranioplasty site. Advantages of this material include a relatively low cost, possibility of in situ contouring, and lack of biodegradation. A prefabricated, customized, modified version of this material (Hard Tissue Replacement, Biomet Corporation, Jacksonville, FL) is composed of polymethylmethacrylate-polyhydroxyethyl methacrylate and available based on preoperative CT data (see below). This form is more porous, allowing for a degree of soft tissue ingrowth. The major drawback to acrylic-based resins, and in particular methyl methacrylate, is the substantial exothermic reaction involved in curing, which in situ can lead to severe thermal tissue injury. The cured, rigid substance has a high bacterial adhesion profile, and thus the high incidence of infected cranioplasties when using this substance.

Medpor

A high-density, porous polyethylene construct (pore size 100–250 mm), Medpor has become versatile in reconstruction of the craniofacial skeleton. Current applications include nasal/malar augmentation, orbital floor reconstruction, ear reconstruction, genioplasty, and cranial augmentation. For the cranium, Medpor has been found to successfully augment resorptive areas of the craniofacial skeleton (e.g., temporal fossa). Due to its porous nature, this implant permits native tissue ingrowth and therefore may provide some resistance to infection. Other advantages include the ability for intraoperative contouring and customized prefabrication based on three-dimensional volumetric data (DICOM) from computed tomography. Despite these benefits, there are clear disadvantages to this material (risk of infection, exposure, extrusion) that limit its use to well-vascularized recipient sites. As with all alloplastic cranioplasties, an irradiated field bears a relative contraindication from the use of this implant.

Conclusions

Alloplastic materials have provided more options when reconstructing the craniofacial skeleton. The advantages and disadvantages of each material must be considered when deciding which type to use, as well as the ability of the material to promote osteoconduction, osteoinduction, and osteointegration. Still, to date, the ideal material has not been developed, and therefore, autologous bone, whether vascularized or nonvascularized, remains the gold standard in bone replacement.

Bibliography

Acarturk TO, Hollinger JO. Commercially available demineralized bone matrix compositions to regenerate calvarial critical-sized bone defects. Plast Reconstr Surg. 2006;118(4):862–73.

Reddi AH, Huggins CB. Citrate and alkaline phosphatase during transformation of fibroblasts by the matrix and minerals of bone. Proc Soc Exp Biol Med. 1972;140(3):807–10.

Urist MR, Strates BS. Bone formation in implants of partially and wholly demineralized bone matrix. Including observations on acetone-fixed intra and extracellular proteins. Clin Orthop Relat Res. 1970;71:271–8.

Part II

Maxillofacial Fractures

10 Clinical Assessment of the Trauma Patient

Anuja K. Antony, Matthew J. Ranzer, and Mimis N. Cohen

Facial injuries result from physical trauma to the face and can manifest themselves with various symptoms such as lacerations, ecchymosis, epistaxis, eye injuries and fractures of the facial bones. These injuries require prompt evaluation and treatment in order to reduce morbidity, minimize disfigurement and loss of function, as well as prevent potential mortality resulting from bleeding and airway interference. It is important to systematically evaluate the patient with facial trauma and establish an accurate and detailed diagnosis before proceeding to definitive care. One should adhere to general trauma management principles and perform a primary and secondary survey to identify potential difficulties with airway, breathing, circulation, neurological function, and any concomitant injuries, as 50–70 % of patients with facial trauma will also have concomitant injuries to other organ systems. Cervical spine injuries can be seen in 4–10 % of patients with a facial fracture, while up to 20 % of patients with a cervical spine injury may have associated facial fractures. Nearly 18–45 % of patients with a facial fracture may have an associated closed head injury. The Advanced Trauma Life Support (ATLS) principles should guide the initial assessment of the facial trauma patient, and once life-threatening injuries have been ruled out or stabilized, a thorough and comprehensive physical examination should ensue to identify maxillofacial injuries. Appropriate radiographic examinations should follow extensive clinical evaluation to confirm suspected injury, delineate the extent of trauma, and guide definitive treatment.

A.K. Antony, MD, MPH, FACS (✉) • M.J. Ranzer, MD
M.N. Cohen, MD, FACS, FAAP
Division of Plastic, Reconstructive and Cosmetic Surgery, University of Illinois, 820 South Wood Street – Suite 515 CSN, Chicago, IL 60612-7316, USA
e-mail: akantony@uic.edu

Initial Emergency Evaluation

The American College of Surgeons (ACS) Advanced Trauma Life Support (ATLS) protocol describes the A, B, Cs of initial trauma management. This includes a rapid and directed assessment (the primary survey) of the critically injured patient to ensure that potential life-threatening injuries are diagnosed and treated in an expeditious manner. The primary survey consists of:

A. Airway
B. Breathing
C. Circulation with control of hemorrhage
D. Disability (mental and neurological deficits)
E. Exposure or environment

Airway

Airway management is the first step in the ATLS primary survey. Facial injuries pose significant threat for airway compromise. Injuries stemming from the nose down to the larynx or trachea can lead to airway obstruction and subsequent death. A patent and protected airway is essential before proceeding with any continued examination of the patient. Loss of airway typically occurs because of injury-related swelling or loss of soft tissue support, as in the case of bilateral mandible or panfacial fractures, bleeding, and/or aspiration. Foreign objects including loose or avulsed teeth, dentures, or bullet and bone fragments may also compromise the airway. Until a cervical spine injury has been ruled out, it is vital to maintain in-line immobilization of the cervical spine while evaluating the patient and obtaining (or maintaining) an airway. Initial maneuvers include suctioning and clearing the mouth of debris. More advanced maneuvers such as a chin lift, jaw thrust or insertion of an oral airway may be required if the tongue or soft tissues are lax or become retropositioned, obstructing the airway.

P.J. Taub et al. (eds.), *Ferraro's Fundamentals of Maxillofacial Surgery*,
DOI 10.1007/978-1-4614-8341-0_10, © Springer Science+Business Media New York 2015

More definitive airway management may be required including insertion of an endotracheal (ET) tube or in some circumstances a surgical airway in the form of a cricothyroidotomy or tracheostomy. There has been some debate over the best way to secure an airway in the patient with significant maxillofacial injury. Historically, significant panfacial or mandibular fractures would warrant eventual tracheostomy. The indications for performing routine tracheostomy, however, have become more specific. As every case is different, clinical decisions need to be tailored for the individual patient being treated, but current indications for insertion of a tracheostomy in the patient with facial fractures are listed in Table 10.1. In fact, for the patient with massive facial injuries, it may actually be *easier* for the anesthesiologist to place an endotracheal tube orally directly into the exposed airway (See Fig. 10.1a, b). Cricothyroidotomy is typically reserved for cases of extreme emergency when other methods of securing an airway have failed.

Breathing

Once the airway has been secured, a focused assessment of breathing is performed. This includes inspection, palpation, and auscultation of the chest to ensure adequacy of ventilation and oxygenation whether by spontaneous respiration, bag-valve masking, or mechanical ventilator support. Many problems with breathing can arise in the general trauma patient including pneumothorax, tension pneumothorax, flail chest, diaphragmatic rupture, and hemothorax. Treatment of these conditions is beyond the scope of this chapter but should be appropriately addressed.

Table 10.1 Indications for emergent cricothyroidotomy

1. Acute airway obstruction and failed oral ET placement
2. Anticipated prolonged intubation and ventilator requirement (or anticipated difficult reintubation)
3. Laryngeal or tracheal injury
4. Intermaxillary fixation in patients with other significant injuries

Specific to maxillofacial trauma is the risk of aspiration. Aspiration can occur in the form of blood, oral secretions, gastric contents, or fractured teeth and is often compounded by concomitant head injury, as these patients are often unable to protect their airway. Signs of aspiration include poor oxygenation, noisy respiration (throat or oral gurgling during respiration), and decreased lung compliance as measured by the mechanical ventilator. Prevention of aspiration is paramount as aspiration-related complications can prolong intubation, hospital length of stay, morbidity, and mortality. Insertion of an ET tube for patients not already intubated may be necessary, as well as oral, endotracheal, or gastric suctioning. Until skull fractures have been ruled out, it is not advisable to blindly place a nasogastric tube into the nares for fear of passage of the tube through the fracture (i.e., the involved cribriform plate) into the cranium. Medical adjuncts include anticholinergic agents for assistance with excessive secretions. Control of aspiration secondary to ongoing maxillofacial bleeding will be discussed in the next section.

Circulation

The next step in the ATLS protocol is control of life-threatening bleeding. In the trauma setting, bleeding can

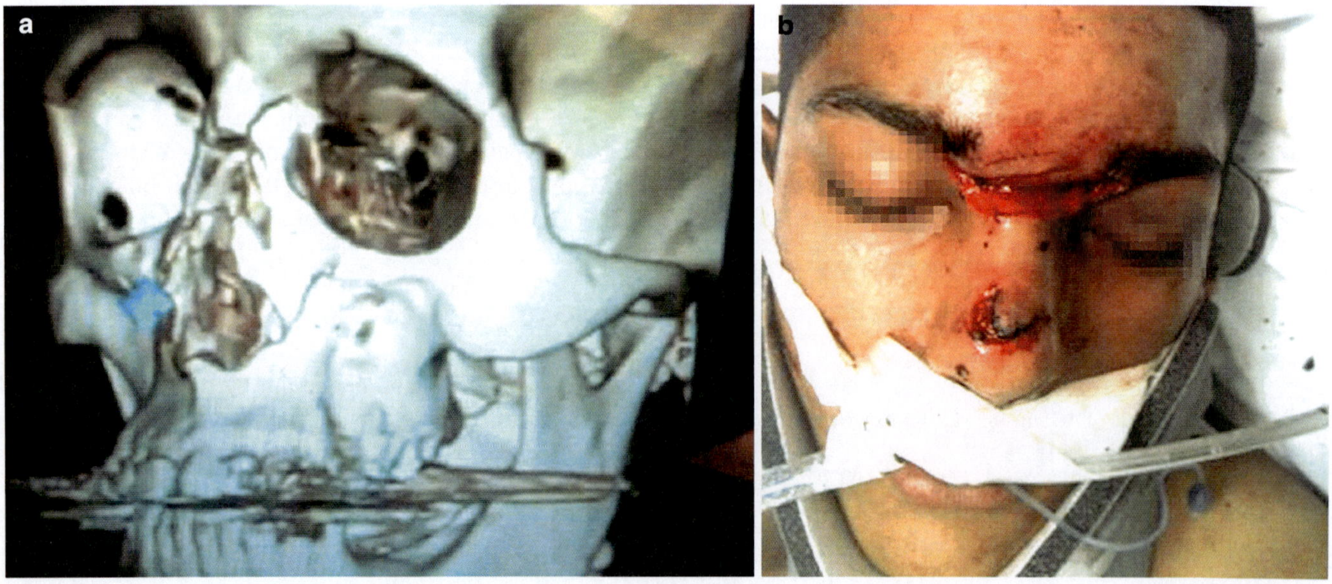

Fig. 10.1 (**a**, **b**) Patient with facial injuries requiring airway management using endotracheal intubation

occur into closed compartments (pelvic, abdominal, thoracic, extremities) or as exsanguinating hemorrhage into the environment. While it is common to defer management of facial injuries until other traumatic injuries have been controlled, life-threatening hemorrhage can also occur in the setting of facial lacerations or maxillofacial fractures. It is imperative that these injuries are controlled as part of the initial ATLS protocol or significant hemorrhage can go untreated while assessing for other sources of bleeding. (See Fig. 10.2a, b.)

Control of Significant Facial Bleeding

Life-threatening hemorrhage in maxillofacial trauma is typically related to either facial lacerations, midface fractures, or closed fractures involving the major sinuses. When presented with bleeding from facial lacerations, initial management of the bleeding is best handled by digital pressure with a sterile glove. Profuse bleeding is often the result of a partially transected artery. However, without direct visualization, it is not advisable to attempt control with blind use of clamps or suture as the risk of injuring the facial nerve branches is high. Once the vessel has been tamponaded with direct pressure, a careful local dissection can be performed to ligate the bleeding culprit vessel. (See Fig. 10.3a, b.)

For bleeding associated with fractures, a systematic stepwise approach to control of hemorrhage is often applied. Initial attempts to control nasal bleeding include anterior and posterior nasal packing and manual reduction of the fracture if possible. Anterior nasal packing is achieved by use of nonadherent petroleum impregnated gauze which is rolled and packed firmly into each nare. Although specialized devices for posterior nasal packing exist, a simpler approach involving use of two 30 cc Foley catheters inserted through the nostrils (one through each nare) to the posterior pharynx, inflation with 10–15 ml of saline, followed by traction to the catheters will enable a tamponade of the posterior choanae. Attention must be paid to avoid pressure necrosis of the septum or columella due to excessive or prolonged compression; this can be mitigated by providing periodic relief of posterior packing after the initial 2 h.

The majority of nasal hemorrhages will be controlled by a combination of anterior and posterior nasal packing and manual reduction of the fracture segments. When these methods are insufficient for control of hemorrhage, additional measures may be necessary. Although not often required, identification of the bleeding vessel by angiogram, embolization, and/or ligation of major vessels may be necessary. Institutional experience varies but when employed, angiography is often successful at locating the culprit vessel and effectively controlling bleeding with subsequent embolization. Occasionally, direct ligation of the offending artery may be required. This may include ligation of the internal maxillary artery (a common source of bleeding after midface injuries), the superficial temporal artery, or rarely the external

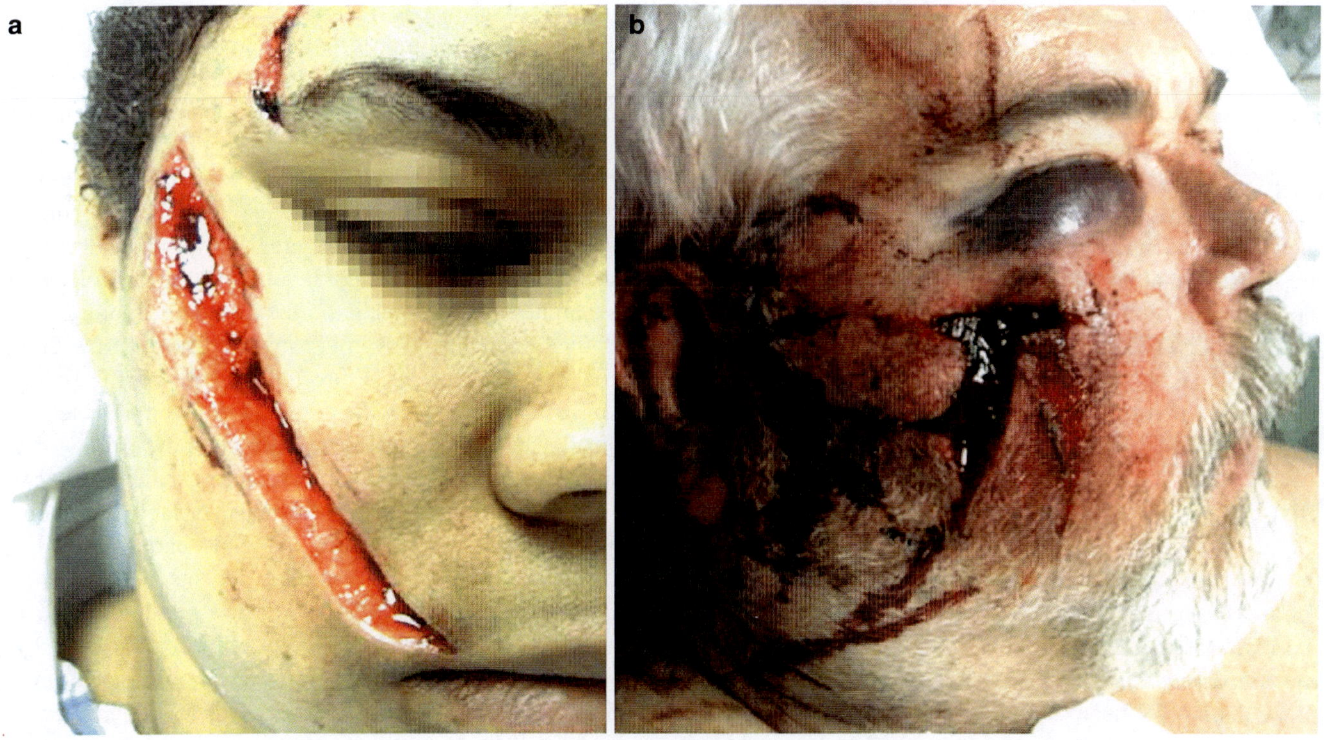

Fig. 10.2 (**a**, **b**) Patients with blood loss from extensive facial lacerations

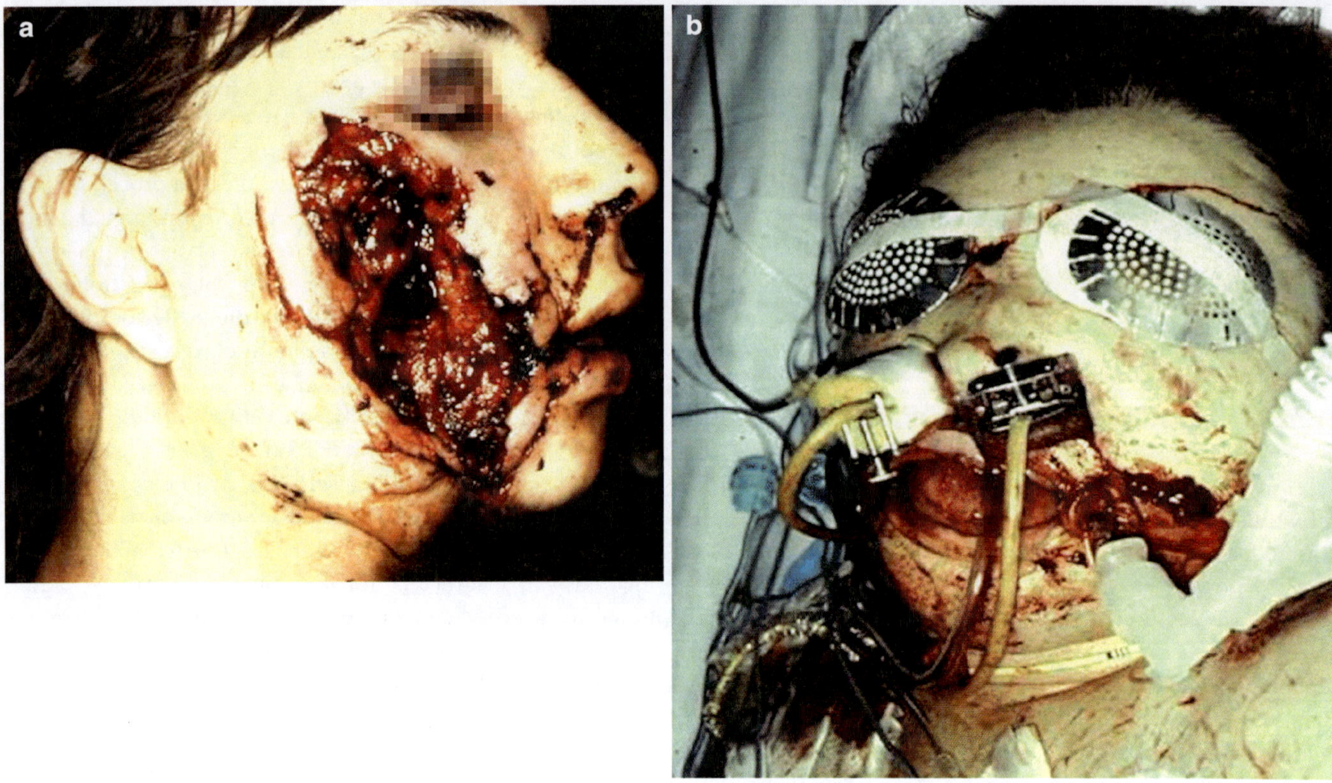

Fig. 10.3 (**a**, **b**) Facial and nasal bleeding; control of nasal bleeding using two Foley catheters

carotid artery. Ligation of the internal maxillary artery (IMAX) can be achieved through the Caldwell-Luc approach (window created through the anterior and posterior maxillary sinus, described by George W. Caldwell in 1893 and Henri Luc in France in 1897) and direct ligation with clips of the IMAX and its branches. It should also be noted that coagulopathy is common in the trauma patient and adequate correction of any clotting disorder is necessary to achieve hemostasis. Many institutions have transfusion protocols that ensures adequate platelets and fresh frozen plasma (FFP) are transfused along with blood when large volume transfusion is anticipated to avoid the dilutional coagulopathy that would otherwise develop. The optimal ratio of packed red cells, FFP, and platelets to be transfused is still under investigation and is institution specific.

History

The mechanism of injury can yield important information for areas to be examined. For example, blast injuries may be the result of fire, explosions, or from high velocity projectiles imparting their energy outside the radius of direct soft tissue damage. Whenever there is suspicion for a blast component to the injury pattern, an otoscopic examination should be performed to evaluate the integrity of the eardrum. The utility of perforated tympanic membranes (TM) as a marker for a blast injury is somewhat in dispute. One report on the incidence of tympanic membrane rupture following blast injury in soldiers from Iraq found that TM rupture was present in 50 % of patients who had sustained blast injuries. When present however, it is a good indicator that a blast injury has occurred and more detailed investigation should be performed outside of the obvious zone of injury looking for occult damage. This may include checking for cerebrospinal fluid (CSF) leaks if there is otorrhea indicating a potential skull base or temporal bone fracture, as well as having a higher index of suspicion for closed head injury.

Other mechanisms of injury may be associated with particular fracture patterns. Protected falls are often associated with fractures involving the zygoma, while unprotected falls typically involve the teeth, nose, or central portions of the mandible and maxilla. Motor vehicle accidents typically involve the midface and frontal sinus. Assaults more commonly involve the nasal bones, mandible, and zygoma.

It should be remembered that patients may have had previous antecedent injuries, asymmetries, or deformities and it is important to ascertain the status of their pre-injury exam. Not all facial asymmetries are the result of an acute injury, especially when they are non-tender or bear no other secondary signs of acute trauma to the aesthetic deformity. While identification of a patient's pre-injury physical exam is help-

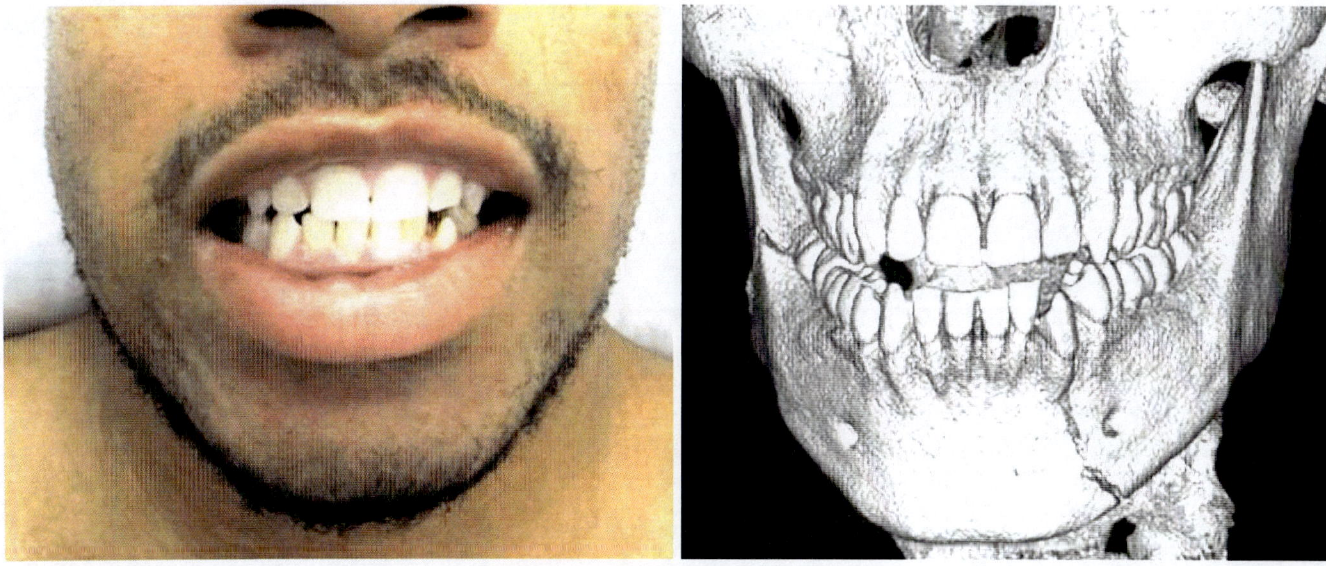

Fig. 10.4 Left parasymphyseal fracture with right open bite

ful, it is not always possible. This can sometimes be accomplished through having family members bring in old photographs, dental records, or orthodontic retainers and models. When possible, pre-injury dental records, photographs, or occlusal splints or models can be useful in surgical planning. When time permits, it may be helpful to take alginate impressions of the patient to assist in operative planning.

Physical Evaluation and Imaging

While the mechanism of injury may assist in suggesting potential injuries that may exist in the patient, it is the physical examination that identifies these injuries to the astute clinician. Once the patient has been appropriately evaluated according to the ATLS protocol and deemed stable, a detailed clinical examination of the facial trauma patient begins. The goals of the clinical examination are to identify soft tissue and underlying bony injuries, to document the patient's presurgical neurological and functional deficits, and to direct additional adjunctive studies including radiological imaging. It is important that the examination be conducted in a systematic fashion so that no injuries are missed. Typically, this is done in a top-down fashion with attention to bruises, pain, step-offs, sensory defects, lacerations, or contour deformities providing clues to the corresponding fractures which underlie these external signs. It is important that all bony surfaces are palpated, dentition (edentulous, teeth in line of fracture, poor status of teeth) and occlusion are documented, the intraoral and intranasal surfaces are examined, extraocular muscle movement and vision are checked, and the facial nerves are tested. Following the physical examination, appropriate imaging studies, typically thin-cut axial, coronal, and sagittal CT scans with 3D reconstructions are often obtained to better understand the fracture patterns and ensure that no other injuries go missed. Thus, the initial clinical examination of the patient will involve close observation and inspection, palpation, evaluation of epistaxis and other sources of bleeding, assessment of dentition, assessment of neurological status and any loss of consciousness, neck stabilization, determination of coexisting head and neck pathology, mechanism of injury, and potential involvement of supportive services and consultation from neurosurgery, ophthamology, ENT, and trauma/general surgery. Clearance from these services is often required prior to definitive fracture management.

While an occasional facial fracture may be isolated (e.g., nasal, mandible), oftentimes there can be concomitant injuries and an extensive physical evaluation will be of paramount importance to determine the true extent of any associated trauma. The frontal, temporal, and orbital bones should be palpated for pain, crepitus, step-offs, or mobility, followed by the zygomatic arches. The bony inspection continues with the nose, maxilla, and mandible. The mandibular condyles should be palpated with opening and closing of the jaw to assess for pain or displacement from the temporomandibular joint (TMJ). A detailed intraoral examination is essential to assess for malocclusion, missing, loose or fractured teeth, intraoral lacerations, mobility of the midface, and alveolar bone step-offs. (See Figs. 10.4 and 10.5.)

A rhinoscopic examination is necessary to ensure that no occult laceration or CSF rhinorrhea is present, as well as identifying if septal hematomas are present and establishing patency of the airway. If septal hematomas are identified, drainage with a #11 scalpel to prevent pressure necrosis of the septum will be warranted. CSF leak is often associated with fractures of the frontal sinus and the anterior cranial base; the

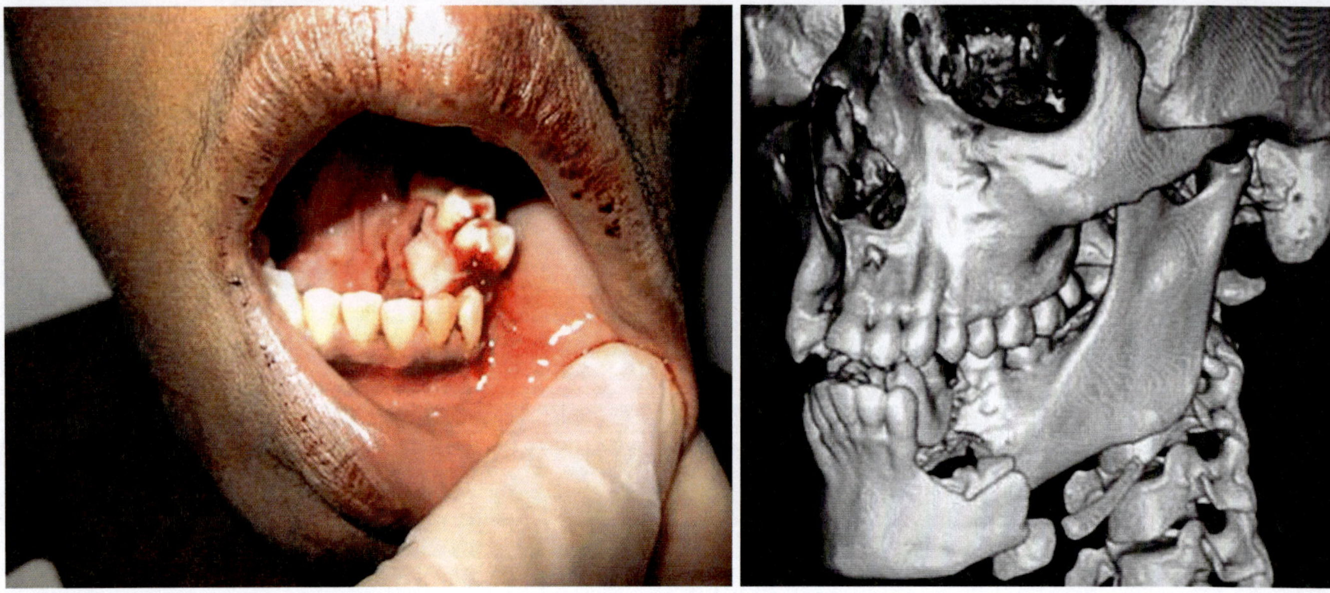

Fig. 10.5 Left mandible fracture with fracture of the alveolar ridge

corresponding work-up should be initiated to identify pneumocephalus, anterior and/or posterior table defects, and brain and/or dural injury, and a neurosurgical consultation will be required. Anterior fossa fractures can lead to rhinorrhea, raccoon eyes, altered vision and oculomotor palsy, and anosmia. Middle fossa fractures will manifest with hemotympanum, otorrhea, Battle's sign (mastoid ecchymosis), and unilateral hearing loss. Posterior fossa fractures are associated with hypotension and alterations in respiration due to brainstem compression. An otoscopic examination should be performed to evaluate for lacerations, perforated TMs, and presence of blood (midfossa bleeding) or CSF indicative of a basilar skull or temporal bone fracture. An ophthalmic examination must be conducted to assess for visual acuity, field defects, pupillary symmetry, hyphema, subconjunctival hematoma, corneal injury, retinal detachment, enophthalmos, diplopia, and extraocular muscle (EOM) function and potential entrapment using forced duction testing. Any suspicion of a globe injury or visual impairment mandates an ophthalmologic consultation.

Appropriate radiographic examinations are performed to confirm suspected injury patterns. Typically, CT scan and 3D reconstructions are performed. Occasionally, panorex or facial x-rays are sufficient for clinical examination findings consistent with isolated mandible or nasal fractures.

Clinical Findings Associated with Facial Fractures

Subsequent chapters are devoted to the evaluation and treatment of each of the specific fracture patterns, so a detailed description of the evaluation of each of them is not included here. However, key findings on physical exam indicative of an underlying fracture are described below and listed in Table 10.2. A practical abbreviated guide to fractures and associated clinical findings follows. Fractures of the frontal sinus may be associated with lacerations of the forehead, ecchymosis of the forehead or periorbital regions, and CSF rhinorrhea. Associated CT findings may include demonstration of anterior or posterior table displacement and pneumocephalus. Supraorbital fractures may have upper lid lacerations, periorbital ecchymosis, anesthesia in the supratrochlear and supraorbital nerve distributions, brow ptosis, step-offs of the superior orbital rim, exophthalmos, and superior gaze paresis. Associated CT findings include displacement of the supraorbital roof or retrobulbar hematoma. (See Fig. 10.6.)

Orbital fractures may be associated with lacerations of the lids or cheek, periorbital ecchymosis, subconjunctival hemorrhage, orbital rim step-offs, diplopia, infraorbital nerve paresthesias, enophthalmos or exophthalmos, and impaired extraocular movements on forced duction testing. CT findings include displacement of fracture segments, herniation or entrapment of orbital contents, and orbital emphysema.

Nasal fractures are associated with nasal and periorbital ecchymosis, nasal deformities, or lacerations, crepitus, and epistaxis. (See Fig. 10.7.) Rhinoscopic examination may demonstrate septal hematomas or dislocation of the septum. CT findings help identify displacement of the various nasal structures and exclude adjacent orbital or ethmoidal fractures. Naso-orbital-ethmoid (NOE) fractures are characterized by the presence of telecanthus with flattening of the nasal dorsum. Other associated findings include periorbital ecchymosis, step-offs of the orbital rims, subconjunctival

Table 10.2 A practical guide to clinical findings associated with facial fractures

Fracture type	Possible associated ecchymosis location	Possible associated laceration location	Physical findings	Other possible associated findings
Frontal sinus	Frontal	Forehead	Palpable deformity of frontal bone	Pneumocephalus
	Periorbital			CSF rhinorrhea
				Epistaxis
				Anosmia
Supraorbital	Periorbital	Upper brow	Step-off of superior orbital rim	Paresthesias in supratrochlear or supraorbital nerve distribution
			Brow ptosis	Superior gaze paresis
			Exophthalmos	
Orbit	Periorbital	Upper or lower lid		Infraorbital nerve anesthesia
	Subconjunctival	Cheek		Visual changes
Naso-orbital-ethmoid (unilateral or bilateral)	Periorbital Subconjunctival	Nasal bridge	Unilateral or bilateral telecanthus	Epistaxis
			Flattening of the nasal dorsum	Visual issues
			Orbital rim step-off	
Nasal	Nasal	Nasal	Crepitus	Epistaxis
	Periorbital		Deformity	Septal hematoma
				Septal dislocation
				Airway obstruction
Maxillary	Lower eyelid	Midface	Malocclusion	LeFort I: mobility of upper jaw
	Midface	Intraoral	Nasopharyngeal bleeding	LeFort II: mobility of upper jaw and nasal bones (pyramidal)
			Crepitus	LeFort III: mobility of face from cranium
Zygoma/ zygomaticomaxillary complex	Cheek, zygoma	Cheek	Malar flattening Infraorbital paresthesia	Trismus
	Orbit	Lateral orbit	Entrapment	Visual changes
			Enophthalmos	
Mandible	Cheek	Intraoral	Step-off deformity	Trimus
	Lower face, neck	Extraoral	Malocclusion	Pain
	Chin		Missing or loose teeth	Intraoral swelling
				Paresthesia in mental nerve distribution

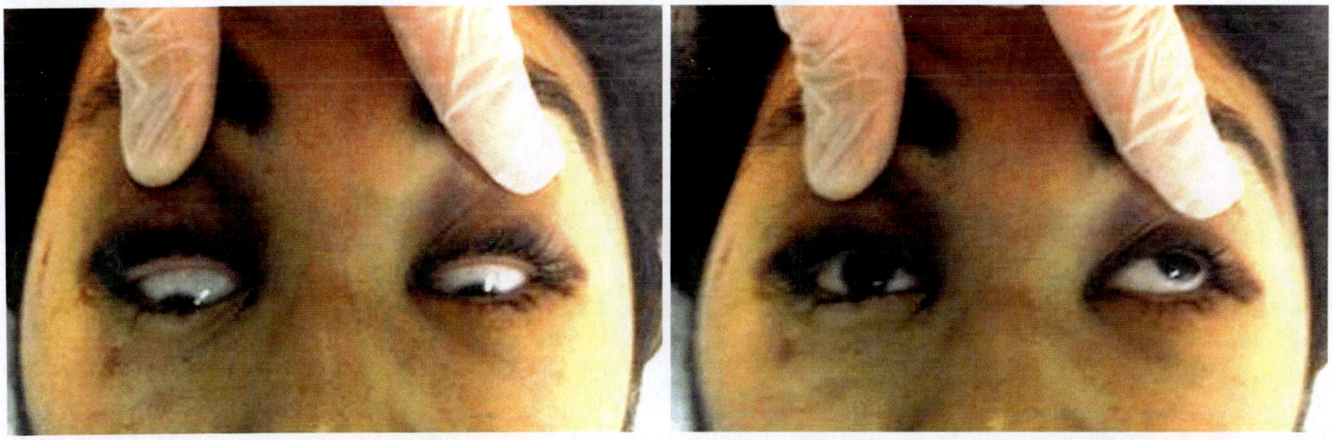

Fig. 10.6 Right orbital fracture with entrapment on upward gaze

hemorrhage, and epistaxis. Associated CT findings include pneumocephalus, orbital emphysema, and frontal sinus involvement. The Brown-Gruss provocation maneuvers can help delineate the condition of the nasal supporting structures with external manual pressure; Brown-Gruss I (upper vault compression) will cause collapse of the upper third of

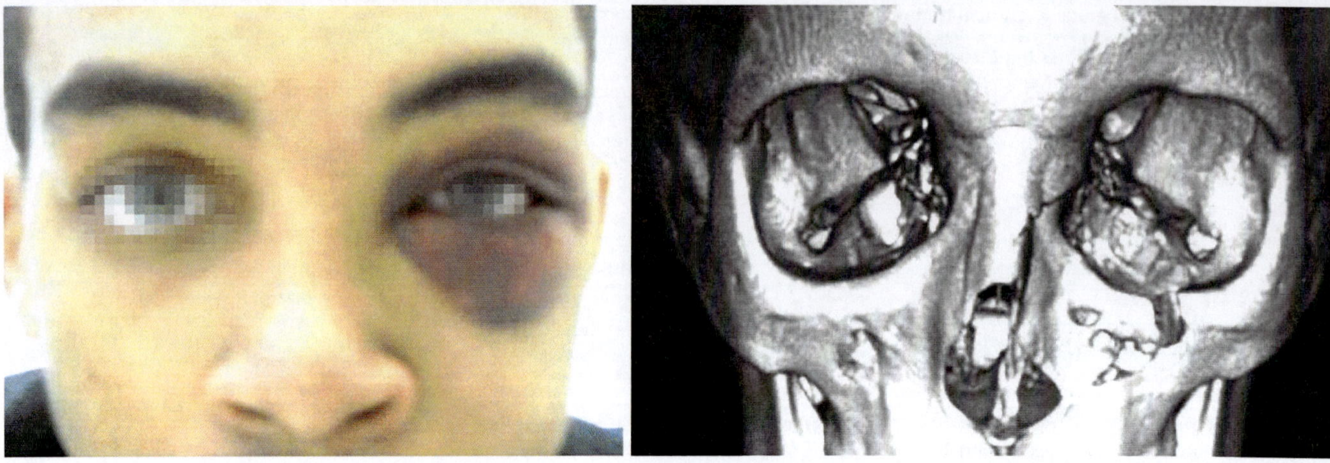

Fig. 10.7 Left nasal and medial orbit fractures with associated periorbital ecchymosis

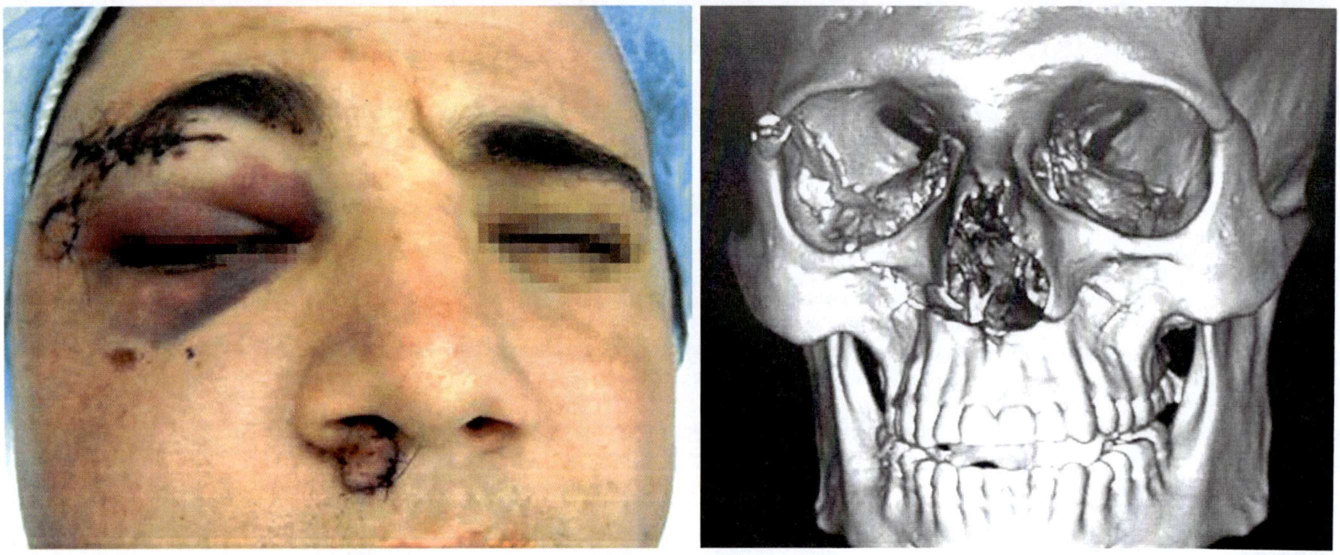

Fig. 10.8 Right zygomaticomaxillary fractures with associated periorbital lacerations and ecchymosis

the nose with severe communition of the nasal bones and frontal processes of the maxilla. More extensive collapse or complete disappearance of the nose may be observed when severe trauma has affected all three vaults of the nose.

Isolated zygomatic arch fractures may display malar flattening, an obvious contour deformity or trismus if the fracture segment is posteromedially displaced and impinges on the coronoid process or temporalis muscle. Zygomaticomaxillary complex fractures may have malar flattening, trismus, infraorbital paresthesias, enophthlamos or step-offs along the inferior orbital rim, zygomatic arch, or zygomaticomaxillary buttress. (See Fig. 10.8.) CT findings may include orbital floor herniation or entrapment, opacification of the maxillary sinus, and displacement of the zygomatic arch.

Maxillary fractures may demonstrate mobility of the upper jaw in LeFort I fractures, mobility of the upper jaw and nasal bones (maxillary pyramid) in LeFort II fractures, and rarely, mobility of the entire face from the cranium in LeFort III fractures (craniofacial dysjunction). (See Fig. 10.9.) Other physical findings include ecchymosis of the lower eyelids and midface, malocclusion, nasopharyngeal bleeding, obvious step-offs, and crepitus. CT findings are dependent on the level of fracture and may include components of zygomatic, orbital, and naso-orbital-ethmoidal fractures including fluid-filled maxillary sinuses, pneumocephalus, orbital emphysema, and palatal disruption.

In addition to obvious step-offs or contour deformities, mandibular fractures typically demonstrate malocclusion, trismus, paresthesias in the mental nerve distribution, missing or loose teeth, and intraoral and extraoral lacerations. CT findings may demonstrate impacted teeth, isolated alveolar fractures, and condylar fractures. Obviously, these fractures need not occur in isolation and many patients will present with a constellation of fracture components from each of the anatomic fracture areas.

Facial trauma often occurs in combination with other traumatic injuries. (See Fig. 10.10.) It should not be taken for granted that when a specialty consultation for facial trauma is called, other injuries have been ruled out. It is important that a systematic approach be used to identify and treat potential life-threatening injuries according to the ATLS protocol, before assessing the patient for facial trauma injuries. Once the patient has been stabilized, a systematic approach to the facial trauma examination should be performed. This ensures that no injuries are missed, pretreatment deficits are documented, and appropriate ancillary studies are performed. There are many potential fracture patterns that occur in facial trauma, and often they do not occur in isolation. Complex combinations of facial fractures are often encountered, but a thorough clinical examination will ensure that each fracture is identified so that optimal treatment can be planned.

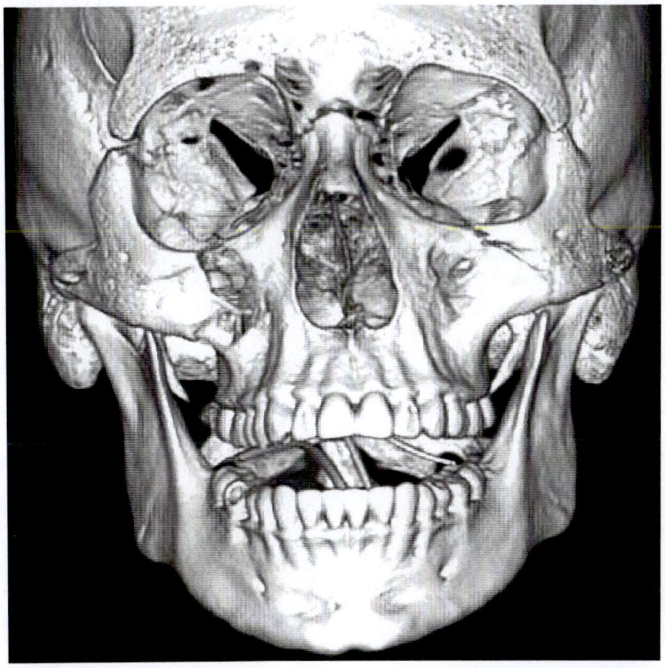

Fig. 10.9 Bilateral LeFort II facial fracture (*right side* complete, *left side* incomplete)

Conclusion

Facial trauma requires a systematic approach to evaluate the extent of injury before proceeding to definitive care. Prompt evaluation and treatment of facial injuries will reduce morbidity with disfigurement and loss of function, as well as potential mortality resulting from bleeding and airway interference. Proper diagnosis using clinical evaluation and appropriate radiographic imaging is critical to implementing treatment with the goal of restoring pre-injury appearance and function.

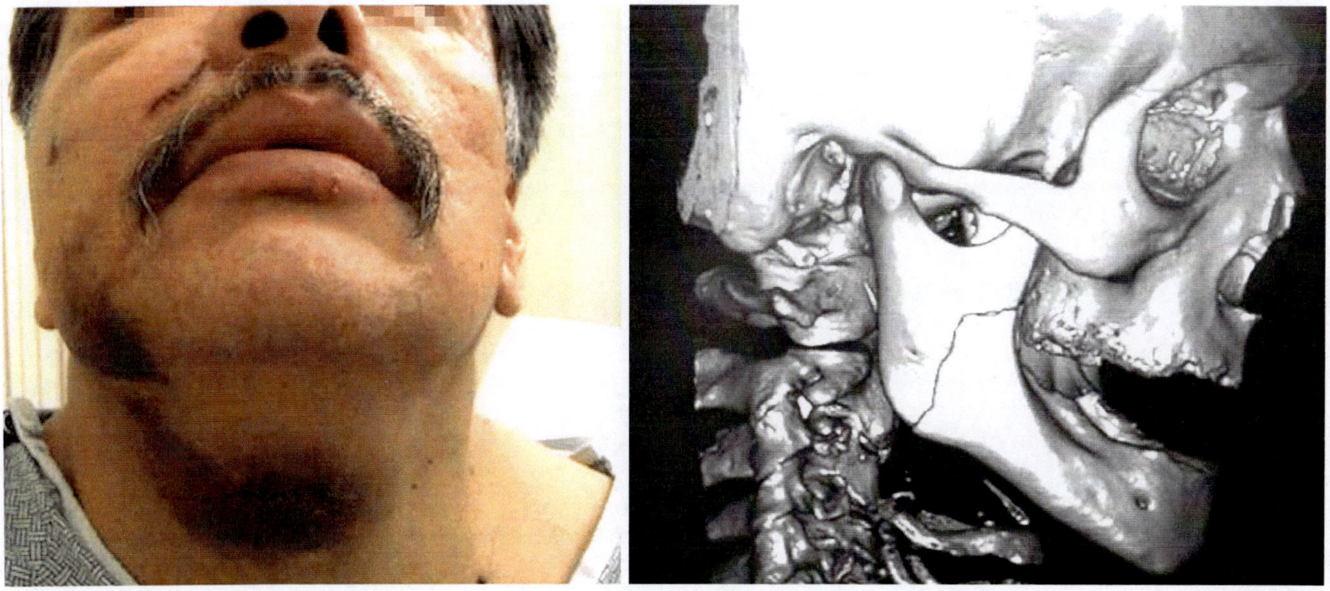

Fig. 10.10 Right mandibular body fracture in an edentulous patient with an associated mandibular and neck contusion

Bibliography

Adamo AK, Katsnelson T, Rodriguez ED, Karasik E. Intraoperative airway management with pan-facial fractures: alternative approaches. J Craniomaxillofac Trauma. 1996;2(3):30–5.

American College of Surgeons. Advanced trauma life support for doctors. 7th ed. Chicago: American College of Surgeons; 2005.

Dean NR, Ledgard JP, Katsaros J. Massive hemorrhage in facial fracture patients: definition, incidence, and management. Plast Reconstr Surg. 2009;123(2):680–90.

Erdmann D, Follmar KE, Debruijn M, et al. A retrospective analysis of facial fracture etiologies. Ann Plast Surg. 2008;60(4):398–403.

Girotto JA, MacKenzie E, Fowler C, et al. Long term physical impairment and functional outcomes after complex facial fractures. Plast Reconstr Surg. 2001;108:312–27.

Hackl W, Fink C, Hausberger K, et al. The incidence of combined facial and cervical spine injuries. Trauma. 2001;59:41–145.

Harrison CD, Bebarta VS, Grant GA. Tympanic membrane perforation after combat blast exposure in Iraq: a poor biomarker of primary blast injury. J Trauma. 2009;67(1):210–1.

Haug RH, Savage JD, Likavek MJ, et al. A review of 100 closed head injuries associated with facial fractures. J Oral Maxillofac Surg. 1992;50:218–22.

Holmgren EP, Bagheri S, Bell RB, et al. Utilization of tracheostomy in craniomaxillofacial trauma at a level-1 trauma center. J Oral Maxillofac Surg. 2007;65(10):2005–10.

Khanna S, Dagum AB. A critical review of the literature and an evidence-based approach for life-threatening hemorrhage in maxillofacial surgery. Ann Plast Surg. 2012;69(4):474–8.

Manson P. Facial injuries (chapter 66). In: Mathes S, editor. Plastic surgery, vol. 3, part 2. New York: Elsevier; 2005.

Manson PN. Facial injuries. In: Cameron JL, editor. Current surgical therapy. 9th ed. Philadelphia: Elsevier; 2008.

Mithani SK, St-Hilaire H, Brooke BS, et al. Predictable patterns of intracranial and cervical spine injury in craniomaxillofacial trauma: analysis of 4786 patients. Plast Reconstr Surg. 2009;123(4): 1293–301.

Orloff G. Management of facial fractures (chapter 19). In: Thaller S, editor. Craniofacial surgery. New York: Informa; 2008.

Pollock R. Nasal trauma: pathomechanics and surgical management of acute injuries. Clin Plast Surg. 1992;19:133.

Raval CB, Rashiduddin M. Airway management in patients with maxillofacial trauma – a retrospective study of 177 cases. Saudi J Anaesth. 2011;5(1):9–14.

Roccia F, Bianchi FA, Zavattero E, et al. Etiology and patterns of facial lacerations and their possible association with underlying maxillofacial fractures. J Craniofac Surg. 2011;22(6):e19–23.

Sargent LA. Nasoethmoid orbital fractures: diagnosis and treatment. Plast Reconstr Surg. 2007;120(7 Suppl 2):16S–31.

Shuker ST. Maxillofacial blast injuries. J Craniomaxillofac Surg. 1995;23(2):91–8.

Management of Soft Tissue Injuries

11

Jordan P. Steinberg, Alexandra Junewicz, and Arun K. Gosain

Initial Assessment and General Principles

Soft tissue trauma constitutes a majority of the injuries of the craniomaxillofacial region that present for urgent management. In adults, motor vehicle collisions or interpersonal violence are the most typical causes of injury, whereas in children and the elderly, slips and falls are more common. Management of craniomaxillofacial soft tissue injuries varies widely depending on the region involved. The extent of injury is also a significant factor and often delineates simple closure of wounds in the Emergency Department from more complex, multistaged reconstructive procedures in the operating room.

Evaluation of the craniomaxillofacial trauma patient should begin with the Advanced Trauma Life Support (ATLS) protocol and immediate interventions to address any life-threatening injuries according to the "ABCs" (*A*irway, *B*reathing, and *C*irculation). Airway compromise due to direct injury, foreign bodies, bleeding, or extensive swelling may necessitate endotracheal intubation or tracheostomy. In-line stabilization of the cervical spine should always be a consideration with such airway interventions, as some 7 % of craniomaxillofacial injuries are accompanied by cervical spine fractures. Assessment of circulation must take into account hemorrhage from facial injury, which rarely, but notably, may be life-threatening due to the robust vascularity of the head and neck region. Hemodynamically, significant hemorrhage may be managed with direct pressure, nasal packing or Foley catheter-based tamponade, angiographic embolization, or direct surgical ligation. Finally, neurologic disability should be evaluated with the Glasgow Coma Scale.

The secondary survey for craniomaxillofacial trauma patients commences with a complete, yet efficiently gathered, history. Any medical history of diabetes, immunosuppression, malnutrition, chronic renal failure, collagen vascular disorders, or other conditions associated with delayed wound healing should especially be noted. Details regarding how the injury occurred may also facilitate predictions of delayed healing, tissue devitalization, and necrosis. Other key items include allergies, current medications, past surgical (including ocular) history, time of last oral intake, and tetanus vaccination status.

The secondary survey continues with a detailed, but focused, physical examination. Physical examination of the head and neck is paramount in cases of craniomaxillofacial bony and soft tissue injuries. While thin slice computed tomography (CT) scans (with or without 3D reconstructions) are easily obtained in many trauma centers today and add valuable information for diagnosis as well as treatment planning, such scans should be viewed as a supplement to the primary physical examination and not a substitute for it. Extensive swelling, distracting injuries, and the psychological impact of the craniomaxillofacial trauma may occasionally render the physical examination difficult or even impossible in the initial setting. Local anesthesia and nerve blocks may be used to alleviate patient discomfort.

Examination generally proceeds in a craniocaudal fashion, beginning with the scalp and continuing down toward the neck. Bony injuries should be assessed with palpation of the orbital rims, zygomatic body, zygomatic arches, and nasal bone for step-offs or relative mobility. Traction on the midface with one hand grasping the palate from an intraoral approach may permit diagnosis of a LeFort fracture. The mandible should likewise be assessed for step-offs or relative mobility. From a soft tissue perspective, the face should be assessed for symmetry from both frontal and worm's eye views and any abnormalities compared, if possible, to

J.P. Steinberg, MD, PhD
Division of Plastic and Reconstructive Surgery, Northwestern University Feinberg School of Medicine, Chicago, IL, USA

A. Junewicz
Case Western Reserve University School of Medicine, 10900 Euclid Avenue, Cleveland, OH 44106, USA

A.K. Gosain, MD (✉)
Division of Pediatric Plastic Surgery, Lurie Children's Hospital and Northwestern University Feinberg School of Medicine, Chicago, IL, USA
e-mail: argosain@luriechildrens.org

P.J. Taub et al. (eds.), *Ferraro's Fundamentals of Maxillofacial Surgery*,
DOI 10.1007/978-1-4614-8341-0_11, © Springer Science+Business Media New York 2015

pre-injury photographs. The extent of facial motor and sensory function should be thoroughly documented. Eyes should be examined independently for visual acuity, relative afferent papillary defects (RAPD), extraocular muscle mobility, and damage to lids, lacrimal canaliculi, or the globes themselves. The oral cavity should be inspected for loose or fractured teeth, foreign bodies, and malocclusion. Finally, any lacerations, avulsions, and crush injuries should be carefully assessed with respect to wound location, size, and shape as well as the presence of foreign bodies and devitalized edges. Photographs can help document features of the latter injuries. When taken, such photographs should be included together with the appropriate consent forms as part of the medical record.

Following documentation of soft tissue injury of the head and neck on secondary survey of the trauma patient, initial plans can be formulated regarding the most appropriate means of repair. General consensus points to irrigation of soft tissue wounds with saline in a pulsatile fashion to lower bacterial counts and closure as early as feasible. The ideal time window for closure of simple soft tissue wounds has been noted to be 8–12 h from the time of injury. It should be recognized, however, that there are no prospective trial data to directly support these recommendations. Because the time of initial injury is often unclear, and because more serious systemic injuries or unavailability of the consultant surgeon may practically limit the ability to repair soft tissue lacerations within this restricted time frame, we favor the more general recommendation of repair within the first 24 h. As discussed in subsequent sections of the chapter, wounds with a high level of contamination (e.g., bites) and those open for greater than 24 h may not be appropriate for immediate closure and be better approached with a strategy of delayed primary repair. Fortunately, the excellent vascularity of the head and neck region renders the chances of infection less likely, and many wounds can be therefore be closed in the immediate setting following local anesthetic infiltration, irrigation, and preparation of the wound bed including trimming of devitalized edges and removal of foreign materials. The ability to perform these tasks effectively in the Emergency Department must be evaluated on a case-by-case basis. When resources are not adequate or cooperation of the patient is a significant factor (i.e., with the pediatric patient, as discussed later in this chapter), the operating room becomes the preferred venue for repair.

A variety of recommendations have been made regarding the selection of suture material and technique of suture closure of head and neck soft tissue lacerations. As with timing of repair, prospective trial data to bolster such recommendations are lacking. While it is often believed that fine, nonabsorbable suture material such as 5–0 or 6–0 polypropylene or nylon will yield the least amount of inflammation and therefore the most optimal scar when used for skin approximation, this must be evaluated in light of potentially longer closure times and the need for subsequent suture removal. As discussed later in this chapter, suture removal, particularly in the periorbital region, may be a challenging and potentially impossible task in a young child without the use of sedation. Although the published literature contains few prospective reports, recent data from the Emergency Department on cosmetic outcomes 9–12 months post-repair indicate no appreciable difference between lacerations closed at the skin level with fast-absorbing catgut, removable nylon, and octyl cyanoacrylate glue.

Following repair of soft tissue wounds, patients should be instructed to clean the site daily with soap and water and keep the area free of heavy crusts that may impede healing. A diluted peroxide solution may help with the removal of crusts and/or dried blood. Permanent sutures on the face should be removed early enough to prevent track marks, which is roughly 4–5 days post-repair for most patients. Antibiotics for facial soft tissue trauma are generally not required, with the exception of wounds at high risk for contamination such as bites. After wound healing is complete, the patient should be advised to massage scars regularly and to apply facial moisturizer and sunblock judiciously. Pressure therapy or silicone gel sheeting may have some efficacy in minimizing scar pending the acceptability of cost of these materials. Patients should be advised of the requisite 6–12 months for full scar maturation before consideration of any surgical revision.

Specific Principles

Scalp and Hairline

The management of traumatic scalp loss depends on the size, location, and depth of the defect and may incorporate all aspects of the reconstructive ladder. After appropriate evaluation and preparation of the traumatized tissue as described above, consideration may be given to closure and reconstruction. The scalp is distinguished from other tissues by its hair-bearing nature, inelasticity, relative thickness, and unique layers. These unique layers consist of the skin, subcutaneous tissue, galea aponeurotica, loose areolar tissue, and pericranium. The thick connective tissue of the galea, in combination with the convexity of the underlying cranium, often makes primary closure difficult and necessitates scoring and/or wide undermining. These characteristics increase with increasing age of the patient, with substantial differences appreciable between the hypermobile scalp of the infant relative to the much stiffer, tethered scalp of the mature adult (see Fig. 11.1). Generally feasible for defects measuring less than 3–4 cm in diameter, primary closure is the simplest option for reconstruction. As illustrated in Fig. 11.1, it

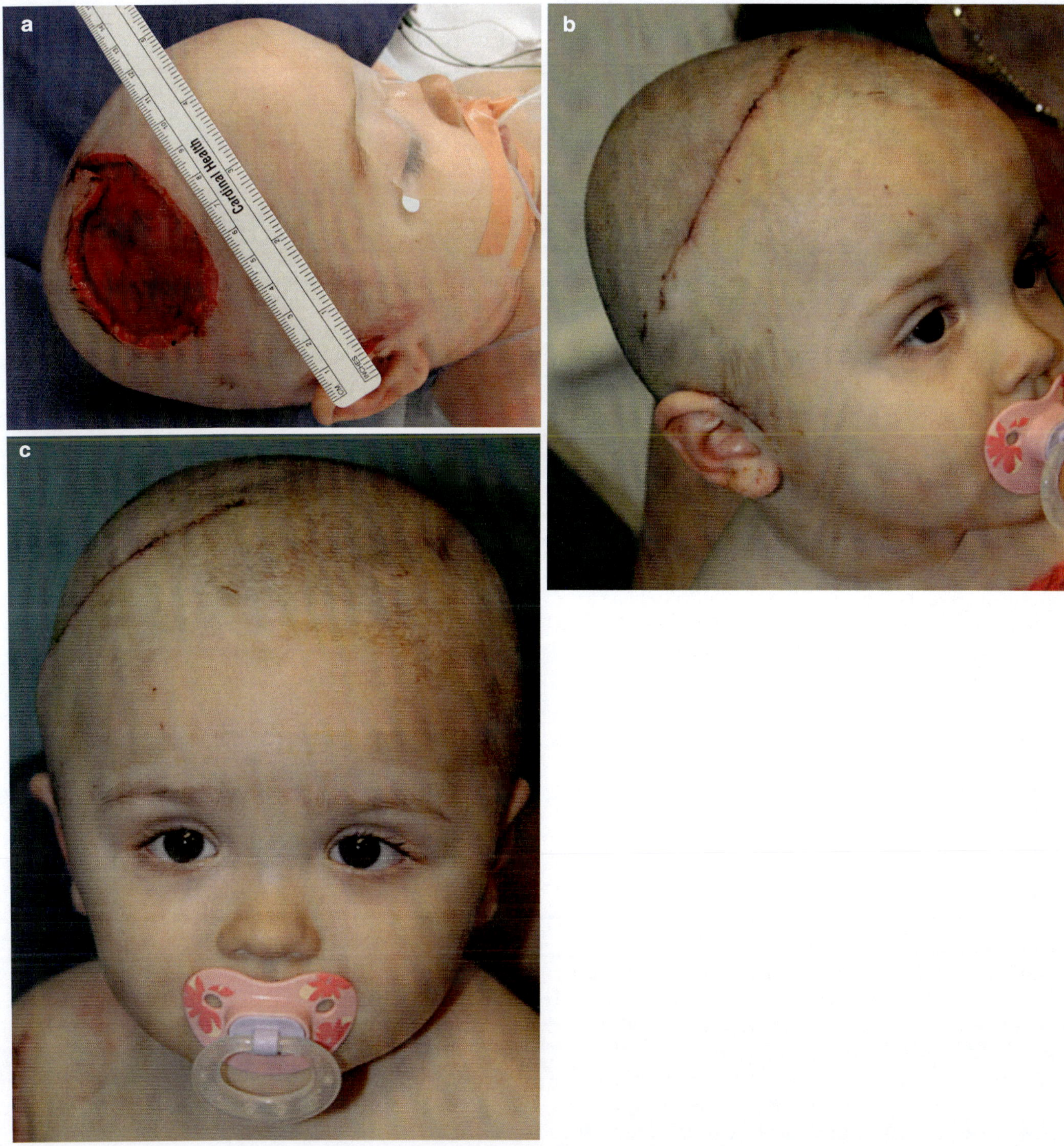

Fig. 11.1 A 13-month-old female with avulsive dog bite wound of the scalp: (**a**) preoperative on-table photograph showing avulsive wound of the right parietal scalp caused by a bite from a pitbull; (**b**) 1-week postoperative result after wound edge debridement, subgaleal undermining, galeal scoring, and primary approximation (profile view); (**c**) 1-week postoperative result (frontal view). Note excellent healing with no appreciable distortion of the hair growth pattern

is also frequently the best option in terms of minimizing distortion of hair growth patterns. Because excessive tension may also damage hair follicles, primary closure should be avoided if significant tension is present despite attempts at galeal scoring and undermining in the loose areolar plane.

Skin grafting and tissue expansion may be used alone or combined with other methods of scalp reconstruction. Skin grafts, whether for primary defects or for donor sites from which local flaps have been taken, require the presence of intact pericranium as an underlying vascularized bed.

Trephination or burring of the outer calvarial table to expose bleeding diploic bone may be performed in the absence of an intact pericranial layer, provided that adequate compression is applied over the skin graft to promote adherence. In both cases, however, grafts often yield a poor cosmetic outcome due to lack of hair, color mismatch, and lack of tissue height and contour restoration. Tissue expansion, although not generally an option in acute, traumatic defects, may be of utility in secondary scalp reconstruction. Despite a complication rate of up to 25 %, it is generally accepted that tissue expansion can allow reconstruction of up to 50 % of the scalp without distorting the hair growth pattern or creating a new donor defect.

Local flaps are a mainstay of reconstruction for moderate-sized traumatic defects of the scalp not amenable to primary closure. As in oncologic reconstruction, large rotational flaps or double hatchet-type flaps are most useful and can allow closure of traumatic defects up to 6 cm in diameter. In combination with skin grafting of donor areas, local flaps may allow coverage of even larger areas. Grafted areas can then be excised secondarily, either with small serial excisions or with tissue expansion. As a general principle, large rotational flaps should include at least one axial scalp vessel and have a length five times the diameter of the defect to enable rotation and advancement. The parietal scalp has the greatest elasticity and should therefore be incorporated whenever possible. Extensive scalp defects may be addressed with the technique of multiple interdigitating flaps as described by Orticochea.

Near-total defects of the scalp are best managed with free tissue transfer. Options include latissimus dorsi and serratus anterior muscle flaps, rectus abdominis muscle or myocutaneous flaps, anterolateral thigh and scapular/parascapular fasciocutaneous flaps, and omental flaps. Flap choice should be dictated by the specific reconstructive needs associated with the traumatic defect. Non-meshed skin grafts are preferred for coverage of free muscle flaps. The latissimus dorsi free muscle flap has been used most commonly for near-total scalp reconstruction because of its large surface area, long pedicle, and overall good aesthetic outcome.

In the case of near-total scalp avulsion, consideration should be given to scalp replantation. In these avulsive injuries, shear forces cause separation of the scalp at the level of the loose areolar tissue. Replantation may be attempted within an 18-h time frame from injury. In general, anastomoses are performed to the superficial temporal system, occasionally with the use of vein grafts to avoid the zone of injury. Multiple venous anastomoses may also be of benefit to avoid congestion.

As a final point of emphasis, when managing soft tissue injuries to the scalp or forehead, efforts should be made to preserve the contour of the patient's natural anterior hairline. The male hairline normally demonstrates frontotemporal recession, represented by the angle between the frontal and temporal hairlines. During reconstructive procedures, orienting incisions perpendicularly with respect to the hairline will avoid contour distortion. Alternatively, incisions may be placed along the hairline in a parallel and beveled fashion to camouflage scars.

Eyelids

The identification of eyelid injuries should be an integral part of the secondary survey discussed earlier for the trauma patient. Because ocular or periocular injuries frequently coexist with other soft tissue injuries of the head and neck, it is incumbent upon the craniomaxillofacial surgeon to appropriately identify and characterize these injuries even if the ophthalmologist has been or will be consulted in addition. Preliminary evaluation should always include an assessment of visual acuity. If a Snellen chart is not available, the examiner may record vision crudely based on finger counting, hand motion, or light perception. Vision should be separately recorded for each eye. Pupils should be assessed for size and symmetry, and the swinging flashlight test should be performed to check for the presence of a relative afferent pupillary defect. This simple test can reveal relative dysfunction of the optic nerve that should prompt the immediate involvement of the ophthalmologist. Finally, the conjunctiva and eyelids should be carefully inspected for signs of trauma including hemorrhage, lacerations, and canthal disruption. As with any facial lacerations, the size and depth should be estimated and photographs taken for documentation. Special attention should be directed to any fat seen herniating through the eyelids, as this may signify violation of the orbital septum and direct injury to the globe. Eyelid lacerations medial to the lacrimal puncta should raise the suspicion for canalicular injury and are discussed in greater detail below.

Many eyelid injuries can be addressed in the Emergency Department with the use of local anesthetic; however, one should always consider the use of the operating room when resources are inadequate (e.g., lighting, instruments, assisting personnel) or patient anxiety is a significant factor. Repair of eyelid trauma in children should be done in the operating room under general anesthesia, with the possible exception of isolated periorbital lacerations for which intravenous sedation may be adequate. The injection of local anesthesia with epinephrine can reduce bleeding and improve visualization during repair, but is counterbalanced by the possibility of introducing excessive edema and tissue distortion. Targeted nerve blocks can reduce the requirements for direct wound edge infiltration and are therefore encouraged. This includes blockade of the supraorbital, supratrochlear, and infraorbital nerves. The supraorbital and supratrochlear nerves can be anesthetized with an injection through the lateral part of the middle third of the eyebrow extending toward the nasal bone in a deep subperiosteal plane. The infraorbital nerve is best anesthetized with a percutaneous injection between the alar rim and the nasolabial fold aimed up at the infraorbital rim along a line dropped vertically from the medial limbus of the eye.

Successful repair of eyelid injuries requires the preservation and/or reapproximation of normal anatomic landmarks including the lid margin, gray line, and lash line. This not only prevents lid inversion and notching but also ensures mobility of both lids and stability of the lid margins. The repaired eyelid should appear similar to the contralateral eyelid in terms of height, contour, and tarsal show. Whenever possible, suture lines should be hidden in the tarsal crease. In the setting of significant bilateral eyelid injury, the ideal aesthetic measurements may guide repair. Specifically, the distance between the lateral and medial canthi should equal the distance between the medial canthi, with the lateral canthi elevated 2° above the medial canthi. When the eye is open, the upper eyelid should rest 1 mm below the upper limbal edge, the lower eyelid should rest at the lower limbal edge, and the supratarsal fold should sit 3–4 mm above the upper lid margin. When the eye is closed, the supratarsal fold should sit 10–11 mm above the upper lid margin.

As with soft tissue defects for other facial subunits, the reconstructive ladder may be applied to eyelid reconstruction. In older patients with partial-thickness lid defects covering less than 25 % of the lid, secondary intention healing may be preferred. This may also be an option for superficial trauma to concave surfaces of the medial canthal region. In other areas, however, secondary intention healing may lead to unacceptable contractures and deformities. Depending on the age of the patient and the degree of eyelid skin laxity, defects of up to 25–40 % of the upper or lower eyelid may be closed primarily in layers. Any necessary incisions to conservatively debride devitalized tissue should be oriented perpendicularly with respect to the lid margin and extend to the tarsal margin to decrease the risk of lid notching, retraction, and lagophthalmos. Vertically oriented repair should be performed in layers, with tarsal plate approximation as the most critical step. This is typically accomplished with partial-thickness interrupted sutures of 5-0 or 6-0 polyglactin through the tarsal plate after preliminary placement of a lid margin retraction stitch for alignment. Care is taken to avoid passing the suture through the conjunctiva on the undersurface to avoid postoperative corneal irritation. Once all sutures have been placed, sutures are tied with buried knots. Additional sutures can then be placed through the lid margin for support, including one anteriorly through the ciliary line and one posteriorly through the gray line if needed. The anterior lamella consisting of the orbicularis muscle and skin is then repaired separately. Absorbable sutures such as fast-dissolving catgut are often preferred for the latter repair, particularly if follow-up in trauma patients is to be a problem.

More extensive eyelid injuries may require skin grafts and flaps for adequate reconstruction. Partial-thickness, superficial defects may occasionally be addressed with full-thickness skin grafts harvested from the contralateral eyelid, preauricular, precervical, or lateral cervical regions. Skin from these areas will provide the best color match for eyelid skin. Full-thickness defects not amenable to primary closure will require more detailed reconstruction. In these cases, attention should be directed to reconstitution of both the anterior lamella, consisting of the skin and muscle, and the posterior lamella, consisting of the tarsal plate and conjunctiva. Posterior lamellar reconstruction in both the upper and lower eyelids may be accomplished with the use of tarsoconjunctival flaps, periosteal flaps, and buccal mucosal or palatal grafts, the latter three potentially in combination with cartilage support grafts. Anterior lamellar reconstruction can be accomplished with the well-described Tenzel semicircular rotational flap in combination with lateral canthotomy, the temporal forehead Fricke flap, or, for lower lids, the Tripier blepharoplasty-type flap or the Mustarde cheek flap. Full-thickness defects of the upper lid may also be repaired with a lid-sharing approach using a pedicled flap from the lower lid as described by Mustarde (and akin to the Abbe lip flap).

Avulsive injuries to the medial canthal region as well as lacerations that extend medial to the lacrimal puncta should prompt careful evaluation for damage to the lacrimal system. The lacrimal system begins at the lacrimal puncta, visible at the medial margins of both the upper and lower eyelids. The upper and lower canaliculi extend from the puncta, initially with a straight vertical path for 2 mm, then with a horizontal path for an additional 8–10 mm, toward the common canaliculus and then into the lacrimal sac. The lacrimal sac lies within the bony depression of the medial orbital wall and drains into the lacrimal duct, which runs within the mucosa of the lateral nasal wall and then exits beneath the inferior nasal turbinate. When injury to the lacrimal system is suspected, two methods may be used to help rule out injury: (1) a Jones test with fluorescein dye and (2) direct probing and irrigation. Both can be performed in a cooperative adult patient under local anesthesia. For children, or other patients in whom initial assessment proves difficult, examination (with potential repair) should be conducted in the operating room, preferably within 48–72 h of the initial trauma. Consultation with an ophthalmologist will generally be required unless the reconstructive surgeon has particular expertise with the techniques described. The Jones test is performed by instilling fluorescein into the affected eye, having the patient occlude the contralateral nasal passage, and then blowing the nose into a tissue and looking for presence of the dye. Direct probing and irrigation requires passage of a lacrimal cannula into the canalicular system followed by irrigation to confirm nasal drainage.

In cases of confirmed canalicular injury, lacrimal system intubation and repair is indicated to prevent epiphora. This is performed most easily under general anesthesia, but may also be performed in the cooperative patient after instillation of topical local anesthetic into the eye and application to the punctum using a cotton-tipped applicator. The nose is also packed with pledgets soaked in oxymetazoline or 0.25 % phenylephrine to promote vasoconstriction in the area of the inferior turbinate. Punctal dilation is performed, after which a Bowman probe is then passed through the proximal canaliculus (first vertically and then horizontally). Once the distal cut end of the canaliculus is identified, the probe is passed through this distal end and continued until the "hard stop" of the bony lacrimal fossa is identified. At this point, the probe is rotated and advanced down the lacrimal sac and duct until exiting the inferior meatus. Using the probe as a guide, the injured canaliculus is then intubated in a monocanalicular fashion with the tube acting to stent the site of laceration. Alternatively, bicanalicular intubation is performed and the tube is secured inside the nose. Suture repair of the stented canaliculus is controversial, but may be performed with the aid of a microscope using fine (8-0) absorbable sutures. As a final step, in cases of medial canthal avulsion, the medial canthal tendon is sewn back to the anterior lacrimal crest with a double-armed suture of 4-0 silk and tied over a bolster.

Ears

Trauma to the auricle warrants specific consideration due to the potential complexity involved in recreating a normal-appearing ear with reasonable overall symmetry to the contralateral side. In most adult and pediatric patients, typical ear trauma can be managed effectively in the Emergency Department. Significant avulsive injuries may require grafts and flaps for reconstruction, however, and these are best managed in the operating room with full control over the patient, proper instrumentation and lighting, and cautery. Simple lacerations of the ear should be approached as for other soft tissue lacerations of the head and neck with infiltration of local anesthetic containing epinephrine, copious saline irrigation, and meticulous layered closure. The commonly relayed admonition against the use of epinephrine in local anesthetic blocks to the ear should be regarded as a myth. A "field block" consisting of local anesthetic infiltration around the perimeter of the ear, coupled with direct injection into the conchal bowl to anesthetize Arnold's nerve, will generally provide complete anesthesia. Suture repair should separately include the posterior skin, cartilage, and anterior skin. Small areas of injured cartilage or exposed cartilage with non-intact periosteum may be conservatively debrided to minimize the chances of chondritis following closure. As discussed in other sections, antibiotic prophylaxis is not generally indicated unless a high degree of contamination is suspected (e.g., in the case of bite wounds to the ear).

Avulsive defects of the auricle are approached according to the location of the defect, similar to oncologic resections. For the conchal bowl, skin defects may be reconstructed with full-thickness skin grafts over intact perichondrium or left to heal by secondary intention. Defects for which the perichondrial layer is absent may be treated with resection of the cartilage followed by skin grafting from pre- or postauricular sites. Defects of the upper auricular third may be treated by conversion to a simple wedge excision for small (< 1.5 cm) defects of the helix and antihelix. To allow tension-free primary closure, the wedge may be extended into the conchal bowl with additional cartilage resection as necessary. Of note, this will generally produce shortening of the ear, but can allow the maintenance of an acceptable ear shape with minimal morbidity. Larger defects of the upper third may be addressed with Antia-Buch chondrocutaneous advancement flaps for the helix, bipedicled postauricular tubed flaps, or, in cases of significant defects, rib cartilage covered by temporalis fascia and a full-thickness skin graft (See Fig. 11.2). Defects of the middle third of the ear may be reconstructed via wedge resection and primary closure or, for larger defects, in a staged manner with a postauricular pedicled flap. Inferior third (i.e., lobule) defects are often treated in a staged fashion with preliminary banking of conchal or nasoseptal cartilage followed by secondary elevation of the composite construct. Traumatic clefts of the earlobe may be repaired with variations of Z-plasty or rolled flap techniques.

Avulsions in which the amputated part has been recovered and preserved deserve specific mention. In children especially, consideration can be given to reattachment of the amputated part as a composite graft. Like reattachment of lip tissue, the success of composite grafting in such cases stems from the exquisite vascularity of the tissue bed. Chances of success are higher in younger patients and for small avulsed segments. Retroauricular banking of avulsed cartilage is another frequently described option, but is subject to multiple complications including resorption of the graft, the need for staged operations to elevate the composite unit, possible infection, and poor overall aesthetic outcomes. This technique has currently fallen out of favor, and traditional reconstructive techniques as discussed above are preferred. Finally, for near-total or total amputations, microsurgical replantation may be considered. This is fraught with considerable challenges, however, and failures are common.

Acute hematoma is another common manifestation of soft tissue trauma to the ear that may be observed in the

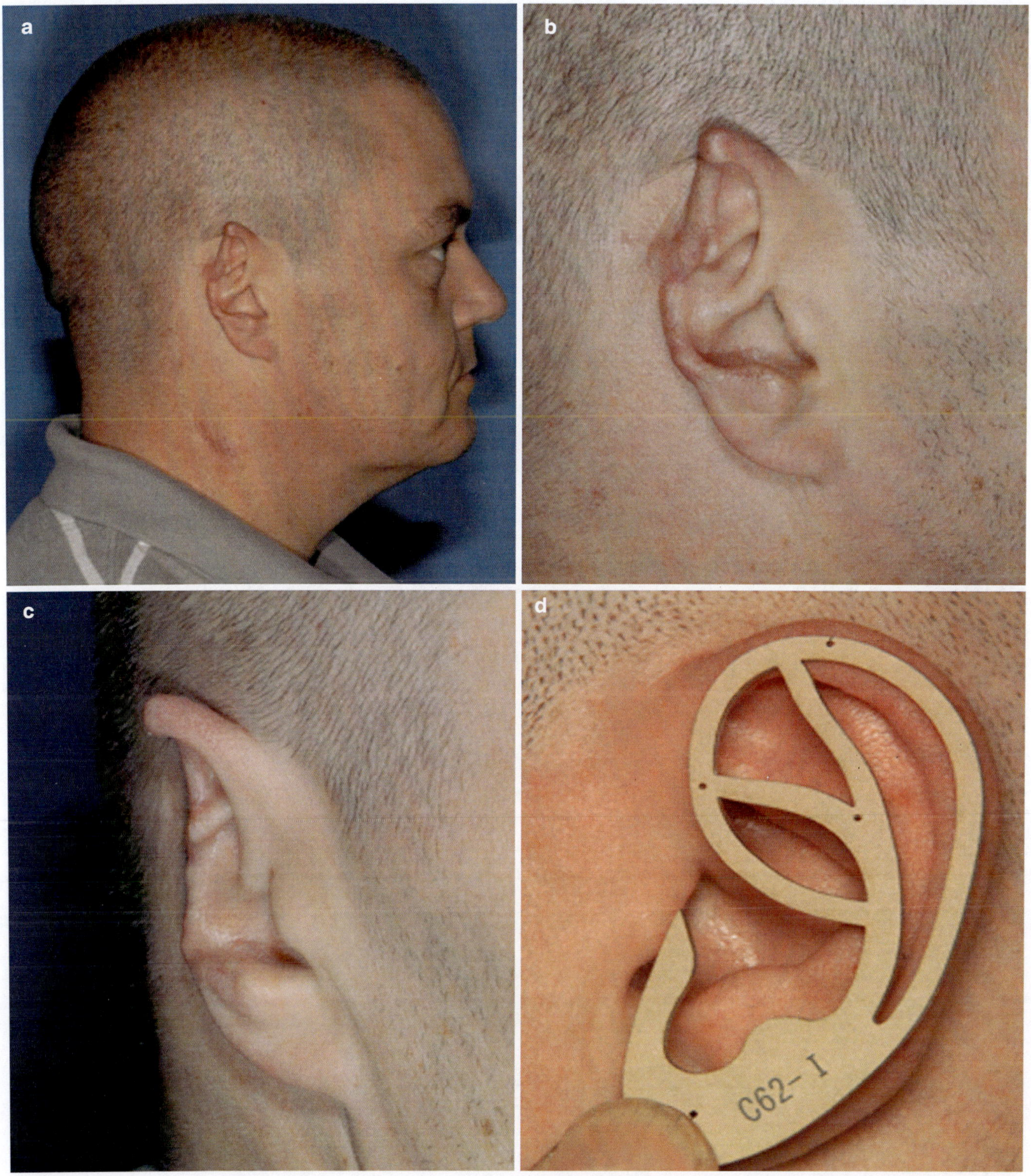

Fig. 11.2 Avulsive injury to the upper and middle thirds of the auricle, treated with rib cartilage graft, temporoparietal fascial flap, and skin graft: (**a**) preoperative photograph of the right ear (lateral view); (**b**) preoperative photograph (lateral view, zoomed in); (**c**) preoperative photograph (oblique view); (**d**) basic framework of ear sized according to the contralateral side; (**e**) construction of the sculpting template based on the upper and middle thirds of the auricular framework; (**f**) sculpting of the rib cartilage graft based on the template; (**g**) marking of the inferiorly based temporoparietal fascial flap (note: incision in *black ink*, flap borders in *green*, and superficial temporal vascular pedicle in *red*); (**h**) elevation of the temporoparietal fascial flap and inset of the cartilaginous graft; (**i**) coverage of the graft with the fascial flap; (**j**) skin grafting of the fascial flap with application of closed suction drainage; (**k**) 2-month postoperative outcome

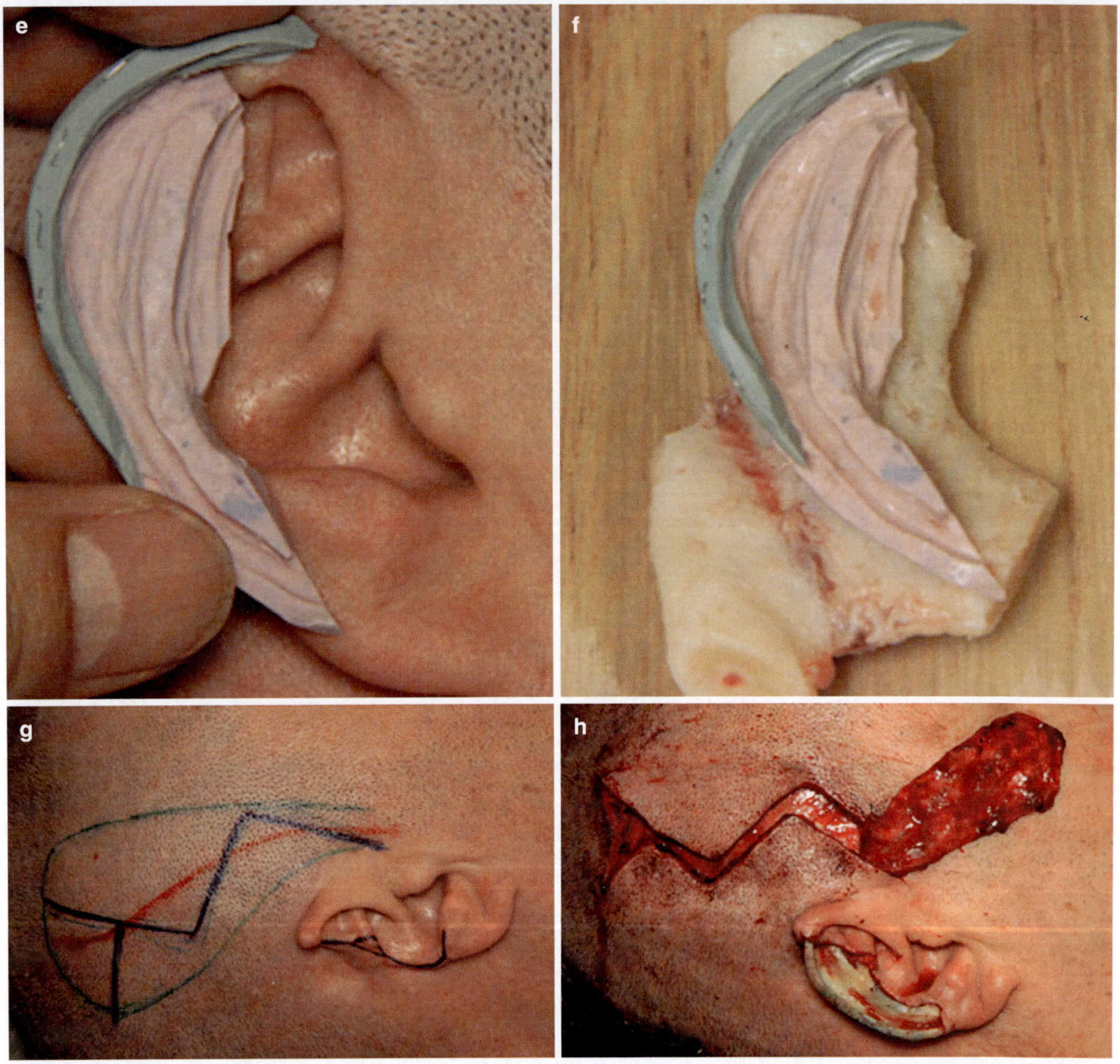

Fig. 11.2 (continued)

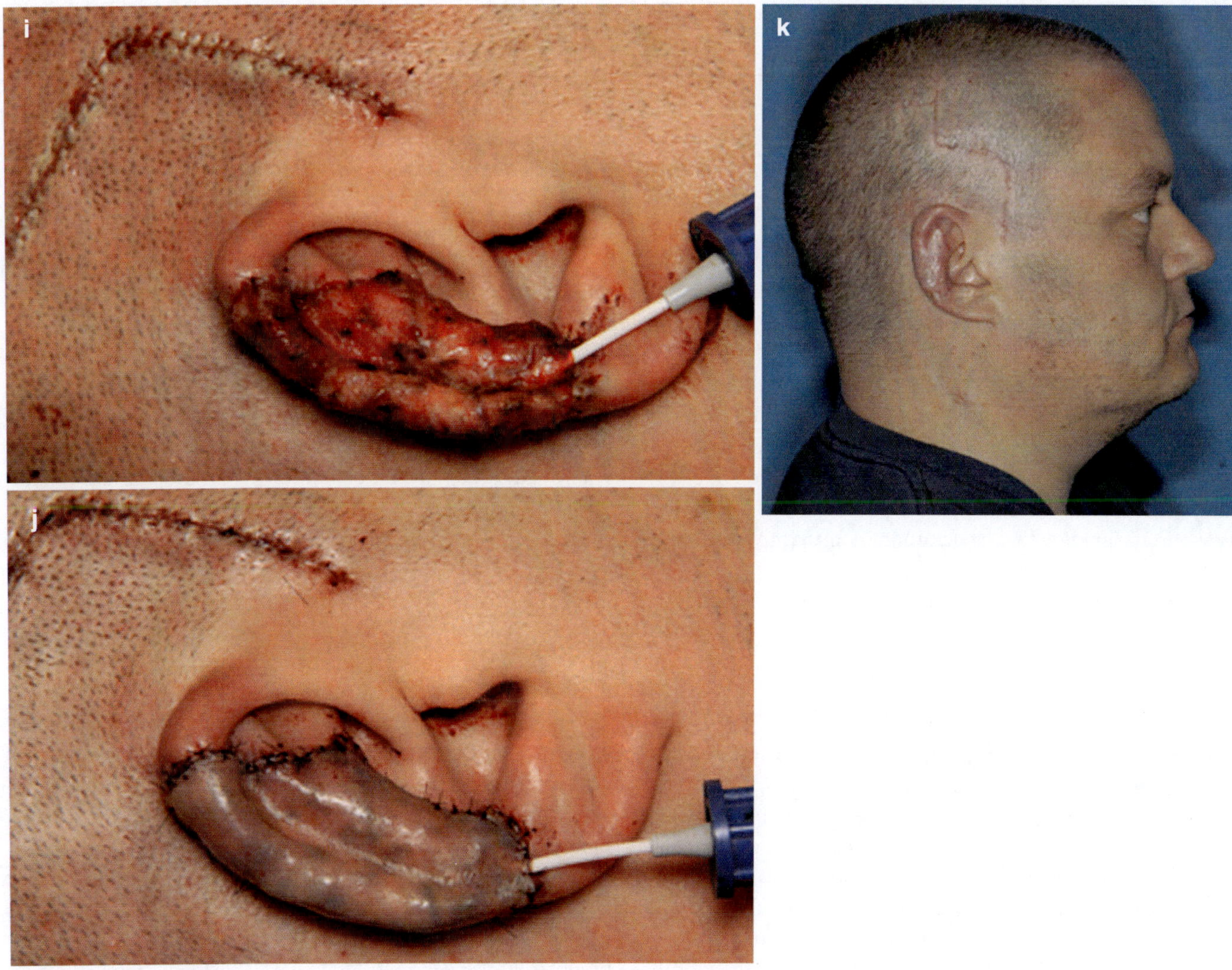

Fig. 11.2 (continued)

Emergency Department setting. Hematomas form when blood pools beneath the perichondrial layer of the cartilaginous framework. Incision and drainage with application of a bolster dressing is necessary to prevent the development of reactive cartilage formation and the "cauliflower ear" deformity.

Lips

Repair of soft tissue injuries to the lips requires meticulous reapproximation of the vermilion border and exquisite attention to anatomic detail, as a misalignment of even 1 mm will lead to a perceivable deformity. In addition to vermilion reapproximation, care must be taken to achieve proper alignment of the white roll along the lip border and the red line between the wet and dry portions of the red lip. Any incisions should be placed within relaxed skin tension lines or between the medial and lateral aesthetic subunits of the upper lip to minimize the appearance of scars. Though reconstructive surgeons should strive to preserve the natural height, balance, and appearance of the lips, ideal aesthetic measurements may be useful in optimizing outcomes. In general, the distance from the columella to the stomion should be one-half the distance from the stomion to the lowest point on the chin. The upper lip should be thinner than the lower lip and contain a defined cupid's bow. On profile view, the lower lip should be slightly posterior to or in line with the upper lip. The lips should seal on repose yet reveal 2–3 mm of the incisors when slightly parted.

Careful inspection of lip and perioral trauma should be followed by formulation of plans for repair either in the Emergency Department or in the operating room as deemed appropriate. The abundant vascularity of the lip makes it helpful to use local anesthetic containing epinephrine to induce vasoconstriction. As with eyelid repair, however, it should be recognized that local infiltration of anesthetic solution into the wound edges may distort key anatomic landmarks. To circumvent this issue, landmarks may be marked in ink prior to the injection of local anesthetic. Alternatively, nerve blocks (e.g., infraorbital or mental) may be used to lessen the requirement for direct infiltration. Because it is generally helpful to anesthetize the tissue prior to saline irrigation of the wound, ink marks made before injection may be washed off by the time repair is ready to commence. Tattooing with a hypodermic needle and methylene blue dye, as done in a cleft lip repair, may therefore be helpful. Although debridement of jagged tissue edges as discussed earlier in the chapter is a typical recommendation for most lacerations, trimming of lip tissue should be done with caution, especially in the pediatric patient. Robust vascularity of lip tissue dictates a much more conservative approach in this case.

Although healing by secondary intention may result in good functional and aesthetic outcomes in the pediatric population, most defects involving less than one-third of the lip should undergo direct primary closure in layers. Partial-thickness defects of less than one-third of the lip, particularly in adult males where adjacent tissue transfer from non-hair-bearing regions would give a suboptimal result, should generally be converted to full-thickness defects by excision and then closed primarily. In children, small partial-thickness defects resulting from avulsion may be addressed with composite tissue grafting of the avulsed part, similar to what may be done in cases of ear trauma. In general, primary repair should be achieved in a layered fashion from an "inside-out" approach, beginning first with the mucosal layer closure with an absorbable suture such as 5-0 chromic gut. The orbicularis oris muscle is approximated next with buried absorbable sutures (e.g., 4-0 or 5-0 polyglactin). Finally, the vermilion and skin are repaired, often with absorbable suture such as 5-0 chromic gut for the vermilion and nonabsorbable 6-0 polypropylene or nylon for the skin. For the lower lip, incisions may be carried down the labiomental groove in manner analogous to the excision of a Burow triangle. Similarly, in the upper lip, perialar crescentic extensions can be carried out to facilitate primary approximation.

Moderate to large lip defects involving up to two-thirds of the lip length typically require more complex reconstructions with flaps (See Fig. 11.3). Due to the time, planning, and resources required for these flaps, they are best performed in the operating room in a delayed fashion rather than immediately at the bedside of the acute trauma patient. Lip-sharing approaches include the Abbe flap or, in the case of commissural defects, the Estlander flap. Pedicle division for Abbe flaps is often performed 10–14 days after flap placement or when perfusion of the transferred segment appears independent of flow through the pedicle; this can be assessed by pinching off the intervening tissue. Estlander flaps may require secondary commissural revision. In general, lip-sharing flaps are designed to be half as long as the defect measured along the vermilion. Alternative approaches for moderate to large defects include the Karapandzic circumoral advancement flap for the central upper or lower lip, the Webster-Bernard cheek advancement for the central lower lip, or the Webster combination procedure for the central upper lip (consisting of bilateral perialar crescentic excisions with a central Abbe flap from the lower lip). Near-total lip loss may require free tissue transfer. The radial forearm free flap has been used most often for this application, often together with the palmaris longus tendon to serve as a sling for lip support. In cases of traumatic amputation of lips where tissue has been well preserved, microsurgical replantation is an option.

Facial Nerve

An understanding of facial nerve anatomy is central to the effective management of facial nerve injuries. After exiting the stylomastoid foramen, the facial nerve divides within the parotid gland into its respective extratemporal branches, which then proceed to innervate the muscles of facial expression. These five major extratemporal branches include the temporal, zygomatic, buccal, marginal mandibular, and cervical branches. Significant crossover between the buccal and zygomatic branches confers a degree of protection from injury. In contrast, the temporal and marginal mandibular branches have been reported to have less than 15 % crossover, which suggests a lower likelihood of spontaneous recovery after injury. Based on the descriptions of Pitanguy and Ramos, the temporal branch is often envisioned along a line extending from 0.5 cm inferior to the tragus to 1.5 cm superior and lateral to the lateral aspect of the eyebrow. However, Gosain and coworkers have shown that the temporal branch appears to consist of multiple rami that fan out over the zygomatic arch rather than a single branch whose path can be easily predicted using two landmark points. The course of the marginal mandibular branch may likewise be harder to predict based on landmarks than originally thought. The classic studies of Dingman and Grabb indicated passage of the marginal branch above the inferior border of the mandible 80 % of the time when posterior to the facial vessels, and 100 % of the time when anterior to the vessels. This was challenged by Nelson and Gingrass in a study involving live surgeries in which the marginal branch could be stimulated as far as 2 cm below the inferior border of the mandible in all cases.

The clinical presentation of facial nerve injury most often consists of functional and aesthetic deficits of the ocular and oral musculature. The ocular effects of facial nerve injury

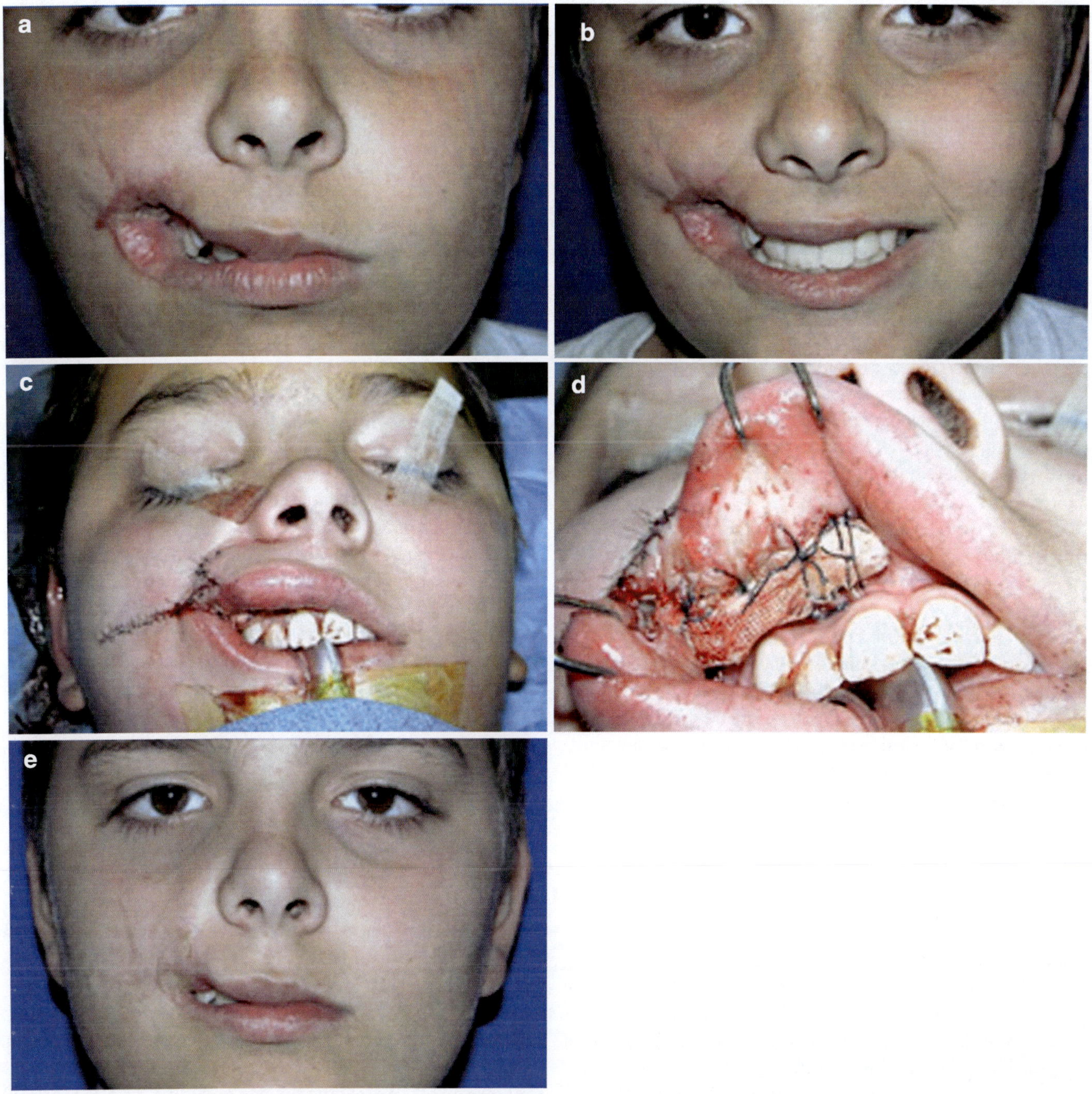

Fig. 11.3 A 6-year-old boy with loss of right lateral commissure from a dog bite injury: (**a**, **b**) the wound had healed by secondary intention at the time of initial presentation; (**c**) initial reconstruction consisted of local tissue rearrangement to reconstruct the lateral commissure; (**d**) a skin graft was additionally placed to deepen the upper labial sulcus (**e**)

include lagophthalmos, dry eyes, inability to blink, and lower lid ectropion. Oral effects include oral incompetence, drooling, and food retention. Facial asymmetry and impairment of emotional expression can significantly impact the psychological well-being of the patient, with the inability to smile as perhaps the most devastating.

As mentioned earlier, secondary survey of the head and neck trauma patient should include a focused assessment of facial nerve function. Because traumatic facial nerve injuries most often result from fractures of the temporal bone secondary to motor vehicle accidents or gunshot wounds, associated injuries may necessarily delay the secondary survey. However, once the patient has been stabilized, he/she should be prompted to elevate the eyebrows, close the eyes forcibly, pucker the lips, and show the teeth. Facial nerve defects should be documented at rest and with movement through photography and videos, which again should become part of the medical record with proper consent from the patient. In the acute phase, specific nerve testing is not useful. However, beginning approximately 14 days post-injury, electromyography (EMG) can help confirm denervation of facial muscle groups in cases of nerve branch transection.

Treatment options for facial nerve injury depend principally on the time elapsed from the initial traumatic event. In cases of complete nerve transection with loss of function, distal nerve branches can be effectively stimulated up to 72 h following injury. Responses, however, may be weakened after only 24 h. Therefore, if direct nerve end coaptation is to be performed using stimulation to help identify the distal branches (in an effort to minimize synkinesis), this should be done as soon as possible after injury and preferably within the first 24 h. Primary neurorrhaphy using 9-0 or 10-0 epineurial sutures is the treatment of choice when nerve ends can be coapted without tension. When tension is present, interposition nerve grafts (e.g., sural or greater auricular), synthetic nerve tubes, or cadaveric nerve matrices should be considered. It should be noted that, in the event facial asymmetry is questionable on examination or cannot reliably be assessed, exploration is warranted if the mechanism of injury suggests possible involvement of the facial nerve. This relates directly to the possibility of performing primary neurorrhaphy should a transected nerve branch be identified. Note that this may influence the decision to repair associated lacerations in the operating room rather than in the Emergency Department under less than ideal conditions. Despite the oft-quoted recommendation that injuries medial to a vertical line dropped from the lateral canthus do not warrant operative exploration, we recommend operative exploration in all cases where the facial nerve may be injured. Even if distal branches are not amenable to surgical repair, operative exploration allows thorough documentation of injury, which becomes important for proper follow-up.

Intermediate facial nerve injuries, namely, those with an elapsed time of less than 12 months, are generally characterized by preserved motor endplates within the distal facial musculature. In the majority of these cases, the nature of the injury is such that the proximal facial nerve branch is unavailable or nonfunctional for reconstruction. As a consequence, reanimation proceeds using the principles of nerve transfer to the distal facial nerve stumps. This may be done with the ipsilateral hypoglossal, spinal accessory, or masseteric nerves. Because the former two options involve weakening of existing cranial nerves as well as reliance on inconvenient cortical associations (e.g., requirement of tongue protrusion for smiling), the option of using the motor nerve to the masseter is preferable. Cross-face nerve grafting is also an option and can allow for bilaterally coordinated movements as well as spontaneity of movement. The technique involves coaptation of sural nerve grafts to branches of the contralateral facial nerve and, once axons have migrated through the grafts, coaptation to the distal ipsilateral nerve stumps. Due to the time required for cross-face axon outgrowth, the procedure is completed in two stages with intermediate banking of the distal sural grafts in the upper lip. With clinical or histologic evidence of regeneration at the ends of the sural grafts, distal coaptation then proceeds. A "babysitter" nerve transfer may be required to the distal ipsilateral facial nerve stumps to prevent motor endplate recession prior to the time required for cross-face axon migration.

When facial nerve injury has persisted longer than 1 year, muscular atrophy and motor endplate loss greatly limit functional recovery and the success of reanimation using nerve repair or nerve graft to existing branches of the facial nerve. In this situation, options are twofold: (1) static procedures to address deficits and asymmetries and (2) dynamic muscle transfers to restore function. The two are not mutually exclusive, as static procedures are frequently used to facilitate eyelid closure, while dynamic reanimation procedures are used to restore the more socially important function of smiling. Static procedures for the eyelids include blepharoplasty, canthoplasty/canthopexy, and placement of gold weights to correct lagophthalmos. Dynamic muscle transfers may include regional muscle transfers such as segmental turnover or transposition of the temporalis or masseter, respectively. Such transfers have often not been effective due to suboptimal vectors of pull, inadequate excursions, difficulty obtaining symmetry, and lack of spontaneity of smile function. Excellent results, however, have been obtained with innervated free muscle transfer using the gracilis muscle. In this procedure, originally detailed by Zuker and Manktelow, a segmental free gracilis muscle flap is harvested along with its obturator nerve and then anchored with the appropriate tension to the deep temporal fascia and to the oral commissure. Microvascular anastomosis is performed as well as neural coaptation, either to the ipsilateral masseteric motor nerve or to a previously placed cross-face sural nerve graft. Superior results have been demonstrated in children using this technique, including the development of spontaneous smiles with both innervation methods and significant improvements in oral competence including drooling, drinking, and speech. Recent comparative results suggest increased excursion of the oral commissure with the use of the ipsilateral masseteric nerve (to within 2 mm of the unaffected side), but less spontaneity of the smile when compared with use of cross-face nerve grafts. A process of cortical reeducation is necessary to dissociate smiling from biting when the masseteric nerve is used.

Outcomes in facial nerve reconstruction may be influenced by a number of factors, and, as stated above, static or nonsurgical measures may be required in addition to surgery to achieve optimal results. The location of the nerve injury relative to the target muscle, the axonal load of the donor nerve, and the duration of target muscle denervation are all key determinants of the success of surgical reconstruction. Younger patients with a greater number of axons in the proximal nerve or nerve graft tend to enjoy better clinical outcomes. Patients with very proximal injuries are prone to errors in nerve regeneration with resultant synkinesis or dyskinesis. Options to improve suboptimal outcomes following facial nerve reconstruction include selective neurectomy or myectomy, brow lifts, face lifts, and static slings or suture suspensions. In addition, botulinum neurotoxin may be administered on the unaffected side to improve facial symmetry and on the affected side to relieve muscle twitches due to synkinesis.

Parotid Duct

The bulk of the parotid gland lies superficial to posterior border of the masseter muscle, while its major duct, Stensen's duct, courses anterior to the masseter and ultimately pierces through the buccinator muscle to enter the oral cavity opposite the second maxillary molar. Facial soft tissue injuries that cross a line from the tragus of the ear to the midportion of the upper lip increase the risk of parotid duct injury. Van Sickels describes three regions of ductal injury: region A, situated posterior to the masseter and involving the gland itself; region B, consisting of the main duct and gland directly overlying the masseter; and region C, representing the distal duct anterior to the masseter and extending medially toward the intraoral papilla. Region B is the most common site of ductal injury. Of note, since the major buccal branch of the facial nerve tends to run with the parotid duct in this region, motor deficits in those muscles innervated by the buccal branches (e.g., weakness of the upper lip on facial animation) should raise the suspicion for injury to both structures. Unlike buccal branch deficits, parotid duct injuries may not be readily apparent on examination. In some cases, saliva may be visualized in the wound at rest or with milking of the parotid gland. In other cases, and particularly in the Emergency Department with limited resources and lighting, confirmation may be difficult or even impossible. A high degree of clinical suspicion must therefore be maintained in the appropriate setting, and the threshold kept low for operative exploration.

As with suspected facial nerve injuries, exploration is best done within 24 h of the initial traumatic event. Ductal injury may be confirmed with introduction of a lacrimal probe through the intraoral papilla and out into the wound or with the introduction of saline or methylene blue dye via angiocatheter injection into the papilla. Dye injection is controversial, as multiple investigators point to generalized tissue staining that may make subsequent ductal repair difficult. Sialography may be useful in cases of delayed diagnosis of ductal injury or in postoperative follow-up assessments, but has no practical role in the setting of acute injury.

Three methods are generally employed in the management of parotid duct injuries: primary ductal repair, creation of a controlled oral fistula, and suppression of salivary gland function. To a large extent, location of the parotid duct injury (according to the Van Sickels classification) influences selection of the appropriate treatment. Isolated parotid glandular injuries in region A can generally be managed nonoperatively with the application of compression dressings to limit the accumulation of saliva, administration of oral anti-sialogogues to suppress saliva production, serial aspiration, antibiotic administration, and avoidance of oral intake for several days to weeks. For ductal injuries in region B, primary anastomotic repair using 8-0 or 9-0 nylon sutures is advocated. This is often performed over a silicone stent to prevent stenosis and maintain ductal patency during a healing period of 1–2 weeks. The stent is sutured to the buccal mucosa just anterior to the papilla to avoid displacement during this time. For distal ductal injuries in region C, primary anastomosis may not feasible. In such cases, the proximal parotid duct may be sutured directly to the buccal mucosa with 8-0 nylon to create a controlled oral fistula for salivary diversion. Lastly, for cases in which distal duct identification is impossible and avulsive tissue damage creates a gap too large for proximal ductal diversion, ligation of the proximal ductal stump is an option. After an initial period of inflammation, swelling, and pain, this method induces parotid glandular atrophy as a result of result of retrograde pressure.

Late complications of parotid duct injuries, whether due to intentional or unintentional delays in treatment, primarily include sialoceles and salivary fistulas. Sialoceles often develop 8–14 days post-trauma and may be confirmed via aspiration and identification of amylase within the specimen. Treatment consists of pressure dressing application, serial aspiration, antibiotic therapy, and anti-sialogogue administration. Fistulas may develop within the first week after trauma and present with salivary drainage into the wound at rest or with milking of the parotid gland or mastication. As with sialoceles, initial treatments are conservative and directed at suppression of saliva production and the promotion of glandular atrophy. If conservative measures fail for either fistulas or sialoceles, surgical intervention may be warranted. Primary repair of the duct at this later stage may not be feasible due to scarring, but proximal duct ligation may be performed. Tympanic neurectomy may allow a reduction of parotid gland secretion via parasympathetic denervation, but results are often short-lived. Presently, the administration of botulinum neurotoxin is favored for parasympathetic blockade and reduction of salivary gland secretions. Using this technique, excellent results have been observed with minimal side effects. In extreme cases of problematic fistula, sialocele, or sialorrhea, superficial or total parotidectomy may be required.

Special Considerations

Bite Wounds

It has been estimated that 50 % of people in the USA will, at some point during their lifetimes, experience an animal or human bite wound. Dogs are by far responsible for the majority of bite wounds and account for an estimated 80–90 % of bites that require medical attention. Recent estimates indicate that nearly 4.7 million dog bites occur annually in the United States and that one out every six patients requires medical attention. Children have been estimated to sustain serious dog bites requiring medical attention three times more often than adults. In one of the largest reported series on pediatric dog bites from the Children's Hospital of Philadelphia recorded over a 5-year period, the highest incidence of injury was found in children aged 6–12 years. Dog bites to the face occurred in approximately 30 % of patients overall, but was the most common site of injury in children up to 5 years of age. The prevalence of facial dog bites in infants and toddlers predominantly reflects their stature, since their faces are often at eye level with the dog and easily accessible upon provocation. Bites are most common in a "central target area" that includes the nose, cheeks, and lips. Biting dogs are typically family pets or neighborhood pets known to the victims. Pitbulls, rottweilers, and German shepherds are the breeds responsible for the majority of documented bites.

In addition to dog bites, which are responsible for most bite wounds, cat bites and human bites may result in soft tissue trauma to the head and neck. Cat bites are the second most common and account for approximately 5–15 % of animal bite wounds. Compared with dog bites, cat bites are believed to carry a higher risk of wound infection, on the order of 30–50 %. This may stem from the long slender teeth of cats, allowing deep inoculation into the tissues, or from the unique oral flora in cats. Human bites are clearly less common than animal bites, but may have the highest rates of infection of all bite wounds. Human bites most typically occur during interpersonal violence, and approximately 15–20 % of the time occur on the head and neck.

Facial bite wound patients should be approached as any other patient with craniomaxillofacial trauma discussed earlier in this chapter. After ensuring the stability of the patient via completion of the primary survey, the secondary survey commences with a focused history. The events leading up to the injury and the time of injury should be documented. For animal bites, descriptions of the perpetrating animal including its ownership, behavior, and immunization status should be chronicled. The local or state health department should be notified regarding any considerations of postexposure prophylaxis for rabies, as discussed in more detail below. Finally, medical history of the bite wound victim should be obtained per usual, including documentation of tetanus immunization status. Physical examination of the bite wound victim should include careful survey of any lacerations, avulsions, crush injuries, and devitalized or infected tissue. The integrity of the facial nerve and parotid duct should be assessed in the setting of cheek trauma. For periorbital bites, integrity of the globe and lacrimal system should be assessed. The latter is especially important for dog bites to the eyelids, particularly the lower eyelids, as the incidence of canalicular injury is significantly higher when compared to eyelid trauma from other etiologies. Finally, in children especially, soft tissue bites near the orbits, nose, and cheeks should be carefully examined for the presence of underlying bony fractures and appropriate supplemental imaging obtained as needed.

Management of bite wounds to the head and neck follows the same principles discussed earlier for injuries of the respective anatomic regions, albeit with an increased vigilance for postoperative infection due to the contaminated nature of the wounds. The risk of infection may be overestimated, however, for bites to the head and neck where vascularity is excellent. The classic study by Guy and Zook indicates a wound infection rate of 1.4 % for dog bites to the head and neck following pressure irrigation and suture repair in the absence of antibiotics. It is important to note that this study excluded wounds more than 6 h old, which calls into the question whether wounds after this time period have a significantly higher risk of infection and whether they should be left open. Although prospective data are lacking, general consensus suggests that bite wounds to the head and neck are appropriately managed with primary closure within 24 h of injury, provided there are no signs of acute infection such as cellulitis, purulence, or fever. In accordance with recommendations of Guy and Zook, wounds should be thoroughly irrigated with sterile saline under pressure and then repaired with as few deep sutures as necessary to reduce tension, followed by fine simple interrupted sutures for the skin to allow potential drainage.

The use of prophylactic antibiotics for bite wounds is controversial, but may be considered for deep tissue injuries with exposed structures such as cartilage, wounds closed after 6–12 h, cat and human bites, and patients with immunosuppressive comorbidities. Prophylactic antibiotics or empiric antibiotics in the case of wound infection should be directed at the common causative organisms, which include *Pasteurella*, *Streptococcus*, *Staphylococcus*, and anaerobes for cat and dog bites and *Eikenella*, *Streptococcus*, *Staphylococcus*, and anaerobes for human bites. Amoxicillin/clavulanate (or intravenous ampicillin/sulbactam) is the most suitable single agent to cover these pathogens. In penicillin-allergic patients, alternatives include clindamycin with a fluoroquinolone (for adults) or clindamycin with trimethoprim/sulfamethoxazole (for children). Treatment duration is generally 5–7 days for prophylaxis and 10–14 days for empiric therapy. Tetanus prophylaxis is recommended if the patient has had fewer than three doses of tetanus toxoid or more than 5 years has elapsed from the last vaccination. In the case of dog bites, rabies prophylaxis is administered if the offending dog was seen to manifest signs of disease at the time of the bite or if any dog placed into a 10-day quarantine period begins to manifest such signs. For bites from stray dogs for which vaccination status and/or behavior is unknown, the local or state public health department should be consulted.

Pediatric Soft Tissue Trauma

Pediatric soft tissue trauma of the head and neck continues to be a common reason for consultation of the craniomaxillofacial surgeon. Primarily a result of rapid brain growth in the early years of life, the disproportionately large head and face of children predisposes to injuries in this region. Underlying bony fractures are less common than in adults due to the relatively elastic nature of the developing facial bones. Although the principles of soft tissue repair do not differ fundamentally from those outlined earlier in this chapter, special consideration must be given to two practical issues in this population: (1) appropriate sedation and anesthesia, and (2) future growth and scar development.

Regarding anesthesia and sedation, it should be recognized that soft tissue injuries that would otherwise require simple repair in the Emergency Department for adult trauma patients may demand considerable efforts for the pediatric patient. Complex lacerations, particularly those of the periorbital region or those for which patient cooperation is paramount, will likely require more than simple infiltration with local anesthetic. Popular options for anesthesia and sedation in the pediatric Emergency Department can be categorized by level of invasiveness and include the following: (1) simple local anesthetic injection (e.g., lidocaine 0.5–1.0 % or bupivacaine 0.25 % with 1:100,000–1:200,000 epinephrine) with or without pre-application of topical skin anesthetic creams (e.g., lidocaine-epinephrine-tetracaine [LET] or lidocaine-prilocaine [EMLA]), (2) intranasal or oral midazolam for anxiolysis in addition to local anesthetic injection, and (3) intranasal or oral midazolam for anxiolysis, insertion of an intravenous line, and intravenous ketamine administered as conscious sedation with appropriate cardiorespiratory monitoring. At the Lurie Children's Hospital of Chicago, we have developed this multi-tiered scheme for anesthesia and sedation as a joint effort between the Division of Plastic Surgery and Department of Emergency Medicine. In general, school-age children (6–12 years) with low complexity lacerations are treated using the first option of simple local anesthetic infiltration, whereas infants (birth to 1 year) and preschoolers (2–5 years) are treated using the second or third paradigms depending on the complexity of the repair. Intranasal midazolam has become a popular option in our Emergency Department in many cases, as this obviates placement of an intravenous line and can often quell patient anxiety to a sufficient degree to enable irrigation and suture repair of a large majority of lacerations. As discussed throughout this chapter, soft tissue injuries which require detailed exploration and major repair, including facial nerve injuries, parotid duct injuries, and lacrimal system injuries, should be addressed in the operating room under general anesthesia where conditions are optimal.

An additional important concern in children with soft tissue injuries of the head and neck is the issue of potential growth disturbances and scar formation resulting either from the trauma itself or from attempts at repair. On the scalp, for example, care must be taken to minimize disturbance to hair growth pattern, particularly in a young girl (See Fig. 11.1). For the ear, attempts at primary layered closure or with local advancement flaps may produce shortening of the auricle, and parents must be counseled regarding the possibility of persistent visible asymmetries in size. A further example is injury to the nasal septum, for which care must be taken during any surgical interventions to preserve the integrity of the growth centers at the bony-cartilaginous junctions. Finally, in regard to scar formation, it should be noted that children often heal with exuberant hypertrophic scars that continue to fade and flatten over time. Parents should be counseled regarding the inevitability of scar despite meticulous attempts at soft tissue repair. The possibility of reduced inflammation and scarring with the use of nonabsorbable sutures must be balanced with the need for subsequent suture removal, which may be difficult or impossible with young children in the office setting. Octyl cyanoacrylate glues or fast-absorbing catgut sutures for the skin layer are popular alternatives that have not been shown to produce inferior scars in the laceration literature. In all cases, scar massage should commence once initial healing is complete, and topical silicone products may be applied to help minimize scar hypertrophy. Topical hydrocortisone, dermabrasion, and pulsed dye laser therapy may ultimately be helpful for scars with early hypertrophy or persistent erythema, respectively. Ultimately, some mature scars will still require surgical revision.

Soft Tissue Trauma Associated with Craniomaxillofacial Fractures

Optimizing the outcome of soft tissue reconstruction after craniomaxillofacial trauma requires the appropriate management of underlying bony fractures. Soft tissue contraction is common after traumatic injuries and may impair the healing and growth of underlying skeletal structures. Bony reconstitution performed simultaneously with soft tissue repair not only prevents extensive scar contractures but also helps the soft tissues retain their volume and degree of expansion. Therefore, adequate skeletal fixation, or skeletal replacement in the case of bone loss, is essential to maximizing the results of soft tissue repair.

During repair of concomitant soft tissue and bony craniomaxillofacial injury, attention should be given to any lacerations that may allow direct operative access to fractures for stabilization. As mentioned earlier, the secondary survey for the craniomaxillofacial trauma patient should include careful documentation of any lacerations, avulsions, or crush injuries to the soft tissues. In selected cases, advantage may be taken of preexisting lacerations adjacent to fractured facial bones for operative exposure and fixation. A commonly encountered example is orbitozygomatic fractures, for which periorbital lacerations may allow direct access to the orbital floor, zygomaticomaxillary buttress, or frontozygomatic suture without the need for additional transcutaneous or transconjunctival eyelid incisions and their attendant risks of lid malposition. Naso-orbito-ethmoid or complex nasal bone fractures may also be approached through advantageous lacerations without the need for coronal incisions.

A final point to make regarding concomitant bony and soft tissue reconstruction relates to the important, but often ignored, effect of extensive tissue dissection on positioning of the soft tissues. As stressed by Gruss and coworkers, wide elevation of the midfacial soft tissues in the subperiosteal plane to expose fractures often contributes to a prematurely aged appearance when the soft tissues are not properly resuspended. This is characterized predominantly by loss of zygomatic projection, fullness in the region of the nasolabial fold, and possible inferomedial displacement of the lateral canthus. Akin to a subperiosteal face lift, midfacial soft tissue can be resuspended using sutures placed through the deep periosteal layer and secured to the inferior orbital rim via simple drill holes. Lateral canthal position can also be reestablished using drill holes through the inner aspect of the lateral orbital rim.

Bibliography

Ambro BT, Wright RJ, Heffelfinger RN. Management of bite wounds in the head and neck. Facial Plast Surg. 2010;26(6):456–63.

Angelos PC, Downs BW. Options for the management of forehead and scalp defects. Facial Plast Surg Clin North Am. 2009;17(3):379–93.

Armin BB, Ruder RO, Azizadeh B. Partial auricular reconstruction. Semin Plast Surg. 2011;25:249–56.

Bruce AM, Spencer JM. Surgical myths in dermatology. Dermatol Surg. 2010;36(4):512–7.

Chandler DB, Gausas RE. Lower eyelid reconstruction. Otolaryngol Clin North Am. 2005;38(5):1033–42.

Codner MA, McCord CD, Mejia JD, Lalonde D. Upper and lower eyelid reconstruction. Plast Reconstr Surg. 2010;126(5):231e–45e.

Coppit GL, Lin DT, Burkey BB. Current concepts in lip reconstruction. Curr Opin Otolaryngol Head Neck Surg. 2004;12(4):281–7.

Dean NR, Ledgard JP, Katsaros J. Massive hemorrhage in facial fracture patients: definition, incidence, and management. Plast Reconstr Surg. 2009;123(2):680–90.

Della Rocca DA, Ahmad SM, Della Rocca RC. Direct repair of canalicular lacerations. Facial Plast Surg. 2007;23(3):149–55.

DiFrancesco LM, Codner MA, McCord CD. Upper eyelid reconstruction. Plast Reconstr Surg. 2004;114(7):98e–107e.

Dingman RO, Grabb WC. Surgical anatomy of the mandibular ramus of the facial nerve based on the dissection of 100 facial halves. Plast Reconstr Surg Transplant Bull. 1962;29:266–72.

Fattah A, Borschel GH, Zuker RM. Reconstruction of facial nerve injuries in children. J Craniofac Surg. 2011;22(3):782–8.

Fisher J. Management of alopecia. In: Guyuron B, Eriksson E, Persing JA, Chung KC, Disa JJ, Gosain AK, et al., editors. Plastic surgery: indications and practice. London, UK: Elsevier; 2009.

Fisher M, Dorafshar A, Bojovic B, Manson PN, Rodriguez ED. The evolution of critical concepts in aesthetic craniofacial microsurgical reconstruction. Plast Reconstr Surg. 2012;130(2):389–98.

Ghali S, MacQuillan A, Grobbelaar AO. Reanimation of the middle and lower face in facial paralysis: review of the literature and personal approach. J Plast Reconstr Aesthet Surg. 2011;64(4):423–31.

Gordin EA, Daniero JJ, Krein H, Boon MS. Parotid gland trauma. Facial Plast Surg. 2010;26(6):504–10.

Gosain AK, Matloub HS. Surgical management of the facial nerve in craniofacial trauma and long-standing facial paralysis: cadaver study and clinical presentations. J Craniomaxillofac Trauma. 1999;5(1):29–37.

Gosain AK, Sewall SR, Yousif NJ. The temporal branch of the facial nerve: how reliably can we predict its path? Plast Reconstr Surg. 1997;99(5):1224–33; discussion 34–6.

Greywoode JD, Ho HH, Artz GJ, Heffelfinger RN. Management of traumatic facial nerve injuries. Facial Plast Surg. 2010;26(6):511–8.

Grunebaum LD, Smith JE, Hoosien GE. Lip and perioral trauma. Facial Plast Surg. 2010;26(6):433–44.

Guy RJ, Zook EG. Successful treatment of acute head and neck dog bite wounds without antibiotics. Ann Plast Surg. 1986;17(1):45–8.

Guyuron B. Patient assessment. In: Guyuron B, Eriksson E, Persing JA, Chung KC, Disa JJ, Gosain AK, et al., editors. Plastic surgery: indications and practice. London, UK: Elsevier; 2009.

Ha RY, Trovato MJ. Plastic surgery of the ear. In: Kenkel JM, editor. Selected readings in plastic surgery. Dallas: Selected Readings in Plastic Surgery, Inc.; 2011.

Hogg NJ. Primary and secondary management of pediatric soft tissue injuries. Oral Maxillofac Surg Clin North Am. 2012;24(3):365–75.

Holger JS, Wandersee SC, Hale DB. Cosmetic outcomes of facial lacerations repaired with tissue-adhesive, absorbable, and nonabsorbable sutures. Am J Emerg Med. 2004;22(4):254–7.

Hollier Jr L, Kelley P. Soft tissue and skeletal injuries of the face. In: Thorne CH, Beasley RW, Aston SJ, Bartlett SP, Gurtner GC, Spear SL, editors. Grabb and Smith's plastic surgery. Philadelphia: Lippincott Williams and Wilkins; 2007. p. 315–32.

Janis JE, Leedy JE. Lip, cheek, and scalp reconstruction. In: Kenkel JM, editor. Selected readings in plastic surgery. Dallas: Selected Readings in Plastic Surgery, Inc., 2006.

Kaye AE, Belz JM, Kirschner RE. Pediatric dog bite injuries: a 5-year review of the experience at the Children's Hospital of Philadelphia. Plast Reconstr Surg. 2009;124(2):551–8.

Klein EJ, Brown JC, Kobayashi A, Osincup D, Seidel K. A randomized clinical trial comparing oral, aerosolized intranasal, and aerosolized buccal midazolam. Ann Emerg Med. 2011;58(4):323–9.

Kretlow JD, McKnight AJ, Izaddoost SA. Facial soft tissue trauma. Semin Plast Surg. 2010;24(4):348–56.

Krunic AL, Weitzul S, Taylor RS. Advanced reconstructive techniques for the lip and perioral area. Dermatol Clin. 2005;23(1):43–53, v–vi.

Langstein HN. Reconstructive lip surgery. In: Guyuron B, Eriksson E, Persing JA, Chung KC, Disa JJ, Gosain AK, et al., editors. Plastic surgery: indications and practice. London, UK: Elsevier; 2009.

Leedy JE, Janis JE, Rohrich RJ. Reconstruction of acquired scalp defects: an algorithmic approach. Plast Reconstr Surg. 2005;116(4):54e–72e.

Lifchez SD, Matloub HS, Gosain AK. Cortical adaptation to restoration of smiling after free muscle transfer innervated by the nerve to the masseter. Plast Reconstr Surg. 2005;115(6):1472–9; discussion 80–2.

Mehrara BJ, Disa JJ, Pusic A. Scalp reconstruction. J Surg Oncol. 2006;94(6):504–8.

Melvin TA, Limb CJ. Overview of facial paralysis: current concepts. Facial Plast Surg. 2008;24(2):155–63.

Morley AM, deSousa JL, Selva D, Malhotra R. Techniques of upper eyelid reconstruction. Surv Ophthalmol. 2010;55(3):256–71.

Murchison AP, Bilyk JR. Management of eyelid injuries. Facial Plast Surg. 2010;26(6):464–81.

Nabili V, Knott PD. Advanced lip reconstruction: functional and aesthetic considerations. Facial Plast Surg. 2008;24(1):92–104.

Nelson DW, Gingrass RP. Anatomy of the mandibular branches of the facial nerve. Plast Reconstr Surg. 1979;64(4):479–82.

Perry M. Maxillofacial trauma – developments, innovations and controversies. Injury. 2009;40(12):1252–9.

Phillips JH, Gruss JS, Wells MD, Chollet A. Periosteal suspension of the lower eyelid and cheek following subciliary exposure of facial fractures. Plast Reconstr Surg. 1991;88(1):145–8.

Pitanguy I, Ramos AS. The frontal branch of the facial nerve: the importance of its variations in face lifting. Plast Reconstr Surg. 1966;38(4):352–6.

Rafii AA, Enepekides DJ. Upper and lower eyelid reconstruction: the year in review. Curr Opin Otolaryngol Head Neck Surg. 2006;14(4):227–33.

Rovak JM, Tung TH, Mackinnon SE. The surgical management of facial nerve injury. Semin Plast Surg. 2004;18(1):23–30.

Savar A, Kirszrot J, Rubin PA. Canalicular involvement in dog bite related eyelid lacerations. Ophthal Plast Reconstr Surg. 2008;24(4):296–8.

Sowerby LJ, Taylor SM, Moore CC. The double hatchet flap: a workhorse in head and neck local flap reconstruction. Arch Facial Plast Surg. 2010;12(3):198–201.

Steinberg MJ, Herrera AF. Management of parotid duct injuries. Oral Surg Oral Med Oral Pathol Oral Radiol Endod. 2005;99(2):136–41.

Terzis JK. Facial reanimation. In: Guyuron B, Eriksson E, Persing JA, Chung KC, Disa JJ, Gosain AK, et al., editors. Plastic surgery: indications and practice. London, UK: Elsevier; 2009.

Terzis JK, Karypidis D. Therapeutic strategies in post-facial paralysis synkinesis in adult patients. Plast Reconstr Surg. 2012;129(6):925e–39e.

Terzis JK, Konofaos P. Experience with 60 adult patients with facial paralysis secondary to tumor extirpation. Plast Reconstr Surg. 2012;130(1):51e–66e.

Terzis JK, Wang W, Zhao Y. Effect of axonal load on the functional and aesthetic outcomes of the cross-facial nerve graft procedure for facial reanimation. Plast Reconstr Surg. 2009;124(5):1499–512.

Thorne CH. Otoplasty and ear reconstruction. In: Thorne CH, Beasley RW, Aston SJ, Bartlett SP, Gurtner GC, Spear SL, editors. Grabb and Smith's plastic surgery. 6th ed. Philadelphia: Lippincott Williams and Wilkins; 2007. p. 297–312.

Tu AH, Girotto JA, Singh N, Dufresne CR, Robertson BC, Seyfer AE, et al. Facial fractures from dog bite injuries. Plast Reconstr Surg. 2002;109(4):1259–65.

Van Sickels JE. Management of parotid gland and duct injuries. Oral Maxillofac Surg Clin North Am. 2009;21(2):243–6.

Vasconez HC, Buseman JL, Cunningham LL. Management of facial soft tissue injuries in children. J Craniofac Surg. 2011;22(4):1320–6.

Wexler A. Posttraumatic facial restoration: a philosophy of care. J Craniofac Surg. 2009;20(1):12–4.

Wright RJ, Murakami CS, Ambro BT. Pediatric nasal injuries and management. Facial Plast Surg. 2011;27(5):483–90.

Zide BM, Swift R. How to block and tackle the face. Plast Reconstr Surg. 1998;101(3):840–51.

Zuker RM, Goldberg CS, Manktelow RT. Facial animation in children with Moebius syndrome after segmental gracilis muscle transplant. Plast Reconstr Surg. 2000;106(1):1–8; discussion 9.

Dentoalveolar Fractures

12

William Hoffman and Peter J. Taub

Each tooth that sits within the maxilla or mandible is surrounded by softer alveolar bone. Dense cortical bone covers the exposed surface of the alveolar process as well as the underlying cancellous bone (see Fig. 12.1). The actual tooth socket is lined with thin, compact bone that is penetrated by blood vessels, lymphatics, and nerves. Connective tissue fibers ("Sharpey fibers") of the periodontal membrane hold the teeth to the surrounding bone. With dental loss, the surrounding alveolar process undergoes atrophy.

Clinical

Fractures may occur in the alveolar segments either in isolation or in combination with other portions of the maxilla or mandible. Teeth associated with alveolar fractures are characterized by mobility of the alveolar process.

While mandible fractures are fairly prevalent, those involving the alveolar process of the mandible are uncommon, accounting for only 1–5 % of all mandibular fractures. Alveolar process fractures are the result of blunt or penetrating trauma. The common causes mirror those of mandible fractures and include motor vehicle accidents, assaults, and accidents (epileptic seizures). Other causes include athletic injuries, falls, iatrogenic injury (dental extraction, endoscopy, or oral intubation), and industrial accidents. Penetrating injury usually results from gunshot wounds. Isolated dentoalveolar fracture is seen among children and adolescents with boys having a three-fold greater risk than girls.

Careful examination is required, since imaging studies may not show the fracture. The anterior teeth are usually injured as a result of a direct impact, while the closing force of the two jaws tends to injure the posterior teeth. Intrusion of the upper teeth is more frequent.

Alveolar fractures may present in conjunction with any fracture of the mandible (or craniofacial skeleton) with localized tenderness, swelling, and malocclusion. One or more teeth may be noted to move as a unit when mobility is checked on bimanual examination. Pre-injury occlusal pattern is often present disrupted.

Dental Injury

The teeth within a dentulous segment may be fractured along with the surrounding alveolar bone. Injury to the actual teeth may occur at the crown or at the root. Looseness and displacement of teeth carries a high risk of subsequent necrosis of the pulp. Secondary complications

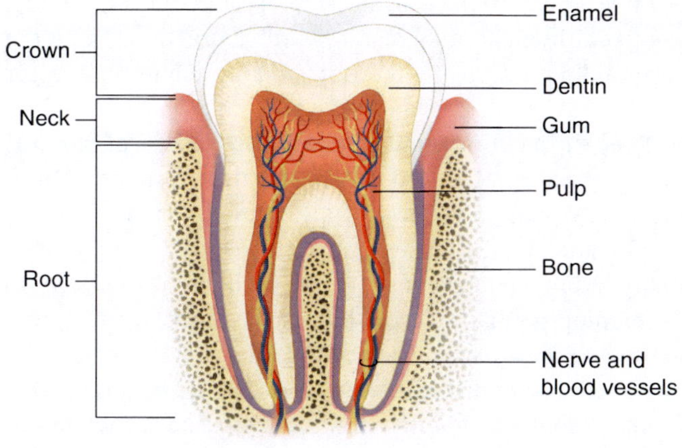

Fig. 12.1 Anatomy of a tooth

W. Hoffman, MD
Division of Plastic and Reconstructive Surgery,
Department of Surgery, University of California, San Francisco,
San Francisco, CA, USA

P.J. Taub, MD (✉)
Division of Plastic and Reconstructive Surgery,
Mount Sinai Medical Center, 5 East 98th Street, 15th Floor,
New York, NY 10029, USA
e-mail: peter.taub@mountsinai.org

P.J. Taub et al. (eds.), *Ferraro's Fundamentals of Maxillofacial Surgery*,
DOI 10.1007/978-1-4614-8341-0_12, © Springer Science+Business Media New York 2015

include resorption, canal obliteration, ankylosis, and loss of alveolar bone. Intact but loosened, laterally luxated or extruded teeth should be repositioned and splinted for 1–3 weeks respectively by semirigid splint (acid-etch composite, arch bar, orthodontic wire, soft stainless-steel wire loop, or vacuum formed splint). Completely avulsed teeth necessitates immediate replacement and semirigid splinting for 1–2 weeks. Prognosis for successful take is dependent on the stage of root development, the length of exposure time, medium in which it is stored, and the way the teeth are handled and splinted. Handling of involved teeth and neighboring healthy teeth includes gently drying the tooth with compressed air or absolute alcohol and keeping the tooth dry during the fixation procedure. If exposed, the root surface of the displaced teeth is cleansed with saline solution. The tooth-bearing alveolus is then repositioned with combined labial and lingual digital pressure until its normal position has been reestablished, indicated by alignment of the dental arch in proper occlusion. Strong force for reduction is usually required. In rare cases, forceps may be needed for reduction.

For a fracture through the crown of the tooth, treatment may include dressing of any exposed dentin, minimal pulpotomy or pulp extirpation, and restoration of damaged part of the tooth. For a fracture of the root fracture (*either oblique, vertical, or transverse*), extraction may be inevitable, but the tooth may be saved by rigid splinting for a minimum of 8 weeks, devitlaiztion (RCT) with eventful apico surgery, and/or orthodontic extrusion or crown lengthening.

A fracture through the root requires consultation with a dentist for possible root canal treatment and may be an indication for extraction. When the apical portions of the tooth roots are completely separated from their blood supply, the affected teeth may become devitalized and result in a periapical abscess. Again, urgent root canal therapy may be indicated to save these teeth and help prevent complication. Attempts should be made to preserve teeth; however, the decision to retain or extract teeth should include a consideration of the surrounding periodontal structures. Poor oral hygiene may lean towards extraction, since the surrounding tissues will offer a poor environment for healing.

Specific mention should be given to injury of the primary dentition. Most (70 %) involve the maxillary central incisors. Common patterns of injury include intrusion, lateral luxation, and avulsion. Intruded teeth are likely to normally erupt spontaneously. One problem is damage to developing permanent teeth by displaced tooth. Fractured, extruded, or grossly displaced primary teeth should be extracted. Minimally displaced teeth with no occlusal interference should be monitored, since extraction carries risk to permanent one.

Diagnosis

The diagnosis of an alveolar fracture is best made on clinical examination. Bimanual palpation of the maxillary and mandibular dentition should reveal areas of tenderness or mobility. In addition, evidence of local gingival ecchymosis, laceration, or bleeding should be concerning for an underlying fracture. This may affect the alveolus alone or the alveolus in conjunction with the maxilla or mandible.

Imaging studies are indicated to better delineate the presence of a fracture and the pattern of the fracture. An orthopantomogram will identify concomitant fracture(s) of the mandible. A cone beam CT scan is more sensitive for both the maxilla and mandible but may not identify dental fractures. In this case, coned down, periapical views of the teeth may be indicated. A chest x-ray is indicated if teeth are absent and cannot be located or the patient is obtunded to rule out aspiration.

Alveolar fractures may be classified by their specific location and amount of displacement (see Fig. 12.2). A *class I* fracture of the alveolar process involves a fracture of the edentulous segment. A *class II* fracture involves a dentulous segment with little, if any, displacement (see Fig. 12.3). A *class III* fracture involves dentulous segment with moderate-to-severe displacement (see Fig. 12.4). A *class IV* fracture shares one or more fracture lines with other fractures of the tooth-bearing facial skeleton.

Management

Treatment is often problematic, since surgeons are unfamiliar with dental structures and tend to underestimate these types of fractures and their problems. Management involves reduction and institution of some form of stabilization. Operative fixation is often not possible, since the amount of bone stock outside the tooth-bearing segments that is available for screws is limited. Even with an edentulous segment, hardware is rarely practical, because it usually ends up under a dental prosthesis and cannot be tolerated. If a splint is necessary, it needs to be fabricated before surgery from alginate impressions and plaster casts. Model surgery on the plaster models is performed to recreate the normal anatomic relationships of the fractured segments and allow fabrication of an accurate splint.

The decision of when and how to treat an alveolar fracture should be made in the context of the patient's overall clinical condition. Immediate care may not be warranted on account of more serious trauma. Maneuvers to reduce and simply stabilize the fractured segment(s) may be performed in the emergency department or the operating room should other treatment be required.

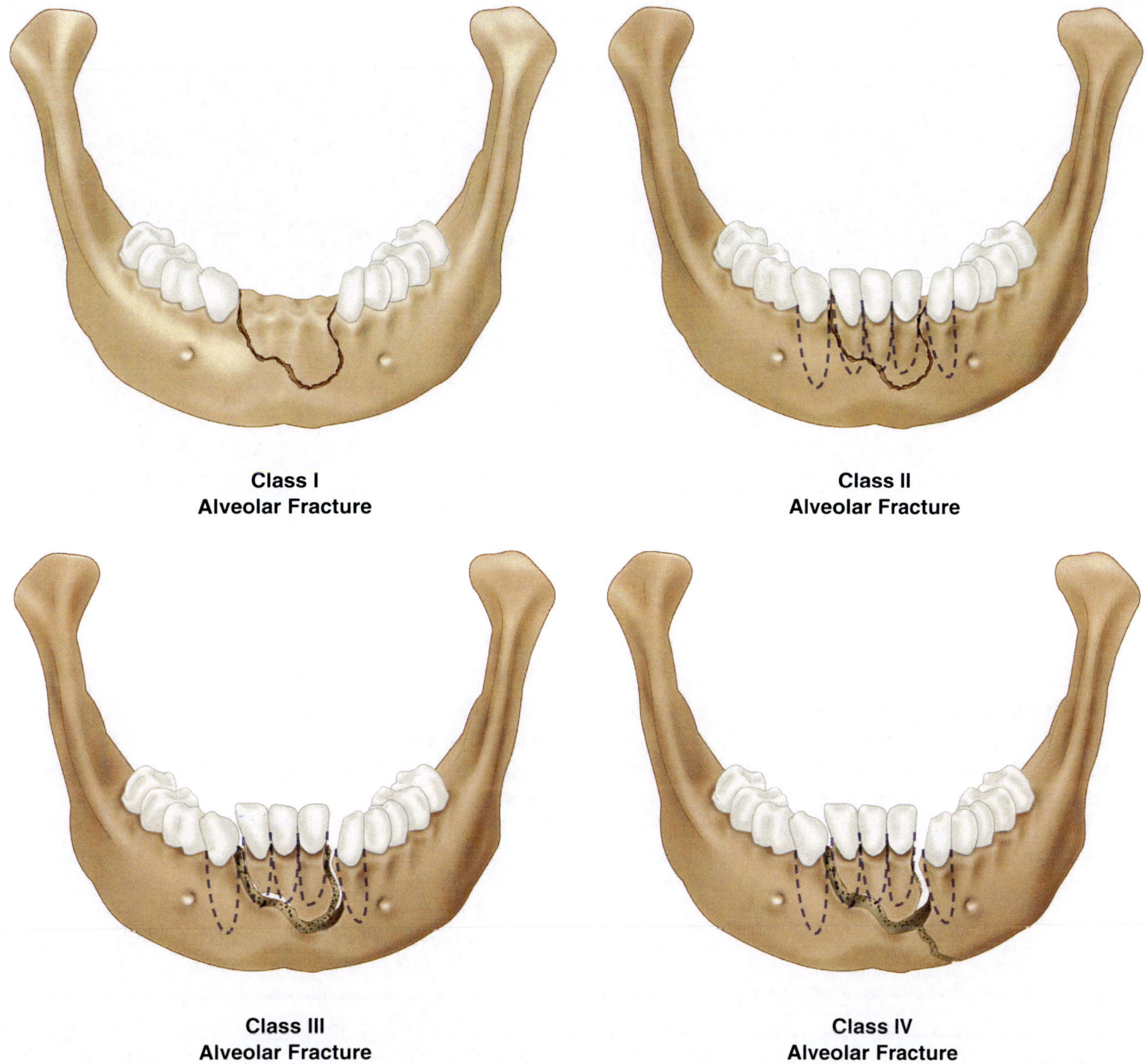

Fig. 12.2 Classification of alveolar fractures

Numerous studies have demonstrated that delays in treatment increase the complication rate and reduce the chance of obtaining the best surgical result. Reduction and immobilization of a displaced alveolar fracture is indicated if the patient will tolerate it. Nasal intubation will be required if the jaws need to be placed into occlusion for adequate fracture reduction.

Soft-tissue repair should precede the splinting of the teeth. Damage to the lip is observed more often with anterior dentoalveolar fractures. A thorough search for teeth or foreign material embedded in the lips should be undertaken. Degloving of the mental region is a common injury to the lower anterior teeth. Lacerations of the gingiva associated with dentoalveolar fracture are repaired with absorbable chromic or Vicryl simple or mattress sutures.

One mode of stabilizing an alveolar segment is the use of an acid-etch wire composite splint. This involves fixing a heavy stainless steel wire across the involved segment as well as several stable neighboring teeth on each side of the fragment. Attachment to the teeth is achieved with a composite dental restorative material/resin that adheres to both

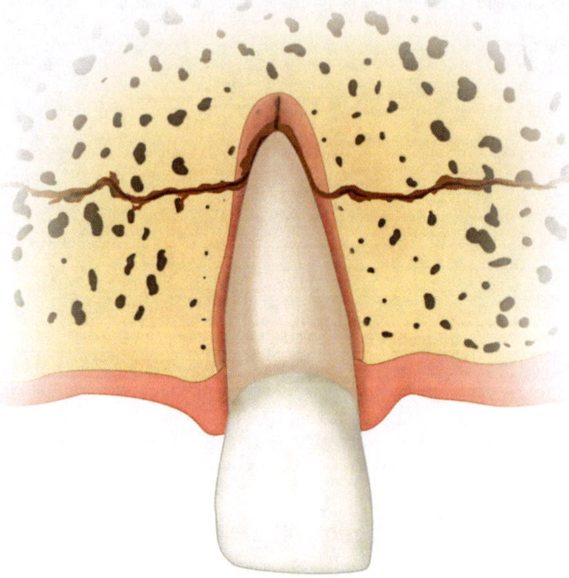

Fig. 12.3 Minimally displaced alveolar fracture

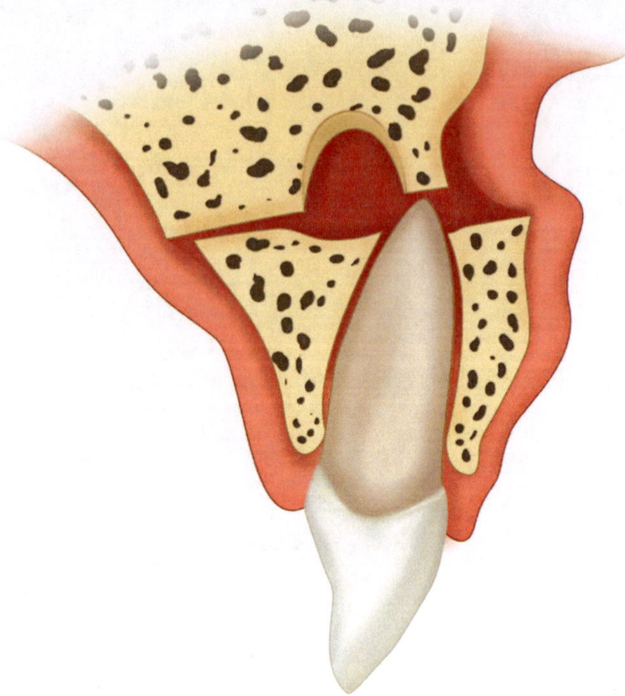

Fig. 12.4 Displaced alveolar fracture

the wire and to the acid-etched dental enamel. It is imperative that the enamel be kept dry until the resin has completely set. The resin material is similar to that used for temporary crowns and bridges and is applied to provide stabilization. The resin material allows a certain flexibility of the splinting and is easy to remove. Occlusion should be checked and no premature occlusal contacts should be permitted. The fixation should be maintained for at least 4 weeks. For removal, the resin can be peeled off with a dental scaler or removed with a burr. The teeth of the fractured segment must be supported with the fingers of the opposite hand during this maneuver to minimize the risk of refracture.

Erich-type arch bars may also be used in a similar manner with the fractured segment attached to the arch bar with thin gauge dental wire. When splints are used, they may be placed on the lingual or the buccal side and ligated to sound teeth and may be further secured by three-point circummandibular wiring.

Specific treatment by class of alveolar fracture is as follows:

Class I fractures that involve a non-displaced, edentulous alveolar segment often do not require treatment other than a soft diet and observation. If there is concern about the stability of the fracture during the healing process, stabilization may be used.

Class II fractures that involve a displaced dentulous segment and need reduction may require a great deal of force to realign the fractured segment. Posterior fragments are almost always displaced to the lingual area. Large forceps may be helpful to apply a force suitable to reduce the bony fragment. Reduced fragments may be held in place by maxillomandibular fixation (MMF) or splints (see Fig. 12.5).

Class III fractures of a moderately or severely displaced dentulous segment may be too difficult to reduce adequately. There may be scant room into which the irregular, displaced segment needs to be replaced. It may be necessary to burr or rasp down the displaced segment or the opening in the remaining bone to successfully reduce the fracture. This is usually best accomplished by use of a power drill with a suitable size bur or a fine rhinoplasty rasp. The amount of tissue that is removed should be limited so that sufficient bone-to-bone contact remains for bony union as the fracture heals. Maintenance of class III fractures in a reduced position may be accomplished with arch bars, maxillomandibular fixation, and/or a variety of splints.

Class IV fractures that extend into one or more non-alveolar fracture lines are usually less challenging than class III fractures because (1) the bone segments are larger, (2) the treatment of the associated fractures gives excellent exposure, and (3) usually no physical barrier exists to reduction. Plates, screws, arch bars, maxillomandibular fixation, and/or a variety of splints may be used.

Postoperative care includes analgesics and antibiotics for several days to provide pain relief and lessen the risk of infection. If maxillomandibular fixation is used, a

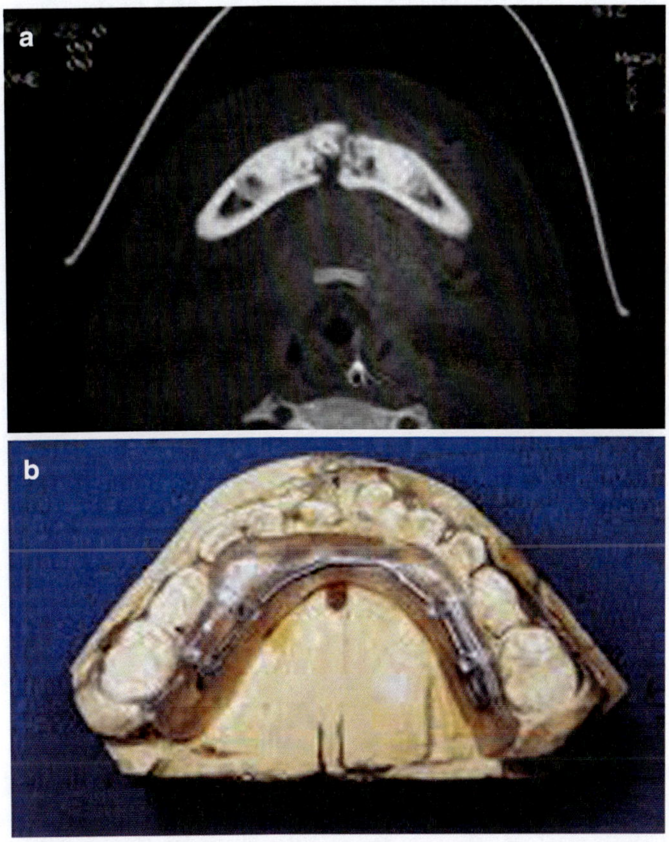

Fig. 12.5 CT scan of a displaced symphyseal fracture involving the alveolar ridge (**a**). Lingual splint used to hold the alveolar segments together (**b**)

wire cutter should be kept with the patient at all times, and attempts to minimize nausea and vomiting should be undertaken. Examination in the office on a weekly basis should monitor weight loss, wound healing, oral hygiene, maintenance of occlusion, and evidence of nonunion and infection. Administration of antibiotics for alveolar fractures reduces the prevalence of infections. Penicillin, or similar agent, is an excellent choice. For the patients who are allergic, clindamycin is a good alternative.

The complications following treatment of an alveolar fracture either in isolation or in conjunction with other craniofacial trauma include malunion, nonunion, and infection, among others. Malunion and malocclusion are the most common major complications. They result from inadequate reduction and/or loss of reduction during the healing process from inadequate stabilization. Infection is usually localized to the traumatized area, since wide exposure is not necessary. It typically responds to oral antibiotics. Frankly purulent material should be evacuated and the area copiously irrigated. If present, hardware may require removal. Nonunion requires debridement of the devitalized bone edges and possibly placement of bone graft.

Bibliography

Kajan ZD, Taromsari M. Value of cone beam CT in detection of dental root fractures. Dentomaxillofac Radiol. 2012;41(1):3–10.

Marão HF, Panzarini SR, Manrrique GR, Luvizuto ER, Evangelista Melo M. Importance of clinical examination in dentoalveolar trauma. J Craniofac Surg. 2012;23(5):e404–5.

Padilla RR, Felsenfeld AL. Treatment and prevention of alveolar fractures and related injuries. J Craniomaxillofac Trauma. 1997;3(2):22–7. Review.

Schmidt BL, Stern M. Diagnosis and management of root fractures and periodontal ligament injury. J Calif Dent Assoc. 1996;24(2):51–5. Review.

Trope M. Clinical management of the avulsed tooth. Dent Clin North Am. 1995;39(1):93–112.

Mandible Fractures

13

Peter J. Taub and Magdalena Soldanska

The mandible is one of the most frequently fractured facial bones and the most commonly fractured bone in the multiply injured patient. Mandibular fractures account for approximately 20 % of all facial fractures. Motor vehicle accidents and physical altercations are the most common causes of mandible fractures. Understandably, they occur more commonly in males and younger patients. Areas of structural weakness in the bone are the neck, the subcondylar region, and the angle, all of which are frequently seen areas of fracture. The presence or absence of teeth will also contribute to the location of the fracture. Greater than one half of all mandible fractures are multiple; therefore, one should always look for a second site of fracture. Mandibular fractures may be closed injuries or open through the skin externally or through the mucosa intraorally (compound fractures). Equally important is the incidence of concomitant cervical spine injury, which may be present in 2–3 % of patients.

Muscle Groups Associated with the Mandible

In treating fractures of the mandible, it is important that one be knowledgeable with regard to the origin, insertion, and action of muscles attached to the mandible (please refer to Fig. 2.16). Displacement of mandibular fractures occurs based on the direction of pull of the surrounding muscles. Therefore, muscle groups that attach to the mandible may be divided according to the displacement produced.

P.J. Taub, MD (✉)
Division of Plastic and Reconstructive Surgery, Mount Sinai Medical Center, 5 East 98th Street, 15th Floor, New York, NY 10029, USA
e-mail: peter.taub@mountsinai.org

M. Soldanska, MD
Division of Plastic and Reconstructive Surgery, Mount Sinai Medical Center, Icahn School of Medicine at Mount Sinai, New York, NY, USA

Suprahyoid Muscles and Mandibular Depressors

The anterior or suprahyoid muscle group (see Figs. 2.14 and 2.15) consists of the *geniohyoid*, *mylohyoid*, and *digastric* muscles. Based on their origin and insertion, these act to rotate the mandible downward to initiate jaw opening. The *geniohyoid* muscles arise from the inferior mental spine and insert into the body of the hyoid bone. The *mylohyoid* muscle is attached to the inner surface of the mandible along the internal oblique or mylohyoid ridge and extends to the hyoid bone to form the muscular floor of the mouth. The *anterior belly of the digastric* muscle extends between the inner side of the lower border of the symphysis and a ligamentous attachment to the lateral cornu of the hyoid bone. The *posterior belly of the digastric* muscle extends between the mastoid notch of the temporal bone and the hyoid bone. The *genioglossus* muscle originates from the superior mental spine on the inner surface of the body of the mandible, spreads out in a fanlike fashion, and is inserted into the body of the tongue and the upper surface of the hyoid bone.

Muscles of Mastication

The posterior group of mandibular muscles consists of the muscles of mastication (see Fig. 2.13). These include the *masseter*, the *temporalis*, the *medial pterygoid*, and the *lateral pterygoid*. The *masseter* arises from the lower border and deep surface of the whole zygomatic arch. The anterior two thirds of the muscle run down and back to insert into the lateral ramus of the mandible close to its lower border. The posterior third of the muscle runs down with a slight anterior inclination to insert deep to the anterior part into the upper part of the ramus. A few of its fibers insert into the capsule of the temporomandibular joint. The *masseter* acts to elevate and pull the mandible upward and forward.

The *temporalis* muscle arises from the skull along the temporal crest. From this wide origin, it narrows to a flat

P.J. Taub et al. (eds.), *Ferraro's Fundamentals of Maxillofacial Surgery*,
DOI 10.1007/978-1-4614-8341-0_13, © Springer Science+Business Media New York 2015

tendon to pass beneath the zygomatic arch and inserts into the margin and deep surface of the coronoid process of the mandible and along the anterior surface of the superior ramus. The anterior fibers act to elevate the jaw, while the posterior fibers act to retract the mandible.

The *medial pterygoid* muscle arises from the medial surface of the *lateral* pterygoid plate. It runs inferiorly, posteriorly, and laterally to insert into the deep aspect of the inferior ramus and form a sling along with the more medial masseter muscle. The *medial pterygoid* acts to place superior, medial, and anterior traction on the mandible.

The *lateral pterygoid* muscle originates from both the lateral surface of the *lateral* pterygoid plate as well as the adjacent part of the undersurface of the skull. Each portion passes inferiorly and laterally and tapers before inserting into the anterior neck of the mandible as well as into the capsule of the temporomandibular joint. The upper portion acts to pull the mandible superiorly, medially, and anteriorly. The external portion acts to pull the condyle inferiorly, medially, and anteriorly. Asymmetric contraction of one side pulls the chin point to the contralateral side. Contraction of both muscles simultaneously produces protrusion of the mandible.

Occlusion

It is important to note that the mandible is composed of two halves firmly united in the midline (symphysis). It articulates at bilateral temporomandibular joints but also with the maxilla by the dental occlusion between the maxillary and mandibular teeth. The nature of the occlusal relationship is described by Angle's Classification (see Figs. 3.13, 3.14, and 3.15). Class I or normal occlusion exists when the mesiobuccal cusp of the maxillary first molar articulates with the buccal groove of the mandibular first molar. Class II occlusion describes an overbite in which the mesial cusp is anterior to the buccal groove, while class III describes an underbite in which the mesial cusp is posterior to the buccal groove. A given patient's preinjury occlusion is usually unknown at the time of fracture repair; however, anatomic reduction in every dimension is extremely important in order to reestablish the preinjury skeletal relationship of the mandible to itself and with the maxilla. Wear patterns, or facets, on the occlusal surfaces of the teeth exist where chronic contact has been made and provide clues to the preinjury occlusion. No attempt should be made to place the patient into class I occlusion if his wear facets dictate a different preinjury pattern.

Diagnosis

The diagnosis of a mandibular fracture at a single site or multiple sites may be made by history, physical examination, and imaging studies. Important points in the history include the presence of prior fractures, the mechanism of injury, including the direction of the force, whether there is any complaint of malocclusion, and whether there is any associated pain, especially in the cervical spine. This is in addition to basic questions about past medical conditions, medications, and use of tobacco, alcohol, or illicit drugs. Physical examination should determine the patient's dental status, any areas of tenderness, crepitance, mobility of the mandible in the horizontal and vertical planes as well as within the bone itself, mucosal injury, and obvious malocclusion. Associated facial trauma and concomitant injury to other anatomic sites should also be sought.

There are several important imaging modalities for the evaluation of mandible fractures, and each has distinct usefulness. A series of plain films may adequately document the pattern of injury but require specific views to examine each side of the bone individually. As such, submental and vertex views are best to evaluate the symphysis and parasymphyseal areas. Lateral oblique views are included to accurately image the body (see Fig. 13.1), and closed and open mouth AP views must visualize each ramus.

Plain films however have been supplanted by orthopantomograms and computed tomography (CT scan). The former is a version of a plain x-ray in which the beam rotates around the stationary patient to produce a flat image of the mandible similar to a two-dimensional map of the world (see Fig. 13.2). It is an excellent modality to evaluate the parasymphysis, body, and ramus but often blurs out any midline structures, such as the symphysis. An adequate orthopantomogram must include the bottom of the chin and both condyles.

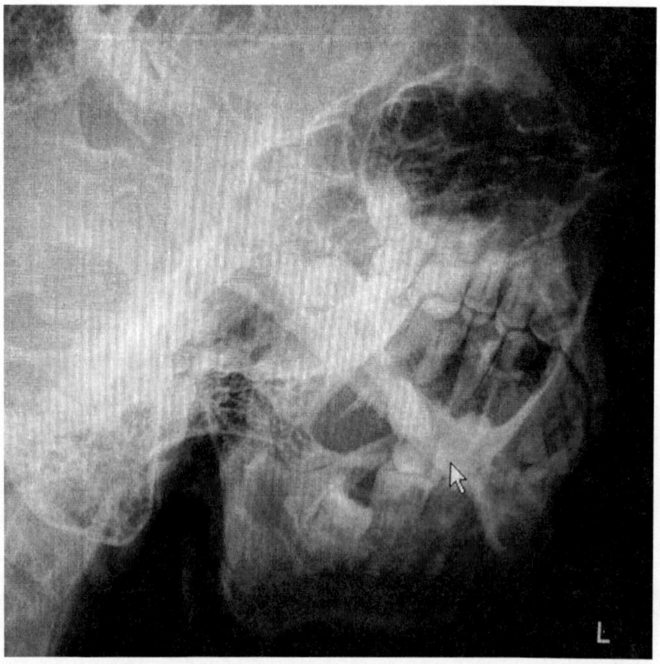

Fig. 13.1 Oblique lateral plain x-ray of the mandible

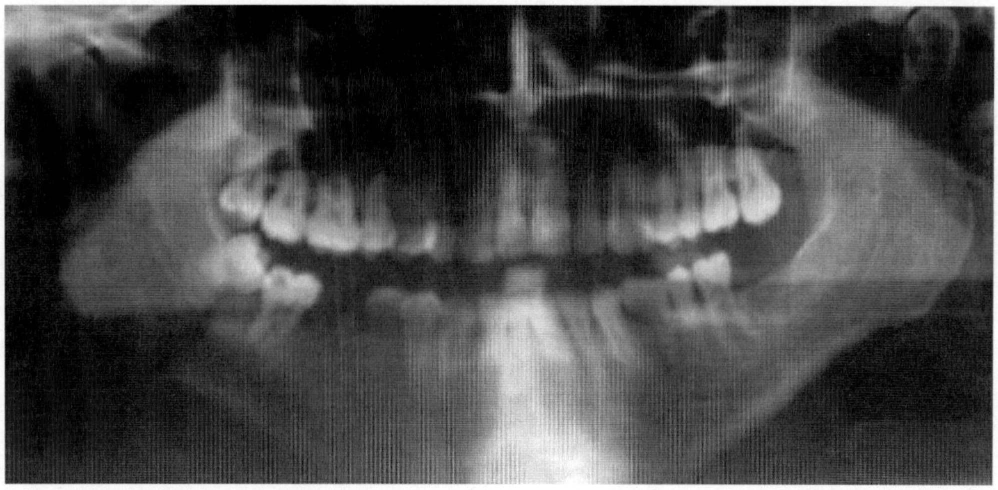

Fig. 13.2 Orthopantomogram

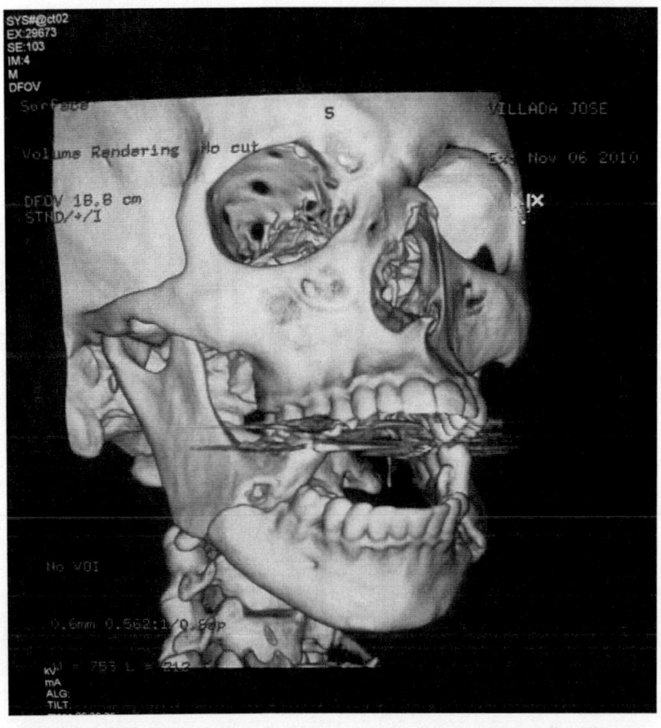

Fig. 13.3 Three-dimensional CT scan of the mandible

CT scanning is able to provide accurate information about every anatomic region of the mandible. They have become easy to obtain in both an emergency and elective setting. Images may be acquired in the sagittal, axial, and coronal planes. A three-dimensional reconstruction of the facial skeleton may then be created to better visualize the fracture pattern (see Fig. 13.3).

Magnetic resonance imaging (MRI) is rarely used for acute trauma of the mandible. It is helpful for soft tissue derangements, including those of the temporomandibular joint. The position and movement of the articular disk can be easily visualized.

Treatment

The most important goal in the treatment of mandible fractures is the reestablishment of the patient's preinjury dental occlusion. If the preinjury occlusion can be recreated, then the skeletal relationship between the components of the fracture will more easily be placed into anatomic reduction. The teeth should be placed into their preinjury relationship by maxillomandibular fixation (MMF). This may be achieved in a number of ways, including Ivy loops, Ernst ligatures, Erich arch bars, MMF screws, and newer screw-retained arch bars. This may serve as the sole treatment or may be used in conjunction with internal fixation. It is perhaps best to leave the arch bars on at the end of the procedure even if accurate reduction and fixation is achieved. This allows the surgeon to reestablish IMF if the patient's occlusion changes in the postoperative period. It may also serve as a necessary component of the fixation. They may then be removed in the office if adequate occlusion is maintained.

The placement of arch bars may be done prior to dissection of the fractures or once the fractures have been exposed and debrided (see Fig. 13.4). Care should be taken when placing them so that their strength and function are maintained during the procedure as well as postoperatively, since they may be required for several weeks. Two participants are usually required with each performing vital roles. The Erich-type arch bar has lugs, which are used to hold the maxilla and mandible together with either surgical wire or dental elastics. They are bound to the teeth with 24-gauge circumdental wires. In the patient with a full complement of teeth, the wires should generally spare the anterior incisors ("show teeth") where injury is more noticeable. They should pass as close as possible to the tooth to avoid injury to the intervening gingiva. The first pass should be on the bone side of the arch bar (inferior for the mandibular arch bar, superior for the maxillary arch bar) so that the second more difficult pass is on the dental side of the bar. As they are tightened, the

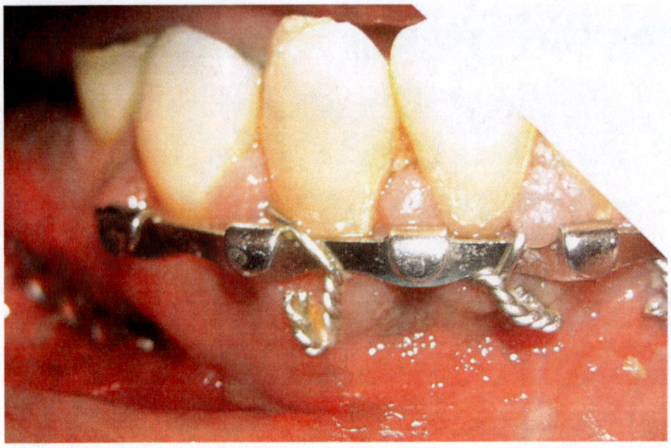

Fig. 13.4 Placement of Erich arch bars with circumdental wires

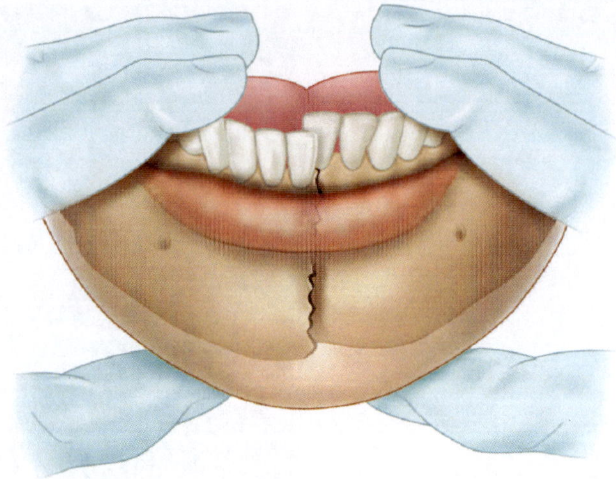

Fig. 13.5 Bimanual examination to diagnosis a symphyseal fracture

wires should be pushed down below the waist of each tooth ("cingulum") to maintain position and avoid breaking off the crown. The amount of tightening requires some experience. It is recommended to twist the wires in a clockwise fashion (by convention) and stop when it starts to turn on itself. At this point, the twisted wire should be shortened to about one inch and then given an extra one and a half turns. To make the wires comfortable to the patient, they are folded on themselves and pushed against the gingiva. As the wires proceed away from the midline, care should be taken that they closely follow the surface of the gingiva and do not leave laxity or gaps above the teeth. Also, the wires should leave the lugs free to receive additional wires or elastics for MMF.

MMF is achieved with similar or slightly thinner surgical wire or ¼″ dental elastics. The latter may be sterilized in a cup of Betadine and passed with a small clamp. They can be easily stretched from a lug on one arch bar around a corresponding lug on the opposite arch bar and hooked backed to the starting point. Multiple elastics along the arch bar provide excellent fixation and stability during fracture plating. Once repaired, they may be left singly looped across two sets of lugs to facilitate occlusion postoperatively. However, they should not be left multiply looped, since their composite strength can lead to extrusion of the teeth over time. If MMF is to be maintained for an extended period of time postoperatively, wire is preferable.

Teeth in the Line of Fracture

There are many instances in which teeth lie along the line of fracture. This most often occurs in the regions of the symphysis and angle. Fractures involving teeth in the line of fracture are considered compound fractures, and as such, patients should probably be covered with antibiotics and oral rinses. As a general rule, those teeth involved in the line of fracture should be extracted. There is a risk in retaining those teeth as they are prone to keep an open conduit from the oral cavity with its high bacterial count into the fracture site. Retention of such teeth should not be done solely the purpose of stabilization and/or maintaining space for anatomic reduction. The decision to retain a tooth in the line of fracture must be made cognizant that there is a risk of developing chronic osteomyelitis at the fracture site. There are instances where teeth, primarily in the symphyseal area involving the mandibular anterior teeth, and also bony impacted posterior teeth (e.g., third molar), can be retained with a somewhat lower incidence of risk. The risk of osteomyelitis should be discussed with the patient prior to surgical intervention.

Symphysis and Parasymphysis Fractures

The anterior regions of the mandible, especially the symphysis, are relatively strong with a great deal of cortical bone and thus less frequently fractured. With fractures of the symphysis, one should always look for concomitant fractures of the condylar area as well as hyperextension injury of the cervical spine due to the force required to produce these injuries. Tenderness over the area, pain with mouth opening, motion of the segments (see Fig. 13.5), and malocclusion are key findings. Paresthesia in the distribution of the mental nerve should be sought and documented in any mandible fracture.

Placement of the teeth into MMF alone may be used to treat nondisplaced or minimally displaced fractures; however, close observation is needed because of significant muscle pull on the anterior mandible. For displaced fractures, open reduction and internal fixation is preferable. Exposure is obtained with a lower gingivobuccal sulcus incision and dissection to the inferior border of the mandible. With the fracture exposed, callus that may have developed following the injury within the fracture site should be removed so that the edges of the bone can be accurately realigned.

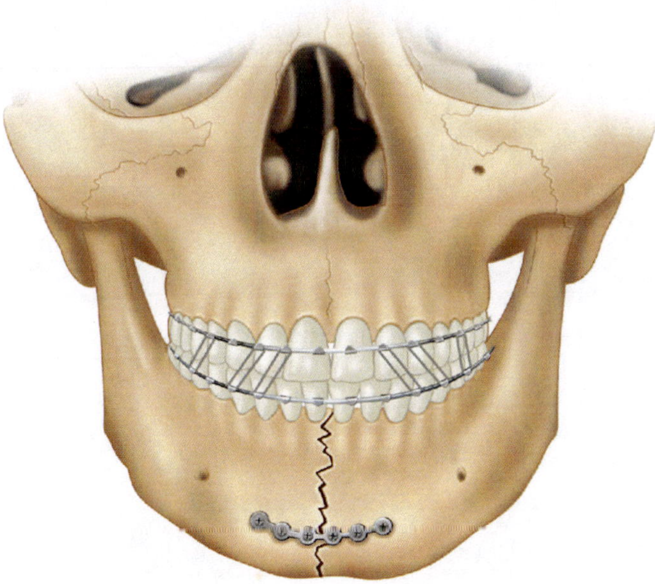

Fig. 13.6 Plate fixation of a symphysis fracture with the arch bar as a tension band

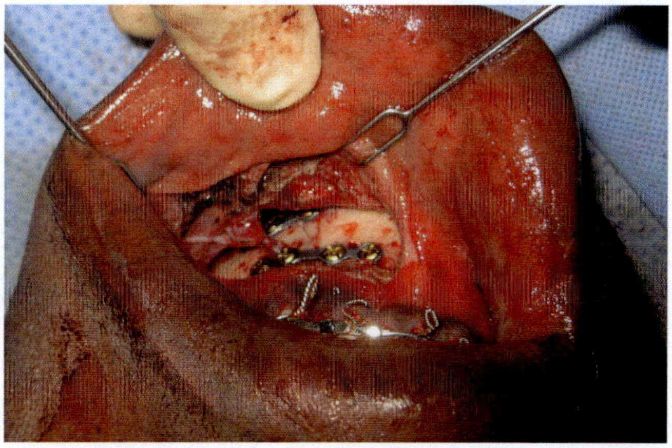

Fig. 13.7 Plate fixation of a parasymphyseal fracture with care taken to avoid injury to the mental nerve during placement of the lower border plate

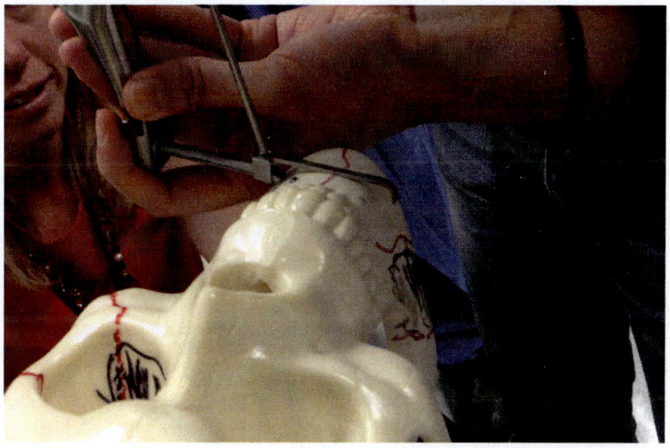

Fig. 13.8 Placement of lag screws across a symphyseal fracture

Following dissection of the fractures, MMF is used to reestablish occlusion. A temporary bridle wire may be placed around the teeth on either side of the fracture to facilitate reduction. In the region of the symphysis and parasymphysis, fixation should be at two different vertical positions in the bone to prevent twisting about any one point of fixation (see Fig. 13.6). This may be achieved with a large inferior border plate, and more superior "tension band" in this region. The inferior border plate is placed low enough to avoid injury to the dental roots, since the screws should be bicortical. In the region of the parasymphysis, careful dissection around the mental nerve is important to permit placement of the plate below the foramen and avoid injury to the nerve (see Fig. 13.7). At least two screws must be placed on either side of the fracture line. This plate will provide much of the strength of the repair but requires a more superior tension band to prevent widening at the superior aspect. The tension band may be a second plate whose screws are monocortical to avoid injury to the dental roots or a mandibular arch bar alone.

Similarly, this may be done with two lag screws that span the fracture from cortical bone on the right to cortical bone on the left. The technique of lag screw placement involves drilling an appropriate diameter hole for the chosen screw across the entire course of the screw then over-drilling the proximal portion up to the fracture line (see Fig. 13.8). The proximal opening is deepened a couple of millimeters with a countersink to accommodate the screw head and avoid being palpable through the skin. As the screw passes easily through the proximal, over-drilled section, it bites into the distal section and effectively pulls the two halves together, compressing the fracture line.

Body Fractures

Fractures of the mandibular body may be diagnosed by point tenderness over the lateral jawline, pain with opening, malocclusion, and mobility. The pterygomasseteric sling, temporalis, and lateral pterygoid muscle will displace the proximal segment superiorly and medially. The mylohyoid and geniohyoid muscles will deflect the distal segment inferiorly and medially (see Fig. 13.9). Additionally, one may note an intraoral communication with a laceration of the gingiva or mucosa. Standard imaging modalities are sufficient (orthopantomogram and CT scan). It is imperative that any tooth in the line of fracture be thoroughly evaluated radiographically. (Further consideration of teeth in the line of fracture is discussed later.) In general, nondisplaced or minimally displaced fractures of the mandibular body may be managed with observation or MMF with a soft diet and close observation. More displaced fractures may require open reduction and internal fixation. A lateral gingivobuccal sulcus incision is preferable, but a submandibular approach

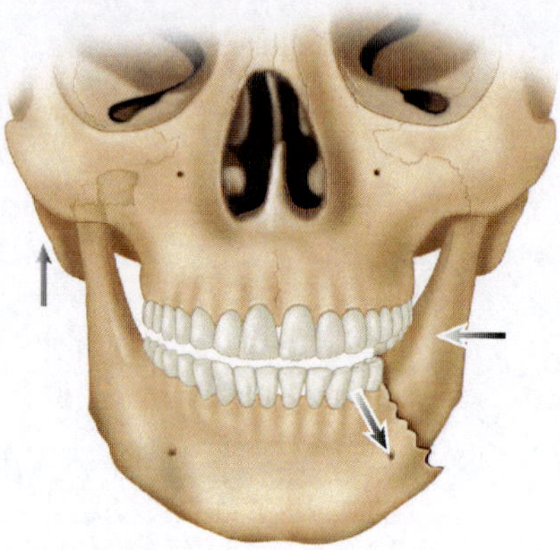

Fig. 13.9 Fractures of the mandibular body

may also be used. Plates and screws are placed along the inferior border of the mandible with a superior tension band provided by the arch bar or a second monocortical plate.

Angle Fractures

The angle of the mandible is a frequently fractured area, due to its thinner cross section and presence of the third molar tooth. The pterygomasseteric sling and temporalis muscle tend to pull the proximal segment superior, whereas the suprahyoid musculature tends to displace the distal segment inferiorly and medially (see Fig. 13.10). Malocclusion due to displacement of the fracture fragments results from the action of the pterygomasseteric sling, which tends to pull the proximal segment superiorly. Attention should be paid to the presence or absence of the mandibular third molar as well as the degree of soft tissue and bony impaction. If any doubt exists as to whether the tooth should be maintained, a general rule is to remove the third molar tooth.

Nondisplaced or minimally displaced angle fractures may be treated with observation and a soft diet or MMF with close observation for possible subsequent displacement. Fractures of the angle usually occur distal to the molar teeth where MMF is not able to serve as a tension band. Therefore, stability must be achieved in other ways. Open reduction and internal fixation may be performed either intraorally, through a modified Risdon, or with a submandibular incision. Once the fracture is reduced, fixation is best achieved with plates and screws. A lag screw technique has been described but is technically more difficult than in the symphyseal region. When a mandibular plate is used along the inferior border, a second plate is usually placed at the superior border to act as a tension band (see Fig. 13.11). Alternatively, a single plate may be placed along the oblique line as described by Champy. Here, a line of tension exists such that a single plate placed along this line is used to hold the segments in the desired position while the natural forces acting on the mandible serve to compress the fracture.

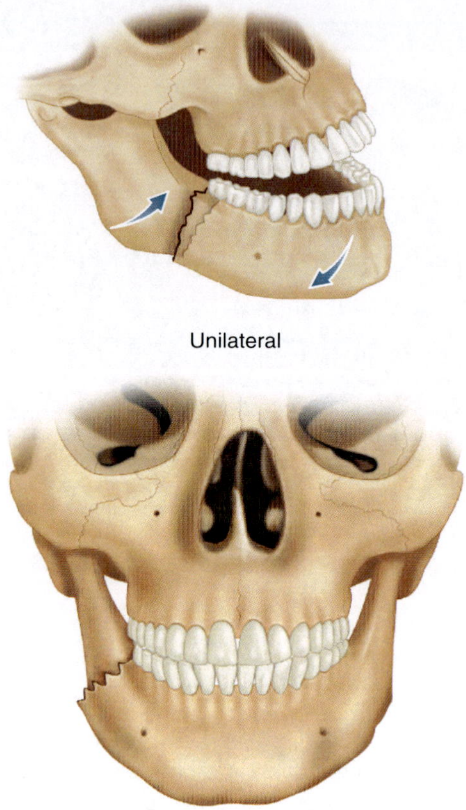

Fig. 13.10 Fractures of the mandibular angle

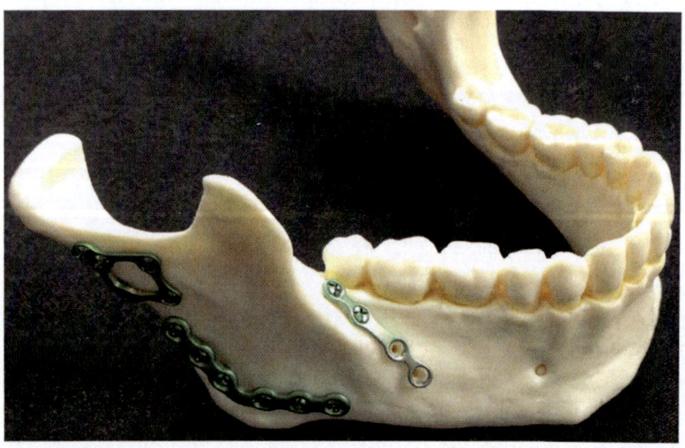

Fig. 13.11 Fixation of a mandibular angle fracture using an anterior Champy plate along the oblique line and a lower border plate (the subcondylar plate would address a separate fracture)

Ramus Fractures

Fractures of the ramus (see Fig. 13.12) are much less common. These may involve the coronoid process as well as sagittal and horizontal portions of the ramus. The diagnosis is made by local tenderness, limited opening, and possible malocclusion. Standard imaging techniques are sufficient. Fractures of the coronoid process may not lead to malocclusion, and conservative treatment may be all that is necessary.

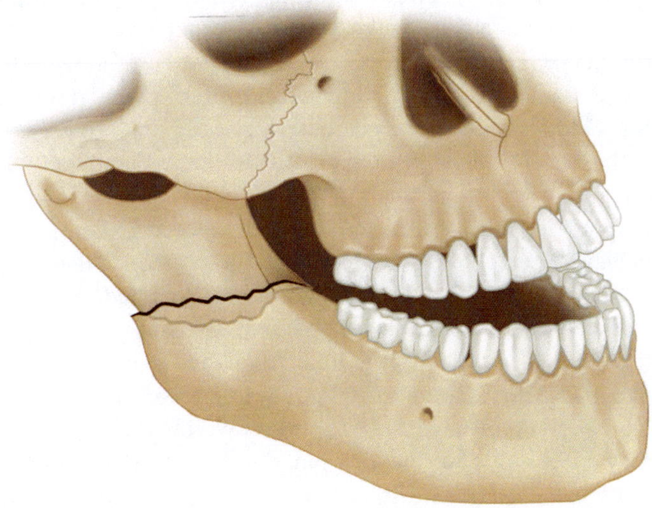

Fig. 13.12 Fracture of the mandibular ramus

The goal in treatment of ramus fractures is reestablishing the patient's occlusion and the vertical height of the mandible. Minimally displaced fractures may be treated with observation and a soft diet or MMF. Fractures that are more displaced and produce malocclusion or reduced vertical height require open reduction and internal fixation via an intraoral approach.

Condylar Fractures

Patients with condylar fractures (see Fig. 13.13) may present with pain or limitation of movement, tenderness in the preauricular region, malocclusion or deviation of mandibular opening, or blood in the external auditory canal. Frequently, there is a history of force directed at the symphyseal region. In addition, the surgeon should palpate the head of the condyle

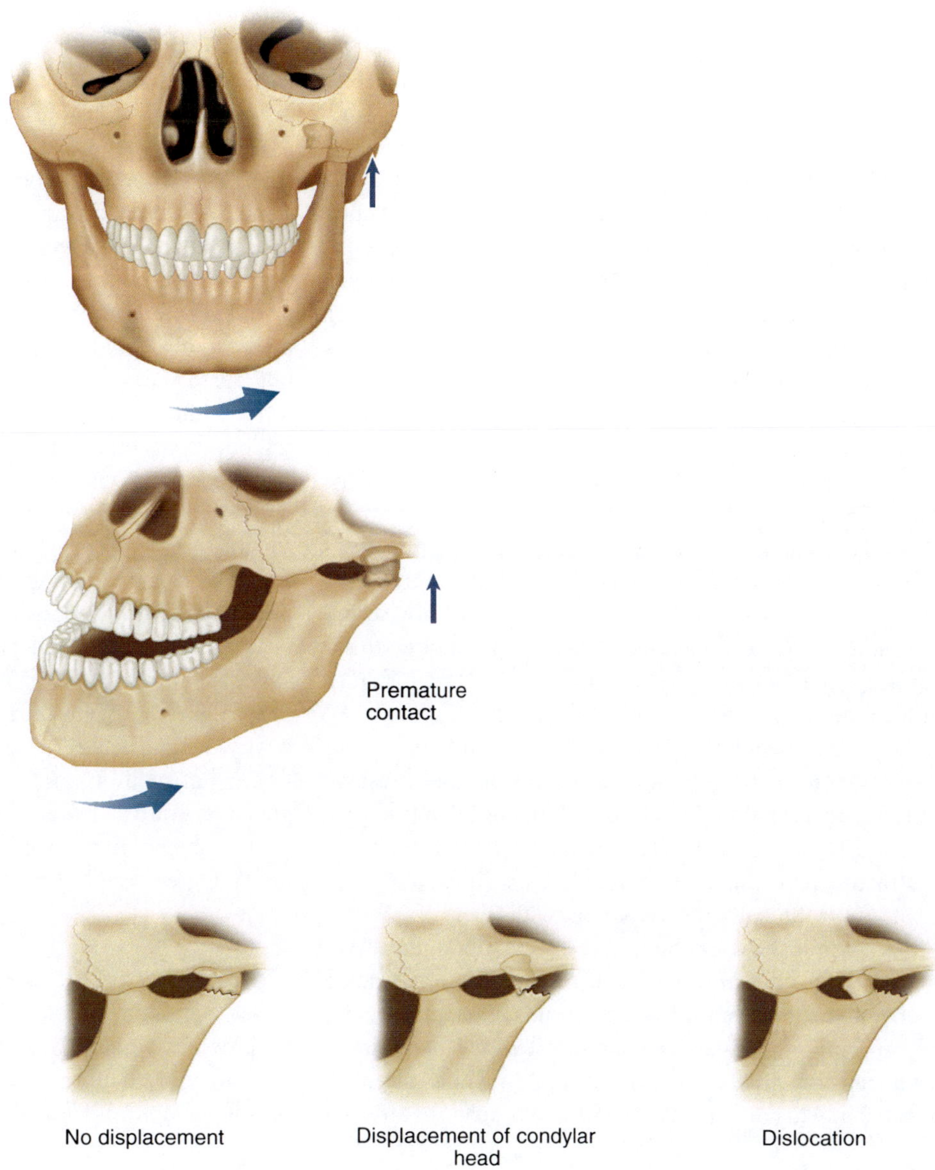

Fig. 13.13 Fractures of the mandibular condyle

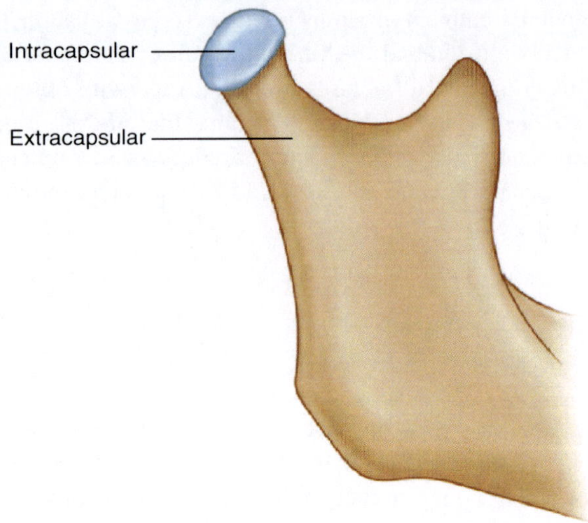

Fig. 13.14 Anatomic division of condylar fractures

within the external auditory canal and ask the patient to open the jaw. For an obtunded patient, this may be done manually. The condylar head should move equally on both sides. Radiographs most helpful in diagnosing fractures of the mandibular condyle include a plain x-ray Towne's view, an orthopantomogram, and a CT scan.

The typical clinical finding of a unilateral displaced condylar fracture is a dental malocclusion, in which the patient occludes prematurely on the maxillary and mandibular posterior teeth on the side of the fracture due to a loss of vertical height of the ramus on the affected side. In patients with bilateral condylar fractures, there is uniform premature occlusion between the maxillary and mandibular posterior teeth, thus leading to an open bite deformity, in which the patient is unable to bring the incisal edges of the maxillary and mandibular anterior teeth together.

Possibly because of the risk of facial nerve injury with open repair, the treatment of mandibular condylar fractures is controversial. Treatment may be divided according to the line of attachment of the capsule, thereby producing either an intracapsular (condylar head) fracture or an extracapsular (condylar neck or subcondylar) fracture (see Fig. 13.14). Generally one should be conservative, with the goal being joint motion, reestablishing normal occlusion, and preserving the vertical height of the ramus. Intracapsular fractures are generally considered best managed conservatively, as these fractures are usually comminuted, and it is frequently difficult to technically do anything with these fractures. There is often insufficient bone stock for fixation, and fixation itself may interfere with joint motion. If conservative (nonoperative) treatment produces an unsatisfactory result, condylar replacement may be contemplated at a later date.

Extracapsular fractures of the condyle involve the neck and subcondylar region. These fractures may be treated closed or open, by either a direct approach or an endoscopic technique. For a closed regimen, the surgeon would place the patient in intermaxillary fixation for 2 weeks followed by release and perhaps guiding elastics during the day and MMF and at night. Physical therapy is essential.

In the course of treating fractures of the condylar area, there may be a time when an intraarticular or subcondylar fracture is noted by history and radiologic examination; however, per clinical examination, the patient will have a normal dental occlusion. When this is encountered, there is a tendency toward treating the apparent undisplaced condylar fracture with analgesics and liquid diet without closed reduction and MMF. The surgeon should be aware that normal mandibular movement with regard to swallowing and speech may cause a displacement by pulling of the lateral pterygoid muscle and eventual displacement of the proximal segment. Thus, what may have been diagnosed as an undisplaced fracture of the condylar area, if not treated appropriately, may result in a displaced condylar fracture. A conservative approach in this type of injury would be to place the patient in MMF with closed reduction.

Open reduction of fractures of the mandibular condyle and neck is more technically difficult as the anatomy in this area is more challenging. Some general indications for considering open reduction include (1) fragments causing functional interference with opening; (2) bilateral fractures with persistent open bite from fracture malposition; (3) limitation of movement of the jaw from the condylar position; (4) fracture, dislocation of the condylar head, medially or laterally out of the glenoid fossa or superiorly into the medial cranial fossa; and (5) bilateral subcondylar and Le Fort fractures. Simple, noncomminuted fractures of the subcondylar region with adequate bone on either side of the fracture line may be treated with an endoscopic approach, which utilizes specialized instruments (see Fig. 13.15). The learning curve for this type of repair is steep but beneficial to the patient. In addition, a preauricular and/or modified Risdon approach provides excellent exposure for open reduction. Care should be taken to protect and prevent injury to the facial nerve. When open reduction of a mandibular condylar fracture is performed, some type of rigid internal fixation is always necessary. A small plate or lag screw provides the best stabilization. Joint mobility and proper occlusion once again is the goal. Generally, a 2-week period of MMF would be indicated prior to beginning movement of the mandible, with subsequent aggressive physical therapy and close observation.

Multiple Mandibular Fractures

As previously noted, over one half of mandible fractures will be fractured at more than one site. Commonly, a fracture of the symphysis or parasymphysis region will produce

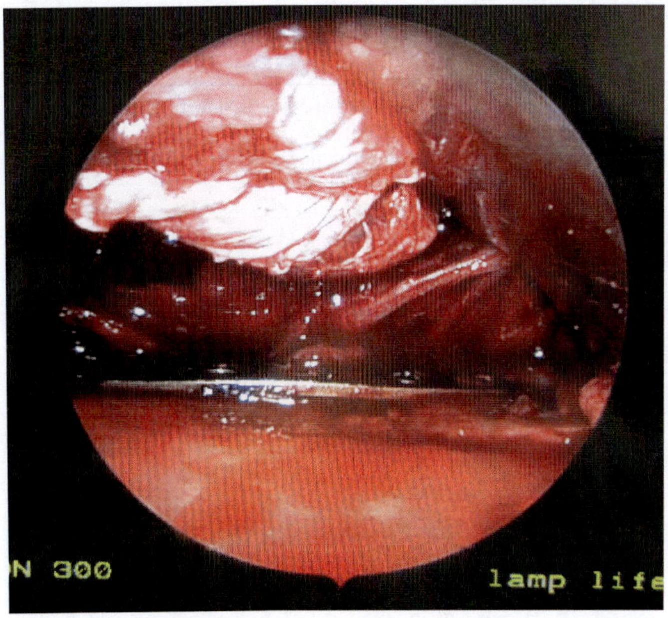

Fig. 13.15 Endoscopic view of a reduced and plated subcondylar fracture

a contralateral angle or peri-condylar fracture. When a severely comminuted fracture is present, the preinjury dental occlusion should be established by placing the patient into intermaxillary fixation with arch bars prior to reducing the multiple pieces with wires or microplates. A large mandibular plate is then applied. If a plating system is used for mandible fractures, one should be exceedingly careful in using plates in the compression mode. One should remember that the goal is to produce the patient's preinjury occlusion, and overzealous compression of fracture segments may be detrimental to obtaining good occlusion. If the fracture is severe enough to produce loss of bone, then immediate bone grafting and/or placement of a long reconstruction plate should be considered to span the defect and maintain space.

Fractures of the Edentulous Mandible

In the presence of a partially or fully edentulous mandible, fractures should be plated in their "dentulous" state. This means that MMF should not juxtapose the two mucosal surfaces of the maxilla and mandible. Space should be left for dentures. In such cases, the patient's own complete or partial denture can be used in the repair. The denture can be affixed with arch bars (see Fig. 13.16) and then secured to the maxilla with drop-down wires from the piriform aperture or the zygomatic arch to the mandible with circummandibular wires.

With the loss of teeth, there is resorption of the alveolar ridge or superior border of the mandible. A long-standing edentulous state may lead to dramatically thin bone, which of course is highly susceptible to fracture. In such cases, the

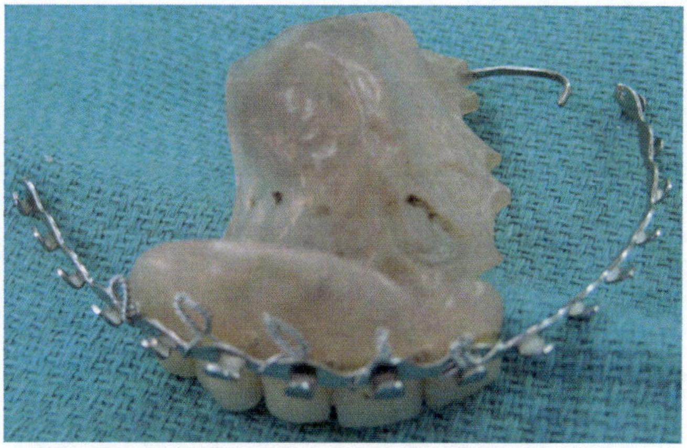

Fig. 13.16 Partial denture fitted with an Erich arch bar

mental nerve may be within the bone or largely outside of it. Fractures that are stable or have minimal displacement may sometimes be treated by soft diet alone. With displacement or mobility, open reduction with internal rigid fixation should be the treatment of choice. Here, larger reconstructive plates are required. When the height of the mandibular body is less than 1 cm, consideration should be given to primary bone grafting. Dental splints may be a useful adjunct in the treatment of edentulous fractures.

Pre- and Postoperative Management

The time for operative intervention of mandibular fractures should take place within 3–5 days after the injury, so that soft tissue scarring does not interfere with anatomic reduction and facial symmetry. Early reduction and stabilization not only initiates healing that much faster; it also reduces the intensity and duration of pain. In the event the patient's medical condition precludes surgery, the application of arch bars and intermaxillary fixation should be performed. One must remember that the goal of treatment of mandibular fractures is to reestablish the patient's preinjury occlusion. Therefore, it is imperative that the preinjury dental occlusion should be established and maintained with adequate intermaxillary fixation prior to the application of rigid internal fixation. It should be noted that once the fracture has been reduced and rigid fixation applied, the fixation should be released intraoperatively to ensure proper occlusion. If the occlusion is not correct, the rigid fixation should be completely redone. If the operator feels that the stability of the rigid fixation is excellent, the patient may be taken out of occlusion at the end of the procedure. Subsequently, light elastic traction may be used for the first week or two to put the muscles at rest. When the surgeon feels less confident about the rigidity of internal fixation, a greater length of time may be required for MMF. One should not hesitate to leave the patient in intermaxillary

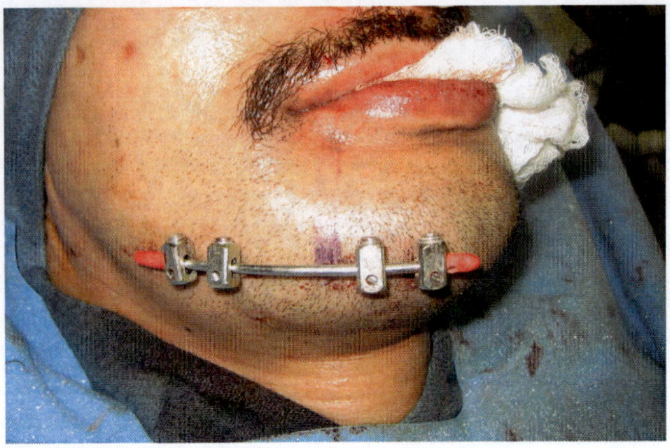

Fig. 13.17 External fixation of a mandible fracture

fixation for 4–6 weeks to ensure proper bone healing. When MMF is being used, careful attention should be paid to good oral hygiene as well as diet. A high-calorie, high-protein diet of blenderized food as well as commercial supplements should be used. Physical therapy is an essential part of the post-MMF period, especially in condylar fractures.

Complications

The major complications of mandibular fractures include paresthesia of the mental nerve, infection, malocclusion (malunion), and nonunion. Patients are normally maintained on antibiotics for at least 1 week. With any sign of a wound infection, the area should be surgically explored and debrided. If the internal hardware requires removal, a means of external fixation may be required. This may be achieved with large Kirchner wires placed into the bony fragments at right angles and joined with either a larger curved rod and fixation clips or a standard chest tube filled with methyl methacrylate if the former is not available (see Fig. 13.17).

Infection may lead to nonunion of a fracture site. With the use of rigid fixation, the diagnosis of a nonunion may be more difficult. Traditionally, the nonunion has been observed with mobility at the fracture site, which may be precluded with the use of the rigid fixation. Therefore, persistent pain or a subsequent wound infection should alert one to the possibility of a nonunion. The lack of evidence of radiographic healing for a period greater than 3 months time may suggest the possibility of a nonunion. The source of nonunion should be identified and eliminated, all necrotic tissue debrided, and then it must be determined whether additional internal fixation or external fixation is indicated. Subsequent bone grafting may be required.

Bibliography

Amanatunga NA. Mouth opening after release of maxillomandibular fixation in fracture patients. J Oral Maxillofac Surg. 1985;45:383.

Amaratunga NA. The relation of age to the immobilization period required for healing of mandibular fractures. J Oral Maxillofac Surg. 1985;45:111.

Bruce RA, Strachen DS. Fractures of the edentulous mandible: the Chalmers J. Lyons Academy Study. J Oral Surg. 1956;34:973.

Chalmers J, Lyons Club. Fractures involving the mandibular condyle: a post-treatment survey of 120 cases. J Oral Surg. 1947;5:45.

Chuong R, Donoff RB. Intraoral open reduction of mandibular fractures. Int J Oral Surg. 1985;14:22.

Chuong R, Piper MA. Open reduction of condylar fractures of the mandible in conjunction with repair of discal injury: a preliminary report. J Oral Maxillofac Surg. 1988;46:262.

Dingman RO, Natvig P. Surgery of facial fractures. Philadelphia: W.B. Saunders; 1964.

Ellis III E, Carlson DS. The effects of mandibular immobilization on the masticatory system. Clin Plast Surg. 1989;16:133.

Ellis III E, Moos KF, El-Attar A. Ten years of mandibular fractures: an analysis of 2,137 cases. Oral Surg Oral Med Oral Pathol. 1985;59:120.

Halazonetis JA. The "weak" regions of the mandible. Br J Oral Surg. 1968;6:37.

Hoopes JE, Wolfort FG, Jabaley ME. Operative treatment of fractures of the mandibular condyle in children: the postauricular approach. Plast Reconstr Surg. 1970;46:357.

James RB, Frederickson C, Kent JN. Prospective study of mandibular fractures. J Oral Surg. 1981;39:257.

Kent JN, Neary CS, Zide MF. Open reduction of fractured mandibular condyles. Oral Maxillofac Surg Clin North Am. 1990;2:69.

Klotch SW, Lundy LB. Condylar neck fractures of the mandible. Otolaryngol Clin North Am. 1991;24:181.

Leonard MS. The use of the lag screws in mandibular fractures. Otolaryngol Clin North Am. 1987;20:479.

Levine PA. AO compression plating technique for treating fractures of the edentulous mandible. Otolaryngol Clin North Am. 1987;20:457.

Marciani RD, Hill JD. Treatment of the fractured edentulous mandible. J Oral Surg. 1979(569).

Melmed EP, Koonin AJ. Fractures of the mandible—a review of 909 cases. Plast Reconstr Surg. 1975;56:323.

Neal DC, Wagner WF, Alpert B. Morbidity associated with teeth in the line of the mandibular fractures. J Oral Surg. 1978;36:859.

Prein J and Kellman RM. Rigid internal fixation of mandibular fractures – basics of AO technique. Otolaryngol Clin North Am. 1987;20(3):441–56.

Robertson BC, Manson PN. Concepts in mandibular fractures. Trauma Q. 1992;9:54.

Schwimmer AM, Greenberg AM. Management of mandibular trauma with rigid internal fixation. Oral Surg Oral Med Oral Pathol. 1986;62:630.

Shetty V, Freymiller E. Teeth in the line of fracture: a review. J Oral Maxillofac Surg. 1989;47:1, 303.

Sinn DP, Pollock RA, Rohrich RJ. Facial fractures II: mandibular, maxillary, and craniofacial. Selected readings. Plast Surg. 1989;5:26.

Woods WR, Hiatt WR, Brooks RL. A technique for simultaneous fracture repair and augmentation of the atrophic edentulous mandible. J Oral Surg. 1979;37:131.

Zide MF, Kent JN. Indications of open reductions of mandibular condyle fractures. J Oral Maxillofac Surg. 1983;41:89.

Midfacial Fractures

14

Joseph L. Hill and Henry C. Vasconez

A complete evaluation of the maxillofacial skeleton is paramount in order to produce the best anatomic and functional results. The aim, then, of the maxillofacial reconstructive surgeon, after a thorough evaluation of the patient, is to properly diagnose the fractures involved, reestablish proper occlusion, provide for proper open reduction and fixation of all fracture sites through adequate exposure, augment with bone grafting those areas of missing bone or skeletal structure, and correct any soft tissue deformities present. The following will be a review of that process.

The face has traditionally been divided into upper face, midface, and lower face. Fractures of the craniofacial skeleton can similarly be divided into these three regions. The upper face consists of fractures involving the frontotemporal bones, including the frontal sinus as well as the orbital roof, while the lower face includes fractures of the mandible. The midface is more complex, secondary to its many and variable components. It involves all entities of the facial skeleton between the upper face and the lower face, including the orbital rims and walls (except the roof), the nasal bones, the maxilla and pterygoids, and the zygoma and its arch.

Buttress System

The skeletal components of the midface, while distinct entities, form a network of reinforced bone that surrounds the pneumatic cavities, the sinuses, and the nasal airway. They also serve as a platform for the globe and surrounding tissues, the nose, and the maxillary dental arch. This reinforced bone is oriented into vertical and horizontal pillars or buttresses (see Fig. 14.1). Vertically oriented buttresses relate the facial bones to the frontal cranium and cranial base. They protect the maxilla from vertically directed forces and provide midfacial height. The horizontally oriented buttresses of the midface protect it against horizontally directed forces and provide the midface with width and projection. There are three pairs of vertically oriented buttresses: two anterior and one posterior. These include the nasomaxillary medially, the zygomaticomaxillary laterally, and the pterygomaxillary posteriorly. The horizontal buttresses of the midface include the zygomaticotemporal (arch) laterally and the orbital rim, maxillary alveolus, and palate medially.

Evaluation

In general, patients with fractures of the midface can present with pain at the fracture site, swelling, paresthesia in the distribution of the infraorbital nerve, periorbital ecchymosis, or subconjunctival hemorrhage. Patients with nasal bone fractures can present with epistaxis and nasal airway obstruction secondary to a deviated septum or a septal hematoma. The nasal bones may also be mobile and/or comminuted. Patients with zygomatic fractures may present with a step-off or tender point at the inferior or lateral orbital rim, globe dystopia, or enophthalmos. The buttress concept explains why these fractures most commonly occur in combination. Hence, a serious zygomatic fracture or zygomaticomaxillary complex (ZMC) fracture will present with at least four breaking points or a quadripod fracture (see Fig. 14.2). Patients with orbital fractures can present similarly to those with zygomatic fractures but also with diplopia and limited extraocular movement with entrapment of periocular tissues. Any periorbital fracture, including zygomatic fractures, demands a thorough evaluation of the globe and its various functions. Finally, those individuals presenting with maxillary fractures cannot only present with similar findings associated with other types of midfacial fractures but also with malocclusion.

In addition to the history and physical examination, a radiographic examination is also of paramount importance. Once considered too costly and unnecessary, spiral computed tomography (CT) has become the gold standard for evaluat-

J.L. Hill, MD • H.C. Vasconez, MD, FACS (✉)
Division of Plastic Surgery,
University of Kentucky College of Medicine, Lexington, KY, USA
e-mail: hcvasc@uky.edu

P.J. Taub et al. (eds.), *Ferraro's Fundamentals of Maxillofacial Surgery*,
DOI 10.1007/978-1-4614-8341-0_14, © Springer Science+Business Media New York 2015

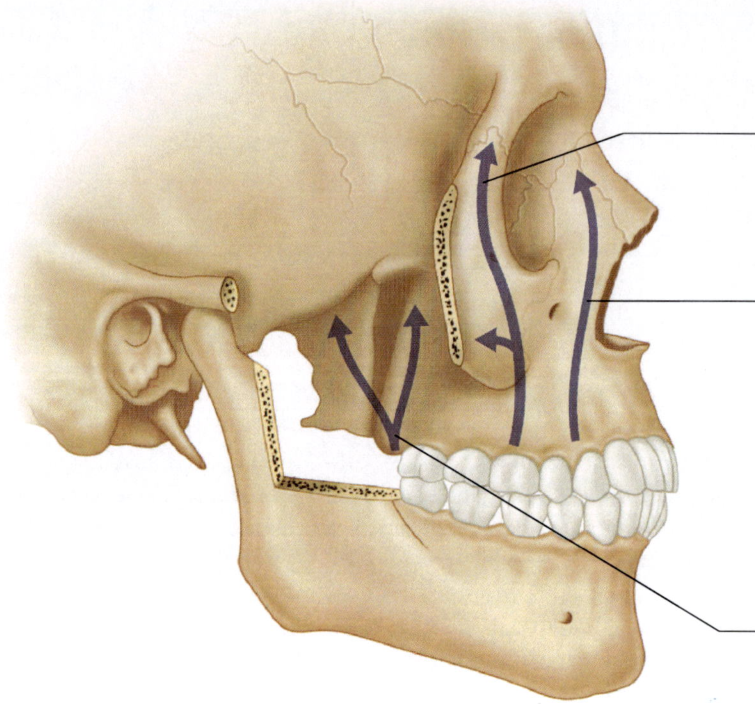

Fig. 14.1 Vertical buttresses of the maxillofacial skeleton

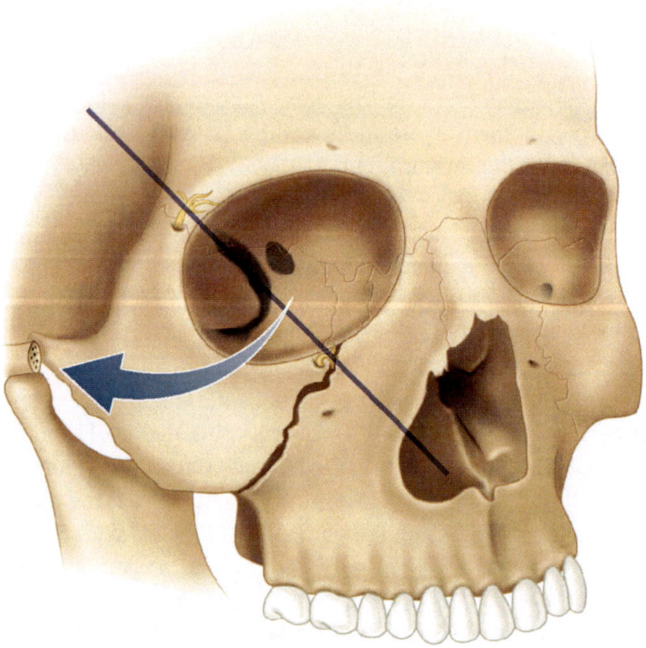

Fig. 14.2 Rotation of the zygomaticomalar complex if fixation is not performed at three points

ing facial trauma with suspected fractures, especially of the midface. Axial and coronal views are indispensable in demonstrating the fracture lines, the degree of displacement, and the associated injuries. In addition, newer high-resolution 3D CT reconstruction aids in understanding the orientation of the fracture, the size and number of broken fragments, and the degree of dislocation, depression, elevation, distraction, and rotation, all of which aid in optimal surgical planning.

Classic patterns of midfacial fractures were originally described by Rene Le Fort in 1901 (see Fig. 14.3). He demonstrated that these common fractures occur along lines or areas of thin and weak bone surfaces due to sinuses or various foramina. The Le Fort type I fracture is a transverse fracture of the maxilla above the dentition extending from the area of the maxillary tuberosity to the nasal aperture. The Le Fort type II or pyramidal fracture extends medially from the nasal bones, down through the medial orbit, the infraorbital rim and foramen, and the zygomaticomaxillary suture or buttress and extending posteriorly to the pterygomaxillary fossa. The Le Fort type III fracture, or craniofacial disjunction, occurs in more severe injuries and separates the facial bones from the attachments to the cranial base.

True and classic Le Fort fracture patterns are rarely seen in modern day clinical practice due to the high impact and velocity injuries that are typically encountered in major medical centers. Depending on the mechanism of injury, the force and direction of the blow, and the position of the craniofacial skeleton, any combination of fracture patterns can occur. The Le Fort classification is still useful to direct the maxillofacial surgeon in a full analysis of the midfacial injury. Typically, one or more of the vertically and/or horizontally oriented buttresses are involved.

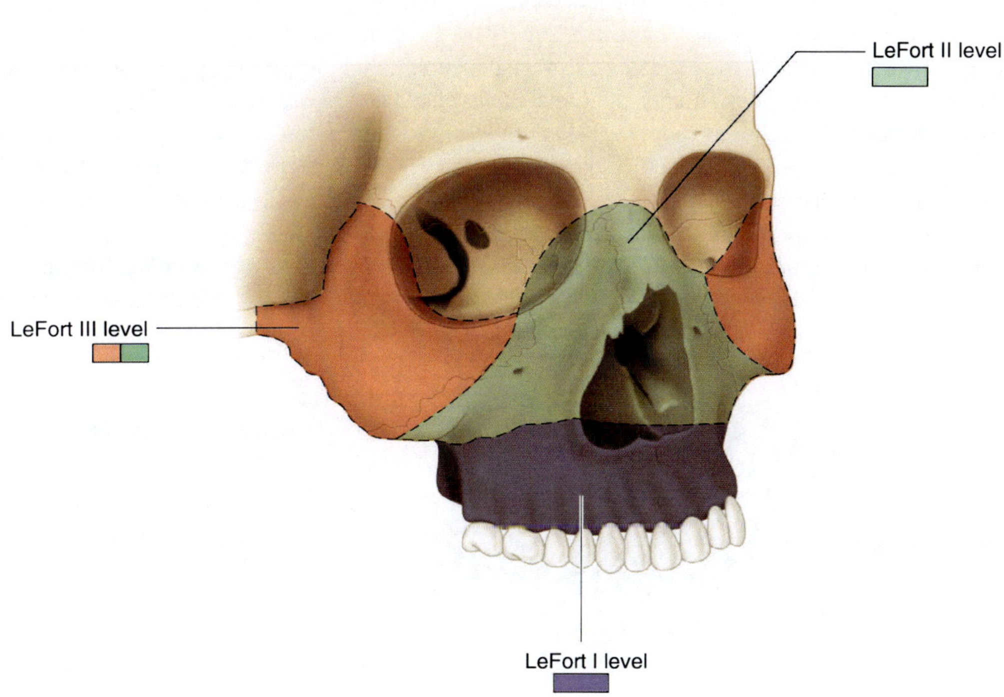

Fig. 14.3 Classification of Le Fort midfacial fractures

Management

Regardless of the fracture pattern, the treatment goal for midfacial fractures is the same: (1) to restore the anatomic relationship between the maxilla and the cranial base above and the mandible below, (2) to reestablish normal midfacial height and projection, and (3) to stabilize the fractures by means of rigid fixation. One of the major objectives in treating midface fractures is to preserve or reestablish the patient's pre-injury occlusion. This is accomplished through mandibulo-maxillary fixation, which reestablishes the relationship between the mandible and the midface. This is accomplished by means of Erich arch bars or direct screw posts with eyelets to provide for wire fixation of the teeth. After doing so, the fracture sites of the midface can be addressed through a combination of an upper gingivobuccal sulcus incision and an eyelid incision – either a subciliary or a transconjunctival incision (see Fig. 14.4). An equally important goal in the treatment of midfacial fractures is to reestablish the patient's pre-injury facial height and projection (see Fig. 14.5). Reestablishing facial height is a product of anatomic reduction of the anterior vertically oriented buttresses. In doing so, the relationship between the cranium and the midface is restored. Treatment of fractures of the posterior buttresses is generally unnecessary. Facial projection and width is a function of the horizontal buttresses, and anatomic reduction helps to reestablish the pre-injury midfacial characteristics and form.

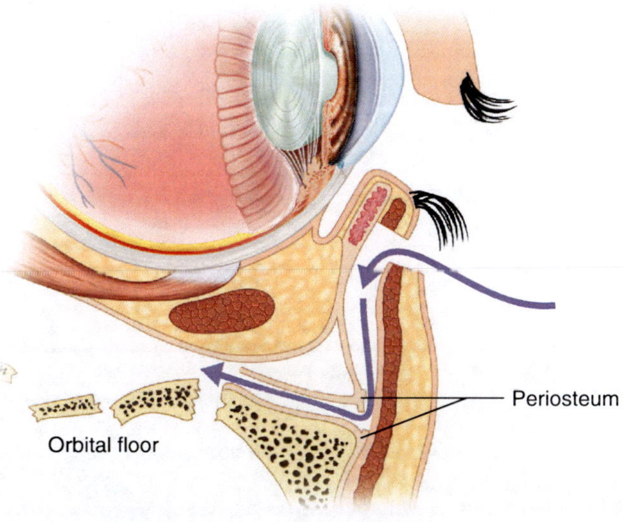

Fig. 14.4 Subciliary approach to the orbital floor

Once the vertical and horizontal buttress fractures have been anatomically reduced, they require fixation. Historically, intraosseous wiring was the preferred fixation technique. Today, rigid or functionally stable fixation with miniplates is the gold standard (see Fig. 14.6a, b). There is currently no consensus regarding the exact size and thickness of plates and screws to utilize within the midface for fixation purposes [4]. This will depend on the nature of the injury and the need for structural support. Different diameter screws are used depending on the thickness of the plate. Newer rigid fixation sets now come with standard diameter screws of different lengths that fit a wide range of plates that vary depending on the thickness of the bone. Thinner more malleable plates are used in thinner bone, usually more cephalad; thicker, stronger plates are used in thicker bone subjected to more forces, such as mastication, that are usually more caudad. The plates are generally non-compression of variable length and configuration depending on the fracture. Newer self-drilling and self-tapping screws and locking screws and plates can be used and may provide the surgeon with several advantages. These advantages may include faster application, less stripping and loosening of the screws, and possibly less compromise of osseous blood supply. The more drill holes and screw fixation on either side of the fracture allows for more load sharing between the plate and the bone and consequently more stable fixation. Further details about rigid fixation can be found in other parts of this book. Bone grafts should be considered for areas of bones loss and bone gaps greater than 0.5 cm. The sources of bone graft are usually from the rib, ilium, or calvarial bone.

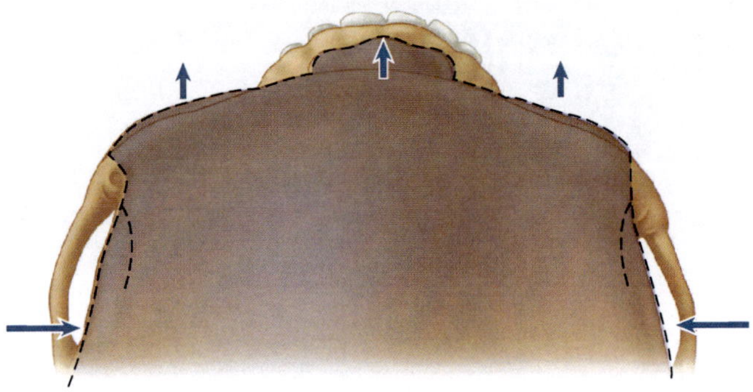

Fig. 14.5 Anterior face demonstrating the importance of reestablishing facial width and projection

Palatal Fractures

Significant forces directed on the midface may also fracture the palate, which, as was noted above, acts as a horizontal buttress of the midface providing for midfacial width. In fact, palatal fractures accompany 8 % of all Le Fort fractures. A common theme with all palatal fractures is the discontinuity of the maxillary alveolus, which permits displacement and rotation of the dental alveolar segments. Because proper reestablishment of pre-injury occlusion is necessary for adequate midface fracture reduction, misdiagnosed or mismanaged

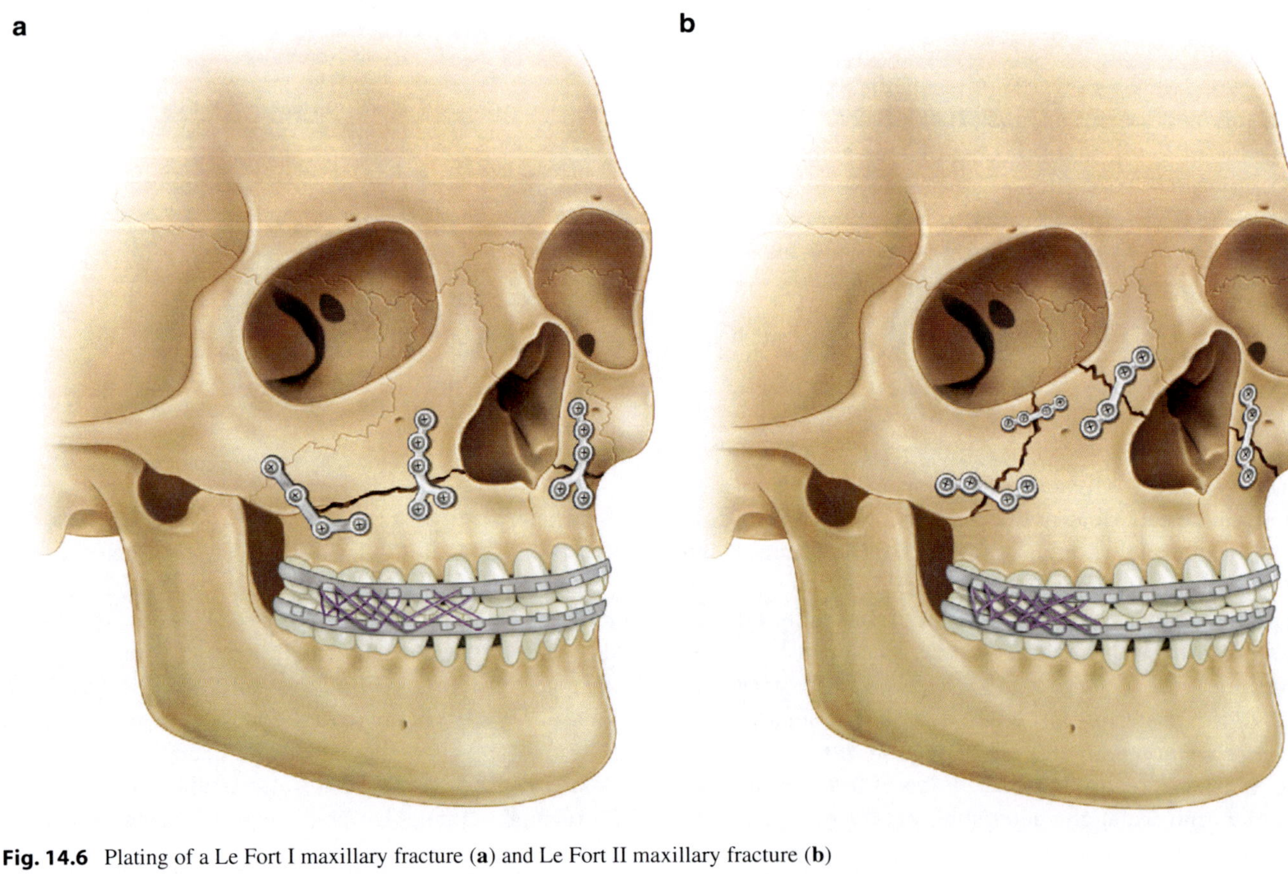

Fig. 14.6 Plating of a Le Fort I maxillary fracture (**a**) and Le Fort II maxillary fracture (**b**)

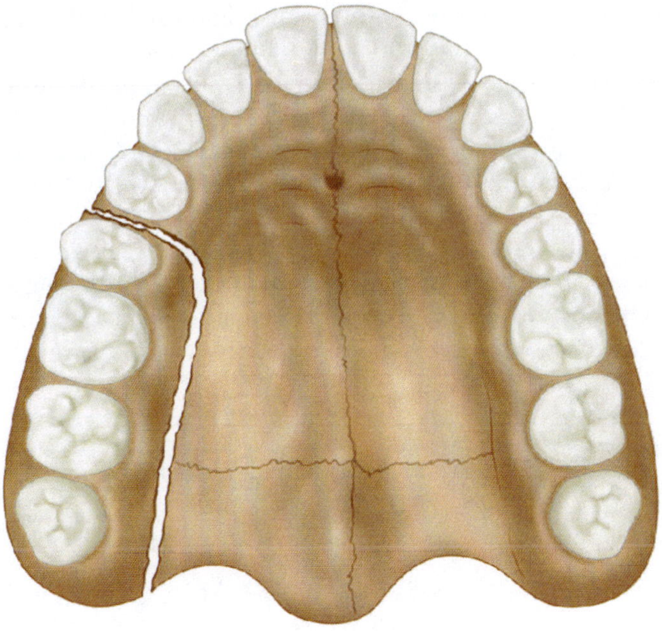

Fig. 14.7 Palatal fracture involving the alveolus

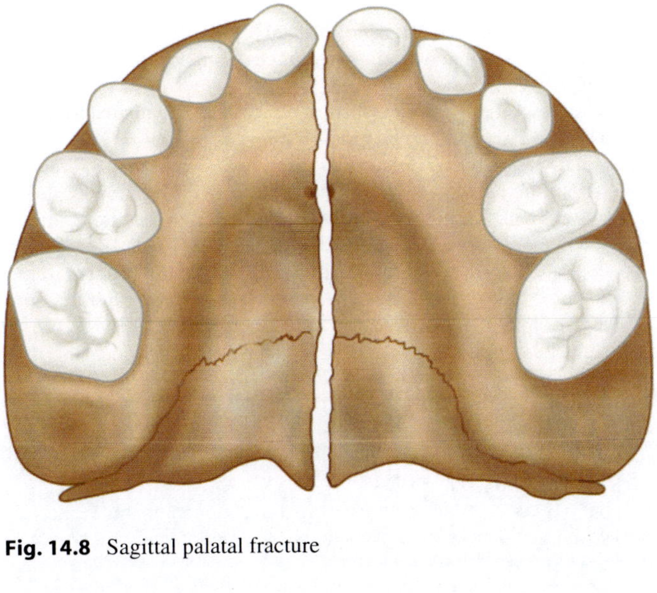

Fig. 14.8 Sagittal palatal fracture

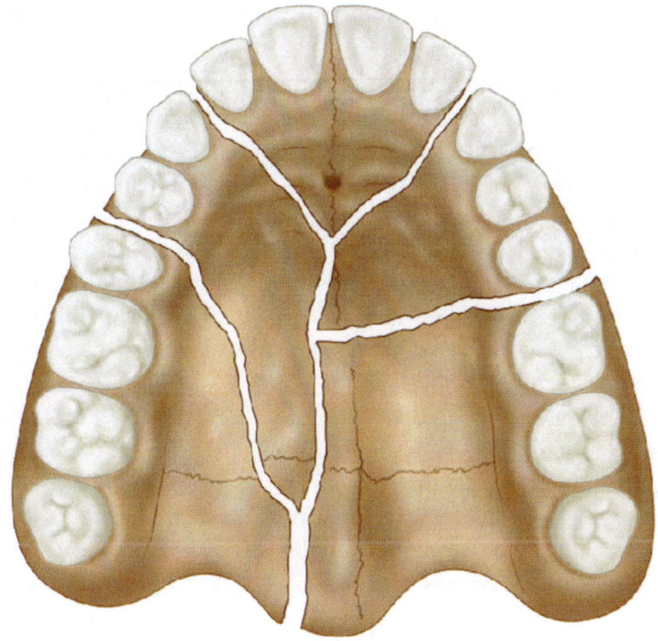

Fig. 14.9 Comminuted palatal fracture

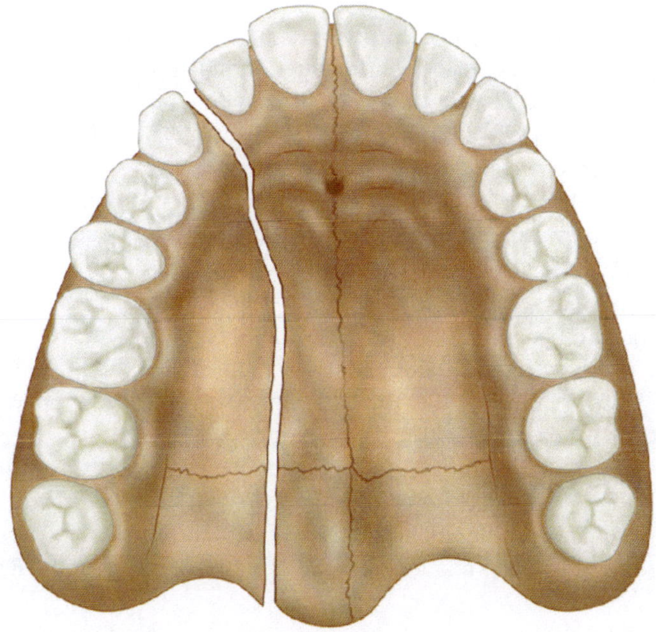

Fig. 14.10 Parasagittal palatal fracture

palatal fractures increase the risk of nonanatomic midfacial fracture reduction and consequently persistent malocclusion.

In addition to involving the alveolus (see Fig. 14.7), palatal fractures commonly occur in a sagittal (see Fig. 14.8) plane. Severe injuries produce complex and comminuted patterns (see Fig. 14.9). Very rarely do they occur in a transverse pattern. Hendrickson et al. classified palatal fractures into six fracture types. Type III (the parasagittal) (see Fig. 14.10) and type IV (the para-alveolar) are the most common types of palatal fractures in adults, while type VI (the transverse) is the least common fracture type. Depending on the location and the vector of force, most involve the alveolus and a sagittally oriented fracture of the palate. In the more severe and complex type V fractures (see Fig. 14.8), oblique or comminuted fracture patterns are present. CT scanning is necessary in the axial, coronal, and sagittal views for determination of the fracture type and pattern. Once the type of fracture pattern is ascertained, the surgical management of the fracture can be determined.

Type I fractures are typically treated with an arch bar with or without mandibulo-maxillary fixation. If the fracture is significantly displaced, small miniplates with unicortical screws may be used to provide supplemental stabilization. Fracture types II, III, and IV may be reduced anatomically by exposure of the palatal vault. Initial alignment with placement of a maxillary arch bar is performed. This also serves as a tension band. Exposure of the palatal vault should be made through traumatic lacerations of the palatal mucosa or through an incision in midline of the palatal mucosa in an anterior-posterior direction in order to optimize the blood supply to the palate. Once the fracture has been reduced, the fracture is rigidly fixated with a medium titanium plate such as a 2.0 mm system. After fixation of the fracture, the maxillary dental segments are intact and can be utilized for mandibulo-maxillary fixation. Commonly, the palatal fracture will be combined with other buttress fractures of the midface that also need to be reduced and rigidly fixated. Complex type V fractures are typically managed with an arch bar, splint, and vertical buttress stabilization.

Pollock noted that despite attempts to avoid malrotation and disinclination of the palato-alveolar segments, this does occur in approximately 1 in 10 patients with standard palatal fracture management. In his opinion, the keys to successful management of palatal fractures include precise fracture pattern classification, anatomical reduction, and instrument stabilization. He describes an instrument similar to a Hayton-Williams forceps used for pelvic reduction (a 205 mm forceps). He proposes rigid fixation with a 2.0 mm locking plate and screws well contoured to the palate. The mucoperiosteum is left intact and lacerations are meticulously repaired. This spares the blood supply to the palate and may aid in fracture healing. This assembly as described provides rigid fixation by acting as an external fixator. The plate and screws can be removed in the office or under conscious sedation at 6 weeks or when proper bone healing has occurred.

In summary, the midface is a highly complex system of bone. Buttresses, or areas of reinforced bone, surround pneumatic cavities, the nasal airway, and the orbit. Adequate reduction and fixation of the vertical and horizontal buttresses is necessary to reestablish midfacial height and width, respectively. In doing so, the anatomic relationship between the maxilla and the cranial base above and the mandible below can be reestablished. Palatal fractures, due to their inherent nature of disrupting the maxillary dentoalveolar segments, can lead to improper anatomic reduction of midfacial fractures if they are not adequately addressed. Adequate identification of the type of palatal fracture is necessary for treatment planning, which commonly requires some form of rigid fixation to avoid malrotation of dentoalveolar segments.

Bibliography

Alpert B, Gutwalk R, Schmelzxeisen R. New innovations in craniomaxillofacial fixation: the 2.0 lock system. Keio J Med. 2003;52(2):120–7.

Erdmann D, Follmar KE, Debruijn M, Bruno AD, Jung SH, Edelman D, Mukundan S, Marcus JR. A retrospective analysis of facial fracture etiologies. Ann Plast Surg. 2008;60(4):398–403.

Gruss JS, Mackinnon S. Complex maxillary fractures: role of buttress reconstruction and immediate grafts. Plast Reconstr Surg. 1986;78(1):9–22.

Hendrickson M, Clark N, Manson PN, Yaremchuk M, Robertson B, Slezak S, Crawley W, Kolk CV. Palatal fractures: classification, patterns, and treatment with rigid internal fixation. Plast Reconstr Surg. 1998;101(2):319–32.

Klenk G, Kovacs A. Do we need three-dimensional computed tomography in maxillofacial surgery. J Craniofac Surg. 2004;15(5):842–50.

Manson PN, Clark N, Robertson B, Slezak S, Wheatly M, Kolk CV, Iliff N. Subunit principles in midface fractures: the importance of sagittal buttresses, soft-tissue reductions, and sequencing treatment of segmental fractures. Plast Reconstr Surg. 1999;103(4):1287–307.

Manson PN, Hoopes JE, Su CT. Structural pillars of the facial skeleton: an approach to the management of Le Fort fractures. Plast Reconstr Surg. 1980;66(1):54–61.

Park S, Ock JJ. A new classification of palatal fracture and an algorithm to establish a treatment plan. Plast Reconstr Surg. 2001;107(7):1669–76.

Pollock RA. The search for the ideal fixation of palatal fractures: innovative experience with a mini-locking. Craniomaxillofac Trauma Reconstr. 2008;1(1):15–24.

Vasconez H. Mid-facial fractures: evaluation and treatment. In: Ferraro JW, editor. Ferraro's fundamentals of maxillofacial surgery. New York: Springer; 1997.

Nasal Fractures

15

Delora L. Mount

Introduction

The nose is the most frequently injured bone of the facial skeleton, in both adults and children. The structural anatomy of the nose includes the nasal and ethmoid bones, the upper and lower lateral cartilage, the septal cartilage, and the lacrimal system, which traverses the lateral nasal cavity. Assessment of each of these structures is imperative in the individual with nasal trauma.

Injury to the nose can occur as an oblique lateral impact or direct frontal blow. This will alter the injury pattern as well as potentially result in other fractures of the facial skeleton. For example, an oblique lateral impact or glancing blow to the nose will likely primarily affect the nasal sidewall(s) and septum, whereas a direct frontal impact may also involve the frontal sinus as well as an ethmoid impaction/fracture of the septum or potentially a combined naso-orbital-ethmoid (NOE) fracture.

Swelling, epistaxis, and contour deformity are frequently immediately noted, although sometimes the resultant deviation may not be evident until edema recedes (48–72 h). Injury to the rich vascular networks supplying the nasal structures may result in severe epistaxis, requiring immediate intranasal packing for control of hemorrhage. A variety of methods for intranasal packing for hemorrhage exist.

In the clinical assessment of nasal trauma, it is important to perform a careful inspection, perform a gentle palpation for bony step-offs, and carry out an intranasal speculum examination to rule out septal hematoma. While the majority of nasal fractures will not require emergency treatment, presence of a septal hematoma requires prompt drainage.

D.L. Mount, MD, FACS, FAAP
Division of Plastic Surgery, University of Wisconsin-Madison, Madison, WI, USA

American Family Children's Hospital, Madison, WI, USA
e-mail: mount@surgery.wisc.edu

Untreated septal hematoma results in septal cartilage necrosis, and dorsal collapse (saddlenose deformity), which will be further described later in this chapter.

Anatomy

Bone

The nasal bones consist of bilateral sidewalls and a dorsal portion. The sidewalls are frequently deviated with fractures, which can constitute a lateral displacement, medial displacement, or impaction. Frequently upon sustaining a nasal fracture, the entire intact pyramid will shift, much like a train jumping the rails, necessitating a reduction of the entire pyramid into position. However, depending on the mechanism of injury, the resultant fracture may impact one sidewall or the other, and a direct frontal injury can yield a fracture in which both sidewalls are displaced laterally, resulting in both a widened bony pyramid and reduced projection. Fractures of the nose may also include extension into the frontal sinus or ethmoid bone; these complex fractures will be discussed in the NOE chapter.

Lacrimal System

The lacrimal crest delineates the nasal bones from the orbit proper. The lacrimal sac, which lies within the palpable depression of the sulcus, provides drainage of tears from the eye to the nose, entering the nose at the inferior aspect of the inferior turbinate. Obstruction, laceration, or disruption of the lacrimal system can lead to epiphora. Rarely, a dacryocystorhinostomy is needed for correction in a simple nasal fracture, although injury to the lacrimal drainage system increases with frequency with the combined naso-orbital-ethmoid (NOE) fractures.

P.J. Taub et al. (eds.), *Ferraro's Fundamentals of Maxillofacial Surgery*,
DOI 10.1007/978-1-4614-8341-0_15, © Springer Science+Business Media New York 2015

Septum

Post-traumatic septal deviation significantly affects nasal airflow by reducing nasal passage size as well as increasing turbulence. Both airway passage reduction and turbulence over an uneven septum increase nasal airway resistance. Individuals with septal deviation and/or fractures frequently subjectively note reduction in ease of breathing and frequently have noisy obstructive nostril airflow. Early following trauma, it is difficult to discern turbulence and obstructed flow from septal origin or secondary to edema. Therefore, it is imperative to carefully examine the septal position in every instance of nasal trauma.

Concepts

Functional

Bony deviation, if significant, may cause airway obstruction by direct narrowing of the nasal air passage (see Fig. 15.1). If medially displaced, the fracture fragment will narrow the ipsilateral passage. If both sides of the nasal bones are deviated, the patient may experience severe obstruction on one side and some reduction of airflow on the other. Comminuted nasal bone fractures are unpredictable in both their presentation and the assessment of both airflow and functional outcomes. The septum will frequently follow the deviation of the bone, particularly with a combined bony and cartilaginous injury. Since early after injury it is often difficult to clinically determine the extent of deviation and the functional restrictions of airflow, it is advisable to wait until early swelling recedes and clinically repeat the examination. If deviation (bony or septal) is clinically present following recession of edema, reduction is indicated. Imaging (plain radiographs) is not very helpful with either the diagnosis or operative planning and therefore should be avoided. Computed tomography (CT) is helpful when clinical diagnosis is unclear or multiple facial fractures or complicated fractures (i.e., NOE) are suspected.

Aesthetic

Aesthetic abnormalities can persist following nonoperative and operative treatment of nasal trauma. Fracture healing in a non-displaced or even properly reduced nasal fracture can result in callus formation, leading to a post-traumatic bump. This is particularly noticeable and frequent at the bone-cartilaginous junction of the dorsum. Early recognition of the callus is important as intralesional steroid injection or digital manipulation/massage/taping can be effective in preventing a permanent aesthetically unacceptable bump.

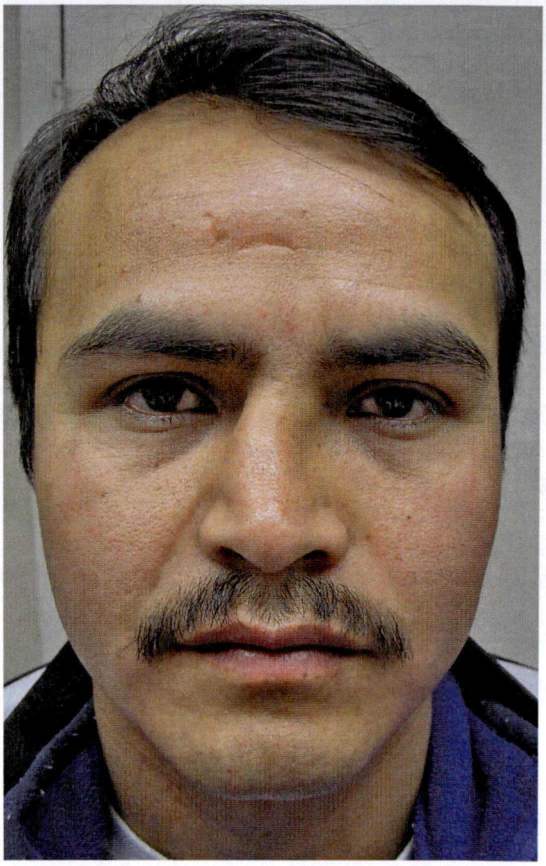

Fig. 15.1 Clinical appearance of a displaced nasal fracture

Aesthetic abnormalities following reduction may include malunion and persistent bone or septal deviation leading to a noticeably deviated nasal pyramid, mid-shaft, or tip deviation. Deviation of the bony pyramid, even slight persistent bony deviation, can result in middle and tip deviation. A poor reduction and resultant malunion of a frontal impact/bilateral nasal fracture may result in a widened nasal contour, which aesthetically is undesirable and secondarily may make the eyes appear further apart (illusion due to decreased projection.) Contour irregularity or a step-off can be particularly noticeable in the individual with thin nasal skin.

Septal Deviation and Projection

A persistent septal deviation secondary to a fracture may result in persistent nasal obstructive symptoms (see Fig. 15.2). If this occurs, secondary treatment with septoplasty (see Fig. 15.3) or submucous resection (SMR) is indicated. If the bone contour is also unacceptably deviated, a complete septorhinoplasty is indicated.

Septal dorsal projection is key for tip projection and dorsal profile contour. Even a subtle septal deviation or intranasal step-off of the septum will reduce dorsal height

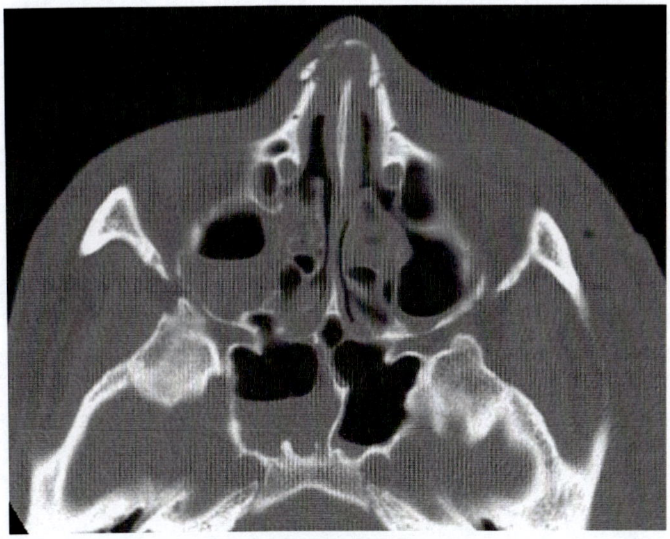

Fig. 15.2 Computed tomogram demonstrating nasal fracture and septal buckling compromising the airway

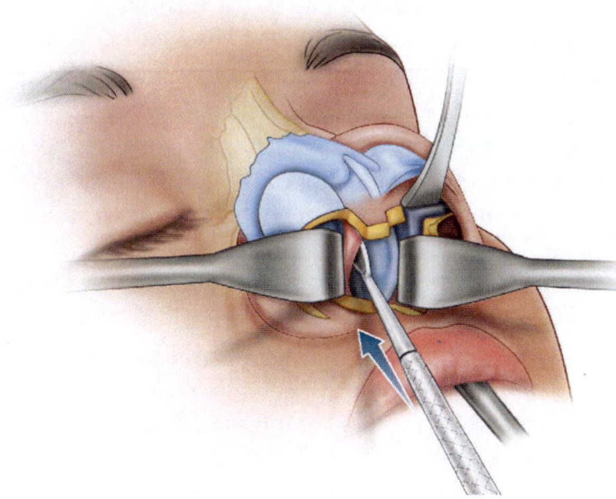

Fig. 15.3 Exposure of the septum for manipulation

and frequently affect the nasal tip projection and dorsal profile. The extreme example of septal dorsal projection abnormality is the saddlenose deformity. In this condition, dorsal collapse of the septum, with intact proximal bony support and intact columellar support, results in a profile of a saddle. In this condition, functional and aesthetic compromise is present. Functionally, airway obstruction and collapse occurs, which is frequently severe. Aesthetically, the dorsal contour collapse is severe, and secondarily, the nasal tip is over-rotated upward also leading to an aesthetic tip deformity. Correction of this deformity is complex, requiring dorsal reconstruction. Avoidance of saddle deformity is paramount.

Reduction

Primary

In treatment of a patient with a nasal fracture in need of a reduction, there are several key considerations:

Timing – In adults with nasal fracture, attention within the first 7–14 days after injury is optimal for a primary reduction. After this point, bony union has begun, and in young healthy individuals in particular, considerable difficulty in adequate reduction is encountered.

Age of patient – In children with nasal fractures requiring reduction, the bony union, "sticky period" of the bone is much earlier. Optimal ease of closed reduction is less than 7 days post-injury.

Open versus *closed reduction* – Early nasal fractures rarely require an open approach for adequate reduction; a closed approach is preferred. This is especially important in children where septal dissection (as through an open approach) can impact midfacial growth.

Location of intervention – Closed nasal reductions can be performed in the emergency department, a well-equipped office setting or in an operating room. In consideration of the location, a few essential tools should be available:

- Anesthetic (local or general) and hemostatic agents (e.g., epinephrine, topical™, liquid cocaine, or other vasoconstrictors)
- Airway monitoring (there will be bleeding with reduction)
- Adequate setup (including lighting, nasal speculum, and adequate suction)
- Postreduction fixation (splint, intranasal packing, or stent)

After careful preparation for the reduction, including intranasal administration of a vasoconstrictor and adequate anesthesia of the area, manual reduction or instrument-assisted reduction is performed. Careful examination, both visually (from all sides and also in profile) and by palpation, is necessary to assure proper reduction. After reduction, intranasal inspection is again necessary to assure septal integrity and absence of septal hematoma. Postreduction fixation by splint, stent, or packing (or combination of the above) is performed. Controversy exists on whether to pack the nasal cavity, due to patient discomfort with packing and the theoretical risk of toxic shock syndrome with a retained pack.

Secondary

Individuals presenting late after nasal fracture (>2 weeks) or inability for proper post-op healing before additional trauma (i.e., athletes in mid-season) may undergo a secondary nasal reconstruction after nasal fracture. Fracture patients with equivocal symptoms early after injury may subsequently experience trauma-related late obstruction or deformity. It is particularly difficult to predict the possible warp or deviation of the septum after seemingly minor septal fracture. In late presentations, independent of etiology, analysis of the position of the bones and septum and the position of the dorsum and width of the nose are instrumental in decision-making for secondary reconstructions. Osteotomies, septoplasty, and dorsal hump reduction are frequently necessary in the secondary treatment of a nasal deformity after trauma.

Potential complications of nasal fracture reduction include incomplete reduction, malunion, persistent deviation and poor aesthetic result. Others relate to function, such as nasal airflow reduction or persistent obstruction. What patients often notice however is a dorsal bump or irregularity at junction of the bone/cartilage interface. Epiphora occurs if there is injury to the lacrimal apparatus.

In conclusion, treatment of nasal trauma requires a systematic and prepared approach. Gone are the days of athletes presenting to the sidelines and undergoing a quick closed nasal reduction and returning to the game. Careful attention to the details of the fracture itself (bone, septum), timing of the injury, the appearance of the nose after edema resolution (widened, deviated in position), and assessment of functional limitations allow proper attention to the fracture and optimal postreduction result.

Zygoma Fractures

16

Kevin J. Kelly and Roop Gill

The zygoma is a sturdy facial bone (see Fig. 16.1). It requires a great deal of force to fracture it. When dealing with zygoma fractures as with all facial fractures, the surgeon should be careful to evaluate the patient for a potential cervical spine injury. A zygoma fracture (see Fig. 16.2) usually extends through the frontozygomatic suture (A) area along the lateral wall of the orbit (B), down through the orbital floor, usually fracturing through the orbital rim along the infraorbital foramen (C), and across the zygomatic maxillary buttress extending along the lateral wall of the maxilla (D). There has to be some disruption between the zygoma and the zygomatic arch (E) to enable the zygoma to become entirely displaced. While this outlined fracture pattern is the most common, multiple more extensive patterns of comminution will result as the severity of the force of impact increases.

Diagnosis

Zygoma fractures can result in a host of clinical findings. Common clinical findings associated with zygoma fractures include edema, periorbital ecchymosis, subconjunctival hematoma, abnormal slant to the palpebral fissure, globe displacement, lower lid retraction, symptoms of orbital floor disruption, infraorbital nerve anesthesia or paresthesia, cheek asymmetry, malocclusion, and pain or restriction when opening or closing the mandible.

Subconjunctival hematoma of the lateral aspect of the globe is pathognomonic of a zygoma fracture (see Fig. 16.3). Any finding related to orbital floor fractures can be seen, such as diplopia or enophthalmos, since a fracture of the zygoma involves the orbital floor. If displacement of the zygoma is severe enough, the globe itself can be injured. On physical exam, a depression of the cheek on the involved side may be evident if edema has not had time to mask this finding (see Fig. 16.4).

On palpation of the region, you may be able to feel a step-off along the orbital rim, at the frontozygomatic suture, and along the zygomaticomaxillary buttress (see Fig. 16.5). A downslanting cant of the palpebral fissure usually occurs if the zygoma fracture is inferiorly displaced. The lateral canthus, which is attached to the fractured segment, will be drawn down with downward displacement of the zygoma (see Fig. 16.6). Patients may also complain of pain on mandibular movement or malocclusion even though the zygoma fracture in its purest

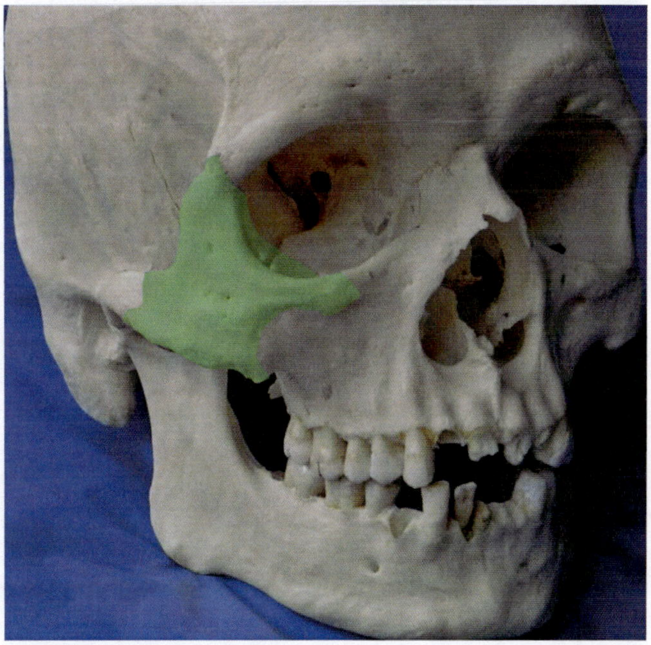

Fig. 16.1 Anatomy of the zygoma

K.J. Kelly, MD, DDS (✉)
Craniofacial Surgery Center, Department of Plastic Surgery, Vanderbilt University Medical Center, Nashville, TN, USA
e-mail: kevin.kelly@vanderbilt.edu

R. Gill, BM, MRCS (Eng)
Department of Plastic Surgery, Vanderbilt University Medical Center, Nashville, TN, USA

P.J. Taub et al. (eds.), *Ferraro's Fundamentals of Maxillofacial Surgery*,
DOI 10.1007/978-1-4614-8341-0_16, © Springer Science+Business Media New York 2015

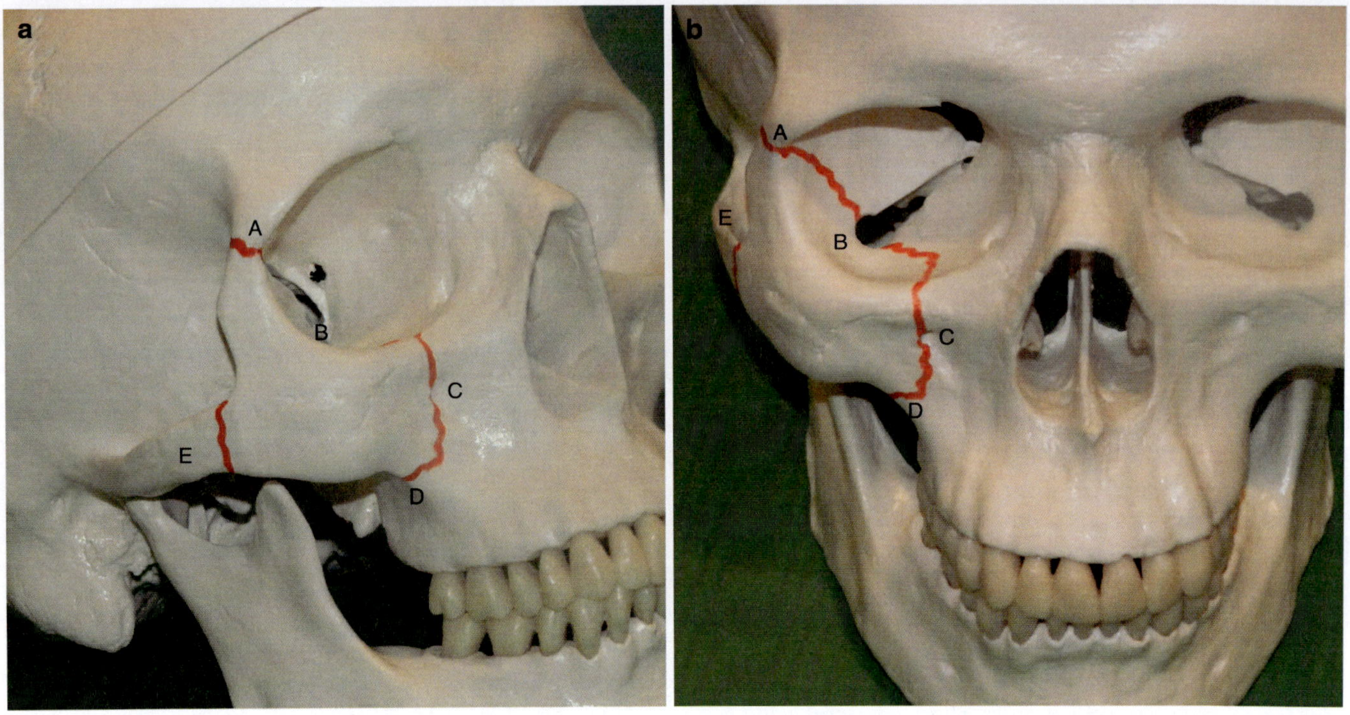

Fig. 16.2 Delineation of zygoma fracture (**a**) Oblique view and (**b**) Anterior view; *A* frontozygomatic suture, *B* lateral wall of orbit *C*, infraorbital foramen, *D* zygomaticomaxillary buttress, *E* zygomatic arch

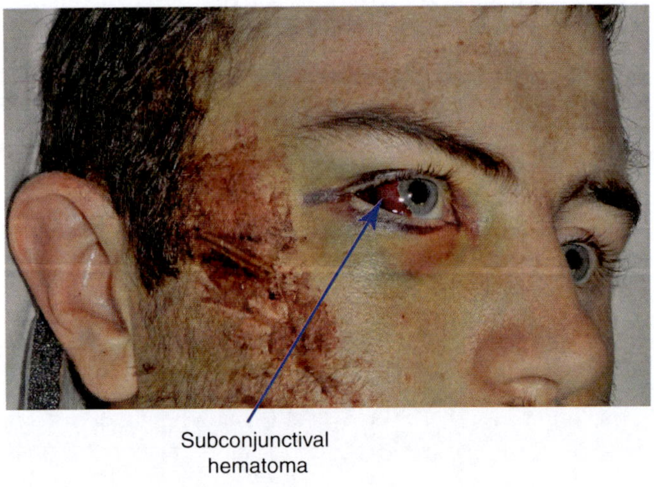

Fig. 16.3 Subconjunctival hematoma

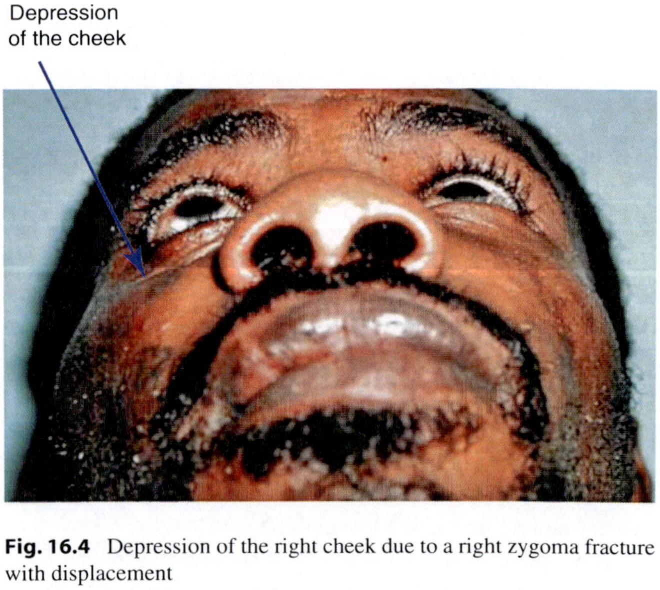

Fig. 16.4 Depression of the right cheek due to a right zygoma fracture with displacement

form does not involve the dentition. A zygoma or zygomatic arch fracture may be displaced enough that it may put some pressure on the temporalis muscle as this muscle passes deep to the zygomatic arch and zygoma (see Fig. 16.7). When the patient is opening and closing his mouth, he may have some compensatory movements to help relieve the pain, and this can result in malocclusion or the inability to open the mouth appropriately. Although impingement of the coronoid is possible, very rarely is the fracture severe enough to actually encroach on the coronoid processes.

Radiographically, these fractures can be diagnosed with a multitude of modalities that include axial, coronal, or three-dimensional CT scans. One of the x-rays most easy to evaluate is the three-dimensional CT scan (see Fig. 16.8). Axial CT scans can also be used (see Fig. 16.9) although these often do not enable clear evaluation of the orbital floor which may need to be assessed with coronal CT images. One of the best signs indicating a zygoma fracture on an axial CT is a disrup-

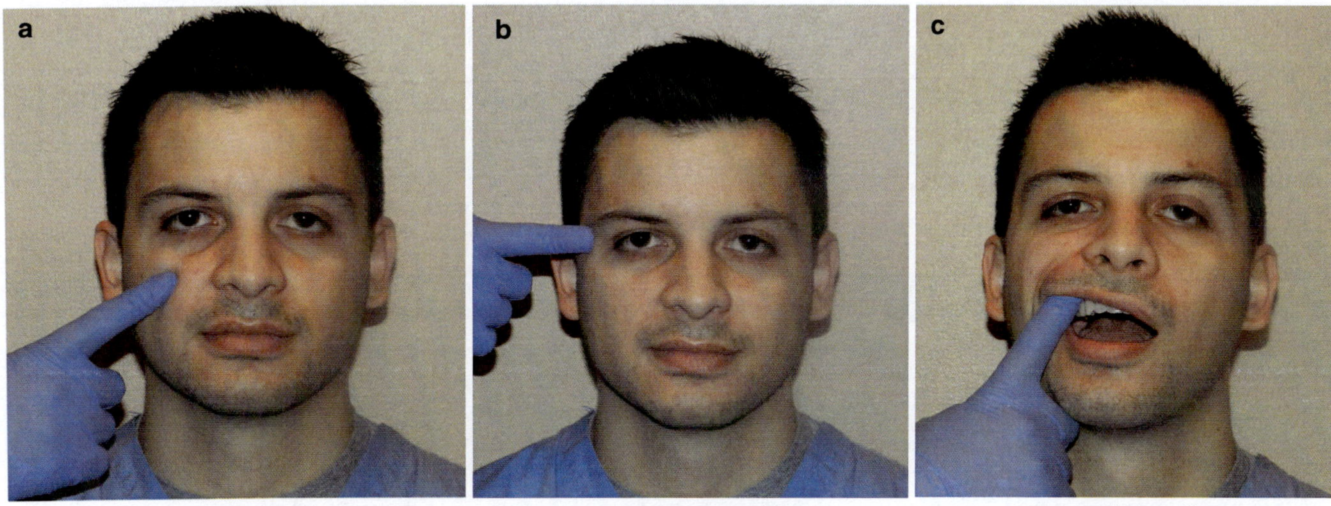

Fig. 16.5 (**a**) Palpation of step-off at infra-orbital rim (**b**) Palpation of suture line step-off at frontozygomatic suture (**c**) Palpation of step-off at zygomaticomaxillary buttress

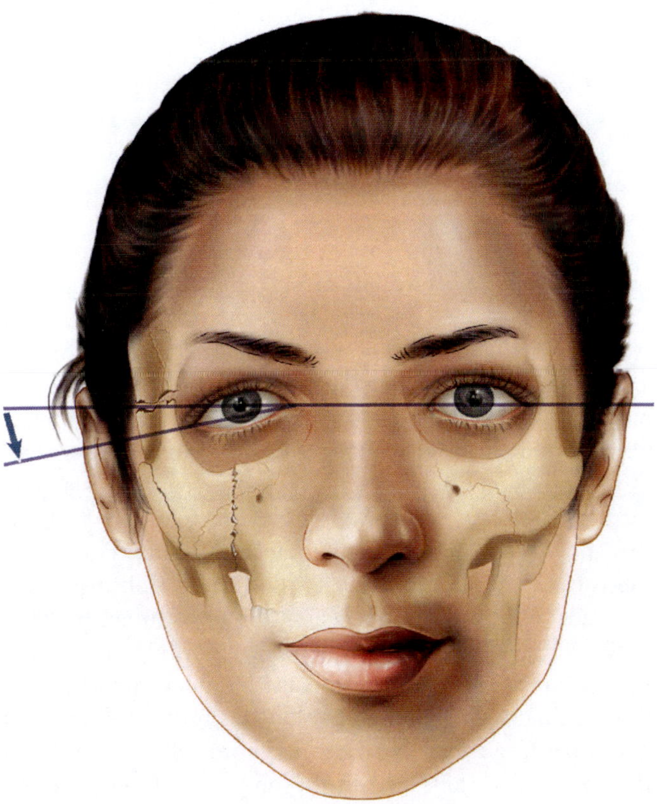

Fig. 16.6 Downward slanting cant of the palpebral fissure secondary to a zygoma fracture

tion at the lateral wall of the orbit (see Fig. 16.10). The sphenoid wing and the lateral zygoma make up the lateral wall of the orbit. Normally the two bones line up to create a straight line. On the patient's right on the CT in Fig. 16.10, you can see the nice alignment between the sphenoid and the zygoma on the non-fractured side. On the patient's left side (fractured side), there is disruption of that orbital lateral wall. For there to be a displaced fracture of the zygoma, there has to be some disruption of that wall, and this is a great clue when evaluating the CT to start thinking of the potential of a zygoma fracture.

A separation of the bones at the frontozygomatic suture can usually be seen. As you continue further through your evaluation of the CT scan, you can see some disruption of the lateral wall of the maxilla (see Fig. 16.11a). The anterior wall of the maxilla will also be disrupted on the CT scan. Often you will find blood in the maxillary sinus on the side of the fracture, easily seen in Fig. 16.11a. Bleeding into the sinus usually results from the orbital floor fracture or maxillary wall involvement. On the CT scan, there has to be some disruption of the attachment of the zygoma to the zygomatic arch or bowing and fracture of the zygomatic arch in order to facilitate significant displacement of the zygoma (see Fig. 16.11b). Coronal CTs may be needed to completely evaluate orbital floor disruption to plan for surgery whether using 3D imaging or axial imaging. Today, plain x-rays are rarely used to diagnose these fractures.

Treatment

If the fracture is a greenstick injury with no displacement, then it is possible just to observe as long as there are no visual symptoms reflecting orbital floor displacement. The masseter muscle is a powerful muscle which extends from the zygoma to the mandible to facilitate chewing (see Fig. 16.12). One has to be very careful to make sure that any greenstick fracture has no displacement at all or as

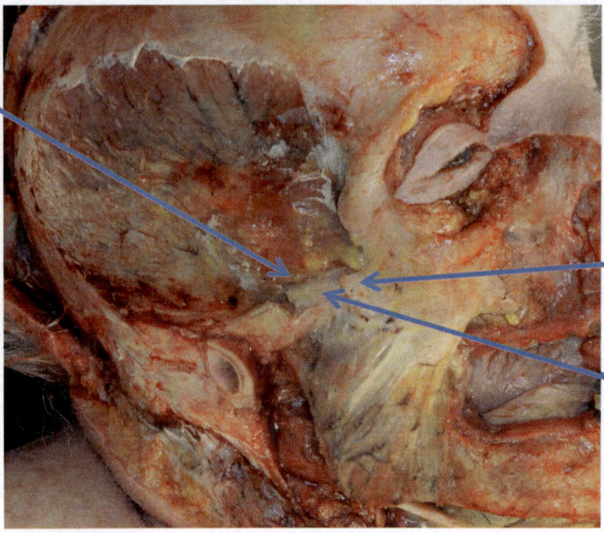

Fig. 16.7 Depression of the zygomatic arch and the body of the zygoma

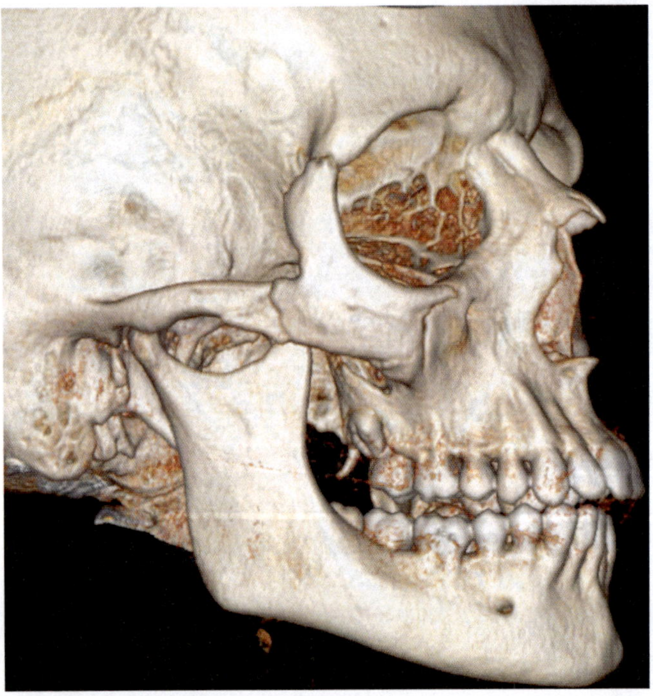

Fig. 16.8 Three-dimensional CT scan of a zygoma fracture

time progresses the masseter can draw the zygoma out of alignment. Therefore the surgeon has to have a low threshold for doing an open reduction and internal fixation of the zygoma with any displacement. If the zygoma is displaced, open reduction and internal fixation to reestablish the alignment to the sphenoid wing, frontozygomatic suture area, orbital rim, zygomaticomaxillary buttress, zygomatic arch, and orbital floor anatomy is imperative. This reestablishes the functional volume of the orbit.

When doing an open reduction and internal fixation, the first goal for the realignment of the zygoma is to reestablish its normal position in the facial skeleton, and therefore this will help to reestablish the orbital volume. A reliable way to do this is to realign the zygoma with the sphenoid wing since the sphenoid wing is not usually involved in the zygoma fracture (see Fig. 16.13a, b). When the alignment of the zygoma and the sphenoid wing makes a straight line, then the surgeon can feel confident that the zygoma has been repositioned properly in relationship to the cranial base, therefore reestablishing the anatomical basis for a normal orbital volume.

A minimum of three-point rigid fixation such as at the frontozygomatic suture, the orbital rim, and the zygomaticomaxillary buttress is often needed to attain full stability (see Fig. 16.14). Fixation at the region of the zygomatic arch to the zygoma can also be stabilized as a fourth buttress. A combination of any three of the zygomatic buttresses will suffice to stabilize the zygoma, but two-buttress fixation is often inadequate to be assured of satisfactory strength. An error that surgeons commonly make is that they will reduce the frontozygomatic suture area and the orbital rim, without the third buttress stabilized they may not recognize an increase in orbital volume. Because of the force of the masseter on the zygoma, a point of rotation at these areas can enable the zygoma to rotate, and this will increase the orbital volume as time goes on. So it is critical to get that third fixation point to be certain that the zygoma is stabilized in the proper position in three-dimensional space securing the orbital volume.

There are several surgical approaches for open reduction and internal fixation of a zygomatic fracture. One is the upper blepharoplasty incision or lateral brow incision to gain access to the frontozygomatic suture area. The second is a lower eyelid incision, such as a subciliary incision or transconjunctival incision. An intraoral incision is used to access the zygomaticomaxillary buttress. For zygoma fractures

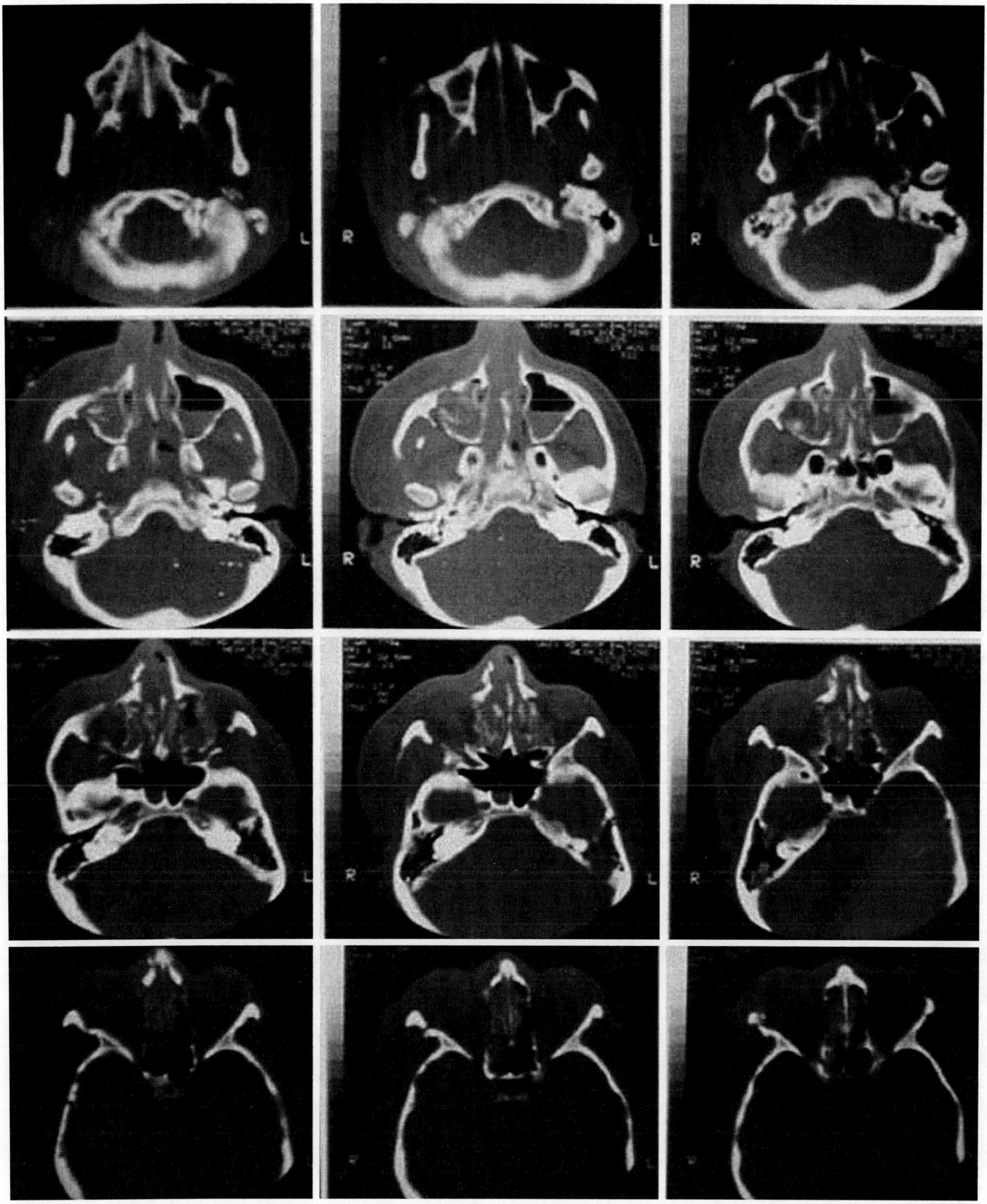

Fig. 16.9 Axial CT scan of a zygoma fracture

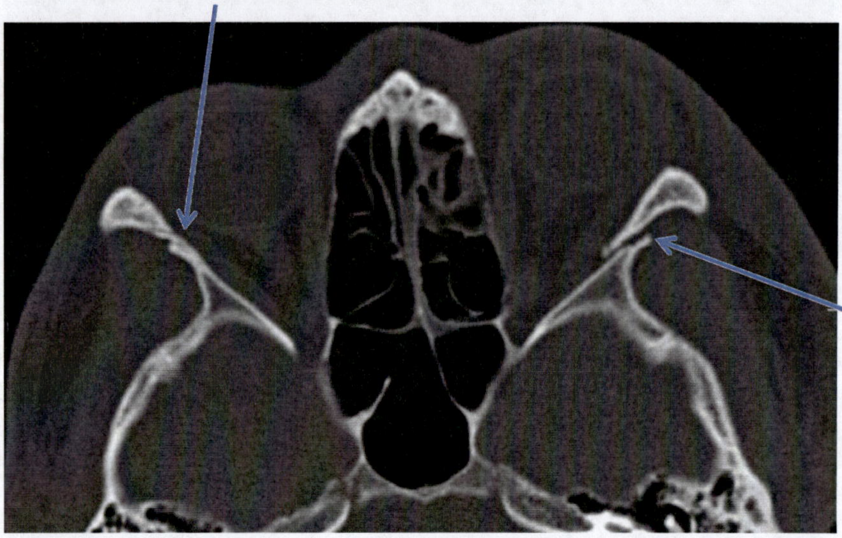

Fig. 16.10 Axial CT showing disruption of the alignment of the lateral wall of the orbit on the fractured side (*patient's left*) compared to the normal side (*patient's right*)

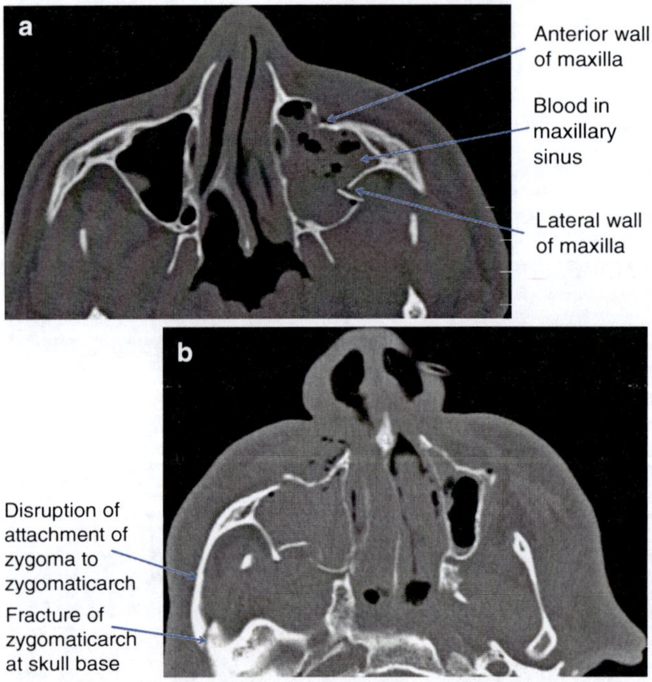

Fig. 16.11 Axial CT showing. (**a**) Disruption of the walls of the maxilla. (**b**) Disruption of the zygoma and zygomatic arch

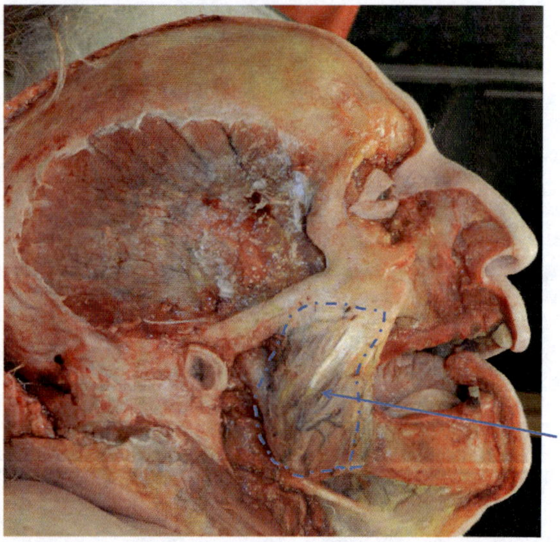

Fig. 16.12 Masseter muscle

that are associated with more extensive injuries, the coronal incision may be necessary.

Figure 16.15a depicts a patient who has had extensive midfacial fractures associated with a zygoma fracture. You can easily see the bowing on the zygomatic arch as it joins the zygoma which has enabled the zygoma to move posteriorly. The coronal incision gives excellent access to this region of the facial skeleton for fixation. The reduction picture (Fig. 16.15b) shows that the frontozygomatic suture is stabilized, and in addition, the zygomatic arch has been reduced and stabilized to the zygoma. The orbital rim is easily exposed through a subciliary incision (see Fig. 16.15c), and the zygomaticomaxillary buttress is approached through an intraoral incision (see Fig. 16.15d). For an isolated zygoma fracture, the coronal approach is often not necessary. A simple fracture can be reduced using the upper blepharoplasty incision, lower lid incision, and an intraoral incision to gain three-point fixation. With more complex facial injuries in conjunction with a zygoma fracture, the coronal approach may be necessary.

The orbital floor is routinely explored when doing open reduction and internal fixation of the zygoma even if the patient does not have eye symptoms at the initial time of injury. It is

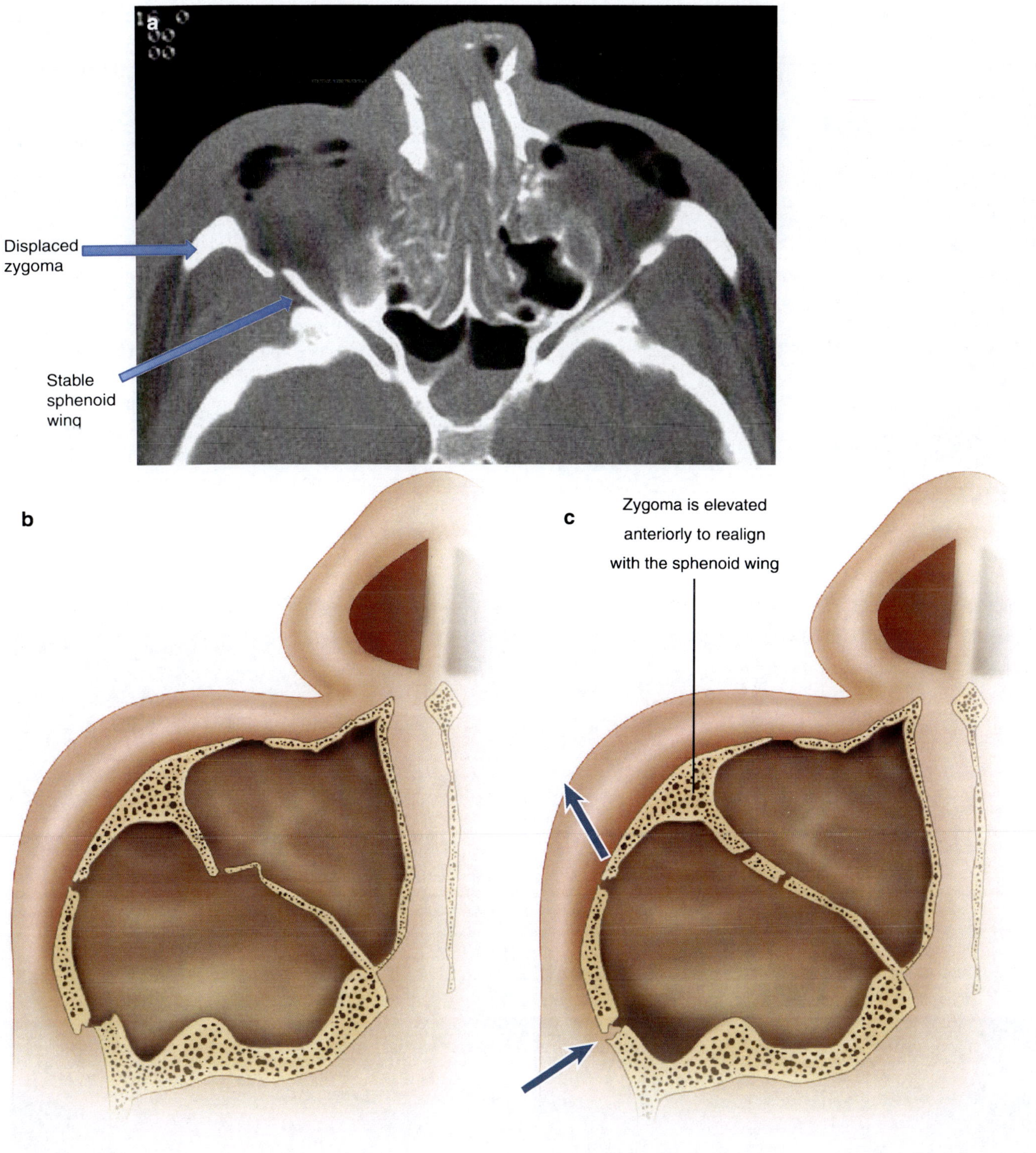

Fig. 16.13 (**a**) Axial CT showing displacement of the sphenoid wing and zygoma. (**b**) Diagram illustrating displacement of the sphenoid wing and zygoma. (c) Diagram illustrating reduction of the zygoma fracture by elevating the zygoma in the direction shown by the *blue arrows*, anteriorly and medially, until it is aligned with the sphenoid wing

possible that the bony support for the orbital floor has been provided by segments of the zygomatic complex being pushed backward. As you reduce the zygoma by drawing it forward, this can result in the loss of support for the floor fragments and allow dropping of the orbital floor segments, which could result in a postoperative orbit volume increase and possible diplopia (see Fig. 16.16). Since a lower lid incision is already being done to reduce the orbital rim, it is a simple matter to sweep

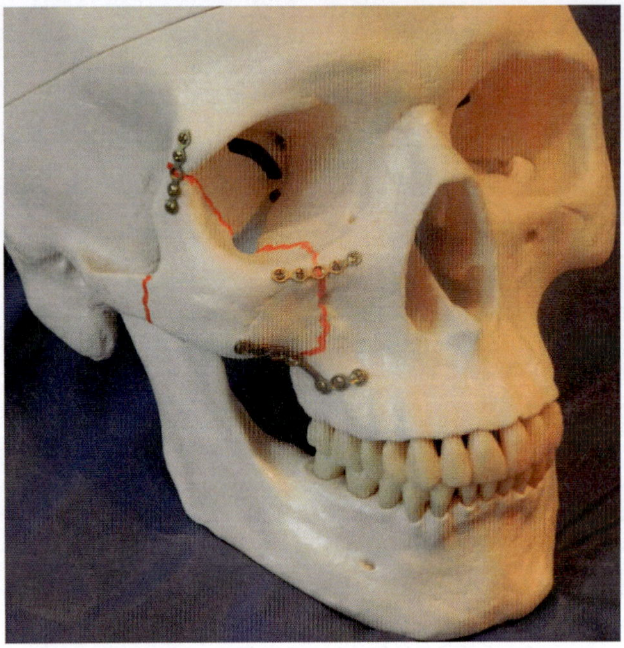

Fig. 16.14 Three-point fixation of a zygoma fracture

posteriorly and examine the floor of the orbit after zygoma reduction and ascertain that the floor is still intact and stable. If it is not, a graft or implant to the orbital floor will be necessary.

Any zygoma fracture having greater than 5 mm of bone loss at any buttress will require bone grafting to allow this buttress to heal properly. Immediate bone grafting right at the time of reduction is best, barring other considerations such as a contaminated wound.

Early treatment is imperative in that a zygoma fracture usually heals in a perior of about 4–6 weeks and more rapidly in children. Therefore, barring any other systemic factors, the surgeon should try to approach this repair as expeditiously as possible. A zygoma that is displaced and starting to form a significant amount of scar makes the reduction more difficult. Contracture of the masseter muscle can make it difficult to manipulate the zygoma as time progresses. If very prolonged displacement of the zygoma has occurred as in a chronic injury, it is possible that part of the masseter may need to be released in order to facilitate bone movement. If allowed to go long enough before reduction, osteotomies

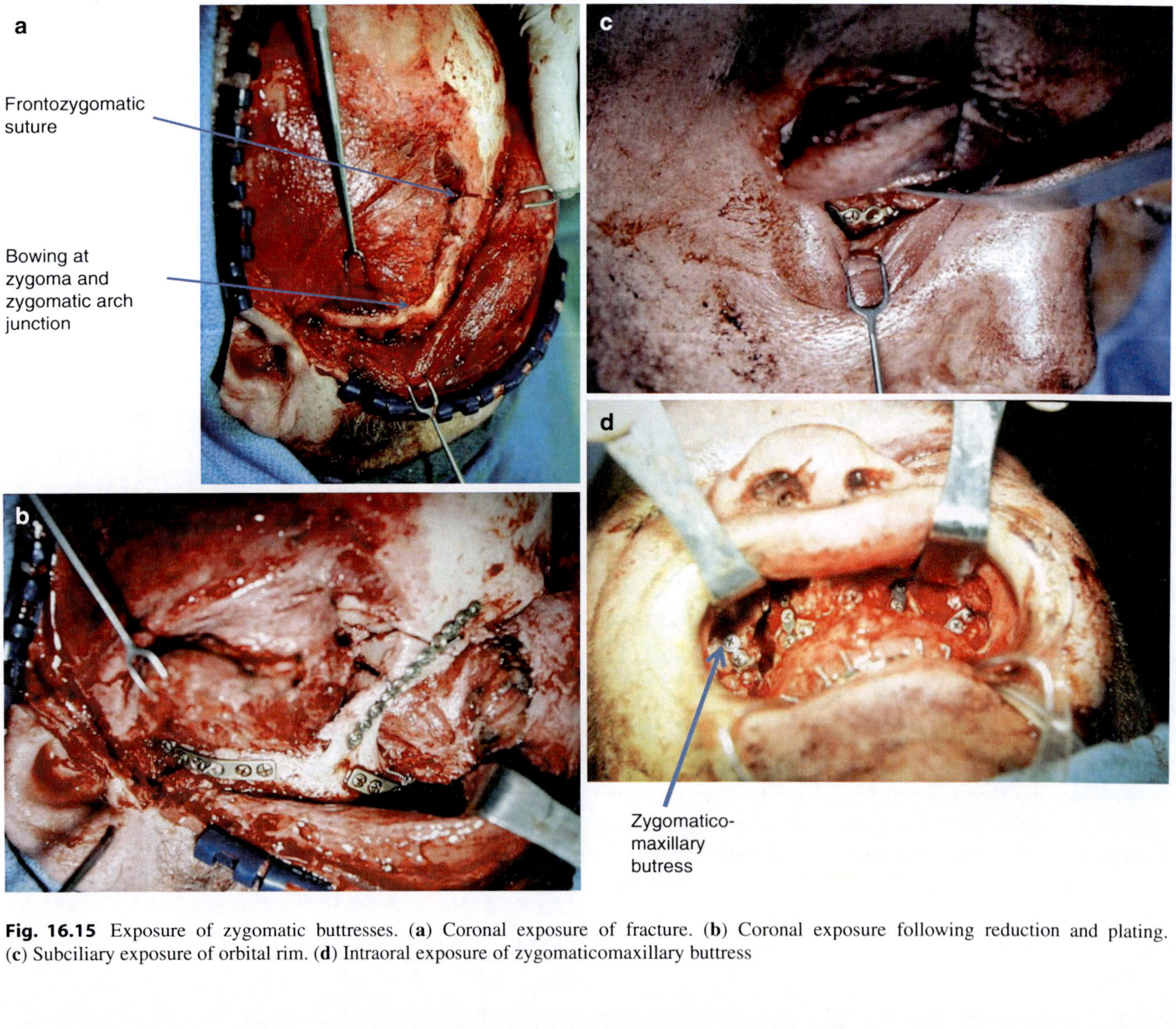

Fig. 16.15 Exposure of zygomatic buttresses. (a) Coronal exposure of fracture. (b) Coronal exposure following reduction and plating. (c) Subciliary exposure of orbital rim. (d) Intraoral exposure of zygomaticomaxillary buttress

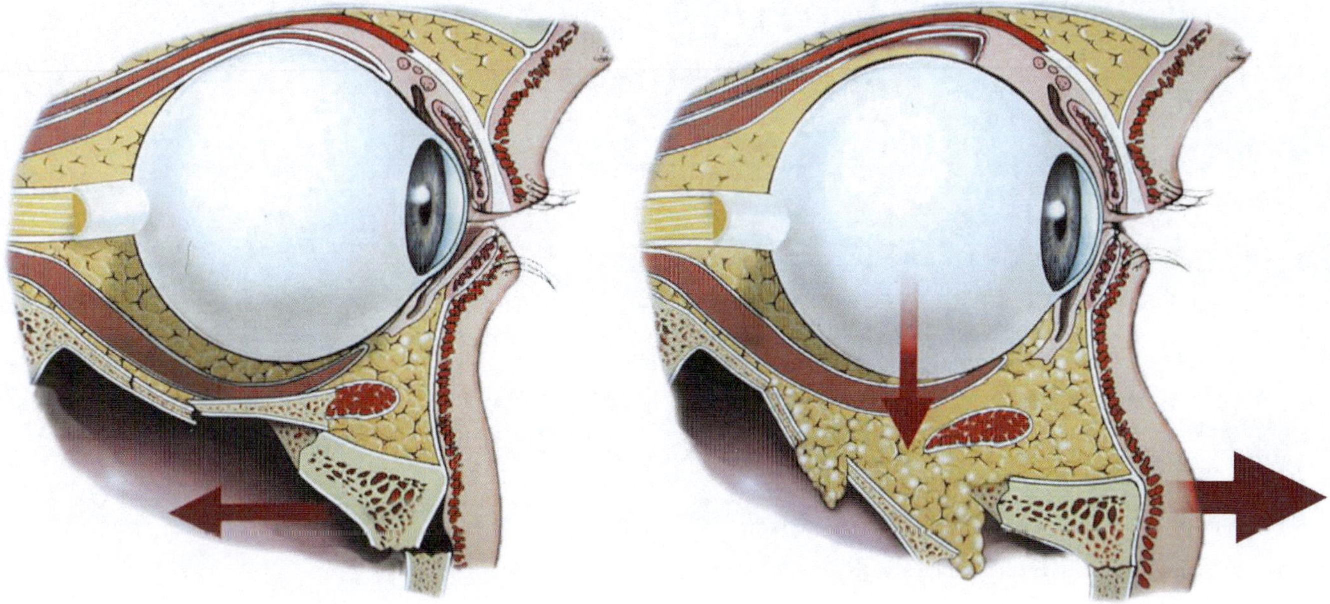

Fig. 16.16 Orbital floor fragments can drop when the zygoma fracture is reduced by drawing forward

may be necessary to facilitate repositioning of the zygoma. In addition, soft tissue around the orbit and zygoma is most likely to drape well over the bone after reduction if the reduction is done early. A prolonged delay will allow this tissue to scar down. The earlier these fractures are repaired the better. Ideally reduction should be done in the first 24–48 h, barring any other systemic factors.

Reducing the zygoma to the pre-injury state in relationship to the rest of the face and skull base will definitely reestablish vertical height, lateral projection, and anterior projection of the face in that region of the skeleton. After doing a reduction, it is imperative that surrounding soft tissue be resuspended to the craniofacial skeleton. This can done by placing a burr hole along the orbital rim or further up along the lateral orbit and through this hole passing a suture to suspend the soft tissue of the cheek and lower eyelid. After reduction, there is a tendency for the soft tissue of the cheek to draw on the lower lid as it heals, and as this contracts, it increases the potential for ectropion.

Suspending the soft tissue to the facial skeleton will reduce that tendency. Fractures of the zygomatic arch are very commonly associated with zygoma fractures. The arch is a thin bone and with a direct blow can be easily fractured. This may be an isolated injury (see Fig. 16.17) or may occur in combination with other facial fractures. The symptoms are usually a noticeable depression in the area, ecchymosis, and pain may be present upon opening and closing the mouth because of the impingement upon the temporalis muscle as it extends from the coronoid process of the mandible to the lateral aspect of the skull as discussed earlier. There are several means to approach this surgically. For an isolated depressed zygomatic arch fracture, a Gillies approach is probably one of the most efficient ways to reduce the fracture. The Gillies approach involves making an incision in the hair-bearing scalp (see Fig. 16.18a), although people have also gone through the lateral brow to approach the zygomatic arch (see Fig. 16.18b). Incising the deep temporalis fascia and dissecting just under the temporalis fascia and over the temporalis muscle will enable the surgeon to slide an elevator under the arch and elevate the bone. The temporalis muscle posses deep behind the zygomatic arch, and a plane just above the muscle enables the surgeon to slide an instrument (Gillies elevator) into the appropriate position behind the arch to reduce it. In order to do this without fixation, ideally this should be done within the first 24–48 h of having an isolated fracture. If delaying reduction beyond that period of time, there is a tendency to start forming fibrotic tissue, and this will make it more difficult to get the reduced bone to stay elevated. After doing the elevation, if it feels that there is still instability, then it may be necessary to open and stabilize it with rigid fixation. Obviously for zygomatic arch fractures associated with other severe midface fractures, access and rigid fixation can be obtained through a coronal incision. After completing a reduction of an arch fracture without fixation, an aluminum finger splint in a jug handle configuration over that region can be used to alert the

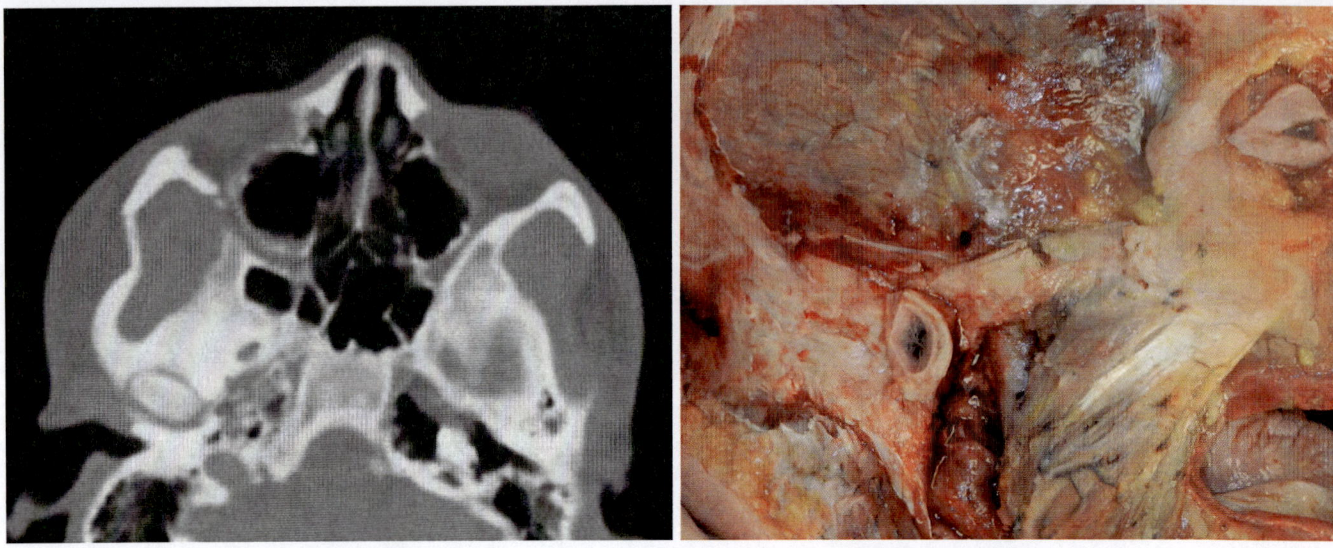

Fig. 16.17 Isolated right zygomatic arch fracture as seen on axial CT scan and prosection

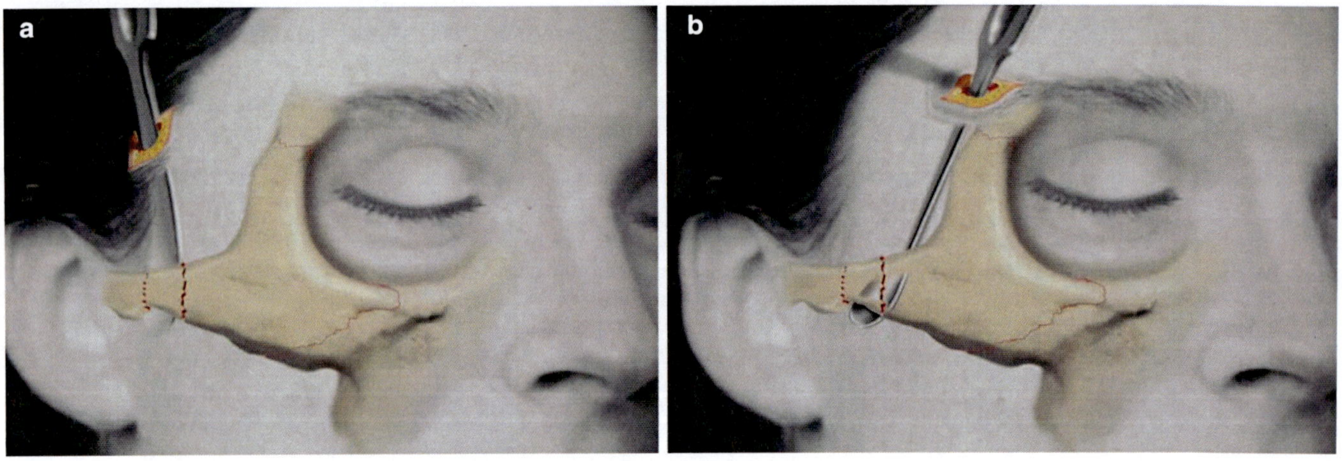

Fig. 16.18 (**a**) Gillies elevation of zygomatic arch fracture. (**b**) Lateral brow approach to the zygomatic arch

nursing staff and the anesthesia staff that the patient should not be lying on that side (see Fig. 16.19). If pressure is placed on that bone after reduction without fixation, it is possible that the zygomatic arch can fall back down.

Complications

Zygoma and zygomatic arch fractures can have certain complications associated with them. If not properly reduced, the orbital rim (lateral portion of the zygoma) remains depressed and it will draw down on the septum orbitale. The septum orbitale is attached to the tarsal plate of the eyelid and the periosteum of the zygoma at the orbital rim and will draw the lid down. Downward tension on this septum increases the chance for ectropion of the lower eyelid. This is one of the reasons ectropion is often a finding of a depressed zygoma fracture clinically on exam of patients at the time of acute injury. Ectropion postoperatively can also occur with a "skin only" flap of the lower lid for exposure of the rim of the orbit. When doing a dissection, it is advantageous to do an orbicularis oculi muscle and skin flap to be certain the lid flap is thick enough to maintain the integrity of the lid. Forty percent of all subciliary "skin only flaps" will result in ectropions. Entropion can also occur postoperatively. Entropion is more common with a transconjunctival approach. Contraction draws the lid inward. There may be interference with mandibular movement due to the impingement on the temporalis muscle if the fracture is not well reduced. Depression of the cheek contour is another complication of an under-reduced fracture. Infection is very rare around the facial region due to excellent circulation but can occur.

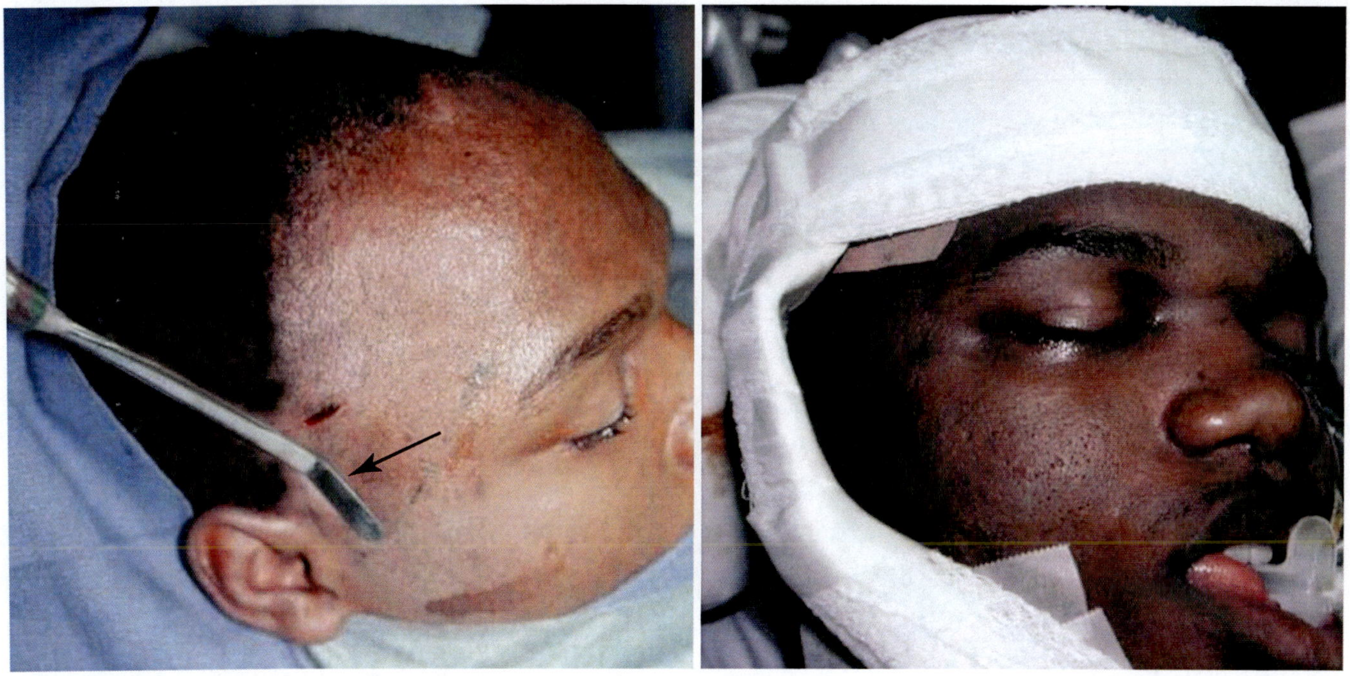

Fig. 16.19 Finger splinting to alert staff of restriction of lying on the fractured side after Gilles reduction with no fixation of an isolated zygomatic arch fracture

Blindness secondary to eye injury can be a complication of the initial injury if there is enough displacement of the zygoma to involve the globe, but blindness can also result from inappropriate care when manipulating the zygoma at the time of surgery. Corneal abrasion can occur while using rotatory instruments when placing plate and screw fixation. Very particular care needs to be taken to avoid injury to the cornea, and scleral shields are very useful. The surgeon must be meticulous in documenting any ocular findings preoperatively (diplopia, blindness, dilated fixed pupil). Any non-documented preoperative conditions may become misconstrued as a postoperative complication! A complete eye exam and vision exam is critical before exploring any region of the orbit.

Bony nonunion and malunion is unusual but can occur. Persistent infraorbital nerve paresthesia may be seen postoperatively. The infraorbital foramen region is a weak area along the anterior wall of the maxilla, and a fracture usually extends through that area. It is common with these fractures for this nerve to be contused resulting in cheek numbness or anesthesia. In most cases, the sensation will return over time after reduction of the bony injury. If the nerve is transected, the nerve can be sutured at the time of surgery. A simple contusion can still result in some nerve paresthesia for 3–6 months, but paresthesia can last up to a year or more. If sensation is not returning after 6 months, some have advocated decompression of the nerve in the infraorbital canal. Once again, it is imperative to document any preoperative sensation deficits and alert the patient of your findings.

Over the years, when plating zygoma fractures as well as all facial fractures, there has been an emphasis on using the smallest and thinnest plates possible. However, it is imperative to make certain the plate fixation is strong enough to stabilize the reduction against the forces of the masseter muscle especially in a patient who may not be cooperative. Figure 16.20 depicts a patient who had a zygoma fracture reduced in conjunction with other injuries through a coronal incision. Several days postoperatively, he had a significant depression of the cheek, despite the fact that on the operating room table at the time of the reduction, it was felt to be well positioned. A repeat CT showed deformity of the plate. On reexploring him it became evident that there was significant displacement of the plate and the bone. It is imperative to be certain that the fixation you are applying to the zygoma is strong enough to do the job of maintaining the bony reduction against the forces exerted on the region.

One of the most common postoperative complications of a zygoma fracture is a change in orbital volume due to inadequate reduction of the zygoma. Figure 16.21 depicts an individual who had open reduction and internal fixation. While the frontozygomatic suture area and orbital rim appeared reduced to the surgeon, in reality there was significant increase in orbital volume resulting from posterior rotation of the zygoma at these points. This resulted in enophthalmos and diplopia. The surgeon must be extremely careful to

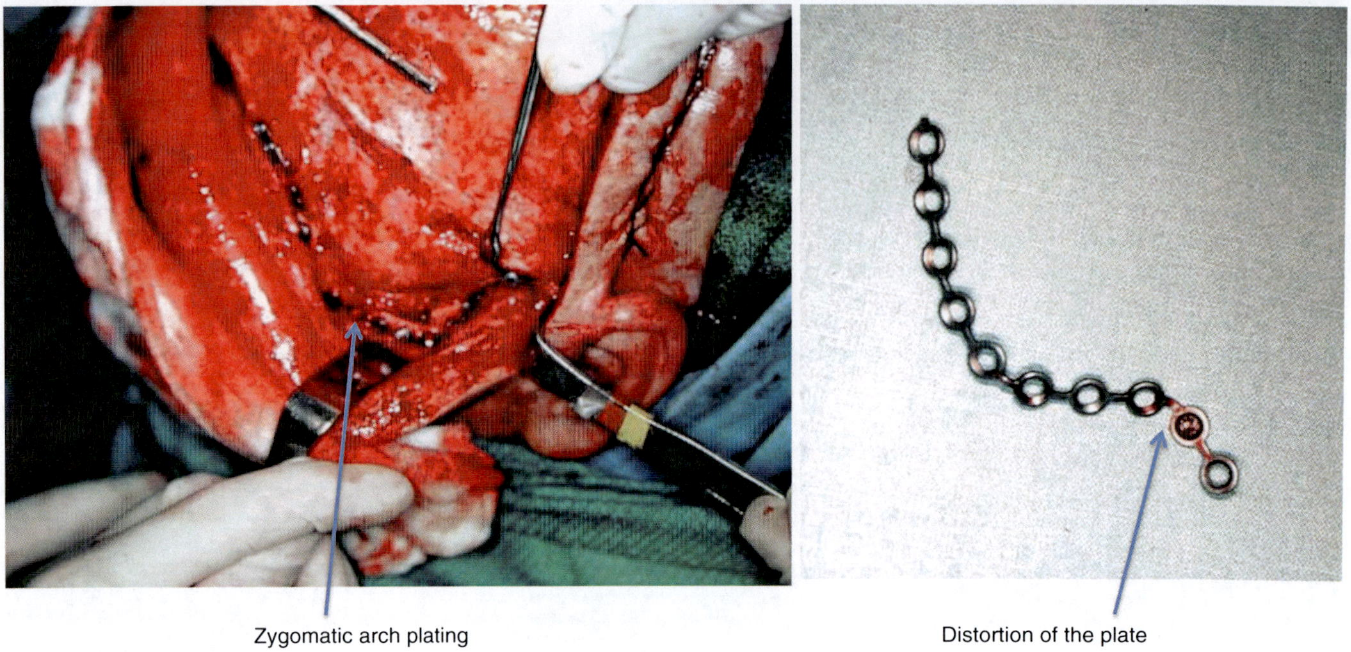

Fig. 16.20 Distortion of a microplate

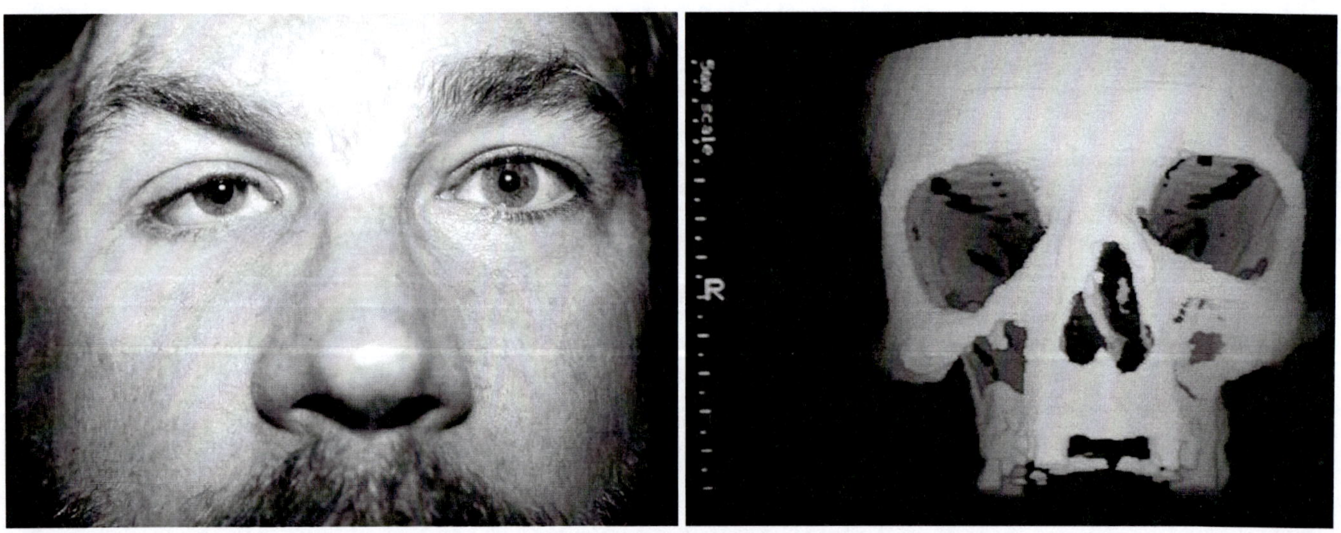

Fig. 16.21 Poor reduction of rigid zygoma fracture resulting in an increased orbital volume

be certain that the orbital volume is reestablished since the zygoma makes up the bulk of the lateral wall of the orbit.

In summary, it is imperative the zygoma be realigned with the cranial base to reestablish its normal 3D position in the facial skeleton to establish form and function of the face in this region. Reestablishing the orbital volume is critical to rebuild the functional unit of the orbit. The alignment of the zygoma (lateral orbit) with the sphenoid wing is an important maneuver utilized to achieve normalization of orbital volume. Early reduction is critical in allowing soft tissue to be able to drape well to the newly reduced bone and will help to decrease soft tissue complications. Reduction of the zygoma fracture as close to the time of injury as is practical as with all facial fractures will result in optimizing the potential for an excellent postoperative outcome.

Bibliography

Alqurainy IA, Stassen LF, Dutton GN, et al. The characteristics of midfacial fractures and the association with ocular surgery: a prospective study. J Oral Maxillofac Surg. 1991;29:302.

Barclay TL. Diplopia in association with fractures of the zygomatic bone. Br J Plast Surg. 1958;11:147.

Barclay TL. Four hundred malar-zygomatic fractures. Transactions of the International Society of Plastic Surgeons, Second Congress. Edinburgh: E & S Livingstone; 1960. p. 259.

Brown MS, Ky W, Lisman RD. Concomitant ocular injuries with orbital fractures. J Craniomaxillofac Trauma. 1999;5:41.

Chen CT. Endoscopic zygomatic fracture repair. Oper Tech Plast Reconstr Surg. 1998;5:282.

Chen CT, Chen YR. Application of the endoscope in orbital fractures. Semin Plast Surg. 2002;16:241.

Dal Santo F, Ellis E, Throckmorton GS. The effects of zygomatic complex fracture on masseteric muscle force. J Oral Maxillofac Surg. 1992;50:791.

Dolynchuk V, Tadjalle H, Manson P. Orbital volumetric analysis: clinical application in orbitozygomatic injuries. J Craniomaxillofac Trauma. 1996;2:56.

Funk GE, Stanley RB, Becker TS. Reversible visual loss due to impacted lateral wall fractures. Head Neck Surg. 1987;113:87.

Furst IM, Austin P, Phardah M, Mahoney J. The use of computed tomography to define zygomatic complex position. J Oral Maxillofac Surg. 2001;59:647.

Girotto J, Gamble B, Robertson B, et al. Blindness following reduction of facial fractures. Plast Reconstr Surg. 1998;102:1821.

Glassman RD, Manson PN, Petty P, et al. Techniques for improved visibility and lid protection in orbital explorations. J Craniofac Surg. 1990;1:69.

Gruss JS. Naso-ethmoid-orbital fractures: classification and role of primary bone grafting. Plast Reconstr Surg. 1985;75:303.

Gruss JS, Hurwitz JJ. Isolated blow in fracture of the lateral orbit causing globe rupture. Ophthal Plast Reconstr Surg. 1990;6:221.

Hakelius L, Ponten B. Results of immediate and delayed surgical treatment of facial fractures with diplopia. J Maxillofac Surg. 1973; 1:150.

Hollier L, Thornton J, Pazmino P, Stal S. The management of orbitozygomatic fractures. Plast Reconstr Surg. 2003;111:2386.

Holt GR, Holt SE. Incidence of ocular injuries in facial fractures: an analysis of 727 cases. Otolaryngol Head Neck Surg. 1983;91:276.

Hwang K, Suh MS, Chung IH. Cutaneous distribution of the infraorbital nerve. J Craniofac Surg. 2004;15:3.

Jackson IT. Classification and treatment of orbitozygomatic and orbitoethmoid fractures: the place of the bone grafting and plate fixation. Clin Plast Surg. 1989;16:77.

Kasrai L, Hearn T, Gur F, Forrest C. A biochemical analysis of the orbital zygomatic complex in human cadavers: examination of load sharing and failure patterns following fixation with titanium and bioresorbable systems. J Craniofac Surg. 1999;10:237.

Kawamoto Jr HK. Late posttraumatic enophthalmos: a correctable deformity? Plast Reconstr Surg. 1982;69:423.

Kelly K, Manson PN, Vander Kolk C, Markowitz B. Sequencing treatment in midface fractures. J Craniofac Surg. 1990;1:168.

Ketchum LD, Ferris B, Masters FW. Blindness in midface fractures without direct injury to the globe. Plast Reconstr Surg. 1976;55:187.

Knight JS, North JF. The classification of malar fractures: an analysis of displacement as a guide to treatment. Br J Plast Surg. 1961;13:315.

Kobayashi S, Sakai Y, Yamada A, Ohmori K. Approaching the zygoma with an endoscope. J Craniofac Surg. 1998;6:519.

Lacy MF, Popisil OA. Lower blepharoplasty post-orbicularis approach to the orbit-a prospective study. Br J Oral Maxillofac Surg. 1987;25:398.

Lederman IR. Loss of vision associated with surgical treatment of zygomatic-orbital floor fracture. Plast Reconstr Surg. 1981;68:94.

Lyon DB, Newman SA. Evidence of direct damage to extraocular muscles as a cause of diplopia following orbital trauma. Ophthal Plast Reconstr Surg. 1989;5:81.

MacKinnon CA, David DJ, Cooter RD. Blindness and severe visual impairment in facial fractures: an 11 year review. Br J Plast Surg. 2002;55:1.

Manson PN. Computed tomography use in repair of orbitozygomatic fractures. Arch Facial Plast Surg. 1999;1:25.

Manson P. Complications of facial fractures. In: Goldwyn R, Cohen S, editors. Complications in plastic surgery. New York: Lippincott-Raven; 2001a. p. 489–513.

Manson PN. Facial fractures. In: Goldwyn R, Cohen S, editors. The unfavorable result in plastic surgery-avoidance and treatment. 3rd ed. Philadelphia: Lippincott Williams & Wilkins; 2001b. p. 489–520.

Manson P. Facial fractures. In: Mathes S, editor. Plastic surgery, vol. 3. Philadelphia: WB Saunders; 2006. p. 77–380.

Manson PN, Iliff N. Surgical anatomy of the orbit. In: Marsh J, editor. Current therapy in plastic and reconstructive surgery. Philadelphia: BC Decker; 1989. p. 117.

Manson PN, Grivas A, Rosenbaum A, et al. Studies on enophthalmos: II. The measurement of orbital injuries and their treatment by quantitative computed tomography. Plast Reconstr Surg. 1986a;77:203.

Manson PN, Clifford CM, Su CT, et al. Mechanisms of global support and post-traumatic enophthalmos: I. The anatomy of the ligament sling and its relation to intramuscular cone orbital fat. Plast Reconstr Surg. 1986b;77:193.

Manson P, Markowitz B, Mirvis S, et al. Toward CT-based facial fracture treatment. Plast Reconstr Surg. 1990;85:202.

Manson P, Clark N, Robertson B, Crawley W. Comprehensive management of pan-facial fractures. J Craniomaxillofac Trauma. 1995;1:43.

Millman AL, Lubkin V, Gersten M. Three-dimensional reconstruction of the orbit from CT scans and volumetric analysis of orbital fractures: its role in the evaluation of enophthalmos (editorial). Adv Ophthalmic Plast Reconstr Surg. 1987;6:265.

O'Hara D, Delvecchio D, Bartlett S, Whitaker L. The role of microfixation in malar fractures: a quantitative biophysical study. Plast Reconstr Surg. 1996;97:345.

Perino KE, Zide ME, Kinnebrew MC. Late treatment of malunited malar fractures. J Oral Maxillofac Surg. 1980;42:20.

Petro J, Tooze FM, Bales CR, Baker CR. Ocular injuries associated with periorbital fractures. J Trauma. 1970;19:730.

Phillips J, Gruss J, Wells M. Periorbital suspension of lower eyelid and cheek following subciliary exposures of facial fractures. Plast Reconstr Surg. 1991;88:145.

Pospisil OA, Fernando TD. Review of the lower blepharoplasty incision as a surgical approach to the zygomatic orbital fractures. Br J Oral Maxillofac Surg. 1984;22:261.

Rinehart G, Marsh J, Hemmer K. Internal fixation of malar fractures: an experimental biophysical study. Plast Reconstr Surg. 1989;84:21.

Rohner D, Tay A, Meng CW, et al. The sphenozygomatic suture as a key site for osteosynthesis of the orbitozygomatic complex in panfacial fractures: a biochemical study in cadavers based on clinical practice. Plast Reconstr Surg. 2002;110:1463.

Rohrich RJ, Watumull D. Comparison of rigid plate versus wire fixation in the management of zygomatic fractures: a long-term follow-up clinical study. Plast Reconstr Surg. 1995;96:570.

Rohrick R, Hollier LH, Watumull D. Optimizing the treatment of orbitozygomatic fractures. Clin Plast Surg. 1992;19:149.

Roncevi R, Stajcic Z. Surgical treatment of post-traumatic enophthalmos: a study of 72 patients. Ann Plast Surg. 1994;32:288.

Schmitz JP, Hollinger JO. The critical size defect as an experimental model for craniomandibulofacial nonunions. Clin Orthop. 1986;205:299.

Sires BS, Stanley RB, Levine LM. Oculocardiac reflex caused by orbital floor fracture: an indication for urgent repair. Arch Ophthalmol. 1998;116:955.

Stanley Jr RB. Use of intraoperative computed tomography during repair of orbitozygomatic fractures. Arch Facial Plast Surg. 1999; 12:523.

Stanley RB, Sis BS, Frank GF, Nerd JA. Management of the displaced lateral orbital wall fractures associated with visual and ocular motility disturbances. Plast Reconstr Surg. 1998;102:972.

Sungeil P, Lindquist C. Paresthesia of the infraorbital nerve following fracture of the zygomatic complex. Int J Oral Maxillofac Surg. 1987;16:363.

Uriens JPM, Vanderglas HW, Bosman F, et al. Infraorbital nerve function following treatment of orbitozygomatic complete fractures: a multitest approach. Int J Oral Maxillofac Surg. 1998;27:27.

Wolfe SA, Davidson J. Avoidance of lower lid contraction in surgical approaches to the lower orbit. Oper Tech Plast Reconstr Surg. 1998;5:201.

Yab K, Tijima S, Imai K. Clinical application of a solid three-dimensional model for orbital wall fractures. J Craniomaxillofac Surg. 1993;21:275.

Orbital Fractures

17

Ivo A. Pestana and Lisa R. David

Introduction

Orbital fractures are some of the most common and challenging midface fractures encountered in emergency departments and, subsequently, by head and neck reconstructive surgeons. The term "orbit" refers to the space formed by the osseous structures that surround the eye. Orbital fractures can occur alone or in combination with other facial injuries or fracture complexes, and the significance of an orbital injury is related to its effect on the orbital contents and/or the space itself. In addition to variations in the type of injury and their association with other facial fractures, debate with regard to indications, timing, and technique of fracture repair exists. Moreover, differences of opinion exist regarding the choice of incision, approach, reconstructive materials, and wound closure.

Regional Anatomy

Bone Anatomy

The bony orbit has a pyramidal shape with a quadrangular base. Seven bones of variable thickness compose the orbital pyramid and include the zygoma, ethmoid, frontal, maxilla, lacrimal, palatine, and greater and lesser wings of the sphenoid (see Fig. 17.1). The bony orbit can be further characterized as having anterior, middle, and posterior thirds. The anterior third includes the stable orbital rim composed of supraorbital, nasoethmoidal, and zygomatic sections. The middle third defines the orbital cavity and its walls are composed of significantly thinner bony elements when compared to the anterior and posterior portions of the orbit. Finally, the posterior third of the bony orbit is the thickest section and is relatively protected from fracture. The bony anatomy of the orbital cavity requires special mention due to its complexity and comparative fragility which predisposes it to fracture as it absorbs forces transmitted through the orbital rim. The orbital cavity is defined by superior, inferior, medial, and lateral walls. The superior wall, or roof, is thin yet protected by a strong superior rim formed predominantly by the frontal bone. The inferior wall, or floor, is defined by the zygoma and maxillary roof. The lacrimal bone and lamina papyracea of the ethmoid compose the medial orbital wall, which is the thinnest area of the orbit. The thicker frontal and zygomatic bones and the greater wing of the sphenoid form the lateral wall.

Nerve Anatomy

Nervous structures pass in proximity to the bony construct of the orbit and may be involved in orbital fracture patterns (see Fig. 17.2). The supraorbital nerve exits the frontal bone through the supraorbital foramen which is located at the level of the eyebrow. The infraorbital nerve travels along, underneath, or through the orbital floor and exits the maxilla just below the infraorbital rim via the infraorbital foramen. The greater wing of the sphenoid houses the superior orbital fissure, through which pass cranial nerves III, IV, and VI, as well as the ophthalmic division of the trigeminal nerve. The infraorbital division of the maxillary segment of the trigeminal nerve and the zygomaticofacial nerve pass through the inferior orbital fissure. The optic foramen, which houses the optic nerve and the ophthalmic artery, can be found in the superior and medial aspect of the orbit, approximately 4 cm from the orbital rim.

Vascular Anatomy

The orbit receives its blood supply from the carotid system. Branches of the internal and external carotid arteries and their anastomoses (see Fig. 17.3) create an intricate vascular

I.A. Pestana, MD • L.R. David, MD (✉)
Department of Plastic and Reconstructive Surgery,
Wake Forest University, Winston-Salem, NC, USA
e-mail: ldavid@wakehealth.edu

P.J. Taub et al. (eds.), *Ferraro's Fundamentals of Maxillofacial Surgery*,
DOI 10.1007/978-1-4614-8341-0_17, © Springer Science+Business Media New York 2015

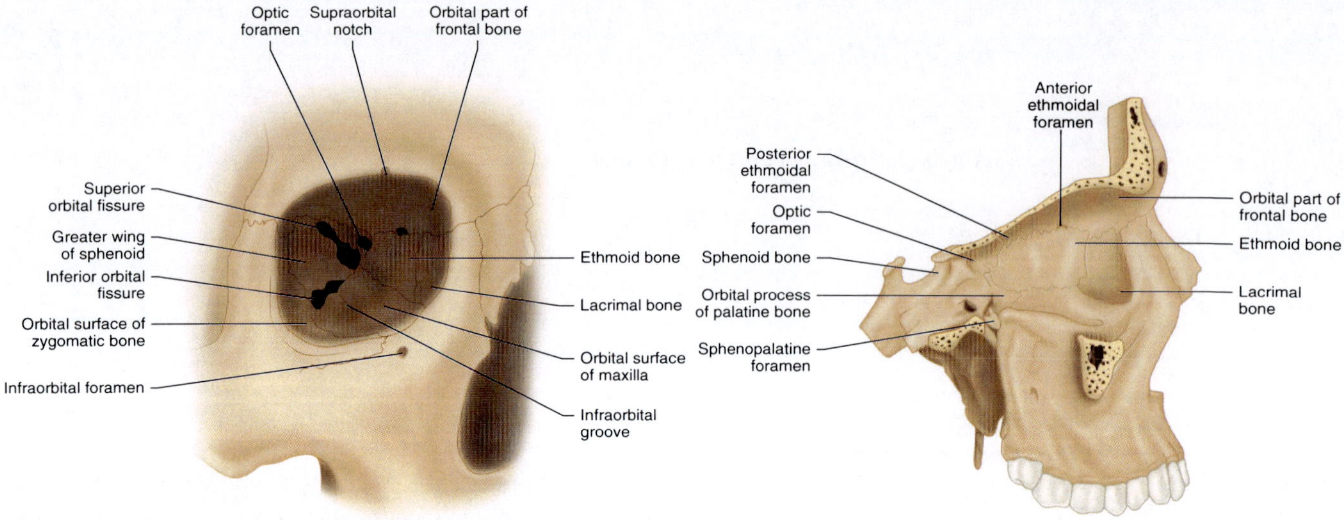

Fig. 17.1 Orbital bony anatomy

Fig. 17.2 Orbital nervous anatomy

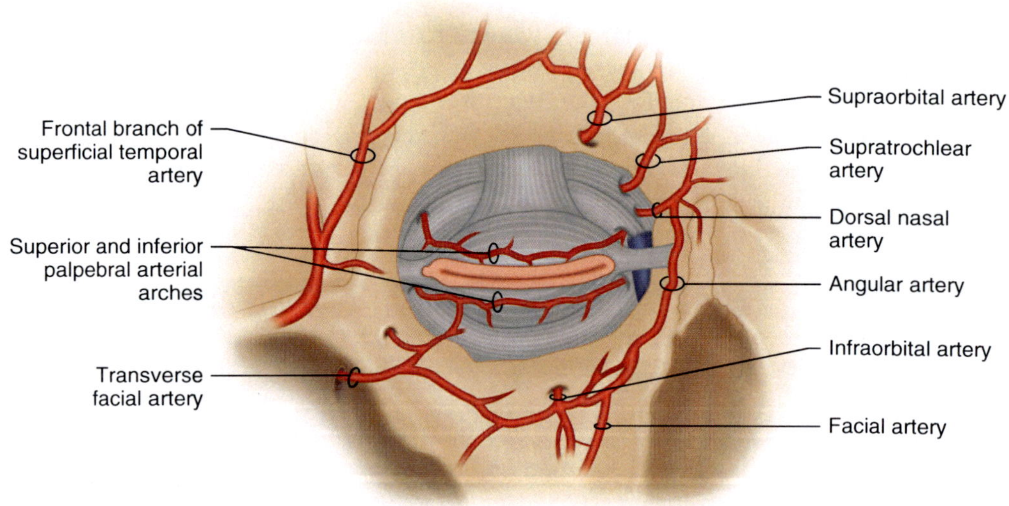

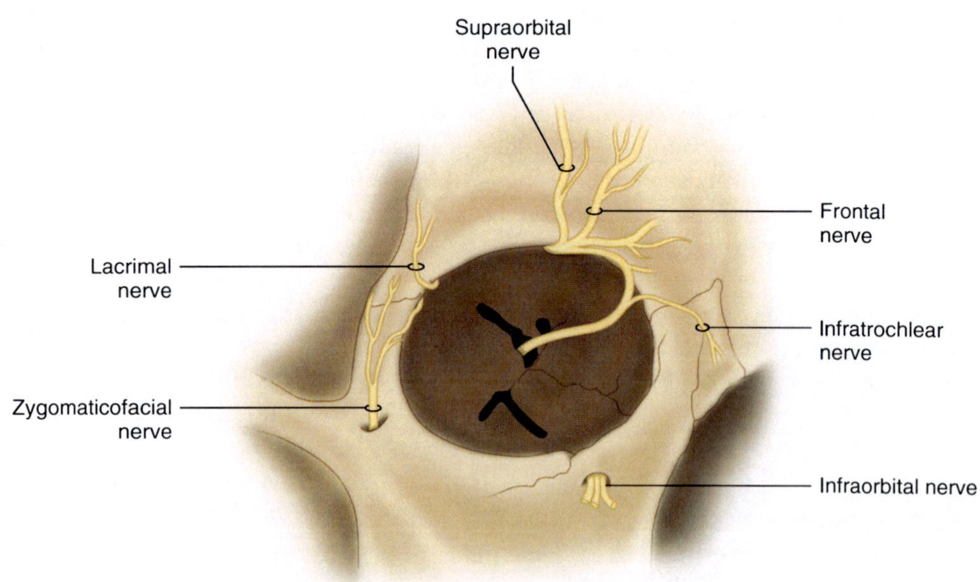

Fig. 17.3 Orbital vascular anatomy

construct supplying the soft tissues of the region. The internal carotid artery gives off the ophthalmic artery, which supplies the eyelid, nasal dorsum, and forehead. The ophthalmic artery branches into the supraorbital, supratrochlear, infratrochlear, anterior and posterior ethmoid, medial and lateral palpebral, and marginal arteries. The anterior and posterior ethmoid arteries, which originate from the internal carotid vascular tree, anastomose with the external carotid system. The external carotid artery gives rise to the internal maxillary artery, which emerges as the infraorbital artery. The infraorbital artery travels a short distance within the pterygopalatine fossa before passing through the infraorbital fissure into the orbit. It continues anteriorly through the infraorbital groove and canal to emerge below the inferior orbital margin to supply the lower eyelid. The superficial temporal artery, just before crossing the zygomatic arch, gives off the transverse facial artery to supply the lateral canthal region.

Eyelid Anatomy

The upper and lower eyelids consist of three lamellae: anterior (skin and orbicularis oculi muscle), middle (orbital septum), and posterior (conjunctiva, capsulopalpebral fascia, medial and lateral canthal tendons, and tarsal plate) (see Fig. 17.4). The orbicularis oculi muscle resides in the anterior lamella. It functions as the primary lid constrictor and is divided into pretarsal, preseptal, and orbital fibers. The middle lamella contains the orbital septum, which consists of a membrane spanning from the tarsus to the periosteum of the orbital rim and separates the orbital contents from the surrounding soft tissues. The levator palpebrae superioris and Müller's muscle, located deep to the levator, serve as the upper eyelid retractors, whereas the capsulopalpebral fascia serves the lower lid in the same capacity. The eyelid tarsal plates are dense, cartilaginous structures that provide vertical support to the eyelid soft tissues. As the tarsal plates progress to the medial and lateral margins of the palpebral fissure, they become confluent with their respective canthal tendons. Ligamentous support of the globe consists of medial and lateral canthal ligaments as well as check ligaments. The lateral canthal tendon is formed by the confluence of the upper and lower crura and Whitnall's ligament. These structures then merge to create the lateral retinaculum, which subsequently inserts onto Whitnall's tubercle of the lateral orbit. The nasoethmoidal region of the medial orbital rim houses the attachments for the levator palpebrae superioris to the medial canthus and Lockwood ligament to the superior aspect of the lacrimal fossa, respectively. Lockwood ligament, which attaches posterior to the lacrimal sac, acts as a suspensory system for the globe. Together with the intermuscular septa

a

b

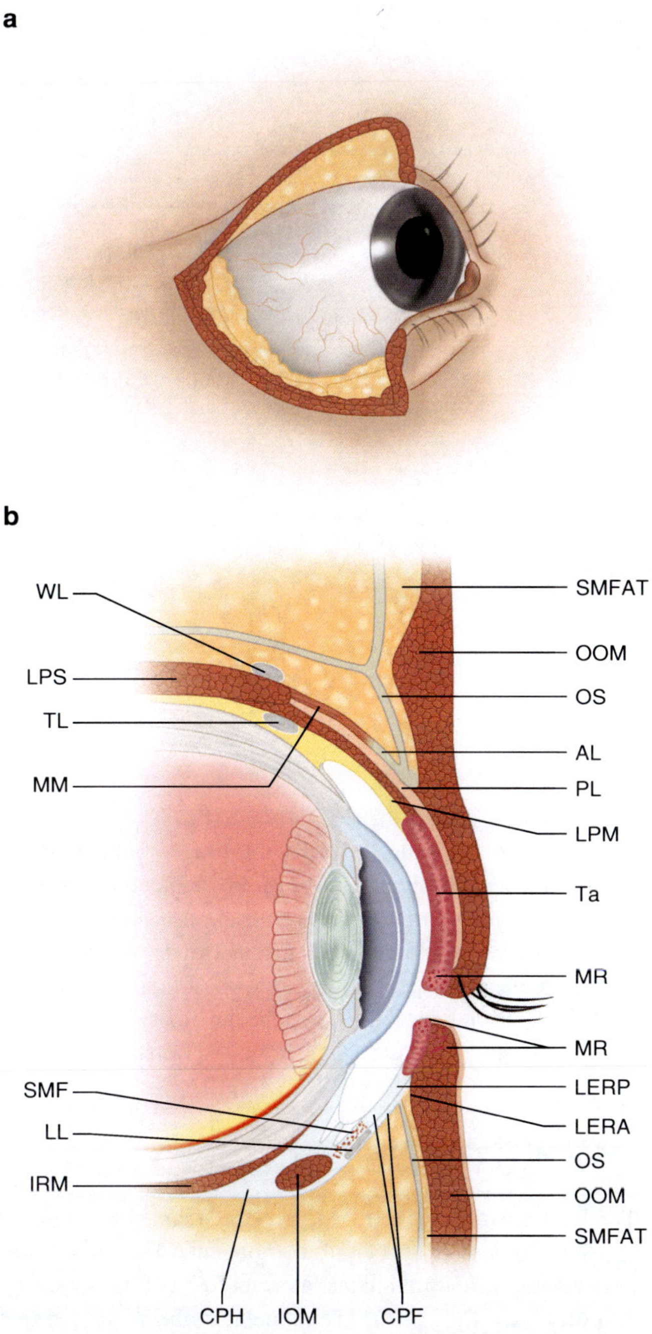

Fig. 17.4 Anatomic structure of the eyelid. *Upper lid*: *MM* Mueller's muscle, *WL* Whitnall's ligament, *LPS* levator palpebrae superioris, *ITL* intermuscular transverse ligament, *LPM* lamina propria mucosae, *MR* muscle of Riolan, *Ta* anterior aspect of the tarsus, *PL* levator aponeurosis – posterior layer, *AL* levator aponeurosis – anterior layer, *OS* orbital septum, *OOM* orbicularis oculi muscle, *SMFAT* submuscular fibroadipose tissue. *Lower lid*: *SMF* smooth muscle fiber, *LL* Lockwood ligament, *IRM* inferior rectus muscle, *CPH* capsulopalpebral head, *IOM* inferior oblique muscle, *CPF* capsulopalpebral fascia, *SMFAT* submuscular fibroadipose tissue, *OOM* orbicularis oculi muscle, *OS* orbital septum, *LERA* lower eyelid retractor – anterior layer, *LERP* lower eyelid retractor – posterior layer, *MR* muscle of Riolan

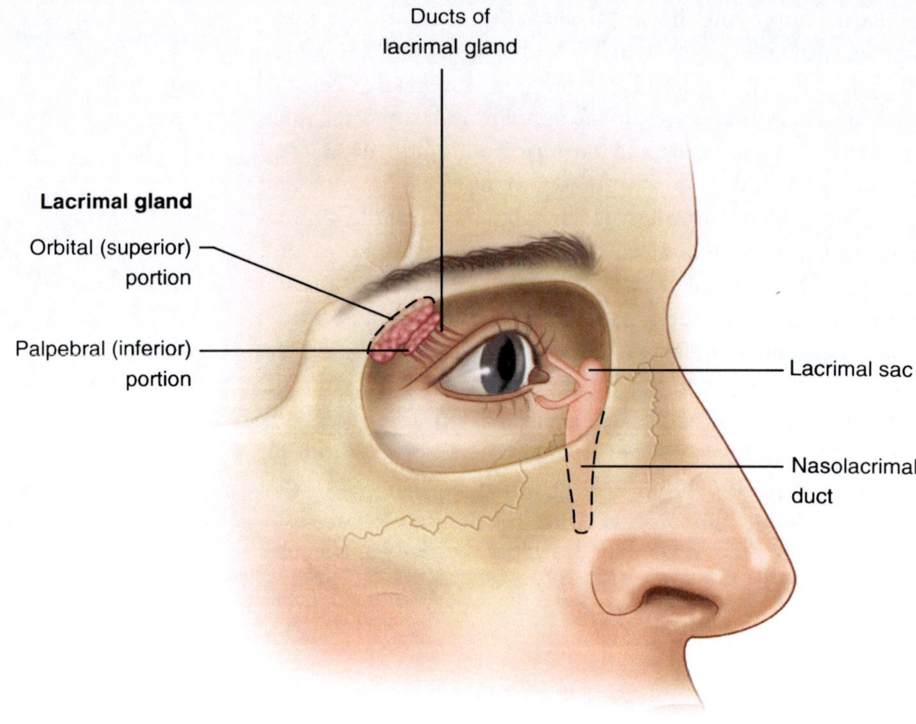

Fig. 17.5 Anatomy of the lacrimal system

and the Tenon capsule, it forms the lower eyelid retractor system. Posteriorly, it arises from fibrous attachments to the inferior side of the inferior rectus muscle and continues anteriorly as the capsulopalpebral fascia (lower eyelid retractors). The medial aspect of the Lockwood ligament attaches to the posterior lacrimal crest, and the lateral retinaculum attaches to the lateral orbital (Whitnall's) tubercle.

Lacrimal System Anatomy

The lacrimal gland functions to produce tears which have an aqueous, mucous, and lipid component. The gland is a bilobed structure found in the lacrimal fossa of the superolateral orbit (see Fig. 17.5). The palpebral lobe of the lacrimal gland is responsible for basal tear secretion and drains into the upper lateral half of the superior fornix. The main orbital lobe of the gland sends ducts through the palpebral lobe for drainage and produces reflex tear secretion. Basal tear secretion provides a constant liquid film for globe lubrication while reflex secretion augments tear flow and may be stimulated by foreign body or emotion. Tears pass from the palpebral fissure through the lacrimal ducts and canaliculi via the puncta lacrimalia. The canaliculi merge as a common canaliculus to empty into the lacrimal sac, which is situated within the bony lacrimal fossa just posterior to the insertion of the medial canthal tendon. The sac joins the nasolacrimal duct, which progresses caudally and drains into the inferior meatus.

Fracture Patterns

Orbital Floor

In the adult population, the orbital floor is most susceptible to injury and is commonly fractured in a craniofacial trauma (see Fig. 17.6). Although many have been proposed, two main mechanisms explain the cause of orbital floor fractures. The *hydraulic mechanism* attributes fractures to the direct transmission of pressure from the intraorbital contents and globe to the orbital floor. In contrast, the *buckling mechanism* implicates osseous conduction, or indirect transmission, of force to the orbital rim as the cause of fracture. The orbital floor is invariably thin, and the presence of the infraorbital foramen and groove makes this site susceptible to fracture from forces applied to the midface. In addition, the contour of the orbital floor changes from concave just behind the infraorbital rim to convex posteriorly toward the apex which may contribute to the high frequency of fracture of the orbital floor in association with midface trauma.

Orbital "Blowout" Fracture

An isolated orbital floor "blowout" fracture involves the internal orbital walls *without* fracture of the orbital rims. On examination, diplopia and enophthalmos are frequently evident. Diplopia is most often the result of edema but can result from

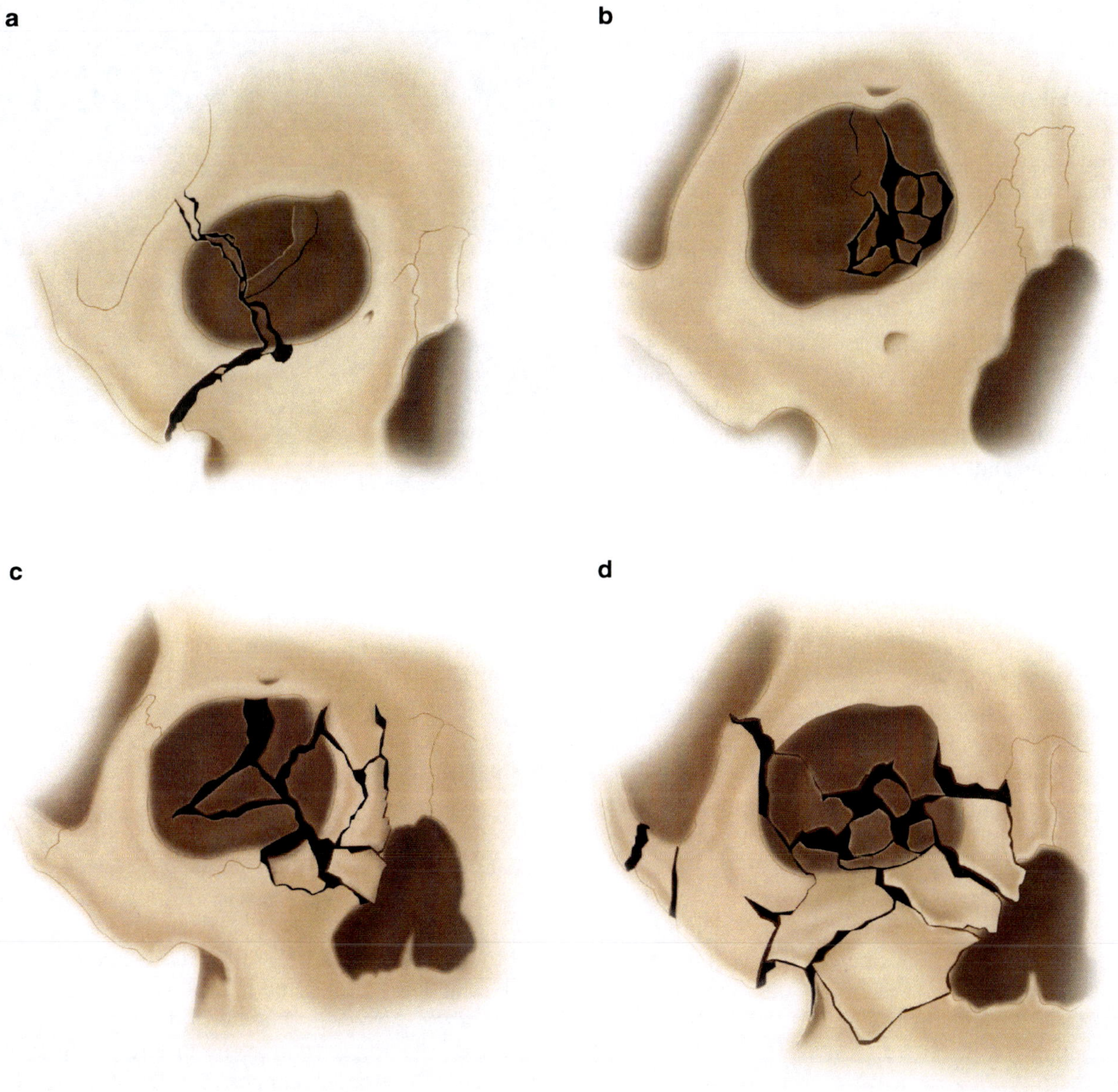

Fig. 17.6 (**a**) Orbito-zygomatic fracture pattern. (**b**) Internal orbital fracture pattern. (**c**) Naso-orbital-ethmoid fracture pattern. (**d**) Complex combined orbital fracture pattern

restricted ocular motion due to incarceration of the inferior oblique or inferior rectus muscles, Lockwood ligament, Tenon capsule, or periorbital fat within the fracture line. Similarly, direct damage to the extraocular muscles, injury to muscular innervation, and hematoma can also lead to diplopia. Orbital floor fractures can occur in combination with zygomaticomaxillary complex (ZMC) or LeFort fractures, each differing in terms of severity and presenting with distinct sequelae. Isolated orbital floor injuries have been demonstrated on CT scan to result in orbital expansion, whereas those occurring in association with ZMC fractures can result in a decreased orbital volume.

Medial Wall

The medial orbital wall is composed of the lacrimal bone and lamina papyracea of the ethmoid. It occupies a vertical position with a slightly lateral tilt. Anteriorly, it houses the lacrimal sac between the frontal process of the maxilla (anterior lacrimal crest) and the lacrimal bone (posterior lacrimal crest). A fracture in this region is typically classified as a nasoorbital ethmoid (NOE) fracture, whereas a fracture of the lamina papyracea connotes a pure medial wall injury. Because the medial wall separates the orbit from the ethmoid sinus spaces, epistaxis and orbital emphysema are commonly seen with floor fractures that involve the medial wall.

Lateral Wall

The lateral orbital wall is formed primarily by the orbital surface of the zygomatic bone and the greater wing of the sphenoid bone. The sphenoid portion of the lateral orbit is separated from the roof of the orbit by the superior orbital fissure and from the floor by the inferior orbital fissure. Isolated fractures of the lateral wall are the least common of all orbital fractures due to the thick and supportive frontal and zygomatic bones. However, fractures of the zygomaticomaxillary complex are common and always involve the lateral wall through articulations with the zygoma and greater wing of the sphenoid.

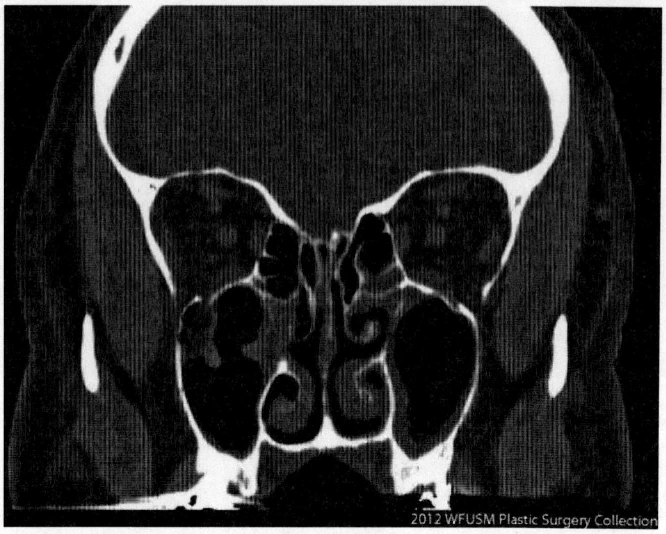

Fig. 17.7 Clinical example of an orbital floor fracture

Orbital Roof

Roof fractures, although rare in the adult population, are the most common orbital fractures seen in children less than 7 years of age. Possible reasons include incomplete pneumatization of the frontal sinus as well as the proportionately larger sized cranium in the pediatric population. After age 7, the orbital floor becomes the most prevalent fracture site since sinus pneumatization, as well as facial development, redirects traumatic forces away from the orbital roof. Incidence of concomitant involvement of the zygomatic complex (50 %), nasoethmoidal region (32 %), and frontal sinus (28 %) are notable, and identification of an orbital fracture on imaging should elicit careful analysis of the remainder of the craniofacial skeleton to rule out commonly associated fracture patterns.

Surgical Indications

General Evaluation

Surgical repair of orbital fractures can be classified as emergent, urgent, or delayed. Indications for repairing orbital fractures include significant structural defects confirmed by imaging, extraocular muscle entrapment, deteriorating visual acuity, persistent diplopia in central gaze, and distortion of globe position (enophthalmos or vertical dystopia). Such fractures are repaired with some urgency, usually within 2 weeks of the injury. If a patient has sustained significant periorbital trauma, an examination by an ophthalmologist should be performed preoperatively and postoperatively to determine the presence of globe injury. This should include an examination of the cornea and anterior chamber to rule out corneal abrasion and hyphema, respectively. A bright-light examination with dilation of the pupil should be conducted for full inspection of the retina to rule out detachment.

Orbital Imaging

The gold standard imaging modality for the diagnosis of orbital fractures is computed tomography (CT) and includes both bony and soft tissue windows (see Fig. 17.7). Thin cuts (1.0–1.5 mm) in the coronal and axial planes are preferable as coronal sections reveal information regarding the status of the orbital floor, roof, and medial wall as well as visualization of the extraocular muscles. CT imaging also allows calculation of orbital volume. In an effort to prevent the incidence of late enophthalmos, defects of approximately 50 % of the orbital floor or a 20 % change in orbital volume are considered to be operative indications. Sagittal images can clarify the position of the injury with regard to the anterior-posterior plane, demonstrate the proximity of injury to the orbital apex, and delineate floor inclination which is critical when prosthetic floor reconstruction is being planned.

Visual Acuity and Visual Field Testing

In the setting of orbital fracture, rates of associated ocular and neurologic injury have been reported as high as 33 and 57 %, respectively. Diplopia can result from muscle or ligament entrapment; evaluation is required. Most commonly, diplopia is elicited on upward gaze but it may also be primary (in the central visual field) or secondary (on extreme peripheral gaze). Long-term follow-up of untreated orbital blowout fractures has demonstrated that, if present on initial presentation, diplopia resolves in over half of patients within 2 weeks of injury and in almost 75 % of patients overall. Several tests have been applied to assess vision, globe mobility, and position. The forced-duction test is a maneuver utilized to differentiate entrapment of the ligaments of the inferior rectus muscle from muscular weakness, contusion, or paralysis. Forced-duction is performed by first instilling a few drops of local anesthetic into the conjunctival sac. The insertion of the inferior rectus onto the globe, which is located at a point approximately 7–10 mm from the limbus, is grasped, and the globe is gently rotated into all cardinal directions of gaze with the patient's head held straight and facing forward. A normal examination result demonstrates unhindered extraocular motion. Duction testing may give spurious results in the first week after injury because of the presence of edema or hematoma and thus should be repeated if results are abnormal or inconclusive, and following any surgical intervention.

Three-Dimensional Volume Assessment

Orbital fractures and associated alterations in orbital structure and volume may produce enophthalmos which is defined as a disturbance of the anterior-posterior position of the globe or the difference between the anterior corneal surface and the lateral orbital rim. It occurs when there has been an increase in orbital volume. Fractures with enophthalmos on initial presentation tend to involve the medial wall as well as the orbital floor. Physical findings associated with enophthalmos include an exaggerated superior sulcus above the upper lid and upper eyelid pseudoptosis (no change in distance between the inferior lid margin and pupil). Using the lateral orbital rim as a reference point, the Hertel exophthalmometer measures the degree of enophthalmos in relation to the normal contralateral orbit. As measurements using this instrument are based on the position of the lateral orbital rim, its measurement will be inaccurate when the lateral orbital rim is displaced or significant posttraumatic edema is present. Enophthalmos or dystopia may only become apparent after 1 or 2 weeks when edema has resolved; thus, a follow-up examination is crucial. A difference between the eyes of more than 3 mm is considered significant displacement. When the lateral orbital rim has been displaced, a Naugle exophthalmometer is preferred, since its reference structures are the frontal and infraorbital structures rather than the lateral orbital rim.

Timing of Surgical Intervention

Emergency Treatment of Orbital Fractures

Emergent operative intervention for management of orbital fractures is indicated for pending partial or complete loss of vision from direct or indirect trauma to the optic nerve.

Retrobulbar Hematoma

Hematoma formation posterior to the globe, or the presence of another acute space-occupying lesion, may result in increased intraocular pressure and compromise neurovascular structures. Vision loss in this scenario may occur within 1 h of onset. The classic presentation of retrobulbar blindness includes proptosis, pain, and oculomotor nerve (CN III) palsy with a progressive decrease in visual acuity. Emergent decompression is indicated with findings of a tense, proptotic globe. Decompression access is obtained through a transcutaneous, transseptal incision (see Fig. 17.8). A transconjunctival pressure release, with or without a lateral canthotomy, is performed and followed by inferior cantholysis. Carotid-cavernous sinus fistulae, presenting with retrobulbar hematoma and pulsating exophthalmos, can be evaluated and ruled out with imaging.

Traumatic Optic Neuropathy

Direct trauma to the optic nerve or optic nerve ischemia from compression in the posterior third of the orbit has been described in association with orbital fracture. Operative fracture reduction itself can also lead to blindness by similar mechanism, confirming the importance of preoperative ophthalmologic examination. The spectrum of physical findings associated with traumatic optic neuropathy range from decreased color perception to total vision loss. In patients with posttraumatic blindness, a high-resolution CT scan can suggest the etiology by demonstrating optic nerve swelling or fracture within the bony canal. Unfortunately, a patient with complete vision loss (absence of light perception) that occurred at the moment of injury is unlikely to recover vision. A patient with progressive loss of visual acuity has a relatively better chance for recovery with appropriate treatment. The use of high-dose steroids has been suggested to be beneficial in all cases presenting with traumatic optic neuropathy. Emergent surgical nerve decompression is reserved for patients with at least some light perception on presentation.

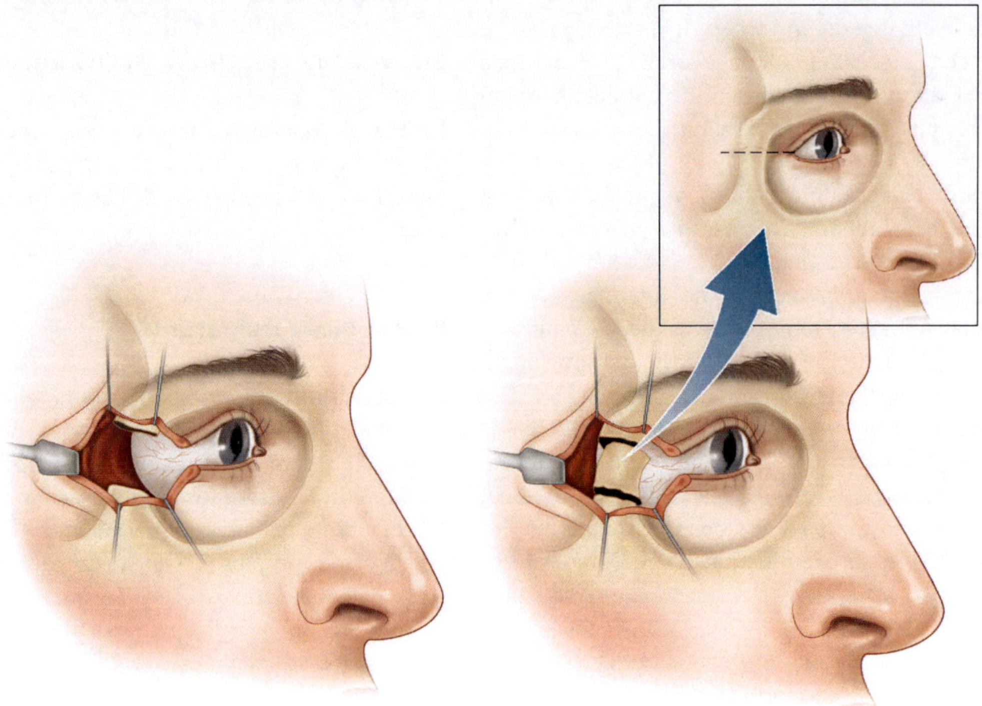

Fig. 17.8 Technique for decompression of a retrobulbar hematoma

Superior Orbital Fissure and Orbital Apex Syndromes

Superior orbital fissure syndrome results from fracture line extension into the superior orbital fissure and subsequent injury to cranial nerves III, IV, VI, and the ophthalmic branch of the trigeminal nerve. Symptoms include ophthalmoplegia, ptosis of the upper eyelid, proptosis, a fixed and dilated pupil, loss of corneal reflex, and sensory loss in the distribution of V1. Orbital apex syndrome results from ischemic optic neuropathy caused by fracture extension into the optic foramen or retrobulbar hematoma. It is similar to superior orbital fissure syndrome, with the distinction that the optic nerve is involved in orbital apex syndrome. A swinging light source moving from one pupil to the other can detect whether a relative afferent pupillary defect exists, often referred to as a Marcus-Gunn pupil. This maneuver can be performed in an unconscious patient. This test is used to identify optic nerve impingement at the orbital apex, which results in a lack of indirect light reaction by the unaffected eye. Visual evoked-potential testing can be employed to confirm unclear results from the physical examination. If it occurs postoperatively, an emergent CT scan is indicated to identify the etiology of the compression followed by operative exploration.

Trapdoor Phenomenon

In the pediatric population, there is a subset of orbital fractures that require emergent repair within the first 24–36 h after injury. A trapdoor fracture refers to an orbital floor fracture that, because of elastic recoil, results in entrapment of orbital contents and/or the inferior rectus muscle (see Fig. 17.9). The recoil occurs as a result of the relatively thick periosteum in children. Examination demonstrates impaired ocular muscle function, pain on attempted range of motion, and possible bradycardia, nausea, and/or syncope resulting from the oculocardiac reflex mediated through the parasympathetic pathway. The recoiled floor often appears uninjured on CT imaging but should demonstrate the entrapped muscle. This ischemic insult to the muscle can progress to myonecrosis, and improved muscle function has been demonstrated with earlier surgical correction.

Nonemergent Treatment of Orbital Fractures

Standard Indications

Most commonly orbital floor fractures present without entrapment and no vision threatening symptomatology. In these cases allowing the edema to resolve and a complete

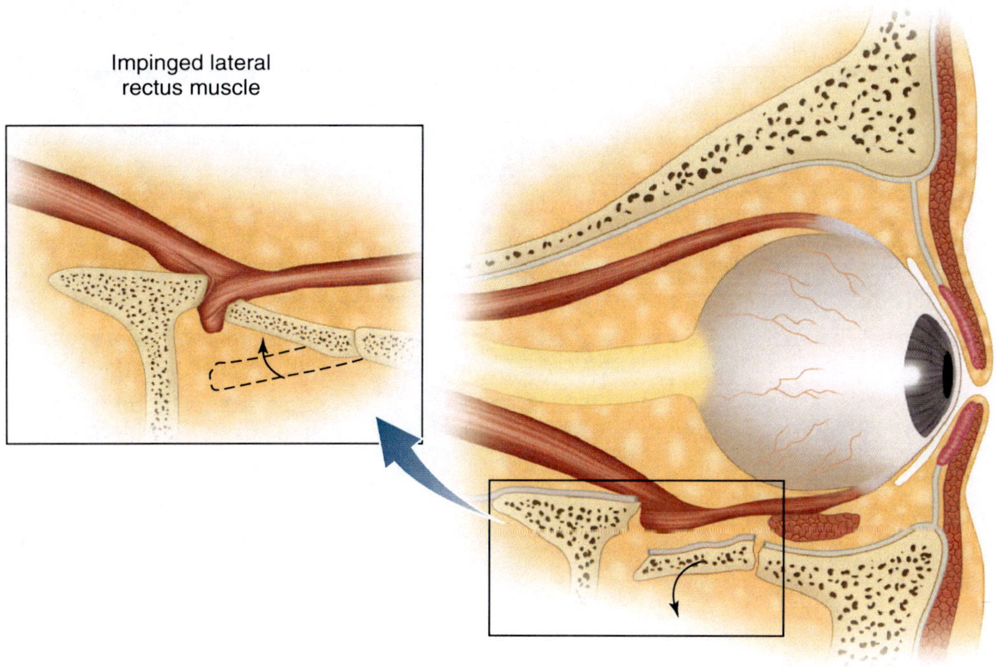

Fig. 17.9 Graphic representation of muscle entrapment with an orbital floor fracture

work-up to be done is in the best interest of the patient. Ideally, the fracture is repaired within a week of the injury.

Symptomatic Orbital Emphysema

Although a common finding with orbital floor and medial wall fractures, orbital emphysema rarely presents with clinical symptoms and usually requires no intervention. However, there are instances in which intraorbital air raises intraorbital pressure and leads to central retinal artery occlusion. Indications for needle aspiration of the air include rising intraocular pressure associated with visual deterioration, pain, and ocular motility impairment. In addition, the patient should be instructed to avoid nose blowing during the acute pressure increase.

Contraindications to Operative Repair

Observation alone is usually adequate for nondisplaced fractures without disturbance of eye motility. However, if the patient's condition prohibits operative intervention, observation may also be necessary in an acute setting. Severe ocular trauma including globe rupture, hyphema (hemorrhage into the anterior chamber), and retinal detachment may also necessitate a delay of bony orbital repair. Severe ocular injury is a contraindication to early surgical intervention because orbital manipulation increases the risk of secondary bleeding into the anterior chamber and the development of acute closed-angle glaucoma. For a globe injury, communication with the ophthalmologist is necessary to develop a consensus plan for the timing of repair. In addition, orbital fracture in a patient's only functional eye remains a relative contraindication to operative reduction and fixation since secondary deformities that result can be challenging to correct and may risk vision in the remnant functional eye.

Operative Intervention

Treatment Goals

Operative intervention is performed to treat symptoms associated with orbital fracture and restore facial appearance. For orbital rim reconstruction, fractured fragments are first aligned with regard to adjacent intact, stable structures. The goal of orbital reconstruction is to restore anatomy in all three dimensions. This begins by addressing the most reliable reference structures on the side with the least comminution. Multiple portions of the orbit are often fractured, and stabilization of both the rim and internal orbital walls must be achieved. The accuracy of the reduction is increased with simultaneous exposure of multiple fracture segments for alignment.

Surgical Techniques

Operative Exposure

Surgical access to the entire orbit is not possible through any single incision. Many incisional techniques have been described for access to the craniofacial skeleton for

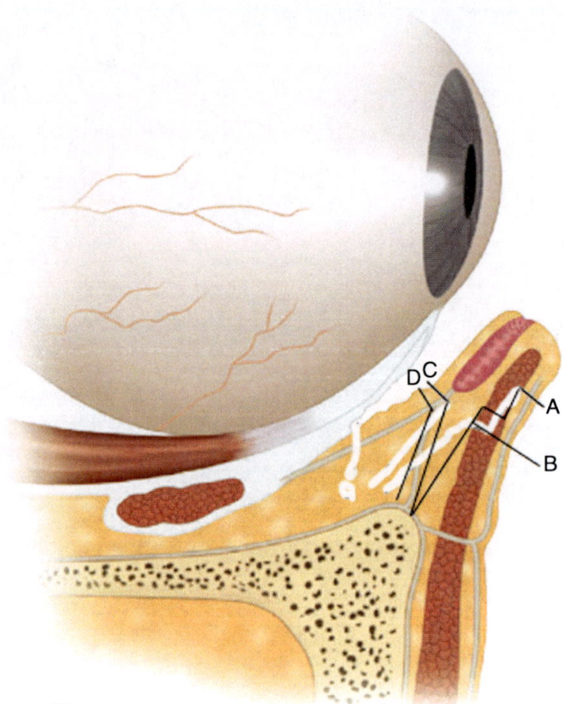

Fig. 17.10 Surgical approaches to the lower eyelid – subciliary (*A*), subtarsal (*B*), and transconjunctival (*C*)

traumatic fracture repair. Three basic approaches through the lower eyelid give access to the inferior, lower medial, and lateral aspects of the orbital cavity. The subciliary, subtarsal, and transconjunctival approaches (see Fig. 17.10) provide adequate orbital exposure for fracture fixation but are each associated with a distinct set of complications. The decision between transcutaneous and transconjunctival incisions reflects a balance between a need for adequate exposure and a desire for an aesthetically acceptable incision. A proper understanding of each technique requires an appreciation of the relevant anatomy and the risk of associated complications.

Subciliary Approach

The subciliary approach was first described for use in orbital trauma by Converse. Originally described as an incision several millimeters below the lash line, currently there are two main variations of this technique: the skin-only flap approach and the skin-muscle flap approach. The skin-only flap approach involves dissection just below the skin and superficial to the orbicularis oculi muscle to the level of the infraorbital rim. It has been associated with skin necrosis and a high rate of ectropion. The skin-muscle flap employs a stepped technique in which the skin flap is elevated for 4–5 mm before splitting the muscle along its fibers and continuing in the preseptal (submuscular) plane to the level of the orbital margin. This technique preserves the integrity of the pretarsal orbicularis oculi musculature which is critical to lower eyelid support and therefore is associated with decreased risk of scar inversion and lower incidence of ectropion.

Subtarsal Approach

The subtarsal approach, popularized in the 1960s, offers direct access to the infraorbital rim with minimal risk of retraction. The appropriate subtarsal wrinkle is infiltrated with local anesthetic, and incision is then made along a natural crease parallel to the ciliary margin at a level just below the tarsal plate. Dissection is carried through the orbicularis oculi in the direction of its muscle fibers, and the orbital septum is exposed down to the infraorbital rim in the preseptal plane. After the orbital rim is identified, an incision is made from the facial side of the rim through the periosteum and above the infraorbital nerve. Following osteosynthesis, the periosteum and skin are reapproximated. The benefits of the subtarsal approach include maintenance of pretarsal orbicularis oculi innervation integrity and thus decreased risk of scleral show and ectropion. It is a valid option for older patients with pronounced wrinkling and skin laxity.

Transconjunctival Approach

The transconjunctival approach was introduced in the early 1920s for use in lower eyelid blepharoplasty. Tessier reintroduced the technique and Converse applied it in the management of facial trauma. Over the past decade, the transconjunctival approach has gained popularity due to the hidden orbital incision and the associated decreased risk of ectropion. It allows for rapid access to the inferior orbital rim and floor, provides adequate exposure for fracture visualization, and eliminates external postoperative scars. A lateral canthotomy can be added for additional exposure, if necessary. The incision site is infiltrated with local anesthetic and followed by application of traction sutures through the lid margin (gray line) to aid in eversion. The incision is carried out at the conjunctival level approximately 5 mm below the level of the tarsus and directed lateral to medial. Dissection is performed sharply in the preseptal plane, between the orbicularis oculi and orbital septum. Blunt dissection with a cotton-tipped applicator is also a useful means to define this avascular plane. Dissection is continued to the infraorbital rim, where the arcus marginalis will be visualized. The periosteum is incised, and a leading edge is elevated and continued onto the floor. An elevator is placed into the defect using an upward sweeping motion to reduce the prolapsed periorbital fat and soft tissues. Regarding closure of operative wounds, minimal to no re-approximation of incised tissues is recommended since closure in traumatically disrupted soft tissue planes may lead to an increase in postoperative eyelid malposition, including entropion.

Superior Orbital Exposure

Exposure to the superior orbit can be achieved through the brow, lateral extension of the upper blepharoplasty incision, canthal detachment with lower eyelid incision, and coronal approaches. The incision is made in a supratarsal upper lid skin crease (at least 10 mm above the upper lid margin). If only the lateral aspect of the superior orbit requires exposure, the incision can be limited to extend from the midpupil level to the lateral orbital rim. A skin-orbicularis flap is then raised with care taken to avoid incising the underlying levator aponeurosis and orbital septum. The periosteum is then incised, and the fracture is exposed. For supraorbital rim fractures, one must be conscious of the supraorbital foramen/fissure to avoid injury to the supraorbital nerve.

Operative Timing and Sequence

Initially, swelling may limit the ability to perform meticulous exposure and to retract the orbital contents; therefore, in nonemergent cases a delay of 1–3 days may be beneficial. Most orbital fractures should be repaired within 2 weeks. Beyond this time, the thin orbital bones become brittle because of the initial osteoclastic response of normal healing. This can lead to further propagation of the fracture during exposure. In isolated orbital floor injuries, exposure is performed using one of the aforementioned techniques. Ideally, a stable shelf will be present surrounding the defect on which a reconstructive implant or graft can rest. Due to the normal inclination of the orbital floor, dissection for orbital floor implant placement should proceed in a superior direction, rather than directly posteriorly, to avoid placing implants into the maxillary sinus. The posterior shelf must be defined to support the implant or graft, but in injuries extending far posteriorly, the posterior ledge of the remnant floor may be difficult to identify. By placing a blunt freer elevator in the maxillary sinus and "walking" up the posterior wall of the sinus, the shelf may be more easily defined. When fractures of the orbital rims occur (such as in panfacial trauma or zygomaticomaxillary complex injury), the orbital exposure is often performed early to allow for more careful dissection of the delicate structures. However, fractures of the orbital walls or floor are generally the last fractures to be plated or repaired following restoration of the buttresses. For the orbital rims, a variety of titanium microplates and miniplates are available for fixation. Low-profile plates (1.0–1.3 mm) are recommended to prevent plate prominence and palpability. Plates should be fixed with at least two screws in each fracture fragment. In some cases, large fragments of the orbital floor or walls may remain stable after reduction. However, comminution frequently results in bone defects that must be reconstituted using some form of implant. The main material distinction is between a graft and an alloplastic implant. Among grafts, options include autogenous grafts, allografts, and xenografts; of these, autogenous grafts are most common and are taken from either the iliac crest or split calvarium. For large defects with involvement of the ethmoid and/or maxillary sinuses, many authors prefer autogenous grafts to reduce the risk of late infection. Depending on the size and location of the defect, alloplastic implants of various materials, sizes, and shapes are also available. There remains a lack of evidence to definitively support the ideal choice for an orbital implant. The options include nonresorbable or resorbable alloplastic materials and composites.

In general, orbital implants should be cut to the minimum size required, fixed with the minimum fixation points required, and contoured to fit the defect. In general, the implant should be fixed behind the internal orbital rim with a screw to prevent migration. The anterior-posterior position of globe should be evaluated after the implant is positioned to ensure correct placement. A narrow elevator can be placed beneath the implant after it has been secured to confirm that its posterior border lies above the posterior shelf. At the conclusion of any orbital reconstruction, a forced-duction test should be performed to ensure free mobility of the globe. Soft tissues are then reapproximated, depending on the type of exposure. Lid support is the final step of the procedure to avoid lid retraction (ectropion or entropion). Support of the lower eyelid can be achieved through lateral canthoplasty or canthopexy, and a variety of techniques may be used. We most frequently employ a lateral retinacular suspension in which the inferior limb of the lateral canthus is secured using an undyed 4–0 or 5–0 braided permanent suture to the inner aspect of the orbit at the level of Whitnall's tubercle. A frost suture is then place using a 5–0 silk along the gray line of the lid, securing it with adhesive and tape to the forehead. It is left in place for 3–5 days.

Postoperative Care

An assessment of gross vision should be performed after the patient has awakened from anesthesia. Postoperative care consists of elevating the head of the bed and using ice packs as needed to control edema. Nose blowing should be avoided for at least 10 days after orbital fracture repair to prevent orbital emphysema. Frost sutures remain in place 3–5 days, and the patient should be reassessed often to confirm that the sutures are in place and the cornea is adequately protected. Ophthalmic ointment may be used to ensure adequate lubrication, although conjunctival irritation with prolonged use has been reported. Some surgeons implement extraocular range of motion exercises postoperatively. Visual acuity should be carefully monitored in all orbital trauma patients, and a prompt CT scan should be performed if any deterioration is noted. Postoperative imaging should be repeated at the surgeon's discretion to evaluate implant position and the accuracy of the stabilization as well as to detect any neurologic or visual abnormalities. No clear data exist to suggest a benefit to perioperative antibiotics. Similarly, although preoperative administration of intravenous steroids has been suggested to decrease swelling and allow better assessment of postoperative globe position, their definitive role in the postoperative period has not yet been established. One suggested regimen recommends dexamethasone 20 mg intravenously on initial presentation, followed by 10 mg every 8 h for three doses total, after which steroids are discontinued. NSAIDs should be avoided in the first postoperative week. Nasal decongestants can be prescribed if symptoms warrant their use. Finally, for a minimum of 6 weeks after trauma, patients should avoid airline travel, scuba diving, and other environments that expose them to changes in air pressure to prevent air embolization.

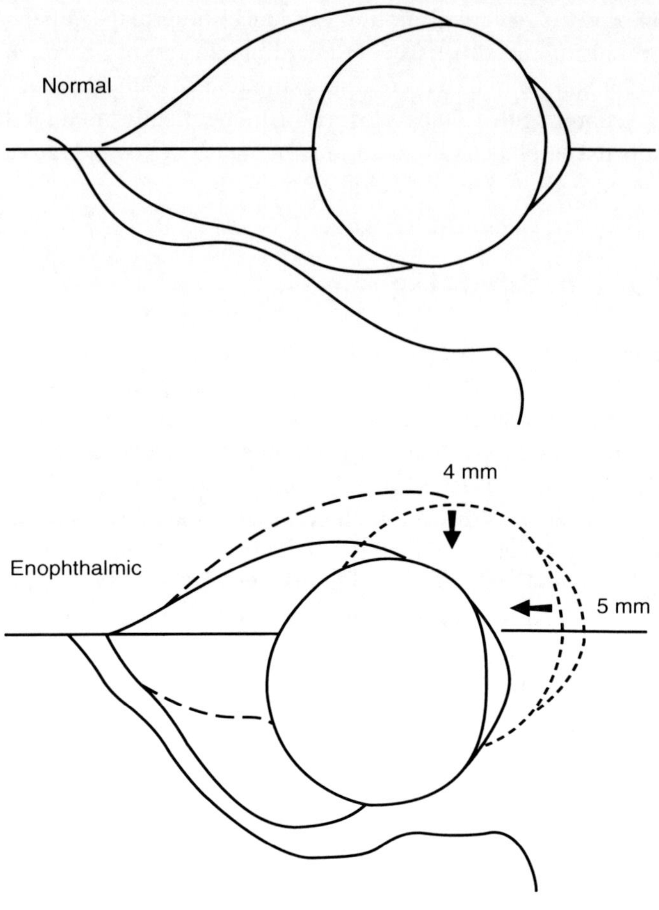

Fig. 17.11 Graphic representation of enophthalmos

Consequences of Injury and Complications

Orbital injuries themselves are associated with a number of possible problematic sequelae regardless of treatment.

Lower Eyelid Malposition

In addition to visual changes/loss, there are a number of known complications related to operative exposure and fixation. Lower lid malposition is a common complication after treatment of orbital fracture. Ectropion, or eversion of the eyelid margin away from the globe, is typically of a cicatricial, paralytic, and/or mechanical nature after orbital trauma, with an overall reported incidence of 5 %. It is seen more frequently with transcutaneous approaches to the orbital floor, notably with the subciliary incision. Cicatricial ectropion results from vertical shortening of the anterior lamella from the lid being tethered to the orbital rim. Postoperative placement of a frost suture can hinder its development. Management ranges from conservative measures, such as corneal lubrication, taping, and massage, to surgical scar release for symptomatic problems that persist without gradual improvement.

Persistent Diplopia

Persistent diplopia following surgical repair may result from persistent or recurrent soft tissue incarceration or implant adhesions. Forced-duction testing should be performed to rule out a mechanical cause, and if test results are normal, conservative management and close follow-up should be performed for up to 6 months, because diplopia resulting from neurapraxia is common. However, diplopia that persists beyond this 6-month observation period warrants surgical re-exploration.

Persistent Enophthalmos

Persistent enophthalmos is caused by increased orbital volume, which can be secondary to inadequate surgical restoration of orbital volume, extraocular muscle contracture and fibrosis, fat atrophy, and ligamentous injury (see Fig. 17.11). The interval between injury and surgical repair is a risk factor for the development of late enophthalmos, since delay in repair beyond the 2-week window has been associated with a greater than threefold increase in the incidence of late enophthalmos. The use of alloplastic implant materials is also associated with a unique set of complications: implant malposition, infection, and extrusion can occur late and may mandate implant removal.

Other Complications

Less common complications and their reported incidences include lower lid edema (1–4 %), hypertrophic scars (1–2 %), entropion (1 %), lower lid retraction, and scleral show.

Recommended Follow-Up

Close follow-up is recommended for fractures treated surgically as well as those treated nonoperatively. Before the patient is discharged, gross vision is assessed. Within 1 week, the patient should be seen for reevaluation and removal of the frost suture. Any early evidence of lower lid retraction is aggressively treated with massage. Tape may be applied to the lateral aspect of the lower lid and retracted superolaterally to support the lower lid to the temple. Clinical signs of visual acuity deterioration or mental status changes at any point should be investigated. Patients should be seen 3 or 4 weeks after the injury or repair to examine vision, lid position, and globe position. Follow-up imaging is performed at the discretion of the treating surgeon. In isolated orbital injuries, a final follow-up visit may be conducted 6–8 weeks after the injury or repair if no specific concerns continue.

Bibliography

AO Foundation. Midface. Available at www.aofoundation.org-midface.

Bourguet J. Notre traitement chirurgical de “poches” sous les yeux sans cicatrice. Arch Gr Belg Chir. 1928;31:133.

Chen YA, Singhai D, Chen YR, Chen CT. Management of acute traumatic retrobulbar haematomas: a 10-year retrospective review. J Plast Reconstr Aesthet Surg. 2012;65(10):1325–30.

Cole P, Boyd V, Banerji S, et al. Comprehensive management of orbital fractures. Plast Reconstr Surg. 2007;120(7 Suppl 2):57s–63s.

Converse JM, Smith B. Blowout fracture of the floor of the orbit. Trans Am Acad Ophthalmol Otolaryngol. 1960;64:676–88.

David LR, Sanger C. Eyelid reconstruction and ptosis repair. In: Serletti JM, Taub PJ, Wu LC, et al., editors. Current reconstructive surgery. New York: McGraw Hill Medical; 2013. p. 355–68.

Elahi E, Spinelli H. Eyelid and orbital surgery. In: Guyuron B, Eriksson E, Persing J, editors. Plastic surgery indication and practice. Edinburgh: Sauders/Elsevier; 2009. p. 851–67.

Emery JM, Noorden GK, Sclernitzauer DA. Orbital floor fractures: long-term follow-up of cases with and without surgical repair. Trans Am Acad Ophthalmol Otolaryngol. 1971;75:802–12.

Fosnot J, Serletti J. Orbital fractures and deformities. In: Serletti JM, Taub PJ, Wu LC, et al., editors. Current reconstructive surgery. New York: McGraw Hill Medical; 2013. p. 233–44.

Frenkel RE, Spoor TC. Diagnosis and management of traumatic optic neuropathies. Adv Ophthalmic Plast Reconstr Surg. 1987;6:71–90.

Gosau M, Schoneich M, Draenert FG, et al. Retrospective analysis of orbital floor fractures-complications, outcome, and review of the literature. Clin Oral Investig. 2010;15:305–13.

Hammer B. Diagnosis and classification. In: Hammer B, editor. Orbital fractures. Seattle: Hogrefe & Huber; 1995. p. 7–17.

Hollier LH, Thornton IF. Facial fractures. Sel Read Plast Surg. 2005;10:1–68.

Manolidis S, Weeks BH, Kirby M, et al. Classification and surgical management of orbital fractures: experience with 111 orbital reconstructions. J Craniofac Surg. 2002;13:726–37; discussion 738.

Raschke GF, Rieger UM, Bader RD, et al. Transconjunctival versus subciliary approach for orbital fracture repair-an anthropometric evaluation of 221 cases. Clin Oral Investig. 2013;17:933–42.

Raskin EM, Millman AL, Llubkin V, et al. Prediction of late enophthalmos by volumetric analysis of orbital fractures. Ophthal Plast Reconstr Surg. 1998;14:19–26.

Steinsapir KD. Treatment of traumatic optic neuropathy with high-dose corticosteroid. J Neuroophthalmol. 2006;26(1):65–7.

Tahernia A, Erdmann D, Follmar K, et al. Clinical implications of orbital volume change in the management of isolated and zygomaticomaxillary complex-associated orbital floor injuries. Plast Reconstr Surg. 2009;123:968–75.

Wang BH, Rrobertson BC, Girotto JA, et al. Traumatic optic neuropathy: a review of 61 patients. Plast Reconstr Surg. 2001;107:1655–64.

18 Nasoorbitoethmoid (NOE) Fractures

Karl C. Bruckman, Thaddeus S. Boucree II, Jose I. Garri, and S. Anthony Wolfe

Introduction

Nasoorbitoethmoid (NOE) fractures comprise a relatively uncommon subset of facial injuries. Although the incidence of NOE fractures varies amongst authors, the occurrence is approximately 5 % in adults. These patients often suffer a significant high-velocity, direct blow to the upper midface. Concomitant injuries to the remainder of the craniofacial skeleton are not uncommon, and a thorough evaluation of such must be carried out. Significant physiologic and cosmetic morbidity can occur with NOE fractures, and delay in their repair can further exacerbate them. Thus, decisions to manage these injuries operatively must be swift and decisive. Multiple surgical approaches exist for the management of NOE fractures, and the choice for such is made on a case-by-case basis.

Anatomy and Pathophysiology

The NOE complex is formed by numerous bony structures in the upper and middle facial third. These articulations are important components of the facial buttresses (see Fig. 18.1). Included in this system are the vertical (nasomaxillary, pterygomaxillary, zygomaticomaxillary) and horizontal (frontal, orbital, maxillary, mandibular, zygomatic) buttresses. These bony structures act as the main supporting framework of the facial skeleton, protecting vital structures in collaboration with the sinus system's force-absorbing function.

Anatomically, the NOE complex can be further subdivided into the nasal unit (nasal bone, paired nasal cartilages, cartilaginous septum), orbital unit (frontal process of maxilla, lacrimal bone, lamina papyracea), and ethmoid unit (orbital plate, ethmoid air cells, crista galli, cribriform plate) (see Fig. 18.2). The bones of the NOE complex are thin and

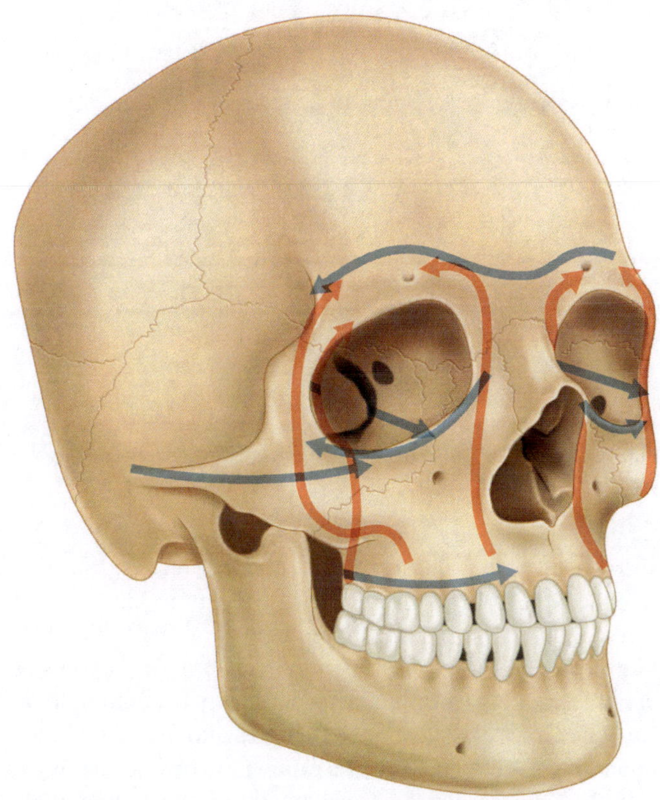

Fig. 18.1 Vertical (*red*) and horizontal (*blue*) buttresses (Courtesy of AO Foundation)

K.C. Bruckman, MD, DDS (✉)
Department of Oral and Maxillofacial Surgery, Thomas Jefferson University Hospital, Philadelphia, PA, USA
e-mail: drgarri@drgarri.com

T.S. Boucree II, MD, DDS
Department of Oral and Maxillofacial Surgery, Larkin Community Hospital, Miami, FL, USA

J.I. Garri, MD, DMD
Department of Plastic Surgery, University of Miami, Miami, FL, USA

S.A. Wolfe, MD
Department of Plastic and Reconstructive Surgery, Miami Children's Hospital, Miami, FL, USA

P.J. Taub et al. (eds.), *Ferraro's Fundamentals of Maxillofacial Surgery*, DOI 10.1007/978-1-4614-8341-0_18,

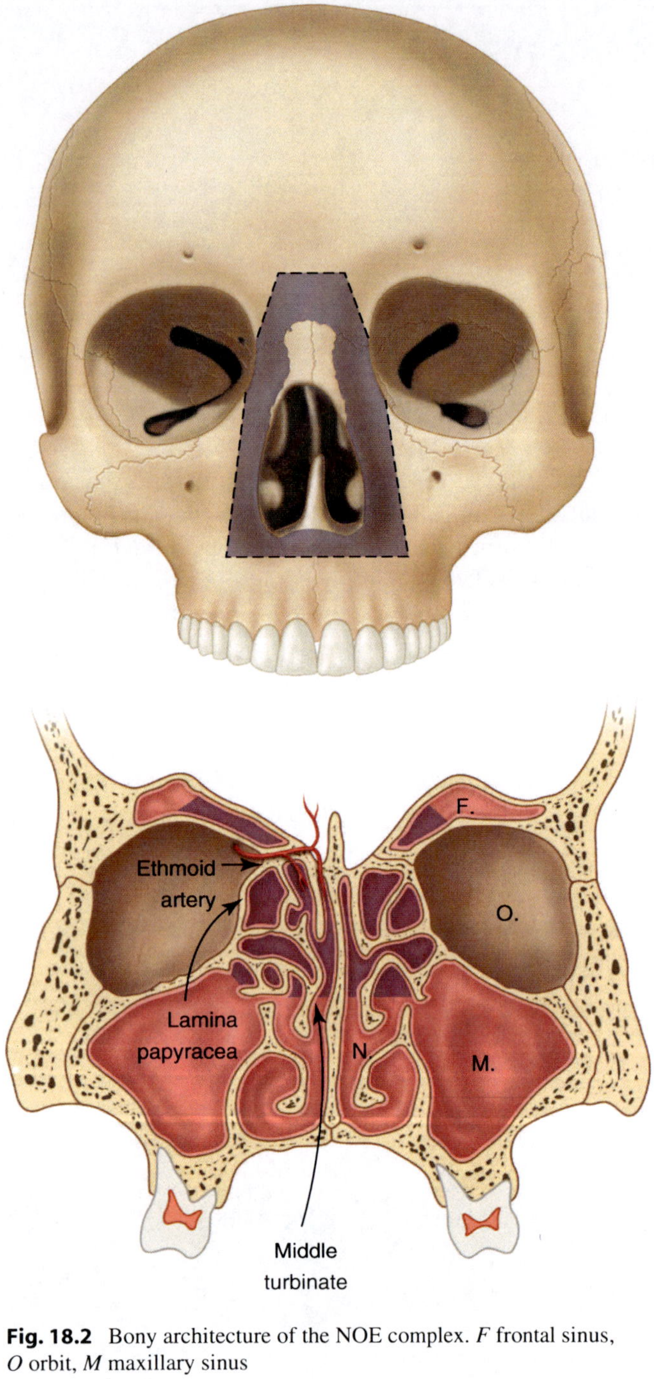

Fig. 18.2 Bony architecture of the NOE complex. *F* frontal sinus, *O* orbit, *M* maxillary sinus

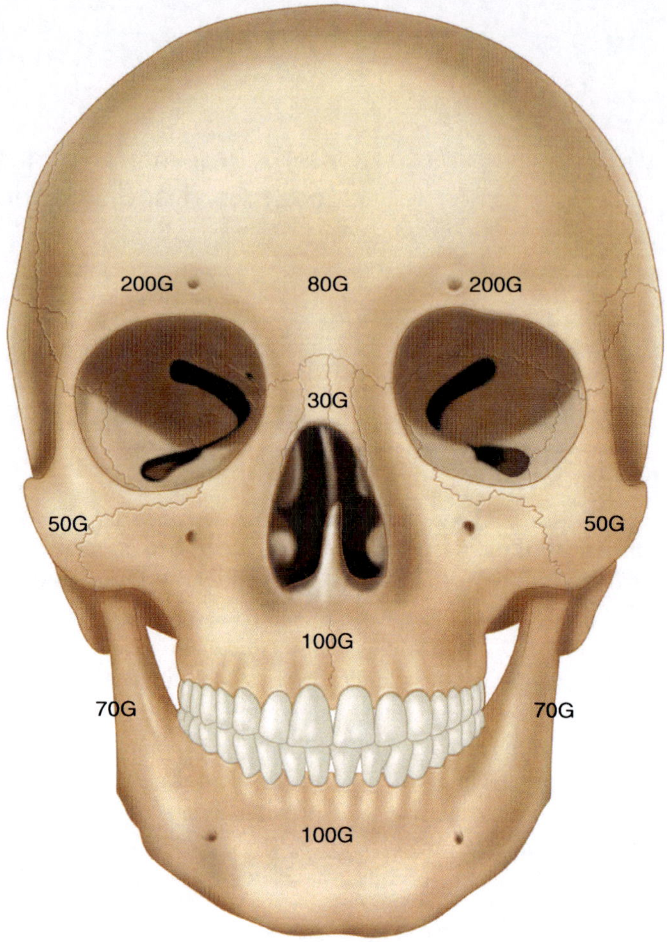

Fig. 18.3 Gravitational forces required to fracture facial bones

surrounded by air sinuses. Thus, the force required to fracture the NOE complex, approximately 30 g (g = gravitational force), is much less than that required for other facial fractures (see Fig. 18.3). The fracture pattern that ensues is variable, ranging from simple displacement to comminution. In 1985, Gruss classified NOE fractures into five types based upon the degree of bony disruption involving the NOE complex and associated facial bones. A more commonly used classification system, perhaps due to its treatment implications, is that of Markowitz and Manson, who further classified these fractures relative to the degree of bony comminution and status of the medial canthal tendon (MCT).

From anterior to posterior, the MCT is situated between the orbicularis oculi and conjunctiva at the medial portion of the orbit. The MCT is a fibrous confluence of the tarsal plates that attaches in three bands (anterior, posterior, and superior). Also situated between the anterior and posterior bands of the MCT is the lacrimal sac. Since the MCT assists in supporting the upper and lower lids, as well as assisting in drainage of the lacrimal system, its disruption can be quite detrimental. Markowitz and Manson explained this traumatic interruption of the MCT and degree of NOE comminution as follows: Type I fractures include one bony segment that contains the attachment of the MCT to the lacrimal crest, Type II involves comminution of the central segment of bone with continued attachment of the MCT to the lacrimal crest, and Type III has bony comminution with dissociation of the MCT and lacrimal crest (see Fig. 18.4). The pattern of NOE fracture is variable, whereas the majority of bilateral fractures are Type II, and nearly an even percentage of unilateral fractures are Types I and II (see Table 18.1).

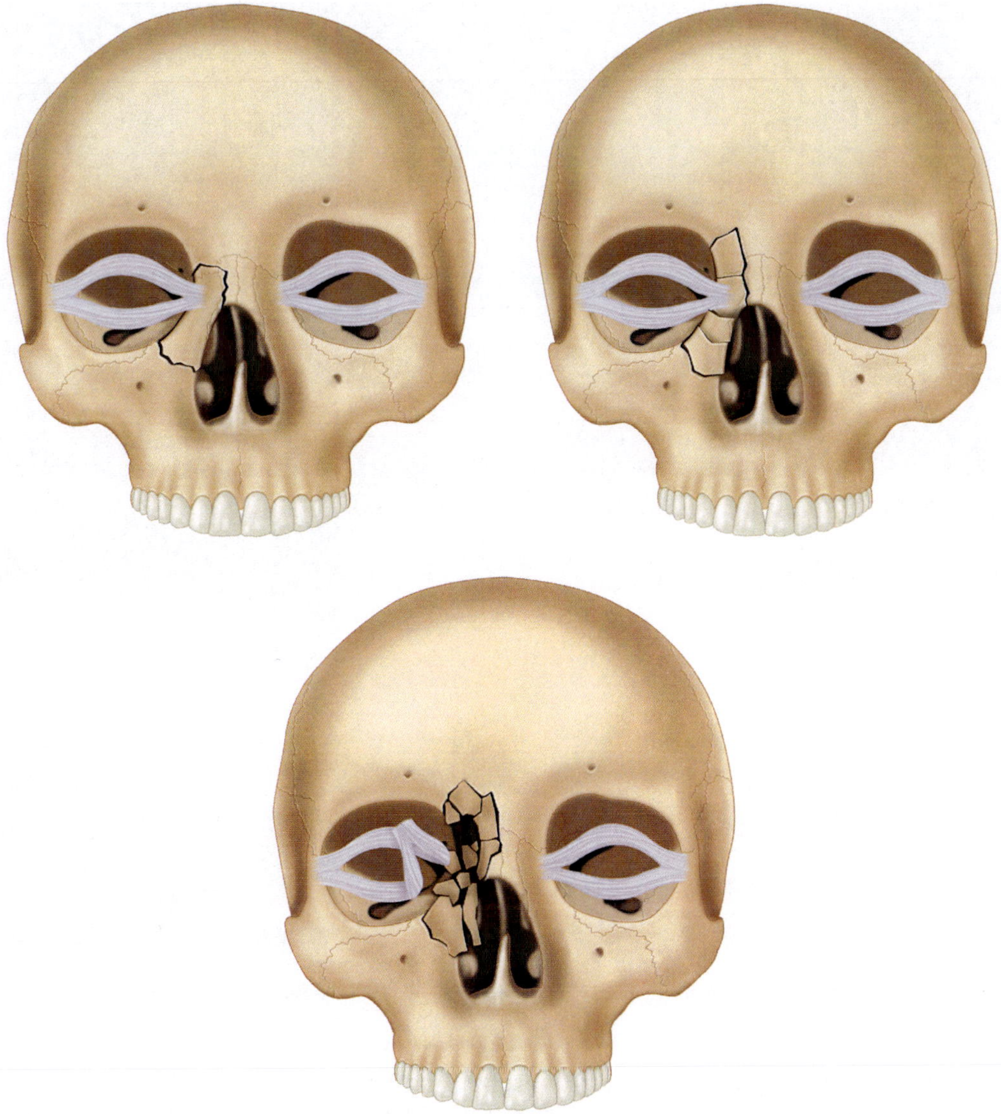

Fig. 18.4 Markowitz and Manson classification of NOE fractures. Type I fracture (*top left*), Type II fracture (*bottom*), Type III fracture (*top right*)

Table 18.1 Percentage of NOE fracture patterns relative to laterality

Fracture pattern	Description	Unilateral (%)	Bilateral (%)
Type I	Single segment	50	13
Type II	Comminuted, MCT attached	44	85
Type III	Comminuted, MCT detached	6	2

Markowitz BL, PN Manson, Sargent L, et al. Management of the medial canthal tendon in nasoethmoid orbital fractures: the importance of the central fragment in classification and treatment. Plast Reconstr Surg. 1991;87(5):843–53

Clinical Presentation

Injuries to the NOE complex are often secondary to motor vehicle accidents or assaults. Therefore, care must be taken to follow a regimented protocol in their initial evaluation to rule out any associated systemic or craniofacial damage. A thorough top-down evaluation of the craniofacial complex should be undertaken once the patient has been stabilized via the primary ATLS survey. Beginning with the cranial vault, close inspection for lacerations and ecchymosis should be followed by palpation for step deformity that would indicate bony fracture. Regions of ecchymosis at the posterior auricular/mastoid region (known as Battle's sign) can be indicative of a skull base fracture. Continuing inferiorly from the hairline, visualize the entire facial skeleton for gross asymmetry. NOE fractures often have significant periorbital edema and ecchymosis (see Fig. 18.5). One may also appreciate telecanthus, which is defined as widening of the medial canthi. It is important to note that widening of the interpupillary distance is hypertelorism—usually a congenital craniofacial condition—which can also be seen in trauma cases, although the two are not mutually exclusive. Anthropometric studies have shown that the normal values for intercanthal

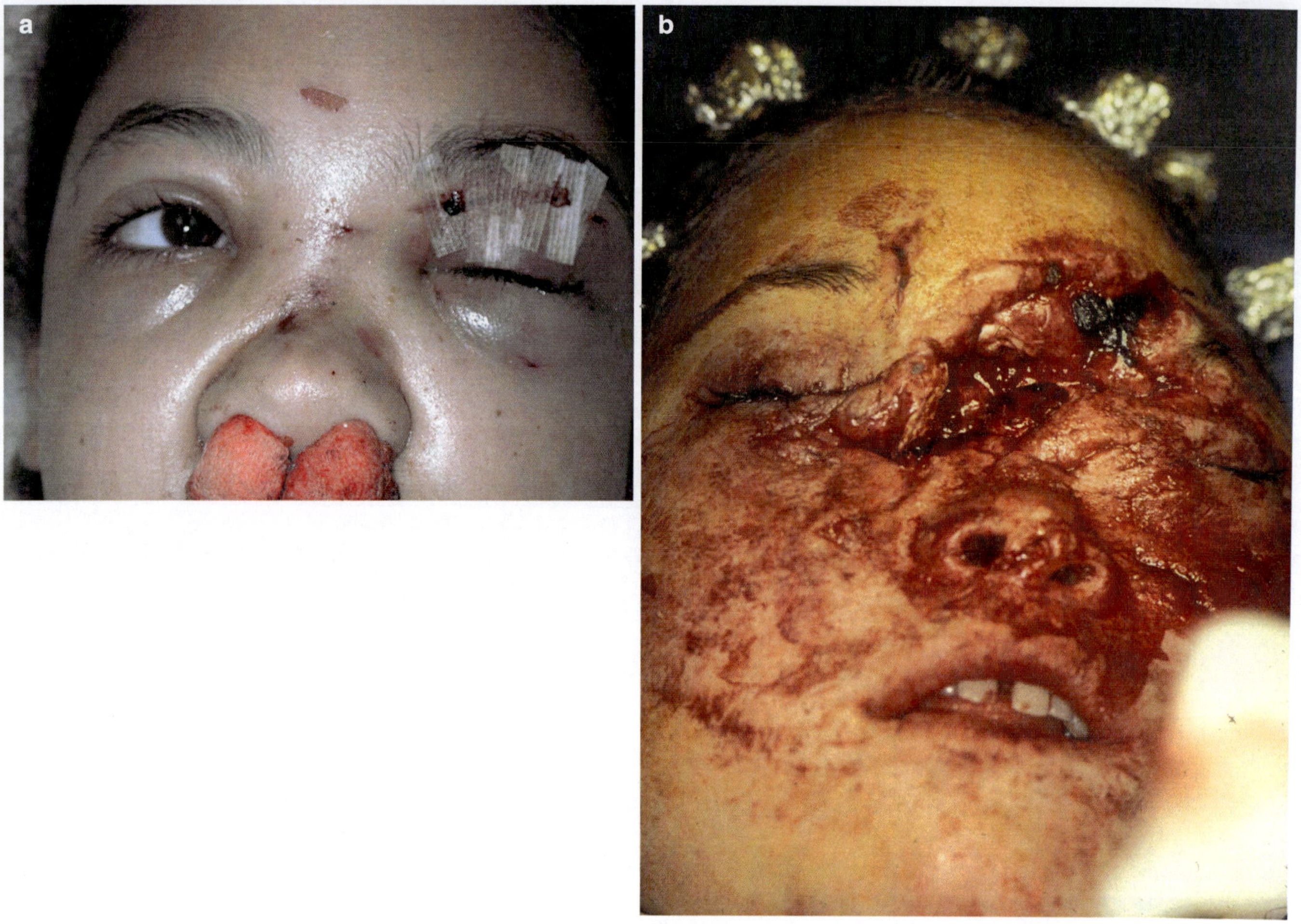

Fig. 18.5 Telecanthus, periorbital and nasal edema, and nasal bone depression associated with NOE fractures [Case #1 (*left*) and Case #2 (*right*)]

distance vary amongst ethnic groups and gender, although little data comparing such exist in the literature. Studies have shown the mean intercanthal distance for Caucasians and mixed populations to be 32 ± 3 mm, whereas the mean for African Americans is 33.9 ± 3 mm. Further bedside examination maneuvers may include the bowstring test. To perform this, on one side of the face, place the index finger over the medial canthal region. While maintaining light pressure over this area, take the other hand and gently retract the outer eyelid in a lateral direction. The ability to feel mobility of the bony structures in the medial canthal region with this maneuver indicates a positive bowstring test, thus a high probability of NOE disruption. Direct digital palpation of the nasal dorsum causing depression and crepitation of the nose can also be indicative of a NOE fracture (see Fig. 18.6). Depression of the nasal dorsum is due to the loss of support from the septal cartilage and associated bony structures. In combination with significant nasal edema, one can also expect to appreciate blunting of the canthal angle. Epiphora can be seen in the acute setting when there is disruption of the nasolacrimal system, although it is not a highly sensitive clinical finding.

Continued evaluation of the midfacial architecture may reveal step deformity about the orbital rims, consistent with fracture. If suspected, careful evaluation of the globe for injury should be undertaken, including gross examination for rupture. Ruling out cranial nerve injury (extraocular movements, visual acuity, pupillary light response) and retrobulbar hematoma (orbital pressures) is important. Consultation with ophthalmology for a formal examination and clearance is highly recommended for all fractures involving the orbit. Careful speculum examination of the nasal cavity should then be performed. Septal hematoma can occur with these injuries, and it should be evacuated as soon as possible to avoid avascular necrosis of the associated cartilage. It is also important to be wary of clear rhinorrhea, a finding significant for cerebrospinal fluid (CSF) leakage. Due to epistaxis, it is often difficult to discern CSF from blood. Thus, sampling the nasal discharge and sending it to the laboratory to identify the presence of beta-2 transferrin is warranted in cases where basilar skull fracture is suspected due to clinical or radiographic findings. This glycoprotein is highly specific for CSF, and its presence in nasal fluid

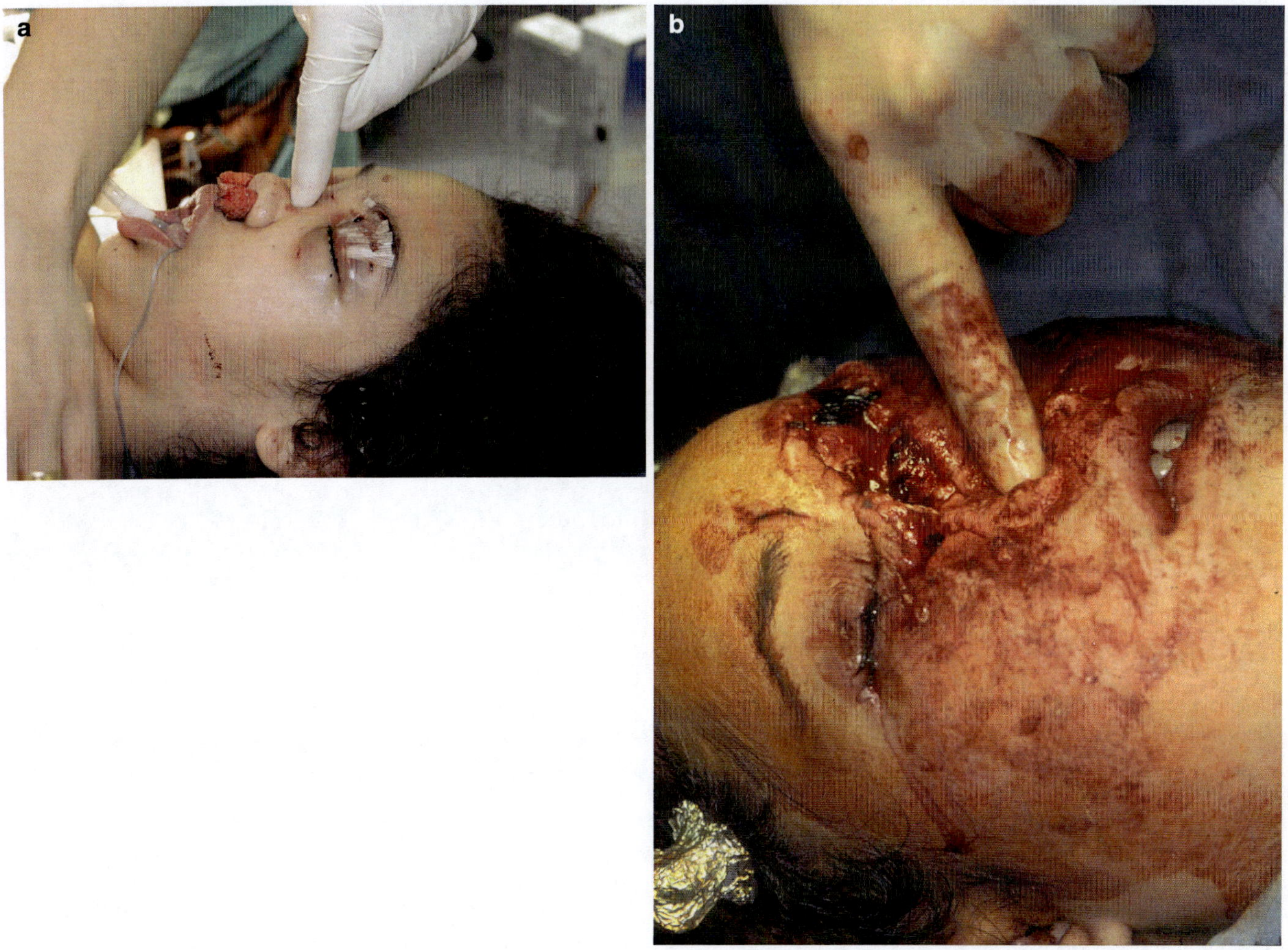

Fig. 18.6 Palpation of nasal dorsum demonstrating lack of nasal support with NOE fracture [Case #1 (*left*) and Case #2 (*right*)]

should prompt consultation with neurosurgery for close monitoring and possible patching of the leak. Further evaluation of the midface, mandible, and neck should be carried out. These examinations are outside the scope of this section.

After completing the physical examination, radiographic imaging should be ordered. Computed tomography (CT) scan of the craniofacial region should include small cuts (1 mm) for close inspection of the NOE complex. These scans should be non-contrast and include axial, coronal, and sagittal sections at minimum. If available, three-dimensional reconstruction of the CT scan is an additional radiographic tool that can show the fracture pattern and degree of bony deformity. When viewing axial sections, attention should be given to displacement of the medial orbital walls, nasal bone, anterior and posterior tables of the frontal sinus, and ethmoid sinus (See Fig. 18.7). With coronal and sagittal views, one can again appreciate the medial orbital walls and ethmoid sinus, as well as damage to the inferior orbital rims, nasal septum, nasofrontal ducts, and cribriform plate/anterior skull base.

Operative Technique

The goals of surgically repairing NOE fractures revolve around the restoration of premorbid form and function. It is important to first note whether or not the NOE fracture is an isolated injury or one of many fractures. In instances with multiple facial fractures, two common, general approaches to repair include reconstruction from the "top-down" or "bottom-up." When approaching the facial fractures from the "top-down," the surgeon should begin with reduction of the calvarium, followed by the orbital rims/NOE complex, zygoma, maxilla (at LeFort I/II/III levels), and mandible. If choosing to repair from the "bottom-up," it is wise to begin with intermaxillary fixation (IMF) and use of the patient's dental occlusion as a guide. This can be accomplished with placement of Erich arch bars, Ivy loops, or IMF screws, followed by maxillomandibular wire fixation. Plating of fractures would then continue in a manner opposite to that of the "top-down" approach. Whichever approach is chosen, it is vital to reestablish the vertical and horizontal buttresses of the facial skeleton.

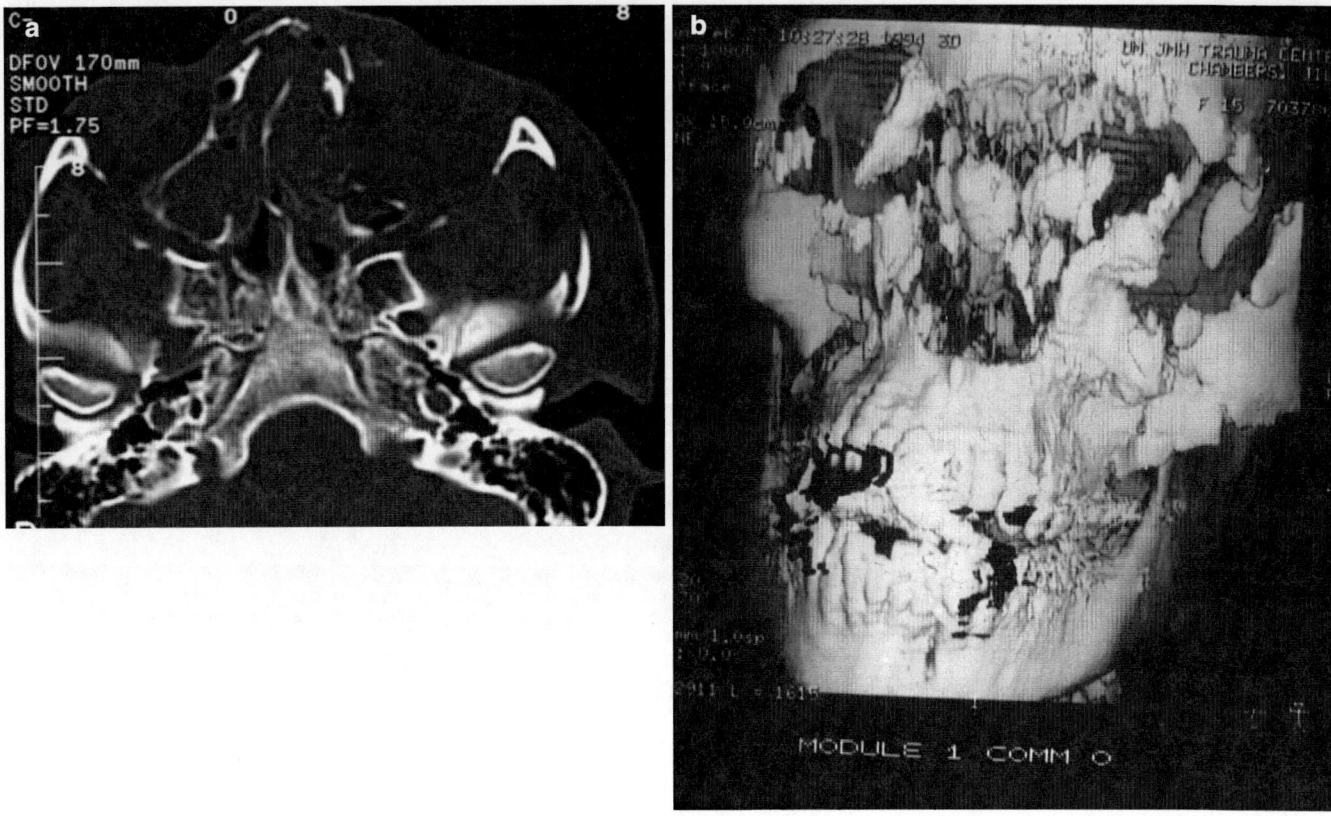

Fig. 18.7 Axial CT section and 3D CT reconstruction demonstrating NOE fractures [Case #1 (*left*) and Case #2 (*right*)]

It is also important to be mindful of the "ideal" facial dimensions. As such, attempts at restoring the appropriate horizontal thirds and vertical fifths of the face are necessary (see Fig. 18.8). The horizontal thirds can be identified when viewing the patient from the side/sagittal view. The upper third should begin at the hairline and end at the glabella, while the middle third would be measured from the glabella to the subnasale region. Finally, the lower third begins superiorly at the subnasale and ends at the pogonion. It is important to note that the lower third is further divided into an upper 1/3 (subnasale to stomion superioris) and lower 2/3 (stomion inferioris to pogonion). When viewing a patient from the frontal/coronal view, the vertical fifths can be appreciated as the width of each eye, the nasal width, and the region lateral to each eye all being equal. One must bear in mind that these ideals are just that, and this may not achievable in each patient. Many ratios also exist for other facial landmarks (including nasal proportions and tip projection, and facial line angles), and they can be referenced separately.

The management of significant NOE fractures has followed a general outline that was described early in the literature. This process involves wide exposure to explore all fractured bony segments and determine the true degree of displacement, thus allowing for adequate reduction and appropriate fixation. If necessary, primary bone grafting can also be accomplished, and the MCT can be resuspended. Finally, the soft tissue envelope is then closed over its reconstructed bony support.

Exposure

Referring again to the Markowitz and Manson classification of NOE fractures, the decision to repair surgically should be based upon the degree of damage to the bony architecture. Many surgical approaches exist for the repair of NOE fractures, and the appropriate choice is dependent on each individual patient, bearing in mind the necessity of wide exposure. If existing lacerations are present, they can be used as found or extended for a broader view of the fractures. Another commonly used approach is the coronal flap. This flap allows bone segment exposure as far inferiorly as the zygomatic arches and nasomaxillary articulation. An additional benefit of the coronal approach is that one can access calvarial bone for use in nasal cantilever grafting. Supplementary exposure of the infraorbital and medial orbital rim region can be accomplished via a transconjunctival or subciliary/subtarsal approach. If the maxillary component of the NOE is significant, a transoral

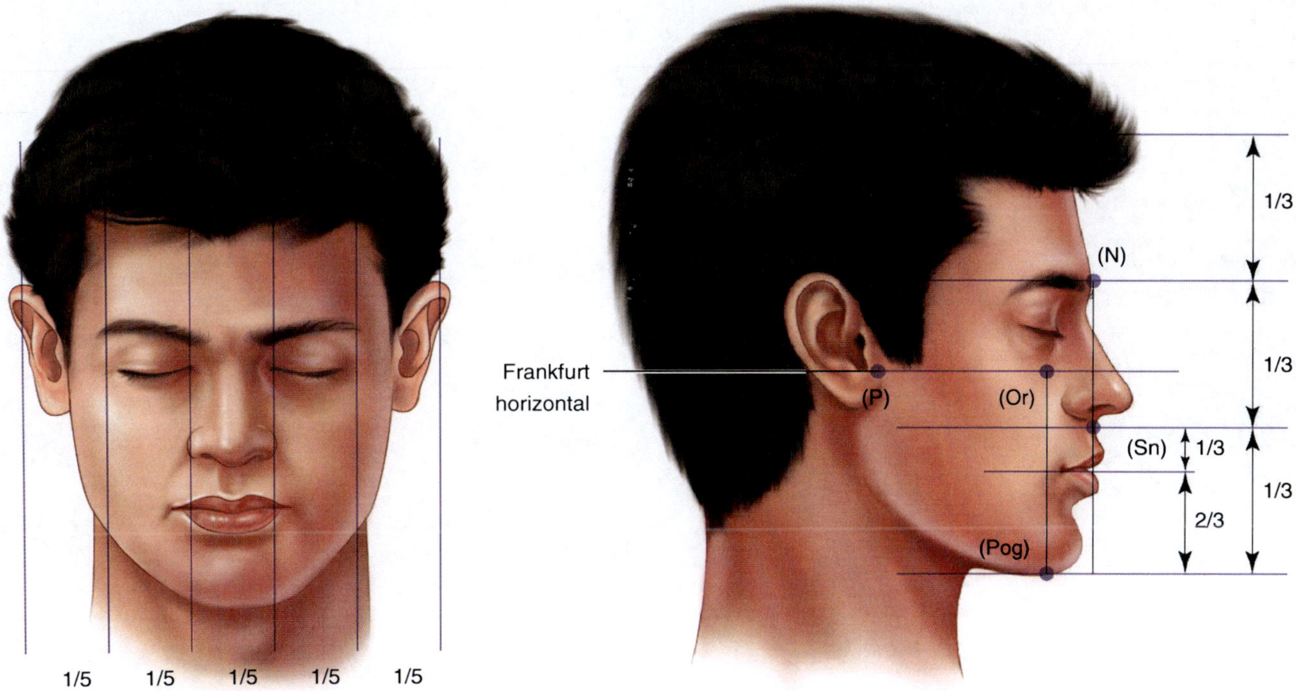

Fig. 18.8 Vertical fifths and horizontal thirds in the operative planning for repair of facial fractures (Courtesy of AO Foundation)

vestibular approach can be made. This will allow visualization of the entire maxillary wall bilaterally, as well as the zygoma. In most NOE fractures, an intraoral approach is not necessary. Care should always be taken to hide any incisions within resting tension lines of the face. Other surgical approaches do exist, although they are not as cosmetically favorable.

Fracture Reduction

After adequate exposure of the fracture segments has been accomplished, any repair to the nasolacrimal apparatus can be performed at this time. Stenting of the lacrimal duct will restore its patency and allow healing to occur. Reduction of fractures with plate fixation can now begin. The first areas of fixation should begin by plating from visibly stable bone to mobile segments. Reestablishment of the buttresses can be carried out in the manner. With reduction of orbital rim components, exploration of the orbital floor should be carried out to determine if any defects are present. If necessary, the orbital floor defect can be repaired with bone grafting (calvarial bone can easily be harvested through coronal approach) or implants (titanium mesh, synthetic material, etc.). With Type I NOE fractures, reduction of the main segment will reestablish the proper anatomic position of the MCT. With Type III fractures, though, the MCT is detached from the lacrimal crest, and it must resuspended via medial canthopexy.

Fracture Fixation

Based on the AO principles of fracture fixation, many different plates can be used for NOE fractures. At present time, titanium plates based upon the following screw diameters can be used: 1.0, 1.3, 1.5, and 2.0 mm. It is best to use low-profile plates in regions of thinner soft tissue (i.e., periorbital structures) to achieve a better cosmetic result. Thicker plates should be used in fixation of the vertical and horizontal buttresses, as more force is distributed to these regions. For example, plating of the inferior orbital walls could be accomplished with a 1.0 mm plate, whereas fixation of the medial orbital wall would be better suited with a larger plate, such as 1.5 mm. Using Crumley's method, nasal projection can be estimated to form a "3-4-5 triangle." Thus, the ratio of nasal proportions is measured as follows: "3" ala to nasal tip, "4" ala to nasion, and "5" nasion to nasal tip. In certain instances, inadequate nasal dorsum support is present after reduction and fixation of NOE fractures. To correct this discrepancy, a cantilever calvarial bone graft can be used. Bone can be harvested from the calvarium (often a the parietal region) via the previous coronal approach. A corticocancellous block can be harvested and used as an onlay graft. If further projection is needed, the two of these blocks can be stacked together and secured with 1 mm screws (see Fig. 18.9). This construct can then be fixated to the nasal dorsum with a 1.5 mm Y-plate to the intact nasal process of the frontal

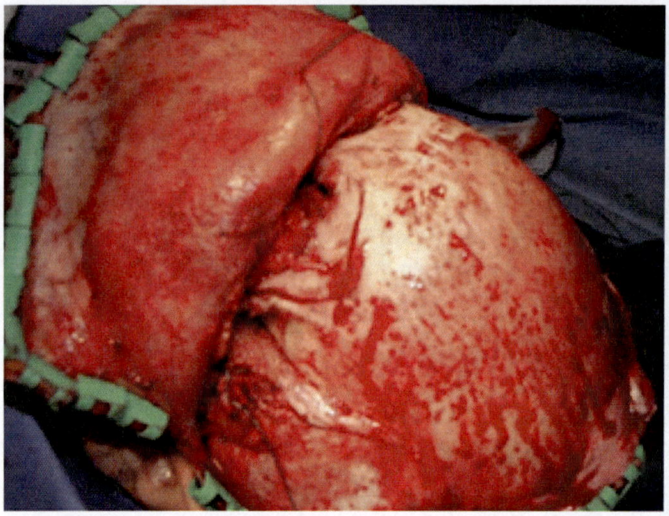

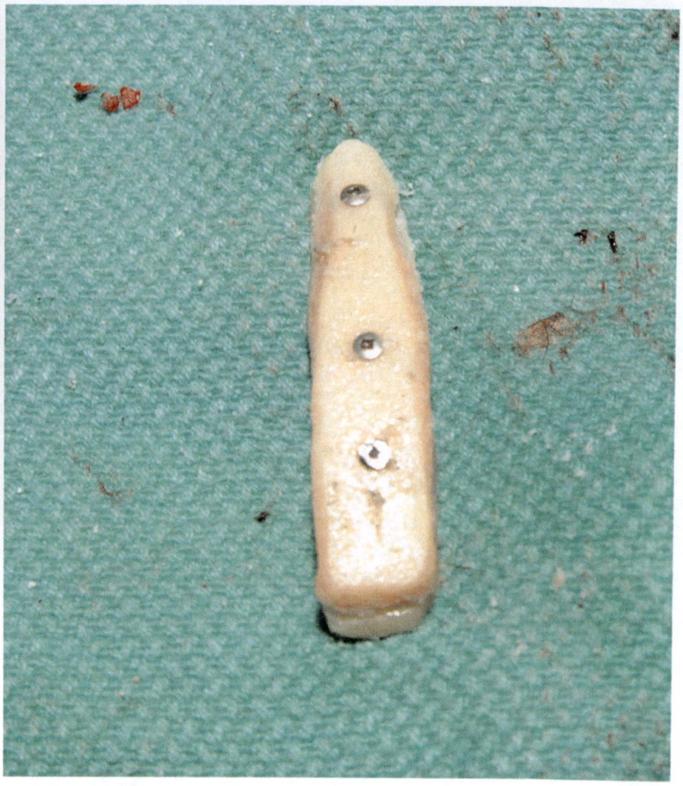

Fig. 18.9 Coronal approach (*left*) to expose fracture and harvest calvarial graft (*right*) (Case #3)

bone (see Fig. 18.10). Cosmetic improvement to the projection and contour of the nose can be noted with this technique (see Fig. 18.11).

Soft Tissue Management

After appropriate reduction and fixation of fractures, the MCT and soft tissue drape can then be addressed. With avulsion of the MCT from the lacrimal crest, it is necessary to perform a medial canthopexy. Once the light-colored tendon fibers of the detached MCT are identified, a figure-of-8 suture is placed through it using a 4-0 suture wire (with a needle). After cutting the needle off, both free ends of the wire suture are passed using either an awl or a spinal needle transnasally. While protecting the globes, the wires are passed in a superior and posterior direction into the opposite orbit in order to "suspend" and fixate the MCT in its proper anatomic position. In order to avoid "chessewiring" through the thin, medial orbital wall, it is best to tie the wires around a one- or two-hole 1 mm bone plate (see Fig. 18.12). It is also important to slightly overcorrect the position of the MCT in order to prevent telecanthus from developing as a late complication.

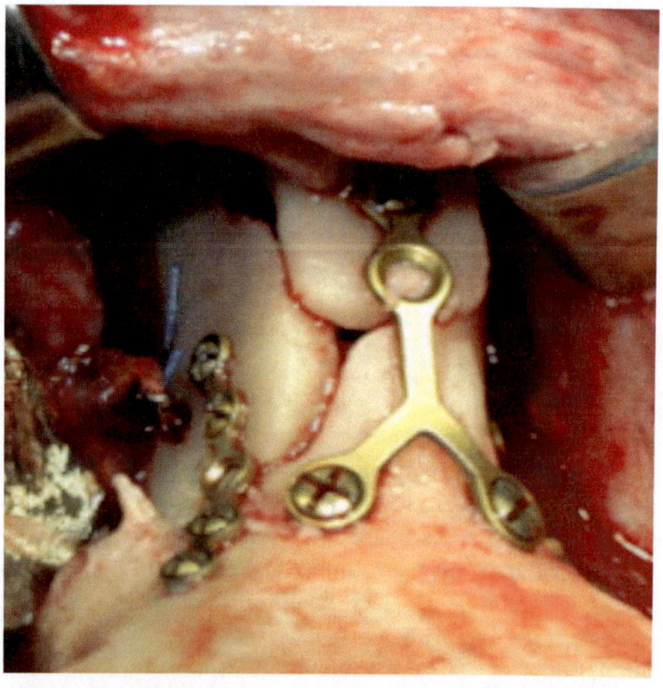

Fig. 18.10 Onlay calvarial bone graft for reconstruction of nasal dorsum with NOE fractures

Due to the increased edema and disruption of bony support, consideration should be given to placement of an external bolster dressing over the nasal dorsum and medial canthal regions. This bolster will help reduce edema and define the epicanthal folds (see Fig. 18.13). Without placement of a

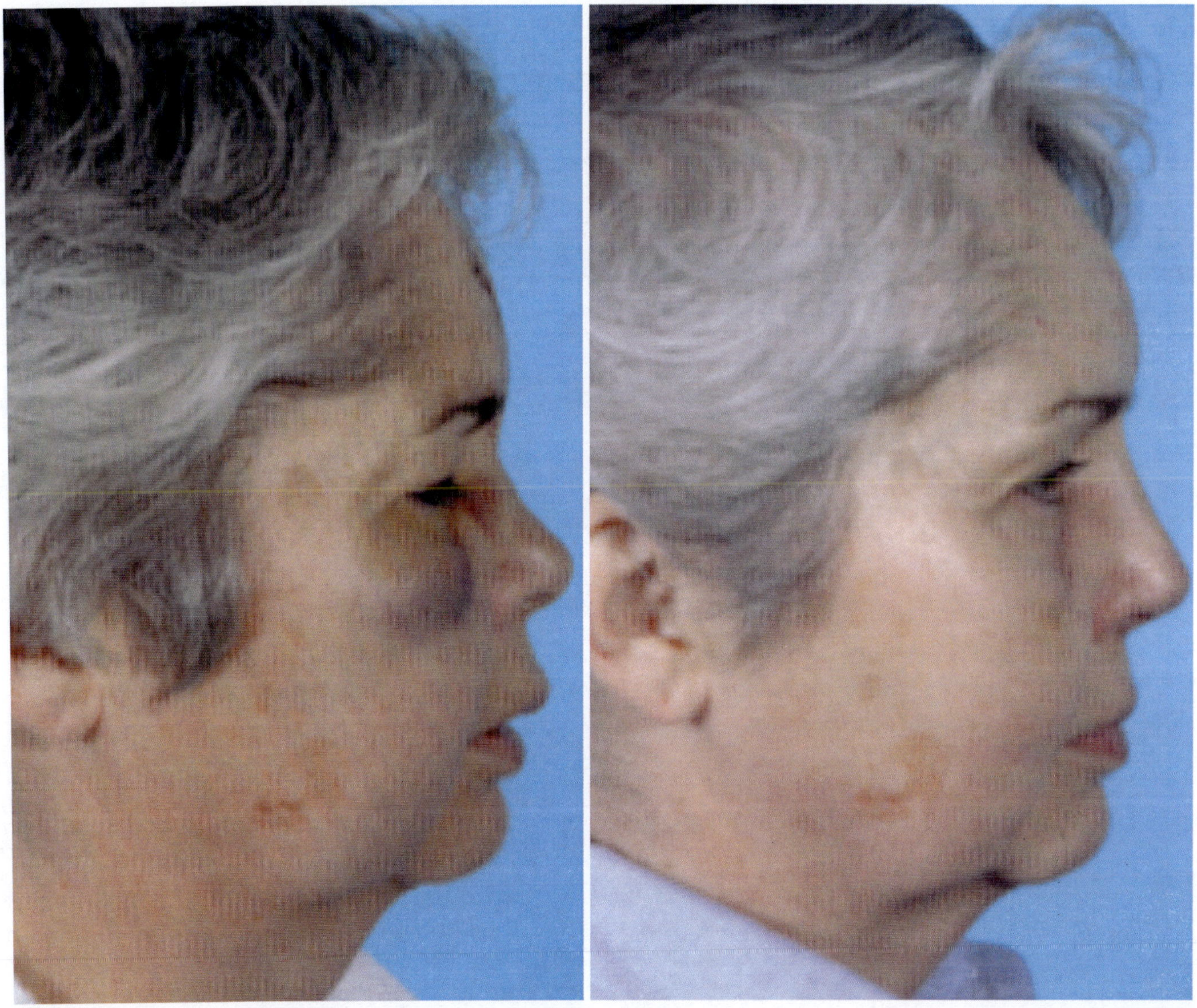

Fig. 18.11 Preoperative (*left*) photograph of patient with loss of dorsal support after NOE fracture and postoperative (*right*) photograph after only calvarial bone graft (Case #3)

bolster, soft tissue tenting can occur and cause a significant cosmetic deformity. The bolster utilizes transnasal sutures and can be fabricated with padded strips of lead (as shown) or with rolled Xeroform gauze. The construct should be rigid enough to cause close adherence of the soft tissue of the medial canthal area and lateral nasal sidewalls to the underlying bony structures. The bolster should remain in place for 7–10 days.

Postoperative Course/Complications

The immediate postoperative course should involve close attention to the patient's ophthalmological exam, with any abnormalities being brought to the attention of the ophthalmologist (see Fig. 18.14). Sinus precautions should also be in place. These include no nose blowing, nasal decongestants and antihistamines, and antibiotics. The patient's head of bed should also be maintained in an elevated position of at least 30°. All wounds should be kept moist and skin sutures removed at an appropriate interval. Late complications include epiphora (uncorrected lacrimal duct repair), telecanthus and pseudotelecanthus (inappropriate resuspension of MCT or nasion repair, respectively), enophthalmos or diplopia (inadequate reduction of orbital fractures), persistent CSF leak and anosmia (unrepaired cribriform plate fracture), and chronic sinusitis. Secondary repair of bony support and soft tissue for cosmetic reasons can be accomplished, although it can be difficult to achieve the same premorbid appearance.

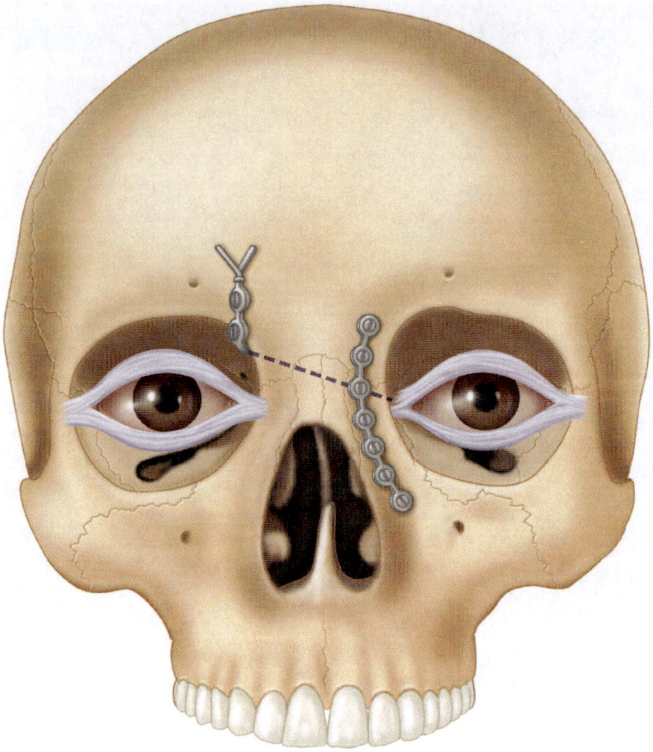

Fig. 18.12 Transnasal canthopexy for resuspension of the medial canthal tendon

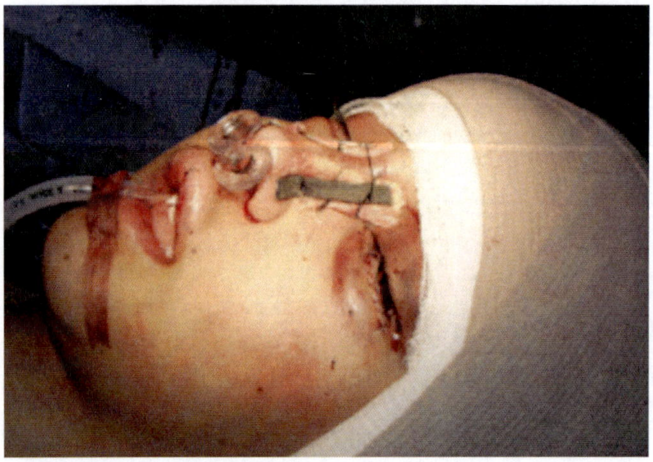

Fig. 18.13 Bolster dressing to maintain soft tissue architecture after NOE repair (Case #1)

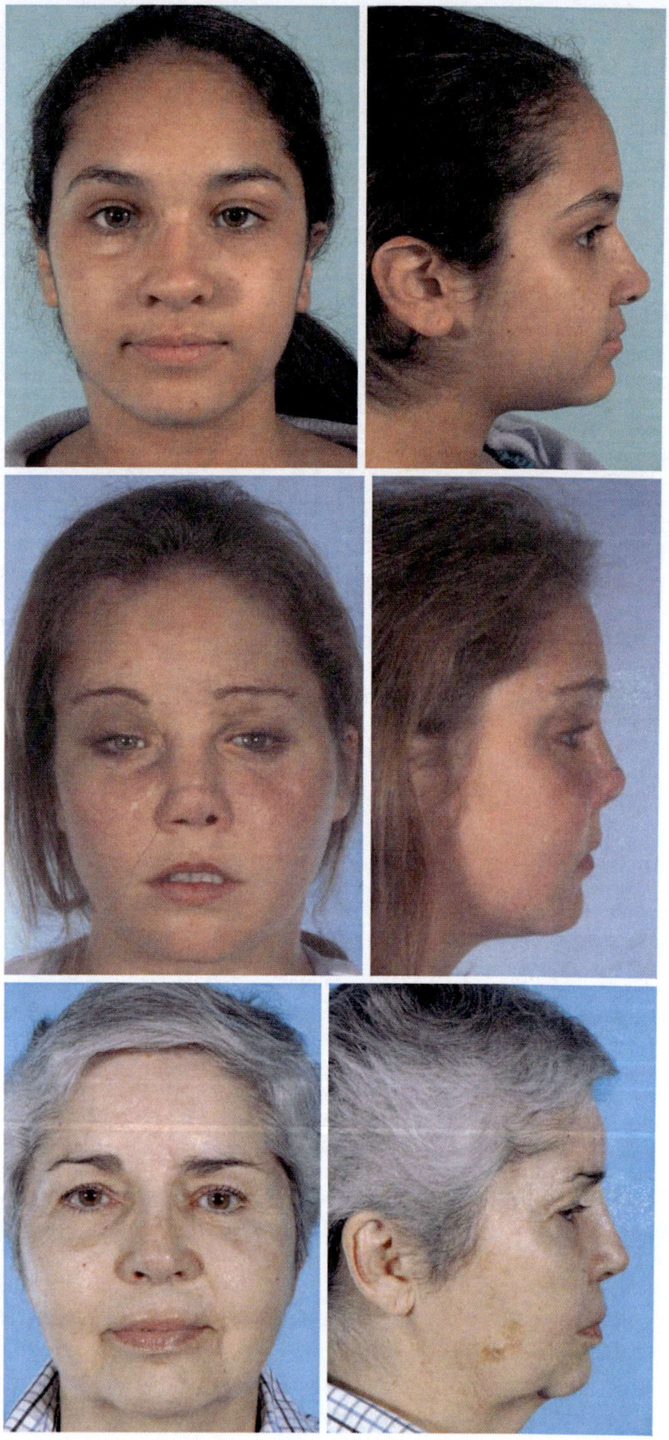

Fig. 18.14 Postoperative follow-up [Case #1 (*top*), Case #2 (*middle*), and Case #3 (*bottom*)]

Bibliography

Bartlett S, Ehrenfeld M, Mast G, et al. AO surgery reference: orthognathic. www.aosurgery.org. July 2012.

Cornelius CP, Gellrich N, Hillerup S, et al. AO surgery reference: CMF – midface. www.aosurgery.org. Dec 2009.

Crumley RL, Lanser M. Quantitative analysis of nasal tip projection. Laryngoscope. 1988;98(2):202–8.

David DJ, Moore MH. Cantilever nasal bone grafting with miniscrew fixation. Plast Reconstr Surg. 1989;83(4):728–32.

Gruss JS. Fronto-naso-orbital trauma. Clin Plast Surg. 1982;9(4):577–89.

Gruss JS. Naso-ethmoid-orbital fractures: classification and role of primary bone grafting. Plast Reconstr Surg. 1985;75(3):303–17.

Gruss JS. Complex nasoethmoid-orbital and midfacial fractures: role of craniofacial surgical techniques and immediate bone grafting. Ann Plast Surg. 1986;17(5):377–90.

Hollier LH, Thornton J. Facial fractures I: upper two thirds. Selected Read Plast Surg. 2002;9(26):1–35.

Leipziger LS, Manson PN. Nasoethmoid orbital fractures: current concepts and management principles. Clin Plast Surg. 1992;19(1): 167–93.

Luce EA, Tubb TD, Moore AM. Review of 1,000 major facial fractures and associated injuries. Plast Reconstr Surg. 1979;63(1): 26–30.

Manson PN, Hoopes JE, Su CT. Structural pillars of the facial skeleton: an approach to management of Le Fort fractures. Plast Reconstr Surg. 1980;66(1):54–62.

Markowitz BL, Manson PN, Sargent L, et al. Management of the medial canthal tendon in nasoethmoid orbital fractures: the importance of the central fragment in classification and treatment. Plast Reconstr Surg. 1991;87(5):843–53.

Murphy WK, Laskin DM. Intercanthal and interpupillary distance in the black population. Oral Surg Oral Med Oral Pathol. 1990;69(6):676–80.

Nguyen M, Koshy JC, Hollier LH. Pearls of nasoorbitoethmoid trauma management. Semin Plast Surg. 2010;24(4):383–8.

Frontal Sinus Fractures

19

Adam J. Oppenheimer, Kristoffer B. Sugg, and Steven R. Buchman

Overview

Treatment of the frontal sinus and its associated pathology is a controversial and highly debated topic in craniomaxillofacial trauma. A lack of consensus exists in the current literature regarding the preferred management of frontal sinus fractures, with contradictory and radically different approaches often made based solely on anecdotal evidence. Most clinical recommendations are derived from single-center retrospective case series with small sample sizes and selection bias. Indeed, there are striking differences between regional and international institutions pertaining to indications for treatment, timing of repair, types of operations performed, use of autogenous versus alloplastic materials, guidelines for prophylactic antibiotics, and appropriate length of follow-up. This chapter attempts to collate the available evidence into a clear and concise format in order to provide clarity to an otherwise confusing domain of fracture management. Our goal is to present a simple treatment strategy that has proven to be safe and reliable in the management of frontal sinus fractures.

A.J. Oppenheimer, MD
Department of Craniofacial Surgery,
Seattle Children's Hospital, Seattle, WA, USA

K.B. Sugg, MD
Division of Plastic and Reconstructive Surgery,
University of Michigan Medical School,
Ann Arbor, MI 48109-4215, USA

S.R. Buchman, MD (✉)
Craniofacial Anomalies Program,
Division of Plastic and Reconstructive Surgery,
University of Michigan Medical School,
1540 E. Medical Drive, 4-730,
Ann Arbor, MI 48109-4215, USA
e-mail: sbuchman@umich.edu

Anatomy and Physiology

The frontal sinus is located within the frontal bone deep to the supraciliary ridge. It is relatively small with an average volume of 5 cm^3 and is considered a tripartite structure consisting of a resilient anterior wall, an intervening air-filled cavity, and a weaker posterior wall (see Fig. 19.1). The average height of the frontal sinus is 24.3 mm (range 5–66 mm), and its average length is 29 mm (range 17–49 mm). The anterior wall (range 2–12 mm) is substantially thicker than the posterior wall (range 0.1–4 mm) with an average thickness of 4 mm. Each sinus cavity is typically described as an inverted pyramid sitting on its point with characteristic scalloping along its borders: easily visualized on plain radiographs due to multiple incomplete septations arising from the sinus walls. The boundaries of the sinus floor include the orbital roof laterally and the cribriform plate medially separated for a short distance by the fovea ethmoidalis. The intersinus septum is an extension of the

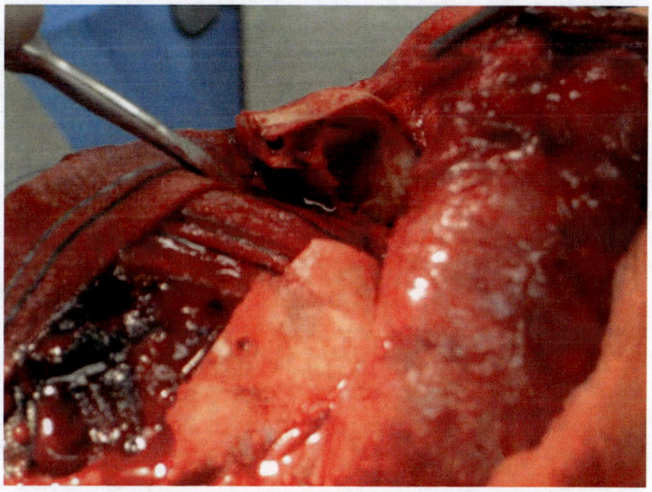

Fig. 19.1 Sagittal view of the frontal sinus intraoperatively. The anterior table is thicker in comparison to the posterior table. The posterior table has been fractured and is in discontinuity (Photograph courtesy of Dr. Joseph S. Gruss)

P.J. Taub et al. (eds.), *Ferraro's Fundamentals of Maxillofacial Surgery*,
DOI 10.1007/978-1-4614-8341-0_19, © Springer Science+Business Media New York 2015

crista galli and contributes to the asymmetric configuration of the sinus cavities by deviating left or right as it courses toward the sinus walls.

The frontonasal ductal system provides the only pathway for drainage from the frontal sinus into the nasal cavity, underscoring its importance in the management of frontal sinus fractures. The hourglass-shaped frontonasal duct has an average diameter of 3–4 mm and consists of three parts: a wide frontal infundibulum that drains into a short, narrow ostium before expanding into the ethmoid infundibulum (see Fig. 19.2). It is located in the posteromedial segment of the sinus floor and travels for up to 2 cm caudally prior to emptying into the middle meatus. Similar to the developmental variability of the sinus cavities, the frontonasal duct is highly inconsistent in its course and may be absent. In these situations, the frontal sinus will drain secondarily into the anterior ethmoid sinus. The frontonasal duct typically opens into the ethmoid infundibulum within the superior portion of the hiatus semilunaris along the lateral nasal wall, which is bound by the uncinate process of the ethmoid bone anteriorly, the bulla ethmoidalis posteriorly, the middle turbinate medially, and the lamina papyracea laterally. In approximately two-thirds of patients, drainage occurs predominantly posterior to the uncinate process.

The mucosa of the frontal sinus consists of a pseudostratified ciliated columnar epithelium interspersed with goblet cells. The goblet cells are responsible for the majority of the mucus production and are primarily located within the caudal portion of each sinus cavity. Mucus production in the frontal sinus is elegantly recycled by flowing in a circular pattern from lateral to medial along the sinus floor. A small bony lip in the frontonasal duct partially blocks the outflow of mucus with only 40 % of all secretions reaching the nasal cavity. Similar to the respiratory tract, synchronized beating of the cilia is crucial to keep the mucus moving in the same direction and to prevent stasis and inspissation of the sinus contents, which is a common source of infection. Finally, the foramina of Breschet are worth recognition due to their

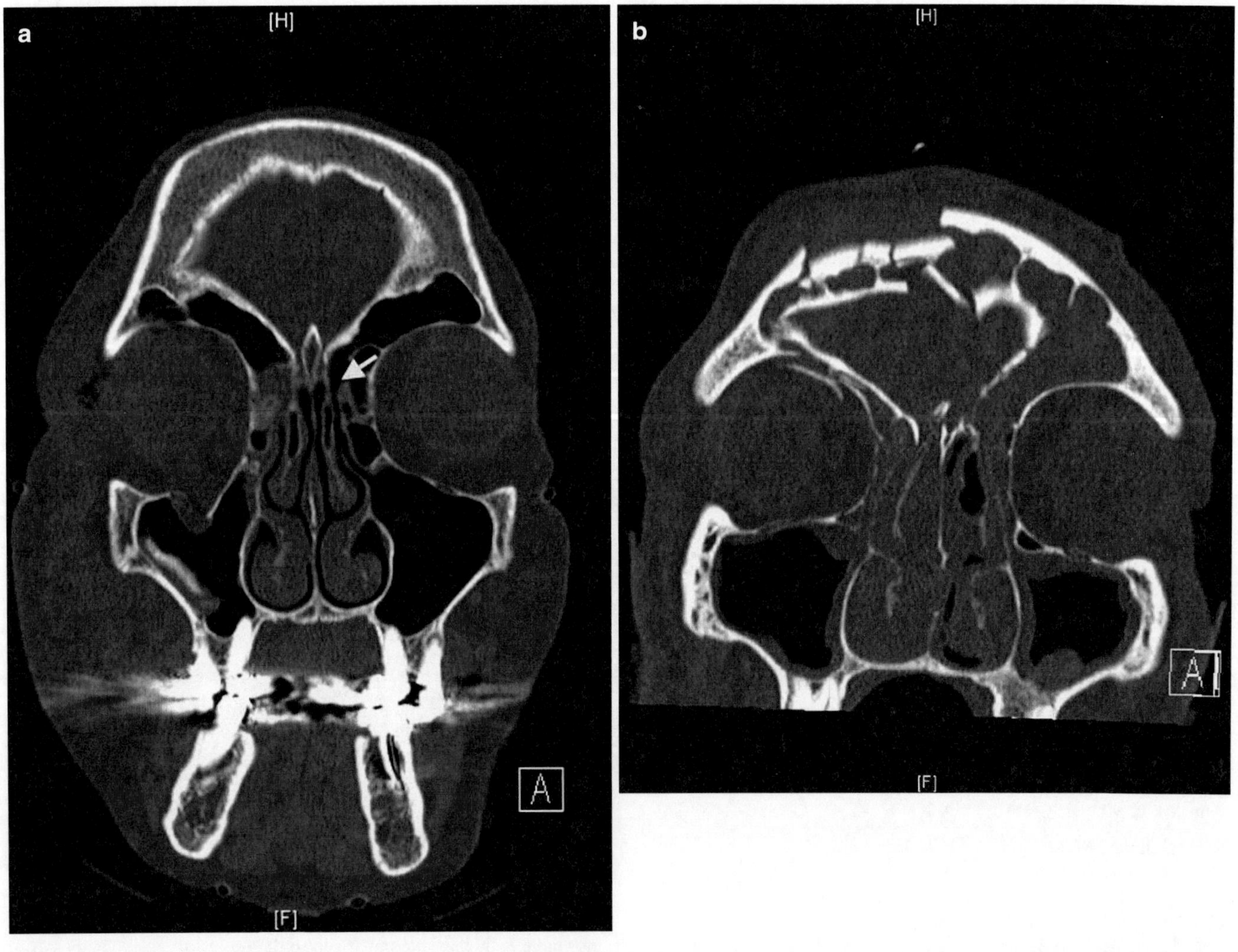

Fig. 19.2 The frontonasal duct. (**a**) Coronal computed tomographic image of patent left frontonasal duct with "hourglass" appearance (*solid arrow*): a wide frontal infundibulum drains into a short, narrow ostium before expanding into the ethmoid infundibulum. Note incidental contralateral orbital floor fracture. (**b**) Coronal computed tomographic image (different patient) with complete bilateral frontonasal duct obstruction in the context of bilateral frontal sinus fractures

clinical significance in mucocele formation. These pseudodiverticulae are located along the posterior wall and contain small evaginations of mucosa whose venules drain directly into the dural veins, serving as potential routes of intracranial dissemination of infection.

The anterior wall contributes to facial contour as it blends caudally with the nasoorbitoethmoid region. Due to similar mesodermal origins, the posterior wall is intimately juxtaposed with the dural lining of the anterior cranial fossa. This dense attachment is loose rostrally but thins out caudally and becomes more adherent as the dura reflects over the fovea ethmoidalis. Unlike the other paranasal sinuses, the frontal sinus firmly approximates numerous intracranial structures including the dura mater, olfactory bulbs, and the frontal lobes. Damage to the frontal bone is readily transmitted to these structures, and their dysfunction in the setting of violent trauma should be expected.

The frontal sinus receives its blood supply from the internal carotid system, namely, the supraorbital, supratrochlear, and anterior ethmoidal arteries. Lymphatic drainage is to the submandibular nodal basin. The ophthalmic division of the trigeminal nerve provides sensory innervation. Venous drainage occurs either intracranially or extracranially, along three independent routes: (1) the angular vein to the facial vein, (2) the ophthalmic vein to the cavernous sinus, or (3) the foramina of Breschet to the dural veins. This complex drainage system explains the risk of infectious complication following frontal sinus fractures, even without disruption of the posterior wall.

The primary function of the frontal bone is to protect the brain. Accordingly, its thick anterior wall makes it the most resistant facial bone to injury; it is capable of withstanding a tolerance band of 800–1,600 lb of peak force under experimental conditions. This equates clinically to a head-on motor vehicle collision in which an unrestrained passenger strikes the windshield traveling approximately 30 miles per hour. For comparison, the mandible is the second strongest bone of the craniofacial skeleton with a tolerance band of 550–900 lb of force, almost half that of the frontal bone. Aside from shielding the brain from injury, many other functions of the frontal sinus have been described, most of which are speculative. These proposed functions include immunological defense through the production of immunoglobulins and nitric oxide, maturation of vocal resonance, warming and filtration of inspired air, olfactory enhancement, assistance with facial growth and development, thermal insulation, reduction in the weight of the cranium for maintenance of equipoise, or its use as a flotation device.

Epidemiology

Frontal sinus fractures only represent 5–15 % of all facial fractures encountered in adult craniomaxillofacial trauma because the increased thickness of the frontal bone confers resistance against most forms of traumatic injury. Therefore, the presence of a frontal sinus fracture is an indicator of significant force. In a recent review of 1,097 patients, Rodriguez et al. reported an average Glasgow Coma Scale score of 12 and an overall mortality rate of 7.9 % in patients with frontal bone fractures. In another study evaluating 21 patients with frontal sinus fractures due to penetrating trauma, 50 % of patients presented in shock, 42 % were comatose, and 25 % died within the first 2 weeks. Additionally, patients with facial fractures exhibit increased injury severity scores, hospital and intensive care unit lengths of stay, number of ventilator days, and hospital charges when compared to those without facial fractures. Unconsciousness has been reported in 20 % of patients presenting with frontal bone fractures, further illustrating the powerful mechanism of injury.

Motor vehicle collisions are the most common culprit, followed by sports-related injuries and interpersonal violence. As previously mentioned, pneumatic expansion of the frontal sinus is not completed until the late adolescent period. Consequently, frontal sinus fractures are rarely seen in children and are seldom diagnosed in adolescents. While frontal *sinus* fractures are not possible in small children, frontal *bone* fractures occur with frequency in this age group because of their high cranium-to-face ratio. Young adults are the most commonly affected group, in which men are predominantly (and predictably) involved.

Physical Examination

As a potential harbinger of life-threatening injury, facial trauma frequently involves collateral damage to the airway, neuraxis, viscera, and axial skeleton.

Initial examination of the facial trauma patient includes simple observation of the craniofacial skeleton for contour deformities, abrasions, and/or lacerations. The most common clinical finding in frontal sinus injuries is a laceration of the forehead. Any hematoma or ecchymosis over the glabellar region should additionally raise suspicion for osseous injury. Patients with frontal sinus injuries will often have visible depression in the supraorbital region that accompanies the soft tissue compromise. Palpation over the suspected site of injury may reveal crepitus, instability, and/or step-off deformities. In a patient with significant swelling, however, these physical findings are often masked and not readily noticeable; thus, a high index of suspicion with close follow-up is required as edema recedes. Sensory disturbances are also commonly reported, indicating neuropraxia of the supraorbital and/or supratrochlear nerves. Although nerve transection is possible, especially if forehead lacerations are present, it is usually not seen in cases of blunt trauma associated with closed frontal sinus injury.

The likelihood of additional fractures to the craniofacial skeleton is high in patients with frontal sinus injuries.

A complete examination of the entire craniofacial skeleton is therefore warranted, including an assessment of the patient's occlusion. Owing to proximity, the clinician should pay particular attention to the ocular examination, including evaluation of globe integrity, extraocular movements (i.e., entrapment), visual fields, visual acuity, and pupillary response. In the unconscious patient, a forced duction test should be performed. While diplopia is defined as subjective double vision, entrapment indicates the limitation of extraocular movements, which can be objectively measured on physical examination by the inability to perform forced duction. Enophthalmos is commonly described in orbital floor fractures, but displacement of the orbital roof and/or the greater wing of the sphenoid bone due to a "blow-in" mechanism is more common with frontal bone fractures. In these cases, proptosis may be seen as well as direct globe injury (e.g., subconjunctival hemorrhage, hyphema, and/or globe rupture). Fractures of the orbital roof that propagate to the orbital apex may demonstrate additional cranial nerve findings consistent with superior orbital fissure and orbital apex syndromes. If the optic nerve is affected, pseudoisochromatic plate testing may reveal color vision deficiency – red color is lost first.

Cerebrospinal fluid (CSF) rhinorrhea may also occur, manifested as clear and persistent nasal drainage. This indicates a combined injury to both the dura mater and the posterior sinus wall and represents a direct communication between the brain and upper aerodigestive tract. The β_2-transferrin test is the gold standard for the diagnosis of CSF leak, but the halo or glucose test may also be used. While quick and relatively easy to perform, they require confirmation due to their low sensitivity and specificity. For the halo test, a "double-ring" sign on filter paper (i.e., an inner ring of blood and an outer ring of CSF) represents a positive test. For the glucose test, a urine dipstick containing glucose oxidase can differentiate between the presence of glucose (i.e., CSF) and the absence of glucose (i.e., normal nasal secretions) based on colorimetrics.

Radiographic Imaging

Advances in the realm of computed tomography have greatly enhanced diagnosis and treatment planning in facial trauma patients. Sections are generally taken 1.25 mm apart for fine detail, but thinner sections (e.g., 0.625 mm) can be obtained if higher resolution is required. Coronal reformatting is crucial for evaluating patency of the frontonasal ductal system (see Fig. 19.2). Three-dimensional computed tomography permits further analysis of fracture patterns, clearly defines the extent of bony injury in the context of the overall craniofacial skeleton, and provides assistance in planning the steps of surgical repair. With this imaging modality, volume and proportionality may be directly assessed. In reviewing two-dimensional computed tomographic images, particular clues to the radiographic diagnosis of frontal sinus fractures include the presence of step-off deformities along the orbital roof and frontal bones, pneumocephalus, and sinus opacification (see Fig. 19.3). Bony displacement in the region of the frontonasal ductal system may have significant impact on the ultimate clinical management of the fracture. In cases of known CSF leak, source localization may be further visualized with computed tomographic or magnetic resonance cisternography, but these tests are rarely used in clinical practice.

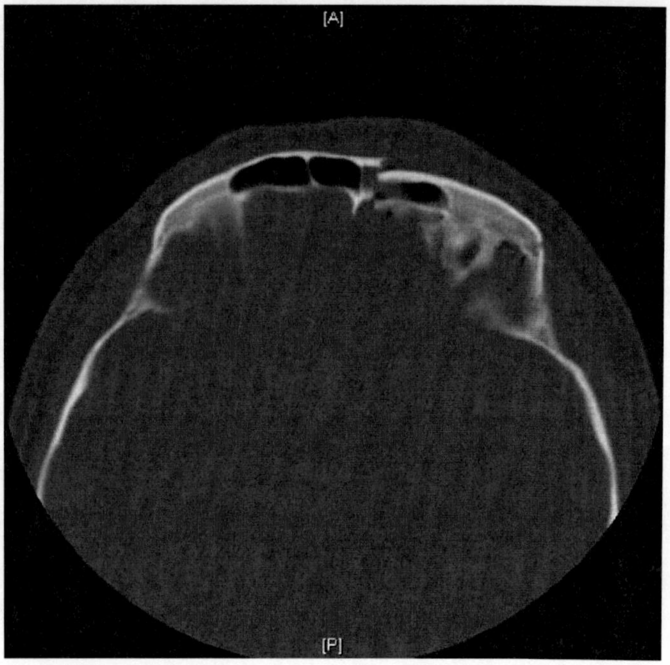

Fig. 19.3 Axial computed tomographic image of a patient with displaced anterior and posterior table fractures, pneumocephalus, and sinus opacification

Operative Treatment

Overview

Most patients with frontal sinus injuries require inpatient treatment at a high-volume tertiary referral center using a multidisciplinary team approach, with coordinated input from the trauma surgeon, neurosurgeon, craniofacial surgeon, and ophthalmologist. The overarching goals in operative treatment of frontal sinus fractures include restoration of forehead contour and structural integrity, evaluation and management of impaired sinus drainage pathways, and reestablishment of the anatomic barrier between the brain and upper aerodigestive tract. With these tenets in mind, a logical and consistent anatomical approach to surgical repair of the frontal sinus can be actualized (see Fig. 19.4).

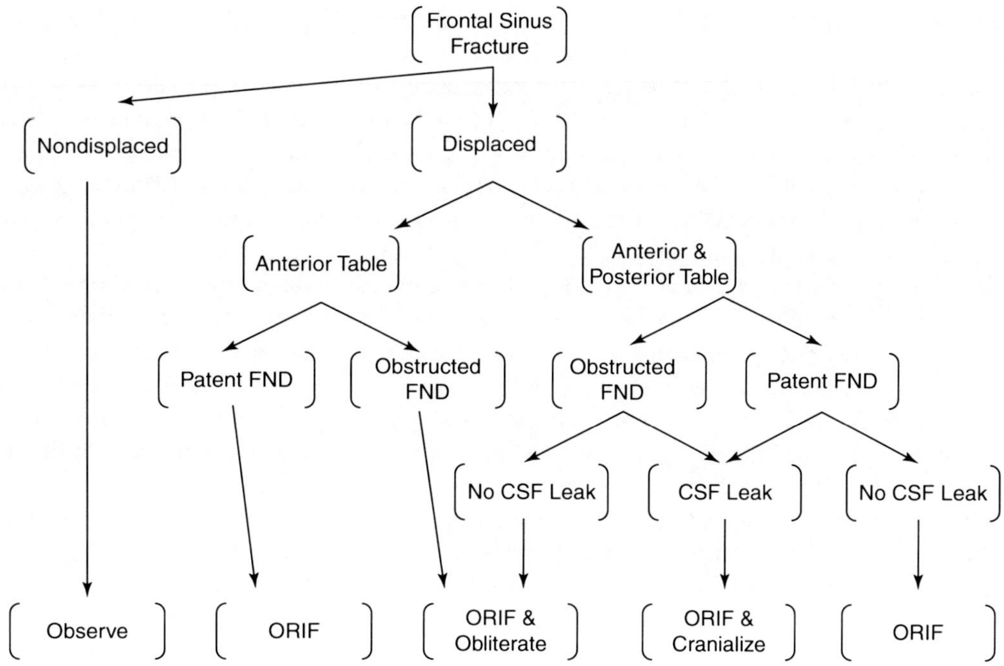

Fig. 19.4 Anatomically-based algorithm to frontal sinus fracture management

Indications

The relative and absolute indications for operative intervention of frontal sinus fractures are listed in Table 19.1. Over the past 20 years, these have resulted in predictable outcomes despite variable clinical presentation. Four anatomical structures dictate the need for surgical repair: (1) the frontonasal duct system, (2) the dura mater (i.e., CSF leak), and (3) the anterior and (4) posterior tables. With strategies geared toward early operative intervention when indicated, adverse sequelae can be avoided.

Contour deformities resulting from isolated fractures of the anterior table are primarily of aesthetic, and potentially of structural, concern. As such, operative intervention is based on clinical severity, and therefore, these types of injuries represent a relative indication for operative correction. Likewise, additional fractures of the craniofacial skeleton often mandate concurrent treatment of the frontal sinus and frontal bone. The restoration of pre-injury facial dimensions requires a stable platform, and the satisfactory reduction and fixation of panfacial fractures relies on anatomic continuity between the cranium and the facial skeleton. Similarly, depressed skull fractures requiring neurosurgical intervention also provide an opportunity to treat injuries of the frontal sinus should there be equivocation in the diagnosis (e.g., uncertain patency of the frontonasal ductal system).

Absolute indications for operative intervention of frontal sinus fractures include persistent CSF rhinorrhea and reasonable suspicion of frontonasal duct injury or obstruction. CSF rhinorrhea denotes disruption of the critical anatomic barrier between the brain and upper aerodigestive tract. While a relatively common complication – occurring in 19 % of cases on presentation – CSF rhinorrhea often resolves without any intervention. For those cases that persist beyond the first 4 days, lumbar drainage is indicated to divert flow of CSF away from the dural tear. If diversion does not ameliorate the leak within 7–10 days, bifrontal craniectomy, dural repair, and sinus cranialization are indicated.

Table 19.1 Frontal sinus fractures: relative and absolute indications for operative intervention

Relative	Absolute
Anterior wall fracture with contour deformity	Persistent CSF rhinorrhea[a]
Concomitant operative correction of additional craniomaxillofacial fractures	Significantly displaced/ comminuted fracture of the posterior wall
Minimally displaced/ comminuted fracture of the posterior wall[b]	Reasonable suspicion of FND injury or obstruction by radiography
Minimally displaced orbital "blow-in" fracture with mild changes in orbital volume, globe function, and/or vision[c]	Significantly displaced orbital "blow-in" fracture with severe changes in orbital volume, globe function, and/or vision

CSF cerebrospinal fluid, *FND* frontonasal duct
[a]Greater than 7 days, despite lumbar drainage
[b]Requires combined neurosurgical and craniofacial consultation
[c]Requires combined ophthalmological, neurosurgical, and craniofacial consultation

Most treatment algorithms for frontal sinus fractures universally use frontonasal duct involvement as one of the key determinants for operative intervention. If outflow obstruction is missed, late complications such as frontal sinusitis, brain abscess, chronic headaches, and mucocele formation can ensue. Frontal sinus obliteration with sinus wall preservation has been advocated for this type of fracture pattern to eliminate all mucus formation. Generally, if a craniotomy is to be performed, cranialization of the sinus is our preferred treatment because obliteration alone always carries a risk of re-mucosalization. We feel that this aggressive strategy (i.e., cranialization) decreases the potential for adverse sequelae by allowing the brain to naturally expand into the previous sinus cavity helping to assure the seal.

Frontal sinus fractures involving the posterior table can be considered either relative or absolute indications for operative intervention depending on the severity of the fracture pattern. Decisions to proceed surgically are not always straightforward: direct communication with a neurosurgeon is advised. Continued observation is often a reasonable alternative with close follow-up for minimally displaced/comminuted fractures of the posterior table. In these cases, our criteria for operative correction include a high likelihood of delayed healing, an inability to form a complete osseous hermetic seal between the brain and the nasal passages, and suspected injury or obstruction of the frontonasal ductal system. The underlying principle is that the sinus is now open to the intracranial cavity, and unless there is a strong prospect that the bony fragments will heal restoring the anatomic barrier, we are biased toward operative intervention to prevent infectious complications; cranialization of the sinus is routinely indicated.

For orbital "blow-in" fractures with minimal changes in orbital volume, globe function, and/or vision, we advise close coordination with ophthalmology and continued observation. If significantly displaced orbital "blow-in" fractures are encountered with severe changes in orbital volume, globe function, and/or vision, the scale will be tipped toward surgical intervention. Accordingly, the superior orbital fissure and orbital apex syndromes provide an absolute indication for surgery.

Some authors have successfully demonstrated conservative management strategies with continued observation. In a series of 675 patients reported by Choi et al., a single death from encephalitis was noted over the 10-year study period in a patient with a gunshot wound. The main arguments for conservative management are that (1) the treatment of frontal sinus fractures is invasive, (2) the infectious complications are rare, and (3) the treatment of said complications involves the same invasive surgical approach as in primary cases. The primary argument against conservative management is the lack of true long-term follow-up with these patients and the significant morbidity associated with those complications.

Timing

Unlike other cases involving injury to the craniofacial skeleton, operative intervention for frontal sinus fractures is preferred within 1 week to reduce the incidence of long-term complications. However, some neurosurgeons prefer to wait longer, especially if there is an associated brain injury with elevated intracranial pressure. All patients with frontal sinus fractures are subjected to bed rest, head elevation, and sinus precautions perioperatively. The use of antibiotic prophylaxis in the management of frontal sinus fractures is controversial and should be considered on a case-by-case basis. Some authors recommend every patient with frontal sinus injury receive antibiotics, whereas others feel that antibiotics outside of the perioperative window offer no additional protection. Indeed, in a retrospective review of 223 facial trauma patients, Lauder et al. demonstrated an overall infection rate of 9 % with no significant difference between groups receiving antibiotics either preoperatively, postoperatively, both pre- and postoperatively, or perioperatively only. A positive correlation between the infection rate and both the number of fractures and open fracture wounds, however, was noted in this study. In our practice, we prefer antibiotic prophylaxis in patients with persistent CSF rhinorrhea or in those patients with significantly displaced/comminuted fractures of the posterior table. Most often, we will defer to the neurosurgeon's preference in this regard.

Exposure

Existing lacerations are only used in cases of isolated fractures of the anterior table. Even in these cases, the laceration may provide insufficient exposure. Instead of extending the laceration, a coronal flap should be utilized. As such, the coronal flap is the standard approach for extensive anterior table fractures and in all obliteration and cranialization procedures. The so-called open-sky approach – a gull-wing incision above the brow – is not recommended. This nonanatomic technique disrupts axial blood supply, causes paresthesia, and yields visible scarring with poor cosmesis.

Coronal flap elevation is performed in the subgaleal plane, and dissection extends down to the supraorbital rims and nasoglabellar junction medially and the frontozygomatic junctions laterally. Preservation of the pericranial layer permits its use as a vascularized flap in cases where obliteration or cranialization is required. Over the temporalis muscle, dissection proceeds directly above the temporalis muscle fascia. This ensures protection of the frontal branch of the facial nerve, which travels within the temporoparietal fascia layer (i.e., superficial temporal fascia).

Endoscopic approaches to the anterior table are mentioned here for completeness sake. While this technique purports decreased operative time and minimal invasiveness, the ability to attain sufficient exposure and fixation limits its utility, and until proven with equal efficacy, should be eschewed.

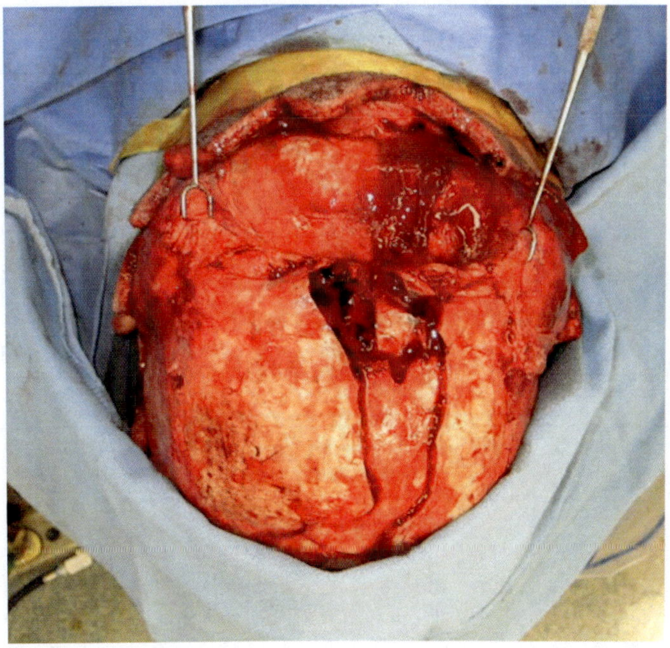

Fig. 19.5 Intraoperative view of frontal sinus with turned coronal flap (double hooks) after removal of comminuted anterior table fragments. A concomitant depressed parietal skull fracture can be visualized (Photograph courtesy of Dr. Joseph S. Gruss)

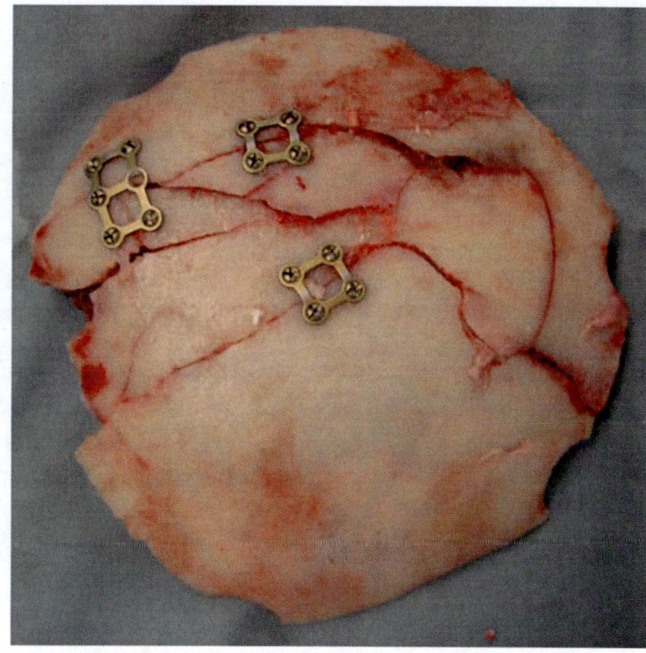

Fig. 19.6 Ex vivo fixation of anterior table fragments using microplates and screws (Photograph courtesy of Dr. Joseph S. Gruss)

Technique

Once the fracture is identified intraoperatively, the fragments are disimpacted (see Fig. 19.5). If the injury is isolated to the anterior table, standard principles of rigid fixation may ensue. The disimpacted fragments may be reconstructed ex vivo using microplates and screw fixation (see Fig. 19.6). In palpable areas, low-profile 1.0-mm microplates are recommended, whereas in non-palpable areas either 1.5-mm, or less commonly 2.0-mm, miniplates can be used. Titanium mesh is also suitable, as the frontal bone is non-load-bearing and the thin soft tissues of the brow may lead to visible and/or palpable hardware. In children, resorbable plating systems may be considered; however, they can be bulky and may be both seen and palpated. Mapping out and carefully removing bony pieces for reorientation during reduction can be quite helpful. Some surgeons utilize a bone pencil in order to establish key relationships prior to disimpaction and removal from the operative field, should this be required. Prior to fixation, any obviously diseased mucosa is removed with a curette, rongeur, or high-speed burr.

If frontonasal duct injury is suspected, the duct is first examined for patency prior to fixation. Fluorescein dye or methylene blue is instilled into the sinus, and a cotton tip applicator is then placed into the nose near the middle meatus. A positive test is when dye is present on the cotton tip applicator. In cases of a negative test and/or if there is significant doubt about frontonasal duct patency or obstruction, the sinus should be obliterated. Of note, cranialization is not required in these cases, as long as the posterior table is intact (see Fig. 19.4). The initial step in sinus obliteration is complete exenteration of all the mucosal lining. Using electrocautery, the plane between the mucosa and the underlying bone is identified. The mucosa is then stripped as a sheet followed by removal of any remaining mucosa using a high-speed contouring burr. The mucosa can be tethered deeply within the bone, especially along the posterior sinus wall in the foramina of Breschet; care should be directed at these particular areas. We prefer to leave a small mucosal sleeve near the sinus infundibulum, which is then turned down into the duct and sewn closed. Finally, we pack either cortical or cancellous bone on top of the mucosal sleeve and then form fit a piece of cortical bone to assure the seal along with a pericranial flap or graft, if a flap is not possible.

Numerous autogenous tissues have been described for utilization in frontal sinus obliteration, including fat, dermis, fascia, pericranium, and galea. Biocompatible compounds such as hydroxyapatite have also been advocated, but we strongly recommend against use of these products because the surgical site is considered a contaminated area, thereby increasing the risk of postoperative infectious complications. Spontaneous osteogenesis without the use of ablative materials has also been noted experimentally. Bone grafts are used exclusively in our practice. We prefer autogenous bone because it is relatively easy to harvest with decreased incidence of infection and extrusion. Fibrin glue, a nontoxic compound with biocompatible properties, can be used to secure bone grafts in place during both obliteration and cranialization procedures (see Fig. 19.7).

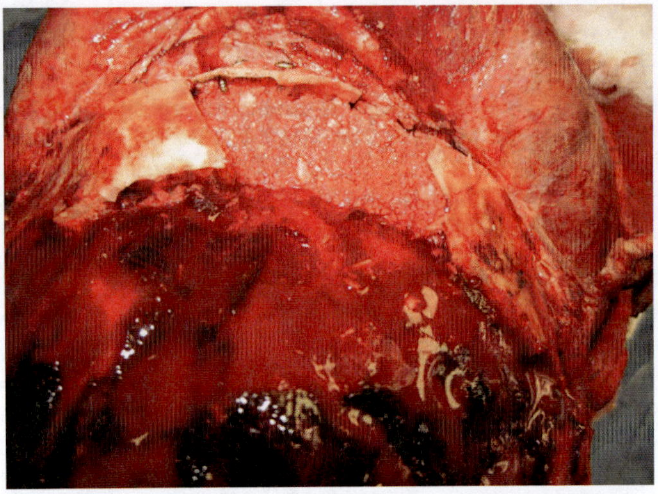

Fig. 19.7 Cranialization of the frontal sinus using morselized bone graft taken from the posterior table. Fibrin glue will be used to seal the graft in place (Photograph courtesy of Dr. Joseph S. Gruss)

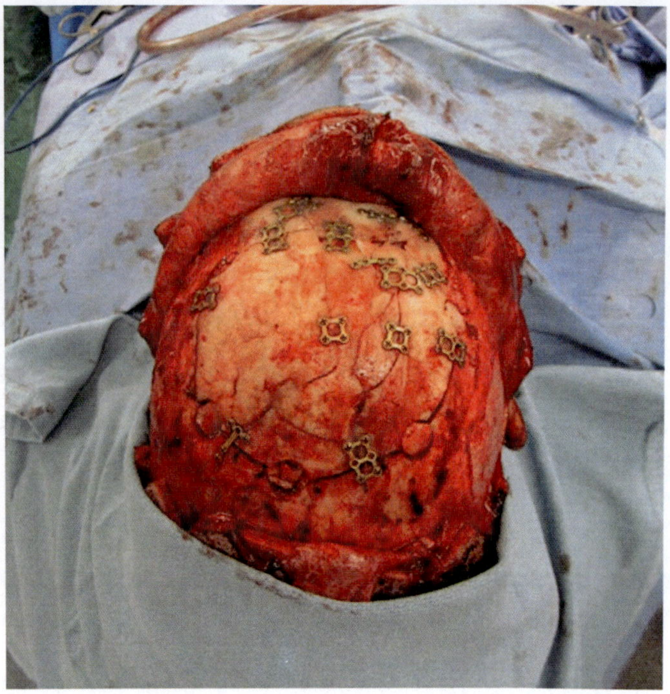

Fig. 19.8 Appearance of patient from Fig. 5.7 following cranialization and rigid anatomic fixation (Photograph courtesy of Dr. Joseph S. Gruss)

Cranialization should be considered when the anatomic barrier between the sinus and intracranial cavity has been disrupted (i.e., significant posterior table comminution/displacement and/or persistent CSF rhinorrhea). Cranialization involves removal of the entire posterior sinus wall and debridement of all sinus mucosa, followed by frontonasal duct blockade. The latter is achieved with bone grafts (see Fig. 19.7), fibrin glue, and an anteriorly based pericranial flap or graft, if a flap is not possible. The galeal-frontalis myofascial flap may also be considered, particularly if the pericranium has been injured and lacks integrity. Dural repair, when required, is performed with a pericranial patch graft secured with braided nylon suture. This "watertight" closure may be checked with Trendelenburg positioning and a ventilator-assisted Valsalva maneuver. The frontal lobe is then allowed to fill the space over time, which further helps to assure the seal; the sinus has now become "cranialized." Reduction and fixation of the anterior table may then proceed as discussed previously (see Fig. 19.8).

Postoperative Care

Postoperatively, patients can undergo radiographic examination to exclude the presence of intracranial bleeding and midline shift, as well as to assess their reduction and fixation. Three-dimensional images are helpful in this regard (see Fig. 19.9). Transfer to the surgical intensive care unit is preferred for regular neurological assessment in the immediate postoperative period (i.e., 24–36 h). The authors prefer head elevation at 30° and propose perioperative antibiotics for 3 days or while the penrose drain is in place. Sinus precautions are recommended for 2 weeks. Due to the high likelihood of coincident traumatic brain injury, referral to physical medicine and rehabilitation specialists is common, as well as physical and occupational therapy. Patients are often discharged to subacute rehabilitation or a skilled-nursing facility for convalescence.

Complications

Despite the many feared complications of frontal sinus injuries, chronic frontal headaches are cited as the most common occurrence. Contour deformities are frequently observed, particularly when observation alone has been used. Paresthesias in the supraorbital and supratrochlear distributions, while present acutely, are rarely permanent, with a long-term incidence of 5 %.

The potential life-threatening infectious complications from frontal sinus fractures, namely, meningitis, encephalitis, brain abscess (see Fig. 19.10), and mucopyocele, have been well described. As previously emphasized, any connection between the brain and upper

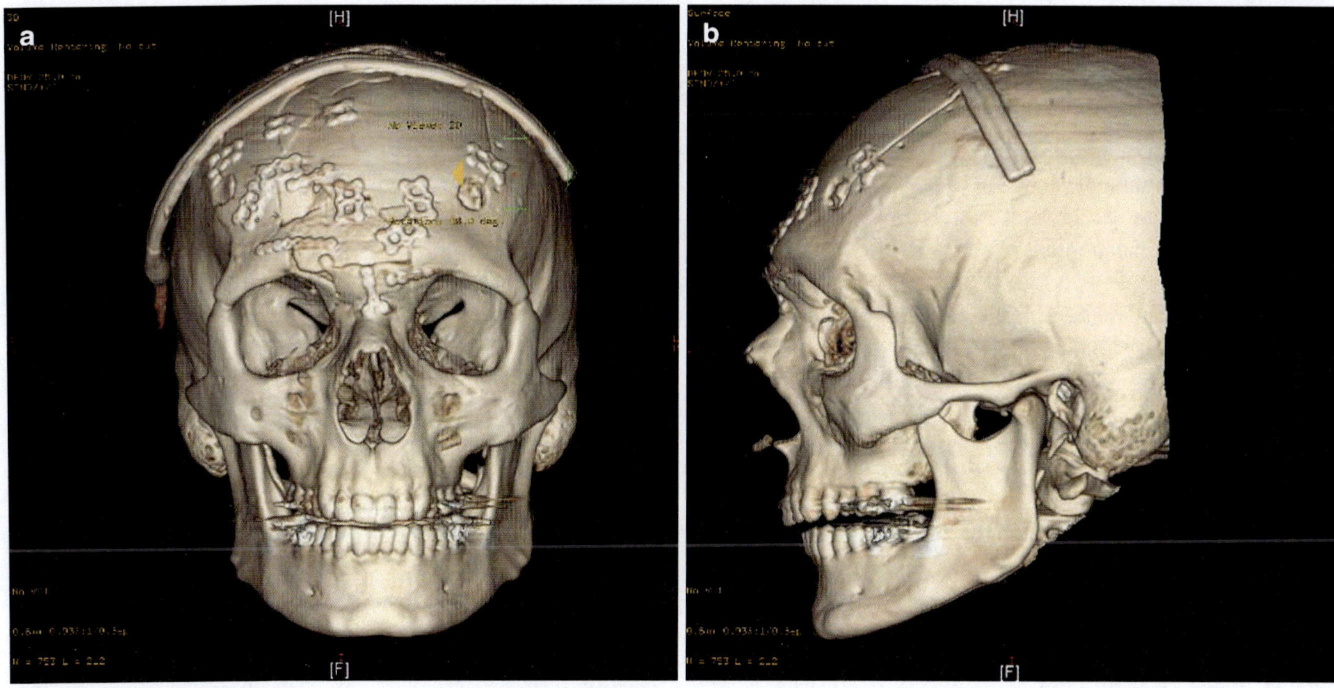

Fig. 19.9 Postoperative imaging: (**a**) anteroposterior and (**b**) lateral views of the same patient following computed tomographic scanning and three-dimensional reformatting. A surgical drain is in place. Satisfactory reduction and fixation has been achieved

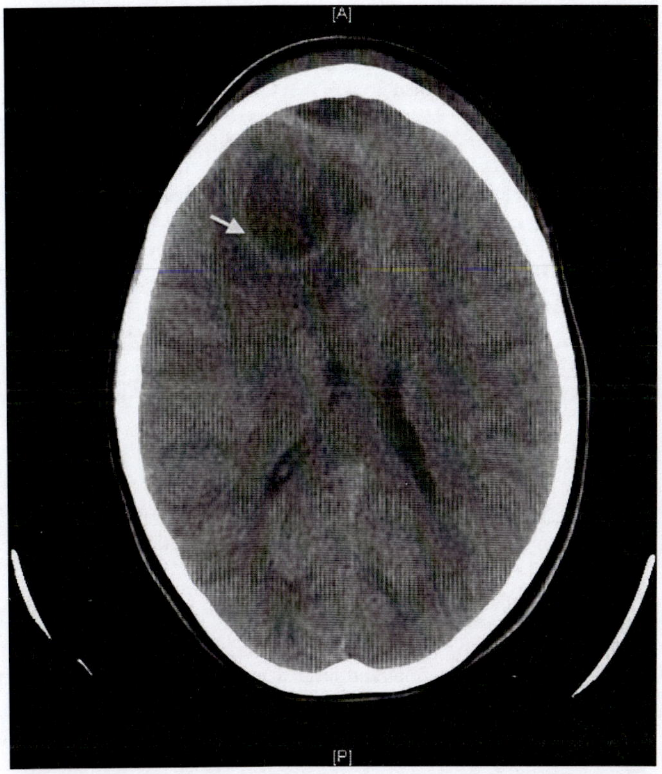

Fig. 19.10 Axial computed tomography with contrast demonstrating rim-enhancing intraparenchymal abscess (*solid arrow*) following untreated frontal sinus fracture with displacement of the posterior table. Mass effect with midline shift can be appreciated

aerodigestive tract is the culprit. Hence, any injury resulting in break in the sinus-osseous barrier should undergo surgical treatment. Rapid infectious spread is possible in cases of relatively minor trauma, even when fracture displacement does not occur, owing to the extensive lymphatic and venous interconnections between the sinus and its surroundings. Meningitis and encephalitis have been documented to occur with expectant and operative management alike, albeit with rare incidence. Mucopyocele, while frequently associated with frontal sinus injury, is relatively uncommon. The pathological mechanism involves mucous production by residual mucosa, which then becomes secondarily infected. The classic presenting sign of mucocele or mucopyocele is progressive proptosis.

The uncommon occurrence of these infectious complications has been used as an argument for simple observation of many frontal sinus injuries. Long-term follow-up with these patients, however, is not routinely observed, making such conclusions of questionable value. The management of these untoward sequelae is a recapitulation of the original reconstructive effort: craniotomy with frontal sinus cranialization. The treating surgeon should maintain a low threshold for restarting antibiotics and/or obtaining repeat imaging when infectious or neurologic signs and symptoms are encountered.

Conclusions

A thorough knowledge of normal anatomy is imperative to the treating surgeon in the case of frontal sinus injury. While the treatment of frontal sinus fractures remains varied and controversial, the aforementioned strategies are based on fundamental anatomical principles. The strategies presented in this chapter have proven to be safe and reliable in the management of frontal sinus fractures.

Acknowledgment The authors wish to thank Dr. Joseph S. Gruss for his clinical expertise and the intraoperative photographs used in this work.

Bibliography

Abiraman S, Varma HK, Umashankar PR, John A. Fibrin glue as an osteoinductive protein in a mouse model. Biomaterials. 2002;23(14):3023–31.

Alvi A, Doherty T, Lewen G. Facial fractures and concomitant injuries in trauma patients. Laryngoscope. 2003;113(1):102–6.

Beirne JC, Butler PE, Brady FA. Cervical spine injuries in patients with facial fractures: a 1-year prospective study. Int J Oral Maxillofac Surg. 1995;24(1 Pt 1):26–9.

Bell RB, Dierks EJ, Brar P, Potter JK, Potter BE. A protocol for the management of frontal sinus fractures emphasizing sinus preservation. J Oral Maxillofac Surg. 2007;65(5):825–39.

Biggs NL, Blanton PL. The role of paranasal sinuses as weight reducers of the head determined by electromyography of postural neck muscles. J Biomech. 1970;3(3):255–62.

Chan DT, Poon WS, IP CP, Chiu PW, Goh KY. How useful is glucose detection in diagnosing cerebrospinal fluid leak? The rational use of CT and Beta-2 transferrin assay in detection of cerebrospinal fluid fistula. Asian J Surg. 2004;27(1):39–42.

Chandra RK, Schlosser R, Kennedy DW. Use of the 70-degree diamond burr in the management of complicated frontal sinus disease. Laryngoscope. 2004;114(2):188–92.

Chen DJ, Chen CT, Chen YR, Feng GM. Endoscopically assisted repair of frontal sinus fracture. J Trauma. 2003;55(2):378–82.

Chen KT, Chen CT, Mardini S, Tsay PK, Chen YR. Frontal sinus fractures: a treatment algorithm and assessment of outcomes based on 78 clinical cases. Plast Reconstr Surg. 2006;118(2):457–68.

Choi M, Li Y, Shapiro SA, Havlik RJ, Flores RL. A 10-year review of frontal sinus fractures: clinical outcomes of conservative management of posterior table fractures. Plast Reconstr Surg. 2012;130(2):399–406.

Davidson JS, Birdsell DC. Cervical spine injury in patients with facial skeletal trauma. J Trauma. 1989;29(9):1276–8.

Davis WE, Templer J, Parsons DS. Anatomy of the paranasal sinuses. Otolaryngol Clin North Am. 1996;29(1):57–74.

Donald PJ. The tenacity of the frontal sinus mucosa. Otolaryngol Head Neck Surg. 1979;87(5):557–66.

Donald PJ. Frontal sinus ablation by cranialization. Report of 21 cases. Arch Otolaryngol. 1982;108(3):142–6.

Donald PJ. Anatomy and histology. In: Donald PJ, Gluckman JL, Rice DH, editors. The sinuses. New York: Raven Press; 1995. p. 25–48.

Donald PJ, Ettin M. The safety of frontal sinus fat obliteration when sinus walls are missing. Laryngoscope. 1986;96(2):190–3.

Donald PJ, Montgomery WW, Calcaterra T. Frontal bone defect with frontal sinus mucopyocele. Head Neck Surg. 1987;10(1):59–62.

Elahi MM, Brar MS, Ahmed N, Howley DB, Nishtar S, Mahoney JL. Cervical spine injury in association with craniomaxillofacial fractures. Plast Reconstr Surg. 2008;121(1):201–8.

Falcone S, Post MJ. Encephalitis, cerebritis, and brain abscess: pathophysiology and imaging findings. Neuroimaging Clin N Am. 2000;10(2):333–53.

Fenton Jr WH, Donald PJ, Carlton 3rd W. The pressure exerted by mucoceles in the frontal sinus. An experimental study in the cat. Arch Otolaryngol Head Neck Surg. 1990;116(7):836–40.

Gaafar H, Abdel-Monem MH, Qawas MK. Frontal sinus outflow tract "anatomic study". Acta Otolaryngol. 2001;121(2):305–9.

Gerbino G, Roccia F, Benech A, Caldarelli C. Analysis of 158 frontal sinus fractures: current surgical management and complications. J Craniomaxillofac Surg. 2000;28(3):133–9.

Gonty AA, Marciani RD, Adornato DC. Management of frontal sinus fractures: a review of 33 cases. J Oral Maxillofac Surg. 1999;57(4):372–9; discussion 380–1.

Gossman DG, Archer SM, Arosarena O. Management of frontal sinus fractures: a review of 96 cases. Laryngoscope. 2006;116(8):1357–62.

Haight JS, Djupesland PG, Qjan W, et al. Does nasal nitric oxide come from the sinuses? J Otolaryngol. 1999;28(4):197–204.

Hardy A. Was man more aquatic in the past? New Sci. 1960;7:642–5.

Harris L, Marano GD, McCorkle D. Nasofrontal duct: CT in frontal sinus trauma. Radiology. 1987;165(1):195–8.

Heller EM, Jacobs JB, Holliday RA. Evaluation of the frontonasal duct in frontal sinus fractures. Head Neck. 1989;11(1):46–50.

Hilding AC. Experimental sinus surgery: effects of operative windows on normal sinuses. Ann Otol Rhinol Laryngol. 1941;50:379–92.

Howell HP. Voice production from the stand point of the laryngologist. Ann Otol Rhinol Laryngol. 1917;408:1–28.

Imahara SD, Hopper RA, Wang J, Rivara FP, Klein MB. Patterns and outcomes of pediatric facial fractures in the United States: a survey of the National Trauma Data Bank. J Am Coll Surg. 2008;207(5):710–6.

Ioannides C, Freihofer HP. Fractures of the frontal sinus: classification and its implications for surgical treatment. Am J Otolaryngol. 1999;20(5):273–80.

Ioannides C, Freihofer HP, Bruaset I. Trauma of the upper third of the face. Management and follow-up. J Maxillofac Surg. 1984;12(6):255–61.

Ioannides C, Freihofer HP, Vrieus J, Friens J. Fractures of the frontal sinus: a rationale of treatment. Br J Plast Surg. 1993;46(3):208–14.

Jackson IT, Adham MN, Marsh WR. Use of the galaeal frontalis myofascial flap in craniofacial surgery. Plast Reconstr Surg. 1986;77(6):905–10.

Keir J. Why do we have paranasal sinuses? J Laryngol Otol. 2009;123(1):4–8.

Kirk NJ, Wood RE, Goldstein M. Skeletal identification using the frontal sinus region: a retrospective study of 39 cases. J Forensic Sci. 2002;47(2):318–23.

Koertvelyessy T. Relationships between the frontal sinus and climactic conditions: a skeletal approach to cold adaptation. Am J Phys Anthropol. 1972;37(2):161–72.

Landsberg R, Friedman M. A computer-assisted anatomical study of the nasofrontal region. Laryngoscope. 2001;111(12):2125–30.

Larrabee Jr WF, Travis LW, Tabb HG. Frontal sinus fractures – their suppurative complications and surgical management. Laryngoscope. 1980;90(11 Pt 1):1810–3.

Lauder A, Jalisi S, Spiegel J, Stram J, Devaiah A. Antibiotic prophylaxis in the management of complex midface and frontal sinus trauma. Laryngoscope. 2010;120(10):1940–5.

Lee D, Brody R, Har-El G. Frontal sinus outflow anatomy. Am J Rhinol. 1997;11(4):283–5.

Lee TT, Ratzker PA, Galarza M, Villanueva PA. Early combined management of frontal sinus and orbital and facial fractures. J Trauma. 1998;44(4):665–9.

Levine SB, Rowe LD, Keane WM, Atkins Jr JP. Evaluation and treatment of frontal sinus fractures. Otolaryngol Head Neck Surg. 1986;95(1):19–22.

Luce EA. Frontal sinus fractures: guidelines to management. Plast Reconstr Surg. 1987;80(4):500–10.

Lundberg JO, Farkas-Szallasi T, Weitzberg E, et al. High nitric oxide production in human paranasal sinuses. Nat Med. 1995;1(4): 370–3.

Malhotra R, Wormald PJ, Selva D. Bilateral dynamic proptosis due to frontoethmoidal sinus mucocele. Ophthal Plast Reconstr Surg. 2003;19(2):156–7.

Manolidis S. Frontal sinus injuries: associated injuries and surgical management of 93 patients. J Oral Maxillofac Surg. 2004; 62(7):882–91.

Manolidis S, Hollier Jr LH. Management of frontal sinus fractures. Plast Reconstr Surg. 2007;120(7 Suppl 2):32S–48.

Mantur M, Łukaszewicz-Zając M, Mroczko B, et al. Cerebrospinal fluid leakage – reliable diagnostic methods. Clin Chim Acta. 2011;412(11–12):837–40.

McHugh HE. Treatment of fractures of the frontal and ethmoid sinuses. Laryngoscope. 1958;68(9):1616–40.

McLaughlin Jr RB, Rehl Jr RM, Lanza DC. Clinically relevant frontal sinus anatomy and physiology. Otolaryngol Clin North Am. 2001;34(1):1–22.

Messerklinger W. On the drainage of the normal frontal sinus of man. Acta Otolaryngol. 1967;63(2):176–81.

Metzinger SE, Metzinger RC. Complications of frontal sinus fractures. Craniomaxillofac Trauma Reconstr. 2009;2(1):27–34.

Mickel TJ, Rohrich RJ, Robinson Jr JB. Frontal sinus obliteration: a comparison of fat, muscle, bone, and spontaneous osteoneogenesis in the cat model. Plast Reconstr Surg. 1995;95(3):586–92.

Millman AL, Lubkin V, Gersten M. Three-dimensional reconstruction of the orbit from CT scans and volumetric analysis of orbital fractures: its role in the evaluation of enophthalmos. Adv Ophthalmic Plast Reconstr Surg. 1987;6:265–8.

Nadell J, Kline DG. Primary reconstruction of depressed frontal skull fractures including those involving the sinus, orbit, and cribriform plate. J Neurosurg. 1974;41(2):200–7.

Nahum AM. The biomechanics of facial bone fracture. Laryngoscope. 1975a;85(1):140–56.

Nahum AM. The biomechanics of maxillofacial trauma. Clin Plast Surg. 1975b;2(1):59–64.

Nambiar P, Naidu MD, Subramaniam K. Anatomical variability of the frontal sinuses and their application in forensic identification. Clin Anat. 1999;12(1):16–9.

Negus V. The function of the paranasal sinuses. AMA Arch Otolaryngol. 1957;66(4):430–42.

Petruzzelli GJ, Stankiewicz JA. Frontal sinus obliteration with hydroxyapatite cement. Laryngoscope. 2002;112(1):32–6.

Plaisier BR, Punjabi AP, Super DM, Haug RH. The relationship between facial fractures and death from neurologic injury. J Oral Maxillofac Surg. 2000;58(7):708–12; discussion 712–3.

Pletcher SD, Goldberg AN. Frontal sinus fractures. In: Lalwani A, editor. Current diagnosis and treatment in otolaryngology – head and neck surgery. 3rd ed. New York: McGraw-Hill Medical; 2012. p. 302–8.

Proetz AW. Observations upon the formation and function of the accessory nasal sinuses and the mastoid air cells. Ann Otol Rhinol Laryngol. 1922;31:1083–100.

Rath SA, Knöringer P. Late brain abscess years after severe cerebrocranial trauma with fronto-orbitobasal fracture. Childs Nerv Syst. 1989;5(2):121–3.

Rhŷs Evans PH. The paranasal sinuses and other enigmas: an aquatic evolutionary theory. J Laryngol Otol. 1992;106(3):214–25.

Rice DH. Embryology. In: Donald PJ, Gluckman JL, Rice DH, editors. The sinuses. New York: Raven Press; 1995. p. 15–23.

Rodriguez ED, Stanwix MG, Nam AJ, et al. Twenty-six-year experience treating frontal sinus fractures: a novel algorithm based on anatomical fracture pattern and failure of conventional techniques. Plast Reconstr Surg. 2008;122(6):1850–66.

Rohrich RJ, Hollier LH. Management of frontal sinus fractures. Changing concepts. Clin Plast Surg. 1992;19(1):219–32.

Rohrich RJ, Hollier LH. The role of the nasofrontal duct in frontal sinus fracture management. J Craniomaxillofac Trauma. 1996;2(4): 31–40.

Rohrich RJ, Mickel TJ. Frontal sinus obliteration: in search of the ideal autogenous material. Plast Reconstr Surg. 1995;95(3):580–5.

Schenck NL. Frontal sinus disease. I. An historical perspective on research. Laryngoscope. 1974;84(6):1031–44.

Schenck NL, Rauchbach E, Ogura JH. Frontal sinus disease. II. Development of the frontal sinus model: occlusion of the nasofrontal duct. Laryngoscope. 1974;84(7):1233–47.

Shapiro R, Schorr S. A consideration of the systemic factors that influence frontal sinus pneumatization. Invest Radiol. 1980;15(3): 191–202.

Sherick DG, Buchman SR, Patel PP. Pediatric facial fractures: a demographic analysis outside an urban environment. Ann Plast Surg. 1997;38(6):578–84; discussion 584–5.

Shetty PG, Shroff MM, Sahani DV, Kirtane MV. Evaluation of high-resolution CT and MR cisternography in the diagnosis of cerebrospinal fluid fistula. AJNR Am J Neuroradiol. 1998;19(4):633–9.

Smith TL, Han JK, Loehrl TA, Rhee JS. Endoscopic management of the frontal recess in frontal sinus fractures: a shift in the paradigm? Laryngoscope. 2002;112(5):784–90.

Snyderman CH, Janecka IP, Sekhar LN, Sen CN, Eibling DE. Anterior cranial base reconstruction: role of galeal and pericranial flaps. Laryngoscope. 1990;100(6):607–14.

Stanley Jr RB. Management of frontal sinus fractures. Facial Plast Surg. 1988;5(3):231–5.

Stanley Jr RB, Becker TS. Injuries of the nasofrontal orifices in frontal sinus fractures. Laryngoscope. 1987;97(6):728–31.

Strong EB, Pahlavan N, Saito D. Frontal sinus fractures: a 28-year retrospective review. Otolaryngol Head Neck Surg. 2006;135(5): 774–9.

Takahashi R. The formation of the human paranasal sinuses. Acta Otolaryngol Suppl. 1984;408:1–28.

Tholpady SS, Schlosser R, Spotnitz W, Ogle RC, Lindsey WH. Repair of an osseus facial critical-size defect using augmented fibrin sealant. Laryngoscope. 1999;109(10):1585–8.

Tiwari P, Higuera S, Thornton J, Hollier LH. The management of frontal sinus fractures. J Oral Maxillofac Surg. 2005;63(9):1354–60.

Tos M, Mogensen C, Novotny Z. Quantitative histologic features of the normal frontal sinus. Arch Otolaryngol. 1980;106(3):143–8.

Treachnor F. Intracranial complications of fracture of skull involving frontal sinus. J Am Med Assoc. 1927;88(13):987–9.

Urken ML, Som PM, Edelstein D, Lawson W, Weber AL, Biller HF. Abnormally large frontal sinus. II. Nomenclature, pathology, and symptoms. Laryngoscope. 1987;97(5):606–11.

Viterbo F, Ranzani F, Campos E. New treatment for frontal sinus hypertrophy. Plast Reconstr Surg. 1990;86(4):776–9.

Wallis A, Donald PJ. Frontal sinus fractures: a review of 72 cases. Laryngoscope. 1988;98(6 Pt 1):593–8.

Weber SC, Cohn AM. Fracture of the frontal sinus in children. Arch Otolaryngol. 1977;103(4):241–4.

Weber R, Draf W, Keerl R, et al. Osteoplastic frontal sinus surgery with fat obliteration: technique and long-term results using magnetic resonance imaging in 82 operations. Laryngoscope. 2000;110(6): 1037–44.

Weitzel EK, Hollier LH, Calzada G, Manolidis S. Single stage management of complex fronto-orbital mucoceles. J Craniofac Surg. 2002;13(6):739–45.

Wenig BM. Atlas of head and neck pathology. 2nd ed. Philadelphia: W.B. Saunders; 2007.

Whatley WS, Allison DW, Chandra RK, Thompson JW, Boop FA. Frontal sinus fractures in children. Laryngoscope. 2005;115(10): 1741–5.

Wilson BC, Davidson B, Corey JP, Haydon 3rd RC. Comparison of complications following frontal sinus fractures managed with exploration with or without obliteration over 10 years. Laryngoscope. 1988;98(5):516–20.

Wolfe SA, Johnson P. Frontal sinus injuries: primary care and management of late complications. Plast Reconstr Surg. 1988;82(5): 781–91.

Wright DL, Hoffman HT, Hoyt DB. Frontal sinus fractures in the pediatric population. Laryngoscope. 1992;102(11):1215–9.

Xie C, Mehendale N, Barrett D, Bui CJ, Metzinger SE. 30-year retrospective review of frontal sinus fractures: the Charity Hospital experience. J Craniomaxillofac Trauma. 2000;6(1):7–15; discussion 16–8.

Yavuzer R, Jackson IT. Coronal incision extending postauricularly. Plast Reconstr Surg. 1999;103(5):1532–3.

Yavuzer R, Sari A, Kelly CP, et al. Management of frontal sinus fractures. Plast Reconstr Surg. 2005;115(6):79e–93; discussion 94e–95e.

Panfacial Fractures

20

William M. Weathers, David Y. Khechoyan, Erik M. Wolfswinkel, Larry H. Hollier, and Edward P. Buchanan

Introduction

A panfacial fracture is a high-energy injury involving bones in all three facial regions – the upper, middle, and lower facial bones. These types of injuries are exceedingly rare, representing only 3.7–15 % of all facial fractures. The fractures can be unilateral or bilateral, oftentimes with significant overlying soft tissue damage. Associated injuries can be severe and life threatening requiring a multidisciplinary team for management. Treatment of these patients should be completed at centers that can provide the complete spectrum of care, including trauma teams, intensive care units, and reconstructive surgeons. A systematic and principled approach, which adheres to the guidelines of modern craniofacial surgery, will aid the surgeon in the successful restoration of pre-injury form and function.

Definition and Presentation

The upper face consists of the frontal bones and the orbits; the midface includes the zygomaticomaxillary complexes (ZMC) and maxilla; and the lower face includes the mandible. Fractures occurring at all three levels of the facial skeleton can be described as panfacial injuries (see Fig. 20.1). It is important to emphasize that not all panfacial fractures are the same or involve every bone in the facial skeleton. Areas that remain unfractured in these injuries assist the surgeon by providing stable landmarks from which to plan the reconstruction. In the rare case that every facial bone is fractured, a consistent reconstructive sequence becomes vitally important for successful restoration.

Most patients with panfacial injuries will present to a major trauma center after an assault, fall, or motor vehicle

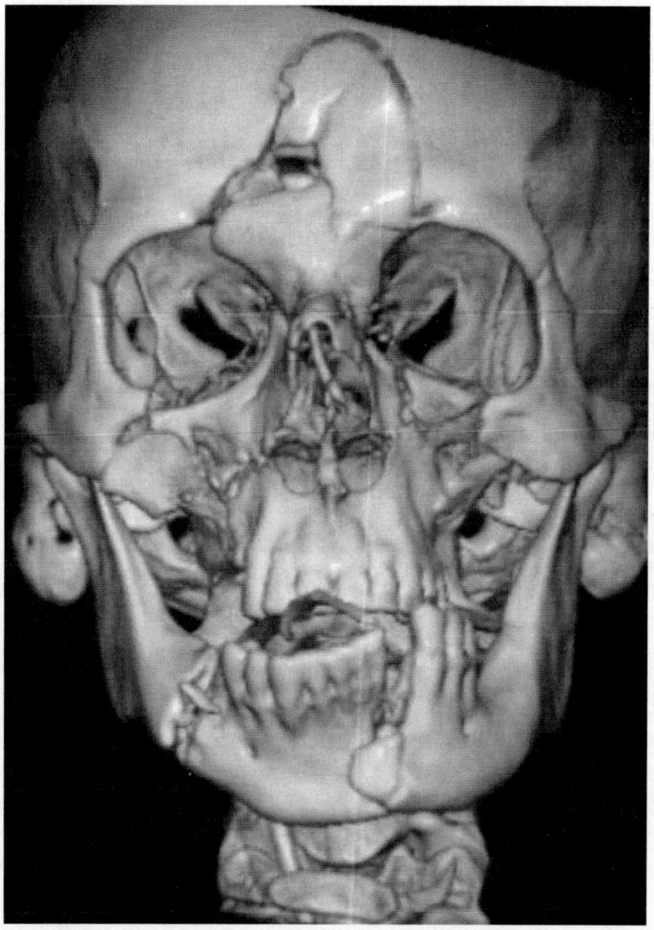

Fig. 20.1 3D CT reconstruction demonstrating a panfacial injury with fractures at all three levels of the face

W.M. Weathers, MD • D.Y. Khechoyan, MD
E.M. Wolfswinkel, MD • E.P. Buchanan, MD
Department of Plastic Surgery,
Baylor College of Medicine, Houston, TX, USA
e-mail: ebuchana@bcm.edu

L.H. Hollier, MD (✉)
Department of Plastic Surgery,
Baylor College of Medicine, Houston, TX, USA

Department of Plastic Surgery,
Texas Children's Hospital, Houston, TX, USA

P.J. Taub et al. (eds.), *Ferraro's Fundamentals of Maxillofacial Surgery*,
DOI 10.1007/978-1-4614-8341-0_20, © Springer Science+Business Media New York 2015

collision. Due to the improvement in motor vehicle safety standards, facial fractures as a result of motor vehicle collisions have been on the decline.

The significant force required to injure multiple levels of the facial skeleton usually results in injuries to surrounding structures, such as the brain, airway, neck, chest, and abdomen. Consequently, these patients are best served at major trauma centers with fully equipped trauma teams. They should be initially assessed in the emergency room via the ATLS guidelines. Their airways are of major importance and concern given the damage that has been done to the surrounding bone and soft tissue. The airway should be stabilized in the field by the paramedics if possible or in the trauma center upon arrival. Disruption of normal bony anatomy, lacerations, and bleeding all can contribute to difficulty obtaining a stable airway. Emergent cricoidotomy or tracheostomy should always be considered in patients with an unsecure airway that cannot be intubated.

Significant facial bleeding should be addressed early to assist with airway evaluation. Significant bleeding in the nasal and oral airways can make visualization impossible. Packing and pressure can help temporarily manage the bleeding until the airway has been secured. Catastrophic arterial hemorrhage from facial injuries is rare. When present, it is best managed by expeditious angiography and selective embolization. Slow, persistent venous bleeding or profuse epistaxis is best managed with direct packing. This can be definitively addressed later, in a more controlled environment, such as the operating room.

It is important for the trauma team to complete their primary and secondary surveys prior to obtaining further subspecialty consultation to rule out potential life-threatening injuries. The most important objective during the initial trauma intake is to determine the extent of the patient's injuries and prioritize their management in an expeditious manner. Once the trauma team has stabilized the patient, other specialties should be consulted for evaluation.

Although any number of the surgical specialties may need to assist with care, otolaryngology, ophthalmology, and neurosurgery are frequently included to assist in the management of the patient with a panfacial fracture. Otolaryngology is frequently needed to assist with the airway or stop significant nasal hemorrhage. Globe rupture, orbital apex syndrome, superior orbital fissure syndrome, and traumatic ophthalmoplegia can all be seen in patients with panfacial injuries. The ophthalmologist should be consulted on admission to perform a thorough exam and obtain a baseline visual test prior to any interventions. Neurosurgical evaluation should be obtained given the proximity of the brain and intracranial contents to the facial skeleton. Some report that up to 45.5 % of facial fractures are associated with head injuries. Any other significant injury should be assessed and evaluated by the appropriate specialty.

Work-Up

Once the primary and secondary ATLS surveys have been completed, and the trauma team has stabilized the patient, a detailed physical examination of the craniofacial region is performed. This includes a systematic approach performed in the same fashion every time so as to prevent any omissions. A top-down approach is generally recommended, starting with the scalp and heading down through the neck. This assessment should include examination of the cranial nerves (especially branches of trigeminal and facial nerve), visual acuity, occlusion, and general mobility of the midface. Scalp lacerations should be addressed early with suture repair so as to prevent significant blood loss during the trauma work-up. Loose dentition and foreign bodies should be removed from the oral cavity to prevent aspiration. Facial lacerations should be carefully inspected and copiously irrigated. If able, these injuries should be closed as soon as possible, either in the trauma bay or in the ICU. If the patient's condition is critical, and they need to go to the operating room, these injuries can be repaired while the patient is under anesthesia. Precise and careful documentation of any physical exam findings during the initial assessment is paramount. Extensive soft tissue trauma is managed by foreign body removal, copious irrigation, and removal of all grossly necrotic and nonviable tissue. These interventions may need to be accomplished over several operative settings to ensure adequate decontamination. Soft tissue lacerations that may be utilized as access points for skeletal reduction and fixation during surgery should be temporarily closed.

A thin-slice computer topography (CT) with three-dimensional reconstructions should be obtained of the head, face, and C spine. This can be done during the initial evaluation by the trauma team in anticipation of facial fractures. Axial, coronal, sagittal and 3D reconstructions should all be obtained to determine the extent of injury and the best surgical approach. Cervical spine clearance should be done by a certified person, either in the emergency room or once on the surgical floor. Reports have shown that up to 9.6 % of facial fractures are associated with cervical spine injuries. CT is the best radiographic modality to assess the patient's fracture pattern and help determine the best treatment course. This imaging modality will provide the surgeon with information regarding fracture patterns, bone quality, displacement, and comminution. It is extremely helpful in understanding the extent of injury during operative repair given the limited view the different surgical approaches provide.

Preoperative records, such as photographs or dental casts, are important to obtain to help the surgeon with the surgical planning. Photographs can be helpful if the fractures are so severe that there are few bony references from which to plan the reconstruction. Furthermore, dental impressions can be extremely important when attempting to restore preoperative dental occlusion in patients with severe maxillomandibular trauma. These things should be obtained from the family when available.

Management

The primary objective in the treatment of panfacial fractures is to safely restore the patient to their pre-injury state. Whether this objective can be achieved completely is dependent on the quality of the structures that have been damaged. There are a few important factors that need to be considered when preparing for these cases. They include timing of repair, airway management, surgical approaches, and operative sequencing. In addition, the basic tenets of surgical repair of facial fractures that have been established over the last 20 years must be strictly adhered to in order to achieve a successful outcome. These include wide exposure of fractures, rigid fixation of fractures from stable to unstable, restoration of facial buttresses, primary bone grafting for segmental defects, and soft tissue resuspension. Each of these points will be addressed to better clarify the operative management.

Timing

One of the first decisions that needs to be made before reconstructing a complex panfacial fracture is when is it appropriate to proceed with operative repair. A number of factors need to be considered. The date of the injury is important to know given the tendency for soft tissue swelling to occur, making dissection more difficult. Facial swelling is usually at its worst 2–3 days after injury, so planning operative repair outside this time frame is recommended to help improve visualization and facilitate repair.

Concomitant injuries should also be considered. As mentioned previously, panfacial fractures are associated with injuries to other parts of the body, both locally and regionally. These injuries should be evaluated and treated by other medical specialties prior to embarking on any surgical reconstruction. Patients should be medically stable and cleared by the treating specialties prior to proceeding with an operative repair. Furthermore, injuries involving the eyes or brain may need operative clearance from the treating specialties prior to surgical intervention. In rare instances, a brain or ocular injury is so severe that treating specialties recommend proceeding with operative repair of the surrounding structures given the risk for further damage. If this is the case, the timing is contingent on these other specialties.

Ideally, facial fractures should be repaired in the first 2–3 weeks. Massive soft tissue swelling is often associated with panfacial injuries. This acute, early swelling may preclude accurate anatomic reduction of fracture fragments. Delaying repair may be necessary in order for the soft tissue swelling to resolve. Further delay may lead to malunion of fracture fragments and contraction of the overlying soft tissue envelope. This makes reduction and fixation more difficult, oftentimes requiring osteotomies. Furthermore, the skin and soft tissue surrounding these fractures will scar over top of the displaced fracture segments. Given the propensity for the soft tissue envelope to contract after injury, if these fractures are not reduced expeditiously, the soft tissue will be more reluctant to return to its pre-injury state. The loss of facial envelope soft tissue laxity will lead to significant difficulty in skeletal fracture reduction and may lead to permanent deformity.

The timing of these repairs often needs to be done in combination with other treating specialties, such as the ophthalmologist or neurosurgeon. If this is the case, long periods of block operative time should be set aside to make it easier for the treating physicians to accomplish their goals. These procedures should be done in the daylight hours with a surgical team who is familiar with the care of facial fracture patients. Undertaking this type of fracture as an add-on case or with unfamiliar staff will result in a significant amount of frustration and poor results. Given the complexity of these cases, a large amount of operative time should be set aside to get all required portions of the case completed. Surgical team members should be given breaks if the procedure lasts greater than 4–6 h, to keep them fresh and ready to make important clinical decisions.

Airway Management

Panfacial fractures involve the bones surrounding the nasal and oral airways. This instability and loss of normal anatomic landmarks makes airway management more difficult. Furthermore, during reduction of fractures, these bones need to be readily visualized without the impendence of an endotracheal tube. A thorough discussion of airway management should be completed prior to any surgical intervention with the intensive care unit physicians as well as the anesthesiologist performing the case. Oftentimes, these patients have received an emergent tracheostomy given their difficult airway on presentation. This is an ideal method to control the airway in the preoperative period, and it can be removed after all acute issues have been addressed. If the patient is intubated, discussion regarding the need for a tracheostomy should be done to determine if this would be beneficial for any other medical problems, such as the need for prolonged intubation. Oral and nasal endotracheal tubes can be used, but they make the operative repair slightly more difficult and increase the risk for extubation during the surgery given their location. Many anesthesiologists will not perform nasal intubations with skull base fractures given the risks of intracranial injury. A third option is the submental intubation, in which the endotracheal tube is brought out in the midline, through the floor of the mouth, and secured into place. This method ensures the tube is away from the surgical field, while providing a secure airway. Whichever method is chosen, the surgeon should be responsible for securing the tube after placement given the amount of head manipulation that occurs during operative repair.

Surgical Approaches

Safely gaining access to the craniofacial skeleton is an important skill set, which should be mastered by any surgeon attempting to repair a complex facial fracture. The common incisions which are the same used for treating less complex facial fractures are often used in conjunction with others. Dissection is performed in a subperiosteal plane, to prevent injury to important facial structures but also to adequately visualize each fracture pattern and completely mobilize and reduce them. It is helpful to break these approaches down according to the areas of the facial skeleton which need to be addressed.

The upper face, including the forehead, supraorbital areas, lateral orbit, medial orbit, zygomatic arch, and naso-orbital-ethmoidal (NOE) areas can all be accessed safely through a coronal incision (Fig. 20.2). The incision extends from just superior to the non-hair-bearing skin above the ear, across the vertex of the scalp, to the same point on the opposite ear. This incision is usually done in a zigzag fashion to prevent unwanted parting once the patient's hair has grown back out. The head does not need to be completely shaved for this to happen, but rather a small strip of hair around the planned incision needs to be cut to make the incisions, closure, and postoperative care easier. The hair that is not cut should be placed in pigtails and bunched together so that it does not become a nuisance during the surgery.

The inferior orbital rim, orbital floor, lower medial orbital wall, and zygomatic body can be accessed through either a midlid (subtarsal incision) or a transconjunctival incision with a lateral canthotomy extension (Fig. 20.3). There are risks and benefits to each incision, and the proper choice depends on the surgeon's skill with either.

The maxilla, lower zygoma, medial and lateral maxillary buttresses, and piriform areas can all be accessed through an upper gingivobuccal sulcus incision. It is important for the surgeon to keep a healthy cuff of sliding gingiva during this approach to ensure watertight closure after the case is completed. This will help prevent plate exposure in the postoperative setting. This incision can be accomplished in one long continuous incision or split into two, with a bridge of gingiva right below the piriform sinus to preserve the ligamentous and muscular attachment to the maxillary crest. If the full incision is needed, an alar cinch suture should be performed to prevent postoperative alar widening.

The mandible can be approached through any combination of the common mandible fracture incisions. These include lower gingivobuccal sulcus incisions to gain access to the symphyseal, parasymphyseal, and mandibular body areas. The oblique ridge incision is used to expose the ramus, angle, posterior body, and low subcondylar areas. This incision along with a transbuccal trocar can be used to help reduce and fixate fractures in the posterior portion of the mandible. For severely comminuted ramus, angle and body fractures, a Risdon, submandibular, or retromandibular approach is usually recommended to ensure adequate reduction and fixation. If the subcondylar region needs to be addressed, a preauricular incision is often preferred to fully visualize these fracture segments and adequately address the loss in lower facial height.

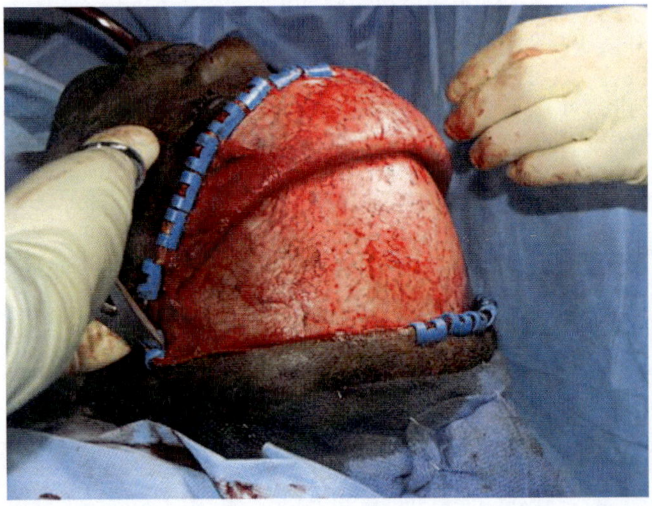

Fig. 20.2 Coronal incision provides access to the upper face

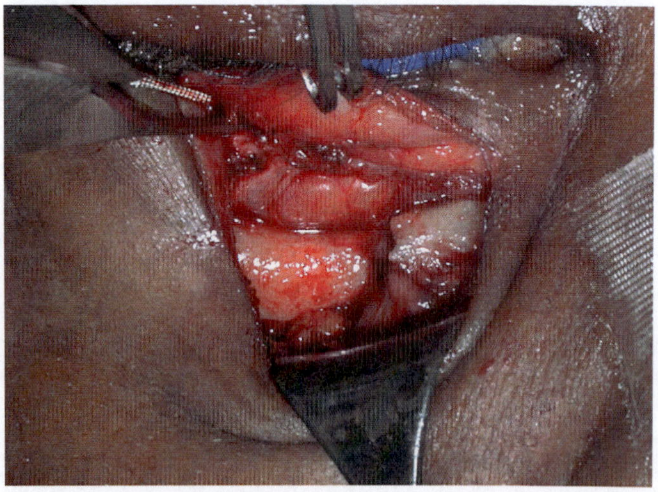

Fig. 20.3 A fractured inferior orbital rim is accessed through a midlid incision

Table 20.1 Commonly used incisions to access the facial skeleton

Surgical incision	Bony access
Coronal	Frontal bone; superior, medial, and lateral orbital rim; zygomatic arch and frontal process of the zygoma; temporal bone; and NOE unit
Lower eyelid	Orbital floor, inferior orbital rim, superior portion of the maxilla, and portions of the zygoma not visualized by the coronal incision
Superior intraoral buccal sulcus	Inferior portion of the maxilla at LeFort I level and body of the zygoma
Gingivobuccal sulcus	Mandible
Preauricular	Mandibular condyles
Submental	Anterior mandible and symphysis
Submandibular	Mandibular body and angle
Retromandibular	Posterior ramus of mandible

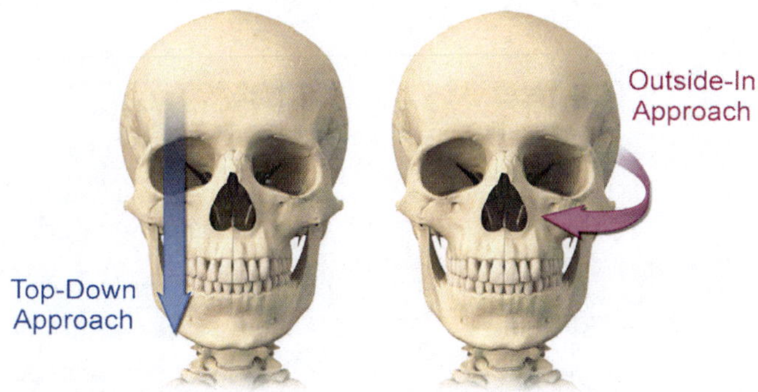

Fig. 20.4 Sequencing of top down and outside-in approach

None of these incisions is specific for panfacial fractures, but they all need to be utilized in order to gain adequate access to the fractures. Table 20.1 presents a summary of incisions and the facial areas they provide access to. Becoming familiar with these approaches is important to treating these injuries in a safe and efficient manner.

Operative Sequence

Because panfacial fractures include almost every bone in the facial skeleton, where to begin rigidly fixating the bone fragments is determined based on one of the operative principles of reconstructive surgery – stable to unstable bone. After the subperiosteal exposure has been completed and the involved fracture fragments have been mobilized, the choice of where to commence with fracture fixation needs to be made. There are two schools of thought regarding sequencing that have become popular over the past 30 years. The goal with either of these approaches is restoration of pre-injury anatomy, including facial fracture reduction, normal occlusion, and soft tissue resuspension. The different sequences are the outside-in approach and the subunit approach.

The outside-in approach is based upon reconstruction of the zygomas and frontal bar to establish an outer frame of the face (Fig. 20.4). Fracture reduction along the outside of the facial skeleton or at the cranial base ensures that the facial fractures are fixated to stable bone. This includes securing the fractures of the upper and medial orbits to the unfractured frontal bones and platting the ZMC fractures to unfractured zygomatic arches. If the zygomatic arches are fractured, then exposure needs to proceed to the temporal process of the zygomatic bone for stable fixation. It is important to understand the shape of the zygomatic arch when using this technique. This structure is a bit of a misnomer, since it does not arch as much as one would think. It actually remains straight until it attaches with the zygoma body, where it takes a gentle curve. Failure to recognize this aspect will result in an overarching zygomatic maxillary complex, loss of facial projection, and excessive facial width. Starting with the zygomatic arches for reconstruction provides the facial width. In untreated panfacial fractures, a "widened" facial appearance and a loss of facial projection is seen. This so-called "dish face" appearance is extremely difficult to correct secondarily given the malunion of bone fragments and loss of soft tissue elasticity. To facilitate three-dimensional reduction of the zygomatic complex, the lateral sidewall of the orbit (zygomaticosphenoid suture) should be used as a bony landmark when intact. However, care should be taken to avoid incorrectly reducing the ZMC anteriorly to a depressed and malpositioned NOE complex. The NOE complex is then reduced with restoration of upper facial width. To achieve correct interorbital distance, an overcorrected reduction of the medial orbital rims may be necessary. The ZMC is then reduced to the anatomically repositioned NOE complexes. Proper positioning of the ZMC helps ensure proper restoration of orbital volume as well. Ultimately, the surgeon must rely on previous experience and judgment regarding the best adjacent bone to use for reduction and fixation of the zygomatic complex for complex panfacial fractures. The rest of the reconstruction can proceed using these stable landmarks to set facial width, projection, and height. This is accomplished by paying specific attention to the facial buttresses (Fig. 20.5). The lower midface at the LeFort I level is then reduced and fixated to the stable, reconstructed upper midface. Mandible reconstruction follows lower midface reconstruction after restoration of occlusion and placement of patient into maxillomandibular fixation.

The subunit method of operative sequencing divides the midface into two halves, an upper and a lower half, separated at the LeFort I level. The lower midface consists of the maxilla, palate, and maxillary arch. The upper midface is made up of the orbits, frontal bone, zygomas, NOE, and anterior

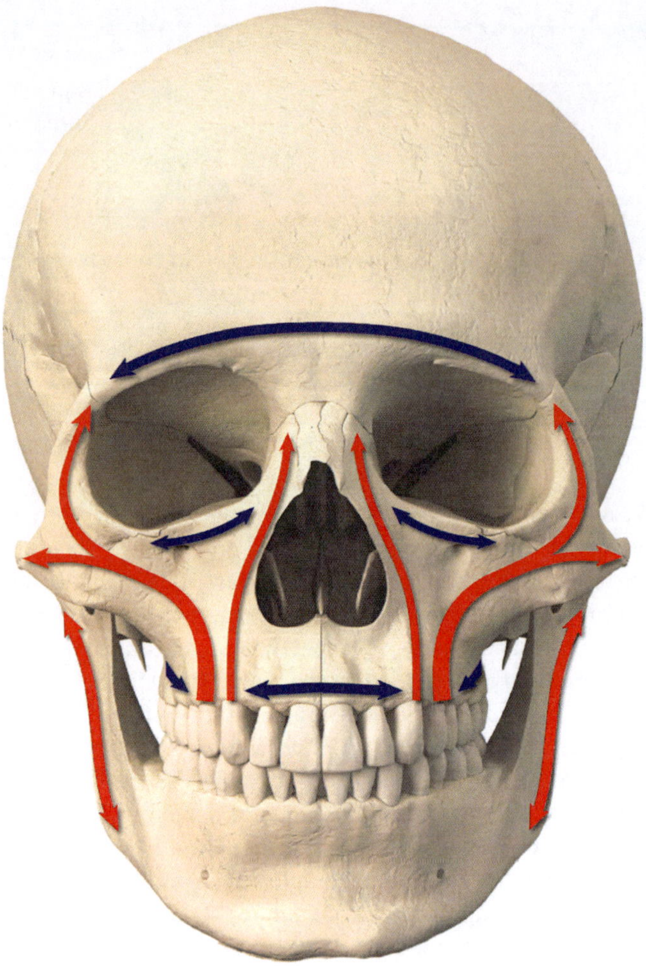

Fig. 20.5 Vertical (*red*) and transverse (*blue*) buttresses are integral to the function and form of the face

temporal bones. This allows the two halves to be reconstructed independently of one another. The lower midface uses the mandible to establish occlusion and its dimensions, while the upper midface uses the frontal bone as its reference for reconstruction. The mandible and the frontal bone make adequate scaffolds for repair of the subunits as both can be rebuilt based upon the skull base. Once these halves are reconstructed and fixated to their respective anchors, they can then be fixated to one another along the vertical buttresses. Addressing the lower midface requires reconstructing the mandible first, to help establish normal occlusion.

Careful positioning of the condyle in the glenoid fossa is required. Assuming the skull base is intact, positioning of the condyles in the mandibular fossa will provide the surgeon with a blueprint for reestablishing posterior facial height. This may be more challenging in patients with associated displaced subcondylar fractures with vertical shortening. In these instances, an open approach with open reduction and internal fixation of subcondylar fracture may be required. Once subcondylar fractures have been repaired and the condyles appropriately seated, mandibular fracture reduction and fixation may be performed. The height and position of the lower midface will then be determined through occlusion of the maxilla with the reconstructed mandible. Plating and fixation of the body, angle, and symphyseal and parasymphyseal regions determines the lower facial width. Facial height and projection are established with repair of the condyles and the ramus. Once the maxillomandibular unit has been repaired and fixated, surgeons will typically proceed with repair of the calvarium followed by the upper midface.

Occlusion

Restoration of occlusion is one of the primary goals of panfacial fracture repair. Given the extent of damage, both dental arches are often disrupted, making restoration of normal occlusion extremely difficult. If one of the dental arches is intact, this will assist the surgeon in establishing proper occlusion. If both dental arches are disrupted, then proper restoration of one arch dictates the repair of the second. It is beneficial for the surgeon to use the arch which is less severe to accomplish this. Alternatively, utilizing pre-injury dental records and impressions is extremely helpful. An occlusal splint can be fashioned to assist the reduction of the fracture segments according to the dental relationship. These are not always available, and oftentimes the surgeon needs to use their clinical judgment and anatomic landmarks intraoperatively.

Preferred Approach

Each panfacial fracture is unique in its own way and should be treated with care and precision during all stages of care. All steps as mentioned in the previous section should be followed to ensure the patient is safe for surgery. Once in the operating room, the airway is secured using either a tracheostomy or a submental intubation to remove this obstruction from the operative field. This tube is secured in place with 2.0 silk sutures so that it is not accidently removed during surgery due to excessive head manipulation. The patient is placed in a supine position with a shoulder to provide for slight neck extension. The eyes are protected with corneal protectors, and the head is shaved in preparation for a coronal incision. For women, the head is shaved only where the incision is made, and the hair is braided and bound together to provide for easy prepping and prevent it from getting in the way during the case. Local anesthetic with epinephrine is injected into the planned out incisions to help with hemostasis during the multiple approaches. The 3D CT scan is

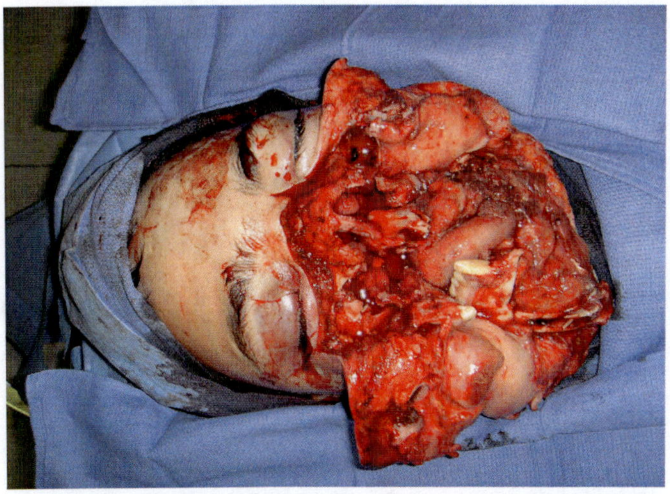

Fig. 20.6 Wide exposure of panfacial fracture using extension of existing soft tissue defects (This defect was a result of a gunshot wound)

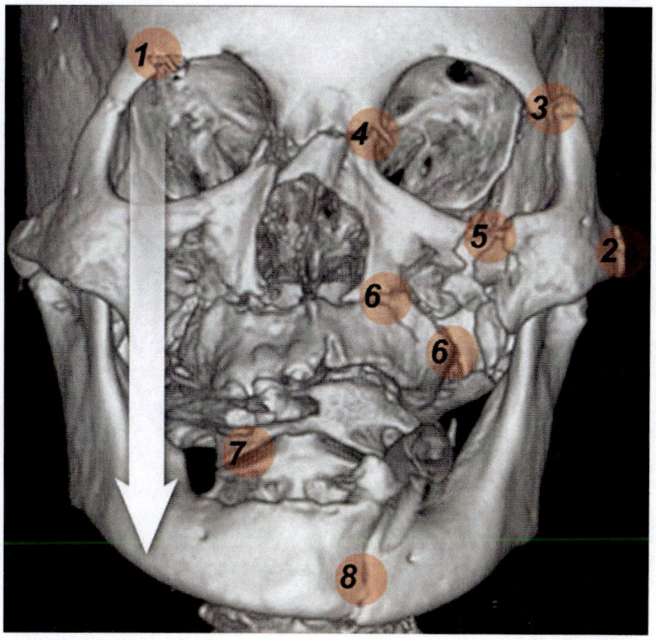

Fig. 20.7 Panfacial fracture with general sequence of fracture fixation

present in the room to help the surgeon with navigation of the fractures during the exposure and reduction. Arch bars are placed prior to beginning the exposure in preparation for maxillomandibular fixation. All approaches are performed wide, in a subperiosteal fashion, to expose each fracture thoroughly. Use existing soft tissue defects to access the facial skeleton when possible (Fig. 20.6). Callus needs to be removed from the fracture sites to facilitate mobilization.

The bicoronal incisions are usually performed first since they require the most time and care around the level of the frontal branch of the facial nerve. Whether the zygomatic arch needs to be dissected out determines the level of dissection around the temporalis muscle. If the arch needs to be exposed, dissection of the deep temporal fascia of the temporal nerve is performed. The surgeon can guarantee they are within this plane and completely below the superficial temporal fascia by using an Adson pickup to make sure all of the loose areolar tissue of the superficial temporal fascia is cleaned off the shiny, tough deep temporal fascia.

Once the bicoronal incision has been performed, the entire upper face should be accessible, including the zygomatic arches. The fracture pattern will dictate which areas of the facial skeleton need to be exposed. Next, the eyelid incisions are made to expose the midface. These are performed through transconjunctival or midlid incisions. The midlid incision is preferred because it gives the surgeon the ability to visualize the entire inferior orbital rim, lateral orbital rim, zygomatic body, and orbital floor. The upper gingival buccal sulcus incisions are performed next to expose the maxilla, and then the necessary mandibular incisions are performed to expose these fractures.

Once all exposure has been completed, the outside-in and top-down approach from the cranial base is the sequence used for fracture fixation (Figs. 20.4 and 20.7). This begins with the reduction of the zygomatic arches, as this sets the facial width. The treating surgeon needs to have detailed and comprehensive understanding of the craniofacial skeleton in all three dimensions, including facial width, height, and projection. The principles of reconstruction for all facial fractures are the same regardless of surgical sequence. Reestablishment of the paired facial buttresses with rigid fixation, restoration of pre-injury occlusion, and resuspension of soft tissue are integral components to any panfacial fracture. Care to plate the arches in a straight configuration and not in an exaggerated bow will prevent the face from being plated too wide.

Surgical repair should begin on the side with the least comminution. This will help establish a facial frame that will serve as a reference for repair of the contralateral side. The arches are then fixated to the frontal bone via plating across the frontozygomatic sutures. The frontal bone is generally intact given its inherent strength and creates a stable fixation point. Fixation to the most stable bone is a key principle in fracture stabilization for panfacial fractures. Next, one should reduce and fixate the NOE and orbital rims proceeding from the zygomatic arches. Trans-nasal wire canthopexy is required to treat posttraumatic telecanthus. Reduction of the NOE and orbital rims will recreate the upper portions of the lateral maxillary and medial maxillary vertical buttresses, along with the upper transverse maxillary buttress.

If the frontal bone is fractured, repair of the frontal bone should precede facial fracture repair. A neurosurgeon may have to be present to help address the frontal sinus if injured.

Frontal bone craniotomies with cranialization are often required. The plastic surgeon has the ability to assist the neurosurgeon obtain a near-watertight closure of the dura and obliterate the frontal sinus by elevating a pericranial flap during elevation of the bicoronal flap. This should always be considered during the preoperative plan.

Once the frontal bone has been addressed and reduced to the stable cranium, the NOE segments are addressed. They are done in conjunction with the ZMC complex. This portion of the procedure requires attention to the anatomic landmarks and requires the surgeon to adequately restore the facial projection. There is a tendency for facial fractures to sink into the midface. The surgeon should be aware of this and attempt to restore preoperative anatomy by correcting for this projection. In extreme cases, this will involve plates that are bent to include the frontal bone and extend to the infraorbital rim along the medial maxillary buttress. These plates should be bent ex vivo and placed through the previous incisions to restore preoperative anatomy. If there is severe comminution in the NOE and maxillary areas, sterilizing a skeleton and bending the plate according this anatomy is helpful. If there is segmental loss of bone in the NOE or maxillary areas, a split cranial bone graft can be harvested from the nondominant parietal bone areas to reconstruct these segmental defects (Fig. 20.8). Any bony gap greater than 3–5 mm will require a bone graft as well. A split rib graft or split calvarial graft in a cantilever fashion may be required to restore projection and definition of nasal dorsum.

The midface, including the maxillary arch, is reconstructed through the gingival buccal sulcus incisions via plates along the medial and lateral maxillary buttresses. These plates are usually 2.0 mm in thickness and help reposition the maxillary arch. Repair of these buttresses will help establish the dimensions of the face.

Once the width of the maxilla has been set, in relation to the vertical buttresses, reestablishment of occlusion of the maxillomandibular unit is undertaken. The mandible is reconstructed using the repaired maxilla as a template for repair. When plating symphyseal and body fractures, care must be taken to apply pressure at the angles bilaterally to prevent widening of the mandible relative to the repaired maxillary segment. Open reduction and fixation is necessary for any subcondylar fractures.

This reconstruction should be done with consideration of the mandibular arch. If the mandible is not severely comminuted, it may be more beneficial to attempt to reduce this prior to plating the maxilla to help establish the normal dental arch. If the maxilla is less comminuted than the mandible, the maxilla should be reconstructed first to help dictate the proper

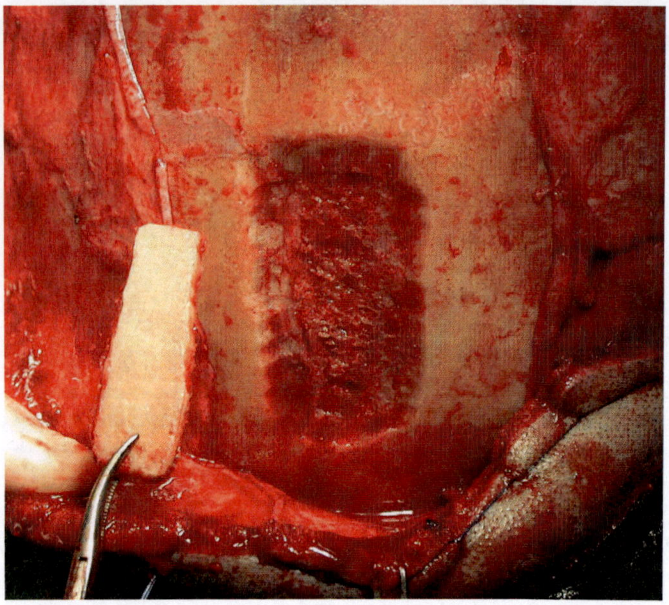

Fig. 20.8 Harvesting of a split calvarial bone graft that can be used to replace bony defects

occlusion. This is where the use of arch bars and occlusion becomes important during fracture reduction. With edentulous patients, this advantage is not available, so bony landmarks need to be followed. If there are bilateral subcondylar fractures, at least one of these needs to be opened, reduced, and plated to reconstruct the posterior facial height. Once the facial buttresses have been rigidly fixed with the appropriate strength plates, the jaws are usually wired shut for a period of 2–3 weeks to allow for bony healing (Fig. 20.9). A throat pack, if used, needs to be removed prior to placing the patient into maxillomandibular fixation.

The orbital walls are then addressed, including the orbital floor and medial orbital walls. Stable medial and posterior ledges should be identified and either autologous or allogenic material is used for reconstruction. Care must be taken not to put too much pressure on the globe during this dissection to prevent ocular injury. Using the oculocardiac reflex can be helpful in knowing if your dissection has created too much pressure on the eye. After placement of the implant, orbital mobility should be checked with a forced duction test, and orbital pressure should be evaluated by examining the reactivity of the pupil. Medpor with a titanium inlay is normally used for these patients, given its convenience and ease of use.

All incisions should be irrigated copiously with antibiotic solution. The incisions are then closed in a sequential pattern. Prior to skin closure, the facial soft tissues should be

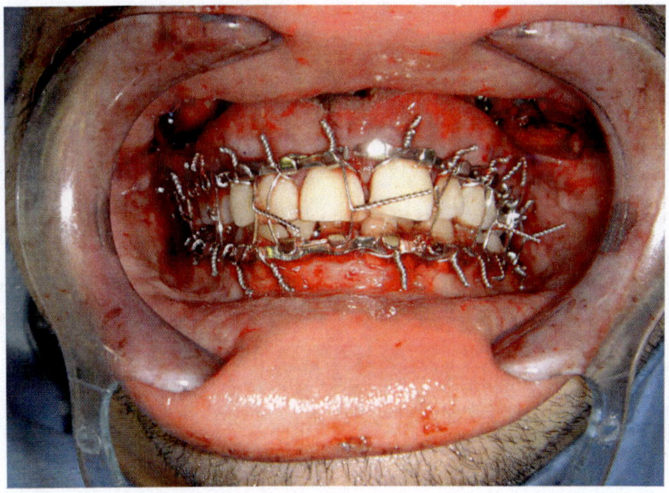

Fig. 20.9 Wiring for intermaxillary fixation

resuspended according to the osteocutaneous ligaments that were dissected off the face. If this is not done, the face will heal with soft tissue ptosis and give the patient an older appearance. Most importantly, the cheeks are resuspended to the infraorbital rims. This can be done by securing the periosteum of the midface to the orbital rim plate or to separate holes drilled in the orbital rims. Once the incisions are closed, the patient is transferred to the intensive care unit for postoperative monitoring. Serial eye exams should be performed when the patient is awake to ensure injury did not occur during repair or there is no pressure on the globe after the reconstruction. Head of the bed should be elevated and intraoperative steroids are often used to help with postoperative swelling.

Conclusion

Panfacial fractures are some of the most difficult injuries to successfully reconstruct in cranio-maxillofacial surgery. Successful outcomes require rigorous planning, flexible thinking, and meticulous surgical technique. Careful, thoughtful sequencing of the repair working from stable to unstable bone is paramount. Always keep in mind the overriding goals of restoration of pre-injury occlusion, orbital volume, facial width, projection, and height.

Bibliography

Buchanan EP, Hopper RA, Suver DW, et al. Zygomaticomaxillary complex fractures and their association with naso-orbito-ethmoid fractures: a 5-year review. Plast Reconstr Surg. 2012;130(6):1296–304.

Erdmann D, Follmar KE, Debruijn M, et al. Concomitant injuries in patients with pan-facial fractures. J Trauma. 2007;63(4):831–5.

Follmar KE, DeBruijn M, Baccarani A, Bruno AD, Mukundan S, Erdmann D. Concomitant injuries in patients with panfacial fractures. J Trauma. 2007;63(4):831–5.

Gruss JS, Van Wyck L, Phillips JH, Antonshyn O. The importance of the zygomatic arch in complex midfacial fracture repair and correction of posttraumatic orbitozygomatic deformities. Plast Reconstr Surg. 1990;85:878–90.

Gruss JS, Bubak PJ, Egbert MA. Craniofacial fractures: an algorithm to optimize results. Clin Plast Surg. 1992;19:195–206.

Guymon M, Crosby DR, Wolford LM. The alar base cinch suture to control nasal width in maxillary osteotomies. Int J Adult Orthodon Orthognath Surg. 1988;3:89–95.

Hopper RA, Salemy S, Sze RW. Diagnosis of midface fractures with CT: what the surgeon needs to know. Radiographics. 2006;26:783–93.

Jack JM, Stewart DH, Rinker BD, Vasconez HC, Pu LL. Modern surgical treatment of complex facial fractures: a 6-year review. J Craniofac Surg. 2005;16(4):726–31.

Kelly KJ, Manson PN, Vander Kolk CA, et al. Sequencing Lefort fracture treatment (organization of treatment for a pan-facial fracture). J Craniofac Surg. 1990;1(4):168–78.

Manson PN, Clark N, Robertson B, et al. Subunit principles in midface fractures: the importance of sagittal buttresses, soft-tissue reductions and sequencing treatment of segmental fractures. Plast Reconstr Surg. 1999;103(4):1287–307.

Markowitz BL, Manson PN. Panfacial fractures: organization of treatment. Clin Plast Surg. 1989;16:105–14.

Mithani SK, St.-Hilaire H, Brooke BS, Smith IM, Bluebond-Langner R, Rodriguez ED. Predictable patterns of intracranial and cervical spine injury in craniomaxillofacial trauma: analysis of 4786 patients. Plast Reconstr Surg. 2009;123(4):1293–301.

Phillips JH, Forrest CR, Gruss JS. Current concepts in the use of bone grafts in facial fractures. Basic science considerations. Clin Plast Surg. 1992;19:41–58.

Roden KS, Tong W, Surrusco M, Shockley WW, Van Aalst JA, Hultman CS. Changing characteristics of facial fractures treated at a regional, level 1 trauma center, from 2005 to 2010: an assessment of patient demographics, referral patterns, etiology of injury, anatomic location, and clinical outcomes. Ann Plast Surg. 2012;68(5):461–6.

Stacey DH, Doyle JF, Gutowski KA. Safety device use affects the incidence patterns of facial trauma in motor vehicle collisions: an analysis of the national trauma database from 2000–2004. Plast Reconstr Surg. 2008;121(6):2057–5064.

Wenig BL. Management of pan-facial fractures. Otolaryngol Clin North Am. 1991;24(1):93–101.

Gunshot Wounds

21

Brent R. DeGeorge Jr. and Kant Y. Lin

Introduction

There is perhaps no greater challenge to the skills and imagination of the reconstructive surgeon than in the management of severe gunshot wounds to the face and neck region. The complexity of the soft tissue injury in combination with the oftentimes massive damage to the underlying bone architecture, resulting from the destructive energy imparted by the penetrating projectile, creates a unique form of injury. Blast wound effects with an evolving zone of injury, pulverized or frankly missing tissue, and exsanguinating hemorrhage in the immediate time frame, coupled with severe and unremitting scar contracture in the long term, make successful reconstruction rare and difficult to obtain. A thorough understanding of ballistics, kinetic energy effects on soft tissue, three-dimensional anatomy, and tissue response to injury during the healing phase is essential if the reconstructive surgeon is to have any chance of a successful repair. As daunting as the physical injury may seem, ultimate success sometimes can only be achieved when the psychic healing is addressed, as the majority of the most devastating injuries are self-inflicted. In the following chapter, we will outline the key elements and principles in the management and reconstruction of gunshot wounds to the face and neck region, as a guide to help the reconstructive surgeon manage these very complex injuries.

B.R. DeGeorge Jr., MD, PhD
Department of Plastic Surgery,
University of Virginia School of Medicine,
Charlottesville, VA, USA

K.Y. Lin, MD (✉)
Department of Plastic Surgery,
University of Virginia Health System,
Charlottesville, VA, USA
e-mail: kyl5s@hscmail.mcc.virginia.edu

Epidemiology of Gunshot Wounds

Firearm-related injuries are among the top 15 leading causes of death in the USA and among the top 10 causes of accidental death [http://www.cdc.gov/traumaticbraininjury/]. According to the most recent data available from the Centers for Disease Control, firearms account for 31,224 fatalities, and for every fatality, there are three nonfatal gunshot injuries [http://webappa.cdc.gov/]. Of the fatal firearm-related injuries in 2007, homicides and suicides were the most common intention of injury, accounting for 12,983 and 17,352 deaths, respectively. Of the nonfatal firearm-related injuries, violence-related injuries and suicide attempts accounted for 80.7 and 6.3 % of injuries, respectively. Firearm-related injuries most commonly involve men, and males account for 86.6 % of fatalities and 89.5 % of nonfatal gunshot-related deaths and injuries, respectively. Firearm-related fatalities are most commonly perpetrated by males aged 20–24; rates were highest among non-Hispanic black males. Gunshot wounds to the head are associated with the highest overall mortality, approximately 75–80 %. Kaufmann et al. estimated that over 90 % of gunshot wounds to the head are ultimately fatal, and two-thirds of these injuries result in mortality at the scene. Indicators of poor ultimate outcome include the following at initial presentation: Glasgow Coma Scale <5, nonreactive pupils, metabolic or lactic acidosis, hypotension, self-inflicted mechanism, and CT pattern consistent with severe intracranial injury. Significant morbidity in the form of cognitive and behavioral impairment, blindness, seizures, and motor dysfunction are commonplace following nonfatal gunshot wounds to the head. Beyond the morbidity and mortality, firearm-related injuries pose a major financial burden on our healthcare system. Cook et al. estimated the cost of acute hospital management of firearm-related nonfatal injuries at approximately $35,000. However, given both the incidence of gunshot wounds in the USA as well as the need for long-term medical care following injury, nonfatal firearm-related injuries account for over $16.2 billion dollars in annual medical costs.

P.J. Taub et al. (eds.), *Ferraro's Fundamentals of Maxillofacial Surgery*,
DOI 10.1007/978-1-4614-8341-0_21, © Springer Science+Business Media New York 2015

Physical Principles of Gunshot Wounds

Gunshot wounds to the face and neck involve varying degrees of soft tissue and bone injury as well as loss, and the degree of total injury is not always apparent on initial evaluation. An understanding of ballistics, the study of the physical principles of a projectile's flight path through space, is required for accurate diagnosis and management of these devastating injuries. Ballistics can broadly be so classified into three main categories: *internal ballistics* deals with the flight of a projectile through the barrel of a gun, *external ballistics* deals with the flight of a projectile through space, and *terminal ballistics* involves the flight of a projectile through its ultimate target. Internal ballistics investigates the interaction of the projectile with the firing chamber and gun barrel, and key concepts in this field are *rifling* and *jacketing*. Rifling refers to the presence of helical grooves in the barrel of a firearm, which impart spin to the projectile to improve aerodynamic stability, accuracy, and reduce drag. Jacketing refers to coating the surface area of the projectile with metal, often copper or nickel alloys, which decreases intra-chamber losses of velocity due to friction and ultimately increases the kinetic energy of the projectile. *Yaw* is a core characteristic of external ballistics and refers to the differential angle of the projectile's flight path with the long axis of the projectile itself. Increasing yaw decreases the aerodynamic stability of the projectile and ultimately increases drag force which acts to reduce the velocity of the projectile in space. Terminal ballistics examines the interaction of a projectile with body tissues and ultimately dictates the degree of traumatic injury following gunshot injury.

Several factors influence the wounding capacity of a gunshot injury, including the physical properties of the projectile, the kinetic energy of the projectile, and the projectile–tissue interaction. The composition of the projectile, its rotational and tumbling velocity, and the diameter and shape of its presenting surface are key determinants in the degree of trauma generated by the projectile. The kinetic energy (KE) of a projectile is described by the equation $KE = 1/2MV^2$, where M represents the projectile's mass and V represents the projectile's velocity. In this relationship, it is apparent that if one were to double the mass of the projectile, the result kinetic energy would be doubled; however, doubling the velocity of the projectile squares the ultimate kinetic energy generated.

The degree of soft tissue and bone injury is determined by the interaction of the projectile with body tissues. Following contact with target tissues, the projectile is deflected, and the immediate pathway of the projectile forms a *permanent cavity*, a finite zone of localized cellular necrosis and tissue cavitation. This is surrounded by a *temporary cavity*, formed by the radially directed distribution of kinetic energy from the projectile which results in displacement of the surrounding tissues. The degree of deflection of the projectile, termed *yaw*, is determined largely by the density and viscoelastic properties of the tissue encountered which imparts frictional or drag force onto the projectile. The drag force increases as the yaw angle approaches a perpendicular orientation to the path of the projectile, which subsequently increases the kinetic energy delivered to the surrounding tissues. This acts to decrease the penetration of the projectile and increase the size of the permanent cavity. The displaced tissues surrounding the permanent cavity contract under negative pressure, potentially drawing in debris and tissue fragments into the permanent cavity. Dense tissues, such as bone, teeth, and cartilage, often fracture in response to projectile entry, and these fracture fragments may generate secondary projectiles which further injure local tissues. For low-velocity projectiles, the entrance wound is typically similar in size to the projectile; however, due to projectile deflection, drag, and secondary projectile formation, the exit wound is typically larger than the entrance wound. If the muzzle of the firearm is in close proximity to the skin upon firing, blast injury will be produced, in which particulates and gases expelled from the firearm directly damage surrounding tissue at the entrance site and increase the size of soft tissue damage at the entrance site. For low-velocity injuries, the zone of injury typically includes both soft tissue and bone; however, significant degrees of soft tissue and bone loss are generally reserved for high-velocity projectile injuries.

Classification of Firearms

Firearms can be broadly classified into three main categories based on the projectile velocity as well as the kinetic energy imparted by the projectile, namely, low-velocity, medium-velocity, and high-velocity firearms. In general, low-velocity firearms generate projectiles of limited mass which typically travel at speeds less than 1,200 ft/s, medium-velocity firearms generate projectiles which travel between 1,200 and 2,000 ft/s, and high-velocity projectiles are typically greater than 2,000 ft/s. Low-velocity firearms include most civilian handguns, whereas high-velocity firearms include hunting and military rifles. Shotguns are typically classified as medium-velocity firearms; however, at close range they can deliver a large mass of pellets over a small distribution of area causing significant tissue damage.

Additionally, firearms and their ammunition can be classified by caliber. *Caliber* refers to the inner diameter of the firearm bore and is typically expressed in fractions of an inch or in millimeters. For example, a .357 Magnum round corresponds to a 0.357-in. or a 9-mm projectile diameter. With respect to shotguns, the internal diameter of the shotgun barrel is referred to as its *gauge* – the larger the gauge of the shotgun, the smaller the internal diameter of the barrel.

Initial Management of Gunshot Wounds

The acute nonsurgical management of gunshot wounds to the face is dictated by the principles of Advanced Trauma Life Support (ATLS) protocols for the trauma patient, including a focused primary survey to assess airway patency and cervical spine stabilization, breathing and ventilation, circulation with hemorrhage control, neurologic disability, and exposure control. This is followed by a secondary survey, including a complete history and head-to-toe physical examination. Airway management is of paramount importance in any trauma scenario. However, following penetrating trauma to the head, face, and neck region, airway patency can be compromised by direct structural injury to the airway; aspiration of soft tissue, bone, and teeth; and/or significant bleeding. In addition, loss of structural support to the tongue and the floor of mouth secondary to fractures of the mandible and maxillofacial skeleton as well as soft tissue swelling may further complicate supraglottic airway management. Therefore, the threshold for securing a definitive airway should be low, and any evidence of apnea, respiratory distress, airway obstruction, depressed level of consciousness, or persistent hypotension should prompt endotracheal intubation or surgical airway management. In a retrospective analysis of 78 craniofacial gunshot wounds, penetrating injuries to the mandible more commonly required emergent airway management (50 %) compared with injuries to the maxillofacial skeleton (25 %). Although cricothyroidectomy or tracheostomy is not required in the urgent setting in the majority of patients (>80 %), approximately 1/3 of patients will ultimately require tracheostomy during their acute hospital admission. Cervical spine precautions must be maintained until cleared both radiographically and by physical examination as concomitant spine fractures can be present. Due to the rich vascular supply in the head and neck region, significant bleeding following penetrating injuries is often encountered. If hemostasis cannot be achieved through focused direct pressure or packing, angiography with selective embolization may be pursued through interventional radiology in the hemodynamically stable patient or through operative exploration in the hemodynamically unstable patient. In the craniofacial trauma patient with significant blood loss, underlying coagulopathy, acidosis, and hypothermia must be identified and promptly corrected. The presence of penetrating trauma to the face requires a thorough neurologic examination, including Glasgow Coma Scale (GCS), cranial nerve evaluation with careful evaluation of pupillary function, visual acuity, extraocular movement, globe and ocular adnexal structural integrity, gross motor and sensory function, and a complete evaluation of the cervical thoracic and lumbar spines for evidence of tenderness, step-offs, malalignment, or deformities. Petridis and colleagues identified several neurologic factors predictive of increased mortality following gunshot wounds to the head, including GCS 3–8, bilateral nonreactive pupils, elevated intracranial pressure greater than 45 mmHg, or radiographic imaging consistent with greater than 10 mm of midline shift of the brain, greater than two cranial bone fragments, or involvement of greater than two brain lobes, the brainstem, or ventricular system. The trajectory of the projectile should be evaluated by physical examination if possible, as a pathway crossing the midline, bi-hemispheric involvement, or extracranial brain tissue all portend a worse prognosis. The location of the entrance wound is also predictive of intracranial injury. Kihtir et al. demonstrated that no patient with an injury to the lower face had evidence of intracranial injury compared with one-third of patients with an entrance wound in the mid- to upper face. Intracranial gunshot wounds mandate neurosurgical consultation to assess indications for ICP monitoring, intracranial decompression, or intracranial wound debridement. Direct palpation of the upper, middle, and lower face should be performed to identify mobile bone fragments, step-offs, or deformities, including an intraoral examination to evaluate for exposed bone fragments, foreign bodies, loose or missing teeth, and the status of occlusion. Projectile trajectories at the level of the lower face or below should raise concern regarding injury to the great vessels in the neck as well as the larynx, trachea, and esophagus – fiber-optic panendoscopy is typically warranted following initial nonoperative stabilization. In general, gunshot wounds to the head are classified as contaminated wounds due to associated damage to the oral and nasal cavities as well as the sinuses; therefore, intravenous antimicrobial prophylaxis providing coverage for cutaneous flora and oral and sinusoidal anaerobes is typically recommended upon arrival. Tetanus prophylaxis should also be administered as appropriate.

Radiographic Evaluation of Penetrating Facial Trauma

Physical examination in the evaluation of craniofacial trauma is hindered by the presence of abrasions and lacerations, soft tissue swelling, and the patient's inability to cooperate due to pain, level of consciousness, or both. Plain radiographs were once considered essential to this evaluation. However, with the evolution of imaging technology, plain radiographs are now thought of as incapable of providing sufficiently detailed information regarding bone injury severity and displacement to be useful for definitive operative planning. Computerized tomography (CT) is currently considered the gold standard for the evaluation of craniofacial trauma, and CT of the head is routinely performed as an adjunct to the initial trauma evaluation to rule out intracranial injury in the presence of facial trauma. Modern multi-detector CT scanners possess excellent spatial resolution characteristics and allow for multi-planar reformatting, in axial, coronal, and sagittal planes, as well as three-dimensional reconstructions for improved diagnostic accuracy and operative planning. CT images must be obtained from the level of the apex of the frontal sinus to the level of the hyoid bone for the evaluation of maxillofacial trauma with images acquired in 1-mm axial sections. 2-D axial CT imaging is more sensitive for the detection of craniofacial fractures; however, 3-D reconstructions assist in the visualization of complex, displaced multi-planar facial fractures, particularly in the zygomatico-maxillary complex and in the naso-orbito-ethmoid complex. For injuries to the lower face, helical CT has now been shown to have superior sensitivity to panoramic tomography in the diagnosis of mandibular fractures. Nevertheless, Panorex x-rays continue to play an important role in operative management of mandibular fractures. Panoramic tomography is still recommended as part of the complete evaluation of the dentition in the line of mandibular fractures and bone loss to assess for dental root involvement. The role of angiography in the setting of penetrating trauma to the neck is well defined. However, its role in the setting of penetrating trauma to the face is unclear, and data supporting its diagnostic and therapeutic efficacy are largely confined to small case reports and case series. Various trauma centers throughout the country perform diagnostic angiography following penetrating trauma to the face and neck. Kihtir et al. reported performing diagnostic angiography in 35 % of patients with gunshot wounds to the face, and in one-third of these patients, a vascular injury was identified. The most common indication for performing diagnostic angiography was missile trajectory where vascular injury is suspected. The most common sites of facial bleeding following penetrating trauma to the face are terminal branches of the external carotid artery – in order of incidence: the maxillary artery followed by the facial and superficial temporal arteries, respectively. These facial vessels are accessible with super-selective embolization performed in stable patients by interventional radiology, providing both diagnostic information and potential therapeutic embolization using coils, PDA foam, gel foam, or other adjuncts. Further clinical investigation will be required before therapeutic application of head and neck angiography can be recommended for penetrating trauma to the face or for acute facial hemorrhage not amenable to standard local control measures.

Classification of Gunshot Wounds to the Face

Several classification schemes for craniofacial penetrating trauma have been developed in the past three decades utilizing anatomic location, degree of soft tissue and bony involvement, and overall severity of trauma in order to better guide operative decision-making. In 1996, Clark et al. described their 17-year experience with 250 civilian handgun, 53 close-range shotgun, and 15 high-energy ballistic injuries to the face at the University of Maryland Shock Trauma Center. Their classification system was based on the anatomic pattern of injury and the ballistic profile of the projectile. Anatomic patterns of injury arose from the projectile path and the zone of tissue damage, both soft tissue *injury* and *loss*, as well as by the components damaged. The ballistic profiles of projectiles were divided into three categories based on the mass and velocity of the projectile, namely, low velocity, intermediate velocity, or high velocity. In their classification schema, low-velocity wounds were best characterized by the location of the exit wound, whereas shotgun and high-energy ballistic injuries were classified by the zone of soft tissue and bone injury and loss. Civilian gunshot wounds to the face were categorized into four general anatomic patterns of involvement: type I, lower face involvement; type II, midface involvement; type III, orbital involvement; and type IV, frontal–cranial involvement. These accounted for 15, 14, 9, and 49 % of the gunshot wounds, respectively, with 24 % of the wounds involving more than one region. Shotgun wounds were characterized by the degree of soft tissue and bone loss, including the lateral mandible, the central face, the lateral midface and orbit, and the lateral cranium and orbit, which accounted for 34, 26, 28, and 11 % of the wounding patterns, respectively. The anatomic pattern of injury for high-energy avulsion wounds were also classified based on the degree of soft tissue and bone loss, namely, the mandible alone, the mandible and maxilla, and the mandible, maxilla, and orbit combined, accounting for 27, 27, and 47 % of the injuries, respectively.

Based on these data, an algorithm for the management of facial gunshot injuries was developed. First, the ballistic profile should be categorized to predict the degree of soft tissue and bone injury. Next, classification of regional anatomic involvement, i.e., cranial, orbital, midface, or mandible, should be accounted. The respective contribution of soft tissue and bone injury and loss in each of these regions should then be estimated. The authors conclude that civilian low-velocity handgun injuries were not associated with significant degrees of soft tissue and bone loss and thus could be managed as facial fractures with overlying lacerations amenable to immediate definitive reconstruction. Intermediate and high-velocity gunshot wounds were associated with a significant degree of soft tissue and bone loss with a higher potential for evolving tissue necrosis. Therefore, these would be best managed by immediate operative stabilization of remaining bone with primary closure of remaining soft tissue. Serial debridement procedures would then be performed every 24–48 h. Only when the extent of evolving tissue necrosis had reached its peak would definitive reconstruction be undertaken.

Several authors have subsequently attempted to classify close-range, high-velocity gunshot wounds to the craniomaxillofacial region to help guide operative decision-making. Vasconez et al. in 1996 developed a classification system based on the kinetic energy of the projectile, the range from weapon to target, and involvement of three anatomic regions – the upper, middle, and lower face, which accounted for 23, 92, and 77 % of gunshot injuries, respectively. In their study cohort, more than 50 % of the gunshot wounds involved multiple facial regions, most commonly the middle and lower face. The authors supported the use of early and aggressive operative intervention including primary bone grafting and early free tissue transfer in order to ameliorate infection, wound contracture, scarring, and maximize overall functional and cosmetic outcome. Vayvada et al. in 2005 described their 10-year experience with close-range, high-energy shotgun and rifle wounds to the face. Their classification system was designed specifically to characterize not only the anatomic area of the face involved in injury but also to describe the severity of injury as well as the composition of tissues involved. Skin, bone, or oral lining involvement, as well as the degree of brain and eye injury, was included. Craniofacial gunshot wounds were subsequently categorized into four groups: cranial, upper face, midface, and lower face. The upper face group was subclassified as with or without eye involvement. The midface group was subclassified as simple, with no tissue loss, or complex, with loss of one component of skin, bone, or oral lining, or compound, with loss of two components, or finally composite, with loss of all three components. The lower face group was subclassified in an analogous fashion to midface injuries. The anatomic distribution of gunshot wounds in their series was predominantly lower face injuries, 93 %, as the etiology of injury was most commonly self-inflicted gunshot wound. However, upper face, midface, brain, and eye involvement were identified in 7, 66, 13, and 13 % of patients, respectively. The authors utilize this classification scheme to help decide whether to proceed with immediate operative reconstruction or to pursue conventional treatment – which included operative stabilization of remaining bone, primary soft tissue closure, serial debridements at 48-h intervals, and delayed reconstruction of bone and soft tissue deficits. Indications for immediate reconstruction included compound or composite tissue loss, insufficient mucosal lining, or insufficient soft tissue coverage for the cranium and brain. The common thread running in all of the classification paradigms is an emphasis on the systematic assessment of the extent of soft tissue and bone deficit, parsed into anatomic subunits, to guide clinical evaluation and facilitate definitive surgical reconstruction.

Stages and Timing of Surgical Management

Once the patient has been stabilized from a trauma and critical care perspective, the treatment plan for management and reconstruction should be dictated by the primary reconstructive surgery team in collaboration with oral surgery, neurosurgery, ophthalmology, trauma surgery, and otolaryngology as appropriate. Several authors have advocated for the use of a staged sequence of operative management with finite goals set at each stage, which must be achieved prior to proceeding to the next stage. Surgical management of gunshot wounds to the face can be partitioned into three phases: initial operative debridement and stabilization, definitive soft tissue and bony reconstruction, and subsequent aesthetic refinement. The goals of the initial operative procedure should include management of any ocular injury or extraocular muscle entrapment, washout and coverage of exposed intracranial contents, early debridement of contaminated and nonviable soft tissue and bone, skeletal fixation of existing bone with restoration of maxillomandibular occlusion, and coverage of soft tissue and bone. Following penetrating trauma to face, the wound bed is often contaminated with nonviable tissue, debris, and foreign bodies. Therefore, the wound needs to be thoroughly decontaminated to prevent future infection or the formation of abscesses or dead space cavities. Initial operative debridement of skin and soft tissues should be conservative and limited to clearly nonviable tissues, as areas of questionable viability should be serially debrided on subsequent operative interventions. Most authors would separate the serial debridements to every 24–48 h, particularly with intermediate-velocity or high-velocity projectile injuries, as the zone of injury and cellular necrosis may evolve over time. In wounds with extensive debris, metallic foreign bodies, and gross contamination, adjuncts such as pulse lavage irrigation and magnetic props should be used to remove all visible evidence of contamination. After decontamination and debridement of all nonviable tissues has been completed, attention should be turned toward skeletal reconstruction and soft tissue coverage. At this point, the reconstructive surgeon must evaluate the ballistic etiology, anatomic location, tissue complexity, and severity of bone and soft tissue injury and loss of the wound, in addition to the patient's overall health status, in order to decide whether to continue with serial operative debridements and delay definitive reconstruction versus proceeding to the immediate reconstruction. Low-velocity civilian handgun injuries are typically associated with minimal soft tissue and bone loss and can typically be managed in the acute setting with debridement, skeletal fixation, and primary closure of the overlying soft tissue defect. However, the potential for evolution of the zone of injury and cellular necrosis in intermediate-velocity and high-velocity projectile injuries renders the decision to proceed with early definitive reconstruction more problematic. Opinions on the timing of definitive reconstruction continue to evolve as the techniques available to the reconstructive surgeon advance. In the 1960s, several groups, including Spira et al., Sherman et al., and Coleman et al., among others, recommended early definitive skeletal stabilization followed by soft tissue wound packing and serial dressing changes. Further operative debridements would be performed on an as-needed basis with definitive soft tissue reconstruction delayed until no evidence of devitalized tissue was present. A major downside with this approach was the significant contracture skin and soft tissues often encountered with the delay. Some authors have advocated the use of temporary plaster or acrylic splinting of the face to combat further contracture of the skin and soft tissue envelope. With the advent of advanced local flap and microsurgical techniques, several authors investigated the use of primary reconstruction of bone and soft tissue deficits utilizing immediate bone grafting and free tissue transfer. Vasconez and colleagues described their experience with high-energy gunshot wounds to the face between 1976 and 1993 and divided their treatment approach into two categories, delayed definitive reconstruction and immediate primary reconstruction. In the former, definitive repair was not performed during the initial surgical debridement, and the resultant deficits were either left open and packed or temporized with skin grafts, local flaps, or external fixators. In the latter, definitive reconstruction with rigid fixation of bony fractures, bone grafting, and coverage of skin and lining defects with grafts, local flaps, or free tissue transfer was performed at the time of initial operative debridement or within the first 24–48 h thereafter. The authors reported no significant difference in rates of infection between the two groups; however, immediate reconstruction was associated with decreased irreversible scarring or contracture and required fewer total operative procedures and fewer secondary refinement procedures. Several authors have reported improved structural, functional, and aesthetic outcomes with aggressive immediate reconstruction. Benefits of an early and aggressive microsurgical strategy include provision of well-vascularized coverage providing for an optimum microenvironment, which promotes both wound and bone healing, as well as immediately addressing three-dimensional deficits in bone and dead space. This prevents subsequent significant contracture and scarring while maintaining normal anatomic projection of the facial skeleton. The decision to proceed with a conservative or aggressive wound management strategy remains an area of clinical debate. The decision should be based on careful evaluation on a case-by-case basis with consideration given to the nature of the wound, the overall health status of the patient, and the past experiences of the reconstructive surgeon.

General Principles of Facial Skeletal Reconstruction

The three principal goals in facial skeletal reconstruction are the establishment of facial projection in the anterior–posterior plane, restoration of facial width in the coronal plane, and realignment of proper maxillary–mandibular occlusion. Techniques of fracture exposure, anatomic reduction, and rigid fixation of the facial skeleton, used in the reconstruction of gunshot wounds to the face, follow the same general principles seen with routine facial fracture management. In low-velocity injuries to the face, extensive bone comminution may be present. However, in general, there is minimal bone loss, and the majority of these fractures can be managed with standard internal rigid fixation techniques. In high-velocity injuries to the face, significant bone comminution is often seen and in combination with significant degrees of bone loss. In order to maximize bone healing and bone structure restoration in this setting, external fixation may need to be utilized. This may be especially useful when adequate soft tissue coverage is present so that further devascularizing of the remaining bone stock during the application of internal fixation can be avoided. In order to restore the proper relation between the facial skeleton, the frontal cranium, and the cranial base, which would allow restoration of midface height, width, and projection, the principle of reestablishing the anatomic relation of the structural pillars of the midface must be adhered to.

The nasomaxillary, the zygomatic, and the pterygomaxillary buttresses constitute the vertical component, and the maxillary arch and palate, fronto-orbital bar, orbital rims, pyriform aperture, and skull base surrounding the oral, nasal, and orbital vaults comprise the system of horizontally oriented buttresses, all of which must be restored. For bony defects larger than 5 mm in both the midface and the mandible, primary bone grafting should be utilized with donor sources including iliac crest, rib, and split cranial bone graft. However, in the setting of significant loss of the craniofacial buttresses particularly in high-velocity gunshot wounds, non-vascularized bone grafts may undergo unpredictable resorption and do not provide sufficient control for rigid fixation. Vascularized bone flaps, including fibula, scapula, radius, ilium, calvaria, and medial femoral condyle, provide more ideal functional skeletal replacement in the setting of significant bone loss (63). The mandible is the primary buttress of the lower face, and proper establishment of occlusion between the mandible and the midface is necessary. Reconstruction of mandibular continuity with locking plates or reconstruction bars followed by maxillomandibular fixation restores the proper vertical distance of occlusion, prevents maxillary rotation, and facilitates reconstruction of proper midfacial height.

Facial Soft Tissue Reconstruction

In the ideal setting, soft tissue reconstruction can be accomplished by direct approximation of the tissues, which is often the case with low-velocity gunshot wounds to the face. These injuries can be managed primarily in a way analogous to a facial fracture with overlying skin and soft tissue lacerations. Soft tissue reconstruction must be designed with layered closure to re-approximate the periosteum, the musculoaponeurotic system, and the skin to prevent malposition and thinning of the soft tissue envelope. Wound re-approximation is facilitated by conservative soft tissue debridement and careful undermining of wound edges. It is critical not to compromise the potential repair with excessive tension on the skin edges. In intermediate-velocity shotgun injury and high-velocity gunshot wounds to the face, massive soft tissue defects oftentimes exceed the capacity for local tissue repair. In the planning of definitive reconstruction, it is of critical importance to appreciate not only the loss of the skin envelope but also the need for lining components, such as conjunctiva, oral mucosa, and nasal mucosa. Failure to recognize this will inevitably lead to contraction, fibrosis, fistula formation, or infection.

With advancements in microsurgical techniques, free tissue transfer has become the gold standard for reconstruction of facial trauma associated with significant tissue loss. Fischer and colleagues reported their experience with the use of free tissue transfer for extensive craniofacial defects. They defined seven critical principles to facilitate improved utilization of free flaps in facial reconstruction. These principles are as follows: use of aesthetic units, identification of defect boundaries, defining precise tissue requirements, establishing a skeletal buttress framework, ensuring ample soft tissue volume, early reconstruction, and use of local provisional procedures. The authors describe the evolution of flap-based reconstruction, from its initial usage in simply filling soft tissue deficits, the so-called defect principle guided reconstruction, to more modern uses of aesthetic and functional subunit soft tissue and bone reconstruction. In their algorithm for facial reconstruction, if defects exceeded greater than 60 % of an individual aesthetic unit, it should be extended both in thickness, contour, and surface area to the nearest anatomic subunit or boundary to optimize ultimate functional and cosmetic outcomes.

Management of Gunshot Wounds to the Neck

Gunshot wounds to the neck pose significant challenges to both the trauma surgeon and reconstructive surgeon alike due to the complex regional anatomy, the superficial location and immediate proximity of vital structures, and the potential for rapid hemodynamic compromise. The local dissemination of tissue imparted by the projectile in addition to the distribution of kinetic energy, through stress waves and cavitation, can cause significant tissue damage both within the immediate projectile path and beyond, capable of causing vascular thrombosis as well as embolism and pseudoaneurysm formation. Historically, the cardinal principle of mandatory exploration of all penetrating injuries to the neck which violated the platysma was derived from the experience of military surgeons during World War II. This principle evolved as the result of the high mortality rate of penetrating neck injury, estimated at approximately 7 %, as well as an unacceptably high rate of unrecognized neurovascular injury following gunshot or shrapnel wounds to the neck. This wartime practice was then extrapolated into civilian trauma centers in the management of penetrating neck injuries. However, in the 1970s, civilian trauma surgeons began to question the appropriateness of this paradigm to civilian practice through recognition that mandatory exploration of penetrating neck injuries led to a significant number of unnecessary surgical procedures. In 1979, Roon and Christensen published the most widely accepted systematic method of evaluation and management of penetrating neck trauma. In their classification scheme, the neck was divided into three anatomic zones anterior to the sternocleidomastoid muscle, including from inferior to superior: zone 1, from the level of the sternal notch cricoid cartilage; zone 2, from the level of the cricoid cartilage to the angle of the mandible; and zone 3, from the angle of the mandible to the skull base. Risk to critical anatomic structures varied based on anatomic zone. In zone 1, the aortic arch and the proximal carotid, internal jugular, and vertebral arteries, the brachiocephalic veins, the esophagus, and the trachea and lung apices were potentially in harm's way. In zone 2, the common carotid and internal and external carotid arteries, the jugular veins, the hypopharynx and esophagus, and the laryngeal structures were at risk, and in zone 3, the internal and external carotid arteries, the vertebral arteries, the facial nerve trunk, and the jugular veins were most frequently injured. Injuries to zone 2 are readily accessed through the area of injury which can also be extended to facilitate exposure through standard neck dissection surgical approaches. The proximity to the thoracic cavity and the skull base limit the ability to readily explore zone 1 and 3 injuries, respectively.

Over the past decade, the advancement of highly sensitive and specific radiologic diagnostic modalities has led to the evolution of protocols which trend toward more minimally invasive diagnostic and therapeutic techniques. The gold standard for radiologic diagnosis of penetrating neck injuries has evolved from standard angiography to computed tomography angiography (CTA) of the neck as the primary screening tool for stable patients with suspected neck injuries. CTA of the neck offers several advantages to conventional neck angiography, including ready availability and ease of use; noninvasive imaging with sensitivity and specificity approaching or equivalent to conventional angiography at 86–100 % and 94–100 %, respectively; the ability to simultaneously detect penetrating vascular injury as well as occult airway and gastrointestinal tract injury; the ability to combine with additional trauma screening imaging; and the ability to provide insight as to the path trajectory of the projectile through the soft tissue. Some authors have advocated the use of CTA of the neck even in the presence of direct evidence of vascular trauma in the stable patient regardless of zone of injury, due to the potential for improved planning of operative management. In addition, a recent study by Steenburg and colleagues identified gunshot wounds to the head and face as an independent risk factor for blunt cervical vascular injury, even when the vessel in question was remote from the path of the projectile. 2.8 % of their 427 patients screened with CTA of the neck following craniofacial gunshot injury displayed indirect cervical vascular injuries.

Even with improved diagnostic imaging techniques, the key question to address when evaluating a patient with penetrating injury to the neck should always be first and foremost whether the patient is stable or unstable. The zone of injury and level of tissue penetration are of secondary importance. Indicators of patient instability requiring urgent operative intervention, either through an open or endovascular approach, include the presence of shock, rapidly expanding hematoma, exsanguinating hemorrhage, acute airway compromise, and massive subcutaneous emphysema. Patients lacking these physical findings can then proceed to CTA of the neck for further diagnostic evaluation. Once the decision to proceed to the operating room or the angiography suite has been made, the zones of the neck guide operative intervention. Currently at our institution, injuries to zones 1 and 3 are most commonly managed through endovascular procedures, as the open surgical approach to these regions is technically difficult and carries significant morbidity, and proximal and distal vascular control is difficult to achieve. Tisherman et al. in the Journal of Trauma in 2008 provide strong evidence supporting selective operative management over mandatory operative management injuries in zone 2 of the neck. When operative intervention is indicated, the current standard of care is to perform open vascular repair ideally via primary repair whenever possible. However, patch angioplasty, interposition vein grafting, or alternative procedures may be performed as needed when appropriate. As the technical capabilities for endovascular repair continue to improve, the management of zone 2 injuries may also continue to evolve accordingly.

Conclusions

The management of gunshot wounds to the head and neck has undergone a significant revitalization over the past half century primarily through improvements in both diagnostic modalities and operative techniques. Recent advances in microsurgical capabilities for free tissue transfer have resulted in a paradigm shift from serial dressing changes and delayed definitive soft tissue reconstruction to immediate bony stabilization and free flap and local tissue rearrangement for soft tissue reconstruction to achieve maximal aesthetic and functional outcomes. Improved imaging techniques including modern multi-planar CT scanners with the capacity for 3-D reconstruction of bone and soft tissue alike have dramatically improved our diagnostic capabilities thus taking guesswork out of the preoperative planning in the management of these injuries. Ongoing evolution of techniques including such promising procedures as composite tissue allotransplantation highlights the fact that our capabilities for reconstruction of devastating gunshot wounds to the head and neck in the future will only get better.

Bibliography

Adams DB. Wound ballistics: a review. Mil Med. 1982;147(10):831–5. Epub 1982/10/01.

Alper M, Totan S, Cankayali R, Songur E. Gunshot wounds of the face in attempted suicide patients. J Oral Maxillofac Surg. 1998;56(8):930–3; discussion 3–4. Epub 1998/08/26.

Arthurs ZM, Sohn VY, Starnes BW. Vascular trauma: endovascular management and techniques. Surg Clin North Am. 2007;87(5): 1179–92, x–xi. Epub 2007/10/16.

Bagheri SC, Khan HA, Bell RB. Penetrating neck injuries. Oral Maxillofac Surg Clin North Am. 2008;20(3):393–414. Epub 2008/07/08.

Baqain ZH, Thakkar C, Kalavrezos N. Superselective embolization for control of facial haemorrhage. Injury. 2004;35(4):435–8. Epub 2004/03/24.

Becelli R, De Ponte FS, Sassano PP, Rinna C. Firearm injuries in maxillofacial region reconstructive surgery. J Craniofac Surg. 1995;6(6):473–6. Epub 1995/11/01.

Bell RB, Osborn T, Dierks EJ, Potter BE, Long WB. Management of penetrating neck injuries: a new paradigm for civilian trauma. J Oral Maxillofac Surg. 2007;65(4):691–705. Epub 2007/03/21.

Caruso RP, Jara DI, Swan KG. Gunshot wounds: bullet caliber is increasing. J Trauma. 1999;46(3):462–5. Epub 1999/03/24.

Chen AY, Stewart MG, Raup G. Penetrating injuries of the face. Otolaryngol Head Neck Surg. 1996;115(5):464–70.

Clark N, Birely B, Manson PN, Slezak S, Kolk CV, Robertson B, et al. High-energy ballistic and avulsive facial injuries: classification, patterns, and an algorithm for primary reconstruction. Plast Reconstr Surg. 1996;98(4):583–601. Epub 1996/09/01.

Coleman Jr CC, Khuri AA, Ruffin Jr W, Hoopes JE. The treatment of maxillofacial injuries. J Trauma. 1963;3:517–26. Epub 1963/11/01.

Cook PJ, Lawrence BA, Ludwig J, Miller TR. The medical costs of gunshot injuries in the United States. JAMA. 1999;282(5):447–54. Epub 1999/08/12.

Demetriades D, Chahwan S, Gomez H, Falabella A, Velmahos G, Yamashita D. Initial evaluation and management of gunshot wounds to the face. J Trauma. 1998;45(1):39–41. Epub 1998/07/29.

Deng W, Huang D, Chen S, Zhang X, Li X, Li J, et al. Management of high-flow arteriovenous malformation in the maxillofacial region. J Craniofac Surg. 2010;21(3):916–9. Epub 2010/05/21.

Dolin J, Scalea T, Mannor L, Sclafani S, Trooskin S. The management of gunshot wounds to the face. J Trauma. 1992;33(4):508–14. discussion 14–5. Epub 1992/10/01.

Evans GR, Clark N, Manson PN, Leipziger LS. Role of mini- and microplate fixation in fractures of the midface and mandible. Ann Plast Surg. 1995;34(5):453–6. Epub 1995/05/01.

Fackler ML. Wound ballistics. A review of common misconceptions. JAMA. 1988;259(18):2730–6. Epub 1988/05/13.

Finch DR, Dibbell DG. Immediate reconstruction of gunshot injuries to the face. J Trauma. 1979;19(12):965–8. Epub 1979/12/01.

Finkle DR, Ringler SL, Luttenton CR, Beernink JH, Peterson NT, Dean RE. Comparison of the diagnostic methods used in maxillofacial trauma. Plast Reconstr Surg. 1985;75(1):32–41. Epub 1985/01/01.

Fisher M, Dorafshar A, Bojovic B, Manson PN, Rodriguez ED. The evolution of critical concepts in aesthetic craniofacial microsurgical reconstruction. Plast Reconstr Surg. 2012;130(2):389–98. Epub 2012/04/13.

Fogelman MJ, Stewart RD. Penetrating wounds of the neck. Am J Surg. 1956;91(4):581–93; discussion, 93–6. Epub 1956/04/01.

Fox CJ, Gillespie DL, Weber MA, Cox MW, Hawksworth JS, Cryer CM, et al. Delayed evaluation of combat-related penetrating neck trauma. J Vasc Surg. 2006;44(1):86–93. Epub 2006/07/11.

Futran ND. Maxillofacial trauma reconstruction. Facial Plast Surg Clin North Am. 2009;17(2):239–51. Epub 2009/04/28.

Futran ND, Farwell DG, Smith RB, Johnson PE, Funk GF. Definitive management of severe facial trauma utilizing free tissue transfer. Otolaryngol Head Neck Surg. 2005;132(1):75–85.

Glapa M, Zorio M, Snyckers FD, Bowley DM, Yilmaz TH, Doll D, et al. Gunshot wounds to the head in civilian practice. Am Surg. 2009;75(3):223–6. Epub 2009/04/09.

Goodstein WA, Stryker A, Weiner LJ. Primary treatment of shotgun injuries to the face. J Trauma. 1979;19(12):961–4. Epub 1979/12/01.

Gruss JS, Antonyshyn O, Phillips JH. Early definitive bone and soft-tissue reconstruction of major gunshot wounds of the face. Plast Reconstr Surg. 1991;87(3):436–50. Epub 1991/03/01.

Hallock GG. Self-inflicted gunshot wounds of the lower half of the face: the evolution toward early reconstruction. J Cranio-maxillofac Trauma. 1995;1(3):50–5. Epub 1995/10/01.

Hogan AR, Lineen EB, Perez EA, Neville HL, Thompson WR, Sola JE. Value of computed tomographic angiography in neck and extremity pediatric vascular trauma. J Pediatr Surg. 2009;44(6):1236–41. discussion 41. Epub 2009/06/16.

Hollerman JJ, Fackler ML, Coldwell DM, Ben-Menachem Y. Gunshot wounds: 1. Bullets, ballistics, and mechanisms of injury. AJR Am J Roentgenol. 1990;155(4):685–90.

Hollier L, Grantcharova EP, Kattash M. Facial gunshot wounds: a 4-year experience. J Oral Maxillofac Surg. 2001;59(3):277–82. Epub 2001/03/13.

Inaba K, Munera F, McKenney M, Rivas L, de Moya M, Bahouth H, et al. Prospective evaluation of screening multislice helical computed tomographic angiography in the initial evaluation of penetrating neck injuries. J Trauma. 2006;61(1):144–9. Epub 2006/07/13.

Karch DL, Logan J, Patel N. Surveillance for violent deaths–national violent death reporting system, 16 states, 2008. MMWR Surveill Summ. 2011;60(10):1–49. Epub 2011/08/26.

Kaufman HH. Civilian gunshot wounds to the head. Neurosurgery. 1993;32(6):962–4. discussion 4. Epub 1993/06/01.

Kaur J, Chopra R. Three dimensional CT reconstruction for the evaluation and surgical planning of mid face fractures: a 100 case study. J Maxillofac Oral Surg. 2010;9(4):323–8. Epub 2011/12/23.

Kihtir T, Ivatury RR, Simon RJ, Nassoura Z, Leban S. Early management of civilian gunshot wounds to the face. J Trauma. 1993;35(4):569–75. discussion 75–7. Epub 1993/10/01.

Kortbeek JB, Al Turki SA, Ali J, Antoine JA, Bouillon B, Brasel K, et al. Advanced trauma life support, 8th edition, the evidence for change. J Trauma. 2008;64(6):1638–50. Epub 2008/06/12.

Kummoona R. Management of missiles injuries of the facial skeleton: primary, intermediate, and secondary phases. J Craniofac Surg. 2010;21(4):976–81. Epub 2010/07/09.

Lichte P, Oberbeck R, Binnebosel M, Wildenauer R, Pape HC, Kobbe P. A civilian perspective on ballistic trauma and gunshot injuries. Scand J Trauma Resusc Emerg Med. 2010;18:35. Epub 2010/06/23.

Maiden N. Ballistics reviews: mechanisms of bullet wound trauma. Forensic Sci Med Pathol. 2009a;5(3):204–9. Epub 2009/08/01.

Maiden N. Historical overview of wound ballistics research. Forensic Sci Med Pathol. 2009b;5(2):85–9. Epub 2009/05/26.

Manson PN, Hoopes JE, Su CT. Structural pillars of the facial skeleton: an approach to the management of Le Fort fractures. Plast Reconstr Surg. 1980;66(1):54–62. Epub 1980/07/01.

Manson PN, Crawley WA, Yaremchuk MJ, Rochman GM, Hoopes JE, French Jr JH. Midface fractures: advantages of immediate extended open reduction and bone grafting. Plast Reconstr Surg. 1985;76(1): 1–12. Epub 1985/07/01.

Manson PN, Clark N, Robertson B, Crawley WA. Comprehensive management of pan-facial fractures. J Cranio-maxillofac Trauma. 1995;1(1):43–56. Epub 1995/04/01.

Manson PN, Clark N, Robertson B, Slezak S, Wheatly M, Vander Kolk C, et al. Subunit principles in midface fractures: the importance of sagittal buttresses, soft-tissue reductions, and sequencing treatment of segmental fractures. Plast Reconstr Surg. 1999;103(4):1287–306. quiz 307. Epub 1999/03/24.

Markowitz BL, Sinow JD, Kawamoto Jr HK, Shewmake K, Khoumehr F. Prospective comparison of axial computed tomography and standard and panoramic radiographs in the diagnosis of mandibular fractures. Ann Plast Surg. 1999;42(2):163–9. Epub 1999/02/24.

McLean JN, Moore CE, Yellin SA. Gunshot wounds to the face–acute management. Facial Plast Surg. 2005;21(3):191–8. Epub 2005/11/25.

Mehta N, Butala P, Bernstein MP. The imaging of maxillofacial trauma and its pertinence to surgical intervention. Radiol Clin North Am. 2012;50(1):43–57. Epub 2011/11/22.

Mohan R, Iyer R, Thaller S. Airway management in patients with facial trauma. J Craniofac Surg. 2009;20(1):21–3. Epub 2009/01/24.

Motamedi MH. Primary management of maxillofacial hard and soft tissue gunshot and shrapnel injuries. J Oral Maxillofac Surg. 2003; 61(12):1390–8. Epub 2003/12/10.

Munera F, Soto JA, Palacio DM, Castaneda J, Morales C, Sanabria A, et al. Penetrating neck injuries: helical CT angiography for initial evaluation. Radiology. 2002;224(2):366–72. Epub 2002/07/31.

Patterson BO, Holt PJ, Cleanthis M, Tai N, Carrell T, Loosemore TM. Imaging vascular trauma. Br J Surg. 2012;99(4):494–505. Epub 2011/12/23.

Pereira C, Boyd JB, Dickenson B, Putnam B. Gunshot wounds to the face: level I urban trauma center: a 10-year level I urban trauma center experience. Ann Plast Surg. 2012;68(4):378–81. Epub 2012/03/17.

Petridis AK, Doukas A, Barth H, Mehdorn M. Outcome of craniocerebral gunshot injuries in the civilian population. Prognostic factors and treatment options. Cent Eur Neurosurg. 2011;72(1):5–14. Epub 2010/03/24.

Ragel BT, Klimo Jr P, Martin JE, Teff RJ, Bakken HE, Armonda RA. Wartime decompressive craniectomy: technique and lessons learned. Neurosurg Focus. 2010;28(5):E2. Epub 2010/06/24.

Robertson BC, Manson PN. High-energy ballistic and avulsive injuries. A management protocol for the next millennium. Surg Clin North Am. 1999;79(6):1489–502, xi. Epub 2000/01/08.

Rodriguez ED, Bluebond-Langner R, Park JE, Manson PN. Preservation of contour in periorbital and midfacial craniofacial microsurgery: reconstruction of the soft-tissue elements and skeletal buttresses. Plast Reconstr Surg. 2008;121(5):1738–47. discussion 48–9. Epub 2008/05/06.

Roon AJ, Christensen N. Evaluation and treatment of penetrating cervical injuries. J Trauma. 1979;19(6):391–7. Epub 1979/06/01.

Rosenfeld JV. Gunshot injury to the head and spine. J Clin Neurosci. 2002;9(1):9–16. Epub 2001/12/26.

Ross AH. Caliber estimation from cranial entrance defect measurements. J Forensic Sci. 1996;41(4):629–33. Epub 1996/07/01.

Roth FS, Kokoska MS, Awwad EE, Martin DS, Olson GT, Hollier LH, et al. The identification of mandible fractures by helical computed tomography and panorex tomography. J Craniofac Surg. 2005;16(3): 394–9. Epub 2005/05/26.

Rowe VL, Lee W, Weaver FA. Acute arterial occlusion secondary to trauma. Semin Vasc Surg. 2009;22(1):25–8. Epub 2009/03/21.

Saigal K, Winokur RS, Finden S, Taub D, Pribitkin E. Use of three-dimensional computerized tomography reconstruction in complex facial trauma. Facial Plast Surg. 2005;21(3):214–20. Epub 2005/11/25.

Sali Bukhari SG, Khan I, Pasha B, Ahmad W. Management of facial gunshot wounds. J Coll Physicians Surg Pak. 2010;20(6):382–5. Epub 2010/07/21.

Santamaria E, Cordeiro PG. Reconstruction of maxillectomy and mid-facial defects with free tissue transfer. J Surg Oncol. 2006;94(6): 522–31. Epub 2006/10/25.

Sherman RT, Parrish RA. Management of shotgun injuries: a review of 152 cases. J Trauma. 1963;3:76–86. Epub 1963/01/01.

Spira M, Hardy SB, Biggs TE, Gerow FJ. Shotgun injuries of the face. Plast Reconstr Surg. 1967;39(5):449–58. Epub 1967/05/01.

Steenburg SD, Sliker CW. Craniofacial gunshot injuries: an unrecognised risk factor for blunt cervical vascular injuries? Eur Radiol. 2012;22(9):1837–43. Epub 2012/05/10.

Suominen E, Tukiainen E. Close-range shotgun and rifle injuries to the face. Clin Plast Surg. 2001;28(2):323–37. Epub 2001/06/13.

Swan KG, Swan RC. Wound ballistics for the civilian surgeon. Surg Annu. 1985;17:163–87. Epub 1985/01/01.

Swan KG, Swan RC. Principles of ballistics applicable to the treatment of gunshot wounds. Surg Clin North Am. 1991;71(2):221–39. Epub 1991/04/01.

Tisherman SA, Bokhari F, Collier B, Cumming J, Ebert J, Holevar M, et al. Clinical practice guideline: penetrating zone II neck trauma. J Trauma. 2008;64(5):1392–405. Epub 2008/05/13.

Van Waes OJ, Cheriex KC, Navsaria PH, van Riet PA, Nicol AJ, Vermeulen J. Management of penetrating neck injuries. Br J Surg. 2012;99 Suppl 1:149–54. Epub 2012/03/28.

Vasconez HC, Shockley ME, Luce EA. High-energy gunshot wounds to the face. Ann Plast Surg. 1996;36(1):18–25. Epub 1996/01/01.

Vayvada H, Menderes A, Yilmaz M, Mola F, Kzlkaya A, Atabey A. Management of close-range, high-energy shotgun and rifle wounds to the face. J Craniofac Surg. 2005;16(5):794–804. Epub 2005/09/30.

Verschueren DS, Bell RB, Bagheri SC, Dierks EJ, Potter BE. Management of laryngo-tracheal injuries associated with cranio-maxillofacial trauma. J Oral Maxillofac Surg. 2006;64(2):203–14. Epub 2006/01/18.

Williams CN, Cohen M, Schultz RC. Immediate and long-term management of gunshot wounds to the lower face. Plast Reconstr Surg. 1988;82(3):433–9. Epub 1988/09/01.

Wilson IF, Lokeh A, Benjamin CI, Hilger PA, Hamlar DD, Ondrey FG, et al. Prospective comparison of panoramic tomography (zonography) and helical computed tomography in the diagnosis and operative management of mandibular fractures. Plast Reconstr Surg. 2001;107(6):1369–75. Epub 2001/05/04.

Ylioja S, Hanks R, Baird A, Millis S. Are cognitive outcome and recovery different in civilian penetrating versus non-penetrating brain injuries? Clin Neuropsychol. 2010;24(7):1097–112. Epub 2010/10/07.

Yuksel F, Celikoz B, Ergun O, Peker F, Acikel C, Ebrinc S. Management of maxillofacial problems in self-inflicted rifle wounds. Ann Plast Surg. 2004;53(2):111–7. Epub 2004/07/23.

Microvascular Reconstruction

22

Emile N. Brown, Mark Fisher, and Eduardo D. Rodriguez

Introduction

The first report of microvascular surgery was in 1960 by Jules Jacobson, a vascular surgeon working at the University of Vermont. At that time, otolaryngologists were using operating microscopes during otologic surgery, but Jacobson was the first to show that a microscope could aid in the anastomosis of blood vessels as small as 1.4 mm in size. In 1963, Kleinert and Kasdan, hand surgeons at the University of Louisville, performed the first successful revascularization of a partial digital amputation. But it was not until 1964 when Buncke reported the replantation of a rabbit ear that the age of modern microvascular surgery was born. By showing that vessels as small as 1 mm could be successfully repaired under the microscope, Buncke opened up the possibility to transfer multiple different free tissues in the human patient. In 1966, he made another landmark achievement when he reported a great toe-to-thumb transfer in a rhesus monkey. Originally working out of his garage, then later at Stanford University and Davies Medical Center, Buncke also furthered the field by developing his own microsurgical instruments and sutures.

Building on the foundation laid by Buncke, multiple types of free flaps were introduced over the next two decades, including the omental flap in 1972, groin flap in 1973, fibula flap in 1975, latissimus dorsi flap in 1976, radial forearm flap in 1978, rectus flap in 1980, and anterolateral thigh flap in 1984. Koshima pioneered the next great innovations in microsurgery in the 1990s including the development of supermicrosurgery techniques and description of multiple perforator-based free flaps. These advances have led to reductions in donor site morbidity and allowed the transfer of increasingly sophisticated freestyle free flaps.

As we move forward, further advances can be made in improving aesthetic outcomes after free tissue transfer. The purpose of this chapter is to outline a list of critical concepts for microsurgical reconstruction of the maxillofacial region developed over the past decade at our high-volume trauma center. These principles are aimed at providing patients with the best possible cosmetic and functional results after composite facial reconstruction. The free flaps most commonly used for maxillofacial reconstruction at our institution will also be discussed.

Critical Concepts in Microvascular Reconstruction of the Maxillofacial Region

Significant advances in microvascular and craniofacial surgery over the past 50 years have resulted in dramatically improved outcomes after maxillofacial reconstruction. Our experience with a large number of free tissue transfers for significant composite maxillofacial defects has led to the development of seven critical concepts that will optimize aesthetic results. They include (1) aesthetic unit appearance, (2) defect boundaries, (3) tissue requirements, (4) provision of vascularized skeletal buttress framework, (5) ample soft tissue volume, (6) early reconstruction, and (7) local revisional cutaneous replacement through multistage planning. While the application of these concepts can make the reconstructive process more complex, they are essential in providing a methodical structure in which to plan and perform optimal reconstruction of composite maxillofacial defects.

E.N. Brown, MD • E.D. Rodriguez, MD, DDS (✉)
M. Fisher, BS
Division of Plastic and Reconstructive Surgery,
University of Maryland R Adams Cowley
Shock Trauma Center, Baltimore, MD, USA
e-mail: erodriguez@umm.edu

P.J. Taub et al. (eds.), *Ferraro's Fundamentals of Maxillofacial Surgery*,
DOI 10.1007/978-1-4614-8341-0_22, © Springer Science+Business Media New York 2015

Aesthetic Unit

In the 1950s, disappointed with his cosmetic outcomes after burn reconstruction, Mexican plastic surgeon Mario González-Ulloa set out to study the variable physical and physiological features of skin in different areas of the body. He performed a series of dissections on cadavers of both sexes and a wide spectrum of ages, from newborn to elderly, going on to describe the variable skin thickness and histology of 40 body regions and 14 facial regions. Building on this work, González-Ulloa argued that the face could be divided into discreet aesthetic units based on variations in skin texture, color, thickness, and histology. He identified lines of demarcation between facial segments and stressed the importance of replacing these aesthetic units in their entirety, using skin grafts from areas with similar characteristics to the site being reconstructed.

Despite the concept of facial aesthetic units championed by González-Ulloa, microvascular reconstruction was initially guided by a more basic "defect principle," in which the goal was to simply fill the entire "hole" with ample soft tissue. During a period when free flap failure rates were as high as 40 %, surgeons were understandably reluctant to adhere to aesthetic unit reconstruction by removing additional native tissues. However, with advances in microsurgical technique and instrumentation, current free flap failure rates have dropped in to the single digits. Therefore, microvascular surgeons need no longer feel precluded from following the principles of aesthetic facial unit reconstruction.

It is important to recognize that aesthetic facial units are not just "skin deep." The vertical and horizontal skeletal buttresses of the face provide critical soft tissue support and provide shape to each facial region. Additionally, the variable distribution of underlying subcutaneous fat makes a significant contribution to overall facial appearance, a concept that has been repeatedly emphasized in cosmetic facial surgery. What we perceive as a facial aesthetic unit actually depends on multiple elements, representing an amalgam of the composite soft *and* hard tissue. Therefore, a "defect-oriented approach" in which a soft tissue-only flap is used to simply solve the immediate goal of wound closure often results in suboptimal aesthetic outcomes. In order to truly rebuild a composite aesthetic unit with free tissue transfer, it is often necessary to include elements that reconstruct the underlying skeletal support in addition to the soft tissue.

Defect Boundaries

The principles of aesthetic unit reconstruction dictate that certain defects be made larger in order to resurface the entire unit and hide the incisions at the borders. When a defect comprises greater than 60 % of an aesthetic unit, resecting the entire unit and using a free flap to reconstruct it as a whole can achieve superior cosmetic results. This approach results in a more uniform color, thickness, and texture match, as well as incisions that are better disguised at the junctions of units. For example, consider a large median forehead defect where resection of the entire forehead unit will allow the scars to be hidden in the pretrichial hairline and just superior to the eyebrows.

However, one should not always adhere to this 60 % rule. Sometimes it is more important to consider the inherent characteristics of the unit that is being reconstructed and the ability of any free tissue transfer to adequately recreate it. For example, no autologous free flap options exist that can recreate a satisfactory semblance of the vermillion lip. In the case of a partial vermillion lip defect, resection and replacement of the entire unit would likely not result in a superior aesthetic outcome. When considering resection of additional local tissue in order to achieve total aesthetic unit reconstruction, the surgeon must also weigh the potential for local cutaneous tissue to be advanced during successive revisionary procedures, which would eventually allow complete excision of the free flap skin paddle. This consideration will be discussed in more detail with the final concept of secondary revisions.

Tissue Requirements

Free flap choice should be based on a careful consideration of the specific tissue types the surgeon is attempting to reconstruct. This concept is particularly important when some form of "lining" tissue (e.g., conjunctiva, nasal mucosa, sinus mucosa, or oral mucosa) is deficient. In Gillies' landmark 1920 textbook *Plastic Surgery of the Face*, he stated "one is struck chiefly with the lack of appreciation of the need for a lining for all mucous lined cavities… No nose, or portion of the nose, can be made without adequate skin for mucous lining." Gillies recognized the paramount need to provide adequate lining in determining outcomes after nasal reconstruction, a concept for which he credited Keegan, a plastic surgeon in India during the late nineteenth century. Despite this early proclamation by the father of plastic surgery, the need for lining reconstruction is still often underestimated by contemporary microvascular surgeons.

Failure to provide an adequate lining can severely compromise results after free flap reconstruction, leading to contracture, fibrosis, and chronic infection. In order to avoid these pitfalls, the surgeon should engage in meticulous preoperative planning in order to truly comprehend the specific tissue types that are deficient. When attempting to reconstruct a composite defect with missing lining, the choice of free flap should include not only the adequate components required for skin coverage, soft tissue bulk, and skeletal support but also a surplus of skin, fascia, or muscle that can be used to provide lining. Intraoperatively, the surgeon should make every effort to fully recreate the defect, especially in cases of delayed reconstruction where scarring and contracture may have further obscured the initial deficiency. In this way, one can be more confident in the true nature of the defect and ensure that the free flap being transferred includes all necessary composite tissue elements.

Bone and Soft Tissue Support

In the past, microsurgeons often failed to address the need for hard tissue reconstruction in free tissue transfer. When facing a large composite facial defect in which both bone and soft tissue were missing, these surgeons would often choose a flap consisting of abundant soft tissue alone. Although this approach succeeded in "filling the hole," it fell short of the fundamental reconstructive goal of replacing "like with like." Conversely, craniofacial surgeons often overemphasized reconstruction of skeletal elements, at the expense of accurate restoration of the deficient soft tissues. With the synthesis of microsurgery and craniofacial surgery, surgeons now recognize the importance of reconstructing both soft *and* hard tissues. It is the rare case when either bone or soft tissue can be substituted for the other without limiting the aesthetic and functional results.

Occasionally, small craniofacial bone defects in which the architectural support is partially deficient but still existent can be camouflaged with soft tissue flaps alone. However, when significant portions of the facial skeletal buttresses are missing, the reconstruction should include an element to restore this structural support. Historically, non-vascularized bone grafts were the mainstay of bony reconstruction and still can serve a limited role in treatment of small skeletal defects. However, non-vascularized bone grafts cannot heal large segmental defects and experience unpredictable resorption, frequently necessitating further reconstructions over time. Additionally, bone grafts generally provide insufficient bone stock to allow placement of osseointegrated implant prostheses. In certain cases, craniofacial bone defects can be reconstructed with an alloplastic implant covered by a vascularized soft tissue flap. However, alloplastic materials are prone to late infection and tend to extrude over time, leading to implant exposure. Like non-vascularized bone grafts, these long-term complications will likely necessitate further surgical interventions down the line. Vascularized bone obviates many of the issues with both non-vascularized bone grafts and alloplastic implants and should therefore be used for hard tissue reconstruction whenever possible. Adequate soft tissue and bone can often be incorporated in the same free flap; however, multiple flaps may sometimes be required to provide sufficient quantities of both types of tissue.

Soft Tissue Volume

The soft tissue volume included in a free flap should be in slight excess of the actual amount that is deficient. In the case of anticipated postoperative radiation, this excess volume should be greater since radiation can result in significant soft tissue contraction. In all cases, long-term soft tissue resorption tends to be unpredictable. It is always easier to debulk excess soft tissue at a later stage, via direct excision and/or liposuction, than to add volume secondarily. The inclusion of ample volumes of well-vascularized fat in particular will minimize subsequent fat necrosis and soft tissue resorption. This healthy adipose tissue will also provide the necessary volume for future revisionary reshaping procedures as the transferred tissue settles. In contrast, denervated muscle flaps tend to atrophy significantly over time, compromising long-term aesthetic outcome and failing to provide durable coverage for alloplastic implants. For instance, while latissimus dorsi muscle flaps have been a traditional choice for scalp coverage of titanium mesh cranioplasties, in our experience these flaps will thin significantly over time, often resulting in tenuous coverage or ultimate exposure of the underlying mesh.

Selection of donor site for free soft tissue transfer must be individualized based on color match and relative relationship between donor site soft tissue volume and recipient site soft tissue deficit. For example, there is wide variability between patients in the subcutaneous fat of an anterolateral thigh (ALT) flap. While some advocate aggressive thinning of the ALT flap at the primary stage, we feel it is preferable to err on the side of a thicker flap that can be debulked secondarily.

Timing

When faced with a traumatic or oncologic defect, free tissue reconstruction should be undertaken as early as possible. By reconstructing the injury acutely, the scar formation associated with the initial injury and the reconstructive procedure is confined to a single period of postoperative wound contracture. The benefits of this approach are twofold. One, dissection of the recipient site and its vessels is simplified when not operating in a scarred bed. Two, the functional and cosmetic results of the reconstruction are improved by reducing the overall scar burden of the soft tissues in that area.

Obviously in cases of congenital deformities, the timing concerns differ since there is no scarring associated with creation of the initial defect. In these instances, reconstruction is often delayed to an extent individualized for each patient. There are multiple issues to contemplate, such as the ongoing development of the child and whether he or she will ultimately "outgrow" their free flap reconstruction. Additionally, the distribution of body surface area differs in the pediatric patient, with the head compromising a greater percentage of the total surface area. This can be an important consideration in free tissue reconstruction of the pediatric craniofacial region. For example, whereas a latissimus dorsi flap can easily cover a large adult scalp defect, it may be of insufficient size for coverage in the pediatric patient. A final concern that may affect timing of reconstruction is the practical consideration of vascular pedicle size in children and the feasibility of successful anastomoses in each individual surgeon's hands.

Secondary Revisions

There is often an impetus to minimize the number of reconstructive procedures a patient requires. As a result, microsurgeons are sometimes tempted to undertake free tissue transfer as a single-stage procedure aimed at definitive reconstruction and plan their free flaps accordingly. However, this approach will generally compromise long-term outcomes due to skin color mismatch and soft tissue contracture. Secondary procedures play a crucial role in microvascular reconstruction and take into account many of the critical concepts discussed previously.

Secondary revisions are fundamental for achieving successful reconstruction of the facial aesthetic units, as outlined in Concept One, and the eventual need for revisionary procedures should be anticipated at the time of the initial free tissue transfer. In accordance with Concept Two, if a defect encompasses more than 60 % of the aesthetic unit, the surgeon should consider extending the defect to the unit border and replacing its entirety. However, when the defect comprises less than 60 % of the unit, it is important to consider the amount of surrounding local tissue available and preserve it maximally, as this can be successively recruited during secondary procedures. Ideally, the initial free flap should include excess soft tissue, as described in Concept Five, which can later be debulked, shaped, and ultimately covered by local cutaneous advancement. For example, consider a cheek defect comprising 40 % of the aesthetic unit being reconstructed with a free ALT flap. It would be unwise to excise the entire unit during the first reconstruction, but the patient will initially be left with an obvious area of color-mismatched and hair-bearing skin, breaking up the cheek aesthetic unit. However, it is important to realize that this distant tissue transfer can be subsequently utilized as a base for local tissue advancement and resurfaced to provide a more favorable cutaneous texture and color match. In this case, the free flap can be selectively de-epithelialized, and the remaining dermis can serve as a substantial anchor from which to resuspend advanced local skin.

Other secondary procedures may include dermabrasion, soft tissue resuspension, suction lipectomy, and fat grafting. In some cases, it may be desirable to directly excise skin from the transferred free flap followed by full-thickness skin grafting from a donor area with more favorable color and texture match, such as postauricular or supraclavicular sites. The intention of all these revisionary procedures is to replace the cutaneous portion of the "unlike" distant tissue with "like" local tissue while further modifying the contour and volume of the underlying hard and soft tissue support in order to better match that which is missing.

Free Flaps for Maxillofacial Reconstruction

Ulnar Forearm Flap (See Fig. 22.1a–d)

History

Following introduction of the radial forearm free flap by Chinese surgeons in 1978, its close relative, the ulnar forearm free flap, was first described by Lovie in 1984. The radial forearm flap has subsequently become a workhorse flap for head and neck reconstruction given its ease of harvest, long vascular pedicle and thin, supple skin paddle. The ulnar forearm flap shares these positive characteristics and also offers some additional advantages over the radial forearm flap, which will be discussed below. However, concerns about donor site morbidity have prevented the ulnar forearm flap from ever achieving the popularity of its radial counterpart.

Anatomy and Surgical Technique

The ulnar forearm flap's blood supply is based on the ulnar artery and its venae comitantes. Alternatively, the basilic vein can be utilized for venous outflow. The arterial and venous pedicles are both approximately 2.5 mm in diameter; however, the venous diameter varies depending on whether the vena comitans or basilic vein is used. The arterial pedicle length is comparable to that of the radial forearm flap (~15 cm) but will always be slightly shorter because the ulnar pedicle is limited proximally by the takeoff of the common interosseus artery, whereas the radial pedicle can be dissected all the way to the brachial bifurcation. The maximum skin paddle size is around 15 × 10 cm and is also similar to that of the radial forearm flap. The medial antebrachial

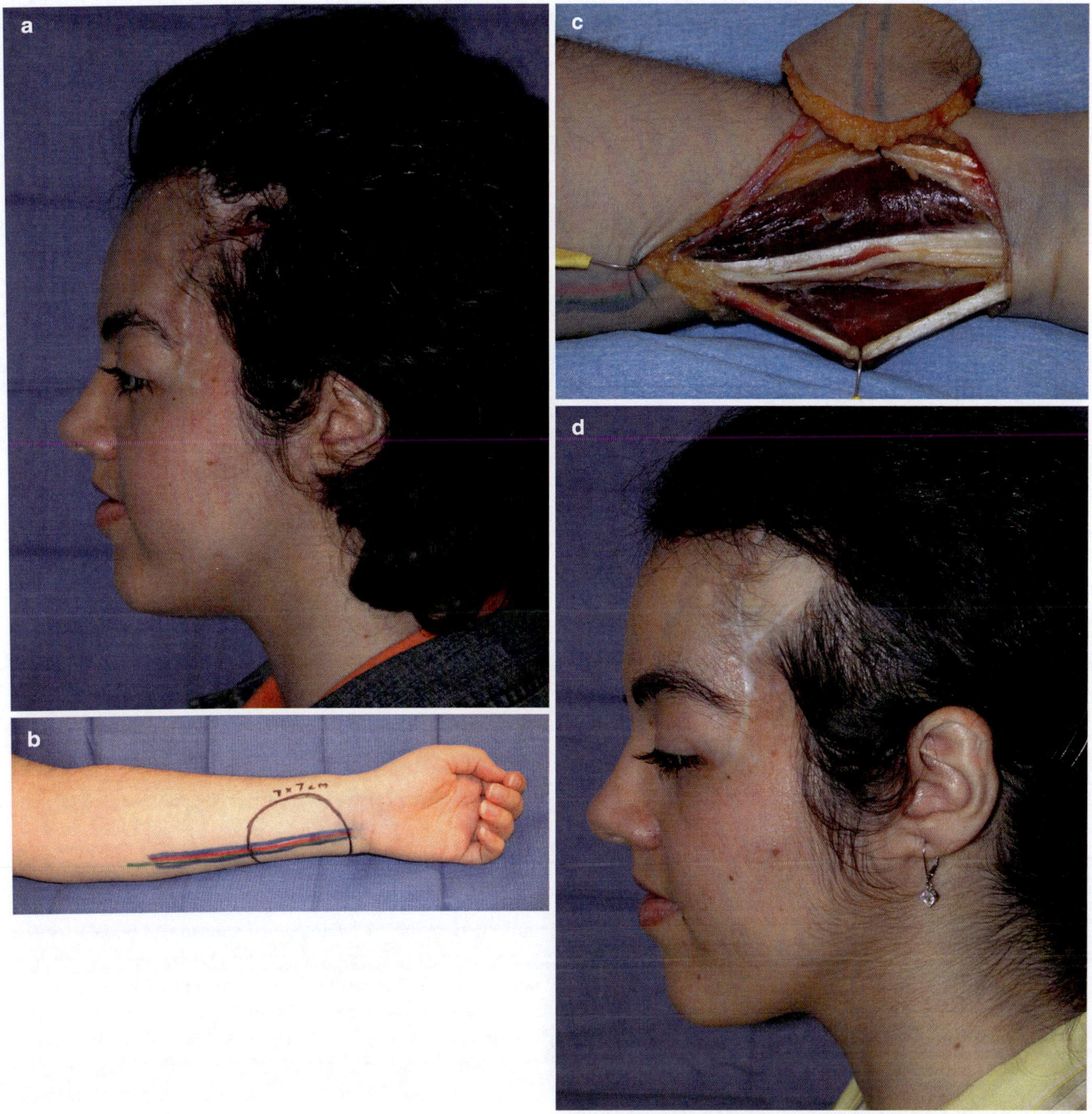

Fig. 22.1 Ulnar forearm flap. (**a**) A 23-year-old woman with history of blunt head trauma to left frontotemporal area presenting with exposed alloplastic cranioplasty. (**b**) Preoperative markings showing vascular pedicle and flap dimensions. (**c**) Flap elevated, prior to pedicle division. (**d**) Postoperative result

cutaneous nerve can be included if a sensate flap is desired for the reconstruction. Although an osteocutaneous ulnar forearm flap incorporating a portion of ulna bone is theoretically possible, it is not commonly described.

The forearm is supplied by the brachial artery, which divides into the radial and ulnar arteries at the level of the antecubital fossa. Anatomic variations in which the ulnar artery arises more proximally or distally are also possible. A short distance after its origin, the ulnar artery gives off the anterior and posterior ulnar recurrent arteries, followed by the common interosseous artery. The ulnar artery courses ulnar and distal, deep to the pronator teres, flexor carpi radialis, and flexor digitorum superficialis to reach the ulnar aspect of the forearm midway along its length. It then travels between the flexor digitorum superficialis and flexor carpi ulnaris muscles until it passes through Guyon's canal at the wrist and divides into superficial and deep palmar branches. The ulnar forearm flap can be drained by the deep or superficial venous systems. The deep system consists of two venae comitantes that accompany the ulnar artery along its course through the intermuscular septum and drain into the median cubital vein near the elbow. The superficial system consists of the basilic vein and its branches. The basilic vein drains the dorsal venous complex of the hand then travels proximally along the dorsal ulnar aspect of the forearm.

The ulnar nerve is closely associated with the ulnar artery along its distal two-thirds and travels just ulnar to the artery. The medial antebrachial cutaneous nerve travels with the basilic vein in the upper arm where it exits the deep fascia above the elbow and divides into anterior and posterior branches. The anterior branch continues with the basilic vein past the elbow and innervates the medial half of the anterior forearm.

Generally, the nondominant hand is the preferred donor site for the ulnar forearm flap. Before attempting to raise the flap, an Allen's test must be performed to ensure sufficient collateral circulation to the hand. Markings begin with a line drawn from the lateral edge of the pisiform bone to the medial epicondyle of the humerus, which approximates the course of the ulnar artery through the mid and distal forearm. Alternatively, the ulnar artery can be traced out with a Doppler probe. The flap is designed with its central axis along the course of the ulnar artery in the mid and distal forearm. The course of the basilic vein through the forearm is also marked.

An upper arm tourniquet is applied and the extremity exsanguinated. Dissection begins at the distal aspect of the skin flap. The skin is incised and dissection proceeds with identification of the ulnar artery and nerve between the flexor carpi ulnaris and flexor digitorum superficialis tendons. The artery is separated from the nerve and ligated distally. The basilic vein can also be located and ligated at this time, if necessary. The skin paddle is then raised in a suprafascial plane from radial and ulnar until the muscular septum between the flexor carpi ulnaris and flexor digitorum superficialis is encountered. At this point, the fascia is incised, and the ulnar vessels are elevated with the skin flap in order to preserve the septocutaneous perforators. The ulnar artery is then dissected proximally (along with the basilic vein if it is being used) until a sufficient pedicle length is achieved or the common interosseous artery is encountered.

A closed suction drain is placed between the muscles. The skin can sometimes be closed primarily, but a skin graft is often necessary. A full-thickness skin graft tends to yield superior cosmetic results and more durable coverage of the exposed tendons; however, a split-thickness skin graft may also be used.

Advantages and Disadvantages

Like the radial forearm flap, the ulnar flap provides a long and reliable vascular pedicle of relatively large caliber and a thin, pliable skin paddle. However, the ulnar forearm flap surpasses the radial flap in terms of both donor and recipient site cosmetic outcomes. The ulnar forearm skin is usually less hirsute than the radial skin, allowing the surgeon to avoid transfer of hair-bearing tissue to reconstruct a defect in a non-hair-bearing region. In terms of donor site, the ulnar forearm flap will generally experience better skin graft take and less tendon glide impairment because there are more underlying muscle bellies as opposed to tendons in this region. The donor site on the ulnar aspect of the forearm is also more easily concealed as it tends to rest along the body in repose.

Many surgeons are reluctant to utilize the ulnar forearm flap out of trepidation about hand perfusion after harvest of the ulnar artery. Additionally, the close relationship of the ulnar artery and nerve has evoked concerns about injury of this critical nerve during flap elevation. However, multiple studies, as well as our own experience, have failed to demonstrate any significant long-term motor, sensory, or vascular impairments after ulnar forearm flap harvest.

Anterolateral Thigh Flap (See Fig. 22.2a–d)

History

The first report of a lateral thigh cutaneous free flap was by Baek in 1983. However, he described a posterolateral skin paddle based off perforators from the profunda femoris artery. In1984, Song was the first to define the true anterolateral thigh (ALT) flap, based off perforators from the descending branch of the lateral femoral circumflex artery. After its introduction, the ALT flap gained widespread popularity due to the relatively large skin paddle and because its components can include muscle, fascia, and skin. Most of the flap's initial proponents were in Asian countries, where the ALT supplanted the radial forearm free flap as the workhorse choice for head and neck reconstruction. Over the past decade or so, use of the ALT flap has become increasingly prevalent in Western countries.

Anatomy and Surgical Technique

The ALT flap's blood supply is based on the descending branch of the lateral femoral circumflex artery. The vascular anatomy is variable, and perforators are predominantly musculocutaneous and less commonly septocutaneous. The vascular pedicle can range from 1.5 to 2.5 mm in diameter and 7–16 cm in length depending on anatomy and flap design. Harvesting the lateral femoral cutaneous nerve can preserve sensory innervation, and motor innervation can be preserved if the vastus lateralis muscle and its motor branch are

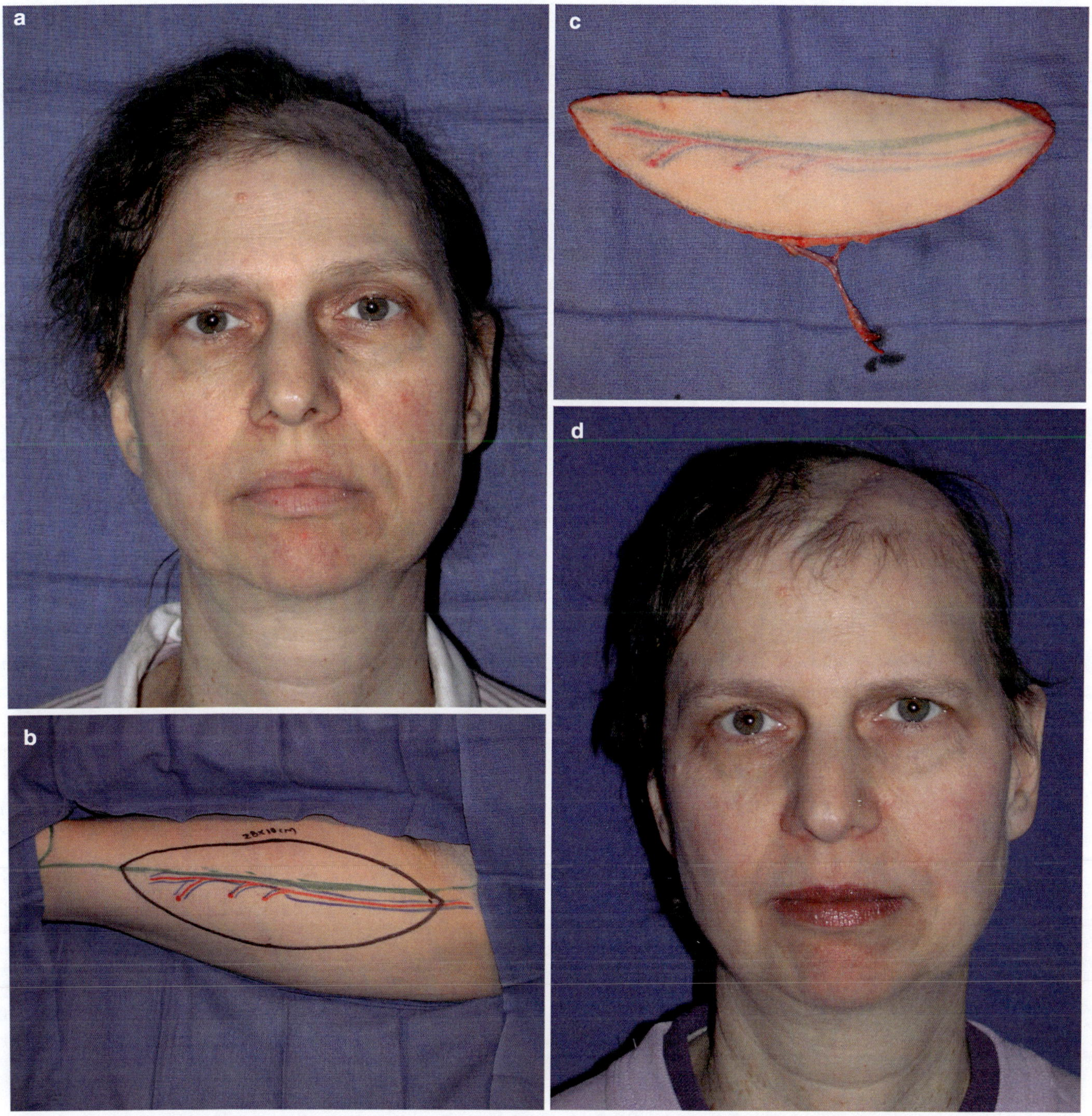

Fig. 22.2 Anterolateral thigh flap. (**a**) A 53-year-old woman with history of left frontal glioma resection presenting with exposed titanium mesh cranioplasty. (**b**) Preoperative markings showing vascular pedicle and flap dimensions. (**c**) Flap elevated, after pedicle division. (**d**) Postoperative result

harvested. A skin paddle of up to 8 × 25 cm can be harvested with primary closure of the donor site or up to 35 × 25 cm if a skin graft is used. The flap can be thinned to as little as 3–5 mm total thickness if minimal tissue bulk is required for reconstruction or retained full thickness for applications where maximal bulk is required. The flap may also be harvested with multiple skin islands to support reconstruction of both skin and lining.

The lateral femoral circumflex artery branches off the profunda femoris and travels laterally, deep to the rectus femoris and sartorius muscles. The artery then divides into descending, transverse, and ascending branches. The descending branch passes along the medial edge of vastus lateralis. In 30 % of patients, the descending branch further divides into the medial and lateral branches. The medial branch continues medially under the rectus femoris to supply the rectus femoris and overlying skin, and the lateral branch continues inferiorly along the intermuscular septum between vastus lateralis and rectus femoris and eventually pierces the vastus lateralis close to the knee. In most patients, the descending branch does not divide and continues along the intermuscular septum, communicating with the lateral superior geniculate artery or profunda femoris above the patella. Venous drainage of the ALT flap is provided by branches of the anterior and lateral cutaneous veins, which drain into the greater saphenous vein before it drains into the femoral vein.

The lateral femoral cutaneous nerve enters the thigh at the lateral end of the inguinal ligament and travels under the tensor fascia lata before piercing it and dividing into anterior and posterior branches that innervate the overlying skin. The motor branch to vastus lateralis branches from the femoral nerve and follows the descending branch of the lateral femoral circumflex artery into the muscle.

Markings for the ALT flap are based on a line connecting the anterior superior iliac spine with the lateral border of the patella. The cutaneous perforators can be located by marking the midpoint of this line and then drawing a circle with a radius of 3 cm that encircles this midpoint. The vessels are most commonly found in the inferolateral quadrant of this circle. A Doppler probe is used to identify vessels within the circle as well as any additional cutaneous perforators. A skin paddle can then be designed (concentrically or eccentrically) around the drawn circle.

A cutaneous flap is elevated by incising along the desired skin paddle markings down to the fascia and dissecting suprafascially in a medial to lateral direction until the vessels to the skin are reached. Alternatively, the initial incision can be made through skin and fascia and dissection carried subfascially to create a fasciocutaneous flap. After identification of the skin perforators medially, the lateral portion of the skin flap can be elevated. Perforator vessels are dissected through muscle if they are musculocutaneous perforators, in which case all branches must be ligated, or if the perforators are septocutaneous, they can simply be followed between the vastus lateralis and rectus femoris to the main pedicle.

A musculocutaneous flap can be harvested by extending the lateral dissection through the fascia down to vastus lateralis. The desired portion of muscle is then elevated, leaving the skin flap and underlying muscle attached. This eliminates the need for isolation of septocutaneous perforators or intermuscular perforator dissection since the portion of vastus lateralis being harvested includes the cutaneous perforator. The vascular pedicle with surrounding cuff of vastus lateralis is dissected, taking care to ligate any small intramuscular branches, until the descending branch of the lateral femoral circumflex artery is reached or proper pedicle length is achieved.

The donor site can be closed primarily if the defect is less than 8 cm wide. Larger defects will require a skin graft for coverage. If the ALT skin paddle is being de-epithelialized for the reconstruction, a split-thickness skin graft can be taken directly from the skin paddle and used to reconstruct the donor site. If muscle was dissected, the muscle edges are reapproximated, followed by closure of the fascia and layered skin closure over a closed suction drain.

Advantages and Disadvantages

The ALT flap can incorporate a skin paddle of variable dimensions and can be made large enough to allow reconstruction of some of the most extensive soft tissue maxillofacial defects. The flap can also include a variety of soft tissue elements in the form of skin, fascia, and muscle and be innervated by incorporation of the lateral femoral cutaneous nerve. It is relatively easy to harvest without significant donor site morbidity. The vascular pedicle is also relatively long, allowing it to easily reach most recipient vessels in the head and neck region.

The main disadvantage to the ALT flap is that it can tend to be bulky, especially in an increasingly obese patient population, often necessitating secondary revisionary procedures to achieve appropriate contour. The skin paddle is also often hirsute, which may result in undesired hair growth at the recipient location.

Groin Flap (See Fig. 22.3a–d)

History

The groin flap has long been used as a random patterned flap for coverage of upper extremity defects. Traditionally, the flap was employed in a delayed fashion, first raising the flap to cover the defect and then later dividing the pedicle. In 1972, McGregor and Jackson were the first to recognize that the groin flap could be designed as an axial patterned flap based on the superficial circumflex iliac vessels. Building on this knowledge, Daniel and Taylor described the first clinically successful cutaneous free flap in 1973, when they reconstructed a lower extremity defect with a free groin flap.

Anatomy and Surgical Technique

The groin flap's blood supply is based on the superficial circumflex iliac artery (SCIA) and the associated cutaneous vein. The arterial pedicle is 1–2 mm in diameter, with the vein generally having a slightly larger caliber. The pedicle length is relatively short, ranging from 2 to 5 cm depending on the size and orientation of the skin paddle. Flaps are commonly designed with a skin paddle of approximately 10×20 cm, while dimensions as large as 22×31 cm have been reported.

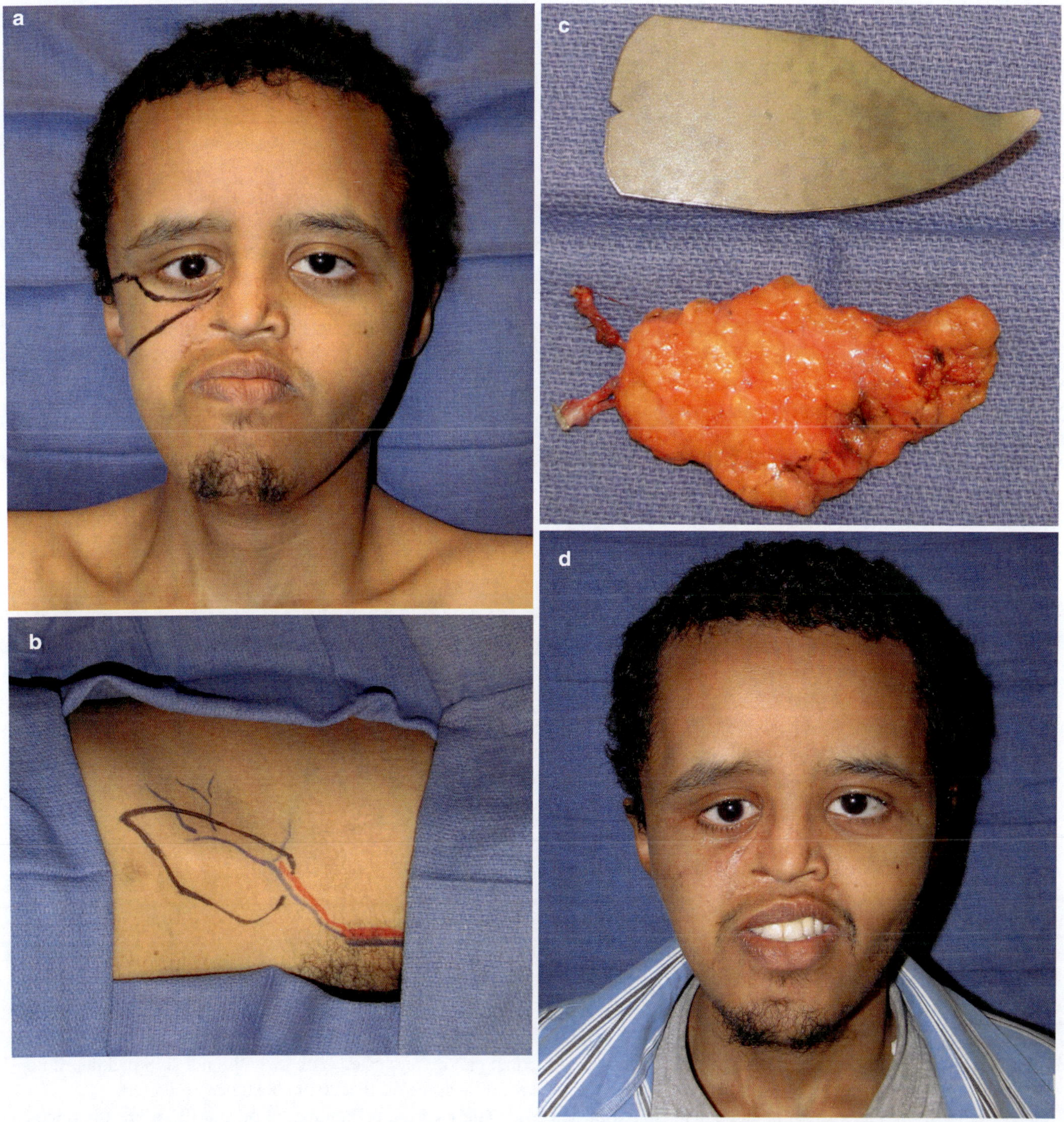

Fig. 22.3 Groin flap. (**a**) A 20-year-old man with history of right facial rhabdomyosarcoma resection and postoperative radiation therapy presenting with hemifacial atrophy. The markings represent the area to be augmented. (**b**) Preoperative markings showing vascular pedicle and flap dimensions. (**c**) Flap elevated, after pedicle division. The defect template is shown above. (**d**) Late postoperative result after revisionary procedure including resection of cutaneous portion of groin flap and advancement of cervicofacial flap

The groin and surrounding tissues are vascularized by both the SCIA and the superficial inferior epigastric artery (SIEA). Both vessels originate from the femoral artery; however, this vascular anatomy is variable with some patients displaying separate origins for both arteries and others originating from a common arterial trunk. Sometimes, a large SCIA alone will perfuse this area and the SIEA will be absent. In most patients, the SCIA branches from the anterolateral aspect of the femoral artery ~2.5 cm below the inguinal ligament and runs laterally towards the anterior superior iliac spine. At a point less than 1.5 cm from its origin, the vessel divides into superficial and deep branches. The superficial branch runs laterally, parallel to the inguinal ligament and superficial to the sartorius muscle. The deep branch runs below the deep fascia and crosses the lateral femoral cutaneous nerve giving off branches to the sartorius, before exiting the fascia at the muscle's lateral border. The deep branch continues to course laterally in the subcutaneous tissues and gives off branches to the iliac crest.

The groin region is drained by both deep and superficial venous systems. The deep system is comprised of venae comitantes of the deep arteries. The superficial system is dominant and consists of the superficial circumflex iliac vein (SCIV) and the superficial inferior epigastric vein (SIEV). In approximately 50 % of patients, the SCIV and SIEV will form a single large vein (saphenous bulb) with an average diameter of 2.5 mm. The SCIV is considered the primary choice for groin flap outflow due to its greater length (2–4 cm) and larger diameter (~2 mm).

Groin flap harvest is begun by marking the anterior superior iliac spine, pubic tubercle, inguinal ligament, and femoral artery. A Doppler probe is used to map out the SCIA. The central axis of the flap runs roughly from the origin of the SCIA ~2.5 cm below the inguinal ligament to the anterior superior iliac spine. The medial extent of the flap will also be located near the origin of the SCIA. The inferior border of the flap is located ~5 cm below and parallel to the inguinal ligament, with the lateral and superior borders tailored to match the defect being reconstructed.

Dissection begins by incising the medial aspect of the flap and identifying the SCIA and SCIV at their origins from the femoral vessels. Once the vessels are isolated and adequate pedicle length is confirmed, the flap is raised lateral to medial until the lateral border of the sartorius muscle is identified. At this point, the deep fascia should be incised and elevated with the flap, in order to include the deep branch of the SCIA. This branch is usually located on the deep surface of the sartorius fascia but may also perforate the muscle, in which case a cuff of the muscle can be harvested with the flap. Larger portions of sartorius can also be included in the flap if muscle is needed for the defect being reconstructed. Groin flaps including tensor fasciae latae muscle, perfused entirely by the SCIA, have also been reported.

The donor site can generally be closed primarily if the defect is less than 10 cm wide. The defect is closed in layers over a closed suction drain.

Advantages and Disadvantages

The free groin flap can supply a large volume of supple cutaneous tissue that tends to be relatively non-hair-bearing. The flap is also unique in that the donor site can be easily concealed and is rarely visible, even in a bathing suit. The main disadvantages of the groin flap are its short pedicle length, small vessel caliber, and variable vascular anatomy. Because of this short vascular pedicle, the surgeon should carefully plan the distance to recipient vessels when planning to utilize a free groin flap.

Deep Circumflex Iliac Artery Flap (See Fig. 22.4a–d)

History

In 1965, Manchester described the use of non-vascularized iliac bone grafts for mandibular reconstruction and noted the anatomic similarity between the iliac and mandibular bones, making it an ideal donor site for these types of reconstruction. After the free groin flap was first described by Daniel and Taylor in 1973, multiple attempts were made to include vascularized iliac bone in the flap. However, these efforts were largely unsuccessful until 1979 when Taylor et al. and Sanders and Mayou accurately defined the vascular anatomy of the iliac bone. These surgeons employed dye perfusion to demonstrate the deep circumflex iliac artery (DCIA) as the main vascular supply to the anterior ilium. Additional studies also showed that perforators from the DCIA perfused both the skin overlying the anterior ilium and the internal oblique muscle. Thus, it was confirmed that the DCIA flap allowed reliable harvest of iliac bone with associated skin and muscle for reconstruction of composite defects.

Anatomy and Surgical Technique

The DCIA flap's blood supply is based on the deep circumflex iliac artery and its vena comitans. The diameter of the arterial pedicle is between 1.5 and 3 mm, with the vein usually slightly larger in caliber. Like the groin flap, the pedicle is relatively short with a maximum length of 5–6 cm. The iliac bone may be harvested as either a bicortical or unicortical bone segment up to 15 cm long and 6 cm wide. The bony component of the DCIA flap includes both cortical and cancellous elements with a robust blood supply that facilitates diminished resorption and allows dental rehabilitation. The flap can be harvested with or without a skin paddle; dimensions as large as 16 × 20 cm have been reported.

The two major landmarks on the ilium are the anterior superior iliac spine (ASIS) and the posterior superior iliac spine (PSIS), which are the most anterosuperior and posterosuperior points of the ilium, respectively. Multiple muscles attach along the lateral and medial edges of the iliac crest. These include the gluteus maximus that attaches along the posterolateral portion and the iliacus that attaches along the medial surface. The transversus abdominis muscle attaches to the anterosuperior border of the crest, ending where the iliacus begins. The internal and external oblique muscles insert along the anterior superior border of the iliac crest, superficial to the transversus abdominis. The transversus abdominis and both oblique muscles also insert on the inguinal ligament.

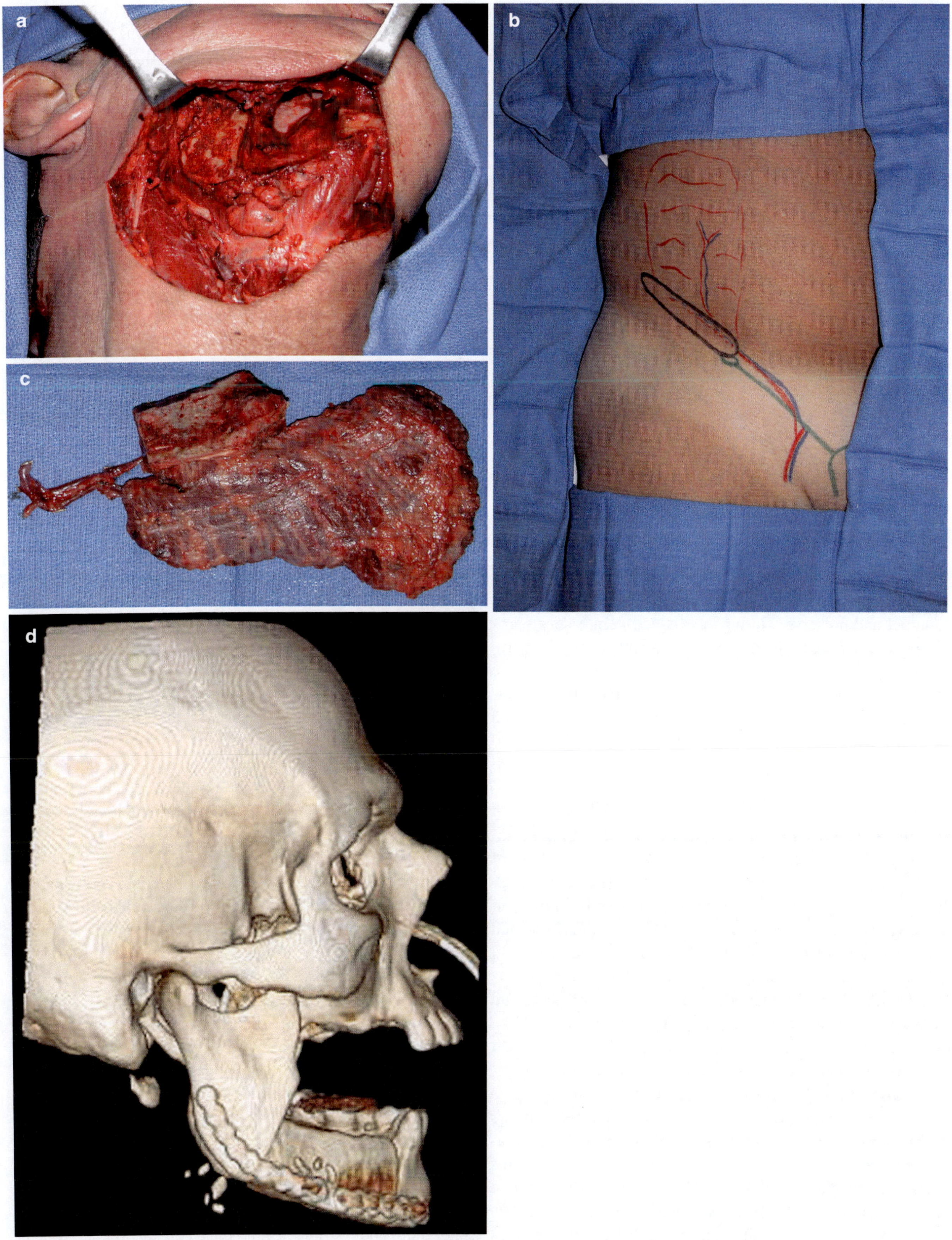

Fig. 22.4 Deep circumflex iliac artery flap. (**a**) A 59-year-old man with history of tonsillar squamous cell carcinoma resection and postoperative radiation therapy presenting with osteoradionecrosis of the right mandibular body. (**b**) Preoperative markings showing vascular pedicle and flap dimensions. (**c**) Flap elevated, after pedicle division. (**d**) Postoperative result

The DCIA takes origin near the junction of the femoral and external iliac arteries and may branch from either one of these vessels. The DCIA may originate alone or share a common trunk with the SCIA. The DCIA then courses laterally parallel to the inguinal ligament within a sheath formed by the junction of the iliac and transversalis fascia. An ascending artery branches off the DCIA close to the ASIS, piercing the transversus abdominis and running superiorly to provide blood supply to the internal oblique muscle. After giving off this ascending branch, the DCIA pierces the transversalis fascia and courses laterally along the medial iliac crest until approximately 6–9 cm past the ASIS where it again enters the transversus abdominis and anastomoses with the iliolumbar and superior gluteal arteries. Venous outflow for the DCIA flap is provided by a vena comitans that courses with the DCIA and drains into either the saphenous, femoral, or external iliac veins.

When choosing the donor side for a DCIA flap, it is important to consider that a hemi-mandibular defect is best reconstructed with iliac crest from the ipsilateral side due to the natural curvature of both bones. Once the donor side is determined, the patient is positioned supine with a bump placed under the ipsilateral buttock in order to elevate and externally rotate the donor site. The iliac crest, inguinal ligament, and femoral artery are palpated and marked. If a skin paddle is desired, the SCIA can also be located with a Doppler and preserved during the dissection in order to provide blood supply to the cutaneous segment.

An incision is made ~2 cm above and parallel to the inguinal ligament. If a skin island is being included, the lateral portion of the incision can include an ellipse based around the location of the SCIA, with its long axis parallel to the superior iliac crest. A skin island less than 10 cm wide will enable primary closure of the donor site.

After dissection down to the abdominal wall, the external oblique aponeurosis is incised parallel to the inguinal ligament in order to access the inguinal canal. The structures of the inguinal canal are retracted and the floor (i.e., transversalis fascia) exposed. The transversalis fascia is incised to identify the DCIA at its origin. The DCIA is then followed on its lateral course towards the ASIS, ligating the ascending branch when it is encountered. The lateral femoral cutaneous nerve will also be found crossing the DCIA in this area, and care must be taken to avoid injury. If a skin paddle is to be included, the superior aspect of the skin paddle is incised and elevated in a plane superficial to the external oblique muscle. After dissection of the skin paddle, the fat deep to the transversalis fascia is retracted and the fascial plane between the iliacus muscle and transversalis muscle identified. The iliacus muscle is divided, leaving a cuff of iliacus that contains the DCIA attached to the ilium. The vascular pedicle is then ligated distally. If a bicortical segment of bone is to be harvested, the gluteus medius and tensor fascia lata muscles must be detached from the outer surface of the ilium in a subperiosteal plane. Once both surfaces of the iliac crest are exposed, osteotomies are performed and the bone segment is removed.

Meticulous donor site closure in multiple layers is important in order to reduce the risk of postoperative hernia. The iliacus muscle and fascia are sutured to the transversalis muscle and fascia, and then the internal and external oblique muscles are sutured to the gluteal and tensor fascia lata muscles. The skin is closed in layers over a closed suction drain.

Advantages and Disadvantages

The DCIA flap can provide a large segment of cortical and cancellous bone that is able to adequately support osseointegrated implants. It can also include a skin paddle if needed. The donor site is easily concealed, but there is a risk of postoperative hernia or numbness due to injury to the lateral femoral cutaneous nerve. Other than potential donor site complications, the main disadvantage is a relatively short pedicle length. Like its relative the groin flap, use of the DCIA flap requires careful consideration of recipient vessel location.

Fibula Flap (See Fig. 22.5a–d)

History

The free fibula flap was originally described by Taylor in 1975 as a method for lower extremity salvage. Then in 1989, Hidalgo was the first to employ a fibula flap for mandibular reconstruction. Over the past two decades, it has become the workhorse option for treatment of segmental mandibular defects. More recently, its application has been extended for reconstruction of multiple other maxillofacial defects including the maxilla, frontal bone, and periorbital areas.

Anatomy and Surgical Technique

The fibula flap's blood supply is based on the peroneal artery and its venae comitantes. The artery is large in caliber with a diameter between 1.5 and 4 mm. The venae are usually similar in size to the artery. The pedicle length is variable depending on how much of the fibula bone is being utilized. A shorter bone segment permits a longer pedicle since the vessels can be dissected free of the proximal bone segment, which is discarded. Conversely, if the entire length of fibula is needed, the pedicle will be relatively short (~5 cm). Depending on patient size, a fibula bone segment up to 30 cm can be obtained. The flap can be harvested with a skin paddle that can also be up to 30 cm in length and should not exceed 14 cm in width.

The fibula is located posterior and lateral to the tibia. It is not involved with the knee joint but does articulate with the lateral tibia below the knee. At the ankle, the fibula forms the

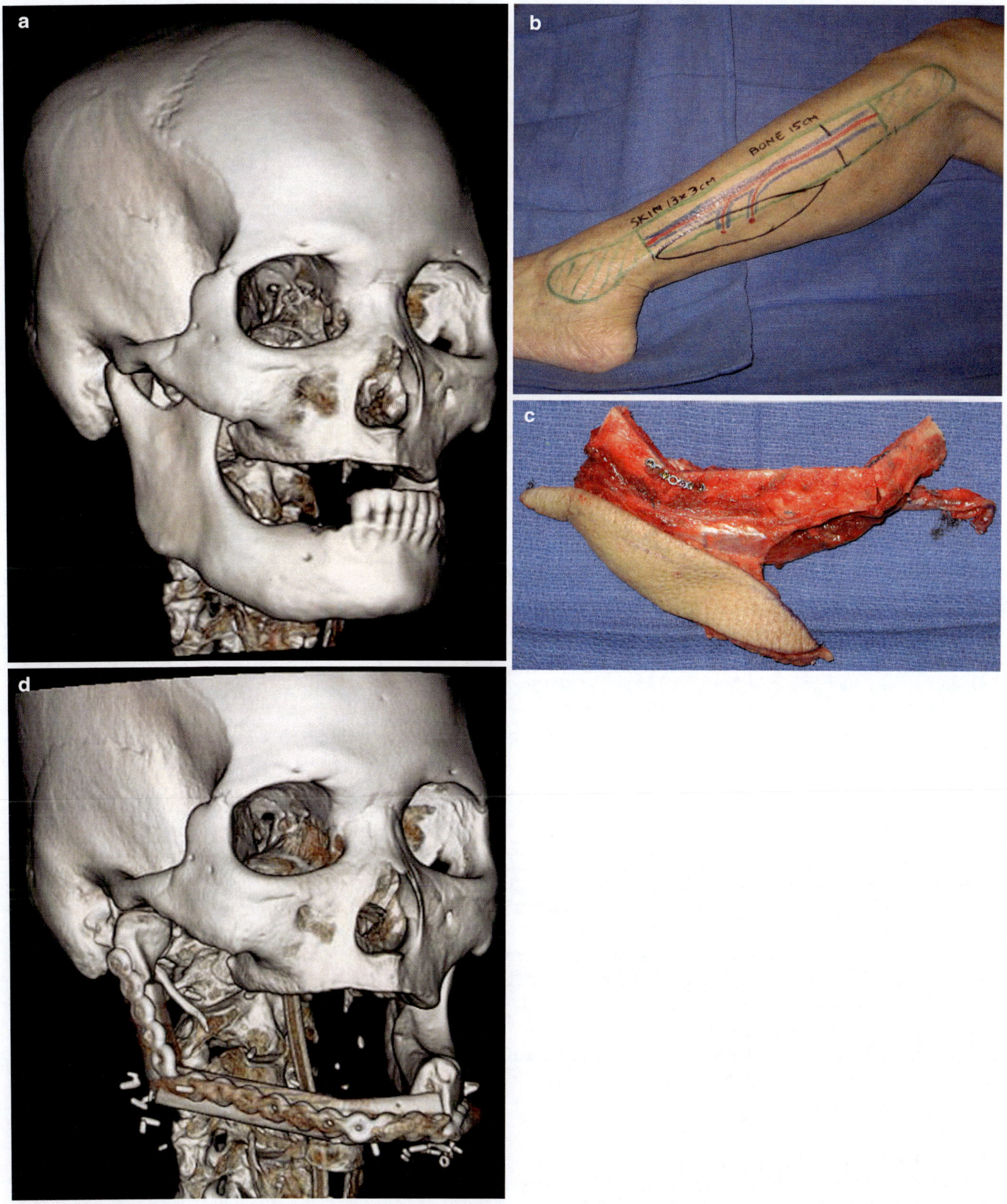

Fig. 22.5 Fibula flap. (**a**) A 72-year-old woman with history of chronic mandibular osteomyelitis presenting with osteonecrosis extending from right subcondylar region to left parasymphysis. (**b**) Preoperative markings showing vascular pedicle and flap dimensions. (**c**) Flap elevated, after pedicle division. The osteotomies and plate fixation were done in situ prior to pedicle division in order to minimize flap ischemia time. (**d**) Postoperative result

lateral malleolus and articulates medially with the talus via the talofibular joint. The fibula acts as an origin and structural support for musculature and helps to stabilize the ankle but plays only a minimal role in weight bearing.

The leg can be divided into four distinct muscular compartments: superficial posterior, deep posterior, anterior, and lateral. The tibia and fibula are connected by an interosseous membrane, which separates the anterior and deep posterior compartments. The anterior intermuscular septum separates the anterior and lateral compartments, while the posterior intermuscular septum separates the lateral and posterior compartments. The transverse intermuscular septum separates the superficial and deep posterior compartments. The peroneal vessels that supply the fibula flap are located in the deep posterior compartment, as is the posterior tibial artery and tibial nerve.

The popliteal artery enters the leg behind the knee and divides into the anterior and posterior tibial arteries. In most patients, the posterior tibial artery then gives off the peroneal artery, approximately 7 cm inferior to the fibular head. In rare cases, the peroneal artery originates from the popliteal or anterior tibial arteries. In ~8 % of patients, the posterior tibial artery is absent and is replaced by the peroneal artery. After its origin, the peroneal artery travels between the tibialis posterior and soleus muscles to reach the medial crest of the fibula. The artery then descends between the tibialis posterior and flexor hallucis longus muscles until it reaches the foot and divides into calcaneal branches. Along its course, the peroneal artery gives off several branches of consequence to the free fibula flap. Approximately 7 cm from the peroneal takeoff, there is generally a nutrient artery that enters the fibula and is directed downward. At intervals of 3–5 cm along the peroneal artery, arcade arteries provide segmental blood supply to the fibula periosteum and then continue on in the posterior intermuscular septum and serves as septocutaneous perforators to the skin. There are also commonly two large muscular branches to the lateral soleus, which allow a cuff of this muscle to be harvested with the fibula flap.

Preoperatively, it is important to examine the lower extremities for any evidence of peripheral vascular disease. The dorsalis pedis and posterior tibial pulses should be palpated, and collateral arterial supply to the foot can be confirmed by performing a foot Allen's test. If there is a concern for peripheral vascular disease, CT or formal angiography studies can be obtained to assess patency of the peroneal artery and the presence of collateral flow from the anterior and posterior tibial arteries.

The patient is positioned supine with a bump placed under the ipsilateral buttock, a tourniquet around the thigh, the knee flexed and hip internally rotated. The outline of the fibula is marked including the fibular head and the lateral malleolus. If a skin paddle is being utilized, the cutaneous perforators are located along the posterior border of the fibula with a Doppler probe and marked. An appropriate skin paddle is outlined based on the location of these perforators.

A straight incision is made along the posterior border of the fibula, diverging to incorporate the skin paddle if necessary. Dissection is carried out down to the muscular fascia, which is incised. The anterior and posterior portions of the skin flap are elevated in a subfascial plane towards the posterior crural septum, identifying and protecting any musculocutaneous or septocutaneous perforators. If there are inadequate septocutaneous perforators, intramuscular dissection through the soleus muscle to preserve the musculocutaneous perforators is essential to maintaining skin paddle viability.

In order to expose the fibula itself, the surrounding musculature is then detached, leaving a very small (<1 mm) cuff of muscle attached to the bone. This involves dissecting the peroneal muscles off of the anterior fibula, taking care to preserve the common peroneal nerve which crosses over the fibula 4–8 cm below the fibular head. The peroneus longus and brevis muscles are reflected anteriorly to expose the anterior intermuscular septum, which is incised to reveal the anterior compartment. The extensor digitorum and hallucis longus are dissected off the anterior fibula. Posteriorly, the soleus muscle must also be detached, revealing the flexor hallucis longus muscle. At this point, an osteomuscular flap can be harvested by instead leaving the lateral half of the soleus attached to the fibula.

The osteotomy sites are selected, and a right angle retractor is placed around the fibula, hugging the bone in order to protect the vascular pedicles. The fibula is osteotomized using a sagittal saw, preserving at least 6 cm proximally and distally in order to maintain stability of the knee and ankle joints. Penetrating towel clamps are used to grasp the bone and retract it anteriorly, revealing the peroneal vessels between the tibialis posterior and flexor hallucis longus muscles. The vascular pedicle is ligated distally, and the fibula is liberated from inferior to superior, dividing the attachments of the interosseus membrane, flexor hallucis longus, and tibialis posterior. The peroneal vessels are dissected to their origin, completing harvest of the fibula flap. While the vascular pedicle is still attached, further defect-specific osteotomies can be performed in situ to minimize flap ischemia. Any required plates can also be adapted and fixated to the fibula at this time.

Once the pedicle is divided and the flap removed, the tourniquet is let down and homeostasis achieved. The muscles are reapproximated over a closed suction drain and the skin is closed in layers. A skin defect up to 5 cm wide can be closed primarily; otherwise, a split-thickness skin graft is required. The ankle is splinted in neutral position, and the patient is allowed to begin full weight bearing within a week postoperatively.

Advantages and Disadvantages

The free fibula flap can provide a longer segment of bone than any other vascularized bone flap and is capable of reconstructing the mandible from angle to angle. It boasts a reliable blood supply, which allows for multiple osteotomies. The flap can also incorporate multiple types of tissue including bone, muscle, and skin. In contrast to the DCIA flap, however, the fibula flap only provides a small volume of cancellous bone stock. Additionally, the pedicle length is variable and can be relatively short if the entire length of fibula is being used. Although it has clearly been shown that the lower extremity can tolerate absence of the fibula, significant donor site morbidity can still result, including decreased ankle mobility, ankle instability, leg weakness, and great toe contracture.

Bibliography

Baek SM. Two new cutaneous free flaps: the medial and lateral thigh flaps. Plast Reconstr Surg. 1983;71(3):354–65. Epub 1983/03/01.

Baudet J, Guimberteau JC, Nascimento E. Successful clinical transfer of two free thoraco-dorsal axillary flaps. Plast Reconstr Surg. 1976;58(6):680–8. Epub 1976/12/01.

Borsuk DE, Christensen J, Dorafshar AH, Bojovic B, Sauerborn PJ, Christy MR, et al. Aesthetic microvascular periorbital subunit reconstruction: beyond primary repair. Plast Reconstr Surg. 2013;131(2):337–47. Epub 2012/10/19.

Bourget A, Chang JT, Wu DB, Chang CJ, Wei FC. Free flap reconstruction in the head and neck region following radiotherapy: a cohort study identifying negative outcome predictors. Plast Reconstr Surg. 2011;127(5):1901–8. Epub 2011/01/14.

Buncke Jr HJ, Schulz WP. Total ear reimplantation in the rabbit utilising microminiature vascular anastomoses. Br J Plast Surg. 1966;19(1):15–22. Epub 1966/01/01.

Buncke Jr HJ, Buncke CM, Schulz WP. Immediate Nicoladoni procedure in the rhesus monkey, or hallux-to-hand transplantation, utilising microminiature vascular anastomoses. Br J Plast Surg. 1966;19(4):332–7. Epub 1966/10/01.

Chen KT, Mardini S, Chuang DC, Lin CH, Cheng MH, Lin YT, et al. Timing of presentation of the first signs of vascular compromise dictates the salvage outcome of free flap transfers. Plast Reconstr Surg. 2007;120(1):187–95. Epub 2007/06/19.

Cigna E, Minni A, Barbaro M, Attanasio G, Sorvillo V, Malzone G, et al. An experience on primary thinning and secondary debulking of anterolateral thigh flap in head and neck reconstruction. Eur Rev Med Pharmacol Sci. 2012;16(8):1095–101. Epub 2012/08/24.

Clark N, Birely B, Manson PN, Slezak S, Kolk CV, Robertson B, et al. High-energy ballistic and avulsive facial injuries: classification, patterns, and an algorithm for primary reconstruction. Plast Reconstr Surg. 1996;98(4):583–601. Epub 1996/09/01.

Daniel RK, May Jr JW. Free flaps: an overview. Clin Orthop Relat Res. 1978;133:122–31. Epub 1978/06/01.

Daniel RK, Taylor GI. Distant transfer of an island flap by microvascular anastomoses. A clinical technique. Plast Reconstr Surg. 1973; 52(2):111–7. Epub 1973/08/01.

Demirkan F, Chen HC, Wei FC, Chen HH, Jung SG, Hau SP, et al. The versatile anterolateral thigh flap: a musculocutaneous flap in disguise in head and neck reconstruction. Br J Plast Surg. 2000;53(1):30–6. Epub 2000/02/05.

Eckardt A, Meyer A, Laas U, Hausamen JE. Reconstruction of defects in the head and neck with free flaps: 20 years experience. Br J Oral Maxillofac Surg. 2007;45(1):11–5. Epub 2006/02/09.

Freshwater MF. Denis F. Keegan: forgotten pioneer of plastic surgery. J Plast Reconstr Aesthet Surg. 2012;65(8):1131–6. Epub 2012/03/17.

Gillies HD. Plastic surgery of the face. London: Oxford Medical; 1920.

Gillies HD, Millard DR. The principles and art of plastic surgery. 1st ed. Boston: Little; 1957.

Gonzalez-Ulloa M. Restoration of the face covering by means of selected skin in regional aesthetic units. Br J Plast Surg. 1956;9(3):212–21. Epub 1956/10/01.

Gonzalez-Ulloa M. Regional aesthetic units of the face. Plast Reconstr Surg. 1987;79(3):489–90. Epub 1987/03/01.

González-Ulloa M, editor. Clinical and experimental research: report on our study of skin thickness of the entire surface of face and body. Transactions of the International Society of Plastic Surgeons, First Congress, Upsalla, 1955.

Gruss JS, Antonyshyn O, Phillips JH. Early definitive bone and soft-tissue reconstruction of major gunshot wounds of the face. Plast Reconstr Surg. 1991;87(3):436–50. Epub 1991/03/01.

Hallock GG. Impact of the successful flap but failed reconstruction on the true rate of success in free-tissue transfers. J Reconstr Microsurg. 2000;16(8):589–92. Epub 2000/12/29.

Harashina T. Analysis of 200 free flaps. Br J Plast Surg. 1988;41(1):33–6. Epub 1988/01/01.

Hidalgo DA. Fibula free flap: a new method of mandible reconstruction. Plast Reconstr Surg. 1989;84(1):71–9. Epub 1989/07/01.

Hidalgo DA, Jones CS. The role of emergent exploration in free-tissue transfer: a review of 150 consecutive cases. Plast Reconstr Surg. 1990;86(3):492–8; discussion 9–501. Epub 1990/09/01.

Hidalgo DA, Rekow A. A review of 60 consecutive fibula free flap mandible reconstructions. Plast Reconstr Surg. 1995;96(3):585–96; discussion 97–602. Epub 1995/09/01.

Higgins KM, Erovic BM, Ravi A, Yeung R, Lee JW, Yao C, et al. Volumetric changes of the anterolateral thigh free flap following adjuvant radiotherapy in total parotidectomy reconstruction. Laryngoscope. 2012;122(4):767–72. Epub 2012/02/02.

Hui-Chou HG, Sulek J, Bluebond-Langner R, Rodriguez ED. Secondary refinements of free perforator flaps for lower extremity reconstruction. Plast Reconstr Surg. 2011;127(1):248–57. Epub 2010/09/28.

Jacobson JH, Suarez EL. Microsurgery – application to organ transplantation. Trans Am Soc Artif Intern Organs. 1961;7(N):301–5.

Kimata Y, Uchiyama K, Ebihara S, Nakatsuka T, Harii K. Anatomic variations and technical problems of the anterolateral thigh flap: a report of 74 cases. Plast Reconstr Surg. 1998;102(5):1517–23. Epub 1998/10/17.

Kimura N, Satoh K. Consideration of a thin flap as an entity and clinical applications of the thin anterolateral thigh flap. Plast Reconstr Surg. 1996;97(5):985–92. Epub 1996/04/01.

Kleinert HE, Kasdan ML. Restoration of blood flow in upper extremity injuries. J Trauma. 1963;3:461–76. Epub 1963/09/01.

Koshima I. Free anterolateral thigh flap for reconstruction of head and neck defects following cancer ablation. Plast Reconstr Surg. 2000;105(7):2358–60. Epub 2001/03/10.

Koshima I, Soeda S. Inferior epigastric artery skin flaps without rectus abdominis muscle. Br J Plast Surg. 1989;42(6):645–8. Epub 1989/11/01.

Koshima I, Soeda S. Free posterior tibial perforator-based flaps. Ann Plast Surg. 1991;26(3):284–8. Epub 1991/03/01.

Koshima I, Soeda S, Yamasaki M, Kyou J. The free or pedicled anteromedial thigh flap. Ann Plast Surg. 1988;21(5):480–5. Epub 1988/11/01.

Lovie MJ, Duncan GM, Glasson DW. The ulnar artery forearm free flap. Br J Plast Surg. 1984;37(4):486–92. Epub 1984/10/01.

Manchester WM. Immediate reconstruction of the mandible and temporomandibular joint. Br J Plast Surg. 1965;18:291–303. Epub 1965/07/01.

Manson PN. Reconstruction of traumatic cutaneous facial defects. Oper Tech Plast Reconstr Surg. 1998;5(4):368–78.

Manson PN, Clark N, Robertson B, Slezak S, Wheatly M, Vander Kolk C, et al. Subunit principles in midface fractures: the importance of sagittal buttresses, soft-tissue reductions, and sequencing treatment of segmental fractures. Plast Reconstr Surg. 1999;103(4):1287–306; quiz 307. Epub 1999/03/24.

McGregor IA, Jackson IT. The groin flap. Br J Plast Surg. 1972;25(1):3–16. Epub 1972/01/01.

McLean DH, Buncke Jr HJ. Autotransplant of omentum to a large scalp defect, with microsurgical revascularization. Plast Reconstr Surg. 1972;49(3):268–74. Epub 1972/03/01.

Momoh AO, Yu P, Skoracki RJ, Liu S, Feng L, Hanasono MM. A prospective cohort study of fibula free flap donor-site morbidity in 157 consecutive patients. Plast Reconstr Surg. 2011;128(3):714–20. Epub 2011/05/17.

Morrison WA, O'Brien BM, MacLeod A. Clinical experiences in free flap transfer. Clin Orthop Relat Res. 1978;133:132–9. Epub 1978/06/01.

Muresan C, Hui-Chou H, Dorafshar AH, Manson PN, Rodriguez ED. Forehead reconstruction with microvascular flaps: utility of aesthetic subunits. J Reconstr Microsurg. 2012;28(5):319–26.

O'Brien BM. Replantation and reconstructive microvascular surgery. Part II. Ann R Coll Surg Engl. 1976;58(3):171–82. Epub 1976/05/01.

O'Brien BM, Morrison WA, Ishida H, MacLeod AM, Gilbert A. Free flap transfers with microvascular anastomoses. Br J Plast Surg. 1974;27(3):220–30. Epub 1974/07/01.

Pennington DG, Pelly AD. The rectus abdominis myocutaneous free flap. Br J Plast Surg. 1980;33(2):277–82. Epub 1980/04/01.

Ramasastry SS, Granick MS, Futrell JW. Clinical anatomy of the internal oblique muscle. J Reconstr Microsurg. 1986;2(2):117–22.

Robertson B, Manson PN. The importance of serial debridement and "second-look" procedures in high-energy ballistic and avulsive facial injuries. Oper Tech Plast Reconstr Surg. 1998;5(3):236–45.

Robertson BC, Manson PN. High-energy ballistic and avulsive injuries. A management protocol for the next millennium. Surg Clin North Am. 1999;79(6):1489–502, xi. Epub 2000/01/08.

Rodriguez ED, Martin M, Bluebond-Langner R, Khalifeh M, Singh N, Manson PN. Microsurgical reconstruction of posttraumatic high-energy maxillary defects: establishing the effectiveness of early reconstruction. Plast Reconstr Surg. 2007a;120(7 Suppl 2):103S–17. Epub 2007/12/27.

Rodriguez ED, Martin M, Bluebond-Langner R, Khalifeh M, Singh N, Manson PN. Microsurgical reconstruction of posttraumatic high-energy maxillary defects: establishing the effectiveness of early reconstruction. Plast Reconstr Surg. 2007b;120(7 Suppl 2):103S–17. Epub 2007/12/27.

Rodriguez ED, Mithani SK, Bluebond-Langner R, Manson PN. Hand evaluation following ulnar forearm perforator flap harvest: a prospective study. Plast Reconstr Surg. 2007c;120(6):1598–601. Epub 2007/11/28.

Rodriguez ED, Bluebond-Langner R, Park JE, Manson PN. Preservation of contour in periorbital and midfacial craniofacial microsurgery: reconstruction of the soft-tissue elements and skeletal buttresses. Plast Reconstr Surg. 2008;121(5):1738–47; discussion 48–9. Epub 2008/05/06.

Rodriguez ED, Stanwix MG, Nam AJ, St Hilaire H, Simmons OP, Manson PN. Definitive treatment of persistent frontal sinus infections: elimination of dead space and sinonasal communication. Plast Reconstr Surg. 2009;123(3):957–67. Epub 2009/03/26.

Rohrich RJ, Pessa JE. The fat compartments of the face: anatomy and clinical implications for cosmetic surgery. Plast Reconstr Surg. 2007;119(7):2219–27; discussion 28–31. Epub 2007/05/24.

Sakai S, Soeda S, Uchida A, Wakabayashi K, Ishikawa A. Use of a combined groin-tensor fasciae latae flap for reconstruction of a full-thickness defect of the abdominal wall. Br J Plast Surg. 1985; 38(4):492–6. Epub 1985/10/01.

Sanders R, Mayou BJ. A new vascularized bone graft transferred by microvascular anastomosis as a free flap. Br J Surg. 1979;66(11): 787–8.

Schusterman MA, Miller MJ, Reece GP, Kroll SS, Marchi M, Goepfert H. A single center's experience with 308 free flaps for repair of head and neck cancer defects. Plast Reconstr Surg. 1994;93(3):472–8; discussion 9–80. Epub 1994/03/01.

Serafin D, Shearin JC, Georgiade NG. The vascularization of free flaps: a clinical and experimental correlation. Plast Reconstr Surg. 1977;60(2):233–41. Epub 1977/08/01.

Sharabi SE, Hatef DA, Koshy JC, Jain A, Cole PD, Hollier Jr LH. Is primary thinning of the anterolateral thigh flap recommended? Ann Plast Surg. 2010;65(6):555–9. Epub 2010/11/03.

Shieh SJ, Chiu HY, Yu JC, Pan SC, Tsai ST, Shen CL. Free anterolateral thigh flap for reconstruction of head and neck defects following cancer ablation. Plast Reconstr Surg. 2000;105(7):2349–57; discussion 58–60. Epub 2000/06/09.

Sieg P, Dericioglu M, Hansmann C, Jacobsen HC, Trenkle T, Hakim SG. Long-term functional donor site morbidity after ulnar forearm flap harvest. Head Neck. 2012;34(9):1312–6. Epub 2011/10/26.

Song R, Gao Y, Song Y, Yu Y. The forearm flap. Clin Plast Surg. 1982;9(1):21–6. Epub 1982/01/01.

Song YG, Chen GZ, Song YL. The free thigh flap: a new free flap concept based on the septocutaneous artery. Br J Plast Surg. 1984;37(2): 149–59. Epub 1984/04/01.

Tan ST, James DW, Moaveni Z. Donor site morbidity of free ulnar forearm flap. Head Neck. 2012;34(10):1434–9. Epub 2011/11/05.

Taylor GI, Miller GD, Ham FJ. The free vascularized bone graft. A clinical extension of microvascular techniques. Plast Reconstr Surg. 1975;55(5):533–44. Epub 1975/05/01.

Taylor GI, Townsend P, Corlett R. Superiority of the deep circumflex iliac vessels as the supply for free groin flaps. Clinical work. Plast Reconstr Surg. 1979a;64(6):745–59.

Taylor GI, Townsend P, Corlett R. Superiority of the deep circumflex iliac vessels as the supply for free groin flaps. Plast Reconstr Surg. 1979b;64(5):595–604.

Wei FC, Mardini S. Free-style free flaps. Plast Reconstr Surg. 2004;114(4):910–6. Epub 2004/10/07.

Wei FC, Jain V, Celik N, Chen HC, Chuang DC, Lin CH. Have we found an ideal soft-tissue flap? An experience with 672 anterolateral thigh flaps. Plast Reconstr Surg. 2002;109(7):2219–26; discussion 27–30. Epub 2002/06/05.

Wong CH, Wei FC. Microsurgical free flap in head and neck reconstruction. Head Neck. 2010;32(9):1236–45. Epub 2009/12/17.

Yang GF, Chen PJ, Gao YZ, Liu XY, Li J, Jiang SX, et al. Forearm free skin flap transplantation: a report of 56 cases. 1981. Br J Plast Surg. 1997;50(3):162–5.

Yim KK, Wei FC. Fibula osteoseptocutaneous free flap in maxillary reconstruction. Microsurgery. 1994;15(5):353–7. Epub 1994/01/01.

Yoshioka N, Haraoka G, Muraoka M, Tominaga S. Single stage reconstruction of scalp and skull using free muscle flap and titanium mesh in patients with epidural infection. J Craniomaxillofac Surg. 1996; 24(2):118–21. Epub 1996/04/01.

Pediatric Facial Fractures

23

Laura A. Monson, Darren M. Smith, and Joseph E. Losee

Introduction

The treatment of pediatric facial fractures can be challenging, stimulating, and occasionally frustrating, especially for those practitioners who only rarely manage these injuries. Difficulties arise from the fact that unlike their adult counterparts, no standardized protocols exist for the management of pediatric facial fractures; there are only broad guidelines and rare case reports. When evaluating a pediatric facial trauma patient, it should be remembered that the same fracture pattern will rarely be seen in a 5-month-old, a 5-year-old, and a 15-year-old due to the inherent differences in craniofacial anatomy, craniofacial proportions, and mechanism of injury. Even if a similar fracture pattern were observed, the treatment for patients of different ages would vary. The differences in craniofacial anatomy, patterns of injury, and capacity for remodeling and future growth must all be considered when determining a specific treatment option. It is paramount to remember that the pediatric patient is not just a small adult. Even with similarly aged patients and fracture patterns, the treatment plan must take into account patient and parent compliance and stage of dentition in that particular child.

L.A. Monson, MD
Division of Plastic Surgery,
Michael E. DeBakey Department of Surgery,
Baylor College of Medicine, Houston, TX, USA

D.M. Smith, MD
Department of Plastic Surgery,
University of Pittsburgh Medical Center, Pittsburgh, PA, USA

J.E. Losee, MD, FACS, FAAP (✉)
Department of Plastic Surgery, University of Pittsburgh
Medical Center, Pittsburgh, PA, USA

Division of Pediatric Plastic Surgery, Children's Hospital of
Pittsburgh of UPMC, Pittsburgh, PA, USA
e-mail: joseph.losee@chp.edu

Demographics

Pediatric facial fractures are an uncommon entity, comprising less than 15 % of all facial fractures. Many studies of pediatric craniofacial injuries have had a significant bias as they were based on inpatient admissions, separated by treating specialty, or restricted to patients undergoing operative intervention. In the authors' series, comprised of all pediatric emergency room visits to a Level 1 pediatric hospital over a 5-year period, a more complete picture of the incidence and demographics of pediatric facial fractures was obtained. In general, these patients were more likely to be older and male (see Fig. 23.1). Fracture pattern, causation, and level of care varied with age, with a general evolution of injury pattern from cranial to caudal (see Fig. 23.2). As age increased, injuries were more often the result of adult behaviors that occurred outside of the home, whereas younger children were more often injured as the result of falls and motor vehicle accidents (see Fig. 23.3).

Although pediatric facial fractures are a rare cause of pediatric trauma presentations (less than 10 %), these

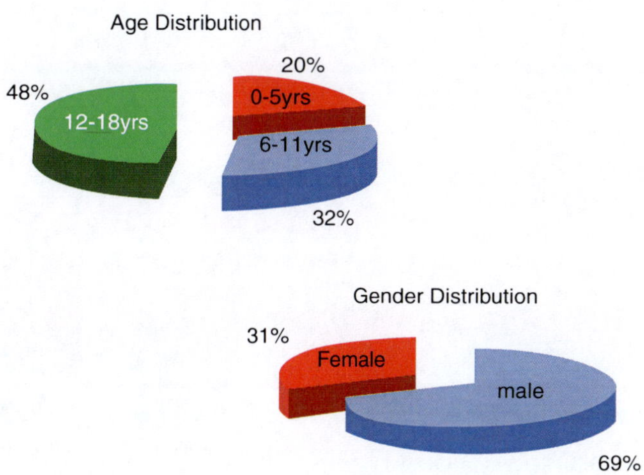

Fig. 23.1 Age and gender distribution of pediatric facial fractures

P.J. Taub et al. (eds.), *Ferraro's Fundamentals of Maxillofacial Surgery*,
DOI 10.1007/978-1-4614-8341-0_23, © Springer Science+Business Media New York 2015

patients tend to have higher injury severity scores, prolonged hospitalizations, and more significant morbidity and mortality. These findings are likely due to the high energy required to overcome the resilience of the pediatric craniofacial skeleton, and it follows that the most common cause of injury in these patients is motor vehicle accidents. Pediatric trauma patients, especially the youngest children, are more likely to require admission to the intensive care unit. Pediatric patients with facial fractures have serious associated trauma in 25–75 % of cases. Brain injury is twice as common in patients with facial fractures as in those without facial fractures. In the authors' series, nearly half of the patients had an associated neurologic injury and 48.6 % suffered a concussion in keeping with the reported literature (see Fig. 23.4). These children require a high index of suspicion for an associated neurologic injury; if a concussion is diagnosed, they require rest and serial testing to chart resolution and prevent long-term impairment. Unlike their adult counterparts, pediatric facial trauma patients are unlikely to suffer cervical spine injuries. In the authors' series, only 2.3 % of patients had an associated cervical spine injury. The most common related facial fracture was an orbital fracture, and all of the patients who had a cervical spine injury were either involved in a motor vehicle collision or a fall.

The incidence of facial fractures increases with age, with the mean age in the author's series being 10.7 years. The greater likelihood of an older child to suffer a facial fracture is due to both the changing anatomy of the child's craniofacial anatomy and the changing environment of the growing child. Small children are more likely to spend the majority of their life in a closely supervised situation, while the teenaged child spends more time unsupervised and partakes in more adult behaviors, such as sports and recreational activities that put them at risk for injury. This pattern was seen in the authors' series as the cause of injury changed from predominantly falls and motor vehicle accidents in the young child to violence, sports, and use of all-terrain vehicles in the older children (see Fig. 23.5). In general, motor vehicle collisions are the most common cause of facial fracture in children across all age groups, and children who are improperly restrained are more likely to suffer facial fractures. Older male patients from lower socioeconomic areas were more likely to have suffered a facial fracture as the result of violence (see Fig. 23.6). Non-accidental trauma is a not uncommon cause of pediatric facial trauma, with an incidence from 4 to 12 % in the literature.

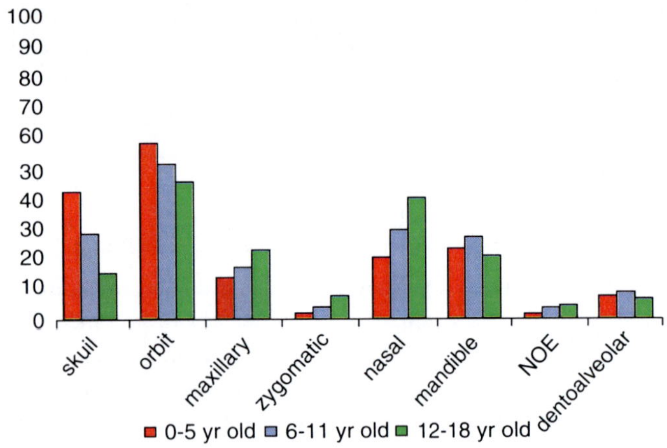

Fig. 23.2 Percent fracture distribution by age

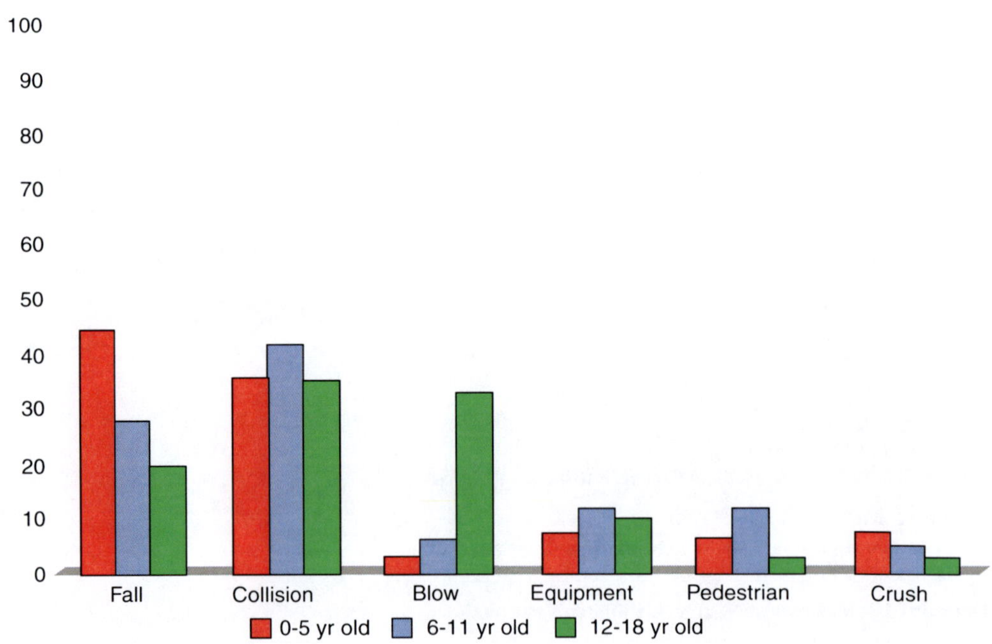

Fig. 23.3 Percent mechanism of injury by age

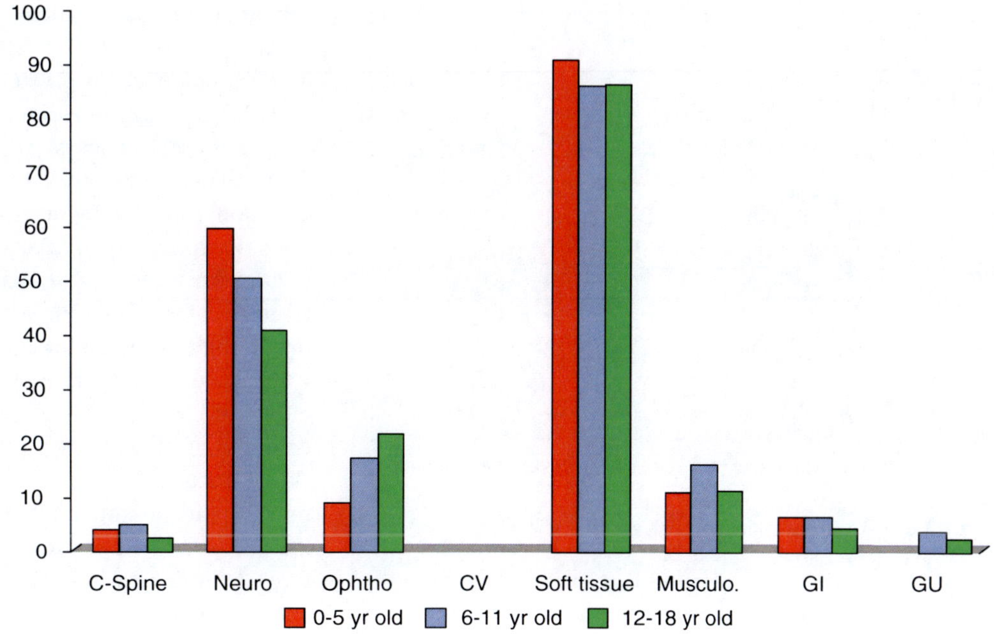

Fig. 23.4 Associated injuries by age

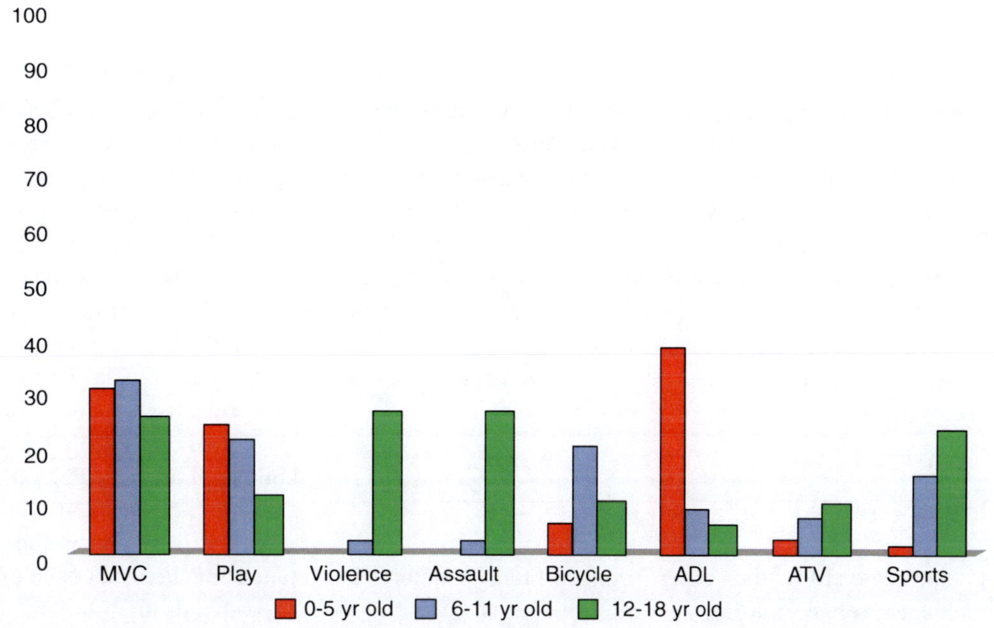

Fig. 23.5 Percent cause of injury by age

Anatomic Considerations

The relatively low incidence of facial fractures observed in the pediatric population is due to both environmental and anatomic factors. The pediatric craniofacial skeleton is unique from the adult craniofacial skeleton in several important facets that impact the patterns of fractures observed as well as the management employed. The infant has a large cranium-to-face ratio, 8:1, at birth that decreases to 4:1 by 5 years of age and progresses to 2.5:1 by adulthood. The growth of the cranium is 75 % complete by age 7 and 95 % complete by age 10. The upper face grows secondary to brain and ocular development and orbital growth is completed by 6–8 years of age. Midface growth follows the development of the nasal capsule and dentition. The palate and maxilla are two-thirds of adult size at age 6 and are largely fully grown by age 12–14, as is nasal growth. The sinuses of the infant are largely undeveloped and poorly pneumatized. The sphenoid sinus begins to develop at age 2 and matures through adulthood. The maxillary sinus develops in parallel with

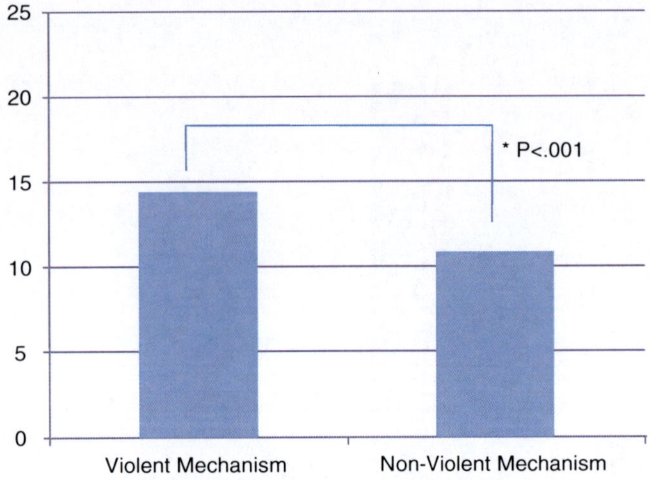

Fig. 23.6 Percent patients living below poverty level

dental eruption, and the frontal sinus does not develop until full facial skeletal maturity is reached. The ethmoid sinus is the first to fully develop and is completed by age 12. The infant mandible is joined in the midline by a cartilaginous symphysis, which ossifies in the first year of life. Unerupted tooth buds form the majority of mandibular volume in early childhood. As the teeth erupt, cortical bone becomes the primary component of the mandible as full growth is achieved. The condyles are a major growth center of the mandible, and development of the mandible is the result of addition of bone at these centers as well as along the posterior border of the ramus. In addition, the overall increase in size of the mandible is the result of surface apposition; the mandible is continuously undergoing changes related to remodeling until growth is complete. In females, adult mandibular size is achieved by age 14–16 and in males by 18–20.

Injury Patterns

Pediatric facial fractures differ from adult facial fractures in incidence, related injuries, and injury patterns. The unique aspects of the pediatric craniofacial skeleton can explain these observed relationships. The pediatric craniofacial skeleton not only differs in the relative proportion of the face to cranium but also in the amount of sinus aeration, buccomaxillary fat pad volume, and cancellous-to-cortical bone ratio. The decreased bone mineral content of the pediatric craniofacial skeleton results in increased tolerance to force without fracture; fractures that do occur are more likely to be unicortical, or greenstick, fractures. Although mandible fractures are widely reported as the most common pediatric facial fractures, cited as anywhere from 20 to 50 % of all pediatric facial fractures, several series have reported that children younger than 5 years of age are more likely to sustain cranial, orbital, and nasal fractures. In one series, cranial vault fractures comprised 54 % of all craniofacial fractures with the highest incidence observed in the youngest patients. In fact, in the authors' series, orbital fracture was the most common fracture observed across all age groups. In children under 6 years of age, cranial and orbital fractures were the most common, followed by mandibular, nasal, and maxillary fractures. Zygomaticomaxillary (ZMC) and nasoorbitoethmoid (NOE) fractures were rare. In children aged 6–11, orbital fractures were again the most common, followed by nasal, mandibular, skull, and maxillary fractures. Again, ZMC and NOE fractures were rare but more frequent with age. In the oldest group, aged 12–18, orbital fractures were the most common, followed by nasal, mandibular, maxillary, and skull fractures. Again, ZMC and NOE fractures were uncommon but more likely in this age group than in either of the two younger age groups (see Fig. 23.2). Mandible fractures demonstrate an age-related distribution; condylar head and subcondylar fractures are the most common (48 %) but decrease with age, while body and angle fractures increase.

Lack of mineralization, increased cancellous-to-cortical bone ratio, incomplete development of sinuses, and dental eruption all lead to different patterns of fracture in the pediatric craniofacial skeleton. Le Fort fracture patterns are rarely observed in the skeletally immature child and, in one series, only seen after 10 years of age. Until 10 years of age, the lack of an aerated maxillary sinus allows forces to be transmitted directly to the alveolus, resulting in alveolar fractures rather than Le Fort I fractures in this age group. Unilateral NOE fractures occur rather than the Le Fort II fractures observed in the mature craniofacial skeleton; oblique craniofacial fractures are the pediatric equivalent of Le Fort III fractures. Oblique craniofacial fractures are observed in the pediatric population as the non-aerated sinuses allow forces to be transmitted easily from the site of impact to the cranium and skull base (see Figs. 23.7 and 23.8).

Another entity to be aware of in the care and treatment of the pediatric patient is the growing skull fracture. Orbital-cranial fractures can develop into growing skull fractures as the brain pulsations are transmitted through dural disruptions and impede healing, leading to a growing bony diastasis. These lesions have been documented in 0.6–2 % of pediatric skull fractures. Children at risk for developing these lesions must be followed long term with a high index of suspicion and a low threshold for repeat imaging to demonstrate complete bony healing (see Figs. 23.9, 23.10, 23.11, and 23.12).

Evaluation

A systematic approach to the evaluation of facial injuries cannot be overemphasized in the pediatric population. Examining an uncooperative child is difficult in itself; if a

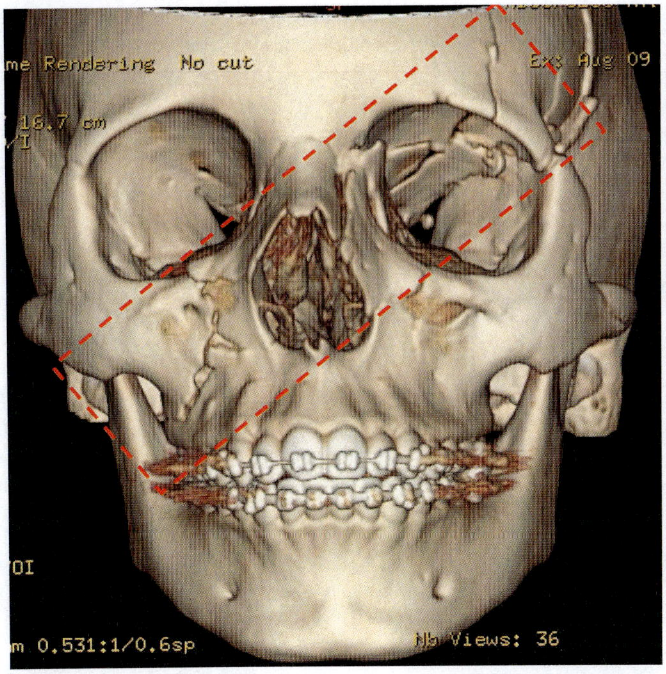

Fig. 23.7 3D CT demonstrating oblique craniofacial fracture pattern (*red hashed box*)

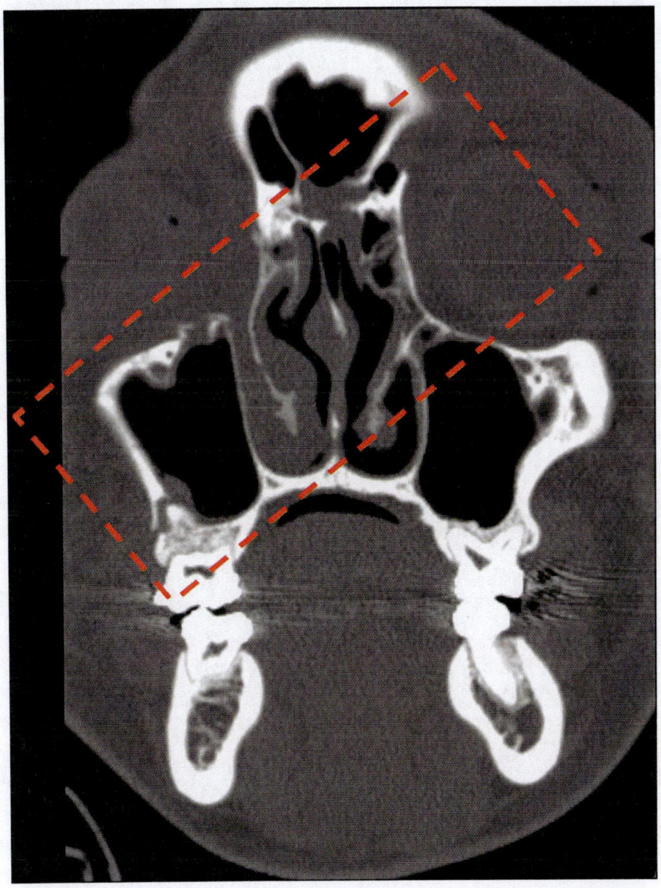

Fig. 23.8 Coronal CT demonstrating oblique craniofacial fracture pattern (*red hashed box*)

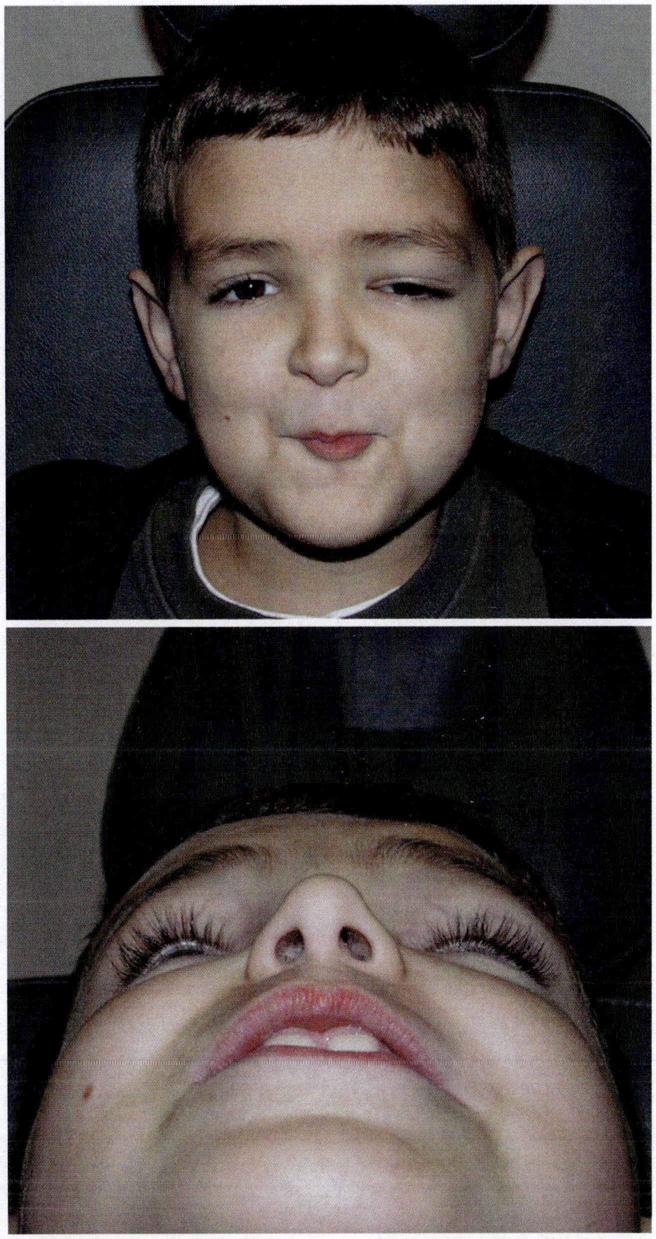

Fig. 23.9 Clinical appearance of growing skull fracture; note left supraorbital fullness

systematic examination is not undertaken, important findings may be missed. A maxillofacial CT scan with fine cuts and 3D reconstructions is invaluable in the full evaluation of a pediatric patient with a suspected facial fracture. Depending upon the fracture pattern present, the examiner should have a low threshold to involve their neurosurgery, ophthalmology, and dental colleagues.

Superior orbital fissure syndrome (internal and external ophthalmoplegia (CN II, IV, VI paralysis), proptosis, and CN V paresthesia) and orbital apex syndrome (superior orbital fissure syndrome with blindness secondary to CN

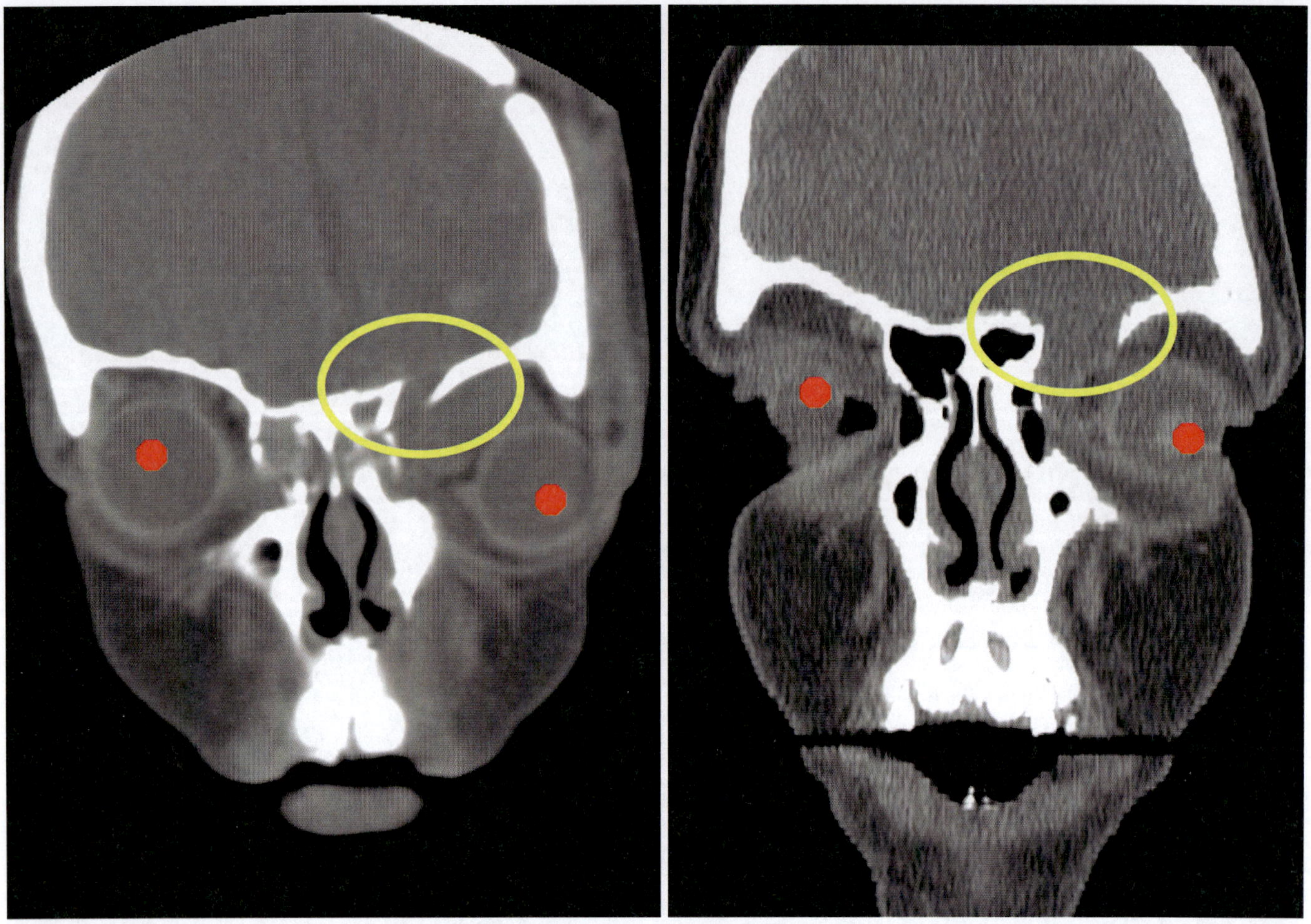

Fig. 23.10 Coronal CT corresponding to clinical photo in Fig. 23.9. The *yellow circle* indicates the growing skull fracture

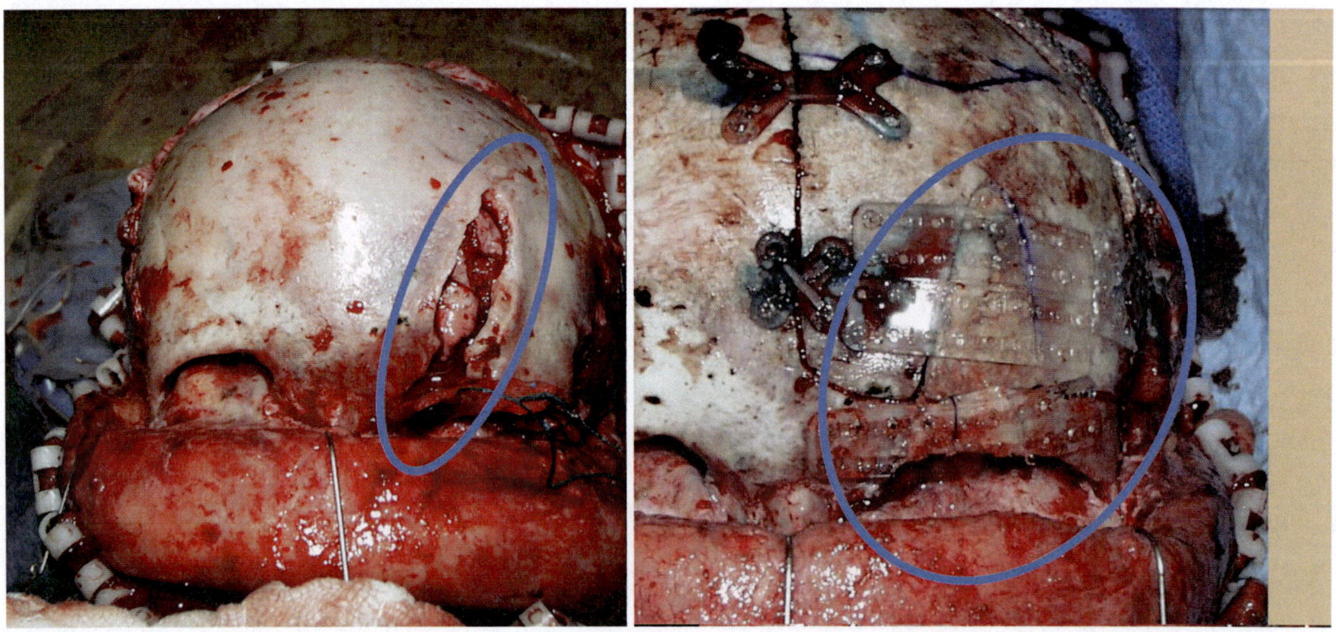

Fig. 23.11 Intraoperative photo of the patient in Figs. 23.9 and 23.10 demonstrating the defect (*left*) and reconstruction (*right*)

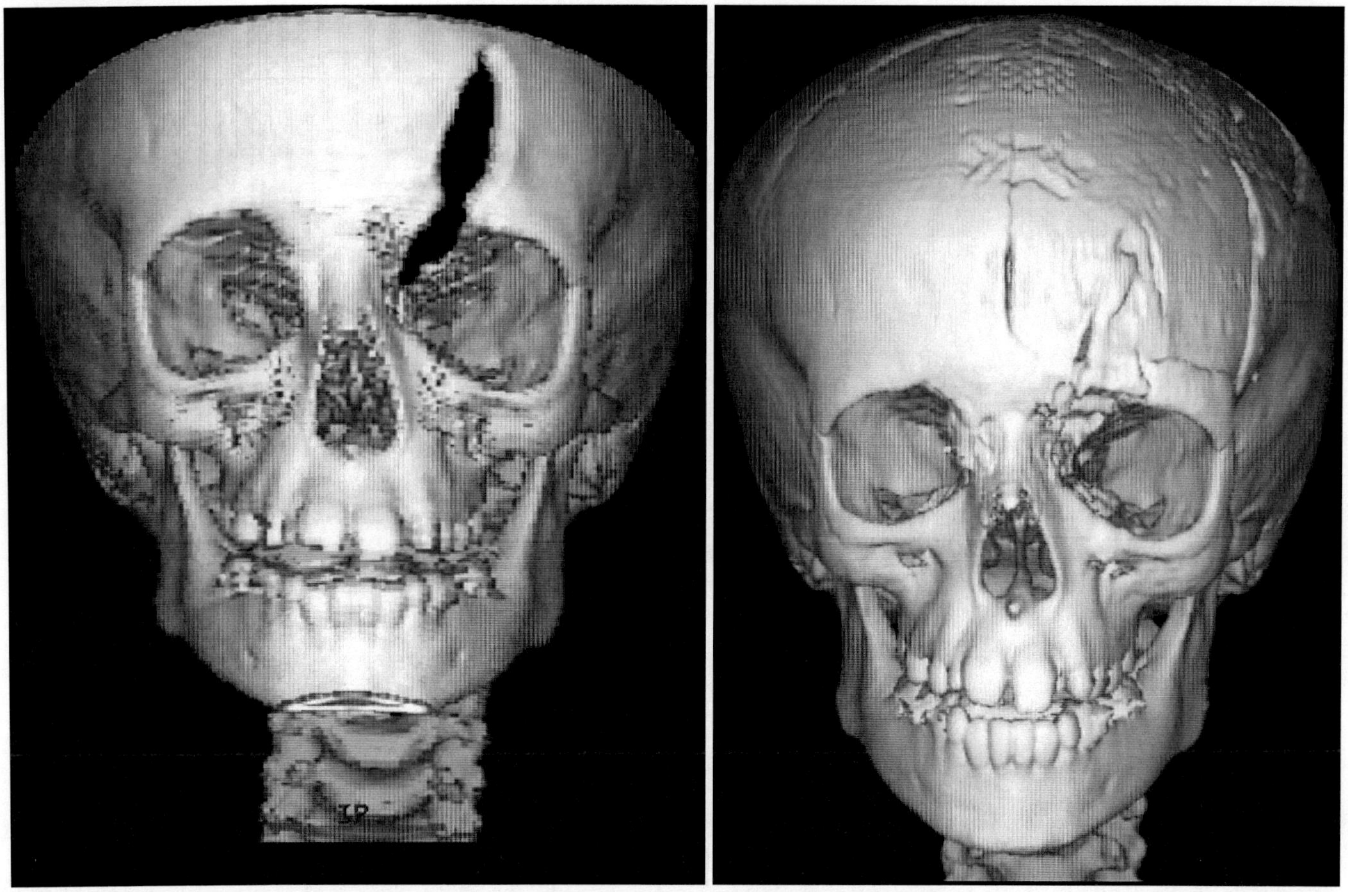

Fig. 23.12 3D CT demonstrating the growing skull fracture pictured in Figs. 23.9, 23.10, and 23.11 before (*left*) and after (*right*) reconstruction

II involvement) must be emergently addressed. Periorbital ecchymosis, hemotympanum, and cranial nerve palsy may indicate a skull base fracture. Ptosis may be secondary to levator paralysis. Exophthalmos and inferior globe displacement point to an orbital roof fracture. Extraocular muscle restriction or globe displacement will cause diplopia. Forced ductions should be performed on the obtunded patient to rule out muscle entrapment. Limitations of gaze, with relatively minimal associated findings, may represent entrapment in the "white-eyed blowout fracture." A bowstring test (palpation of the bony medial canthal attachment with distraction on the lower eyelid) should be performed to assess the integrity of the medial canthal tendon in NOE fractures.

Maxillary mobility and malocclusion may indicate a midface fracture just as in an adult patient, but it should be remembered that true Le Fort fractures are rare and the younger patient is much more likely to have sustained an alveolar fracture. ZMC fractures can be indicated by an upper buccal sulcus hematoma, a preauricular depression, cheek flattening, or lateral canthal dystopia. Impingement of a depressed zygomatic arch on the coronoid will give the patient trismus. Nasal fractures in children are not uncommon and can be associated with nasal deviation, compressibility of the dorsum, as well as septal hematoma, which must be ruled out.

Evaluation of the occlusion in a pediatric patient can be difficult, especially in mixed dentition. Attention must be paid to the wear facets; preinjury dental records and parent input can be helpful as well. Physical exam findings consistent with a mandible fracture include drooling, trismus, decreased maximal incisive opening, discomfort on excursion, and dental step-offs. Evidence of an anterior open bite is indicative of bilateral condylar fractures. A unilateral condylar fracture will result in a contralateral posterior open bite.

Indications for Treatment

In regard to operative intervention for pediatric facial fractures, the decision to intervene is essentially a judgment call with the practitioner weighing the benefits of precise reduction and fixation against the risk of future growth disturbance. It is the senior author's opinion that the younger the

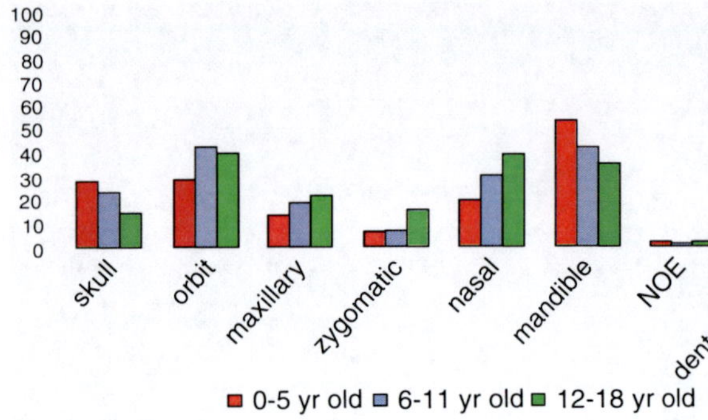

Fig. 23.13 Percent operative fractures by age

patient, the higher the threshold should be for operative intervention. The literature reports rates from 25 to 78 % operative intervention for pediatric facial fractures. In the authors' series, 36 % of all patients went on to undergo operative intervention (see Fig. 23.13). Older children, and those with multiple facial fractures, were more likely to undergo surgery, a finding consistent with the published literature. When the decision is made for operative intervention, surgery should be performed in a more acute fashion than in the adult population as long as the degree of swelling is not prohibitive and the overall patient's status allows. Converse advocated for prompt repair in the 1960s, and others note the propensity of the pediatric patient for rapid adherence of loose fragments within 3–4 days of injury. When operative intervention is undertaken, periosteal stripping should be minimized in order to have minimal impact on growth and development in keeping with Moss and Salentijn's "functional matrix" principle. While the care of pediatric facial fractures can be considered "treating a moving target," the following is a fracture-specific discussion of anatomic and developmental factors to guide the clinician in making informed decisions on a patient-by-patient basis.

Cranial Base and Skull Fractures

Indications for operative intervention for cranial base and skull fractures include a cerebrospinal fluid (CSF) leak that persists despite conservative management, significant displacement, deformation of facial contour, and growing skull fractures. The goals of cranial base and skull fracture repair include protection of the cranial contents, dural reconstruction, control of CSF leaks, prevention of infection, and restoration of craniofacial contour. In older patients with a developed frontal sinus, Rodriguez et al. have presented an algorithmic approach. With obstruction of the nasofrontal duct, obliteration or cranialization of the frontal sinus is indicated. Cranialization allows for single-stage elimination of the sinus as a potential site of infection. With a traumatized but patent duct, nondisplaced fractures of the anterior and posterior tables can be managed conservatively with close follow-up. Significantly displaced isolated anterior table fractures, with resulting contour deformities, can be reconstructed. However, in the child with an immature and underdeveloped frontal sinus, self-correction, with continued growth and development of the sinus, may correct contour deformities. The authors have reported a particularly illustrative case involving an 11-year-old struck in the forehead with a hockey stick. CT scan demonstrated a comminuted, depressed fracture through the left superior orbital rim extending cephalad through the anterior wall of the frontal sinus, as well as caudally into the ethmoids. No radiographic evidence of injury to the nasofrontal duct or extension of the fracture through the posterior table of the frontal sinus was present. Although there was palpable irregularity of the forehead on exam, no visible deformity was present. Therefore, the fracture was managed conservatively with close radiographic follow-up to ensure maintenance of a "safe sinus" where mucus from the frontal sinus would be able to drain into the nose. A repeat CT scan 6 weeks post-trauma demonstrated significant fracture healing and sinus remodeling. On a 1 year follow-up scan, the frontal sinus had completely remodeled with normal aeration, and there was in fact no evidence of prior fracture.

Alternatively, if a CSF leak is present, this finding will direct management. Observation and strict bed rest, with or without lumbar drain, may be pursued for 4–7 days. If the leak is persistent after this course, cranialization may be performed. If the leak resolves with conservative management and the nasofrontal duct is not obstructed, the sinus can be preserved. However, if the leak resolves but the duct is obstructed, then the sinus may be treated with "partial obliteration" (obliteration of the ducts and base of the sinus) and complete removal of the sinus mucosa.

Bone loss is a difficult problem in those patients too old to heal large calvarial defects spontaneously and too young to yield high-quality split calvarial grafts. Autogenous bone grafts are associated with potential donor site morbidity including pain, hemorrhage, nerve injury, and infection in up to 8 % of patients. Artificial bone substitutes are not biocompatible and are susceptible to infection. For these reasons, in donor sites of the calvarium, the authors prefer a bilaminate construct composed of intra- and extracranially placed bioresorbable mesh with interposed demineralized bone matrix mixed with the patient's own bone shavings harvested with a Hudson brace (Medicon, Germany) from the inner cortex of the graft.

Orbital Fractures

In the management of adult patients with orbital fractures, there exist relatively succinct criteria for operative intervention (fracture area greater than 1 cm^2 or involvement of more than 50 % of an orbital wall). Other indications include immediate enophthalmos, vertical ocular dystopia (VOD), superior orbital fissure syndrome, and frontal-temporal-orbital fractures with resulting exophthalmos. In the pediatric population, these indications are less straightforward. The more robust orbital periosteum and supporting ligaments in the pediatric orbit are believed to make enophthalmos and VOD less likely. These sturdier supporting structures may make open reduction and internal fixation (ORIF) less necessary. The authors evaluated operative necessity in a three-group orbital fracture classification system ($n=81$): type 1, pure orbital fractures; type 2, craniofacial fractures (oblique fractures extending from the skull into the orbital roof); and type 3, orbital fractures associated with classically described patterns (blowout, ZMC, NOE). On retrospective analysis, type 1 fractures were treated nonoperatively (88 %) unless there was acute enophthalmos, VOD, or muscle entrapment. Type 2 fractures were managed conservatively with serial scans until an absolute operative indication developed; 17 % were ultimately treated operatively. Type 3 fractures were more likely to undergo operative intervention (72 %). Overall, 23 of 81 (28.3 %) of orbital fractures underwent operative intervention. Based on this data, the authors recommend that all isolated (type 1) pediatric orbital fractures be treated conservatively, despite the findings on CT scan, unless there are clinical indications for perusing an operative approach, such as acute enophthalmos, acute VOD, or muscle entrapment.

For those fractures requiring operative intervention, either to restore globe position, to correct diplopia, or to relieve an entrapment, the transconjunctival approach is preferred due to a generally perceived lower risk for ectropion. A transcaruncular approach to the medial wall can be used as well. All tissues are cleared from the fracture site, and care is taken so that the entire circumference of the defect is visualized. In the case of a "trap-door" fracture with entrapment of the muscle and/or periorbita, the fracture fragment may require further displacement into the maxillary sinus in order to fully mobilize all soft tissues back into the orbit. The residual defect is repaired with resorbable mesh or split calvarial graft depending on the surgeon's preference.

Nasal Fractures

Nasal fractures, with associated septal hematomas, warrant immediate intervention. Closed reduction of nasal fractures often fails to completely correct the deformity secondary to inadequate release; however, aggressive open treatment in children has the potential to affect facial and nasal growth adversely. Hence, the authors recommend that, for all children presenting with a nasal fracture resulting in an obvious deformity, a closed reduction be offered, with the intention of at least improving the deformity. Patients and families should be informed that the option of pursuing definitive open management at skeletal maturity to address any residual deformity or airway obstruction is a possibility. The maneuvers for closed reduction in children are similar to those in adults: an elevator or knife handle may be passed endonasally to outfracture depressed nasal bones, or digital manipulation can be utilized to infracture laterally displaced nasal bones. The septum can be reduced/relocated with Asch forceps. If necessary, internal splints are used in addition to external splints. Septal hematomas, if present, should be addressed with incision, drainage, and then elimination of the dead space with either quilting sutures or internal splints.

NOE fractures are uncommon in the pediatric patient but become more common with advancing age. The age-specific norms for intercanthal distance must be kept in mind when evaluating and treating these patients: newborn = 10–15 mm, 2-year-old = 20 mm, 12-year-old = 25 mm, and adult = 35 mm. Several classification schemes for NOE fractures have been used; however, the one developed by Markowitz et al. is probably the most widely employed as it defines pathology as well as treatment plan. This classification system is more relevant to the adult craniofacial skeleton and does not take into account the higher likelihood of pediatric NOE fractures to be associated with skull base fractures. A separate classification system, developed by Burstein et al., incorporates these differences and can be useful to the pediatric maxillofacial surgeon. The literature is sparse in regard to treatment and long-term follow-up of pediatric NOE fractures. One review of 20 patients who had midface fractures with an NOE component found a rate of 40 % requiring revisional surgery, with younger children being more likely to require additional procedures when compared with older children.

Midface Fractures

Nonoperative management is advocated for minimally displaced or greenstick midface fractures, particularly in the younger child. Dentoalveolar fractures are typically nonoperative and treated with splinting by the pediatric dentists. Palatal fractures may require ORIF or splinting with mandibulomaxillary fixation (MMF). The pediatric patient in primary or mixed dentition presents a challenge to the operating surgeon to achieve appropriate MMF; classically, circummandibular wiring and piriform suspension wiring have been very useful options (see Fig. 23.14). The authors have found, however, that – despite dogma advising against the use of arch bars in mixed and primary dentition for fear of disrupting the development of permanent dentition – arch bars in this population are quite efficacious and benign. Specifically, in 21 such patients with 34 fractures, no adverse effects on permanent dentition were seen after rigorous dental and radiographic assessment. Regardless of the method of MMF employed, the younger the patient, the shorter the

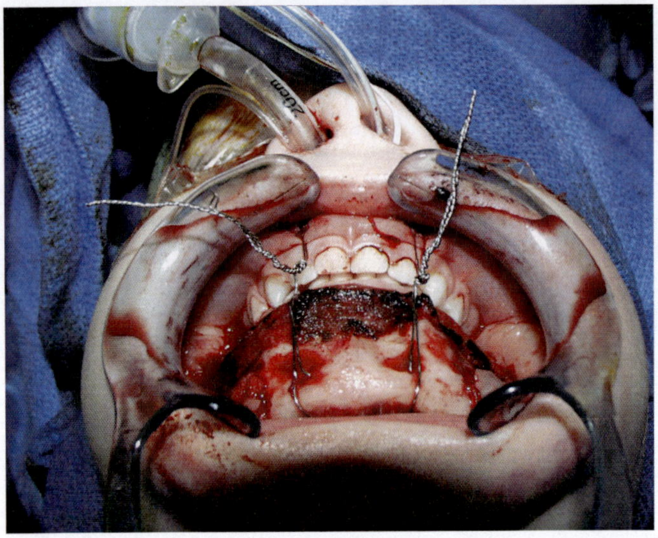

Fig. 23.14 Circummandibular wiring and piriform suspension wiring

course of MMF required; some authors advocate 1 week or less, followed by dental elastics. The unerupted tooth buds must always be kept in mind when performing ORIF in these young patients.

The goals in operative treatment of zygomaticomaxillary complex (ZMC) fractures include correction of VOD or enophthalmos, restoration of occlusion, and preservation of facial appearance. Flattening of the malar eminence can occur secondary to a ZMC fracture, as well as inferior displacement of the lateral canthal tendon due to its attachment to Whitnall's tubercle. This constellation can cause significant cosmetic deformity if left untreated or if treated inadequately. The zygoma can be approached via an upper buccal sulcus and eyelid incision; isolated arch fractures may be approached with a Gillies incision. The zygomaticofrontal (ZF) suture can be accessed through a subciliary incision and a subconjunctival incision with a lateral cantholysis or through the lateral portion of an upper lid blepharoplasty incision. Adequate reduction at the lateral wall of the orbit, or the greater wing of the sphenoid, is essential to proper reconstruction. Reduction must also be achieved at the ZF suture, the inferior orbital rim, and the zygomaticomaxillary (ZM) buttress. The surgeon must ascertain that orbital volume is not altered by the reduction, and reconstruction of the orbital floor may be required.

Mandible Fractures

The pediatric mandible fracture may represent the most challenging pediatric facial fracture to treat. In an attempt to direct therapy, the authors have organized the treatment of pediatric mandible fractures into 4 levels of intervention as follows

Table 23.1 Treatment classification

Treatment level	Description
Non-operative	
Level 1	Physical therapy and/or mandible rest
Level 2	External stabilization (C-collar or ACE wrap)
Operative	
Level 3	CREF ± MMF
Level 4	ORIF ± MMF

(see Table 23.1). *Level 1: conservative management such as soft diet to avoid fracture displacement, rest, and physical therapy.* Level 1 management is indicated for mandibular fractures that are isolated and minimally displaced and that do not disrupt occlusion or mandibular function such as a nondisplaced and nonmobile parasymphyseal fractures (see Fig. 23.15). *Level 2: nonsurgical stabilization with a C-collar or ACE wrap.* Level 2 management is employed when a short course of immobilization is desired (condylar head or neck fractures) or when some degree of mobility is appreciated in a displaced fracture that does not significantly disrupt occlusion or mandibular function (e.g., isolated parasymphyseal fractures). Nonoperative stabilization is appropriate even for the multiply fractured mandible if stability can be maintained with ACE wrap or C-collar and occlusion is preserved. *Level 3: operative CREF with arch bars and elastics or MMF.* Level 3 management is indicated if fracture displacement or significant mobility interferes with occlusion or mandibular function such as a significantly displaced condylar neck fracture affecting occlusion. *Level 4: ORIF ± arch bars and elastics or MMF.* Level 4 management is performed most frequently for displaced mobile fractures of the non-condylar region that affect function or occlusion. Level 4 management is also indicated for the common presentation of a condylar head/neck fracture treated best with physical therapy, combined with a parasymphyseal fracture requiring rigid fixation.

The pediatric condyle warrants special mention as it is an important growth center of the mandible, sensitive to disruptions in blood supply which can result in ankylosis and altered development. Pure intracapsular injuries should be provided Level 1 conservative management to minimize growth disturbance and TMJ ankylosis. Some advocate for more aggressive treatment of dislocated condylar neck fractures in older patients as the condyles are less likely to regenerate in children over 7 years of age. These injuries, in very rare circumstances, may progress to require osteotomy and cartilage grafting for TMJ function and restoration of occlusion. In patients with unilateral condylar neck fractures affecting occlusion, Level 3 treatment with arch bars and contralateral elastics is preferable (see Figs. 23.16, 23.17, and 23.18). The elastics can overcome the patient's trismus and close the open bite while allowing early motion in order to avoid ankylosis. During healing, the occlusion can be

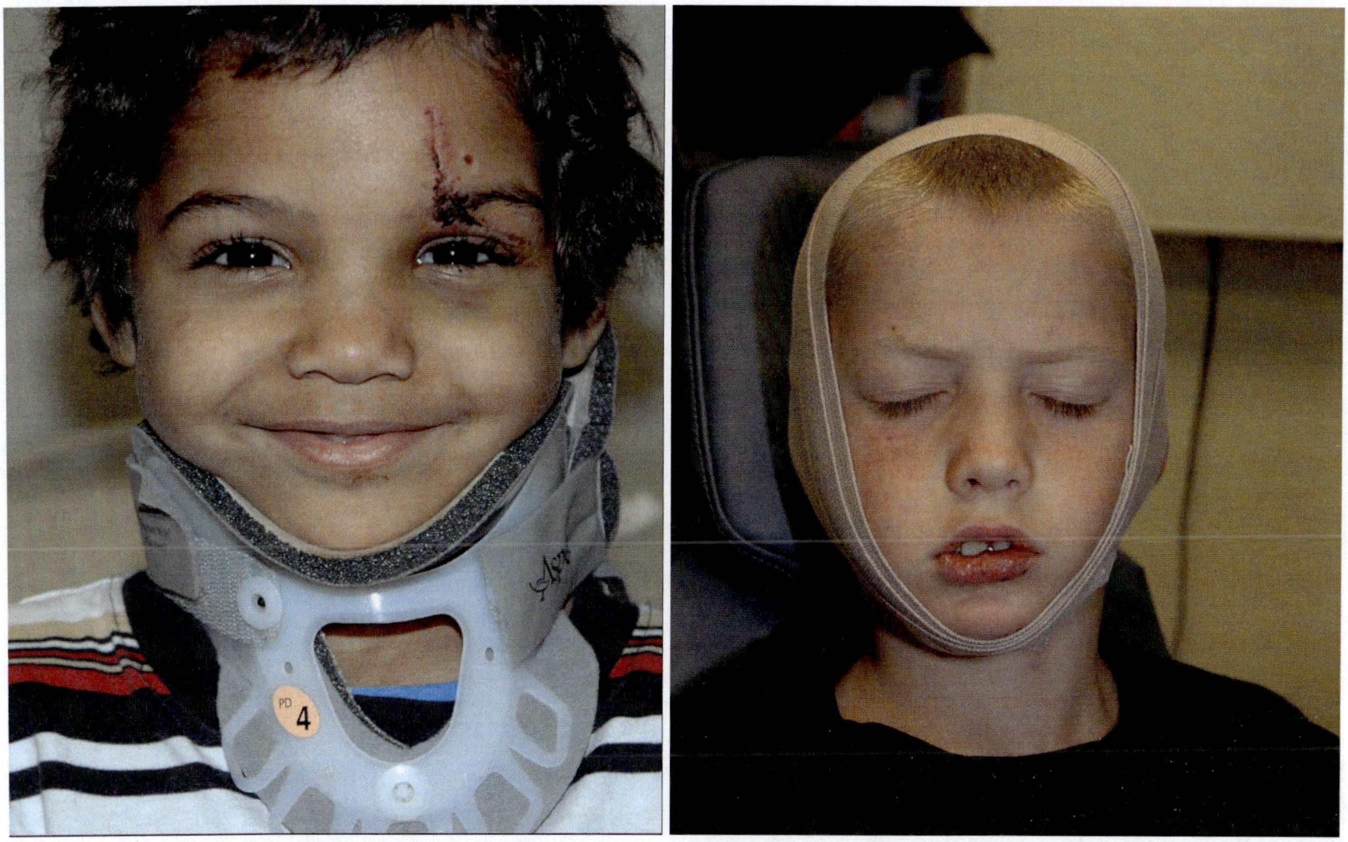

Fig. 23.15 Conservative management of mandible fractures; external stabilization with C-collar (*left*) and ACE wrap (*right*)

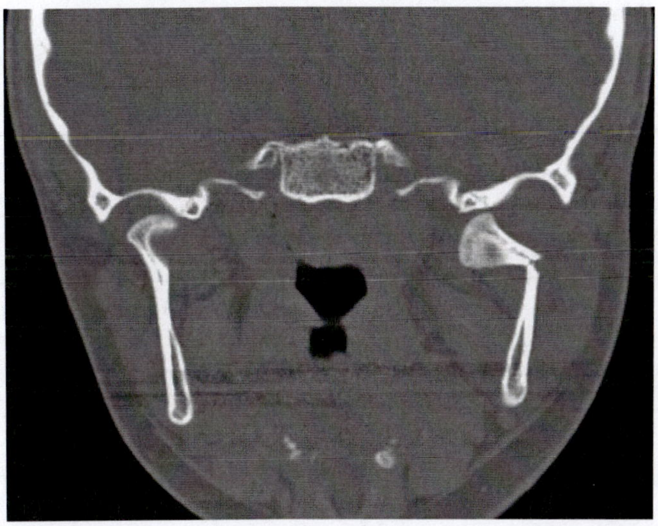

Fig. 23.16 Coronal CT demonstrating left condylar neck fracture

fine-tuned by adjusting the vector of the elastics. In the case of bilateral condylar neck fractures, particularly in the older child with a resultant anterior open bite, Level 4 management with ORIF of one side, along with a short course of intermaxillary fixation, is reasonable. The alternative approach in the immature skeleton would be to perform Level 3 management with IMF, with the understanding that elective orthognathic surgery may be required secondarily if an anterior open bite results. A condylar head fracture, in the presence of another mandible fracture, is an indication for Level 4 management with ORIF of the non-condylar fracture, along with elastic therapy allowing for early TMJ range of motion. Further indications for open treatment include a foreign body in the TMJ, inability to normalize occlusion with closed management, and displacement of a condyle into the middle cranial fossa. Open treatment should be avoided in intracapsular fractures, high condylar neck fractures, coronoid fractures, and any injury where occlusion is preserved and the patient is able to return to early range of motion.

Again, it should be noted that creativity may be required in placing the pediatric patient in primary or mixed dentition into adequate MMF. After 11 years of age (8 years for symphysis fractures), transosseous wiring and bicortical screws can be used. In managing postreduction malocclusion, it should be remembered that the primary teeth will exfoliate and that subsequent orthodontics can improve residual occlusal discrepancies. It is likely prudent to accept a slight malocclusion rather than risk injuring a permanent tooth bud with an attempt at ORIF.

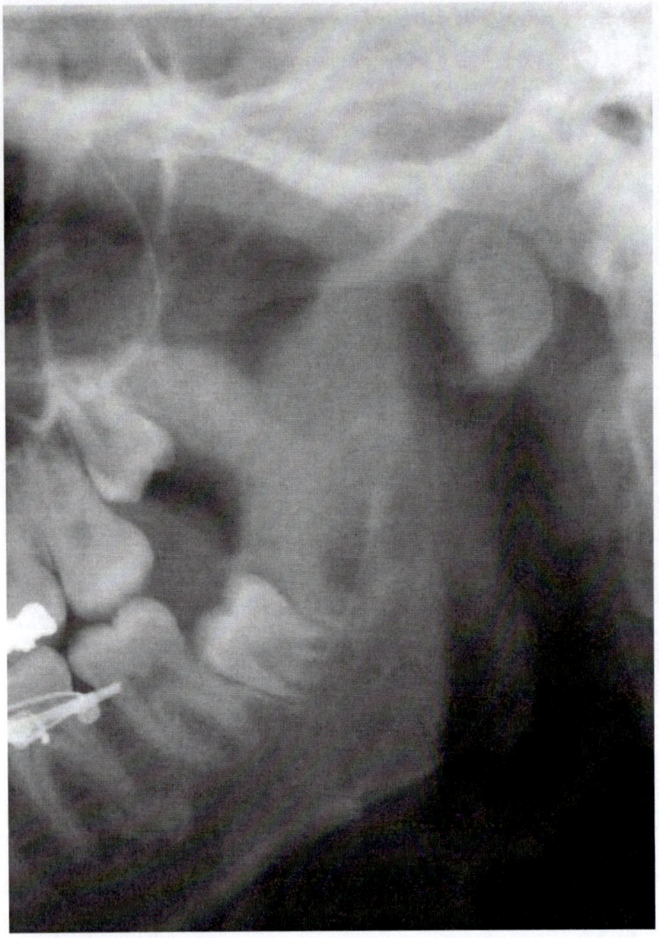

Fig. 23.17 High condylar neck fracture on panorex

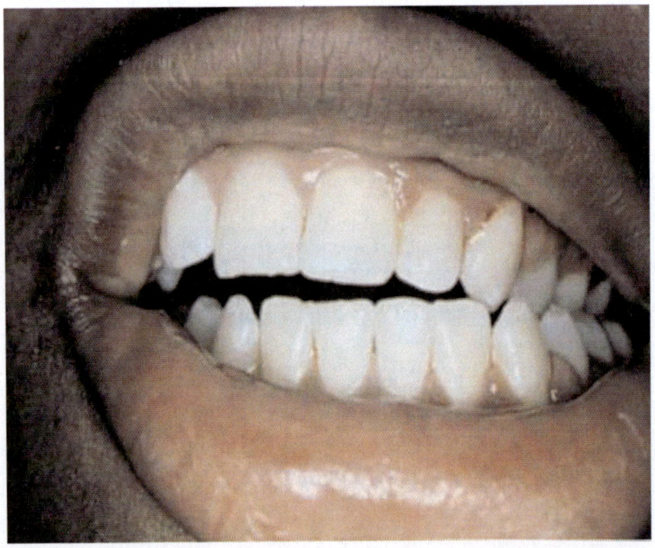

Fig. 23.18 Crossbite and premature contact associated with left condylar neck fracture

Growth Concerns, Outcomes, and Complications

Our understanding and management of pediatric facial fractures are ever-evolving. Imaging modalities and anatomical understanding continue to improve, while reporting of treatment strategies, complications, and adverse outcomes continues to progress. The literature varies widely in the reported rates of complications associated with pediatric facial fractures (anywhere from 7.4 to 27.8 %). This fact underscores the variability both in definition and follow-up of pediatric fractures.

In an effort to clarify the discussion of adverse outcomes in pediatric facial fractures, our group developed and reported the following classification system of adverse outcomes: type 1, adverse outcomes related to the fracture itself (i.e., the loss of a permanent tooth with a mandible fracture); type 2, adverse outcomes secondary to intervention and surgical management (i.e., nerve injury after open reduction and internal fixation of a fracture); and type 3, adverse outcomes that may result from a combination of the fracture, its management, and subsequent growth and development (i.e., asymmetric mandibular growth). In the authors' series of 177 pediatric patients with facial fractures, 32.2 % had an adverse outcome (see Fig. 23.19).

In general, the complications associated with pediatric facial fractures follow a different pattern of distribution than that in adult facial fractures. The more common complications seen in adults (infection, nonunion, and malunion) are rarely seen in the pediatric population. Here, the main concern is for long-term growth disturbances. The actual potential for this adverse outcome is incompletely understood. The relative contributions of open reduction (and associated

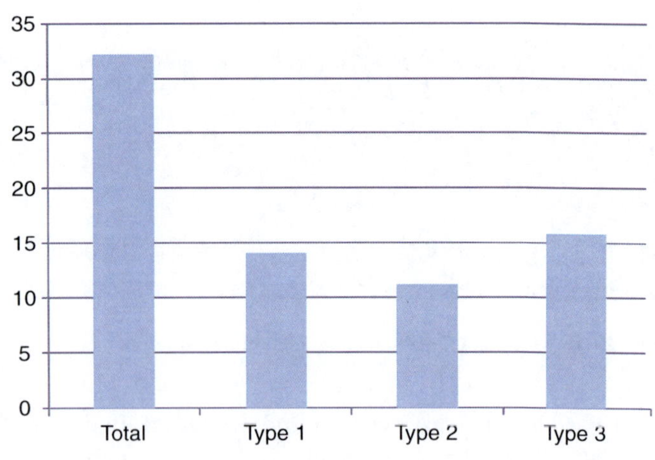

Fig. 23.19 Percent adverse outcomes

periosteal stripping), placement of hardware, and injury to growth centers are all still undergoing investigation.

In cranial- and skull-based fractures, complications can include meningitis, sinusitis, mucoceles, mucopyoceles, brain abscesses, and CSF leaks. Often, a CSF leak will resolve with conservative management within 1 week, and persistent leaks can be treated with lumbar drain prior to surgical intervention. A growing skull fracture can occur in 0.03–1 % of skull base fractures associated with a dural disruption, especially if they occur during the period of rapid skull growth, i.e., less than 3 years of age. These growing skull fractures can lead to further complications. In the authors' series, 40 % of skull fractures had an adverse outcome. Of these adverse outcomes, 1.5 % were type 1, 20 % were type 2, and 35 % were type 3. The complications included growing skull fractures, CSF leaks, enophthalmos, vertical orbital dystopia, ptosis, amblyopia, and exophthalmos.

Orbital fractures can be complicated by diplopia and enophthalmos, both of which may require further reconstruction. In the authors' series, 10.7 % of isolated orbital fractures had an adverse outcome. Of those, 3.6 % were type 1, 3.6 % were type 2, and 3.6 % were type 3. Three patients had enophthalmos, which was not clinically significant (less than 2 mm). While no persistent diplopia was reported in this series, it has been reported in as many as 36 % of cases in other series.

When considering the complications related to nasal deformity, these can be functional, aesthetic, or both. Nasal deviation can result from inadequate reduction and cartilaginous changes. Callous formation and bony deposition can lead to a dorsal hump. The untreated septal hematoma can lead to cartilage destruction and ultimately to a saddle nose deformity. When considering NOE fractures, damage to the lacrimal system can lead to persistent obstruction, necessitating dacryocystorhinostomy. In the authors' series, 21.7 % of nasal fractures exhibited adverse outcomes; 8.7 % of those were type 1 and 17.4 % were type 3, related to persistent deformity and airway obstruction. Corrective rhinoplasty is typically delayed until skeletal maturity in these instances, unless nasal airway obstruction is severe.

In reviewing a series of 215 mandible fractures in 120 patients under 18 years of age, the authors have found that adherence to the treatment guidelines described above results in largely uncompromised mandibular function and growth. Adverse outcomes assessed in this series include dental trauma, restricted maximal incisive opening, mental nerve paresthesia, hardware problems, TMJ deviation, TMJ ankylosis, TMJ pain, TMJ click, and growth disturbances. Of the 56 patients in this series with at least 1 year of follow-up, 14.3 % had a type 1 adverse outcome, 8.9 % had a type 2,

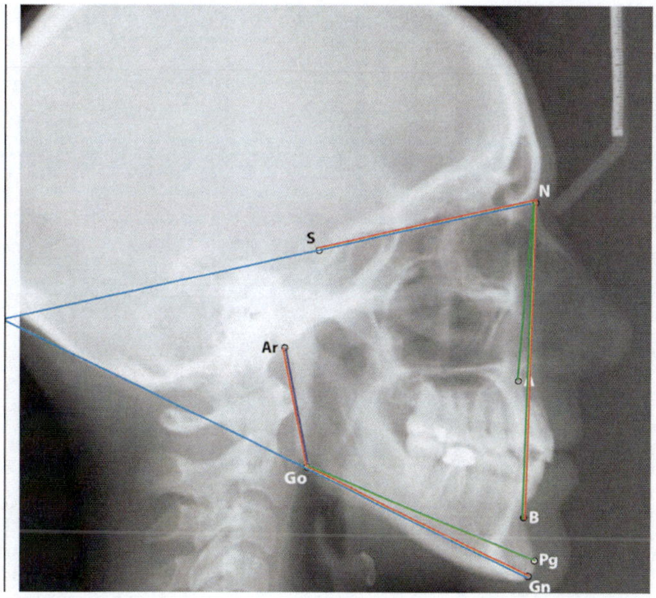

Fig. 23.20 Lateral cephalometric measurements

and 25.0 % had a type 3. None of these adverse outcomes were clinically significant, where "clinical significance" was defined as a functional or aesthetic concern for the patient, family, or treating practitioner. All type 1 outcomes encountered were dental injuries. The most commonly reported type 2 adverse outcome was hardware failure. Type 3 adverse outcomes included primarily TMJ symptoms and disturbances in mandibular morphology. The chances of an adverse outcome increased significantly with having either multiple mandible fractures or mandible fractures requiring operative intervention ($p<0.05$). While there was a trend towards increasing adverse outcome rates with increasing age (0–5-year-olds had a 35.0 % chance of an adverse outcome, 6–12-year-olds had a 40.0 % chance of an adverse outcome, and 12–18-year-olds had a 45.5 % chance of an adverse outcome), these values were not statistically significant ($p>0.05$, chi-square). With respect to postoperative growth and development, there were no significant differences between lateral cephalometric measurements (SNB, ANB, SN-GoGn, Ar-Go-Gn, Go-Pg, Ar-Go) in our cohort of pediatric mandible fractures when compared to age-/sex-matched Bolton norms (see Fig. 23.20). As well, no significant differences were found on posterior-anterior cephalometric measurements (Ar-Go, Go-Me, Ar-Me) (see Fig. 23.21) of injured and uninjured hemi-mandibles. These findings held when the data were stratified by age at injury and by fracture type. In another report, patients who sustained mandible fractures between the ages of 4 and 7 were most likely to have growth

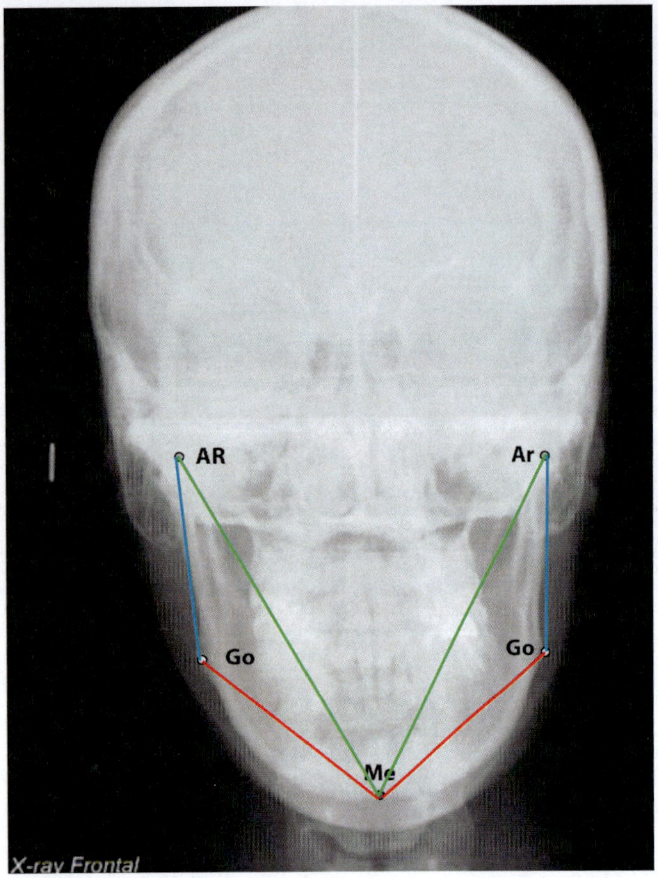

Fig. 23.21 PA cephalometric measurements

disturbances and facial asymmetry, and mandible fractures occurring prior to 4 years of age were least likely to have a growth disturbance.

Conclusions

The pediatric craniofacial skeleton is structurally unique from its adult counterpart. This distinct structure yields specific injury patterns in response to trauma, and these diagnoses must be astutely recognized to facilitate appropriate management. One must exercise special caution in managing pediatric facial fractures such that growth potential is not unnecessarily sacrificed in efforts to achieve perfect reduction and rigid fixation. This growth potential, if protected, lends a powerful plasticity to the pediatric craniofacial skeleton allowing for inherent compensation to the traumatic insult. An increasing recognition of this resilience and an expanding appreciation for the role post-traumatic orthodontics can play in rehabilitating these injuries are coalescing to favor less invasive management of many pediatric craniofacial fractures.

Bibliography

Anderson FM, Geiger L. Craniosynostosis: a survey of 204 cases. J Neurosurg. 1965;22:229–40.

Bite U, Jackson IT, Forbes GS, Gehring DG. Orbital volume measurements in enophthalmos using three-dimensional Ct imaging. Plast Reconstr Surg. 1985;75:502–8.

Burstein F, Cohen S, Hudgins R, Boydston W. Frontal basilar trauma: classification and treatment. Plast Reconstr Surg. 1997;99:1314–21; discussion 1322–3.

Chao MT, Losee JE. Complications in pediatric facial fractures. Craniomaxillofac Trauma Reconstr. 2009;2:103.

Chao MT, Jiang S, Smith D, DeCesare GE, Cooper GM, Pollack IF, Girotto J, Losee JE. Demineralized bone matrix and resorbable mesh bilaminate cranioplasty: a novel method for reconstruction of large-scale defects in the pediatric calvaria. Plast Reconstr Surg. 2009;123:976–82.

Chen KT, Chen CT, Mardini S, Tsay PK, Chen YR. Frontal sinus fractures: a treatment algorithm and assessment of outcomes based on 78 clinical cases. Plast Reconstr Surg. 2006;118:457–68.

Cho YR, Gosain AK. Biomaterials in craniofacial reconstruction. Clin Plast Surg. 2004;31:377–85, v.

Cole P, Boyd V, Banerji S, Hollier Jr LH. Comprehensive management of orbital fractures. Plast Reconstr Surg. 2007;120:57S–63.

Converse JM, Smith B, Obear MF, Wood-Smith D. Orbital blowout fractures: a ten-year survey. Plast Reconstr Surg. 1967;39:20–36.

Cope MR, Moos KF, Speculand B. Does diplopia persist after blow-out fractures of the orbital floor in children? Br J Oral Maxillofac Surg. 1999;37:46–51.

David L, Argenta L, Fisher D. Hydroxyapatite cement in pediatric craniofacial reconstruction. J Craniofac Surg. 2005;16:129–33.

Demianczuk AN, Verchere C, Phillips JH. The effect on facial growth of pediatric mandibular fractures. J Craniofac Surg. 1999;10:323.

Dufresne CR, Manson P. Pediatric facial injuries. In: Mathes SJ, editor. The head and neck, part 2, vol. 3. Philadelphia: Elsevier; 2006.

Eggensperger Wymann NM, Holzle A, Zachariou Z, Iizuka T. Pediatric craniofacial trauma. J Oral Maxillofac Surg. 2008;66:58–64.

Farkas LG, Posnick JC, Hreczko TM. Growth patterns of the face: a morphometric study. Cleft Palate Craniofac J. 1992;29: 308–15.

Ferreira PC, Amarante JM, Silva PN, Rodrigues JM, Choupina MP, Silva AC, Barbosa RF, Cardoso MA, Reis JC. Retrospective study of 1251 maxillofacial fractures in children and adolescents. Plast Reconstr Surg. 2005;115:1500–8.

Gassner R, Tuli T, Hachl O, Moreira R, Ulmer H. Craniomaxillofacial trauma in children: a review of 3,385 cases with 6,060 injuries in 10 years. J Oral Maxillofac Surg. 2004;62:399–407.

Grunwaldt L, Smith DM, Zuckerbraun NS, Naran S, Rottgers SA, Bykowski M, Kinsella C, Cray J, Vecchione L, Saladino RA, Losee JE. Pediatric facial fractures: demographics, injury patterns, and associated injuries in 772 consecutive patients. Plast Reconstr Surg. 2011;128:1263–71.

Hatef DA, Cole PD, Hollier Jr LH. Contemporary management of pediatric facial trauma. Curr Opin Otolaryngol Head Neck Surg. 2009; 17:308–14.

Havlik RJ, Sutton LN, Bartlett SP. Growing skull fractures and their craniofacial equivalents. J Craniofac Surg. 1995;6:103–10; discussion 111–2.

Holland AJ, Broome C, Steinberg A, Cass DT. Facial fractures in children. Pediatr Emerg Care. 2001;17:157–60.

Imahara SD, Hopper RA, Wang J, Rivara FP, Klein MB. Patterns and outcomes of pediatric facial fractures in the United States: a survey of the national trauma data bank. J Am Coll Surg. 2008;207:710–6.

Jordan DR, Allen LH, White J, Harvey J, Pashby R, Esmaeli B. Intervention within days for some orbital floor fractures: the white-eyed blowout. Ophthal Plast Reconstr Surg. 1998;14:379–90.

Kaban LB, Mulliken JB, Murray JE. Facial fractures in children: an analysis of 122 fractures in 109 patients. Plast Reconstr Surg. 1977;59:15–20.

Lehman Jr JA, Saddawi ND. Fractures of the mandible in children. J Trauma. 1976;16:773–7.

Losee JE, Jiang S. Pediatric facial trauma. In: Chung K, Disa J, Gosain AK, et al., editors. Plastic surgery. New York: Saunders Elsevier; 2009. p. 645–55.

Losee JE, Smith DM. Pediatric facial fractures. In: Neligan P, editor. Plastic surgery, vol. 3. 3rd ed. London: Elsevier; 2012. p. 671–85.

Losee JE, Afifi A, Jiang S, Smith D, Chao MT, Vecchione L, Hertle R, Davis J, Naran S, Hughes J, Paviglianiti J, Deleyiannis FW. Pediatric orbital fractures: classification, management, and early follow-up. Plast Reconstr Surg. 2008a;122:886–97.

Losee JE, Jiang S, Deleyiannis FW. Craniofacial fractures. In: Bentz M, Bauer B, Zuker R, editors. Principles and practice of pediatric plastic surgery. St. Louis: Quality Medical Publishing; 2008b. p. 1047–72.

Manson PN, Iliff N. Management of blow-out fractures of the orbital floor. II. Early repair for selected injuries. Surv Ophthalmol. 1991;35:280–92.

Manson PN, Grivas A, Rosenbaum A, Vannier M, Zinreich J, Iliff N. Studies on enophthalmos: II. The measurement of orbital injuries and their treatment by quantitative computed tomography. Plast Reconstr Surg. 1986;77:203–14.

Markowitz BL, Manson PN, Sargent L, Vander Kolk CA, Yaremchuk M, Glassman D, Crawley WA. Management of the medial canthal tendon in nasoethmoid orbital fractures: the importance of the central fragment in classification and treatment. Plast Reconstr Surg. 1991;87:843–53.

Mathes SJ, editor. Plastic surgery, vol. 3. 2nd ed. Philadelphia: Elsevier; 2006.

Mathog RH, editor. Maxillofacial trauma. Baltimore: Williams & Wilkins; 1983.

McCoy FJ, Chandler RA, Crow ML. Facial fractures in children. Plast Reconstr Surg. 1966;37:209–15.

Mericli AF, DeCesare GE, Zuckerbraun NS, Kurland KS, Grunwaldt L, Vecchione L, Losee JE. Pediatric craniofacial fractures due to violence: comparing violent and nonviolent mechanisms of injury. J Craniofac Surg. 2011;22:1342–7.

Messinger A, Radkowski MA, Greenwald MJ, Pensler JM. Orbital roof fractures in the pediatric population. Plast Reconstr Surg. 1989;84:213–6; discussion 217–8.

Moss ML, Salentijn L. The primary role of functional matrices in facial growth. Am J Orthod. 1969;55:566–77.

Naran S, Afrooz PN, Bykowski MR, Smith DM, Rottgers SA, Losee JE. Arch bar use in primary and mixed dentition: feasibility, safety and outcomes. Plast Reconstr Surg. 130:100. Abstract 34p.

Pappachan B, Alexander M. Correlating facial fractures and cranial injuries. J Oral Maxillofac Surg. 2006;64:1023–9.

Parsons GS, Mathog RH. Orbital wall and volume relationships. Arch Otolaryngol Head Neck Surg. 1988;114:743–7.

Perheentupa U, Kinnunen I, Grenman R, Aitasalo K, Makitie AA. Management and outcome of pediatric skull base fractures. Int J Pediatr Otorhinolaryngol. 2010;74:1245–50.

Roaten JB, Partrick DA, Nydam TL, Bensard DD, Hendrickson RJ, Sirotnak AP, Karrer FM. Nonaccidental trauma is a major cause of morbidity and mortality among patients at a regional level 1 pediatric trauma center. J Pediatr Surg. 2006;41:2013–5.

Rodriguez ED, Stanwix MG, Nam AJ, St Hilaire H, Simmons OP, Christy MR, Grant MP, Manson PN. Twenty-six-year experience treating frontal sinus fractures: a novel algorithm based on anatomical fracture pattern and failure of conventional techniques. Plast Reconstr Surg. 2008;122:1850–66.

Rottgers SA, DeCesare G, Chao M, Smith DM, Cray JJ, Naran S, Vecchione L, Grunwaldt L, Losee JE. Outcomes in pediatric facial fractures: early follow-up in 177 children and classification scheme. J Craniofac Surg. 2011;22(4):1260–5.

Sherick DG, Buchman SR, Patel PP. Pediatric facial fractures: a demographic analysis outside an urban environment. Ann Plast Surg. 1997;38:578–84; discussion 584–5.

Singh DJ, Bartlett SP. Pediatric craniofacial fractures: long-term consequences. Clin Plast Surg. 2004;31:499–518, vii.

Smartt Jr JM, Low DW, Bartlett SP. The pediatric mandible: II. Management of traumatic injury or fracture. Plast Reconstr Surg. 2005;116:28e–41.

Smith DM. Mandible fractures in 96 children: demographics, treatment, early outcomes and a prospective analysis of growth and development. Oxford: Society of Craniofacial Surgery XIII Biennial International Congress, 2009; 2009.

Smith DM, Bykowski MR, Cray JJ, Naran SS, Rottgers A, Shakir S, Vecchione L, Schuster L, Losee JE. 215 mandible fractures in 120 children: demographics, treatment, outcomes, and early growth data. Plast Reconstr Surg. 2013;131(6):1348–58.

Thaller SR, Huang V. Midfacial fractures in the pediatric population. Ann Plast Surg. 1992;29:348–52.

Thoren H, Iso-Kungas P, Iizuka T, Lindqvist C, Tornwall J. Changing trends in causes and patterns of facial fractures in children. Oral Surg Oral Med Oral Pathol Oral Radiol Endod. 2009;107:318–24.

Vyas RM, Dickinson BP, Wasson KL, Roostaeian J, Bradley JP. Pediatric facial fractures: current national incidence, distribution, and health care resource use. J Craniofac Surg. 2008;19:339–49; discussion 350.

Ziccardi VB, Ochs MW, Braun TW, Malave DA. Management of condylar fractures in children: review of the literature and case presentations. Compend Contin Educ Dent. 1995;16:874, 876, 878–80 passim; quiz 888.

Zimmermann CE, Troulis MJ, Kaban LB. Pediatric facial fractures: recent advances in prevention. Diagnosis and management. Int J Oral Maxillofac Surg. 2006;35:2–13.

Secondary Bone Reconstruction

24

Reza Jarrahy

Secondary reconstruction of craniofacial skeletal defects represents a particularly challenging subset of maxillofacial surgery. Whether planned as part of multistage procedures or to address complications from primary reconstructive procedures that result in full-thickness bone defects or other suboptimal outcomes, secondary cases of maxillofacial reconstruction are typically more complicated than the initial reconstructive procedure. These surgeries are often associated with hostile wound environments that may be characterized by hypoxia, poorly compliant soft tissue envelopes (e.g., restrictive scar tissue burden), and, in certain cases, radiation injury. Not uncommonly, complex defects of the craniofacial skeleton require recruitment of soft tissue as well as bone to reestablish stable form and function.

Autologous bone grafting represents the gold standard for secondary bone reconstruction, but this approach is not without its own limitations. These include the addition of a secondary operative site, pain and morbidity from this additional surgical site, prolongation of procedure and anesthesia time, the risk of infection or resorption of the graft, and the fact that the number of available donor sites for autologous bone are, by definition, limited. Nevertheless, secondary reconstruction of complex bone defects can be successfully accomplished with autologous bone grafts, yielding excellent and stable long-term results.

When autologous bone proves not to be an optimal solution, alloplastic materials can be used as alternatives. Options include methylmethacrylate, porous polyethylene, ceramics, plastics, and metallic alloys. Below we present an overview of strategies for surgical planning and operative techniques to address reconstruction of complex secondary bone reconstruction, with a focus on the use of autologous bone in craniofacial reconstruction of the upper, middle, and lower thirds of the craniofacial skeleton.

R. Jarrahy, FACS, FAAP
Division Plastic and Reconstructive Surgery, David Geffen School of Medicine at UCLA, Los Angeles, CA 90095, USA
e-mail: rjarrahy@mednet.ucla.edu

Cranial Vault and Upper Facial Third

Full-thickness bone defects of the upper third of the craniofacial skeleton and the cranial vault result from significant blunt or penetrating traumatic injury, composite oncologic resection, neurosurgical intervention, or radiation injury (e.g., osteoradionecrosis). The indications to repair full-thickness calvarial defects depend to some extent on the size of the defects themselves. Not all patients who are missing bone require reconstruction. Small defects with stable soft tissue coverage can be safely managed with observation. Larger defects, however, have been shown to alter regional CSF and cerebral blood flow; abnormal intracranial fluid hydraulics may result in cognitive deficits and other degenerative symptoms referred to collectively as the "syndrome of the trephined." Because there is no commonly accepted standard defect size greater than which cranioplasty is absolutely indicated, clinical judgment based on a thorough history, physical exam, and radiographic evaluation is the most important determinant in selecting patients who are candidates for bone reconstruction.

The list of materials that have been successfully used for cranioplasty is a lengthy one. Most recently, descriptions of innovative biomaterials combined with stem cells have been successfully used in experimental and clinical models to repair cranial vault defects. Such regenerative medicine approaches, however, are still considered to be experimental. While tissue engineering solutions may represent the wave of the future, current choices available to maxillofacial surgeons include autologous and alloplastic materials.

In the modern era, the most commonly used alloplastic materials are metal, acrylic, calcium phosphate, or polymers. The primary benefit to these materials is that they are readily available "off the shelf." Each has the potential for customization to suit the needs of each individual patient. Stereolithographic mapping of the cranial defect with computed tomography can be used to prefabricate implants of various compositions. Methylmethacrylate and viscous hydroxyapatite cements can be molded at the time of surgery

P.J. Taub et al. (eds.), *Ferraro's Fundamentals of Maxillofacial Surgery*,
DOI 10.1007/978-1-4614-8341-0_24,

to accurately conform to the architecture of the defect. Various uniplanar and bilaminate resorbable and non-resorbable composites have been developed. Some of these are being used within a tissue engineering paradigm, incorporating stem cells or potent growth factors, such as bone morphogenetic protein (BMP), to stimulate bone regeneration.

The most common sources for non-vascularized autologous bone graft are the calvarium, ribs, ilium, and tibia. Bone grafts may be harvested at the time of the secondary reconstruction *de novo* or might be otherwise accessible: in the setting of a traumatic or hemorrhagic craniectomy where a decompressive craniectomy is performed, for example, the neurosurgeon may store the removed cranial bone in the patient's subcutaneous tissue or in cryopreservation units for delayed use in secondary cranioplasty. Autologous bone grafts serve as osteoconductive lattices, allowing for migration of surrounding bone cells into the defect and subsequent deposition of mineralized tissue (see Fig. 24.1). The ultimate "survival" of the graft (or more precisely, its replacement with *de novo* bone) provides a distinct advantage over alloplastic material. Alloplasts are never incorporated into the surrounding soft tissue milieu; this is likely the leading factor contributing to infectious and exposure complications associated with the use of alloplastic materials in this setting.

The decision on which type of material to use in cranioplasty and when to perform the reconstruction is ultimately left up to the discretion of the surgical team and is largely subject to personal biases that are based on each surgeon's training and experience. The choice should not be strictly arbitrary, however; several principles apply to the decision-making process. The location and three-dimensional anatomy of the defect should be primarily considered. The integrity of the soft tissue envelope must be closely examined. If indicated, soft tissue coverage may be a necessary component of the plan for cranial or frontal bone reconstruction, either in a staged or combined procedure. Unfavorable soft tissue conditions, including a history of chronic infection or irradiation of the defect site, warrant a strong consideration for delaying cranioplasty until optimal wound conditions are established.

The timing of reconstruction must also be logical. No attempt at primary calvarial reconstruction should be made in the setting of an oncological resection when there is a reasonable suspicion that bone margins may be positive. There is no specific amount of time that should pass between resolution of an acute or chronic wound infection and placement of an implant or bone graft, but stable soft tissue coverage over a healthy defect site is a prerequisite before attempted

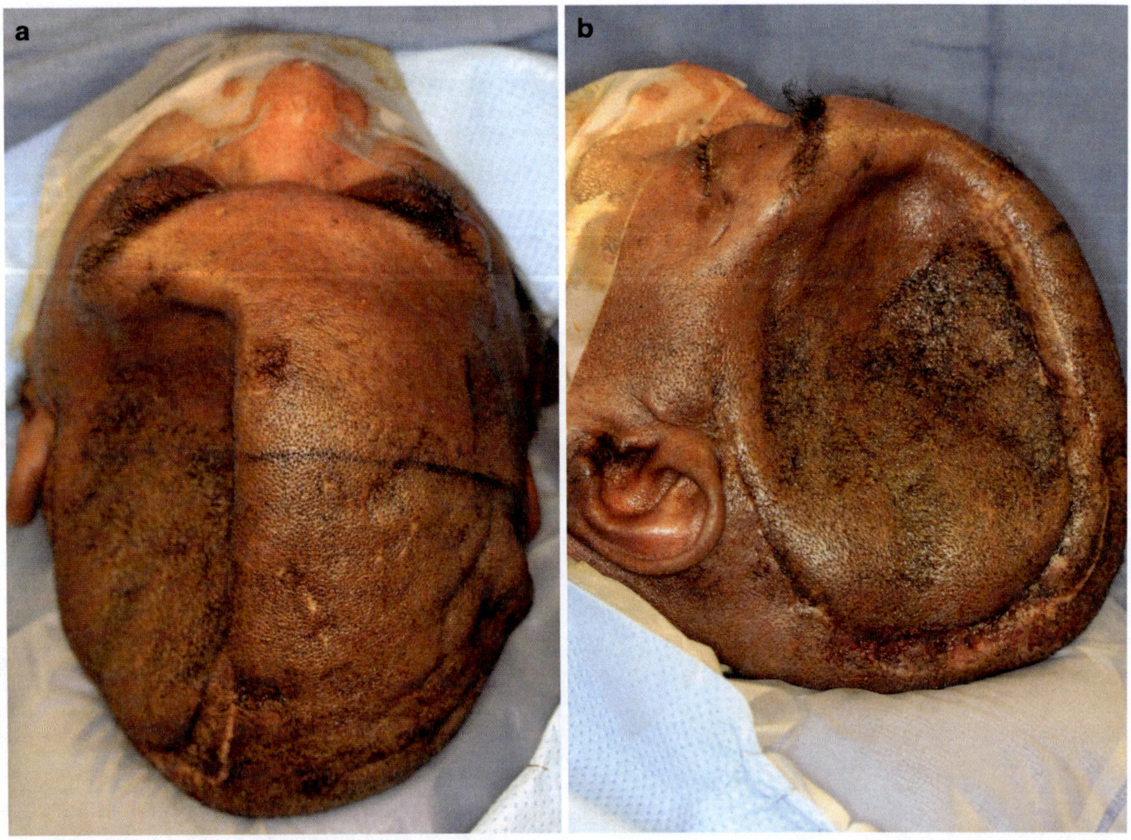

Fig. 24.1 A hemorrhagic cerebral infarct with associated cerebral edema necessitated decompressive craniectomy in this patient. The cryopreserved cranial bone flap was replaced 3 months after the acute event, but subsequently became infected and was removed. The resulting hemicraniectomy defect was repaired with autologous grafts. Due to the magnitude of the defect, a combination of split cranial bone and split rib grafts were necessary. (**a, b**) Immediate preoperative vertex and lateral views; (**c, d**) Intraoperative views demonstrating grafts and fixation; (**e, f**) Immediate results with restoration of cranial vault contour

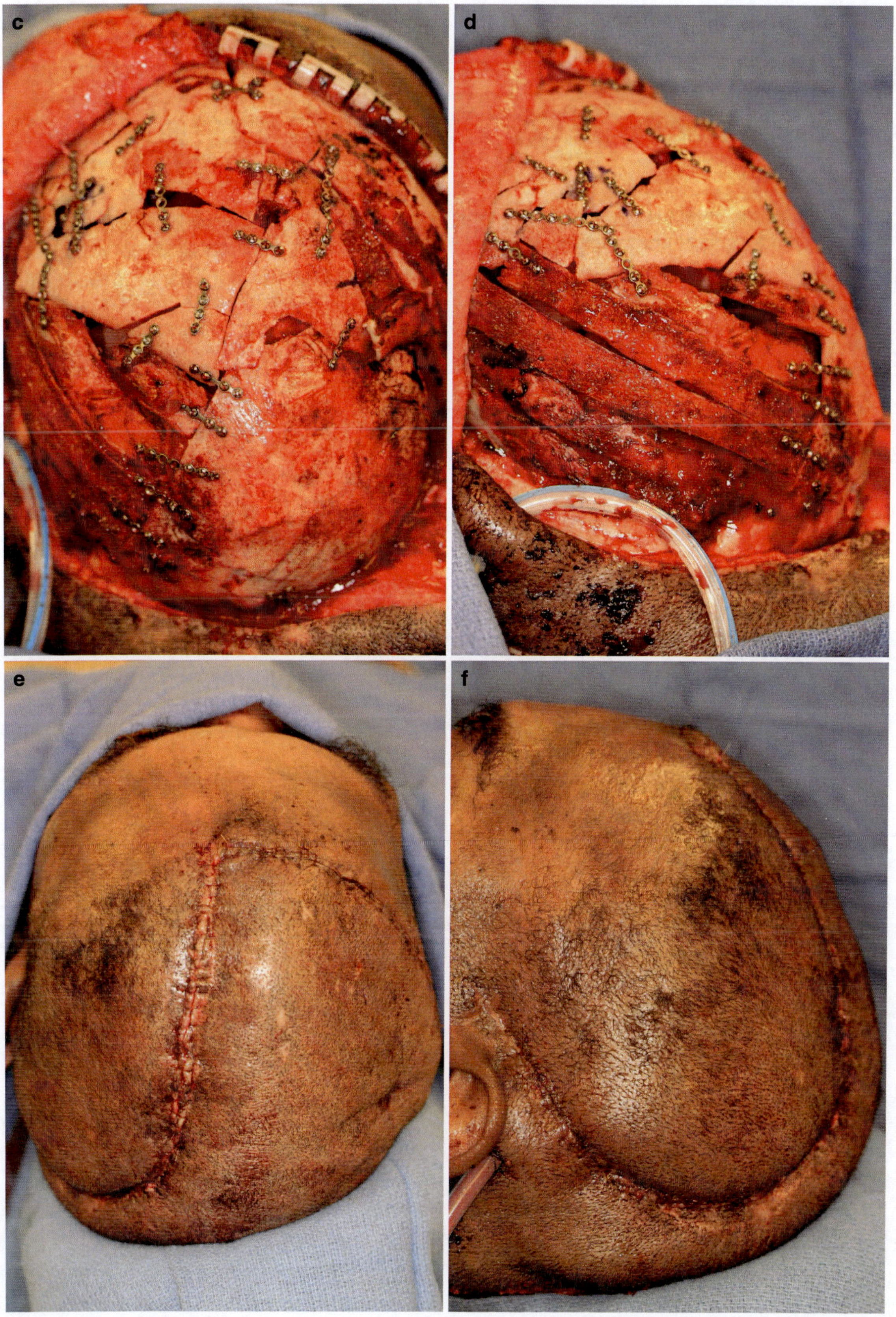

Fig. 24.1 (continued)

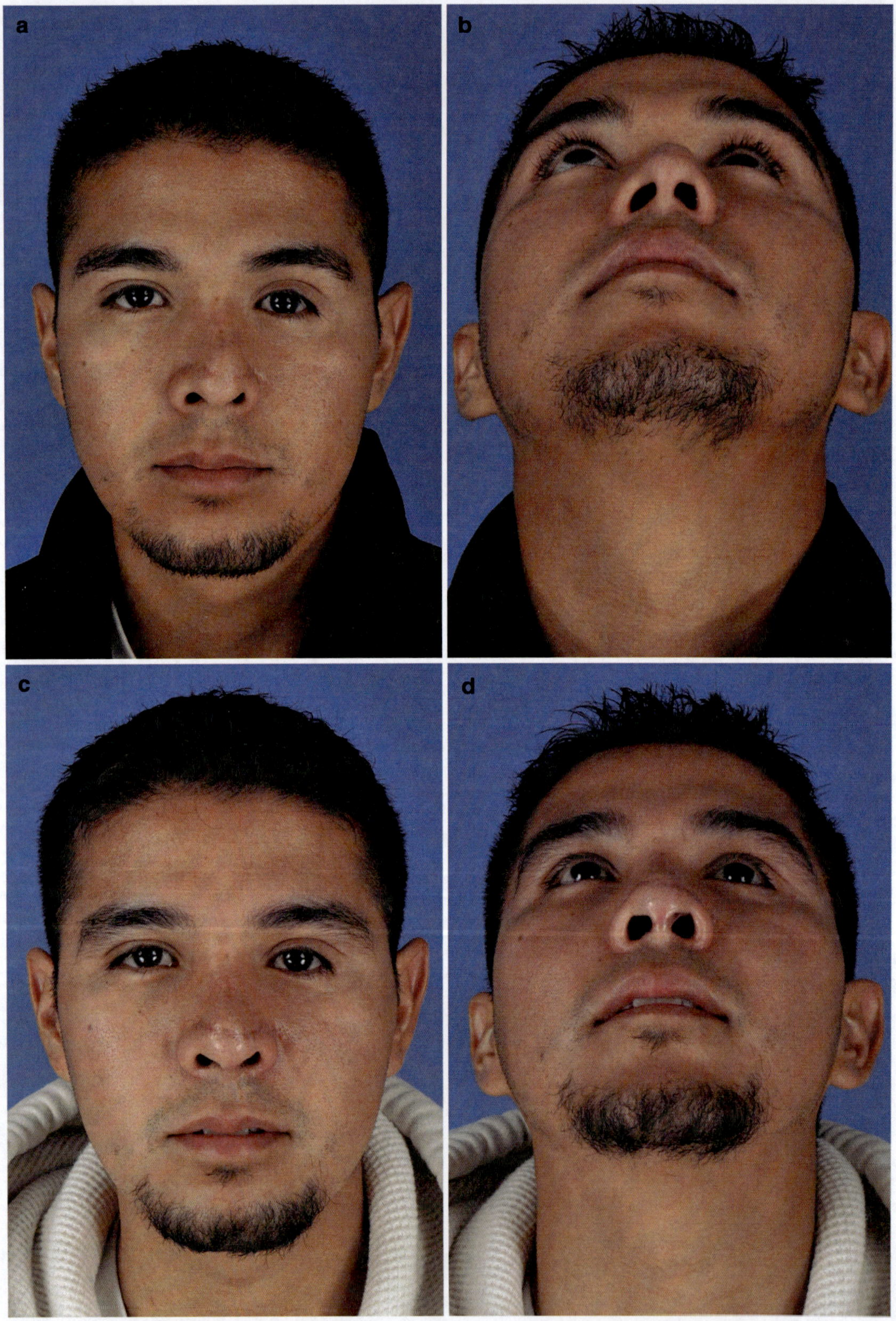

Fig. 24.2 This patient was referred after undergoing repair of a blunt traumatic injury to his left ZMC, orbit, and nose in an industrial accident. Initial treatment resulted in malunion of the ZMC fracture, increased right orbital volume, hypoglobus, enophthalmos, and nasal asymmetry with associated nasal airflow obstruction. He underwent refracture and repositioning of the ZMC, cranial bone graft to the right orbit, and septorhinoplasty, with subsequent improvement of his malar projection, ocular asymmetry, septal deviation, and nasal form and function. (**a**, **b**) Patient appearance at presentation following initial repairs; (**c**, **d**) patient at two year follow up after secondary correction; (**e**, **f**) preoperative CT scan showing inferior displacement of malar process and increased right intraorbital volume; (**g**, **h**) postoperative CT scan showing improved position of ZMC and normalization of orbital volume with removal of titanium plate and replacement with cranial bone graft

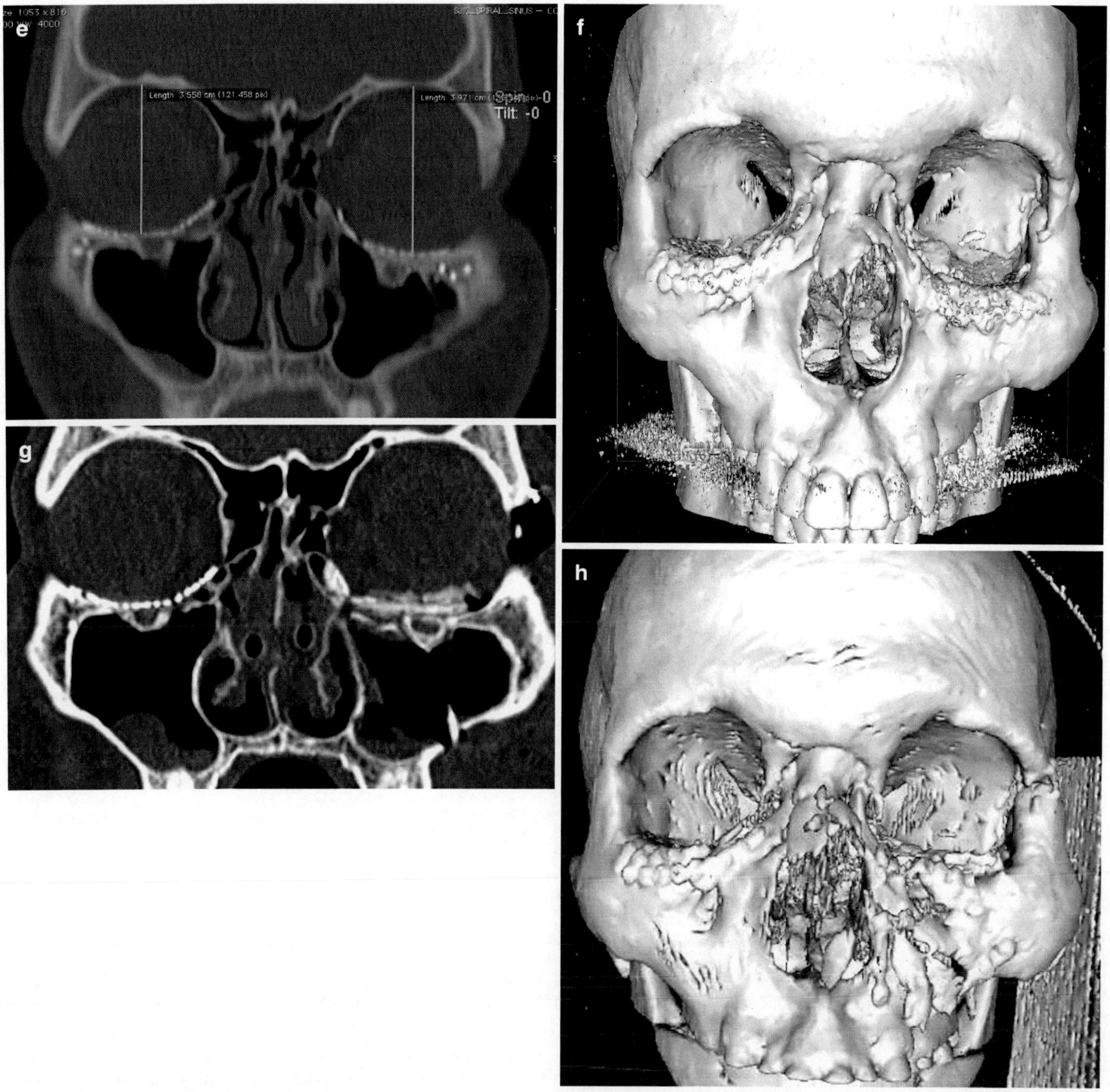

Fig. 24.2 (continued)

secondary reconstruction. Non-vascularized autologous bone covered by free muscle flaps has been successfully used to cover irradiated wounds, as have free muscle flaps in combination with alloplastic material. Large bony defects that have been complicated by significant infection or irradiation can be reconstructed with vascularized bone grafts. Primary one-stage full-thickness reconstruction, including replacement of scalp, skull, and dura, can be safely performed in both pediatric and adult patient populations when wound conditions are favorable.

Middle Facial Third

The middle third of the craniofacial skeleton includes the maxilla, zygoma, orbits, and related maxillary and ethmoid sinuses. The horizontal and vertical buttresses of the midface, including the maxillary alveolus and palate, the inferior and superior orbital rims, the nasomaxillary and zygomaticomaxillary buttresses, the nasofrontal and zygomaticofrontal processes, and the pterygomaxillary buttresses, provide structural support to the midface, determine contours, and support the soft tissues that account for vision, olfaction, speech, deglutition, and mastication. Injury to midface structures can adversely affect any of these functions and result in contour irregularities, decreased midface projection, and abnormal facial width.

Primary surgical reconstruction of the midface is performed in the setting of trauma, oncologic resection, or congenital lesions. Secondary reconstruction is indicated when primary results are suboptimal or associated with complications, including infection, malunion, nonunion, malocclusion, contour irregularities, orbital deformities, or issues of asymmetric facial projection or width. Complex composite midface defects, particularly in patients whose comorbidities make them poor candidates for lengthy reconstructive procedures, are amenable to reconstruction (or rather, coverage) with lifelike prosthetics borne upon osseointegrated implants, should the appropriate resources and a skilled anaplastologist be available. What follows below, however, is a discussion of principles and options in the setting of surgical correction.

Zygomaticomaxillary Complex

The zygomaticomaxillary complex (ZMC) is the most anteriorly projecting bony structure of the lateral midface. As such, it is often vulnerable to blunt traumatic forces originating from the side of the head. The zygomatic arches determine the facial width due to their lateral positioning and are therefore susceptible to trauma directed from the side of the face. Fractures of the ZMC are best treated by open reduction and internal fixation. The three-dimensional anatomy of the ZMC, however, coupled with its complex spatial relationships to the neighboring inferior and superior structures of the midface, renders its accurate repair in the primary setting particularly challenging, especially in complex, high-energy, or comminuted injuries. Because of the relationship of the ZMC to the orbit, malunion of even a few millimeters can result in noticeable asymmetries in the position of the globe on the affected side, such as enophthalmos, or other visual disturbances. Moreover, failure to accurately reduce and fixate the ZMC during primary repair can lead to loss of malar projection (with subsequent ptosis of cheek soft tissues) or asymmetries in facial width.

Management of secondary deformities of the ZMC, regardless of the indication for the initial surgery, is determined by the deformity itself. In the setting of trauma, correction will often include concurrent repair of associated orbital abnormalities. Traumatic zygomatic arch depression can in most cases be treated via a closed temporal or intraoral approach, with or without the use of intraoperative imaging to confirm reduction. Secondary asymmetries of facial width, however, are best treated with open exposure of the arch via a coronal approach with precise anatomical fixation. Loss of malar projection or inferior displacement of the malar complex that is associated with fracture malunion requires an accurate preoperative diagnosis that is complemented by three-dimensional radiographic imaging and an operative plan that involves repositioning of the entire complex. In order to accomplish this, the ZMC must be iatrogenically refractured and repositioned to its correct anatomical location. This can be accomplished via a combination of intraoral and periorbital incisions or through a coronal approach. Once the skeletal anatomy is corrected, the soft tissue envelope, including the malar fat pad, must be assessed for ptosis. If present, the midface soft tissues should be suspended and fixed to the orbit or fixation hardware. Once the ZMC is restored to its anatomical position, exploration of the orbit is mandatory to confirm concomitant correction of orbital volume discrepancies (see Fig. 24.2).

Loss of malar projection can occur due to tumor resection, congenital anomalies, or from symptomatic resorption of the zygoma following attempts at implant-based malar augmentation. Onlay grafting to the malar complex using autologous bone is an effective means of restoring projection, regardless of the etiology of the deformity. The use of implants has also been advocated in the secondary correction setting, although this approach requires careful preoperative planning and specific implant design and selection for success. With either approach, the management of the soft tissue and any evident ptosis must also be addressed at the time of the skeletal reconstruction.

Orbit

The specific goals of orbital reconstruction might vary depending on the indication for the primary procedure, but a common overarching goal exists: to restore normal orbital anatomy and volume. The volume of the orbit is determined by the morphology of its four walls. Alterations to that morphology, whether acquired or congenital in nature, can result in improper positioning of the globe and periorbital soft tissues and subsequent deficits in appearance or function, including enophthalmos, exophthalmos, hypoglobus, hyperglobus, diplopia, and other dysfunction of the rectus muscles.

The need for secondary bony corrections can be avoided during initial reconstruction by an intimate knowledge of orbital anatomy. Without reiterating the discussion on anatomy of the orbit that is presented elsewhere in this text, it bears repeating that the relationship of the bony orbital pyramid and the soft tissues it contains determines the position and function of the eye. Specifically, the contours of the bony orbit need to be replicated in any attempt at primary repair in order to avoid the most common secondary deformities: enophthalmos and diplopia. These are almost universally due to inadequate restoration of intraorbital volume during the initial attempt (see Fig. 24.3). Posterior to the equator of the globe, the orbital floor slopes up in a convexity toward the ledge of the orbital apex. Similarly, the medial orbital wall demonstrates a slight convexity in the posterior orbit. If these contours are not replicated in reconstruction, the relative volume of the orbit is increased, and the soft tissue contents of the orbit, including the globe and periorbita, will reoccupy the new (abnormal) three-dimensional anatomy. The resulting displacement of the globe into the ethmoid or maxillary sinuses results in its posterior displacement, with or without inferior translocation of the axis of the globe. This disequilibrium between injured and uninjured orbits can lead to intractable diplopia.

The goal of secondary orbital surgery, then, is to reposition the globe and visual axis to their natural positions by restoration of normal orbital contours and volume. This is most successfully achieved by an accurate diagnosis: Where is the specific orbital abnormality located and what precisely must be repaired? Knowledge of the initial injury mechanism and details of the technique used in the primary reconstruction are of great assistance in answering these questions preoperatively. As opposed to other regions of the craniofacial skeleton, three-dimensional CT scan renderings are of limited use in the preoperative evaluation. Rather, review of biplanar axial, coronal, and sagittal reformatted images are of greater value. In addition, a detailed ophthalmological evaluation is a prerequisite to any attempt at secondary reconstruction. Any preexisting visual field or rectus muscular deficit must be documented prior to undertaking a secondary intraorbital surgery, as the risk of ocular injury during revision is not insignificant.

One specific challenge facing the surgeon attempting secondary orbital surgery is the manipulation or removal of alloplastic implants placed during primary reconstructive procedures. Perhaps the most commonly used implant in orbital surgery is titanium alloy, as it is readily available in most medical centers, is malleable, and has adequate strength. More recently, a wider array of implants has been

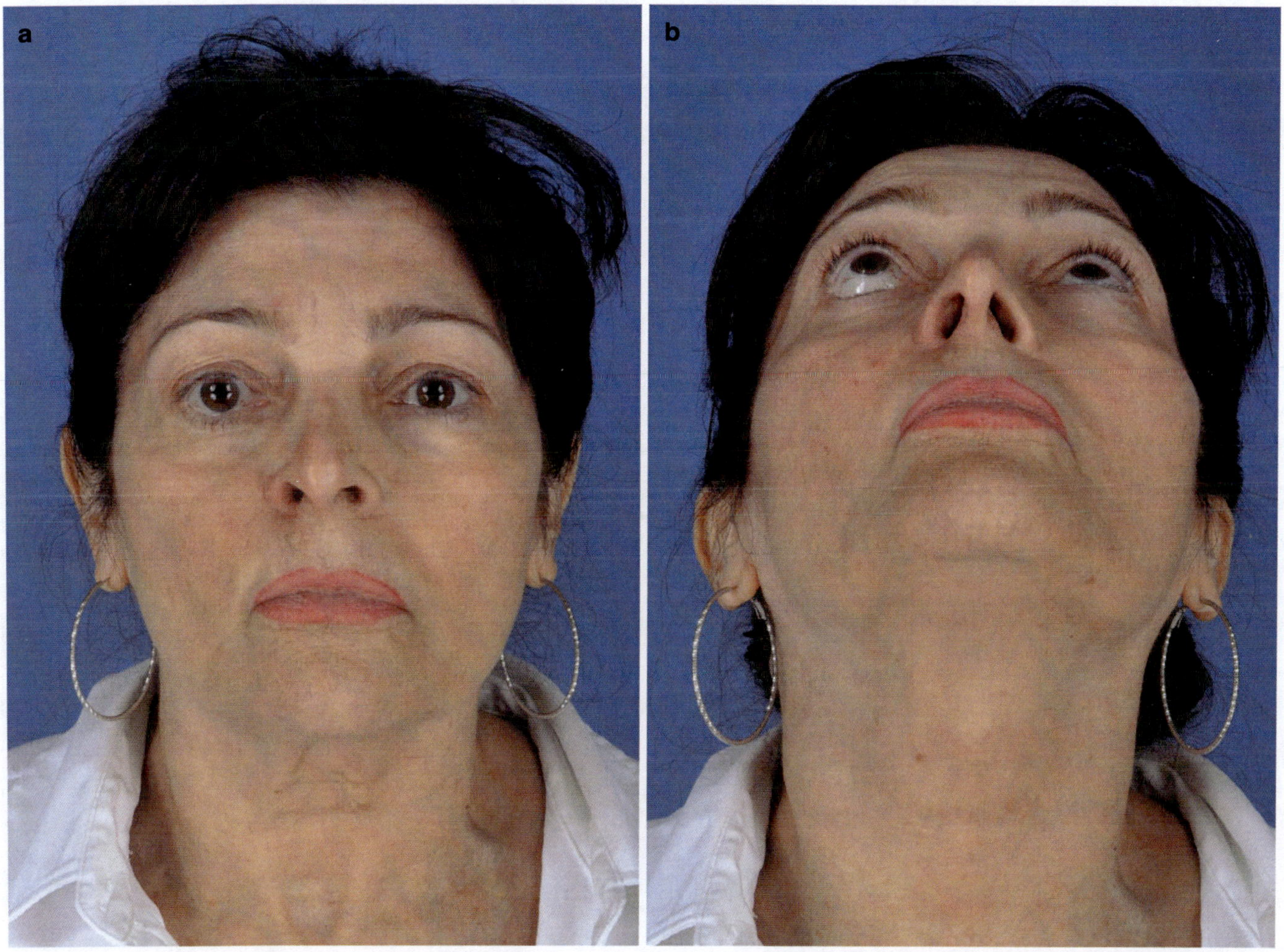

Fig. 24.3 Blunt trauma to the right orbit resulted in an orbital fracture in this patient. The injury was treated with a titanium plate. She presented six weeks after the repair with exophthalmos and diplopia, as well as lagophthalmos due to lower lid malposition. (**a**, **b**) Radiographic investigation revealed displacement of the globe by a superiorly positioned reconstruction plate. (**c**) The globe position, appearance and visual function were significantly improved with plate removal and canthopexy. (**d**, **e**) Postoperative CT confirms improved shape of the orbit and position of the globe. (**f**)

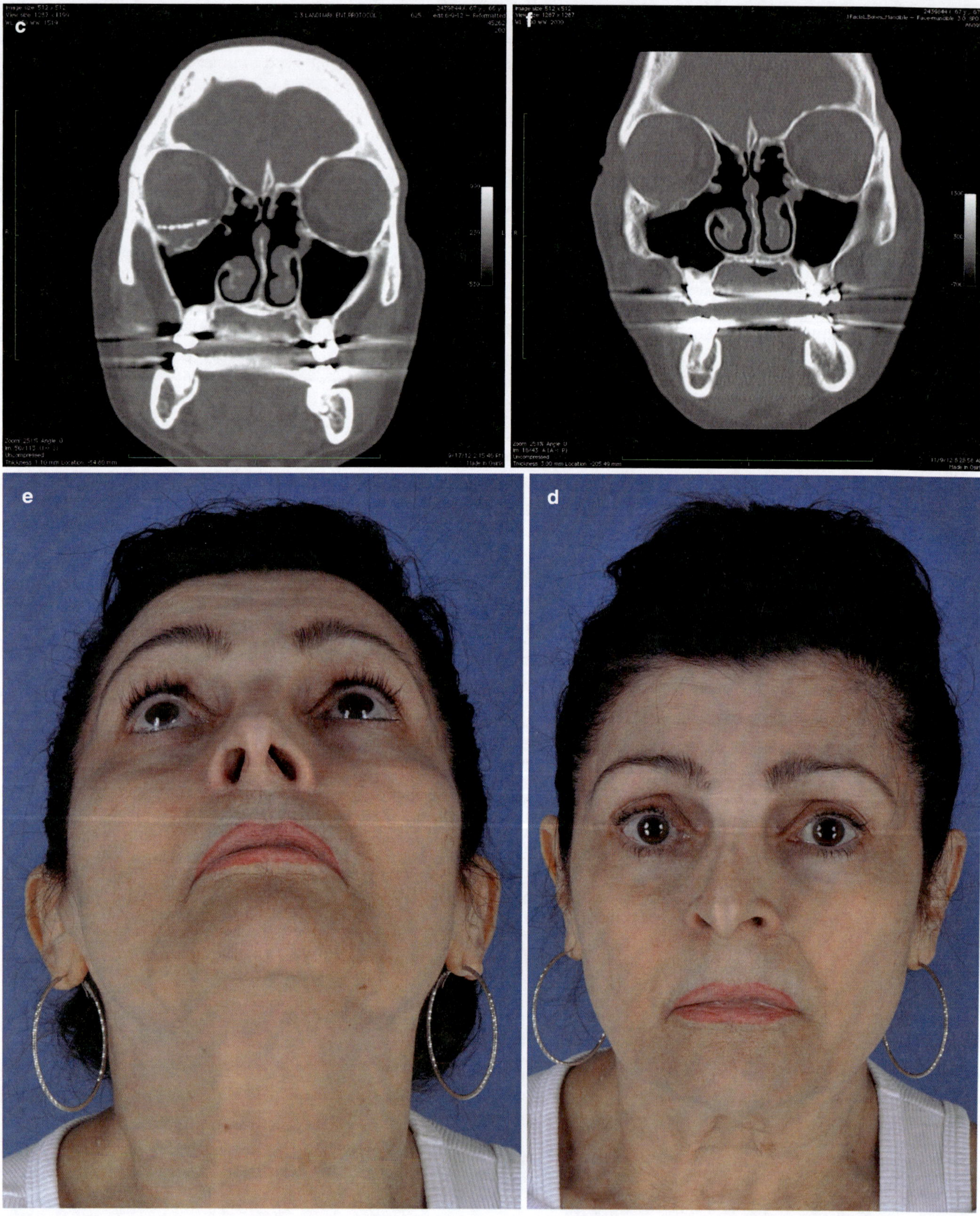

Fig. 24.3 (continued)

implemented in orbital surgery, with porous polyethylene-based alloplastic materials gaining increasing popularity. The major drawback associated with this material, and others such as titanium, is lack of incorporation into the native orbital bones and the tissue ingrowth into the implant itself. While this trait is lauded as a reason for low rates of infection, it also increases the technical difficulty and level of risk associated with secondary revision. Delicate periorbital tissues, including the rectus muscles, are often scarred down to the implants and need to be dissected free prior to implant removal and orbital recontouring. By comparison, autologous bone graft from any source handles much more favorably in the secondary setting, typically requiring no more than the periosteal elevation similar to a primary intervention.

Surgical principles of secondary reconstruction are basic: removal of all foreign material, wide subperiosteal undermining of the involved osseous structures, identification of the defect, replacement of all soft tissues into the orbit, and reestablishment of the appropriate bony volume. If placement of additional materials is needed to maintain volume, autologous tissues such as bone or cartilage grafts are preferred in the setting of revision, particularly if malposition, infection, or extrusion of an implant used in primary repair is the indication for the secondary surgery. Revision surgery in the orbit may be associated with more bleeding that the primary setting, so an appropriate level of perioperative monitoring for complications such as retrobulbar hematoma must be implemented.

In addition to skeletal irregularities that may require secondary correction, the soft tissue structures that surround the orbit and contribute to its proper functioning may be injured and also require revision if not adequately addressed during primary surgery. While an exhaustive discussion of these soft tissue abnormalities is beyond the scope of this chapter, issues such as entropion, ectropion, canalicular and tear duct injuries, and malposition of the medial and lateral canthi can cause significant deformity and discomfort. Repair of these can be especially challenging in the delayed setting due to the nonpliable nature of associated scar tissue.

Maxilla

Planning for secondary maxillary reconstruction must include consideration of related structures, including the maxillary and ethmoid sinuses, the nose, the orbits, and the tooth-bearing segments of the maxillary alveolus. As with secondary reconstruction of the upper facial third, other structures of the middle third, and the lower facial third, the goal of revision maxillary surgery is restoration of form and function. The maxilla provides the platform of the nose and the central and lateral midface vertical buttresses, as well as the occlusal surfaces provided by the upper dentition. Loss of integrity of these structures can have devastating effects on occlusion, support of the soft tissues of the midface, and the overall shape of the face, including the "golden triangle," which is the central facial anatomical unit through which most human beings interact with one another. By extension, poor primary maxillary reconstruction can have a significant deleterious effect not only on form and function but also on more fundamental human processes such as communication.

From a functional standpoint, restoration of dental occlusion is of paramount importance, as malocclusion can subject a patient to lifelong debility if not appropriately corrected. In the setting of trauma where a true LeFort I, II, or III fracture is present in the acute injury, failure to accurately diagnose, reduce, and fixate the fracture will inevitably result in a deformity that will require secondary correction of the malocclusion. This is a complicated process, involving radiographic evaluation (e.g., PA and lateral cephalograms, pantomography, or cone beam CT), cephalometric analysis, taking of dental impressions and surgical planning with dental stone models, and pre- and postsurgical orthodontic therapy.

From a structural standpoint, secondary surgeries should focus on reestablishing the integrity of the vertical and horizontal buttresses, including the nasomaxillary and zygomaticomaxillary buttresses, the hard palate and alveolus, and the inferior orbital rims. The most effective strategy in this, and almost all secondary procedures, is to recreate the original defect. This may involve excision of hypertrophic, disfiguring, or aberrantly located scar tissue, debridement of alloplastic implants or fixation hardware, or resection of adjacent mucosa. When there is bone loss, autologous bone grafting is indicated. Split calvarial bone provides an excellent substrate for reconstruction, but rib or iliac crest can also be used in this setting. Use of free bone grafts must be accompanied by recruitment of adequate lining to avoid graft exposure, infection, and resorption. Depending on the anatomy of the defect, such lining might need to come in the form of a microvascular free flap.

Primary attempts at maxillary reconstruction that make use of viable tissues that are available at the time of initial repair often result in failure. In particular, the residual maxillary alveolus may be inadequate to provide support for soft tissue of the midface or lack the amount of bone stock necessary for dental rehabilitation with implants. Alternatively, immediate reconstruction of composite oncologic resection of a complicated midface lesion, as seen in a partial or total unilateral or total maxillectomy, may be deferred until clear margins are confirmed and any adjunctive therapy is completed. Whether planned or not, definitively secondary reconstruction of these complex defects almost always requires the recruitment of distant osseous and soft tissues using microsurgical techniques. A free fibula flap, for example, can simultaneously provide structural support for the soft tissues of the midface, replace some of those same tissues, and offer adequate bone stock for placement of osseointegrated dental implants.

The Nose and Nasoorbitoethmoidal (NOE) Complex

The evaluation and management NOE fractures is extensively discussed in the trauma sections of this text, but due to the potentially severe consequences associated with malunion of displaced NOE fractures, a brief discussion of the management of secondary deformities is warranted. The NOE complex represents the intersection of the various segments of the midface that have been independently considered above. By extension, secondary NOE deformities may involve any of the aesthetic and functional deficits associated with bony and soft tissue injuries involving the orbits and maxilla, particularly if there is an associated LeFort fracture. In addition, injury to the bony nasal pyramid complicates the management of NOE fractures both in the acute and delayed settings.

As with other secondary midface deformities, any surgical plan must derive first from accurate diagnosis and assessment of the three-dimensional defect. Lack of nasal projection due to inadequate reduction at the nasion can be treated with dorsal augmentation, ideally with cranial bone or rib. Malunion of major NOE fragments may require refracture, repositioning, and internal fixation, as with malunion of ZMC fractures. Significant orbital deformities may call for major orbital reconstruction to restore anatomical positioning or intraorbital volume. Soft tissue correction must also be considered when skeletal revision is required. Most commonly, telecanthus or medial canthal asymmetries following Type 2 and 3 NOE fractures may require medial canthopexy.

More simple injuries limited to the nose and nasal passages may require nasal osteotomies or formal septorhinoplasty with or without spreader graft or spreader flap placement to both reposition the nasal pyramid for optimal symmetry and improve any symptoms of nasal airflow obstruction associated with posttraumatic deformities.

Lower Facial Third

The primary roles of the mandible are to drive mastication, to support the soft tissues of the lower third of the face—both intraoral and extraoral—and their proper function, and to provide lower facial third projection. Because of this latter role, the mandible, like the nose and zygoma that provide anterior and lateral projection to the midface, is often susceptible to blunt traumatic forces. The mucosalized surfaces of the intraoral soft tissues, and our propensity to subject those surfaces to toxins such as tobacco, predispose the mandible to injury from within as well. Mandibular trauma is often performed in the setting of gingivoperiodontal disease, poor dental hygiene, and delayed primary treatment of open fractures due to management of concomitant life-threatening injuries. Oncologic resection of mandibular neoplasms is often undertaken in chronically malnourished patients. Moreover, even the most effective primary reconstructive techniques might be compromised by adjuvant radiation therapy. Within these clinical contexts, complication rates from primary mandibular surgeries that require secondary revision are not insignificant.

Trauma

The goal of mandibular fracture repair is to reestablish appropriate occlusal relationships to allow for normal mastication, speech, deglutition, lip function, and appearance. Failure to establish premorbid occlusion at the time of initial repair, or complications related to poor technique, inaccurate diagnosis, delay in treatment, infection, or poor wound healing, can result in malunion, nonunion, malocclusion, temporomandibular joint (TMJ) dysfunction, and facial asymmetry. The goal of secondary revision, then, is to restore proper occlusion, consolidate the mandibular arch, and reverse any functional deficits. Surgical techniques must be tailored to specific indication for the correction.

If a diagnosis of infection or infected nonunion is confirmed, surgical management should include establishment of premorbid occlusion, incision and drainage, debridement of all infected and devitalized tissues—including proximal and distal fracture edges—and rigid internal fixation. Both immediate and delayed cancellous bone grafting to the area of nonunion have been implemented in this setting with success. Although placement of a non-vascularized bone graft into an infected field eliminates the need for a second stage, it should be done only under optimal wound conditions and in conjunction with appropriate antibiotic therapy and close postoperative monitoring. If drainage and debridement of the area of infection is limited to less than 6 cm in length, nonvascularized bone grafts can be used with a reasonable anticipation of success. For larger defects, free tissue transfer will provide a more predictable and stable outcome.

The approach to malunion with associated malocclusion must include a plan to reestablish the appropriate occlusal relationship with orthognathic surgery. This approach is similar to the refracture and reposition strategy that is recommended for ZMC malunions but must incorporate detailed presurgical planning to ensure success. The patient is best served by multidisciplinary input from dentists, orthodontists, and plastic surgeons. The malocclusion must be accurately detailed in dental records, including photographs, radiographs, impressions, and dental stone models. Surgical planning should be collaborative, particularly on the part of the treating orthodontist and plastic surgeon. A preoperative phase of orthodontia should be implemented to optimize the relationships of the upper and lower dental occlusal surfaces. Patients should also anticipate several months of orthodontic therapy following surgery to perfect the occlusion. The exact placement of corrective osteotomies will depend on the anatomy of the original fracture but may include refracture at the initial site or bilateral sagittal split osteotomy. Basic principles of orthognathic surgery, as detailed in this text, should guide the surgical correction.

In anticipation of orthognathic correction, any issues with limited TMJ motion should be addressed with aggressive physical therapy to mitigate the possibility of long-term TMJ dysfunction following surgery.

Neoplasm

Although the source of the initial insult is different in the setting of neoplasia compared to trauma, the goals of secondary reconstruction are similar: to identify and treat the source of the complication and to establish a functional occlusal relationship. Once reserved for salvage, primary free flap reconstruction of the mandible has evolved into a first-line therapy for large oral cavity tumors that invade the lower jaw. Depending on the anatomy of the defect, either fasciocutaneous or osteocutaneous flaps might be favored. Common fasciocutaneous flaps used in the setting of mandibular reconstruction are the radial forearm and anterolateral thigh flaps. Osteocutaneous flap options include the fibula, scapula, and iliac crest free flaps. Of these, the free fibula flap is the most commonly used, primarily due to its length, thickness, and versatility. The fibula can be designed with multiple osteotomies to reestablish the precise contour of the native mandible or as a "double-barrel" to maximize height of the flap. In addition, it can accommodate implant-based dental rehabilitation and can support or replace existing soft tissues of the lower third of the face with its skin paddle.

Complications from primary free flap reconstruction include infection, hardware failure, plate exposure, graft resorption, soft tissue deficiency, contour irregularity, intraoral contracture, and osteoradionecrosis. Secondary revisions must be tailored to the cause of failure and resultant symptoms. When the primary reconstruction is based on the combination of reconstruction plate and fasciocutaneous flap, hardware removal, debridement of the flap and any irradiated tissues, and replacement with an osteocutaneous flap are indicated. If the primary reconstructive choice was an osteocutaneous flap, alternative donor sites for a replacement osteocutaneous flap should be explored. Regional flaps including the pectoral, deltopectoral, and supraclavicular island flaps can be used in the event of primary and secondary free flap failure.

Distraction Osteogenesis

Distraction osteogenesis (DO) has been widely applied to all regions of the craniofacial skeleton since its description two decades ago. Its main application is in the primary setting, but it can also play a valuable role in secondary reconstruction of mandibles injured by trauma or oncological resection or that have undergone reconstruction due to congenital hypoplasia.

Distraction is commonly used to augment a free fibula flap that is too deficient in the vertical dimension to accommodate a dental implant. This secondary procedure is a valuable technique that allows the patient and surgeon to achieve the ultimate goal of dental restoration and a normal occlusion following mandibular resection and reconstruction. The use of DO has also been described in the setting of posttraumatic malocclusion or other post-ablative deformity treated with a non-vascularized bone graft. Rib grafts used for correction of congenital, posttraumatic, and oncological conditions are also amenable to lengthening with DO. Despite the deleterious effects of radiation therapy on wound healing and tissue regeneration, DO has been used in the secondary setting to provide vertical or horizontal length to a reconstructed or native mandible that has undergone radiation therapy. While initial reports are encouraging, the long-term efficacy of distraction in the setting of irradiated bone is as of yet unclear. The potential benefit of DO in the setting of radiation injury, however, currently drives a robust field of research geared toward developing clinical interventions with improved outcomes.

Transport distraction osteogenesis (TDO) involves the separation of a bloc of bone that is adjacent to an area of defect via a mandibular osteotomy, the distraction of that bony segment along a desired vector, and subsequent bone formation along that path. This approach to mandibular reconstruction can be used in the secondary setting to repair defects caused by infection, nonunion, and bone graft resorption and can potentially obviate the need for free tissue transfer.

Future Directions

The way in which we treat secondary deformities of the craniofacial skeleton in the future (and, in all likelihood, how we acutely manage these injuries) is rooted in the technological and research advances that are being developed today. Once dependent on hand-drawn cephalometric analyses, orthognathic surgery has entered the digital age: Electronic cephalometrics are generated based on digital cephalograms, "model surgery" is performed virtually, and computer-aided design/computer-aided manufacturing (CAD/CAM) processes fabricate occlusal splints and even implantable hardware to facilitate surgical execution. It is almost inconceivable that reconstruction of complex maxillofacial defects in either the primary or, certainly, the secondary setting will not be driven by CAD/CAM technology in the near future.

As promising as the use of CAD/CAM in facial reconstruction is, the potential of developing 3D printing technology combined with our ever-increasing experience with tissue engineering. As our experience with 3D printing increases, we will be able to develop methods to imprint biocompatible polymers with living cells.

If CAD/CAM, 3D printing, and tissue engineering technologies are the building blocks of the reconstructive paradigm of the future, facial composite tissue allotransplantation (CTA) is the last stop on the reconstructive ladder today. To date, over two-dozen face transplants have been performed, with the reconstructed defects becoming more and more complex. The rate-limiting factor associated with the growth of face CTA lies in postoperative immunosuppression protocols. Despite the amount of international attention being given to face transplantation and the growing number of medical centers developing CTA programs, the volume of cases of facial CTA is likely to remain low until research efforts can generate less toxic immunosuppressive agents that can be used in monotherapy protocols. Nevertheless, face transplantation represents current state of the art in complex secondary maxillofacial reconstruction and sets the bar for what our advances in biotechnology must achieve.

Bibliography

Aboul-Hosn Centenero S, Hernández-Alfaro F. 3D planning in orthognathic surgery: CAD/CAM surgical splints and prediction of the soft and hard tissues results – our experience in 16 cases. J Craniomaxillofac Surg. 2012;40(2):162–8.

Baek RM, Kim J, Kim BK. Three-dimensional assessment of zygomatic malunion using computed tomography in patients with cheek ptosis caused by reduction malarplasty. J Plast Reconstr Aesthet Surg. 2012;65(4):448–55.

Baumeister S, Peek A, Friedman A, Levin LS, Marcus JR. Management of postneurosurgical bone flap loss caused by infection. Plast Reconstr Surg. 2008;122(6):195e–208e.

Becking AG, Zijderveld SA, Tuinzing DB. The surgical management of post-traumatic malocclusion. Clin Plast Surg. 2007;34(3):e37–43.

Benson PD, Marshall MK, Engelstad ME, Kushner GM, Alpert B. The use of immediate bone grafting in reconstruction of clinically infected mandibular fractures: bone grafts in the presence of pus. J Oral Maxillofac Surg. 2006;64(1):122–6.

Biller JA, Pletcher SD, Goldberg AN, Murr AH. Complications and the time to repair of mandible fractures. Laryngoscope. 2005;115(5):769–72.

Bogusiak K, Arkuszewski P. Characteristics and epidemiology of zygomaticomaxillary complex fractures. J Craniofac Surg. 2010;21(4):1018–23.

Cheung LK, Chua HD, Hariri F, Pow EH, Zheng L. Alveolar distraction osteogenesis for dental implant rehabilitation following fibular reconstruction: a case series. J Oral Maxillofac Surg. 2013;71(2):255–71.

Chien KB, Makridakis E, Shah RN. Three-dimensional printing of soy protein scaffolds for tissue regeneration. Tissue Eng Part C Methods. 2013;19(6):417–26.

Ciocca L, Fantini M, Marchetti C, Scotti R, Monaco C. Immediate facial rehabilitation in cancer patients using CAD-CAM and rapid prototyping technology: a pilot study. Support Care Cancer. 2010;18(6):723–8.

Czerwinski M, Parker WL, Correa JA, Williams HB. Effect of treatment delay on mandibular fracture infection rate. Plast Reconstr Surg. 2008;122(3):881–5.

De Souza M, Oeltjen JC, Panthaki ZJ, Thaller SR. Posttraumatic mandibular deformities. J Craniofac Surg. 2007;18(4):912–6.

Dean D, Min KJ, Bond A. Computer aided design of large-format prefabricated cranial plates. J Craniofac Surg. 2003;14(6):819–32.

Deshpande SS, Gallagher KK, Donneys A, Tchanque-Fossuo CN, Sarhaddi D, Sun H, Krebsbach PH, Buchman SR. Stem cell therapy remediates reconstruction of the craniofacial skeleton after radiation therapy. http://www.ncbi.nlm.nih.gov/pubmed/?term=23282102. Stem Cells Dev. 2013;22:1625–32.

Dorafshar AH, Bojovic B, Christy MR, Borsuk DE, Iliff NT, Brown EN, Shaffer CK, Kelley TN, Kukuruga DL, Barth RN, Bartlett ST, Rodriguez ED. Total face, double jaw, and tongue transplantation: an evolutionary concept. Plast Reconstr Surg. 2013;131(2):241–51.

Elsalanty ME, Taher TN, Zakhary IE, Al-Shahaat OA, Refai M, El-Mekkawi HA. Reconstruction of large mandibular bone and soft-tissue defect using bone transport distraction osteogenesis. J Craniofac Surg. 2007;18(6):1397–402.

Fedorovich NE, Schuurman W, Wijnberg HM, Prins HJ, van Weeren PR, Malda J, Alblas J, Dhert WJ. Biofabrication of osteochondral tissue equivalents by printing topologically defined, cell-laden hydrogel scaffolds. Tissue Eng Part C Methods. 2012;18(1):33–44.

Foster RD, Anthony JP, Sharma A, Pogrel MA. Vascularized bone flaps versus nonvascularized bone grafts for mandibular reconstruction: an outcome analysis of primary bony union and endosseous implant success. Head Neck. 1999;21(1):66–71.

Frodel Jr JL. Management of the nasal dorsum in central facial injuries. Indications for calvarial bone grafting. Arch Otolaryngol Head Neck Surg. 1995;121(3):307–12.

Furr AM, Schweinfurth JM, May WL. Factors associated with long-term complications after repair of mandibular fractures. Laryngoscope. 2006;116(3):427–30.

Gallagher KK, Deshpande S, Tchanque-Fossuo CN, Donneys A, Sarhaddi D, Nelson NS, Chepeha DB, Buchman SR. Role of parathyroid hormone therapy in reversing radiation-induced non-union and normalization of radiomorphometrics in a murine mandibular model of distraction osteogenesis. Head Neck. 2013. http://www.ncbi.nlm.nih.gov/pubmed/23335324. doi:10.1002/hed.23216.

González-García R, Rodríguez-Campo FJ, Naval-Gías L, Sastre-Pérez J, Díaz-González FJ. The effect of radiation in distraction osteogenesis for reconstruction of mandibular segmental defects. Br J Oral Maxillofac Surg. 2007;45(4):314–6.

Granthan E, Landis H. Cranioplasty and the post- traumatic syndrome. J Neurosurg. 1947;5:19–22.

Gruss JS, Van Wyck L, Phillips JH, Antonyshyn O. The importance of the zygomatic arch in complex midfacial fracture repair and correction of posttraumatic orbitozygomatic deformities. Plast Reconstr Surg. 1990;85(6):878–90.

Herford AS, Ying T, Brown B. Outcomes of severely comminuted (type III) nasoorbitoethmoid fractures. J Oral Maxillofac Surg. 2005; 63(9):1266–77.

Higuera S, Lee EI, Cole P, Hollier Jr LH, Stal S. Nasal trauma and the deviated nose. Plast Reconstr Surg. 2007;120(7 Suppl 2):64S–75S.

Hussussian CJ, Reece GP. Microsurgical scalp reconstruction in the patient with cancer. Plast Reconstr Surg. 2002;109(6):1828–34.

Iwama T, Yamada J, Imai S, Shinoda J, Funakoshi T, Sakai N. The use of frozen autogenous bone flaps in delayed cranioplasty revisited. Neurosurgery. 2003;52(3):591–6.

Jamal BT, Pfahler SM, Lane KA, Bilyk JR, Pribitkin EA, Diecidue RJ, Taub DI. Ophthalmic injuries in patients with zygomaticomaxillary complex fractures requiring surgical repair. J Oral Maxillofac Surg. 2009;67(5):986–9.

Jarrahy R, Vo V, Goenjian HA, Tabit CJ, Katchikian HV, Kumar A, Meals C, Bradley JP. Diagnostic accuracy of maxillofacial trauma two-dimensional and three-dimensional computed tomographic scans: comparison of oral surgeons, head and neck surgeons, plastic surgeons, and neuroradiologists. Plast Reconstr Surg. 2011;127(6): 2432–40.

Jones NF, Johnson JT, Shestak KC, Myers EN, Swartz WM. Microsurgical reconstruction of the head and neck: interdisciplinary collaboration between head and neck surgeons and plastic surgeons in 305 cases. Ann Plast Surg. 1996;36(1):37–43.

Kaufman Y, Stal D, Cole P, Hollier Jr L. Orbitozygomatic fracture management. Plast Reconstr Surg. 2008;121(4):1370–4.

Kobienia BJ, Sultz JR, Migliori MR, Schubert W. Portable fluoroscopy in the management of zygomatic arch fractures. Ann Plast Surg. 1998;40(3):260–4.

Leonhardt H, Pradel W, Mai R, Markwardt J, Lauer G. Prefabricated bony radial forearm flap for secondary mandible reconstruction after radiochemotherapy. Head Neck. 2009;31(12):1579–87.

Li L, Blake F, Gbara A, Gudewer E, Schmelzle R. Distraction osteogenesis in secondary microsurgical mandible reconstruction: report of seven cases. J Craniomaxillofac Surg. 2008;36(5):273–8.

López-Arcas JM, Arias J, Del Castillo JL, Burgueño M, Navarro I, Morán MJ, Chamorro M, Martorell V. The fibula osteomyocutaneous flap for mandible reconstruction: a 15-year experience. J Oral Maxillofac Surg. 2010;68(10):2377–84.

Losee JE, Karmacharya J, Gannon FH, Slemp AE, Ong G, Hunenko O, Gorden AD, Bartlett SP, Kirschner RE. Reconstruction of the immature craniofacial skeleton with a carbonated calcium phosphate bone cement: interaction with bioresorbable mesh. J Craniofac Surg. 2003;14(1):117–24.

Manolidis S, Weeks BH, Kirby M, Scarlett M, Hollier L. Classification and surgical management of orbital fractures: experience with 111 orbital reconstructions. J Craniofac Surg. 2002;13(6):726–37.

Matsumura H, Yakumaru H, Watanabe K. Temporal approach for reduction of zygomatic fractures. Clinical results and advantages of the technique. Scand J Plast Reconstr Surg Hand Surg. 1994;28(1):49–53.

McCombe D, Donato R, Hofer SO, Morrison W. Free flaps in the treatment of locally advanced malignancy of the scalp and forehead. Ann Plast Surg. 2002;48(6):600–6.

Moreira-Gonzalez A, Jackson IT, Miyawaki T, Barakat K, DiNick V. Clinical outcome in cranioplasty: critical review in long-term follow-up. J Craniofac Surg. 2003;14(2):144–53.

Mortellaro C, Rimondini L, Farronato G, Garagiola U, Varcellino V, Berrone M. Temporomandibular disorders due to improper surgical treatment of mandibular fracture: clinical report. J Craniofac Surg. 2006;17(2):373–82.

Movassaghi K, Ver Halen J, Ganchi P, Amin-Hanjani S, Mesa J, Yaremchuk MJ. Cranioplasty with subcutaneously preserved autologous bone grafts. Plast Reconstr Surg. 2006;117(1):202–6.

Nagashima LK, Rondon-Newby M, Zakhary IE, Nagy WW, Zapata U, Dechow PC, Opperman LA, Elsalanty ME. Bone regeneration and docking site healing after bone transport distraction osteogenesis in the canine mandible. J Oral Maxillofac Surg. 2012;70(2):429–39.

Oppenheimer AJ, Mesa J, Buchman SR. Current and emerging basic science concepts in bone biology: implications in craniofacial surgery. J Craniofac Surg. 2012;23(1):30–6.

Reiffel AJ, Kafka C, Hernandez KA, Popa S, Perez JL, Zhou S, Pramanik S, Brown BN, Ryu WS, Bonassar LJ, Spector JA. High-fidelity tissue engineering of patient-specific auricles for reconstruction of pediatric microtia and other auricular deformities. PLoS One. 2013;8(2):e56506.

Sacco AG, Chepeha DB. Current status of transport-disc-distraction osteogenesis for mandibular reconstruction. Lancet Oncol. 2007;8(4):323–30.

Sahoo N, Roy ID, Desai AP, Gupta V. Comparative evaluation of autogenous calvarial bone graft and alloplastic materials for secondary reconstruction of cranial defects. J Craniofac Surg. 2010;21(1): 79–82.

Sawhney R, Ducic Y. Management of pathologic fractures of the mandible secondary to osteoradionecrosis. Otolaryngol Head Neck Surg. 2013;148(1):54–8.

Seitz IA, Adler N, Odessey E, Reid RR, Gottlieb LJ. Latissimus dorsi/rib intercostal perforator myo-osseocutaneous free flap reconstruction in composite defects of the scalp: case series and review of literature. J Reconstr Microsurg. 2009;25(9):559–67.

Soon Sung K, Hak C. Staged reconstruction of infected dura mater using vascularized rectus abdominis muscle. J Craniofac Surg. 2012;23(6):1741–3.

Stockmann P, Park J, von Wilmowsky C, Nkenke E, Felszeghy E, Dehner JF, Schmitt C, Tudor C, Schlegel KA. Guided bone regeneration in pig calvarial bone defects using autologous mesenchymal stem/progenitor cells – a comparison of different tissue sources. J Craniomaxillofac Surg. 2012;40(4):310–20.

Stueber K, Salcman M, Spence RJ. The combined use of the latissimus dorsi musculocutaneous free flap and split-rib grafts for cranial vault reconstruction. Ann Plast Surg. 1985;15(2):155–60.

Tessier P, Kawamoto H, Matthews D, Posnick J, Raulo Y, Tulasne JF, Wolfe SA. Autogenous bone grafts and bone substitutes-tools and techniques: I. A 20,000-case experience in maxillofacial and craniofacial surgery. Plast Reconstr Surg. 2005a;116(5 Suppl):6S–24S; discussion 92S–4S.

Tessier P, Kawamoto H, Matthews D, Posnick J, Raulo Y, Tulasne JF, Wolfe SA. Taking long rib grafts for facial reconstruction-tools and techniques: III. A 2900-case experience in maxillofacial and craniofacial surgery. Plast Reconstr Surg. 2005b;116(5 Suppl):38S–46S.

Thaller SR, Reavie D. Refracture reposition of mandibular malunion. Ann Plast Surg. 1990;25(3):188–92.

Thaller SR, Zarem HA, Kawamoto HK. Surgical correction of late sequelae from facial bone fractures. Am J Surg. 1987;154(1): 149–53.

Thesleff T, Lehtimäki K, Niskakangas T, Mannerström B, Miettinen S, Suuronen R, Ohman J. Cranioplasty with adipose-derived stem cells and biomaterial. A novel method for cranial reconstruction. Neurosurgery. 2011;68(6):1535–40.

Ueda K, Oba S, Omiya Y, Okada M. Cranial-bone defects with depression deformity treated with ceramic implants and free-flap transfers. Br J Plast Surg. 2001;54(5):403–8.

Vega LG. Reoperative mandibular trauma: management of posttraumatic mandibular deformities. Oral Maxillofac Surg Clin North Am. 2011;23(1):47–61, v–vi.

Wang G, Li J, Khadka A, Hsu Y, Li W, Hu J. CAD/CAM and rapid prototyped titanium for reconstruction of ramus defect and condylar fracture caused by mandibular reduction. Oral Surg Oral Med Oral Pathol Oral Radiol. 2012a;113(3):356–61.

Wang JJ, Chen J, Ping FY, Yan F. Double-step transport distraction osteogenesis in the reconstruction of unilateral large mandibular defects after tumour resection using internal distraction devices. Int J Oral Maxillofac Surg. 2012b;41(5):587–95.

Wei FC, Celik N, Yang WG, Chen IH, Chang YM, Chen HC. Complications after reconstruction by plate and soft-tissue free flap in composite mandibular defects and secondary salvage reconstruction with osteocutaneous flap. Plast Reconstr Surg. 2003;112(1): 37–42.

Yaremchuk MJ. Secondary malar implant surgery. Plast Reconstr Surg. 2008;121(2):620–8.

Zinser MJ, Mischkowski RA, Sailer HF, Zöller JE. Computer-assisted orthognathic surgery: feasibility study using multiple CAD/CAM surgical splints. Oral Surg Oral Med Oral Pathol Oral Radiol. 2012;113(5):673–87.

Secondary Soft Tissue Reconstruction

25

Bassan J. Allan, Robert M. Van Haren, Bo Wang, and Seth Thaller

Abbreviations

ALT	Anterolateral thigh
CNS	Central nervous system
CT	Computerized tomography
LCFA	Lateral circumflex femoral artery
MRA	Magnetic resonance angiography

Soft Tissue Analysis

First step of reconstruction is always the assessment of the defect and its relationship to the face as an aesthetic unit. Face and neck can be generally divided into six anatomical entities: skin and soft tissue, intraoral, mandible, midface, cranial base, and scalp. Available reconstructive options include healing by primary closure, secondary intention, skin grafts, local flaps, pedicled flaps, and free tissue transfer. Selection of the reconstructive modality to use is made based on anatomical, physiological nature of the defects (size, location, function) and the patient's condition. For large and complex facial and neck defects, free tissue transfer has proven to be the best aesthetic and functional reconstructive option. Major factor that allows wide use of free tissue transfer in reconstruction is the advancement in microvascular surgery. In past decades, an ample amount of experience regarding each flap's potential in reconstruction has been accumulated, including flap size, pedicle length, and vessel diameter and associated donor morbidities.

B.J. Allan, MD, MBA • R.M. Van Haren, MD, MsPH
B. Wang, MD
Department of Surgery,
University of Miami, Miami, FL, USA

S. Thaller, MD, DMD (✉)
Division of Plastic and Reconstructive Surgery,
Department of Surgery, University of Miami, Miami, FL, USA
e-mail: sthaller@med.miami.edu

Small *cutaneous and soft tissue* defects can be repaired by primary closure and local tissue flaps. Local flaps such as nasolabial, paramedian forehead, and dorsonasal can be employed. Using local tissue flaps gives the advantage of maintaining similar skin color, texture, and thickness, and scars can be easily hidden in wrinkles and shadows. Skin grafts either partial or full thickness can also be used for larger wounds. Disadvantage of skin grafting includes discoloration, less than ideal contour, and graft contracture. Pedicled flaps such as the pectoralis major flaps, latissimus dorsi flaps, and trapezius flaps are more appropriately used in the neck region. Limited by the length of the pedicles, they should not be used in mid- and upper face defects, and instead, free tissue transfer can be utilized.

Intraoral area serves the function of conduit for food, airflow, and speech and contains important structures including, tongue, pharynx, larynx, and esophagus. Majority of small defects can be repaired primarily without causing anatomical constrictions that may affect speech and articulation. For partial glossectomy, the radial forearm free flap has emerged as the standard for most surgeons because it provides desired bulk and contour for reconstruction. However, in total glossectomy, the more bulky anterolateral thigh (ALT) flap and rectus abdominis are able to provide more volume to compensate for the lack of motor function by assisting the propulsion of food into the pharynx during swallowing. Radial and ALT flaps have emerged as the workhorses for intraoral, pharyngeal, and hypopharyngeal reconstruction. Their thin and pliable tissues can be easily contoured, making the radial and ALT flaps good candidates for reconstruction of tubular structures. Conversely, the jejunal free flap is the flap of choice for circumferential cervical esophageal reconstruction. Even though the jejunal flap is technically challenging due to its low tolerance to ischemia, its exceptional motility, low stricture, and fistula formation rates make it the best candidate for cervical esophageal reconstruction.

Mandible can be divided into symphysis, parasymphysis, body, angle, ascending ramus, and condyle. An understanding

P.J. Taub et al. (eds.), *Ferraro's Fundamentals of Maxillofacial Surgery*,
DOI 10.1007/978-1-4614-8341-0_25,

of the physiological demands of each segment of the mandible and adequate selection of reconstruction is key to ensure a long-lasting repair. Use of nonvascularized bone graft requires a well-vascularized recipient bed and a watertight mucosal coverage to prevent the erosion by saliva. Nonvascularized bone usage should be limited to small defects (less than 5 cm) and avoided in previously irradiated fields where vascularized bone graft should be used instead. Fibular free flap has become the dominant candidate in reconstruction of tissue losses with associated with mandibular defects. Fibular free flaps are long, thin, and durable which allow multiple osteotomies in order to form the ideal contour for mandibular reconstructions. Other donor sites for reconstruction include scapula osteocutaneous free flap, iliac crest, and radial forearm; however, all of them have inferior bony components compared to fibular free flaps and may not tolerate multiple osteotomies. Only concern before the use of a fibula flap is in patients with severe peripheral vascular disease, which may compromise both the donor site and the flap repair. Lastly, the anterior mandible is subjected to the highest amount of stress, and the use of metal plates for the reconstruction of this area is not recommended due to its high failure rate. Conversely, the lateral and posterior mandible are the less stressed areas, therefore, prosthetic plates are acceptable options for reconstruction.

Major components of the *midface* include the nose, orbits, maxilla, palate, and paranasal sinuses. Challenge of reconstructing the midfacial defects relates to its three-dimensional nature and its location at the center of the face. Important considerations during reconstruction also include the creation of a barrier between the CNS and aerodigestive tract as well as elimination of dead space. Vascularized bone flaps from iliac crest, scapula, and fibula have been used to establish the bony support required for adequate reconstruction in combination with osteo-integrated devices or prosthesis. Muscle flaps such as the rectus abdominis and radial forearm or anterolateral thigh can be used to fill the dead space after total maxillectomy and orbital exenteration.

Main concern with the repair of *cranial base* defects is to reestablish the barrier between CNS and the external environment. Temporoparietal fascial flaps or pericranial flaps in combination with calvarial bone grafts can be used for small-size defects. Rectus abdominis, radial forearm, and anterolateral thigh are all options for larger defects that cannot be reached by local flaps. Choices depend on the required flap volume to fulfill the dead space.

Local rotational or advancement flaps are the main modalities for closure of small- and moderate-size *scalp defects*. Tissue expanders and pedicled flaps such as the trapezius and latissimus dorsi flaps are options if larger defects are encountered. However, both options are less than ideal. Former requires multiple procedures and is at increased risk for infection. Latter is restricted by its pedicle length and ability to reach the defect without compromising the blood flow. Latissimus dorsi muscle free flaps combined with skin graft or parascapular fasciocutaneous free flap are both good options to cover large areas for scalp defects. Bony defects are generally reconstructed with autologous split-thickness calvarial grafts or titanium meshes and then adequately covered with soft tissue.

Surgical Techniques

Historically pedicled flaps were used for soft tissue reconstruction of head and neck defects. Commonly used flaps included pectoralis major musculocutaneous flap, lateral forehead flap, and deltopectoral flap. Tissue expanders are another option for reconstruction and were first described in 1957 by Neumann. This technique creates a local supply of skin and subcutaneous tissue, as saline is sequentially injected via a port. Tissue expanders are a functional technique that offers acceptable cosmetic results; however, very large defects (>100 cm^2) have a higher rate of failure.

Since the development of microsurgery and free tissue transfer, microsurgery free flaps are considered the standard of care for head and neck secondary soft tissue reconstruction. Free flaps offer significantly more tissue and volume that can be brought into the head and neck for reconstruction. The free flap technique has improved over time in terms of tissue selection, surgical technique, and outcomes. Excellent success rates (91–99 %) have been reported by numerous institutions solidifying the role of free flaps and microsurgery.

Surgical Principles

Similar surgical principles apply to a variety of free flaps that can be used to reconstruct soft tissue defects of the head and neck. After soft tissue analysis has been performed, at least one artery and vein are carefully mobilized for microsurgical anastomosis. Two major sources of recipient arteries of the head and neck are the branches of the external carotid artery and thyrocervical trunk. Four pairs of arteries are usually preferred: superficial temporal, facial, superior thyroid, and transverse cervical vessels. Choices of recipient vessels are based on the length and size of the pedicles and the proximity to the defect in order to ensure a tension-free anastomosis. Ipsilateral vessels should always be considered first, but are not necessarily a requirement. Use of flaps with long pedicles allows anastomosis to be performed on more distant vessels and contralateral vessels without compromising the blood flow. Previous dissection and irradiation impose challenges on surgeons; however, careful preoperative planning and careful dissection allows one to find good recipient vessels for tissue transferring. In order to preserve all available vessels for reconstruction, it is of utmost importance to have a clear plan during the primary surgery for tumor resection.

Keep in mind that reoperation and simultaneous double flaps may be needed to fully reconstruct the defect, and unnecessary sacrifice of vessels may lead to much difficulty during the reconstructive part of the surgery. Interpositional grafts and sequential linked flaps are usually considered as less than ideal options when access to recipient vessels are limited, because of their association with increased failure rates and flap necrosis. Same concepts can be applied when choosing recipient veins. Branches of internal jugular vein and smaller-sized external jugular veins are available options.

Next, the resection site is covered with moist gauze while the flap is prepared. After the flap is harvested, it is inserted with the deepest or the most difficult to reach location first. Tension-free repair is paramount, and the neck should be passively rotated through its range of motion bilaterally to avoid pedicle complications. Arterial anastomosis is generally performed prior to venous anastomosis, because it allows for evaluation of the venous system. A drain is placed in dependent areas to prevent fluid collections per a surgeon's discretion.

Free Flap Selection

There are numerous options for flaps used in head and neck reconstructions, and the selection depends on the soft tissue deficit analysis, individual anatomic considerations, and surgeon preference (see Table 25.1). In this chapter, we will discuss soft tissue, bone, and visceral free flaps.

Soft Tissue Flaps: Anterolateral Thigh Flap (ALT) and Radial Forearm

Two commonly used soft tissue flaps are the radial forearm and anterolateral thigh flap (ALT). Radial forearm flap is one of the most frequently used flaps, and its main advantage is its reliability. It generates a thin, malleable flap with a long pedicle (Fig. 25.1). Its use is limited by the small amount of soft tissue it produces and donor-site morbidity; however, these complications can be limited with a suprafascial technique. Liu et al. compared 53 radial forearms to 21 ALT flaps for head and neck reconstruction and found equivalent survival rates between the flaps. Although, radial forearm flaps had significantly more complications such as numbness and weakness and less patient satisfaction.

ALT flap provides an excellent volume of tissue, and it can be harvested in several variations including subcutaneous, fasciocutaneous, musculocutaneous, or adipofascial. The availability of skin, fascia, and muscle allows for excellent versatility based on the type and quantity of tissue required. ALT flap is generally supplied by the descending branch of the lateral circumflex femoral artery (LCFA) system. However, anatomic variations of the pedicle are seen with the absence of a lateral branch and a replacement with a medial or oblique branch. ALT have utility in a variety of head and neck reconstructions including oral cavity, laryngopharyngeal, skull base, and parotid defects. (See Fig. 25.2.)

Bone Flap

Fibula osteoseptocutaneous flap is ideal when vascularized bone is required, as in cases of mandibular reconstruction. (See Fig. 25.3.) It is a single flap with a bone and soft tissue component. The flap pedicle is supplied by the peroneal artery. The fibula functions well for contouring and can undergo multiple osteotomies. Another advantage is its large size and ability to support dental implantation. Double-barreling of the fibula can help restore mandibular height, especially in the anterior segment. If additional soft tissue is required, a double free flap technique combing the fibula osteoseptocutaneous with the ALT flap is useful. Most common morbidity is great toe flexion contracture or weakness, and less likely lower extremity compartment syndrome or ischemia can develop.

Table 25.1 Description of most commonly used free tissue flaps in the head and neck

Flap type	Characteristics[a]	Pedicle size	Common applications
Anterolateral thigh flap	Length: 5–30 cm Width: 4–22 cm Height: 0.2–1 cm	Length: 7–15 cm Diameter: 1.8–2.4 mm	Intraoral, pharyngeal, and hypopharyngeal reconstruction
Radial forearm flap	Length: 5–30 cm Width: 5–14 cm Height: 0.8–1.2 cm	Length: 15–20 cm Diameter: 2.0–3.0 mm	Intraoral, pharyngeal, and hypopharyngeal reconstruction
Fibula osteocutaneous flap	Length: 12–28 cm Width: 4–12 cm Height: 1–3 cm	Length: 5–12 cm Diameter: 1.2–2.2 mm	Mandibular reconstruction
Visceral (jejuna) flap	Length: 5–30 cm Lumen: 2.5–4.5 cm	Length: 4–7 cm Diameter: 1.0–2.5 mm	Pharyngoesophageal reconstruction

[a]Size of individual components (bone, muscle, skin) may vary depending on reconstructive requirement

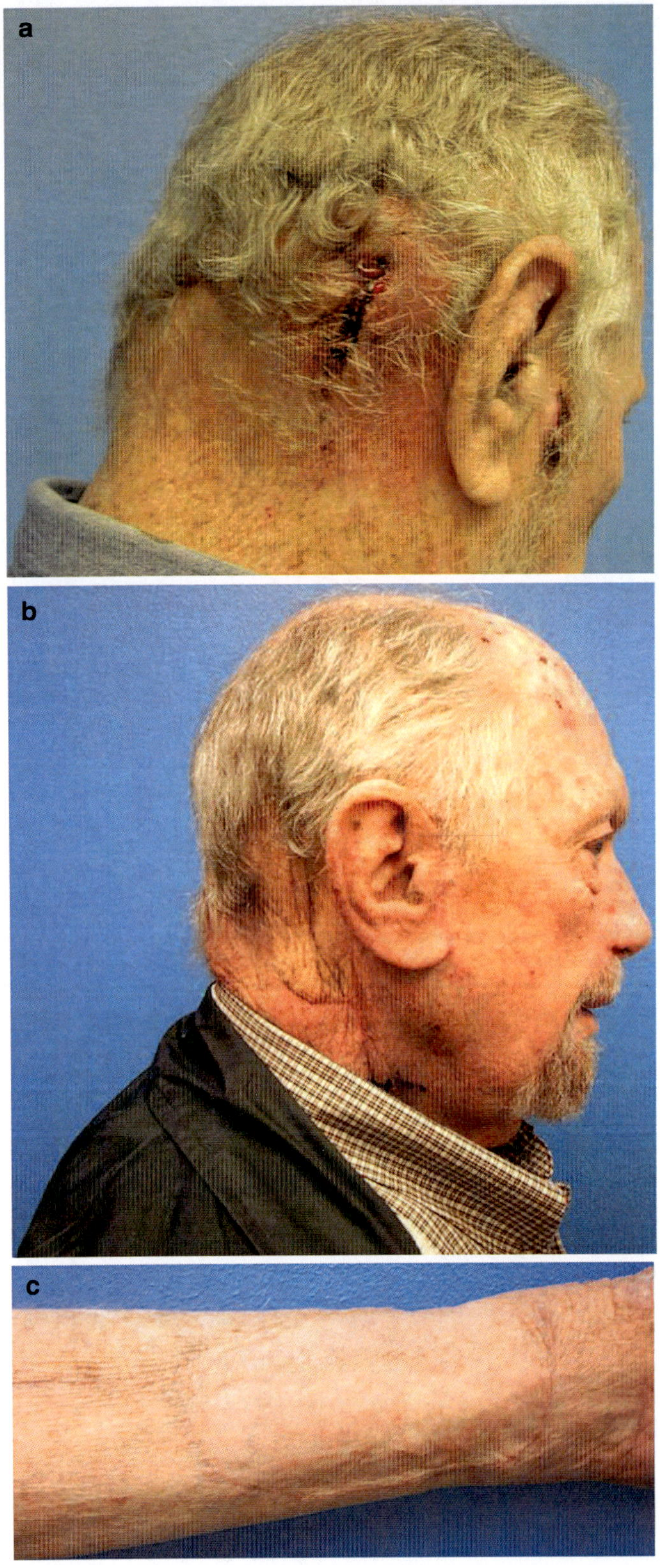

Fig. 25.1 A 58-year-old male with biopsy-proven squamous cell carcinoma of the right posterior scalp (**a**). Defect reconstructed using a radial forearm fasciocutaneous free flap with results for defect (**b**) and donor site (**c**) at 4 months post-op (Courtesy of Dr. Christopher J. Salgado)

Visceral (Jejunal) Flap

Jejunum free flaps can be used with complex pharyngo-esophageal defects. This flap allows for the reconstruction of partial or circumferential defects of the cervical esophagus. It is technically demanding and susceptible to ischemic injury. The jejunum free flap provides good results with return of the swallowing function; however, significant complications are not uncommon. Ikeguchi et al. reviewed various institutions' operative experience and found the rate of anastomotic leakage ranged from 0 to 35 %, necrosis/loss of jejunal graft 0–10 %, and mortality 0–17 %.

Postoperative Care

Basic surgical principles should be followed in postoperative care, including pain and blood pressure control. It is also important to avoid compression of the flap by any medical tubing such as tracheostomy or oxygen tubes. The flap should be exposed and examined frequently. Hourly monitoring is performed immediately postoperatively; however, the duration of hourly monitoring depends on surgeon and institutional policy. Clinical examination is paramount; however, additional monitoring techniques such as Doppler can be employed. Complications and surgical re-exploration are seen in 5–25 % of cases, with a majority of cases ending with successful flap salvage. Venous thrombosis is the most common complication identified at re-exploration. Nonthrombotic vascular events are also common with causes including inappropriate flap inlay, external pedicle compression, and vasospasm. Adequate flap monitoring should include assessment of both tissue and vascular supply integrity. Flap tissue is assessed by its color (pink, not pale or cyanotic), temperature (warm, not cool), and by the tissue turgor (not flat or tense). Vascular anastomosis is evaluated by Doppler monitoring (pulsatile signals present) and capillary refill (normal ≤ 2 s). Lastly, infection should be treated with antibiotics and debridement of devitalized tissue as indicated.

Special Considerations

Large tissue defects in the head and neck may require the use of multiple techniques for adequate coverage. One important technique, although technically demanding, is the use of *double free flaps*. Use of the fibula osteoseptocutaneous flap in conjunction with ALT flap can be used for reconstruction of extensive oromandibular defects with concomitant extensive soft tissue/skin requirements. The ALT flap's primary

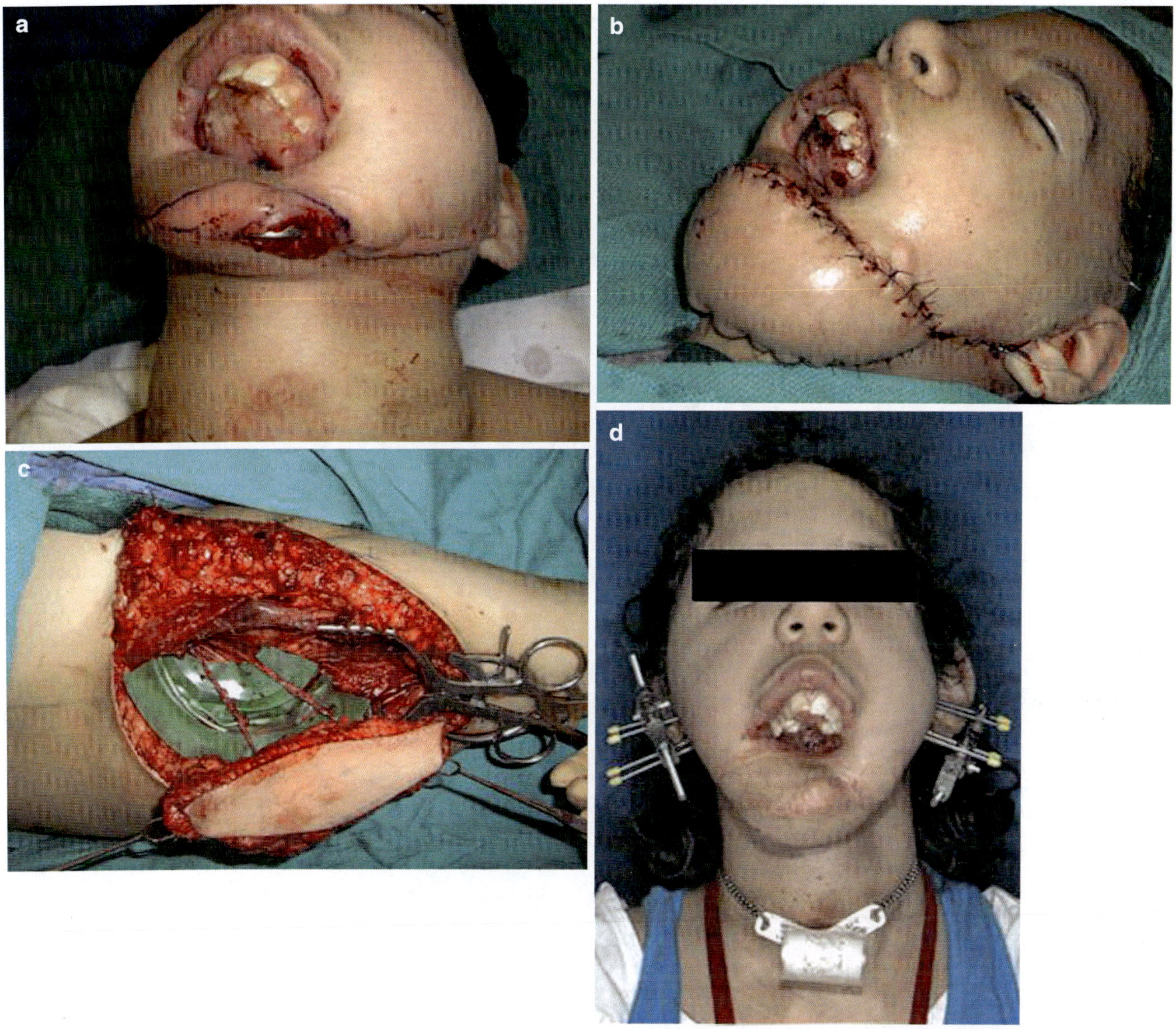

Fig. 25.2 A 10-year-old child with congenital absence of the mandible, both hands, and the right lower extremity below the knee presented after multiple failed mandibular reconstructive procedures. She underwent reconstruction of the mandible using a free fibula osteoseptocutaneous flap. It was found that the skin paddle of the fibula was insufficient to provide stable coverage of the lower facial skin, and the patient suffered from chronic skin breakdown with exposure of the reconstruction plate (**a**). A free anterolateral thigh flap was used to resurface the unstable area. The flap was 18 × 10 cm in size and raised on two musculocutaneous perforators from the thigh affected by the congenital failure of formation (**b**, **c**). The donor site was closed directly and the postoperative course was uneventful. Two years after the soft tissue reconstruction, the patient underwent distraction osteogenesis of the previous fibula bone flap. The ALT flap provided stable coverage of the reconstructed mandible throughout the distraction process (**d**) (Courtesy of Dr. Christopher J. Salgado)

advantage as a secondary flap is the obliteration of dead space, especially in patients expected to complete adjuvant radiotherapy, with minimal donor-site morbidity. Other commonly used flap combinations include the following: the fibula osteoseptocutaneous and radial forearm fasciocutaneous flap or fibula osteoseptocutaneous and rectus abdominis myocutaneous flap.

Depending on the type of reconstruction and the extent of the facial defect, most patients require some form of preoperative radiography. Adequate assessment of recipient vessels correlates with increased reconstructive success. Plain films of the face are historically important to evaluate for fractures and for those reasons more commonly used in

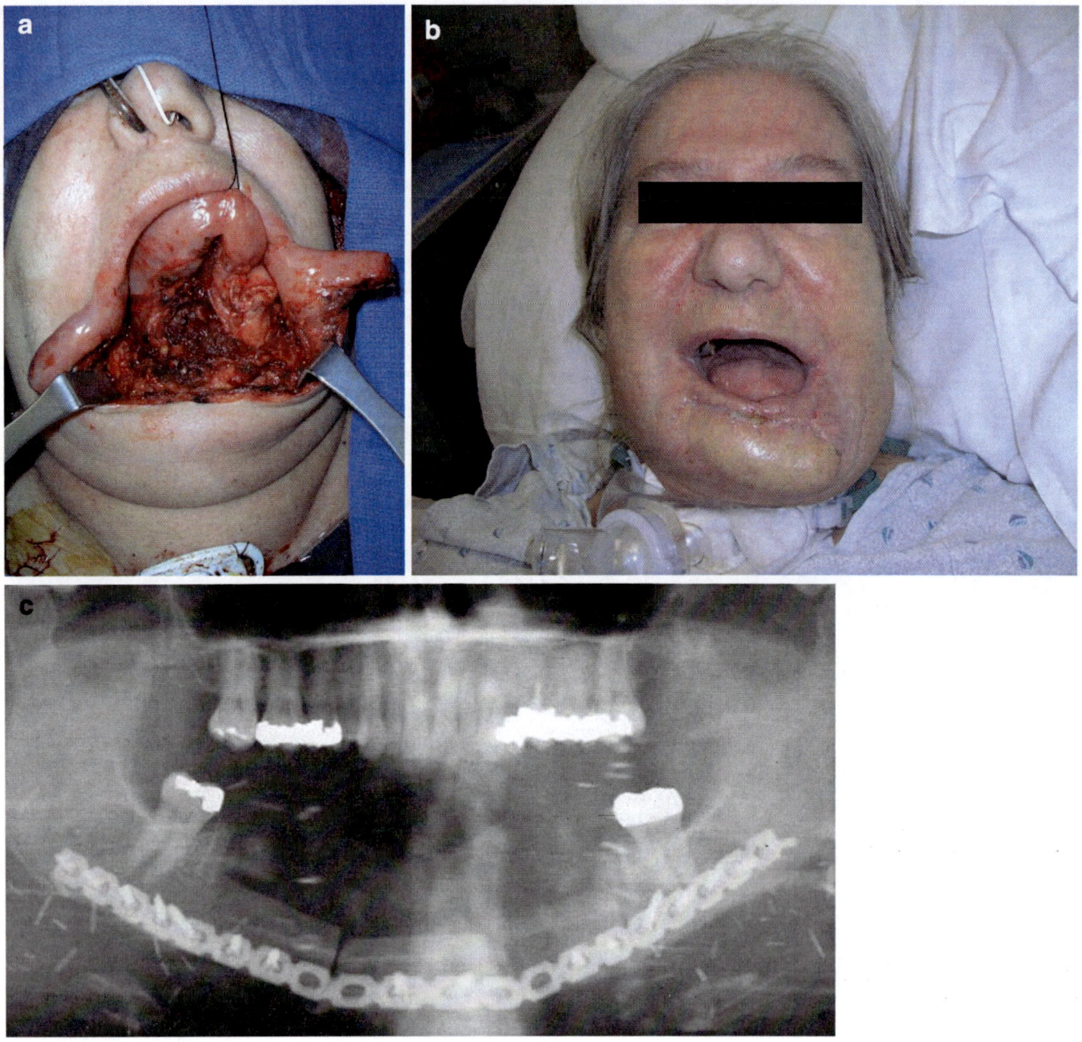

Fig. 25.3 Reconstruction of mandibular and soft tissue defect after resection of a mandibular ameloblastoma (**a**). Plain film demonstrates the bony segment of the fibula osteoseptocutaneous flap used for reconstruction (**b**). Follow-up at 3 months post-op with revision of lower lip (**c**) (Courtesy of Dr. Christopher J. Salgado)

trauma victims. CT angiography allows for visualization and *selection of target vessels* and 3-D reconstruction of adjacent anatomical structures. Other preoperative imaging options include the following: magnetic resonance angiography (MRA), high-resolution ultrasonography, and less commonly used conventional angiography.

Bibliography

Ariyan S. The pectoralis major myocutaneous flap. A versatile flap for reconstruction in the head and neck. Plast Reconstr Surg. 1979;63:73–81.

Cannady SB, Seth R, Fritz MA, Alam DS, Wax MK. Total parotidectomy defect reconstruction using the buried free flap. Otolaryngol Head Neck Surg. 2010;143:637–43.

Chang SC-N, Miller G, Halbert CF, Yang KH, Chao WC, Wei F-C. Limiting donor site morbidity by suprafascial dissection of the radial forearm flap. Microsurgery. 1996;17:136–40.

Chen KT, Mardini S, Chuang DC, Lin CH, Cheng MH, Lin YT, et al. Timing of presentation of the first signs of vascular compromise dictates the salvage outcome of free flap transfers. Plast Reconstr Surg. 2007;120:187–95.

Gurtner GC, Evans GR. Advances in head and neck reconstruction. Plast Reconstr Surg. 2000;106(3):672–82; quiz 83.

Hanasono MM, Sacks JM, Goel N, Ayad M, Skoracki RJ. The anterolateral thigh free flap for skull base reconstruction. Otolaryngol Head Neck Surg. 2009;140:855–60.

Handschel J, Schultz S, Depprich RA, Smeets R, Sproll C, Ommerborn MA, et al. Tissue expanders for soft tissue reconstruction in the head and neck area-requirements and limitations. Clin Oral Investig. 2013;17(2):573–8.

Horiuchi K, Hattori A, Inada I, et al. Mandibular reconstruction using the double barrel fibular graft. Microsurgery. 1995;16:450–4.

Hurvitz KA, Kobayashi M, Evans GR. Current options in head and neck reconstruction. Plast Reconstr Surg. 2006;118:122e–33e.

Ikeguchi M, Miyake T, Matsunaga T, Yamamoto M, Fukumoto Y, Yamada Y, Fukuda K, Saito H, Tatebe S, Tsujitani S. Free jejunal graft reconstruction after resection of neck cancers: our surgical technique. Surg Today. 2009;39:925–8.

Karonidis A, Yao SF. Chimeric anterolateral thigh free flap for head and neck reconstruction. J Plast Reconstr Aesthet Surg. 2009;62:e85–6.

Kim EK, Evangelista M, Evans GR. Use of free tissue transfers in head and neck reconstruction. J Craniofac Surg. 2008;19:1577–82.

Kuo YR, Seng-Feng J, Kuo FM, Liu YT, Lai PW. Versatility of the free anterolateral thigh flap for reconstruction of soft-tissue defects: review of 140 cases. Ann Plast Surg. 2002;48:161–6.

Liu WW, Li H, Guo ZM, Zhang Q, Yang AK, Liu XK, Song M. Reconstruction of soft-tissue defects of the head and neck: radial forearm flap or anterolateral thigh flap? Eur Arch Otorhinolaryngol. 2011;268:1809–12.

Lorenz RR, Alam DS. The increasing use of enteral flaps in reconstruction for the upper aerodigestive tract. Curr Opin Otolaryngol Head Neck Surg. 2003;11:230–5.

Lutz BS, Wei FC. Microsurgical workhorse flaps in head and neck reconstruction. Clin Plast Surg. 2005;32:421–30.

Marques Faria JC, Rodrigues ML, Scopel GP, Kowalski LP, Ferreira MC. The versatility of the free lateral arm flap in head and neck soft tissue reconstruction: clinical experience of 210 cases. J Plast Reconstr Aesthet Surg. 2008;61:172–9.

McGregor IA. The temporal flap in intra-oral cancer: its use in repairing the post excisional defect. Br J Plast Surg. 1963;16:318–35.

Neumann CG. The expansion of an area of skin by progressive distention of a subcutaneous balloon; use of the method for securing skin for subtotal reconstruction of the ear. Plast Reconstr Surg. 1957;19:124–30.

Park CW, Miles BA. The expanding role of the anterolateral thigh free flap in head and neck reconstruction. Curr Opin Otolaryngol Head Neck Surg. 2011;19:263–8.

Pohlenz P, Klatt J, Schon G, Blessmann M, Li L, Schmelzle R. Microvascular free flaps in head and neck surgery: complications and outcome of 1000 flaps. Int J Oral Maxillofac Surg. 2012; 41:739–43.

Saleem M, Hashim F, Babu MM. Compartment syndrome in a free fibula osteocutaneous flap donor site. Br J Plast Surg. 1998;51: 405–7.

Schrag C, Chang YM, Tsai CY, Wei FC. Complete rehabilitation of the mandible following segmental resection. J Surg Oncol. 2006;94: 538–45.

Schusterman MA, Miller MJ, Reece GP, Kroll SS, Marchi M, Goepfert H. A single center's experience with 308 free flaps for repair of head and neck cancer defects. Plast Reconstr Surg. 1994;93: 472–80.

Swanson E, Boyd JB, Manktelow RT. The radial forearm flap: reconstructive applications and donor site defects in 35 consecutive cases. Plast Reconstr Surg. 1990;85:258–66.

Tan O, Kantarci M, Parmaksizoglu D, Uyanik U, Durur I. Determination of the recipient vessels in the head and neck using multislice spiral computed tomography angiography before free flap surgery: a preliminary study. J Craniofac Surg. 2007;18:1284–9.

Timmons MJ, Missotten FEM, Poole MD, Davies DM. Complications of the radial forearm flap donor sites. Br J Plast Surg. 1986;39: 176–8.

Webster HR, Robinson DW. The radial forearm flap without fascia and other refinements. Eur J Plast Surg. 1995;18:11–6.

Wehage IC, Fansa H. Complex reconstructions in head and neck cancer surgery: decision making. Head Neck Oncol. 2011;3:14.

Wei FC, Santamaria E, Chang YM, Chen HC. Mandibular reconstruction with fibular osteoseptocutaneous free flap and simultaneous placement of osseointegrated dental implants. J Craniofac Surg. 1997;8:512–21.

Wei FC, Yazar S, Lin CH, Cheng MH, Tsao CK, Chiang YC. Double free flaps in head and neck reconstruction. Clin Plast Surg. 2005;32:303–8.

Wong CH, Wei FC. Anterolateral thigh flap. Head Neck. 2010a;32: 529–40.

Wong CH, Wei FC. Microsurgical free flap in head and neck reconstruction. Head Neck. 2010b;32:1236–45.

Wong CH, Wei FC, Fu B, Chen YA, Lin JY. Alternative vascular pedicle of the anterolateral thigh flap: the oblique branch of the lateral circumflex femoral artery. Plast Reconstr Surg. 2009;123:571–7.

Yazar S. Selection of recipient vessels in microsurgical free tissue reconstruction of head and neck defects. Microsurgery. 2007;27: 588–94.

Yu P, Hanasono MM, Skoracki RJ, Baumann DP, Lewin JS, Weber RS, et al. Pharyngoesophageal reconstruction with the anterolateral thigh flap after total laryngopharyngectomy. Cancer. 2010;116: 1718–24.

Part III

Orthognathic Surgery

26 Facial Evaluation in Orthognathic Surgery

Donald R. Mackay and Cathy R. Henry

Patients with dentofacial deformities are best cared for by a multidisciplinary team, a comprehensive care setting with orthodontics, dentistry, speech therapy, social services, and internal medicine or pediatrics working along with the plastic surgeon. Orthognathic surgery does not eliminate the need for orthodontic intervention, but instead works in concert with the orthodontics to create the optimal outcome. The goal is an optimal dental relationship and facial aesthetic. Design of the surgical plan often starts with an accurate evaluation of the facial aesthetic relationships.

Preoperative Evaluation

History

All patient interactions begin with a complete history and physical examination. The patient's chief complaint will be a concern over his/her appearance and/or occlusion, as well as the patient's perception of the problem. If the surgeon has the benefit of being part of the multidisciplinary team taking care of the patient from the time of diagnosis, this understanding of the patient perception and expectation is a bit easier to ascertain.

Important details of the past medical history include conditions which would impact surgical management and the recovery process. In congenital dentofacial anomalies, the patient is evaluated for possible syndromes which can have associated abnormalities affecting the renal, cardiovascular, and/or other organ systems, all of which may have implications for their care. Diagnosis of potential genetic syndromes can be aided by the remainder of the physical exam looking for characteristic features as well as probing into family history looking for similarly affected children. Patients with cardiac conditions at risk for infective endocarditis should receive antibiotic prophylaxis according to the American Heart Association guidelines. For patients with immune system compromise such as diabetes, recent chemotherapy, or congenital/acquired immunodeficiency should be counseled regarding an increased risk of operative complication. Patients with diabetes will require strict perioperative glucose control. Those with severe immune deficiency are poor operative candidates. Orthognathic surgery is often completed under relative hypotensive anesthesia to minimize bleeding. Patients with preexisting renal conditions will not tolerate a low blood pressure during surgery. Another important consideration is the presence of conditions that would predispose to excessive bleeding perioperatively. This includes hemophilia or von Willebrand disease. Patients are counseled to cease any aspirin- or NSAID-containing products at least 1 week prior to surgery.

Dental History

A dental history is equally as important. A history of prior tooth extraction, periodontal disease, chronic poor oral hygiene, multiple dental caries, and previous orthodontic work will all impact the outcome of orthodontic and surgical treatment. Any orthognathic patient must have good oral hygiene and healthy habits before any orthodontic preparation can start.

The timing of orthognathic surgery is determined by a plan coordinated with the orthodontist and surgeon. All orthognathic patients by definition will have a skeletal imbalance. They will also have dental compensations as a result of this skeletal imbalance. An example of this is the retroclined mandibular incisors and proclined maxillary incisors one encounters in patients with Class III skeletal deformities. Many of these patients may have had orthodontic treatment

D.R. Mackay, MD, FACS, FAAP (✉)
Department of Surgery, Penn State Hershey, College of Medicine, Hershey, PA, USA
e-mail: dmackay@psu.edu

C.R. Henry, MD
Division of Plastic Surgery, Penn State Hershey Medical Center, Hershey, PA, USA

P.J. Taub et al. (eds.), *Ferraro's Fundamentals of Maxillofacial Surgery*,
DOI 10.1007/978-1-4614-8341-0_26, © Springer Science+Business Media New York 2015

alone in an effort to avoid surgery. This will often produce even more pronounced dental compensations. In order to correct these dentofacial deformities, the dental compensations have to be undone with orthodontia prior to the orthognathic surgery. Patients need to be warned that they will look worse as these compensations are corrected before the surgery.

A history of temporomandibular joint (TMJ) disease should be identified preoperatively. The patient may describe pain in the joint, headaches, and locking or clicking. This can be secondary to the dentofacial abnormality or intrinsic joint disease. TMJ disease can have a significant impact on success or failure of treatment. Additional imaging, specifically MRI of the joint, can detail the anatomy of the joint region and identify dislocation of the meniscus.

Speech evaluation is part of the comprehensive assessment. In cleft lip and palate cases, patients may present with a history of velopharyngeal insufficiency (VPI) treated successfully with palatal lengthening or pharyngoplasties. A maxillary advancement in these patients can result in recurrent VPI. A prior pharyngeal flap will restrict maxillary movements especially any advancement. In any patient, maxillary or mandibular setback can aggravate or create obstructive symptoms leading to sleep apnea.

Preoperative Psychological Assessment

Orthognathic surgery has the ability to lead to a dramatic change in a person's appearance. The patient expectations are key to satisfaction. Changing the relationship of the facial skeleton to cranial base significantly alters the appearance of the face. Although surgery may improve appearance as defined by the conventions of accepted aesthetic norms, the patient may find adjusting to the change very difficult. If any doubt exists as to the patient's ability to adjust, psychological counseling may be necessary.

Clinical Evaluation: Anatomic Assessment of Facial Aesthetics

In evaluating a patient for orthognathic surgery, it is easy to focus on the occlusion and lose sight of the patient's facial aesthetics and facial proportions. A single-minded focus on the occlusion can lead the surgeon and orthodontist to decide on a surgical plan that compromises aesthetics and proportions. A full evaluation of facial aesthetics and proportions is an essential part of every patient's examination and requires a systematic approach. The occlusion is then evaluated within the framework of the interrelationships of the skeletal and soft tissue components. After full analysis, the patient's main concern is identified to ensure that this is considered in the treatment plan. Examination includes assessment of the skin quality including color, thickness, and consistency and for any scars the patient has.

One commonly accepted method of analysis divides the face into upper, middle, and lower thirds. The upper third extends from hairline to eyebrows. The middle third extends from the eyebrows to the subnasale, which is the junction of the nose and the lip. The lower third extends from the subnasale to the menton, which is the lowest point of the chin. Each third is then analyzed from a frontal and profile view and compared to accepted aesthetic norms.

Upper Third

From the anterior view, the length of the forehead is determined. The forehead height varies from 6 to 10 cm. In general, the three zones of the face should be similar in height to give a sense of equal proportions. A high forehead, whether it is congenital or the result of hair loss, can give an aged appearance to the face, particularly if the hairline is posterior to the point of the forehead where the slope decreases and the scalp begins to flatten. It is also important to assess skin quality and the presence of transverse rhytids related to the frontalis muscles and glabellar vertical rhytids secondary to the procerus and corrugator muscles.

The eyebrows are examined for symmetry, hair direction, and position in relation to the superior orbital rim and the medial and lateral canthi of the eye. The medial eyebrow should be at or below the level of the orbital rim. The medial border of the eyebrow should be above the medial canthus. The eyebrow should rise gently, with a gentle peak at least two-thirds of the way to its lateral end and with this peak usually above the lateral limbus. The lateral tail of the brow should be higher than the medial end. The lateral brow terminates at a point in line with the diagonal line drawn from the alar rim through the lateral canthus of the ipsilateral eye. The male brow should be lower and less peaked. From the profile view, it is possible to assess for forehead prominence and the presence of frontal bossing or posterior sloping, all of which can disturb the facial harmony.

Middle Third

From the frontal view, the eyes are examined for symmetry of size and position. The palpebral fissure follows a pattern similar to the eyebrow, meaning the lateral canthus is slightly cephalad to the medial canthus. There is some ethnic variation in the degree of tilt. Certain syndromes can have significant impact on eye position with displacement of the lateral canthus. Treacher Collins syndrome leads to caudal displacement of the lateral canthus and adds to the visual stigmata of

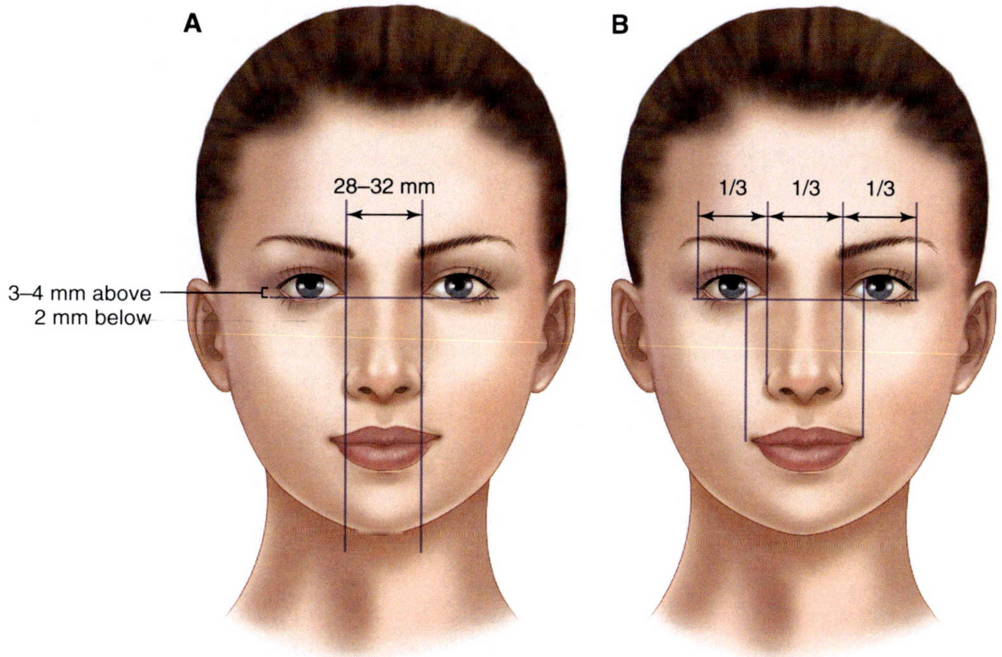

Fig. 26.1 Frontal view of the face demonstrating intercanthal distance and vertical location of the lateral canthi and the relationship of the canthi to the oral commissures

the deformity. The intercanthal distance is measured, and in the adult this normally 28–32 mm and is equal to the palpebral fissure distance from the medial to lateral canthus (See Fig. 26.1). Reduction of the intercanthal distance is usually due to hypotelorism. Increased intercanthal distance may be a result of telecanthus or hypertelorbitism. The distinguishing factor between the two differentials is the interpupillary distance. If the inter pupillary distance is normal, telecanthus due to disruption of the medial canthal ligament is the cause of the increased intercanthal distance. If the interpupillary distance is also increased, then hypertelorbitism is the cause, with the interorbital distance also increased.

The eyelids are examined closely for incisions caused by prior blepharoplasty, prominence of supraorbital fat, and position in relation to the globe. To evaluate eyelid position, the examiner must ensure that the eyebrow is in a neutral position. The patient should relax the forehead so any effort by the frontalis muscle does not mask a potential ptosis. In general, the upper eyelid will overlap the pupil by 1–2 mm. Another commonly evaluated parameter is the distance from the upper lid margin to the light reflex over the pupil with the patient gazing straight ahead. A normal value is less than 2 mm. Ptosis is diagnosed when the margin to light reflex interval is less than 2 mm. Levator function should be evaluated, which will include the point of insertion into the lid (seen by the symmetry of the supratarsal crease bilaterally) and the degree of excursion. Excess supratarsal skin, known as dermatochalasis, may obscure the palpebral fold and give the eyes a hooded appearance. The presence of any eyelid clefting and/or absence of eyelashes should also be noted.

On the profile view, the relationship of the superior and lateral orbital rims to the anterior surface of the cornea should be evaluated. The superior ridge normally projects 8–10 mm anterior to corneal surface. The lateral orbital rims are normally 12–16 mm posterior to the corneal surface (see Fig. 26.2). In males, the average nasofrontal angle is 130°, while in females, it is 134°. The characteristics of a masculine face include a greater incline to the forehead with a more prominent supraorbital ridge and glabellar region. The frontal sinuses do not form until around age 7 when pneumatization begins. Hyperpneumatization can lead to glabellar prominence in either sex with accentuation of the nasofrontal junction.

The nose is also prominent in the middle division. It may be divided into nine anatomic subunits (dorsum, lateral sidewalls, tip, alae, columella, soft triangles) and evaluated for symmetry and proportion. From the anterior view, overall symmetry is assessed by dividing the face in half with an imaginary line that bisects the glabella, nasal tip, upper lip, and chin. Further assessment of proportion occurs with division of the face into fifths (see Fig. 26.3). In general, the alar bases are in line with medial canthus of each eye and each fifth is approximately the width of the intercanthal distance.

The nasal profile is evaluated for nasal projection, the nasofrontal angle, the presence of a dorsal hump, the degree of projection of the nasal bridge, the amount of tip projection and rotation, and the nasolabial angle. The nasofrontal angle ranges from 115° to 130°, with the location of this junction at the approximate level of the superior eyelid sulcus. The amount of tip rotation determines the nasolabial angle. In males, the nasolabial angle is generally 90–95°. In females, it is closer to 95–105°. The position of the nasal spine is impacted by the

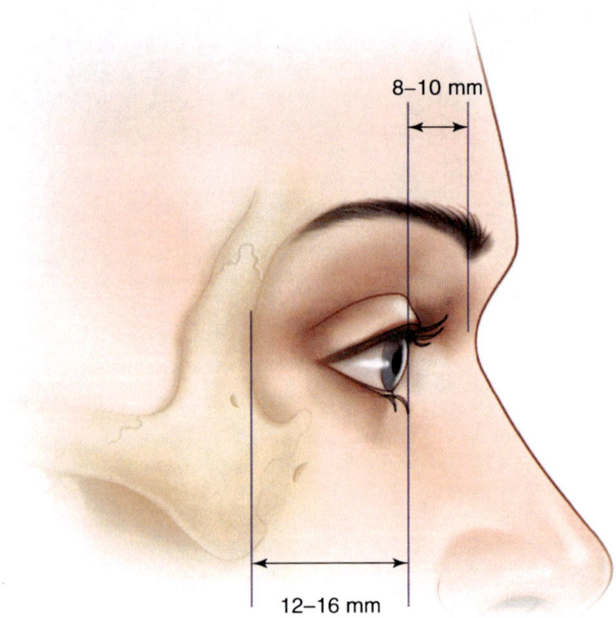

Fig. 26.2 Evaluation of facial symmetry. (**a**) Right to left symmetry is checked by holding an object so it bisects the glabella, nasal tip, upper lip, and chin. (**b**) The face may also be divided approximately into fifths

presence of maxillary excess and deficiency, which are far more common than an actual deformity of the nasal spine itself.

Lastly, in the middle third is the ear. The ears are checked for symmetry of formation, prominence, visibility, location, and direction. In general, the antihelix is slightly visible from the anterior view with helix running almost parallel to the rest of the head. The helix projects 10–15 mm from the mastoid bone. The length of the ear should equal approximately the length of the nose. The inferior border of the ear lobule lies at the horizontal level of the subnasale. The long axis of the ear should form an approximately 30° angle with the axis of the body (see Fig. 26.4).

Lower Third

The upper lip is normally about half the length of the nose and about one-third of the total length of the lower division of the face. When the upper lip is either too short or too long, this can be a reflection of a skeletal abnormality such as vertical maxillary deficiency or excess. Although there can be ethnic variations, the upper lip should have a defined Cupid's bow with distinct philtral dimple. The oral commissure should extend to equal distance on either side of the midline and extend laterally in a direction parallel to an imaginary

Fig. 26.3 Lateral view of the face demonstrating vertical and sagittal relationships

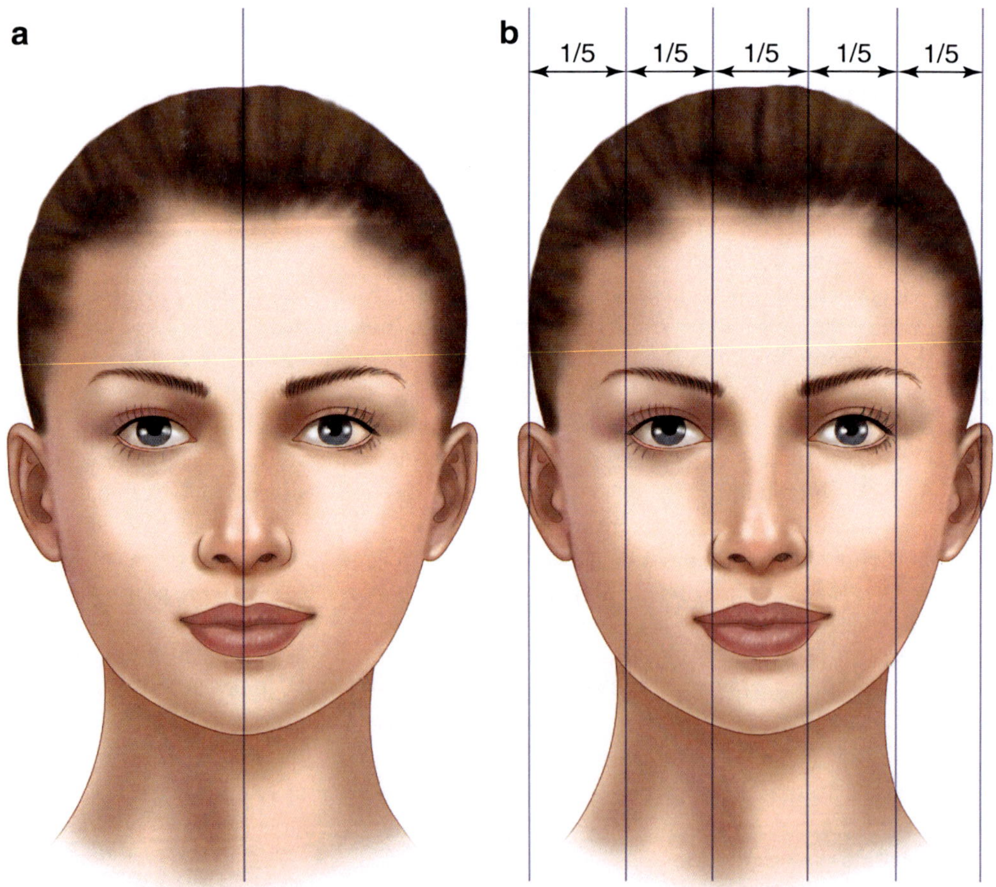

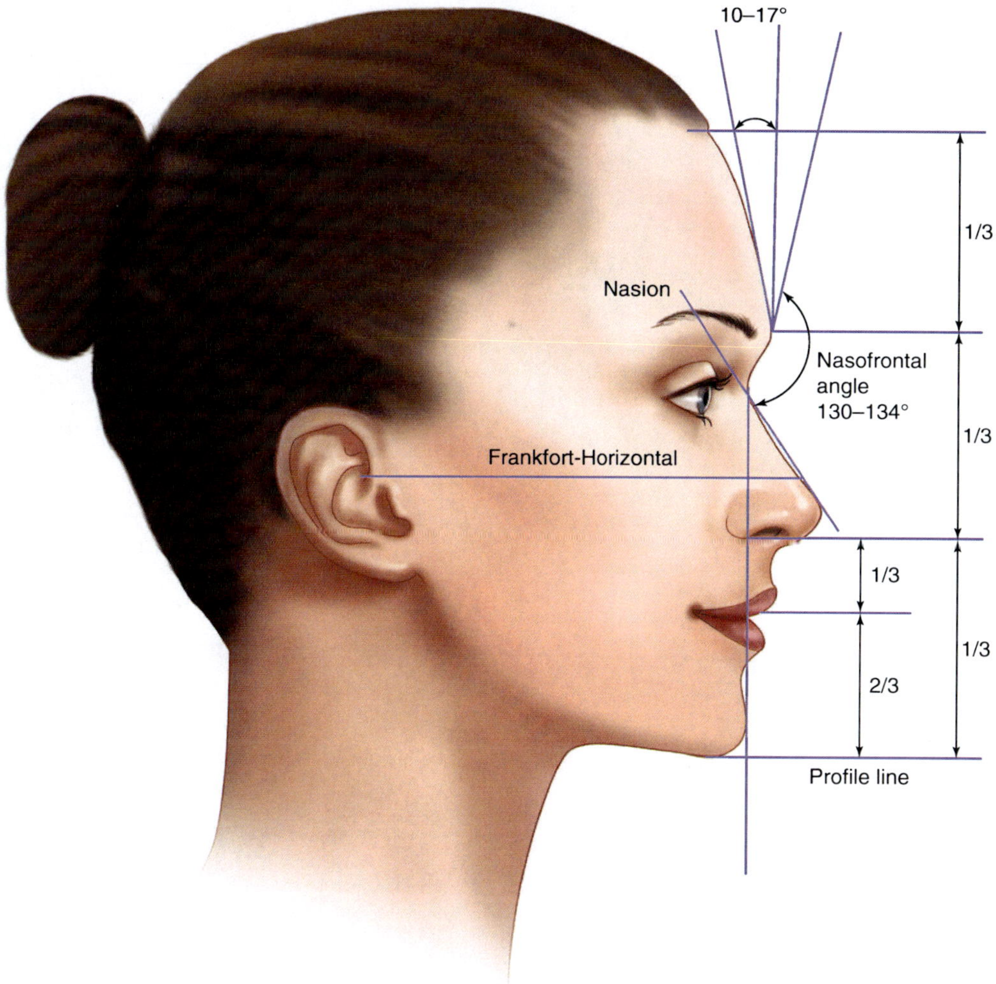

Fig. 26.4 Close-up of profile view demonstrating the relationship of the anterior cornea to the supraorbital ridge and lateral orbital rim

line that connects the lateral canthi. If the facial musculature is functioning properly, an abnormal tilt to the oral commissure signals a skeletal abnormality. The width of the oral opening should equal the distance from one medial limbus of the iris to the other. Significant decrease in the width is termed microstomia and increased width is termed macrostomia. These variations can be found with trauma, after cancer resection and reconstruction or on a genital basis, possibly as part of a larger syndrome.

The chin is analyzed for symmetry of position and shape. An imaginary midline should bisect the chin, but the mandibular angle position should also be symmetric. The submental area is examined for the presence of excess fat, skin, or ptosis of the submandibular glands. From the profile view, the overall projection of the lower third of the face in comparison to the remaining upper and middle thirds is analyzed. Lip competence is easier to appreciate on profile, as the presence of any lip strain required to achieve full closure of the lips is more readily identified on this view.

Facial Width, the Malar Complex, and the Gonial Angle

Horizontal measurements of the face have the greatest variation among different populations. As such, there are standard, accepted facial proportions for facial width, but these should in no way form the only basis for analysis of this dimension. Midface width from zygoma to zygoma is divided into fourths, with each quarter approximately equal to the width of the alar base. The bimalar distance, measured from one malar eminence to the other, is approximately equal to the bitemporal ridge and bigonial distance. The bizygomatic arch distance is the widest part of the face and is located just lateral to the zygomaticotemporal suture. The malar-midface inclination is identified by extending a line from the zygomaticotemporal suture to the nasolabial fold and measuring the angle the line makes with the Frankfort horizontal, and the normal value is about 45°. In the ideal face the gonial angle is 105–115°. From a profile view, the nasofrontal angle, lower lip, and chin point should form a vertical line.

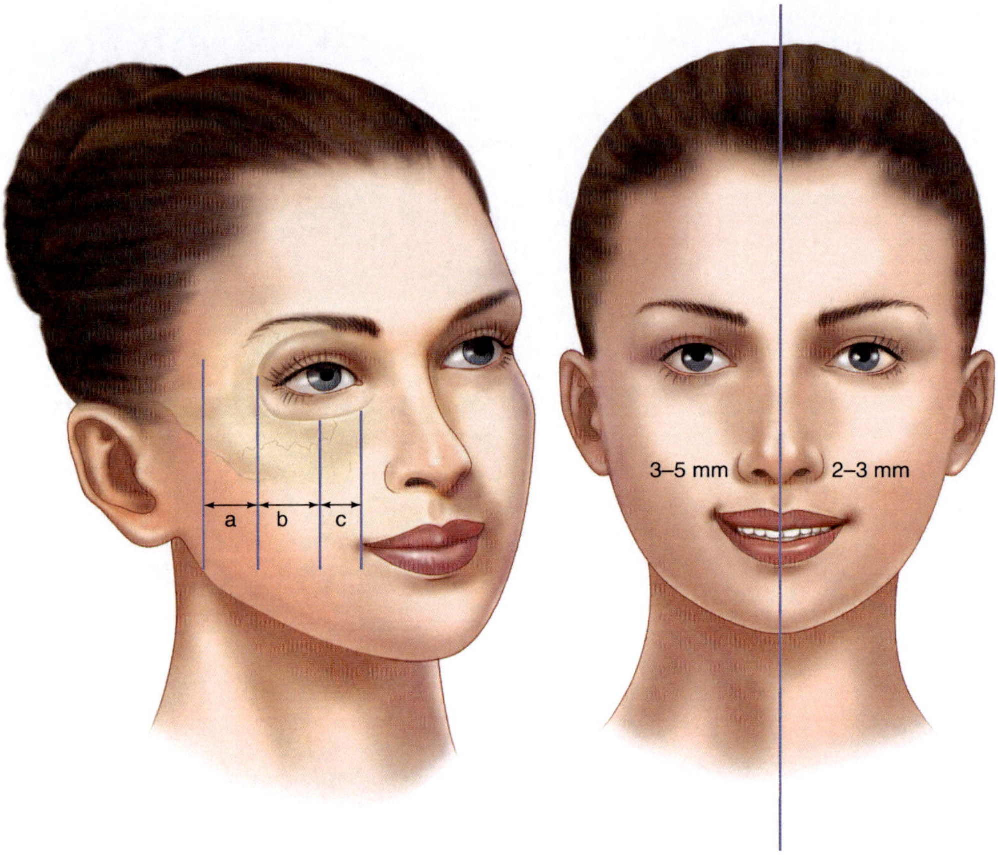

Fig. 26.5 Ideal normal tooth show is approximately 2–3 mm at rest. Up to 4–6 mm of show may be attractive in some patients if mentalis strain to achieve lip competence is not present

Areas of Contrast

Soft tissue overlying the bony prominences reflects light in variable patterns to create areas of the face that are highlighted and lowlighted. Preserving this contrast during surgical planning aids in maintaining a natural appearance and aesthetically pleasing outcome. Highlight areas include the temporal ridge, supraorbital ridge, malar eminences, and the mandible angle to the chin. The lowlight areas are those in between the abovementioned regions. During the execution of the surgical plan, the highlight areas are further accentuated, and the lowlight areas can be de-emphasized with relatively simple maneuvers such as a buccal lipectomy to add perceived projection to the malar eminence.

Intraoral Examination

Intraoral examination should not be omitted. It begins with assessing the relationship of the upper lip to the central incisors with lips slightly parted and relaxed. This is also referred to as assessing the amount of tooth show with the lips in repose. In the classically aesthetically pleasing face, with normal maxillary growth and occlusion, 2–3 mm of the upper central incisors are visible with the lips in repose. In some women, 4–6 mm of tooth show is acceptable as long as mentalis strain is not required to achieve full lip closure, also known as lip competence (see Fig. 26.5). Tooth show is also assessed with the patient smiling. With this action, the full length of the upper central incisors is visible, with minimal or no showing of the gum. A gummy smile indicates vertical maxillary excess or deficiency of upper lip soft tissue. Deficient show of the central upper incisors during full smile signals vertical maxillary deficiency. The form and size of the upper lip must be kept in mind during treatment planning. The appearance of a patient with a thin vermillion at baseline may worsen with maxillary repositioning.

Alignment of the teeth is assessed. The midline of the upper and lower central incisors should lie along a vertical line connecting the midline face, upper lip, and chin. Crowding of the teeth can result from inadequate arch space or abnormal dental inclinations. Dental hygiene is paramount to achieving good outcomes in orthodontic and orthognathic treatment. Active periodontal disease is a contraindication to orthodontic treatment. As orthodontic care is a major part of the planning and execution of orthognathic surgery, the dental hygiene issues must be addressed prior to undertaking the major surgery. Areas of inadequate gingival attachment may need the attention of a periodontist prior to performing orthognathic surgery. Occlusion is examined in great detail and can often be the leading factor in a patient pursuing orthognathic surgery. The dental arch relationship is the standard of evaluating orthodontic outcomes. A patient may have a functional slide of the mandible from centric relation to centric occlusion. Horizontal incisor overjet and vertical overbite are noted. Occlusion is evaluated at the molar and canine levels (angle classification figure). The presence of either an anterior or posterior open bites or crossbites should be noted. Tongue size can affect the formation of the palatal arch. The presence of an occlusal cant is identified by having the patient place a tongue blade horizontally between the teeth. The blade should form a line parallel to an imaginary line through the lateral canthi or pupils. A canted occlusion signals differential growth of the two sides.

Masticatory Function

Temporomandibular joint (TMJ) disorders often coexist with dentofacial anomalies. It is important to elicit symptoms from the patient by inquiring about clenching or grinding of teeth, headaches, jaw muscle pain, and locking or popping or limited opening of the jaw. The examination must include palpation the TMJ and muscles of mastication while at rest and with jaw excursion. Note clicking, crepitus, locking of the joint with range of motion. Inter-incisal opening, lateral excursion, and ability to protrude the mandible are all indicators of TMJ mobility. Any deviation from midline that occurs when opening or closing the jaw will key the examiner to TMJ dysfunction in the opposite joint. The normal inter-incisal opening distance, including about 2 mm of overbite, is 40–56 mm. The normal maximal lateral movement with jaw open about 1 cm is 9–13 mm.

Radiologic Examination

Radiographs are used to supplement the physical examination. Standard radiographs for patients considering orthognathic surgery include lateral and posterior/anterior cephalograms and an orthopantomogram. Cephalograms are used to create prediction tracings of the bony movement and resultant impact on the overlying soft tissue when performing orthognathic surgery. The orthopantomogram provides general information on the state of the TMJ, the number or erupted and unerupted teeth, and the position of the third molars. If a potential problem is noted on the orthopantomogram, more detailed films including periapical views for teeth or CT scans of the TMJ can be ordered. When planning a maxillary osteotomy, it is necessary to identify the position of the tooth roots in the proximity of the osteotomy to avoid damage. Also, the presence or absence of the third molar teeth, which lie along the osteotomy lines for a LeFort I osteotomy of the maxilla and a sagittal split osteotomy of the mandible, should be noted and extracted if still present. Further advances in technology show an increasing reliance on advanced imaging and surgical planning techniques such as cone-beam CT scanning and 3D imaging.

Bibliography

Aston SJ, Martin J. Section 9: Rhinoplasty, Chapter 37: Primary closed rhinoplasty. In: Aston S, Steinbrech DS, Walden JL, editors. Aesthetic plastic surgery. Philadelphia: Saunders/Elsevier; 2009.

Cottrell DA, Edwards SP, Gotcher JE. Surgical correction of maxillofacial skeletal deformities. J Oral Maxillofac Surg. 2012;70(11 Suppl 3):e107–36.

Farkas L. Anthropometry of the head and face. 2nd ed. New York: Raven Press; 1994.

Guyuron B, Behmand RA, Green R. Shortening of the long forehead. Plast Reconstr Surg. 1999;103(1):218–23.

Powell N, Humphreys B. Proportions of the aesthetic face. New York: Thieme-Strattion, Inc; 1984.

Rees T, LaTrenta GS. Aesthetic plastic surgery. Philadelphia: Saunders; 1994.

Van Steenbergen E, Litt MD, Nanda R. Presurgical satisfaction with facial appearance in orthognathic surgery patients. Am J Orthod Dentofacial Orthop. 1996;109(6):653–9.

Warren R. Section 5: Browlift, Chapter 23: Non-endoscopic limited incision browplasty. In: Aston S, Steinbrech DS, Walden JL, editors. Aesthetic plastic surgery. Philadelphia: Saunders/Elsevier; 2009.

Wilson W, et al. Prevention of infective endocarditis: guidelines from the American Heart Association: a guideline from the American Heart Association Rheumatic Fever, Endocarditis, and Kawasaki Disease Committee, Council on Cardiovascular Disease in the Young, and the Council on Clinical Cardiology, Council on Cardiovascular Surgery and Anesthesia, and the Quality of Care and Outcomes Research Interdisciplinary Working Group. Circulation. 2007;116(15):1736–54.

Zide BM. The temporomandibular joint. In: McCarthy JG, editor. Plastic surgery. 3rd ed. Philadelphia: W.B. Saunders; 1990.

Surgical Planning: 2D to 3D

27

Pravin K. Patel, Linping Zhao, and James W. Ferraro

Introduction

Surgeons and orthodontists are faced with the practical problem of objectively assessing a patient's dentofacial skeletal deformity, developing a "blueprint" of maxillofacial surgery to execute, and predicting the possible surgical outcome prior to the operation. Maxillofacial surgical planning is a multilevel process. It involves incorporating the clinical assessment of the soft-tissue envelop, the underlying facial skeletal structures, and the dentition. All three elements must be assessed independently and then as a composite to understand the deformity and the reconstruction required.

The surgeon needs to determine which components of the skeletal structure need to be separated and repositioned and then placing each of the elements in a new spatial position relative to the cranial base and relative to the alteration of the soft-tissue envelop to optimize aesthetic appearance and functional outcome. Cephalometric analysis has been the "tool" for abstracting the complexity of the human craniofacial skeleton into a geometric scheme that would allow comparison to normative data and to the ideal surgical-orthodontic treatment goal. For more than half a century, this involved (1) obtaining 2D profile lateral radiographs using a standardized cephalostat machine, (2) marking the key anatomy landmarks, (3) measuring linear distances and angles, and (4) comparing those measured to a specific population norm.

The orthodontist and surgeon would then determine the ideal skeletal position and incisor relations. The treatment is then based on the mechanics needed to move the dentition using orthodontic appliances and surgery to move the skeletal bases to the desired geometric pattern.

However, this approach reduced the complexity of the 3D craniofacial problem to a 2D planar problem in the sagittal plane, and the assumption was patients had an acceptable degree of facial symmetry. While single profile assessment was sufficient for the vast majority of the patients who presented with the developmental dentofacial deformities, the treatment planning became less reliable with patients with significant component of facial asymmetry. This included patients with condylar hyperplasia, hemifacial microsomia, skull base asymmetries, and congenital cleft and craniofacial conditions. In such cases, surgeons and orthodontists would incorporate frontal cephalometric radiographs with the lateral cephalometric radiographs to add a third dimension in their planning. Nevertheless the use of 2D radiographs in orthogonal planes remained less reliable, and frequently surgical repositioning depended more on the surgeon's assessment in the operating room. Consistent results were difficult to obtain. Today, surgical-orthodontic management has become increasingly reliable with the ability to visualize using 3D radiologic cone beam CT scans and software that allows the surgeon to simulate surgery with 3D movement of the dental-skeletal components.

While clearly the next generation of maxillofacial surgeons will be fully immersed in 3D virtual surgical simulation, this chapter at the transition will begin with the traditional 2D approach that has been well tested for more than half a century. Understanding how to develop a surgical-orthodontic plan in 2D lays the foundation for addressing the complexity of a deformity that exists in all three planes and the value of 3D technology to assist the surgeon.

P.K. Patel, MD, FACS (✉)
Pediatric Plastic and Craniofacial Surgery,
University of Illinois, Division of Plastic, Reconstructive and Cosmetic Surgery, Chicago, IL 60612, USA
e-mail: pkpatelmd@gmail.com

L. Zhao, PhD
Division of Plastic, Reconstructive and Cosmetic Surgery, Department of Surgery, University of Illinois, Chicago, IL 60612, USA

J.W. Ferraro, DDS, MD
Franklin Park Physical Medicine, Department of Surgery, 750 E Broad St., Suite 200, Columbus, OH 43205, USA

P.J. Taub et al. (eds.), *Ferraro's Fundamentals of Maxillofacial Surgery*,
DOI 10.1007/978-1-4614-8341-0_27, © Springer Science+Business Media New York 2015

Conventional 2D Image-Based Surgical Planning for Orthognathic Surgery

Cephalometry and Cephalometric Analysis

Cephalometry, as defined by Dorland's Illustrated Medical Dictionary, is the scientific measurement of the dimensions of the head. Broadbent in 1931 described a "new x-ray technique" that would allow the clinician to consistently obtain a skull radiograph. The cephalostat was designed to consistently position the patient with their head oriented at 90° to the x-ray beam at a distance of 5 ft from the x-ray tube and 11 in. from the film (Fig. 27.1). This became the standard under which all cephalometric radiographs were taken, and it ensured that radiographs taken at different centers and institutes could be directly comparable. Once standardized radiographs (Fig. 27.2) could be reliably obtained, anatomic structures could be outlined (Fig. 27.3), anatomic landmarks could be defined (Fig. 27.4), and various linear and angular distances could be measured (Fig. 27.5). This then converted the complex 2D shape of the facial skeleton into a series of numbers, a cephalometric analysis. It allowed the clinician to follow growth and development of the craniofacial skeleton and the ability to compare a given patient against a population norm, and it gave the clinician the ability to surgically plan and objectively assess the outcome of treatment. As data was gathered on the effect of treatment, it then gave the clinician the ability to do predictive treatment planning.

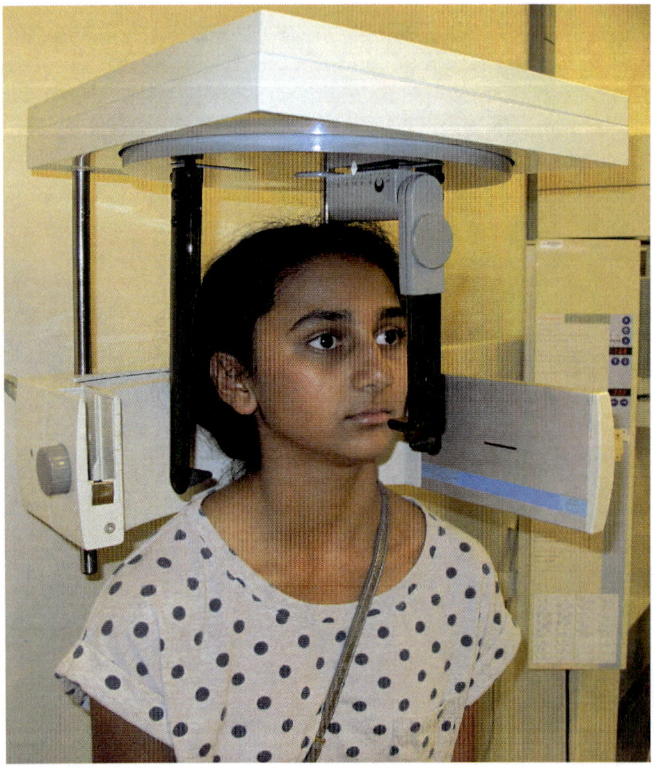

Fig. 27.1 X-Ray unit used for obtaining standardized lateral and frontal cepahlometric radiographs and panoramic radiographs

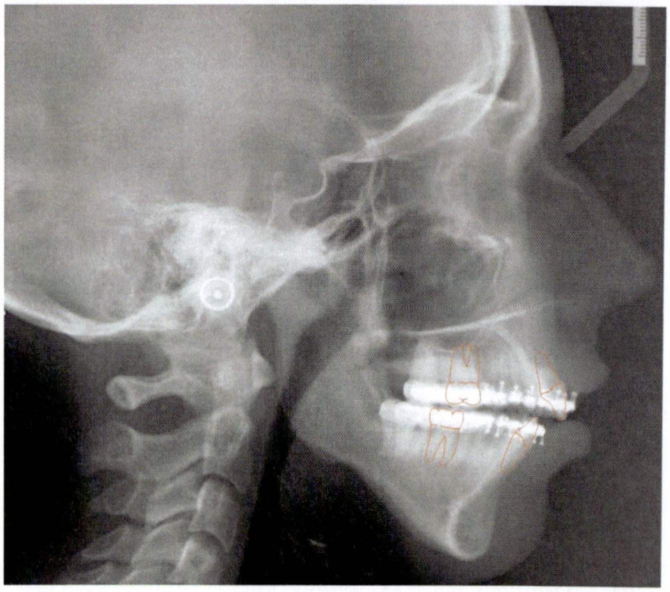

Fig. 27.2 Standardized lateral cephalometric radiograph. Overlapping structures between the left and right may be difficult to distinguish as are the dentition. In this particular radiograph, the central incisor and first molar are marked. There is a soft-tissue filter in the modern units that enhances the profile. Notice also that the posterior airway space can be identified

When properly obtained, the cephalometric x-rays yielded a wealth of information for the clinician. From a single radiograph, an analysis of not only the dentofacial skeleton was obtained but also the overlying soft-tissue profile and the nasopharyngeal airway space was now accessible for quantification by the clinician. Additionally, a phonation cephalometric radiograph could be obtained in which the soft palate can be traced. Therefore, if the patient was asked to phonate, the degree of elevation of the palate could be assessed.

Cephalometric analysis (Fig. 27.6) began with the studies by William Downs in the 1940s followed by Reidel, McNamara, Steiners, Rickets, Tweed, Sasouni, Burstone, and others. Over succeeding decades, a multitude of analysis, each depended on the area of interest of the orthodontist for whom it was named after, came into being. While it is beyond the scope of this chapter to review pros and cons of the various analyses, we will present a composite analysis that will provide the beginning orthognathic surgeon sufficient understanding of the value of analysis and its role in surgical planning. The reader is asked to refer to the 2D cephalometric section at the end of this chapter with the following remarks.

The Skeletal Profile Analysis

The fundamental question for a surgeon is to determine which jaw(s) to operate on since the surgeon has the ability to reposition the maxilla via a LeFort procedure, the mandible via a BSSO, and the chin via genioplasty. Specifically, the surgeon needs to determine spatially the anterior–posterior translation, the vertical translation, and the rotation of

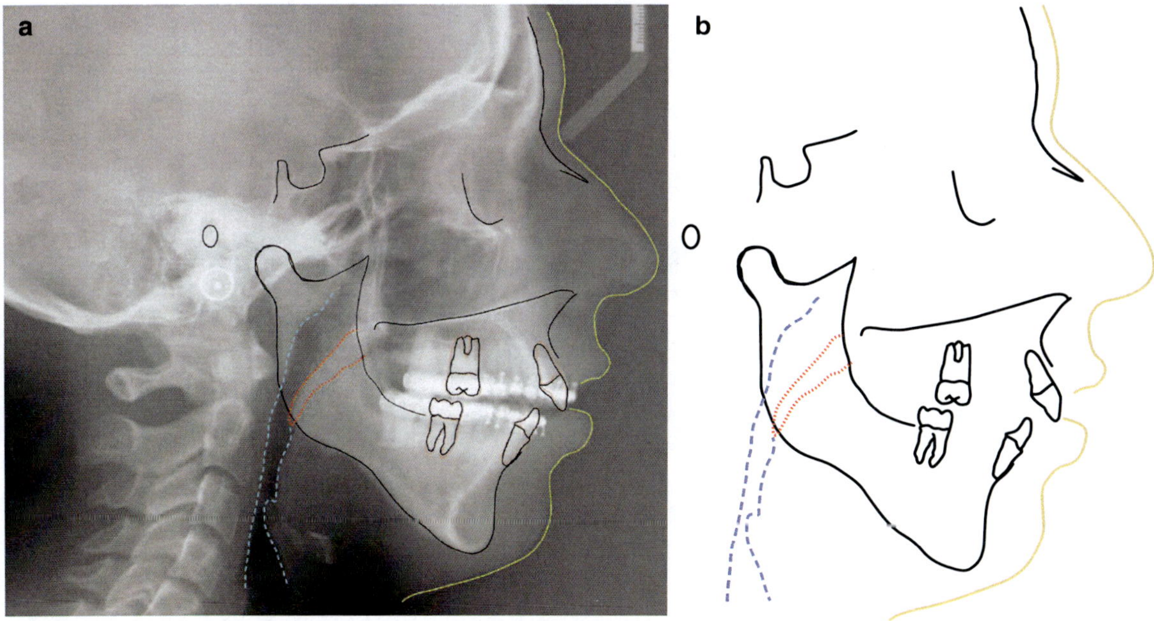

Fig. 27.3 (**a**) Frosted acetate paper is placed on top of the radiograph and key structures are marked: skeletal, dentition, soft-tissue profile, airway and soft-palate. (**b**) The radiograph itself is no longer needed. After tracing the key structures, the frosted acetate paper is removed from radiograph and placed on top of a sheet of white paper to enhance the outlines and analysis

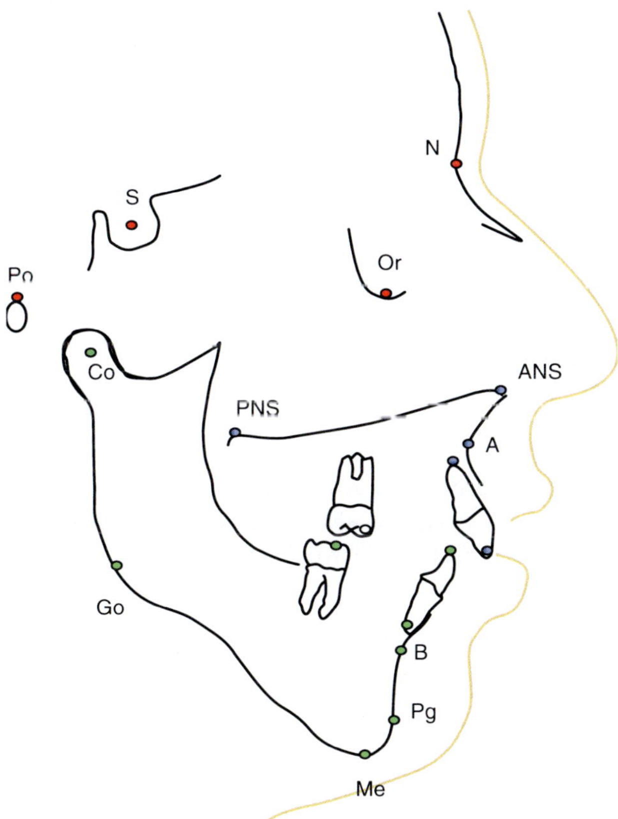

Fig. 27.4 The key anatomic landmarks are marked. The Sella (*S*), Nasion (*N*), Orbitale (*Or*) and Porion (*Po*) defines the cranial base and reference structures. The Posterior Nasal Spine (*PNS*), the Anterior Nasal Spine (*ANS*), and the A point (*A*) defines the maxilla. The B point (*B*), the Pogion (*Pg*), the Menton (*Me*), the Gonion (*Go*), and the Condyle (*Co*) define the mandible. The axis of the maxillary and mandibular central incisors is defined by their incisal tip and their root. The first maxillary molar is marked by the lingual cusp and the mandibular molar by the lingual groove

each of the skeletal elements in a 2D plane. There are two horizontal planes that can be used as a "fixed" reference for the maxilla and the jaw: (1) the anterior cranial base SN and (2) the Frankfort Horizontal plane.

If we assume that the cranial base is normal, then the question becomes relating the spatial position of the maxilla to the cranial base, the mandible to the cranial base, and the mandible to the maxilla relative to each other. We then need anatomic landmarks that can be reliably visualized on the radiograph that represent each of the structures: the sella (S) and the nasion (N) for the cranial base and A point for the maxilla and B point for the mandible. Thus, knowing only 4 anatomic landmarks begins to help us objectively quantify the facial skeleton. Based on normative angles, then the surgeon can determine whether it is the maxilla (SNA), the mandible (SNB), or both are spatially in an abnormal position. To determine whether the chin is in an appropriate position, a fifth anatomic landmark is needed, the pogonion (Pg). The pogonion can then be related to the cranial base as an angular measurement (SN–Pg).

The addition of an anatomic landmark at the inferior orbital rim orbitale (O) referenced to SN is a useful measure of the level of the midfacial involvement. If SNO is within a normal range and SNA is more acute, then a midfacial skeletal repositioning at the LeFort I level would be indicated. However, if both SNO and SNA are more acute than the normal range, consideration should be given to midfacial advancement at either an upper level modified LeFort I or the LeFort III level that would include advancement of the orbital rim.

Thus far we have defined the maxilla and mandible relative to the cranial base. However, there are instances where the relationship of the jaws is better defined by a horizontal reference plane not influenced by the cranial base. This is the

Skelettal analysis		
Sagittal analysis		CASE
Maxilla to cranial base		
SNA	82 ± 3°	82°
NA-FH	90 ± 4°	92°
Mandible to cranial base		
SNB	79 ± 3°	72°
Go-Me to FH	24 ± 3°	38°
Chin to cranial base		
SnPg	80 ± 3°	82°
NPg-FH	88 ± 3°	73°
Mandible to maxilla		
ANB	~ + 2°	+9°
Convexity at A Point	0 ± 8°	+17°
Chin to Mandible		
Pg - NB	3 ± 2 mm	0 mm
Vertical analysis		
UFH		54.5 mm
LFH		60 mm
UFH/LFH	0.9–51.0	0.91

Dental analysis		
Maxillary incisor		
U1 to SN	103 ± 6°	102°
U1 to NA	22 ± 6°	20°
Mandibular incisor		
L1 to NB	21 ± 7°	23°
Interincisal relationship		
Overjet	+ 2 mm	+7 mm
Overbite	+ 2 mm	+2 mm
Occlusal plane		
OP-FH	8 ± 4°	10°
Dental Display*		
Repose*	M +2 mm ± 2 mm F +3.5 mm ± 2 mm	F +4.5 mm
Smile*	Full crown + 2 mm gingiva	+3 mm

*Measured clinically

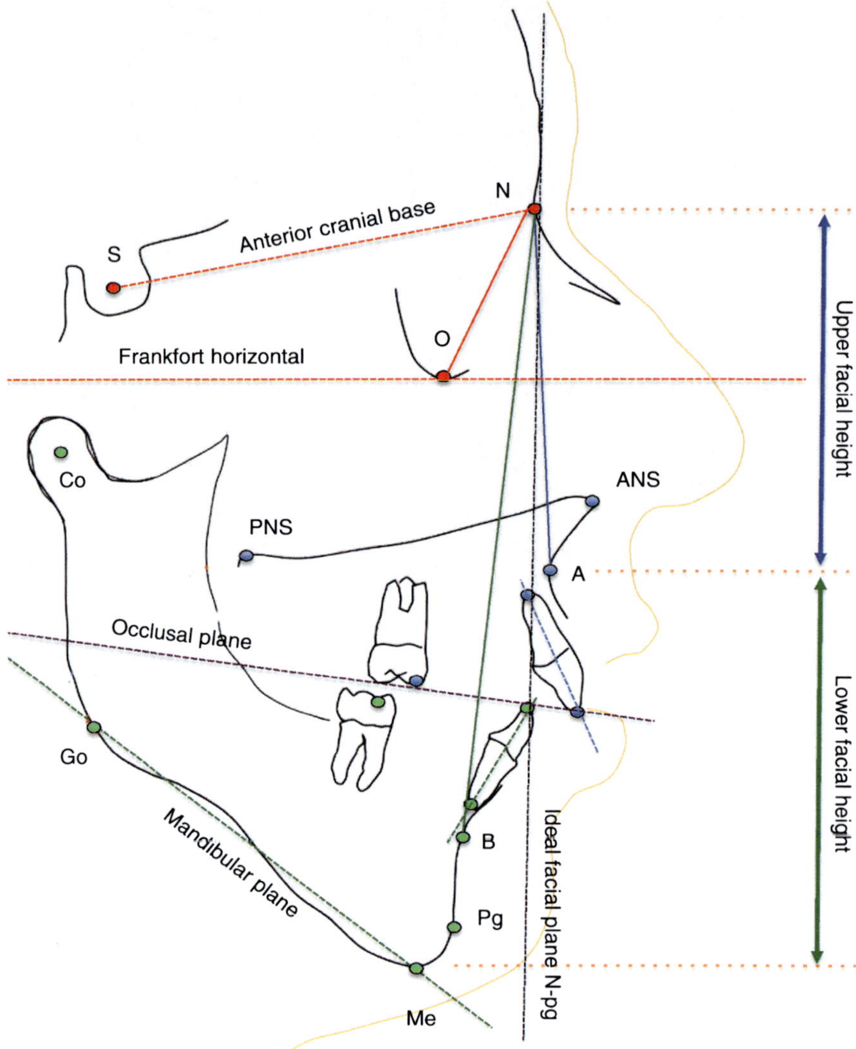

Fig. 27.5 Basic dentofacial skeletal analysis that is sufficient for the majority of cases. Note that the 'Ideal Facial Skeletal Plane' is marked to indicate the deviation from of the maxilla and mandible from the "ideal." This is the skeletal equivalent of the soft tissue Ulloa-Gonzalez 0. Meridian is the perpendicular from the glabella

case in craniofacial conditions in which the anterior cranial base is foreshortened and/or has steeper or flatter inclination than normal. The maxillary–mandibular angles measured relative to the SN plane that is assumed to be "normal" but which is not will mislead the clinician.

The Frankfort Horizontal plane is used commonly as a second reference plane. This plane was established by anthropologists to allow comparison of dry skull specimens independent of the skull base. It was defined in 1884 at the World Congress of Anthropology at Frankfurt, Germany, as the plane passing through the inferior margin of the orbit (orbitale, Or), and the upper margin of the ear canal or external auditory meatus, a point called the porion (Po), best approximated the position of the head normally carried in a living subject when looking at a distant horizon or themselves in a mirror. Using the Frankfort Horizontal plane to orient the skull in 3D space allowed the anthropologists a consistent methodology for comparative study of dry skull specimens and the orthodontists an approach to a consistent cephalometric analysis as 2D planar radiographs were obtained in a consistent manner relative to the FH plane in living subjects.

The relationship between the two reference planes—the SN plane and the FH plane—provides an important check that the cranial base is within an acceptable range, and thus the surgeon and orthodontist can be confident that the deformity can be addressed with maxillofacial surgery alone. The angle between the two horizontal reference planes should be approximately 7°, and the length of the anterior cranial base—the SN distance—should measure approximately 72 mm for an adult male and 67 mm for an adult female.

Using the Frankfort Horizontal plane, similar angles can be defined for the maxilla and mandible using N, A, and B. As

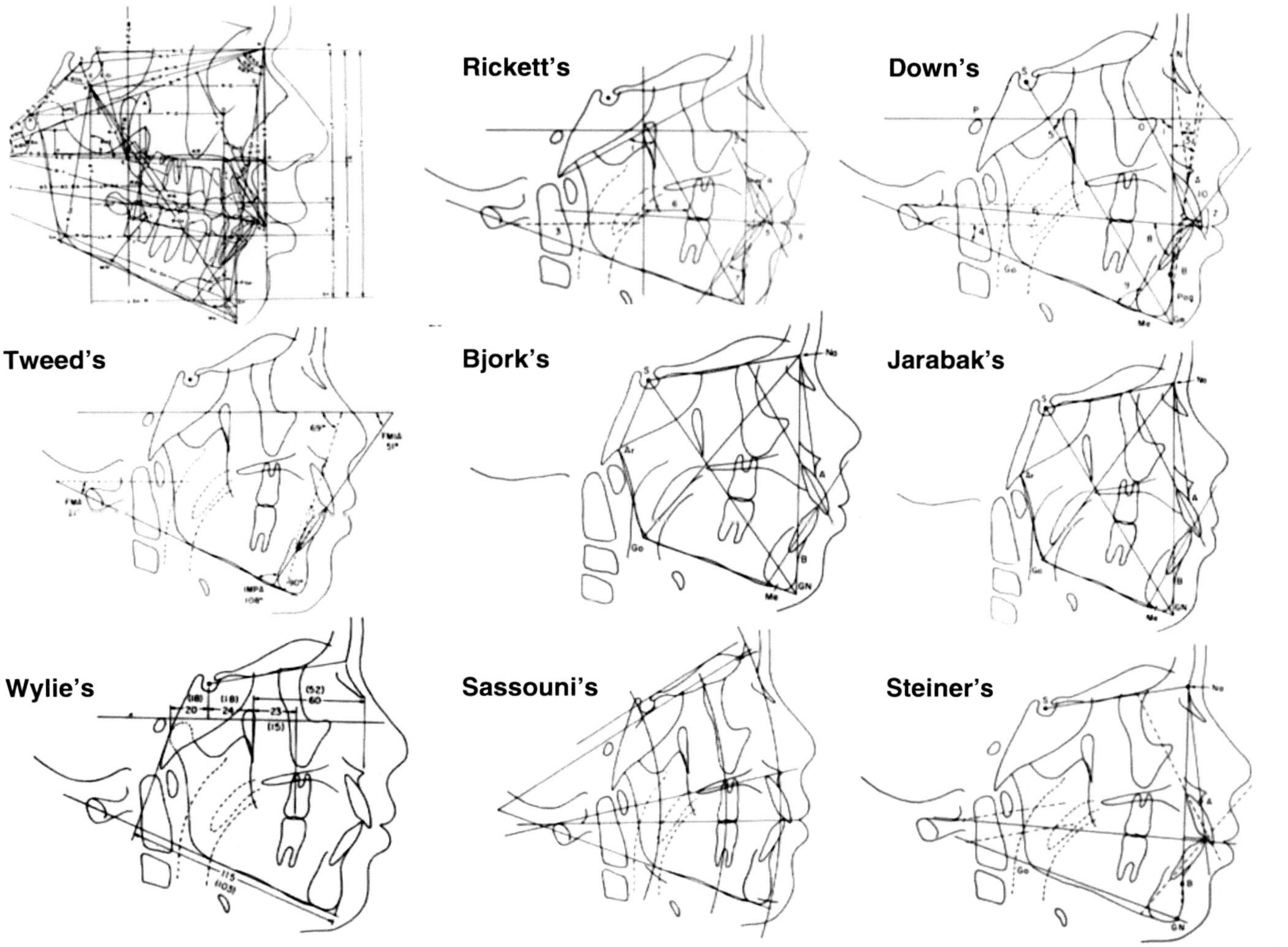

Fig. 27.6 Illustration of the multitude of analysis that can be performed depending on the clinical and research interests

with the cranial base SN reference, the surgeon then has another guide to reposition the maxilla and mandible knowing the normative values relative to the FH plane. However, with the understanding that even orbitale may be malpositioned in subjects with craniofacial dysostosis conditions and therefore both the SN and FH planes are affected, the surgeon and the orthodontist must make adjustments in the analysis to achieve an optimum outcome.

In terms of vertical planes, the facial plane is the most important. It best anatomically defines the face by the line (plane) passing through the nasion and the pogonion. Irrespective of the position of the maxilla and mandible, it is the relative importance and position of the chin that dominates face and thus defines the facial plane.

To determine the vertical relationships of the facial height, then a sixth point is needed, the menton (Me). The vertical facial relationship can then be determined by measuring the distance between nasion and A point, measuring the distance between A point and menton and then calculating the ratio of the two measurements. The proportionality of the upper facial height relative to the lower facial height is more important than the absolute measurements.

These five points—N, A, B, Pg, and Me—define only the anterior relation of the facial skeleton. Angulation or rotation of the maxilla/mandibular complex relative to the cranial base is equally important as it defines the palatal plane angulation, inclination of the occlusal plane, and the steepness of the mandibular plane. Thus, additional anatomic points are needed to help define the spatial rotation of the maxilla and the mandible that are under the control of the surgeon. For the maxilla, the palatal plane defined by the line that passes through the anterior nasal spine (ANS) and the posterior nasal spine (PNS) will guide the rotation of the maxilla. For the mandible, the mandibular plane defined by the line passing through the Me and gonion (Go) defines the steepness of the mandible.

As with the anterior facial height, analysis of the posterior facial height is important and is under the control of the surgeon. The posterior facial height is a combination of the maxilla and the mandible. The posterior height of the maxilla is measured as a distance from PNS to the Frankfort

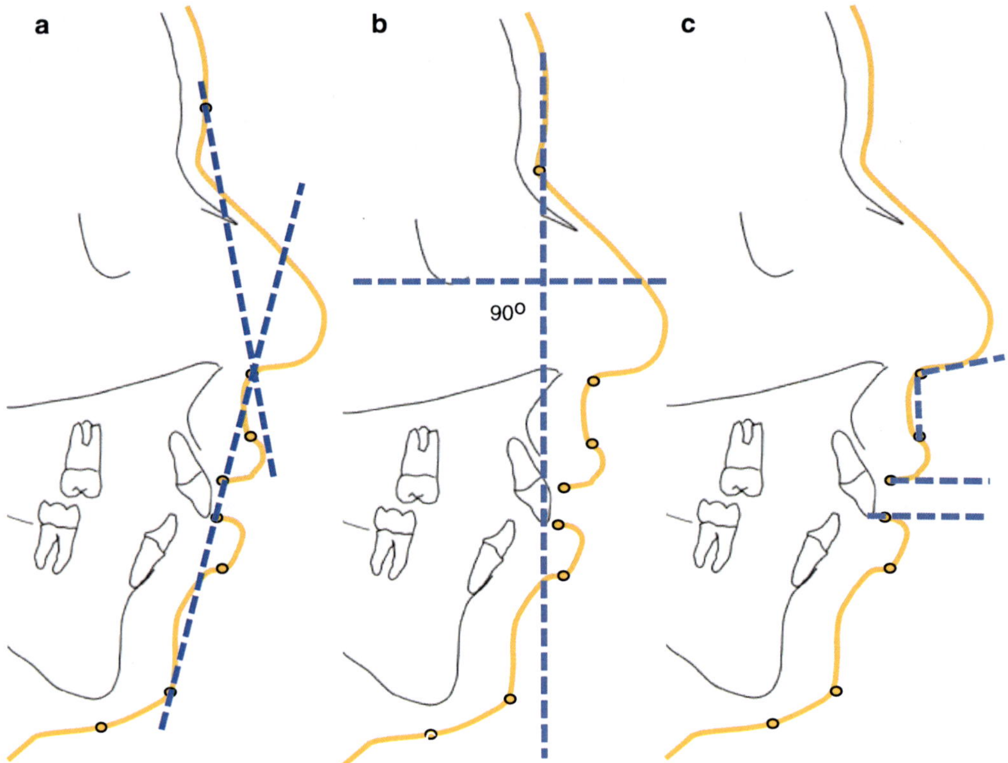

Fig. 27.7 Soft tissue cephalometric analysis. (**a**) The Facial Convexity at Sn, (**b**) The Gonzalez-Uolla zero meridian line and (**c**) Naso-labial angle and Dental Display

Horizontal plane. The posterior mandibular height measured as the ramal height is from the condyle (Co) to gonion (Go).

Thus, 12 anatomic landmarks—S, N, Or, ANS, PNS, A, B, Pg, Me, Go, Co, and Po—with relevant angular and distant measures are sufficient for the maxillofacial surgeon to guide the repositioning of skeletal elements (maxilla, mandible, and chin) to optimize facial skeletal morphology based on population normative data and aesthetic ideals established by personal preferences of the patient.

The Dental Analysis

As with skeletal analysis, dental analysis needs to be incorporated as an integral component. For the surgeon, the relevant landmarks are the maxillary and mandibular incisor tip and roots and the molar relationship. Using these landmarks, critical measurements include overjet, overbite, the incisor inclinations, and the occlusal plane angulation. In surgical-orthodontic planning, the desired skeletal movements will be dictated by the incisor relation. As an illustration, a patient may require significant mandibular skeletal advancement for airway and to improve the lower third facial aesthetics. However, the degree of advancement may not be achievable if the overjet is not significant. The orthodontist will need to maximize the amount of overjet by retroclining the mandibular incisors maximally and may require extractions of the lower first bicuspids to retract the anterior dentition. The maxillary incisors may require to be bought into a proper relationship by proclining the incisor axis. Maximal decompensation is required. A similar situation may occur in patients with midfacial deficiency, where the maxillary incisors are needed to be maximally decompensated to allow sufficient midfacial skeletal advancement. The angulation of the maxillary incisors plays an important role in upper lip support and aesthetics. The appropriate incisor angulation needs to be planned with both orthodontic treatment and maxillary rotation. Finally, the angulation of the occlusal plane is important as it relates to the TMJ rotation to optimize occlusal function. Thus, both the surgeon and orthodontist must closely plan the final position of both the facial skeleton and the dentition.

The Soft-Tissue Analysis

Ultimately it is the soft-tissue envelope that the patient sees, and the goal of the dentofacial surgery is to achieve the optimal soft-tissue form and aesthetic smile. A well-taken cephalometric radiograph will reveal simultaneously the facial skeleton and the soft-tissue profile of the face. Soft-tissue landmarks that are relevant are illustrated in Fig. 27.7.

An overall assessment of the face can be obtained by measuring the convexity of the face, the deviation face plane from a line perpendicular to the soft-tissue Frankfort Horizontal plane dropped from the nasion, and the vertical proportions of the face.

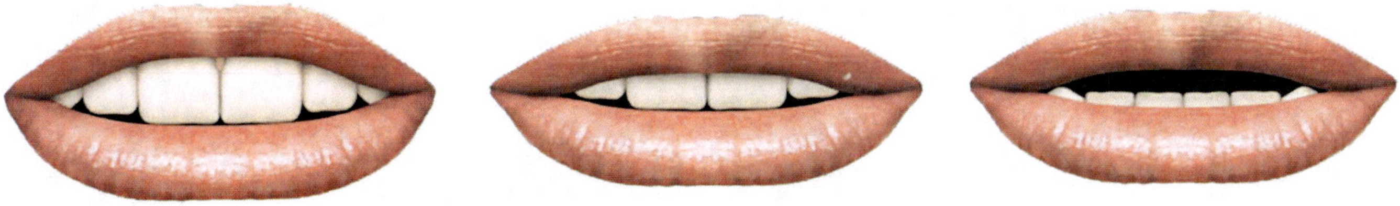

Fig. 27.8 Illustrates the relationship between the upper lip and amount of dental display from excess to insufficient. Orthodontic treatment and maxillary surgery can alter the amount of dental display to improve the aesthetic appearance of the smile

The upper facial assessment includes the frontonasal angle, the nasal length and columella height, and the nasolabial angle and the upper lip length.

For the lower face, the components of the soft-tissue analysis include the projection of the lower lip, the depth of the labial-mental sulcus, the projection of the chin, and the cervical-mental contour. If the radiograph is taken with the lips in a relaxed position, then distance between the lips may reveal the degree of lip incompetence. If the radiograph is taken with the lips closed, then the lower third contour may reveal the strain to bring the lips together.

The Smile Analysis

An important component in any orthognathic surgical procedure and orthodontic management is analyzing the lips as they rest on the dentofacial skeleton and the dynamic nature of the smile. Teeth, lips, and the soft tissue (gums) surrounding the teeth together make up a smile. If any of these three components deviate from an accepted norm, the smile may appear to be unsightly, even if the dentition is straight and white. All three components can be altered by treatment.

The assessment begins with the lips at rest without strain. The average lip length is 23 mm in men and 20 mm in women. What is critical is the relationship of the upper lip to the maxillary central incisors and the labial commissure. The appropriate dental display is typically between 2 and 3 mm in males and 3 and 4 mm in female at rest. The lip length should be approximately equal to the commissure height, defined as the vertical distance from a horizontal at the subnasale. Figure 27.8 illustrates the relationships and shows the variation between an excess of dental display and insufficient dental display and variation in commissure heights relative to the central lip. Ideal relationship is achieved at rest.

When patients are asked to smile, there is a broad range from a voluntary social smile to an involuntary smile of laughter. The social smile is a "controlled" smile as when greeting friends or posing for a photograph. The full 10 mm of dental crowns are displayed with 1–2 mm of gingival display. Excess gingival display at repose and in a social smile becomes unattractive. Such patients will typically avoid smiling in social situations.

The curvatures of the arcs of the lips and its relationships to the dentition play an important role in aesthetics. The smile arc is the relationship between a curve drawn along the edges of the maxillary anterior teeth and the inner contour of the lower lip in the posed smile. Figure 27.9 illustrates the ideal and variations that can occur. With the ability of the surgeon to alter the occlusal plane and the incisor angulation, the smile arc can be impacted. If the maxillary occlusal plane is canted excessively upward anteriorly, the incisal edges will move away from the lower lip, resulting in a less attractive smile arc and a reduced dental display. Conversely, if the occlusal plane has an excessive clockwise rotation, the upper incisal edges will be covered by the lower lip, resulting in a less attractive smile and an increased dental display.

The relationship between orthodontic dental movement, surgical dentoalveolar movement en block, and the soft-tissue lip dynamics is complex and requires careful planning between the surgeon and the orthodontist to optimize the perioral aesthetics both in repose and in a dynamic smile.

The Airway Analysis

The nasopharyngeal airway space can be assessed using the lateral cephalometric x-ray with the understanding that it represents a 2D projection of a 3D structure. Studies have shown there is a good clinical correlation between direct endoscopic examination and the morphologic assessment. Various analyses exist and are beyond the scope of this chapter. Figure 27.10 illustrates one such analysis that focuses on the relevant measurements that involve in determining the nasopharyngeal, oropharyngeal, and hypopharyngeal airway space at determined levels. Additional relevant intraoral structures including the tongue and palate are as illustrated.

Asymmetry Analysis

If there is any significant facial asymmetry, then a frontal PA cephalometric radiograph is obtained. The key anatomic points are illustrated in Fig. 27.11, and the deviation from symmetry

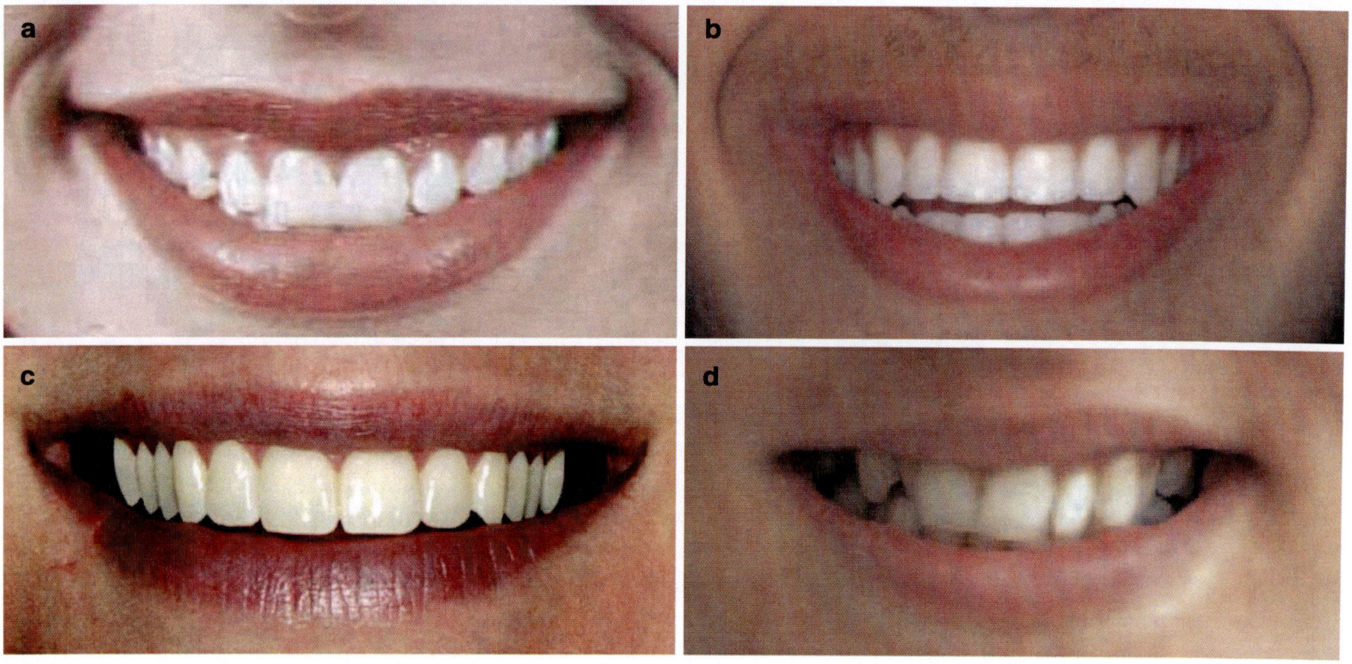

Fig. 27.9 The smile arc can be controlled by orthodontic treatment and maxillary orthognathic surgery in controlling the occlusal pitch, yaw and roll. (**a**) The arc of the maxillary incisal edges should follow the lower lip arc in an ideal smile. (**b**) The maxillary dental arc has been unintentionally flattened by treatment resulting in a less ideal aesthetic appearance. (**c**) While the smile arch is acceptable, the lateral buccal corridor space is enlarged resulting in a less than ideal smile. (**d**) An asymmetric smile arc

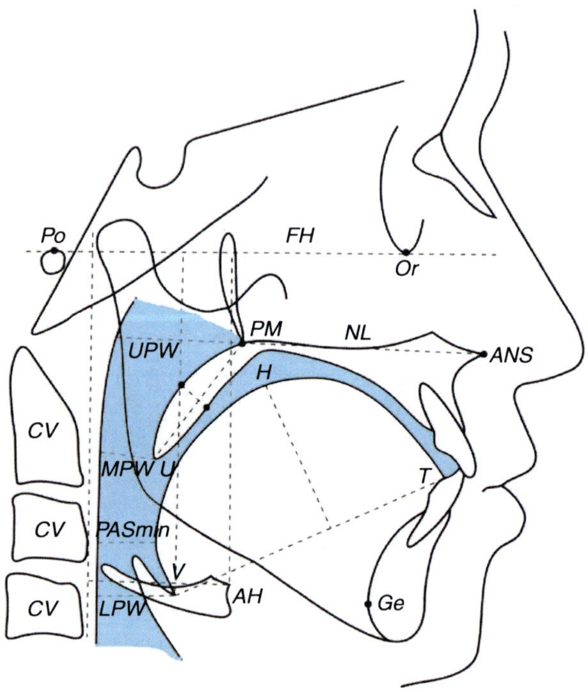

Fig. 27.10 Cephalometric analysis for airway space. *AH* anterior hyoid, *ANS* anterior nasal spine, *CV* Cervical vertebrae, *FH* Frankfurt Horizontal plane, *Ge* Genital tubercule, *H* superior part of tongue, *LPW* lower pharyngeal wall, *MPW* middle pharyngeal wall, *NL* nasal line, *PM* pterygo-maxillare, *Or* Orbitale, *Po* Porion, *T* tip of tongue, *U* uvula, *UPW* upper pharyngeal wall, *V* vallecula, the junction of the epiglottis and the base of the tongue, *PASmin* The shortest distance between the base of the tongue and the posterior pharyngeal wall, the narrowest sagittal airway space

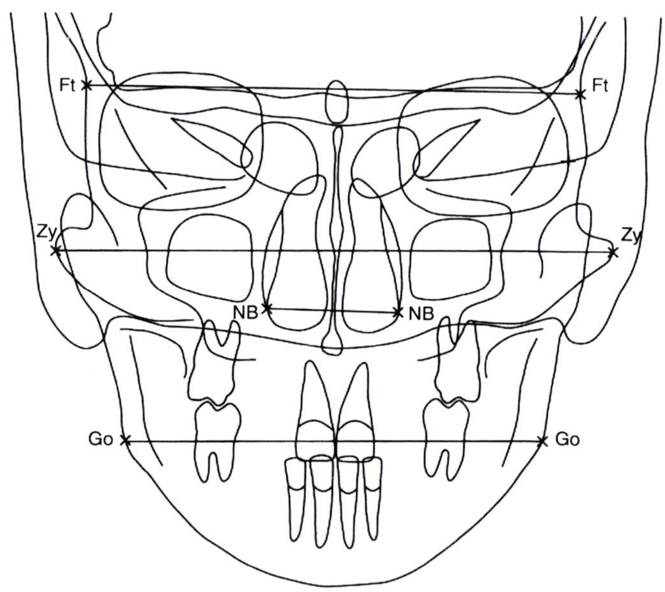

Fig. 27.11 Frontal analysis from a PA cephalometric radiograph. *Ft* Frontozygomatic suture, *Go* Gonion, *NB* nasal butress, *Zy* lateral of the zygomatic arch

can be quantified. However, the practical clinical application of frontal cephalometry to surgical planning is limited. Many of the patients will present with complex asymmetry in not only the coronal plane captured by the PA frontal cephalometry but also rotational asymmetries in the transverse plane that cannot be captured accurately with radiographs.

2D Prediction Tracings and Cephalometric Surgery

Once the analysis is completed, central to the surgical-orthodontic planning is a visual treatment objective (VTO) in determining where each of the components—the skeletal bases, the dentition, and the soft tissue—should be positioned to the fixed reference structure (skull base) and relative to each other. Essentially the VTO is a simulation of the surgery on paper in 2D. Construction begins with knowing where to place the skeletal bases in an "ideal" position based on normative data but tempered more importantly on the aesthetic goals of the patient and the clinician rather than achieving a population mean. The fallacy with cephalometrics is the failure to understand that no patient comes wanting treatment to look average, and the clinician who treats such patients to the normative data fails to understand the variance to the mean. There is a broad range to normative data to achieve an aesthetically pleasing outcome. The mean data should be used as a guide, a first approximation of the planned surgical-orthodontic treatment to be refined to achieve patient-specific goals.

There are different approaches to a VTO, and we will describe one of the simplest approaches that will be useful to the beginning orthognathic surgeon. As a first approximation, cephalometric surgery begins in a stepwise manner beginning with placement of the maxilla in the sagittal plane (A-P vector). A LeFort I osteotomy is done on paper by tracing the maxilla on a clear acetate paper. This paper LeFort I segment can then be repositioned. If we would like the final SNA angle to be 82°, then a line is constructed at that angle with respect to the SN plane, and the A point of the repositioned maxilla can be positioned anywhere along the constructed line (Fig. 27.12). To determine where on that line the A point should be positioned of the paper LeFort I segment, the surgeon needs to know the desired vertical height of the upper facial skeleton based on the amount of the desired dental display. For example, in a female patient with midfacial class III skeletal deficiency in the sagittal and in vertical plane, a dental display at rest is −2 mm, but the desired dental display may be +4 mm. This means that the vertical distance at the incisal edge and the A point should increase by+6 mm in the vertical dimension. This then positions the maxilla both in the sagittal and vertical planes (Fig. 27.13). Next the rotation of the LeFort I segment needs to be determined. This is based on the desired incisor inclination (and the occlusal plane) to optimize the lip support and smile arc as discussed above (Fig. 27.14). The LeFort surgery is completed and is the intermediate position without the mandibular surgery. These changes in the *X* and *Y* direction in the maxilla are then recorded and will be used in the dental model surgery for the intermediate splint fabrication. Next the mandibular sagittal split of the ramus is performed on paper by tracing the distal segment with the dentition. The mandible is now

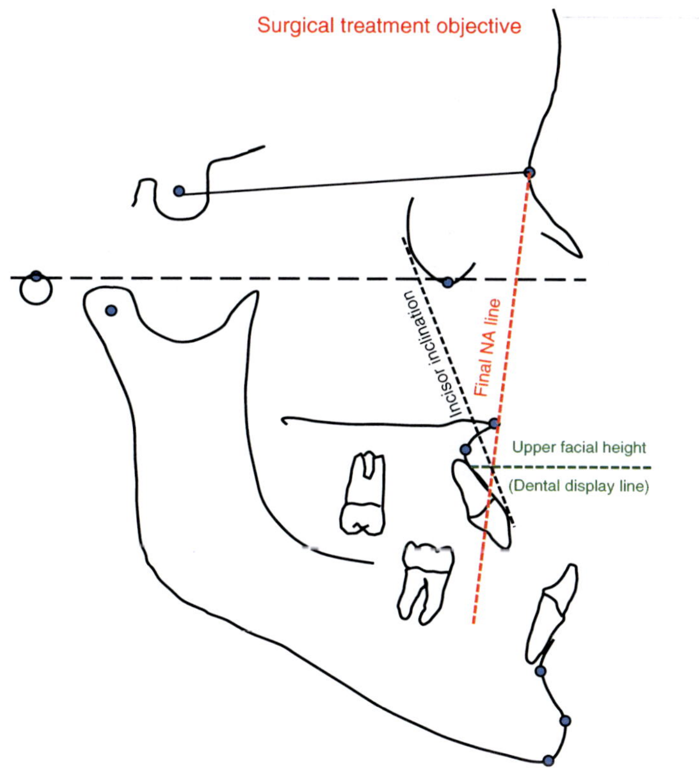

Fig. 27.12 To determine the final position of the maxilla at A point, the surgeon and the orthodontists needs three lines: the amount of desired maxillary projection determined by the the NA line (SNA angle), the amount of desired maxillary dental display determines the upper facial height (UFH), and the desired inclination of the maxillary incisors determined by the incisor axis

repositioned based on the position of the LeFort I segment so that there is an appropriate overjet and overbite anteriorly and molar relationship posteriorly (Fig. 27.15). With the LeFort I and BSSO completed, a final occlusal splint can be fabricated using dental models. To position the chin, an ideal facial plane is constructed by dropping a vertical line from the nasion (Fig. 27.16). The pogonion then can be positioned either at the "ideal" facial plane, a few millimeters posterior for female, or a few millimeters anterior for male based on the patient's aesthetic goals. This determines only the sagittal position of the chin. To determine the vertical position of the chin, vertical analysis is used. The position is based on the vertical height of the upper facial skeleton, the distance between nasion and A point. Depending on the patient's desires, the lower facial height can be equal to or greater than the upper facial height. Once the paper orthognathic surgery is completed, the soft-tissue predictions based on the new skeletal contour are drawn. The predictions are based on historical collection of records, and the surgeon uses a table of ratios that indicate how much soft-tissue change for each millimeter change in the skeleton. A cephalometric analysis is done of the completed VTO. The final skeletal and soft-tissue prediction tracing should be carefully reviewed, and if

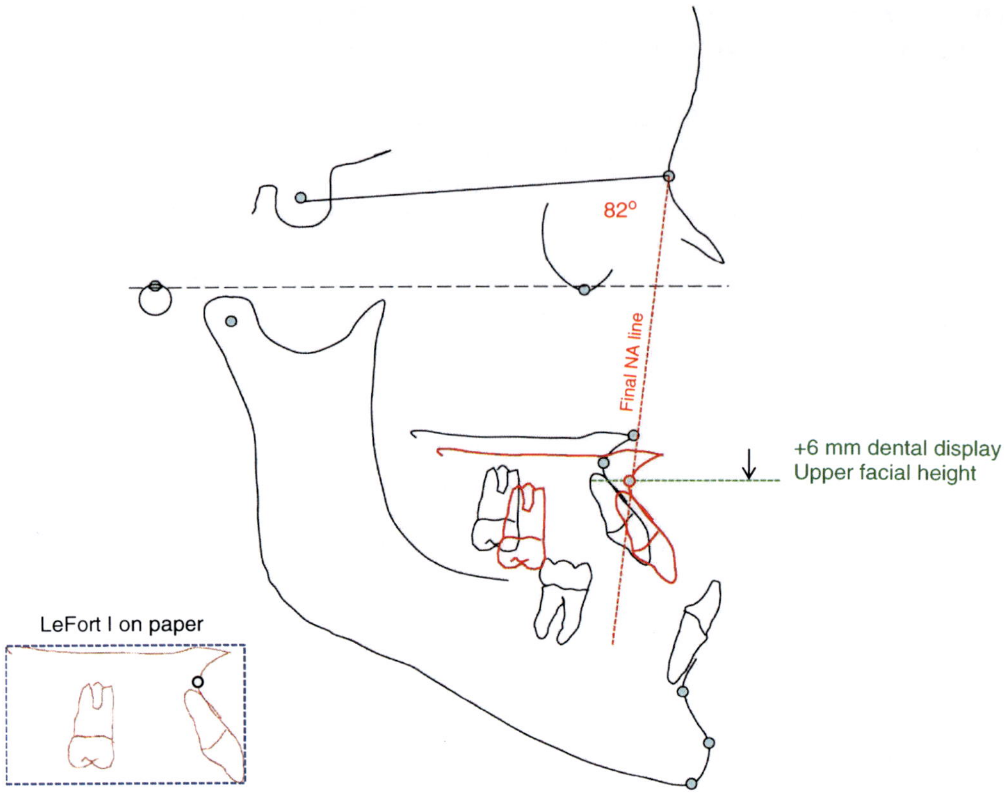

Fig. 27.13 A LeFort I is carried out on paper. This is done by tracing the maxilla on frosted acetate paper and repositioning the maxilla to the final position. For instance, the surgeon and orthodontist may determine that they would like the maxillary projection to be an SNA of 82°. The A point should be on the NA line. In addition, the decision is to increase the dental display by 6 mm, then the change in A point should be + 6 mm down in the *Y* direction. This would be the position of the maxilla without changing the incisor inclination

	Pre Op	Max →	Md ←	Chin
Facial convexity 0 ± 8°	−30°	−11°		
Facial plane 90°	95°	95°		
SNA 82±–4°	74°	84°		
SNB 80±3°	88°	88°		
ANB ~2°	−14°	−4°		
UFH/LFH 0.95–1.0	0.90	+5 mm		

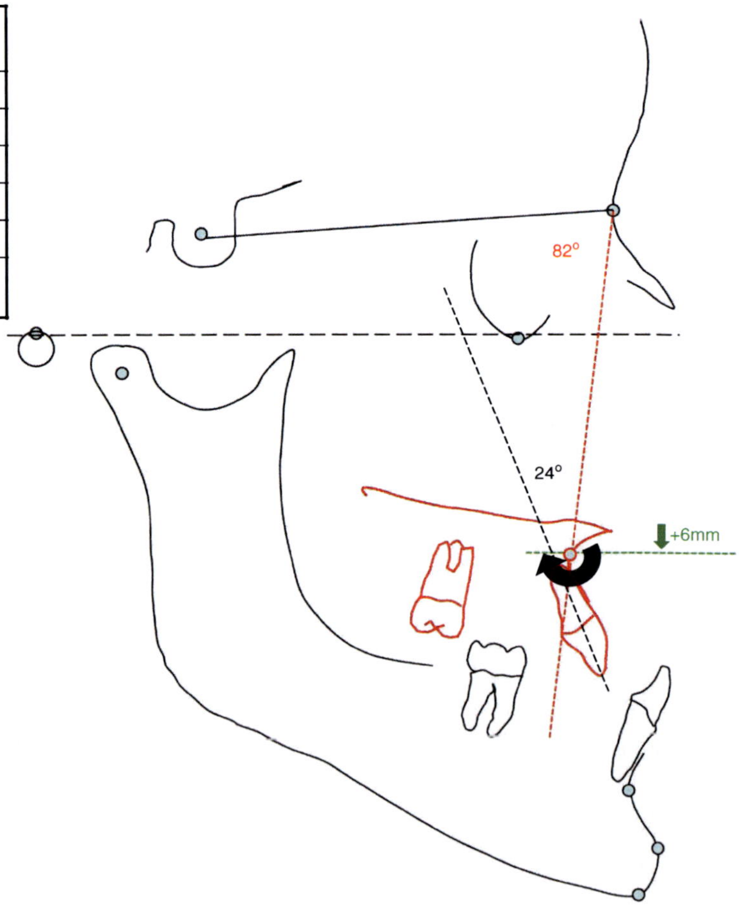

Fig. 27.14 Next, the LeFort I segment is rotated about the A point so that the incisor inclination is optimized. This final placement of the maxilla results in the intermediate position (i.e., after the LeFort I, before the BSSO). This maxillary–mandibular relationship is what the surgeon should see in the operating room. The changes in the *X* and *Y* vectors of the maxilla is translated to the facebow mounted maxillary dental model (model surgery). An intermediate splint is made

	Pre Op	Max →	Md ←	Chin
Facial convexity 0 ± 8°	−30°	−11°	+2°	
Facial plane 90°	95°	95°	88°	
SNA 82 ± 4°	74°	84°	84°	
SNB 80 ± 3°	88°	88°	82°	
ANB ~2°	−14°	−4°	+2°	
UFH/LFH 0.95–1.0	0.90		1.0	

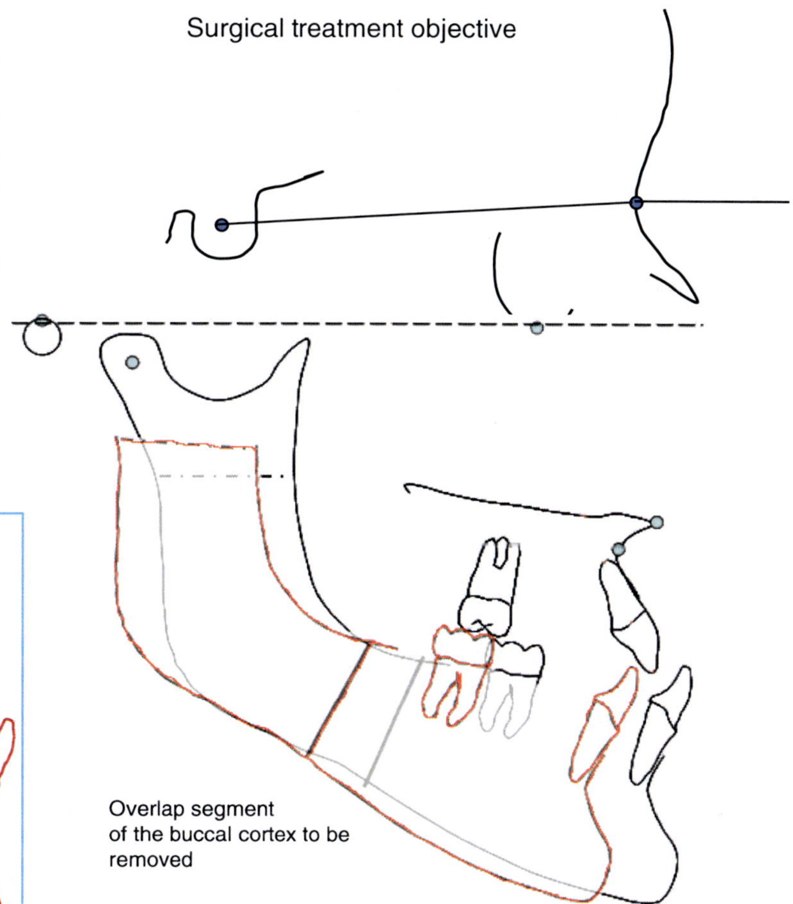

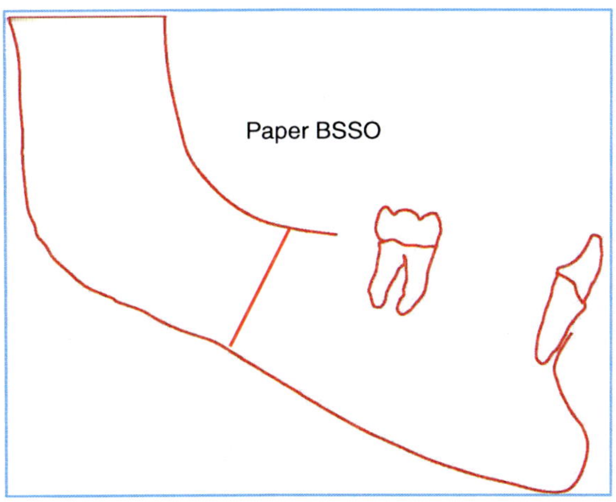

Fig. 27.15 The mandible is setback. Its position is entirely determined by the position of the maxilla. The occlusal plane of the mandible matches that of the maxilla and the overjet, and overbite relationship is set to 2 mm. The SNB is then measured. This should be the final position of the maxilla and the mandible in the operating room. Note that the tracing indicates how much bone will need to be resected (overlapped segment) to set the mandible back. A final occluasl surgical splint is made using the dental models. This will index the dental arches

needed, re-doing the cephalometric surgery above to achieve an optimal prediction.

It maybe that maxillary surgery alone is needed. One way of determining would be to perform a LeFort I paper osteotomy as indicated above. The maxilla and mandible are positioned together (placed in maxillary–mandibular fixation). The complex is then rotated with regard to the condyle (Fig. 27.16). With the rotation of the complex to achieve an ideal dental display (upper facial height), cephalometric analysis will then reveal whether or not an acceptable outcome can be achieved based on the angulation of occlusal plane, SNA, SNB, and the facial plane (N–Pg). If not, then a double jaw procedure is needed.

It may be that the maxilla is in an acceptable position, and only mandibular surgery is needed. A paper mandibular BSSO is performed. The distal segment is then repositioned to an appropriate overjet/overbite relationship and along the occlusal plane of the maxilla. To determine if an osseous genioplasty is desired, an ideal facial plane is constructed by dropping a vertical line from the nasion (Fig. 27.17). If the pogonion is within an acceptable distance to the "ideal" facial plane and the vertical height is acceptable, then osseous genioplasty is not needed. Otherwise, a genioplasty will allow the surgeon to establish the facial plane at the pogonion and the lower facial height by the menton as described above.

Instead of the SN anterior cranial base plane as the "fixed" reference for the VTO, the surgeon and the orthodontist can use the Frankfort Horizontal plane for the VTO in a similar manner as described above. The important principle is that the clinician must know the desired final position of the facial skeleton based on the patient's desires and the achievable surgical-orthodontic goals that can be delivered. The cephalometric analysis and VTO provides a structured approach to treatment planning for the beginning orthognathic surgeon.

Once the final skeletal position is completed, then a soft-tissue prediction is accomplished based on available tables that indicate the approximate change in millimeters of the soft-tissue landmark per the change in millimeters of the skeletal landmark. As an illustration, a maxillary advancement of 10 mm results in an advancement of subnasale (SN) by 6 mm, labrale superius (LS) by 9 mm, and the nasal tip by 3 mm. Soft-tissue prediction is an art in itself and has a

	Pre Op	Max →	Md ←	Chin
Facial Convexity 0 ± 8°	−30°	−11°	+2°	
Facial Plane 90°	95°	95°	88°	
SNA 82 ± 4°	74°	84°	84°	
SNB 80 ± 3°	88°	88°	82°	
ANB ~2°	−14°	−4°	+2°	
UFH/LFH 0.95 −1.0	0.90		1.0	

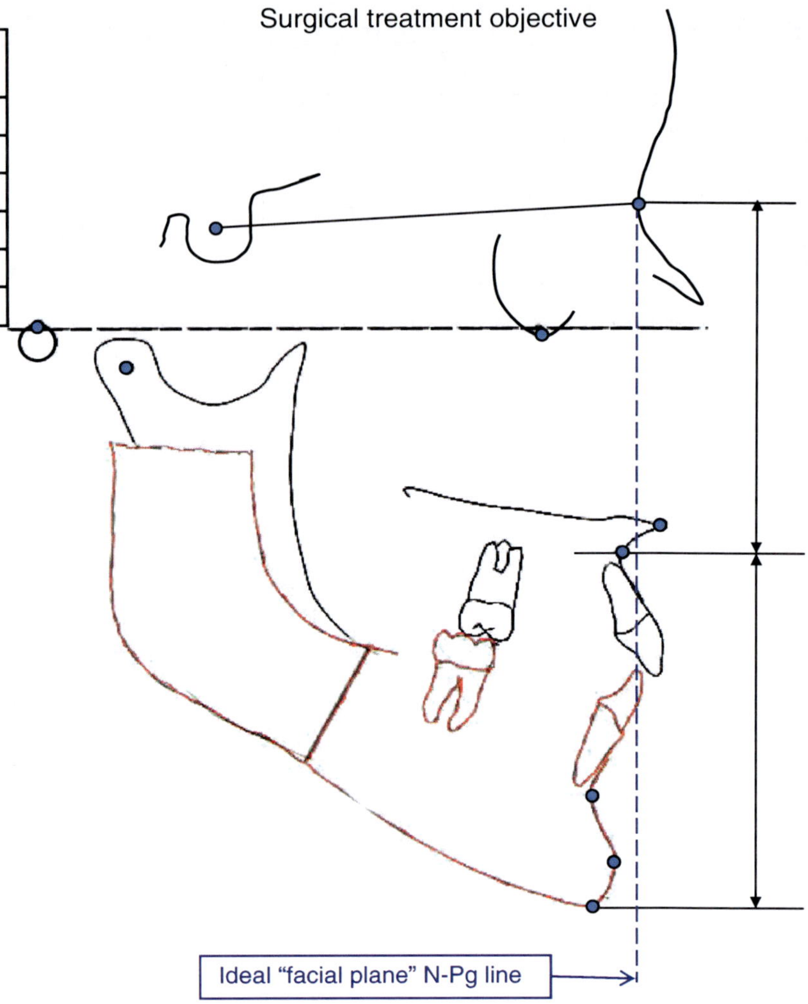

Fig. 27.16 Finally, a decision is made whether a genioplasty would be of benefit. There are two lines that are needed: the desired Facial planes (N-Pg) angle relative to the Frankfort Horizontal (FH) and the desired Lower Facial Height(LFH). Both these lines are drawn on the VTO. An osseous genioplasty on paper can be done and repositioned so that the chin Pg in on the N-Pg line and the chin Me is on the LFH line

variability of accuracy. It is dependent on the qualitative properties of the soft tissue. The prediction of a patient with a dentofacial deformity with facial cleft would be different than the patient without a facial cleft. Moreover, the skeletal repositioning is in multiple planes, and so simple ratios as indicated in the tables are approximations at best. Their value is understanding the qualitative response: a maxillary advancement will increase the nasolabial angle and the upper lip length. The basic rule is that if the skeletal framework is placed in the appropriate position within an acceptable range of norms, then an acceptable soft-tissue profile will follow.

Dental Model Surgery

Once the cephalometric surgery on paper is completed and the final positions of the maxilla and mandible are determined, the challenge for the surgeon is to translate this to the operating room. The paper osteotomies are converted to physical models through the use of dental stone models. The maxillary and mandibular dentition is then moved in 3D space to match that of the movement of the maxilla and mandible that was planned based on the VTO described in the previous section. This is done by mounting the dental casts in an articulator which is a mechanical device that allows the dental casts to be moved to match that planned by the VTO.

There are two articulators that are useful for the surgeon: a Galetti articulator and a semi-adjustable articulator that utilizes a facebow. When the VTO involves movement of only a single jaw, either the maxilla or mandible, a Galetti articulator (Fig. 27.18) or a simple hinge articulator (Fig. 27.19) is used. The Galetti articulator is a plasterless articulator that allows quick mounting of casts essentially for study purposes and for single jaw surgery. The hinge point of the articulator that represents the TMJ is fixed and is not anatomical. Model surgery with a Galetti articulator can be

	Pre Op	Md →	Chin →	
Facial Convexity 0 ± 8°	+17°	+12°		
Facial Plane 90°	84°	86°		
SNA 82 ± 4°	82°	82°		
SNB 80 ± 3°	73°	76°		
ANB ~2°	+9°	+6°		
UFH/LFH 0.95–1.0	0.90	0.93		

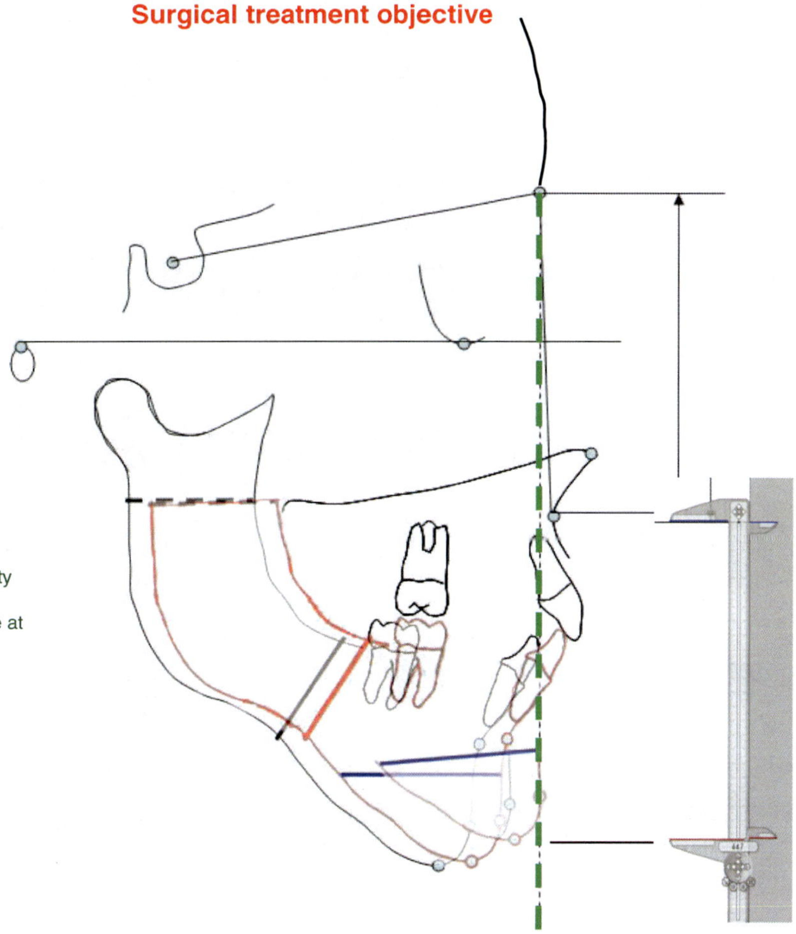

Paper genioplasty

1. Using a Black Pencil, mark osteotomy of the chin.
2. Using a small piece of tracing paper, trace out the genioplasty with a Blue Pencil
3. Advance the chin so that Pg is at the facial plane and the Me at the appropriate vertical height
4. Tape the paper genioplasty using celephane tape (Fixation)
5. Re-do the cephalometric analysis.

Fig. 27.17 Positioning the chin allows the surgeon to control the Facial Plane (N-Pg) in the sagittal plane and the Lower Facial Height (LFH) relative to the upper facial height (UFH) to achieve acceptable facial proportions. This is illustrated in a patient with a Class II dentofacial skeletal deformity. Mandibular advancement alone is insufficient to correct the excess the facial convexity angle

quickly done simply repositioning the dental casts in their final occlusal position with the use of the device's set screws. An acrylic splint, the occlusal guide, is fabricated using this position to index the dental arches to each other (Fig. 27.20). The acrylic splint is then used in the operating room as a surgical guide to index the maxillary dentition to mandibular dentition as if it were on an articulator. The occlusal guide is an integral component of the procedure to properly position the jaws through the use of the dental arches.

When the VTO involves movement of both the maxilla and mandible, then a semi-adjustable articulator is used (Fig. 27.21), as these articulators can better reproduce the centric relation and centric occlusion to an acceptable anatomic average. The spatial position of the dental casts within the articulator must match that of the spatial position in the lateral cephalometric radiograph and then be able to be moved physically to match the movements in the VTO. This is achieved through a facebow registration that fixes the maxillary cast in the same 3D plane in relation to the condyles as it exists in the patient and thereby reproduces the patient's upper teeth position with regard to the Frankfurt Horizontal Plane and Porion. This is best illustrated in Fig. 27.22 that shows the facebow registration and the transfer to the semi-adjustable articulator. Once the maxillary cast is fixed in position, the mandibular cast is fixed using a bite-wax registration of the initial occlusion. Once both the maxillary and mandibular dental casts are plaster mounted in the articulator, then a spatial correlation of the dental arches is established between the lateral cephalometric x-ray and the physical models (Fig. 27.23). In a two-jaw surgery, the maxillary dental cast is sectioned (LeFort I) and moved based on the VTO. The maxillary dental cast is then replastered in the final planned position of the maxilla (Fig. 27.24). This then is the intermediate position in the VTO and what would be expected in the operating room after the maxillary surgery. In this intermediate position, an acrylic occlusal splint (Fig. 27.25) is made. This splint is then used in the operating room to guide the final position of the maxilla. Similarly, the plaster-mounted mandibular dental cast can be sectioned (BSSO) and repositioned and plaster mounted into the final

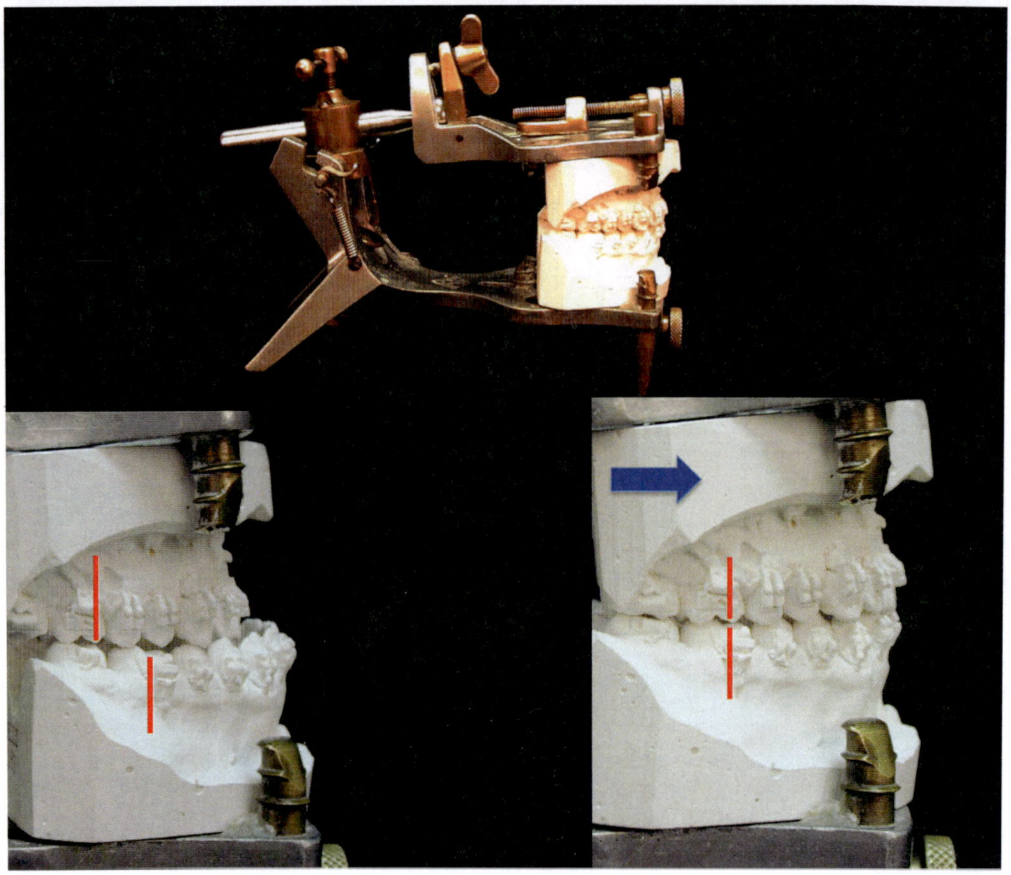

Fig. 27.18 Model surgery using a Galetti – type articulator for a single jaw procedure. The occlusal splint is then fabricated and used in the operative procedure to guide the position of the maxilla relative to the mandible based on the desired occlusion. *Blue arrow* indicates the movement of the maxilla, while *red line* marks the same point on the casting and indicates the maxillary movement

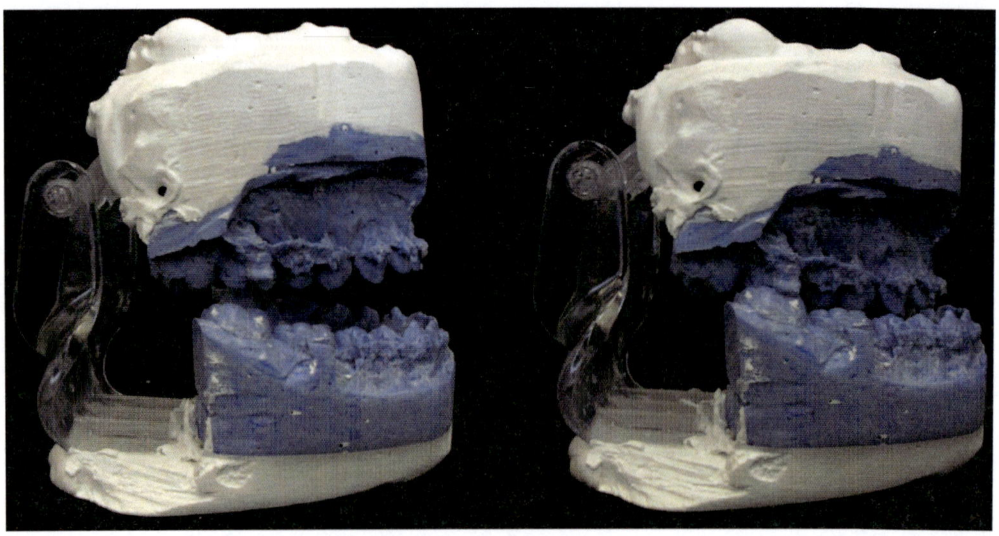

Fig. 27.19 A simple hinge articulator can be used for a single jaw surgery. It requires mounting the dental arches using plaster. The disadvantage is that it does not allow the surgeon to easily reposition the dental arches for model surgery. This illustrates the initial Class III dental model mounting

occlusal position. A final acrylic splint can be fabricated. However, much less laboratory time is needed if the surgeon has duplicate dental models to work with. One set can be used to be facebow mounted in a semi-adjustable articulator to fabricate the intermediate splint. Simultaneously, the remaining set can be used to make a final occlusal splint with a Galetti articulator. Thus, with two occlusal guides (acrylic splints), the planned VTO can be reproduced in the operating room.

In the situation where there is benefit to reposition the mandible first, then both the VTO and the mandibular dental model surgery are performed first so that the intermediate occlusal guide would match that of the operative sequence.

Caveat in 2D Cephalometric Planning and Plaster Model Surgery

Errors in cephalometric technique that include 3D projection of x-rays on to the 2D plane, accurate and consistent location of the landmarks, accuracy of prediction tracings (VTO), facebow recording errors, inaccurate prediction of the autorotation of the mandible, the difference in mandibular position in upright and supine patients, and inaccurate dental model surgery are possible causes of the inaccuracies of orthognathic surgery planning. Moreover many patients who need accurate surgical planning present with facial asymmetry in all three planes, and thus 2D analysis in the orthogonal planes, are difficult to integrate in the surgical planning with sufficient degree of confidence. While the facebow transfer provides some guidance, many of the patients will have auricular asymmetry, and the reference planes for the VTO must be decided based on clinical exam. With each step of the planning—from cephalometric analysis to dental

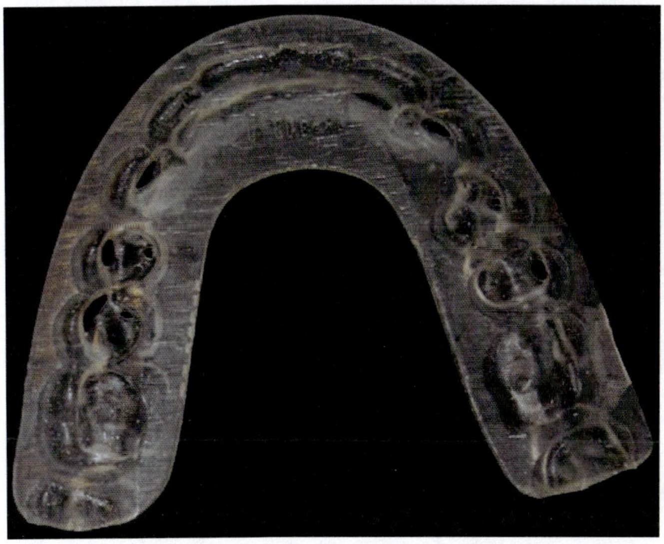

Fig. 27.20 An acrylic occlusal guide is fabricated using the articulator with the dental arches coordinated in the final position. This occlusal guide is used in the operating room to 'index' one jaw against the other

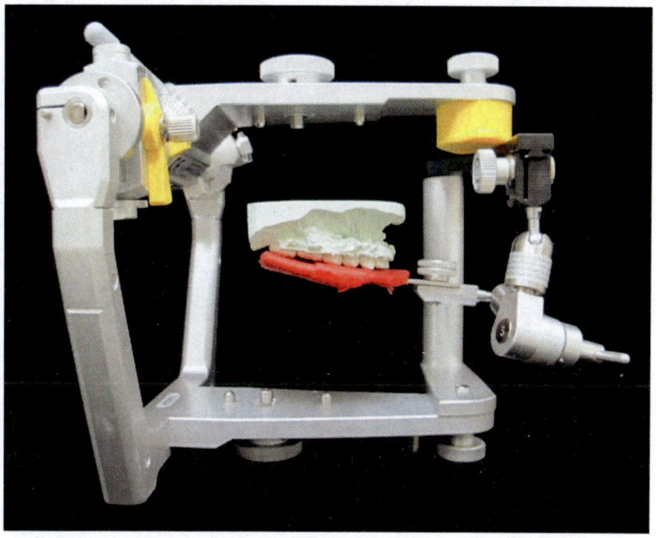

Fig. 27.21 A semi-adjustable articulator

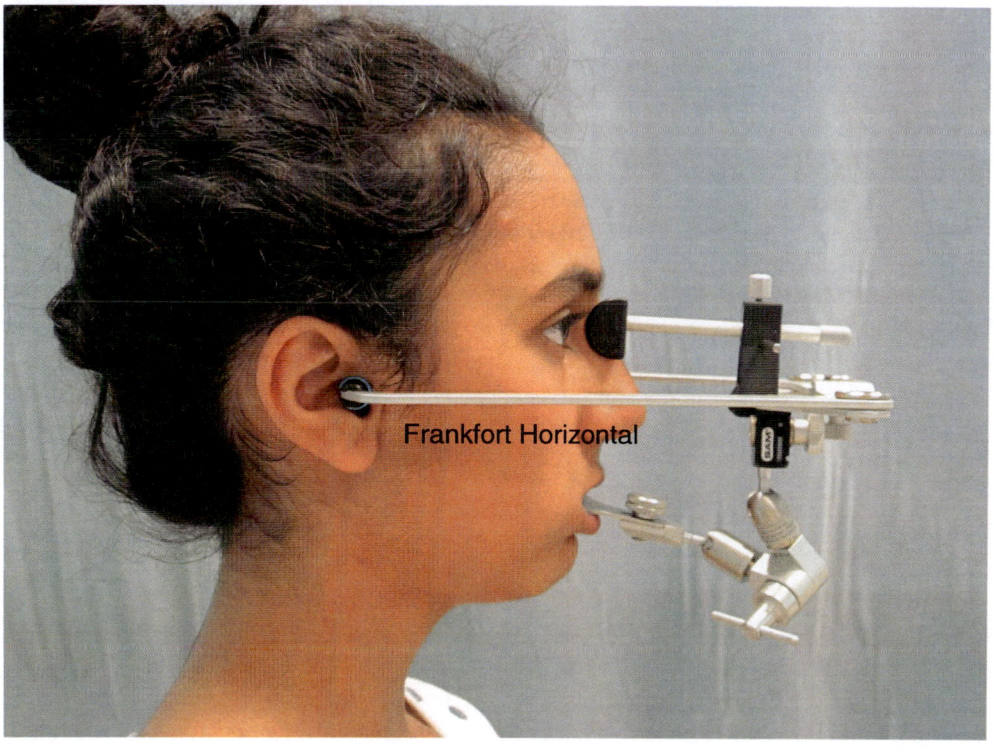

Fig. 27.22 Facebow transfer. This allows the surgeon to transfer the maxillary dental position relative to the Frankfort Horizontal to the semi-adjustable articulator in Fig. 27.21

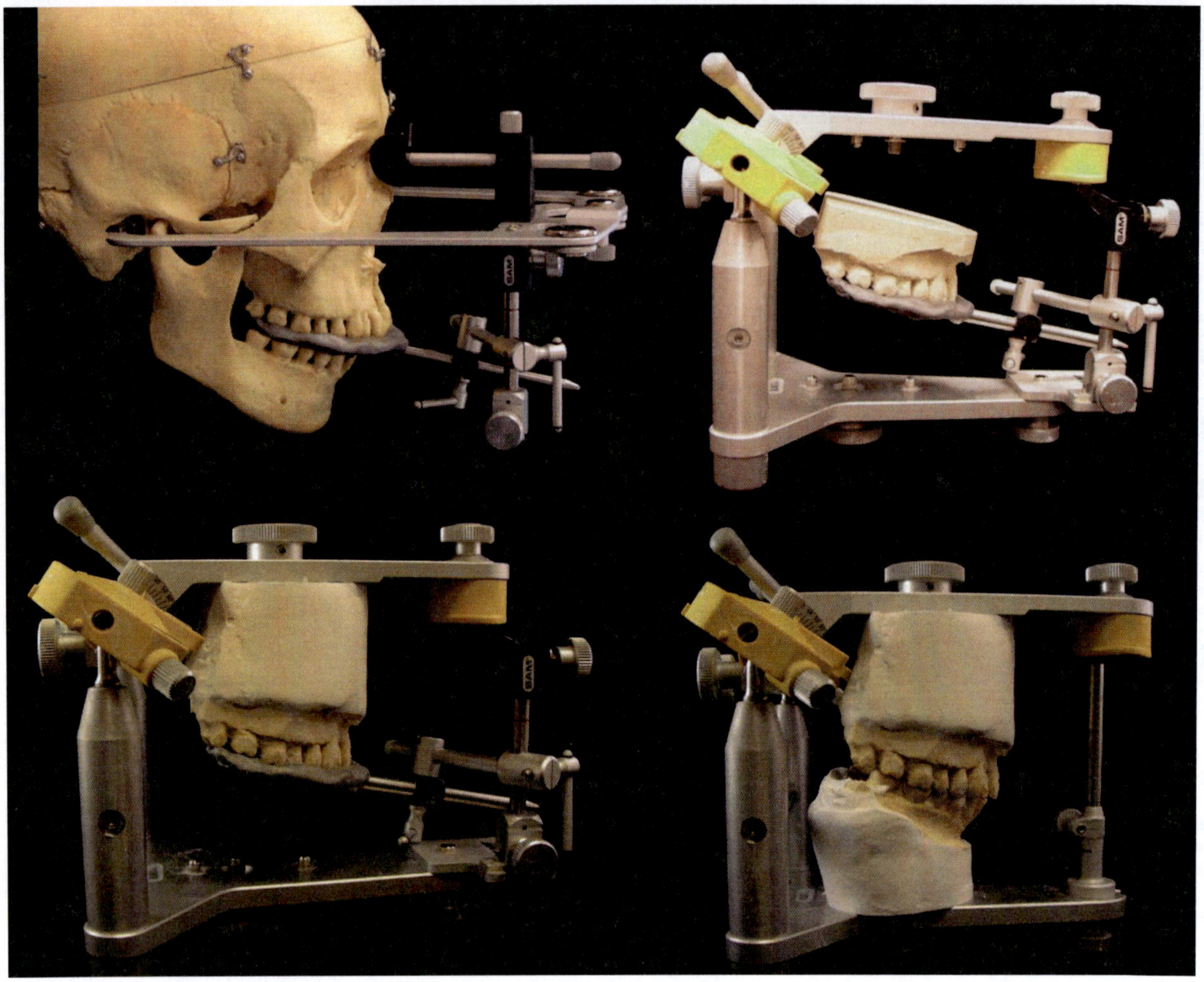

Fig. 27.23 This illustrates the mounting of the dental casts. *Top left* facebow registration; *Top right* facebow transfer; *Bottom left* mount maxilla; *Bottom right* mount mandible. The plaster mounted dental casts spatially positioned in the articulator simulate the true dental arches in the skull illustration

model surgery—the errors accumulate and are then built into the occlusal splint fabrication. Thus, the surgeon may find him or herself frequently in the operating room with an undesired clinical outcome. Ultimately, the surgeon must then eliminate the occlusal splint and rely on intraoperative clinical assessment to execute the surgery. Inaccurate surgical planning leads to inaccurate surgery. Surgical planning at best should be considered as a guide, and the final judgment of the planning is an intraoperative assessment that requires judgment from surgeon during the operation. Thus, conventional 2D orthognathic surgery planning is limited for all but the simplest cases in which there is an acceptable degree of symmetry and a single jaw movement is preferred.

While digital available software may eliminate many of the errors with hand tracing and measurements, the inherent limitation of the basis of the surgical planning in 2D radiographs remains. Moreover, the VTO using digital software and soft-tissue predictions treats all LeFort I osteotomies as the same as with conventional physical plaster-mounted models. There was no correlation of the surface skeletal anatomy, and thus the surgeon relied only on the spatial relationships of the dental arches. It is only with the ability of capturing the 3D surface facial skeletal anatomy with initially the conventional medical grade CT and more recently the lower radiation dosage cone beam CT scan that accurate surgical planning came within the reach of the surgeon.

Emerging 3D Image-Based Virtual Surgical Planning for Orthognathic Surgery

Overview

Since the 1990s, 3D CT imaging with reconstruction of stacked 2D-acquired data has become routinely available in the clinical setting. Compared with conventional 2D dentofacial cephalometric films, the 3D images provided considerably better visualization and detail of the morphology of the

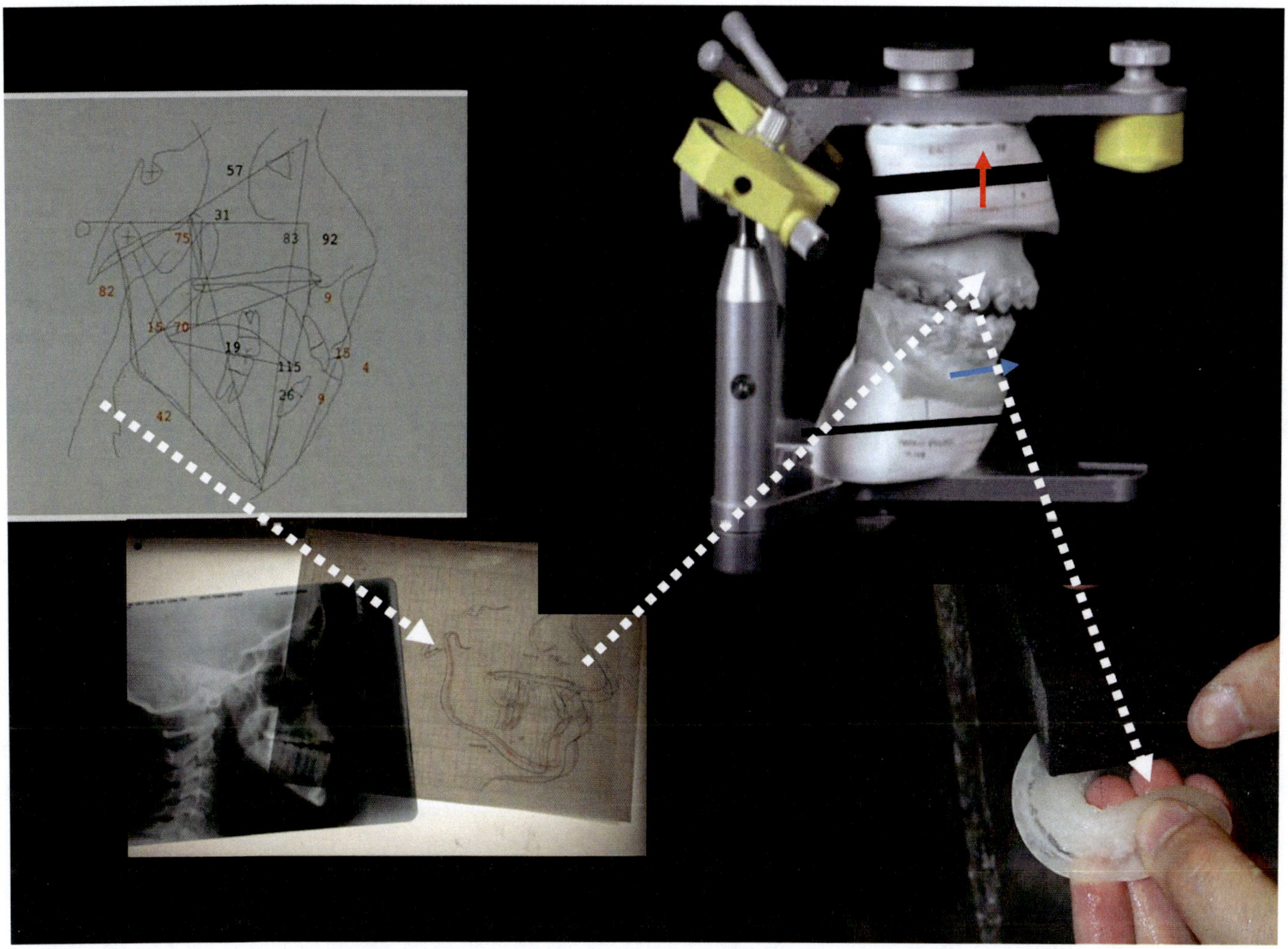

Fig. 27.24 The sequence of model surgery: from tracing, surgical simulation or VTO, model surgery to fabricating an occlusal splint

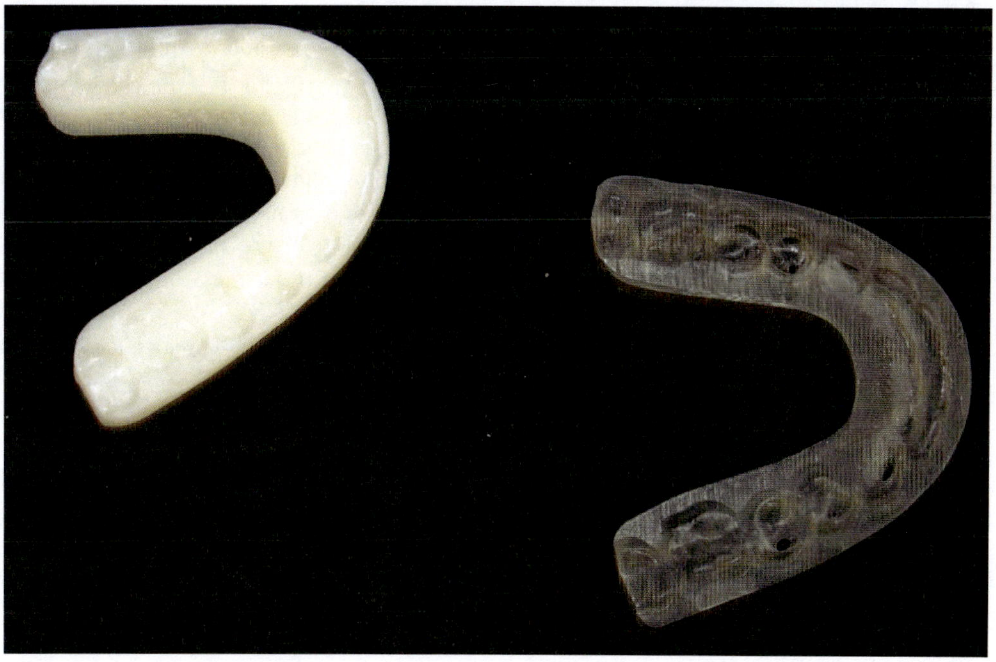

Fig. 27.25 The intermediate (*left*, white) and final (*right*, clear) splint fabrication

skeletal structure, the dental arches, and the overlying soft tissue. With the availability of 3D volumetric images, new tools were developed that allowed the surgeon to navigate away from the limitations of conventional 2D cephalometry.

In the last two decades, significant technical developments further enhanced the 3D medical imaging technology: multi-detector spiral CT scan with less capture times and with higher resolution, cone beam CT (CBCT) scan with significantly less radiation and the ability to capture the data in the natural head position of an upright patient, and 3D optical and laser surface image capture of the color and texture of the facial appearance within milliseconds.

Advances in both the computer hardware and software within the last decade enable interactive display of the data on personal computers, with the ability to selectively view soft tissue or skeletal hard tissues from any angle as cross-sectional images and 3D surface planes. Recent developments in the 3D medical image analysis software make it possible to build accurate 3D patient-specific virtual anatomical models from the high-resolution medical images including CT and CBCT scans. Both in plane and in 3D, measurement tools allow clinicians to extract useful information conveniently. The anatomic landmarks can now be more accurately located without the averaging of a 3D projection on to a 2D cephalometric radiograph. Cephalometric analysis no longer needed to be confined to the midsagittal plane. Analysis can now be performed in 3D to allow the surgeon and the orthodontist to address asymmetry in all three planes.

Today software for virtual surgical planning (VSP) is capable of simulating surgical procedures with ever-increasing user applicability: from the imaging research lab to routine daily clinical application. The facial skeleton is treated as a solid 3D object in virtual space that can be digitally manipulated. Osteotomy planes can be defined, and the 3D facial skeletal object can be digitally sectioned into two separate solid objects, where each can now be moved independent of the other. The software treats the CT data set as solid objects on which Boolean algebra can be performed. Thus, 3D visual objects can be added and subtracted digitally. The registration and superimposition technique makes it possible to build a composite model based upon both volumetric information from CT/CBCT scan and surface information of the dentition from laser or optical scans with greater clinical accuracy that can be integrated. Surgical planning can now be performed in 3D space instead of in planar projection 2D cephalometric films. The complex facial skeletal asymmetries can be addressed. Moreover the conventional inaccuracies and the time-consuming laboratory process of facebow transfer, plaster mounting of dental casts, sectioning, repositioning, and remounting of the dental casts are all eliminated. The surgeon now has the ability to easily execute various surgical options to optimize outcome. 3D anthropometric analysis is available to the surgeon and the orthodontist dynamically as the skeletal segments are manipulated. Regions of interference during the skeletal movement can be assessed and detected (such as with maxillary impaction and mandibular rotation cases), the dental roots can be visualized within a skeletal framework for interdental osteotomies, and the course of the inferior alveolar nerve can be visualized for mandibular osteotomies.

While 3D VSP is increasingly becoming the new standard in the surgical planning, the real breakthrough is transferring the virtual surgical plan to the operating room. For this, the VSP technology has been integrated with established CAD/CAM technology with state-of-the-art additive manufacturing technologies, such as stereolithography (STL), 3D printing, and electronic beam melting (EBM). Virtual surgical planning integrated with CAD/CAM system is capable to design and fabricate patient- and procedure-specific physical instruments, osteotomy guides, various templates, and intermediate and final occlusal guidance or splints. The traditional location-specific dental laboratory for orthognathic surgery is being transformed to a digital lab that is accessible at any location where Internet access gives the surgeon the software tools to plan the procedure.

However, current limitations of the technology at this writing include the difficulty for the surgeon who is used to the tactile sense of physically manipulating solid stone dental models. Without the physical tactile sense, virtual manipulation digital dental models and the skeletal elements as in a solid 3D model are difficult to assess the collision. Many surgeons used to the conventional plaster model surgery will continue to rely on the final surgical splint to be fabricated from the physical stone models because of the lack of confidence in the collision detection software and the lack of tactile haptic feedback to the surgeon with the currently available software. There is an acceptable tolerance limit to the fabrication of digital occlusal splints for the intermediate position in a two-jaw surgery but not necessarily acceptable for the final occlusion. Additionally there is reluctance on many surgeons with multi-segmental maxillary surgery that is planned virtually without the surgeon physically sectioning and repositioning the dental arches in a lab. An additional limitation is the predictive 3D soft-tissue algorithms for the skeletal surgery. Unlike the half century of 2D soft-tissue data for which predictive algorithms had been worked out with the available vast amount of experience, the 3D soft-tissue data is lacking and remains a topic of research for the future with increasing accumulation of such data. It would be expected that soft-tissue predictive algorithms will be improved over time.

Our current protocol is described as follows:

1. Clinical examination and 3D data acquisition
2. Building a composite 3D virtual model
3. Quantification of the deformity via 3D anthropometric analysis
4. Interactive surgical simulation including osteotomy and repositioning

5. Soft-tissue prediction and 3D visual treatment objective (VTO)
6. Design of the virtual occlusal guide, or splint
7. Delivery of the surgical plan to the operating room

Clinical Examination and 3D Data Acquisition

As with conventional orthognathic surgery planning, thorough physical examination and clinical anthropometric measurements are essential in the decision-making process involved in the planning. It must always be remembered that technology, no matter how advanced, can never be a substitute for a surgeon's clinical examination and judgment. The outcome rests on this foundation. Clinical examination is the only way to obtain information regarding the patient, the quality of the tissues, and their dynamic deformation with function (oral, airway, speech, smile, and facial expression). This is essential to guide the process of the VSP accurately, efficiently, and economically. During the physical examination, critical areas of concern should be head orientation (natural head position, or NHP), the occlusion (centric relation, centric occlusion, and habitual occlusion), dynamics of the smile, and temporomandibular joint motion. This dynamic information is critical as the planning is based on static CT images that displays on a 2D screen from which alone the surgeon does not have depth perception. In addition to the above clinical data, there are three additional components needed for VSP: the cone beam CT data (CBCT), 3D photos, and the 3D dental casts.

3D VSP begins with acquiring CBCT scan in a consistent manner as a replacement for the conventional 2D radiographs. The patient is positioned sitting upright in the natural head position as depicted in Fig. 27.26. The patient is asked to close his/her eyes at time of the scan to reduce motion artifact. For the currently available CBCT scanner, the largest field of view needs to be employed so as to include the full face from inferior to the chin to the mid-head forehead. The patient should be in a centric relationship with the condyles positioned within the glenoid fossa. A thin bite wafer may be utilized to help the patient maintain centric relation at the time of the scan. The scan protocol should be 0.3 × 0.3 mm × 0.3 mm voxel mm with a field of view of 22 cm (minimum) in height.

3D surface color and texture images (3D photos) are taken in the NHP, as shown in Fig. 27.27. In addition to the neutral or relaxed facial expression, other facial expressions can be taken such as (1) eye closed, (to match the CBCT scan for fusion), (2) smiling (to document the dental display then), (3) lip repose and smile (to document the soft tissue), (4) mouth open (to document the oro-motor function), among others.

The stone dental casts are digitized using a laser scanner to document the upper and lower dental arches and the interdental arch relationship. Alternatively the dentition can be scanned in vivo using an optical scanner without the need for stone casts. It should be noted that CBCT scan cannot be utilized accurately for the dental arches because of the artifact from the orthodontic appliances.

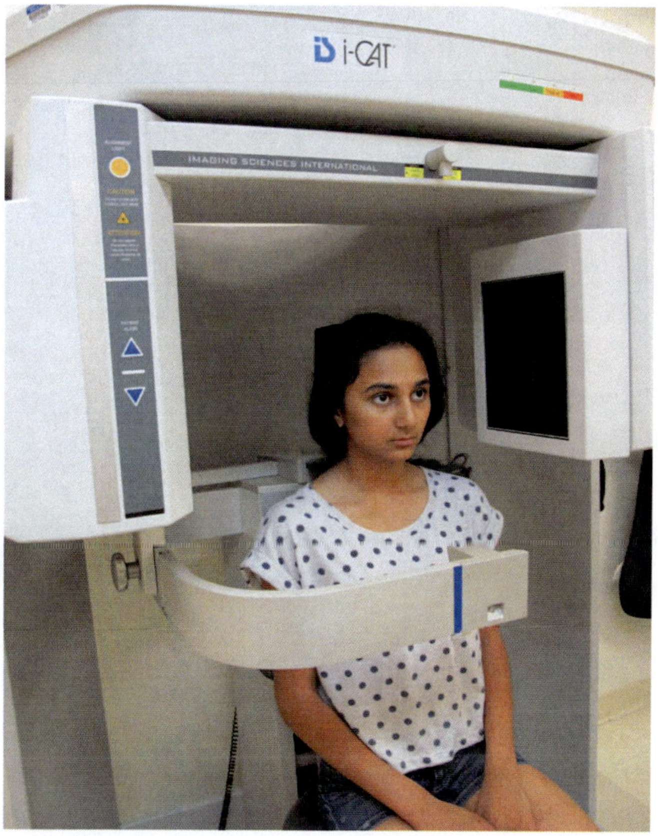

Fig. 27.26 Cone beam computerized tomography (CBCT) acquisition using iCAT Next Generation system (Imaging Sciences International, Hatfield, PA). The extended view is necessary to capture the largest field of view for maxillofacial/orthognathic surgery. The patient is in a upright position unlike the recumbent positioning in medical CT scans

The acquired 3D images are viewed using visualization software that can range from a limited viewer to the full capability of allowing the surgeon and orthodontist to manipulate the data set for planning. However, any 3D images used for virtual surgical planning must maintain the original resolution and accuracy without artificial manipulation and compression of the data. In addition, it is critical that the image data files are in a proper format. The CBCT data must be in uncompressed DICOM (Digital Imaging and Communications in Medicine) format, the 3D surface image photos must be in obj format (object) and the conventional jpg or bmp format, and the scanned dental arches in stl (stereolithography) or obj format.

Building a Composite Model

A composite digital 3D facial skeletal model is required for accurate virtual surgical planning. This requires building a

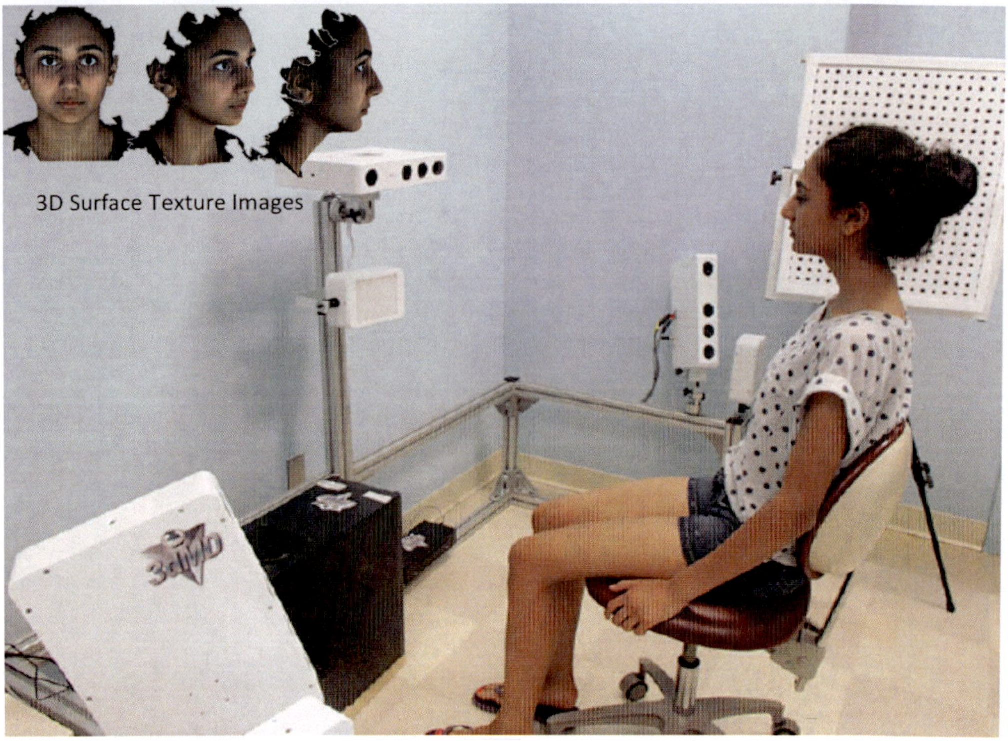

Fig. 27.27 3D surface color and texture image acquisition using 3dMd Trio system (3dMD, Atlanta, GA)

composite model of the acquired 3D data sets described in the previous section: the CBCT, the 3D photos, and the 3D dental arches.

We begin with importing the CBCT scan into the virtual surgical planning (VSP) software. We then segment the anatomical structures. This involves outlining the shape of structures visible in the cross sections of a volumetric data set. Based upon the Hounsfield unit and anatomical characteristics of the CBCT, hard and soft tissues are separated. Anatomical components such as skull, mandible, soft tissue, nerve canal, and the airway are structurally defined as independent elements. The dental arches with their artifact caused by the braces are subtracted because of the inaccuracy.

We now fuse the more accurate digital dental models with the above-segmented 3D CBCT model without the dental arches. The two separate digital data sets, the digital dental models and the 3D CT, are merged with or without fiducial markers (common reference points) depending upon the capabilities of the superimposition software and skill of the technician.

To provide a more realistic facial appearance with color and texture, lacking in CBCT scan, 3D photos are now mapped onto the surface of the above CBCT with fused dental casts.

Thus, a patient-specific 3D composite model is built, as shown in Fig. 27.28. This virtual model displays an accurate rendition of the patient for VSP.

Anthropometric Analysis

3D anthropometry, or 3D anthropometric analysis, is the extension of the conventional 2D cephalometric analysis using 3D digital model based upon the 3D medical images (CBCT/CT) with life-size scale (1:1). It uses anatomical landmarks and linear and angular measurements but in 3D space. The analysis extends to cross-sectional and longitudinal comparison of 3D distances, linear projections, orthogonal measurements, the surface distances, surface area, and volume of anatomical elements.

Although the anthropometric analysis can be performed in an internal coordinate system, it is convenient to align the internal coordinate system to an external system that is conventionally used in clinics by both orthodontists and surgeons. This process starts with the reorientation of the 3D composite model to the natural head position (NHP).

Ideally, the 3D model aligns with the external coordinate system and positioned in a reference coordinate system: the Frankfort Horizontal plane is parallel to the horizontal plane (X-Y plane), the midsagittal plane is parallel with the vertical plane (*X-Z* plane), and sella (or another specific landmark such as soft-tissue nasion) is set as the origin. While the *X*-axis is defined as from posterior to anterior direction, *Z*-axis from bottom to the top, the *Y*-axis is defined from right to the left to following the right-hand rule. The deviation of the NHP from the ideal alignment is quantified as (1) roll, the

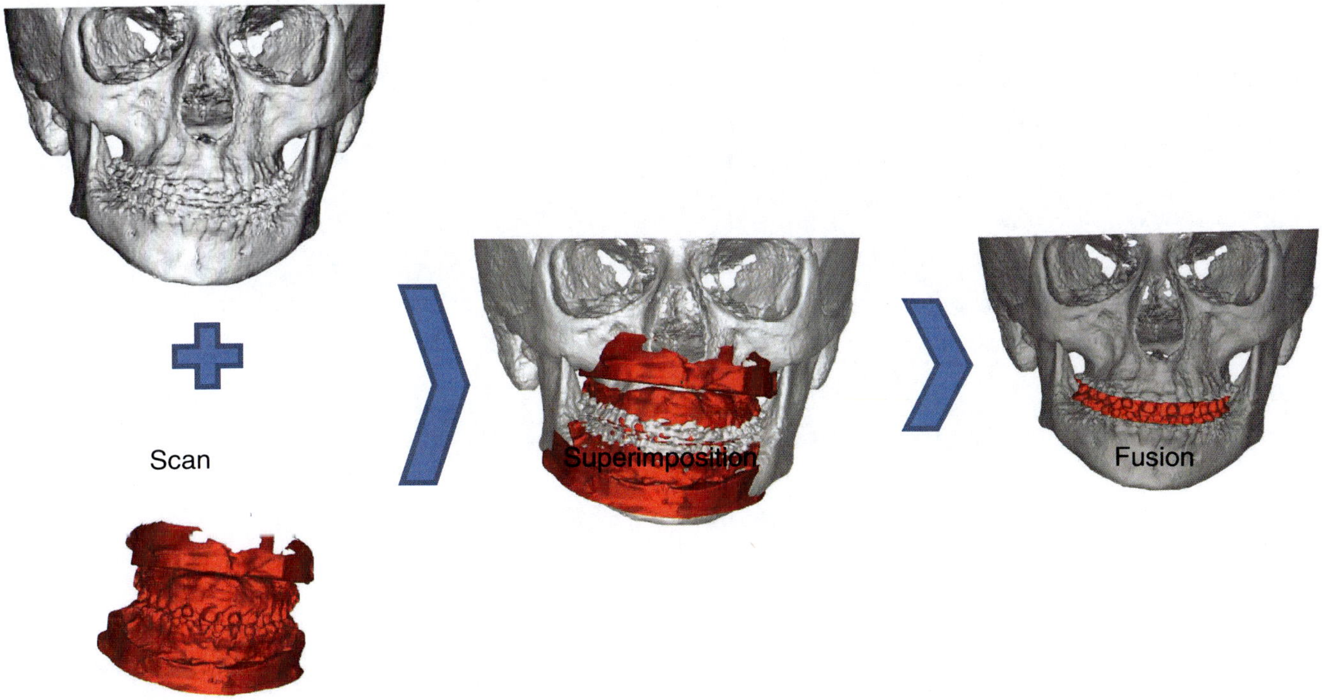

Fig. 27.28 Built the composite model that consists of skull from CBCT and teeth from laser scan of the dental casts

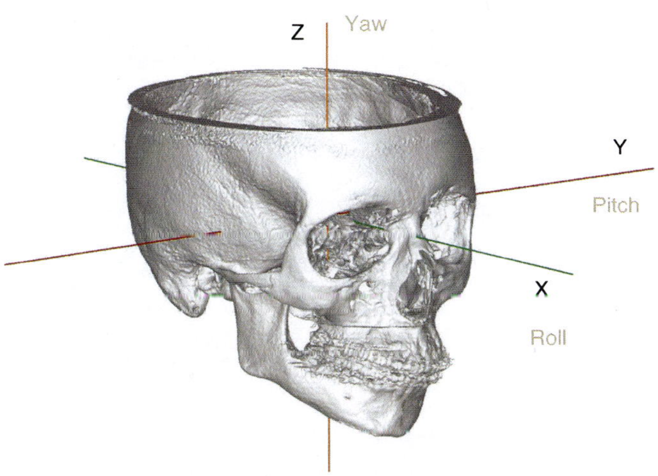

Fig. 27.29 Internal Cartesian coordinate system: origin at Sella. Roll-rotation around *X*-axis, Pitch-rotation around *Y*-axis, and Yaw-rotation around *Z*-axis

rotation around the *X*-axis; (2) pitch, the rotation around the *Y*-axis; and (3) yaw, the rotation around the *Z*-axis. Such deviations can be measured and applied in the model reorientation. These definitions are illustrated in Fig. 27.29.

Once the composite model is positioned in the 3D reference system, anatomical landmarks are selected, and the desired analysis is performed. Accurate identification of landmarks requires anatomic knowledge and experience in landmark definition. Landmarks at the cranial base, foramina, canals, and sutures are used. Well-defined landmarks in 2D cephalometric x-rays, as introduced in previous sections, can be employed. However, caution needs to be made with the following considerations:

1. Some landmarks (e.g., anterior nasal spine or ANS) are easier to identify, whereas others (e.g., sella or S) more difficult. Multi-view technique that includes both 3D and 2D views is needed to accurately identify a landmark.
2. Bilateral landmarks, such as porion (Po), orbitale (Or), and gonion (Go), are separated as individual landmarks (left, right). This allows for a more accurate assessment of the asymmetries involved when planning the surgical correction.
3. Many landmarks have to be redefined (e.g., pogonion) based upon 3D anatomical features instead of characteristics in projected 2D x-ray.
4. Some conventional 2D landmarks disappeared, while new 3D landmarks (e.g., posterior maxillary point) have to be defined.

From the 3D anatomical model that aligned with certain external coordinate system, it is possible to regenerate 2D virtual cephalogram that is comparable with the conventional 2D cephalogram.

When a landmark is indicated on the 2D cephalogram image generated from CT scan, the point should be positioned

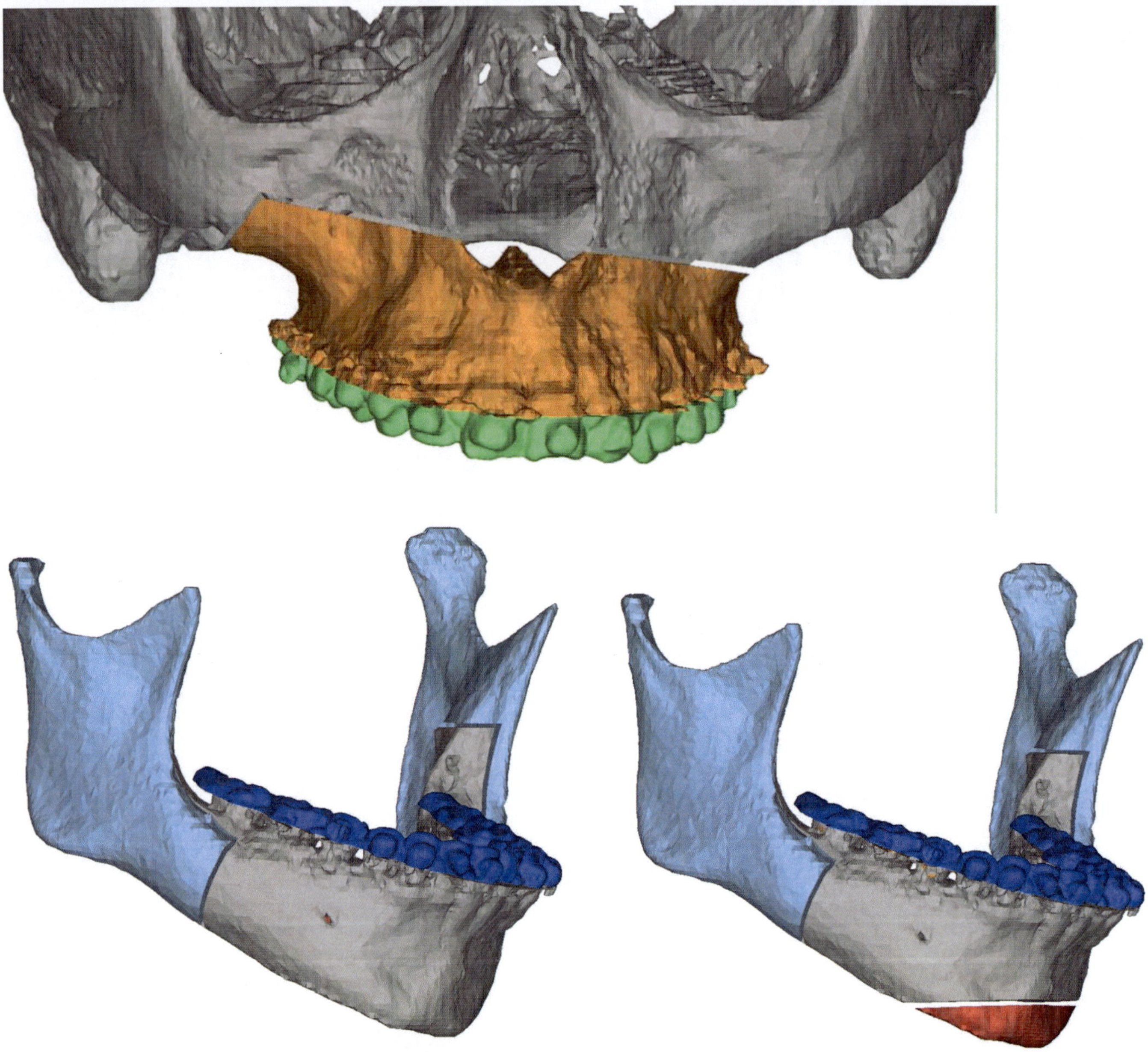

Fig. 27.30 Simulation of an asymmetric modified LeFort, BSSO and genioplasty

on the bone surface in 3D space. Therefore, the geometrical relationship between cephalogram and CT image volume is a prerequisite if one is to benefit from the combination of CT and virtual cephalograms. This combination of 2D and 3D information is the key to accurate indication of landmarks in a repeatable way and, to larger extense, in consistent with conventional cephalometric analysis.

This virtual 2D cephalogram and corresponding 2D measurements (actually the projection of the 3D measurements on the mid sagittal plane) can be used to compare with conventional 2D cephalometric analysis data, which many clinicians are more familiar with.

The symmetric analysis, in addition to the mirror image, is generally performed first to identify and quantify the asymmetry. Additional reference points and measurements are also defined and identified based upon the procedure to be simulated.

Surgical Simulation: Osteotomy and Reposition

The osteotomy is simulated via separation of the bone defined as an object using various cutting tools from free form to pre-setup tools such as sagittal split tool. Nearly any type of osteotomy can be simulated that is tailored to the patient's deformity. Figure 27.30 demonstrates the simulated Le Fort osteotomy, BSSO, and genioplasty.

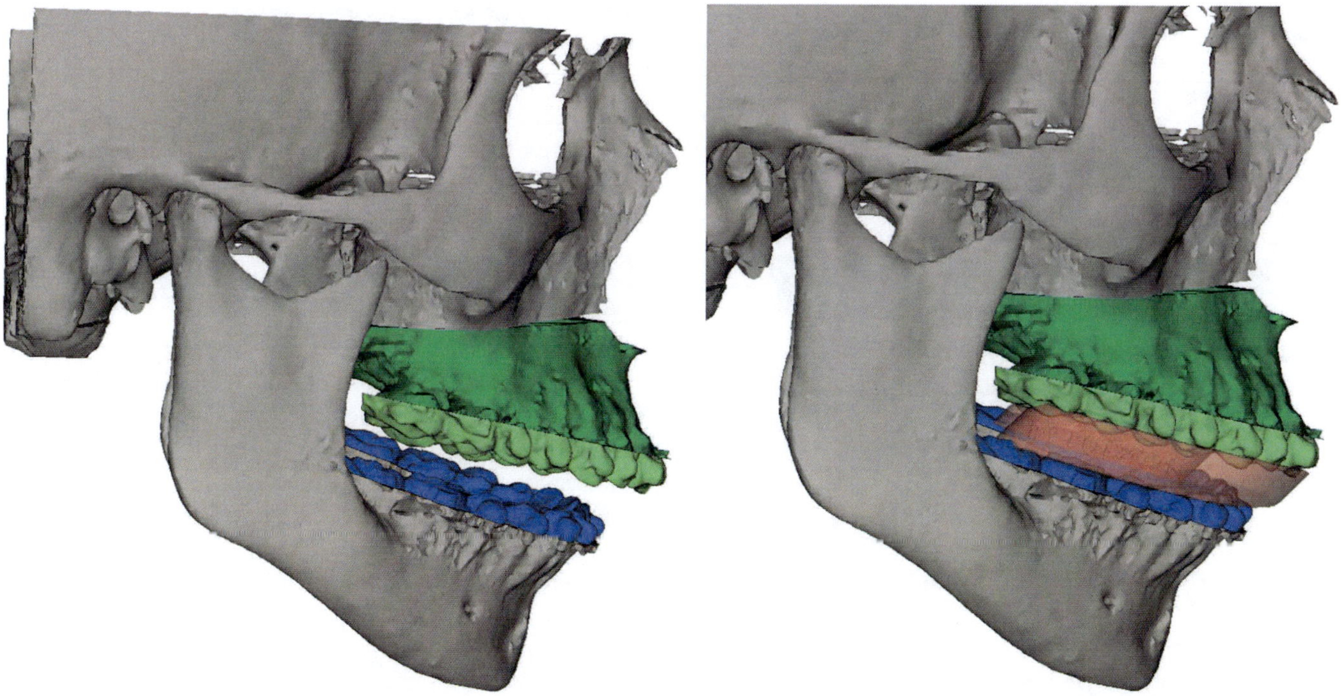

Fig. 27.31 Intermediate position and the intermediate splint after maxillary reposition

After the facial skeleton is virtually sectioned, the user can reposition the various bony elements to their desired position. The user has the ability to reposition each element with six degrees of freedom: three translations and three rotations. The available software has the ability to detect interferences with the bony movements which does not prevent collision but provides feedback to the surgeon as an alert. The anthropometric analysis is calculated dynamically, and the user is given feedback with comparison to available normative data. The user then has the ability to revise the surgical plan in terms of redefining the osteotomies and the repositioning to achieve the desired outcome.

In patients requiring both maxillary and mandibular surgery, the maxillary movement is usually simulated first. The level of the osteotomy is first tailored to the patient's deformity and may be asymmetric so that the final position is optimally symmetrical. The maxilla is then repositioned to correct rotational asymmetry by correcting the roll (cant), then lateral translation to align the upper dental midline with facial midline. With the dental midline as the center of rotation, the yaw is then corrected. We then correct the anterior–posterior (sagittal plane) discrepancy to the desired midfacial projection (SNA or maxillary depth) and the midfacial vertical height based on the desired dental display. We then correct the pitch (occlusal plan angle) to optimize the incisor inclination for upper lip support and smile dynamics described above. With the maxilla in the desired and final position, this defines the intermediate surgical position in which the upper jaw surgery is completed and the lower jaw surgery remains to be executed. The intermediate surgical occlusal guide is then virtually defined, as shown in Fig. 27.31.

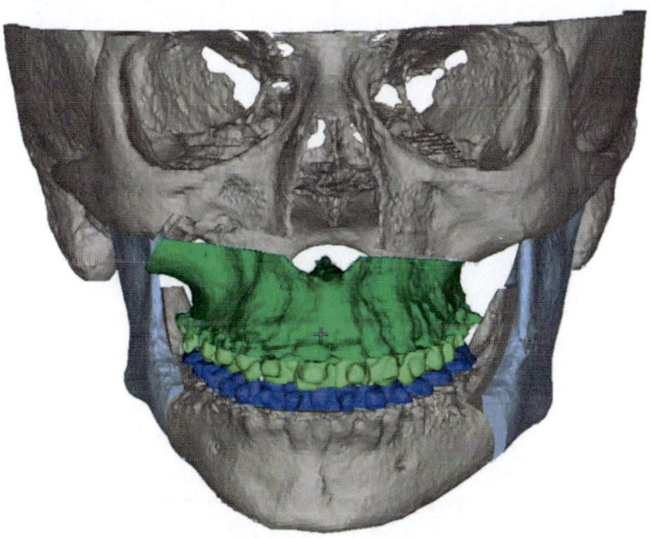

Fig. 27.32 Predicted spatial position of the skeletal components as a consequence of the double jaw surgery

Mandibular osteotomies are then made virtually and the mandible repositioned using the maxillary dental arch as its reference in 3D space. The relationships between the proximal ramal and distal body segments are assessed. This may require repositioning to minimize the interferences and may require redesigning the ramal osteotomies. Once the mandible is in the final position, a final surgical occlusal guide is virtually defined, as shown in Fig. 27.32. Finally an osseous genioplasty can be virtually performed, as shown in Fig. 27.33.

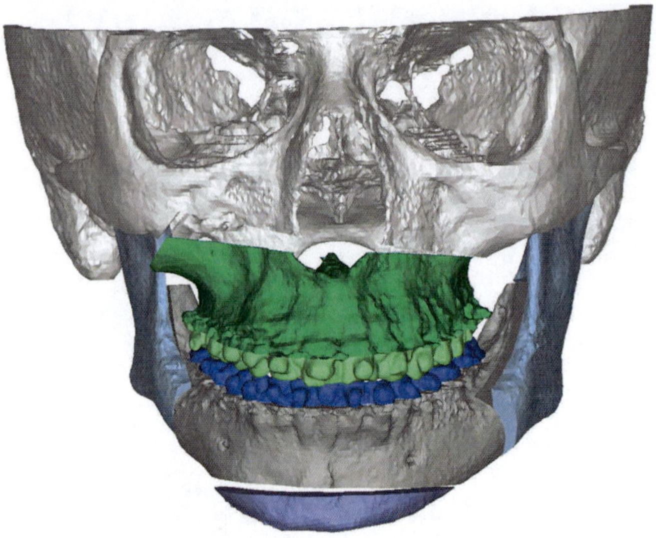

Fig. 27.33 Simulation of the genioplasty together with maxillary and mandibular repositioning

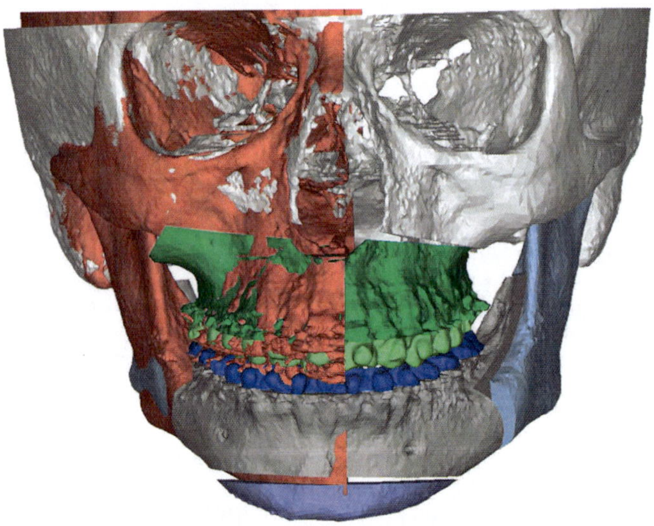

Fig. 27.34 Mirror function of the simulation that allows the surgeon to reposition various skeletal components

In some instances, the repositioning of the osteotomized segments is not sufficient to recreate facial symmetry since the skeletal structure differs in size, shape, and volume. The mirror imaging tool can assist the surgeon to improve the facial symmetry. With this tool, one half of the face is selected, copied, mirror-imaged, and superimposed on the contralateral side, as shown in Fig. 27.34. The differences between the two sides can be calculated using a Boolean operation in volumes, surfaces, and dimensions. Based on this information, the surgeon may decide to add volume (grafting), remove volume (ostectomy), or adjust the position of the segments (camouflage).

Simulation of Soft-Tissue Response

Eventually, the outcome will be evaluated by the facial appearance. Therefore, the prediction of the soft-tissue response to the dental-skeletal movement is important. Soft-tissue simulation can be performed to predict the outcomes of the surgical procedure (Fig. 27.34). However, the reliability of the soft-tissue prediction remains to be evaluated, and there is insufficient accumulation of data to refine the algorithms at this evolutionary stage.

Under such circumstances, the 3D virtual treatment objectives (3D VTO) are presented in the following aspects:

1. Visualization of the reconstructed dental-skeletal structure in 3D space
2. Anthropometric analysis that includes necessary 3D measurements and their projection to the midsagittal plane that can be used to compare with existing 2D cephalometric analysis data
3. The movements of each segments
4. Simulated soft-tissue response to the dental-skeletal reconstruction with the superimposition of soft-tissue images or 3D photo over the skeletal framework

Each surgical plan should be evaluated in all aforementioned aspects.

In general, the 3D VTO can be approached through multiple surgical options. With multiple copies of the 3D composite model conveniently available without additional cost, various options can be and should be explored, simulated, and compared. Consequently, their outcomes can be assessed and compared virtually. Eventually, a treatment option with optimal outcome can be approached.

Transfer Virtual Surgical Plan to the Operating Room

After the surgical plan is finalized, it is necessary to transfer the plan to the patient at the time of the surgery. Surgical occlusal guides or surgical templates can be created for this purpose. Surgical occlusal guides are used to reposition the dentate bony segments, while surgical templates are used to reposition skeletal components.

Both intermediate and final surgical occlusal guides can be defined virtually based upon the 3D VTO from the VSP. The guides are created by a Boolean operation which generates a digital wafer between the maxillary and mandibular dental arches. The surgical templates record the 3D surface geometry of the area of interest so that they fit on the bone in an unique position. These digital constructs are then exported to a CAD object and fabricated using a rapid prototyping machine with additive manufacture technology such as acrylic-based stereolithography (Fig. 27.35).

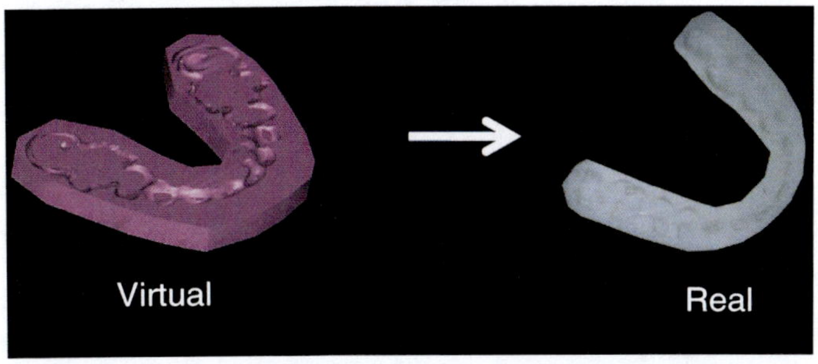

Fig. 27.35 The virtual splint (*left*) can then be printed (*right*)

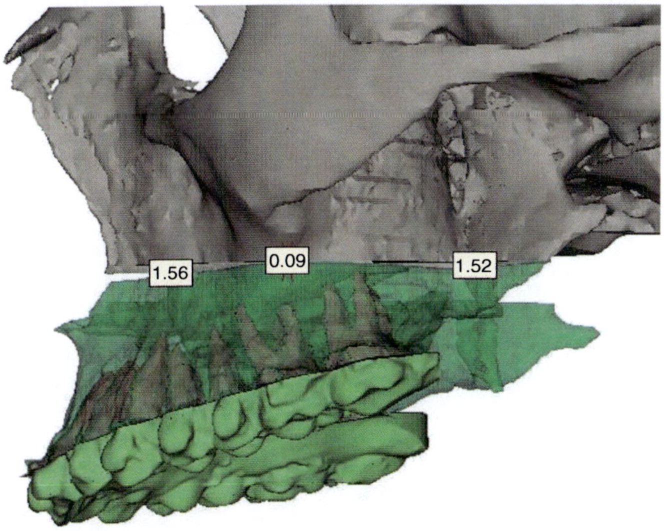

Fig. 27.36 Prediction of the bony interference on the posterior aspect of the maxilla that must be resected. While the anterior gap of 1.56 mm is acceptable, the gap of 0.09 mm in the middle and 1.52 mm overlap in the posterior portion requires resection

What are then available to the surgeon are the surgical guides which translate the virtual VTO to the physical intra-operative guide. In addition the 3D nature of the surgical simulation provides the surgeon with critical information. This may include the depth of the lateral nasal wall for the osteotomy, the anatomy of the pterygoid region, the dental roots, and the nerve canal. In addition the virtual simulation would provide information to the surgeon areas of bony interferences with maxillary impaction and with mandibular setback and rotation (Figs. 27.36 and 27.37).

Moreover, the surgical simulation can be accessed remotely in both the clinical site and the operating room via a hospital-wide network or the Internet. This implementation allows the surgical planning to be conducted in a team conference with the attendance of surgeons, orthodontists, and other clinicians in the clinic sites or each of the individuals at different locations.

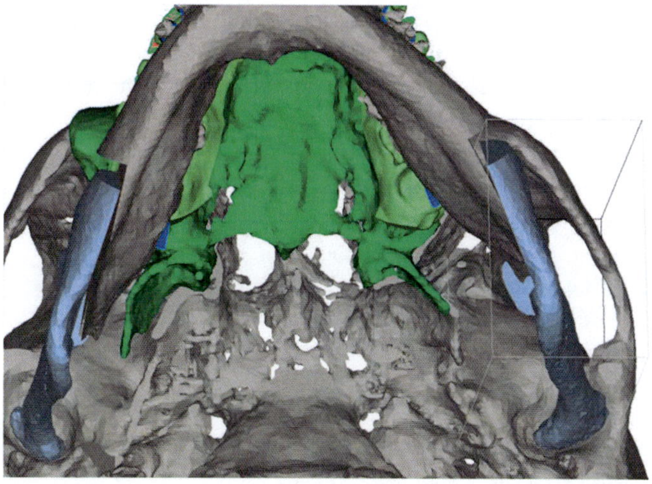

Fig. 27.37 Simulation of the lateral rotate of the ramus to avoid the bony interference. left ramus is highlighted and rotated clockwise with regard to the left condyle hinge point, resulting in displacement of the left ramus

Summary

3D volumetric imaging allows accurate visualization of the morphologic deformity, planning the surgical approach, and evaluating the response not visualized previously with 2D dentofacial records and surgical planning. Virtual surgical planning replaces the conventional 2D cephalometric planning and plaster cast model surgery. 3D craniofacial imaging requires application of various techniques from applied mathematics, computer sciences, and bioengineering to additive manufacturing. 3D virtual surgical planning accurately simulates the operative experience for surgical planning, with predictable morphologic outcomes. Technological evolution will overcome current limitation as a generation of surgeons will be brought up with digital planning as comfortable as the previous and current generations of surgeons with plaster models and conventional model surgery.

Appendix

2D Cephalometric Analysis

A cephalogram (cephalometric x-ray) is a two-dimensional projection of the skull/face. The film is taken in a *cephalostat*, which is a specialized x-ray unit that captures the skull/facial skeleton and soft-tissue profile in a reproducible and standard manner. This allows comparison with time in the same individual and comparison to a population. Anterior–posterior cephalometric x-ray may also be needed to evaluate asymmetry.

Various *cephalometric analyses* exist to describe the craniofacial complex. No analysis is considered superior to another. Most analyses rely on the relatively stable elements in the cranial base to serve as *reference points* and *planes* by which to measure the facial structures relative to the reference structures. Important elements in cephalometric analyses are:

1. Maxillary position relative to the cranial base
2. Mandibular position relative to the cranial base
3. Maxillary position relative to the mandibular position
4. Chin position relative to the cranial base
5. Chin position relative to the mandible
6. Facial proportions/vertical relationships
7. Incisor positions (maxillary and mandibular)

Based on the above, the surgeon and orthodontist can determine the degree of deviation of the dentofacial skeleton from normative data and can serve as a guide to reposition the skeletal bases and the dentition to defined goals.

Performing a cephalometric analysis requires you to trace the x-ray onto a piece of frosted acetate with a pencil. Capturing necessary details in the cranial base, maxilla, mandible, dentition, and soft tissue allows you to measure the various elements. Accurate tracings may also be superimposed on subsequent or previous films to reveal growth or treatment changes.

How to Trace a Cephalogram

Step 1. Trace the cranial base, nasal bones, orbital rims, and porion.

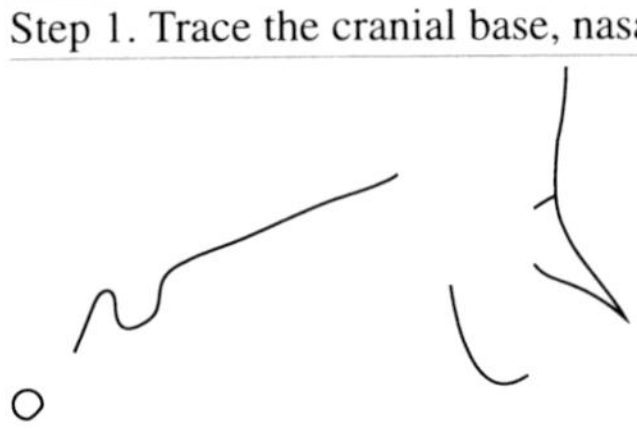

Step 2. Add the maxilla and dentition.

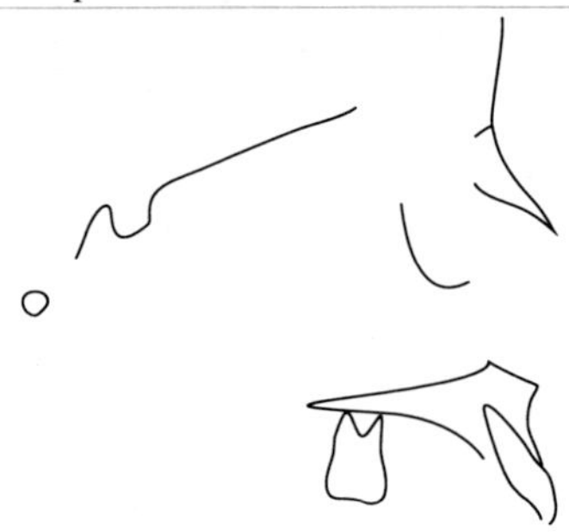

Step 3. Trace the mandible and dentition.

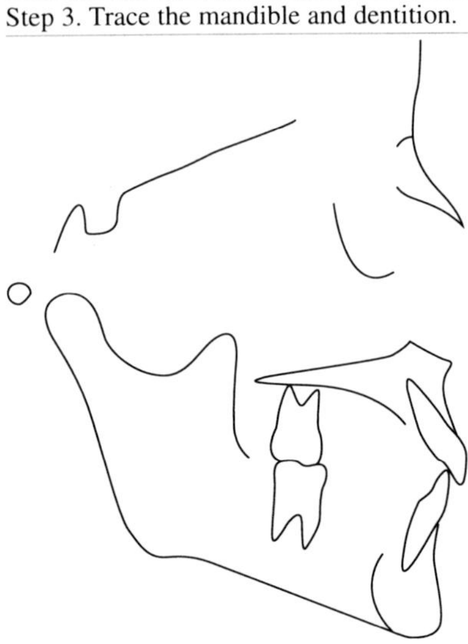

Step 4. Trace the soft-tissue profile.

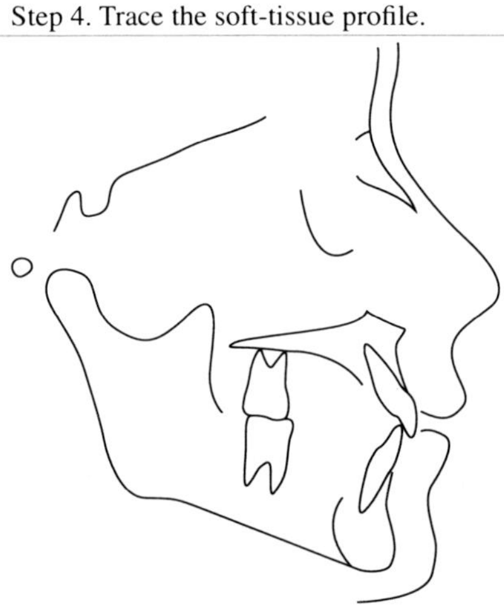

Identify Skeletal Anatomic Landmarks

1. Sella (S): The geometric center of the hypophyseal fossa (sella turcica).
2. Nasion (N): The junction of the nasal and frontal bones at the most posterior point on the curvature of the bridge of the nose.
3. Orbitale (Or): A point midway between the lowest point on the inferior margin of the two orbits.
4. Porion (Po): The midpoint of the upper contour of the external auditory canal (anatomic porion) *or* a point midway between the top of the image of the left and right ear rods of the cephalostat (machine porion).
5. Anterior nasal spine (ANS): The most anterior point on the maxilla at the nasal base.
6. A point (A): An arbitrary measure point on the innermost curvature from the maxillary anterior nasal spine to the crest of the maxillary alveolar process. A point is the most anterior point of the maxillary apical base.
7. Posterior nasal spine (PNS): The tip of the posterior nasal spine of the palatine bone, at the junction of the soft and hard palate.
8. B point (B): An arbitrary measure point on the anterior bony curvature of the mandible. B point is the innermost curvature from chin to alveolar junction.
9. Pogonion (Pg): The most anterior point on the contour of the chin.
10. Menton (Me): The lowest point on the symphysis of the mandible.
11. Gonion (Go): The point midway between the points representing the middle of the curvature at the left and right angles of the mandible.
12. Co (Co): The geometric center of the condyle (rotation).

Identify Soft-Tissue Anatomic Landmarks

1. Glabella (G): The most prominent point in the midsagittal plane of the forehead
2. Nasion (N): The deepest point at the bridge of the nose
3. Columella point (Cm): The most anterior point on the columella of the nose
4. Subnasale (Sn): The point at the junction of the columella and the upper lip
5. Labrale superius (Ls): The vermilion–cutaneous junction of the upper lip
6. Stomion superius (Stms): The lowermost point on the vermilion of the upper lip
7. Stomion inferius (Stmi): The uppermost point on the vermilion of the lower lip
8. Labrale inferius (Li): The vermilion–cutaneous junction of the lower lip
9. Labial-mental sulcus (S): The deepest point between the Li and Pg
10. Pogonion (Pg): The most anterior point of the chin soft tissue
11. Menton (Me): The lowest point on the contour of the chin

How to Trace a Cephalogram

Step 6. Identify the skeletal anatomic landmarks.

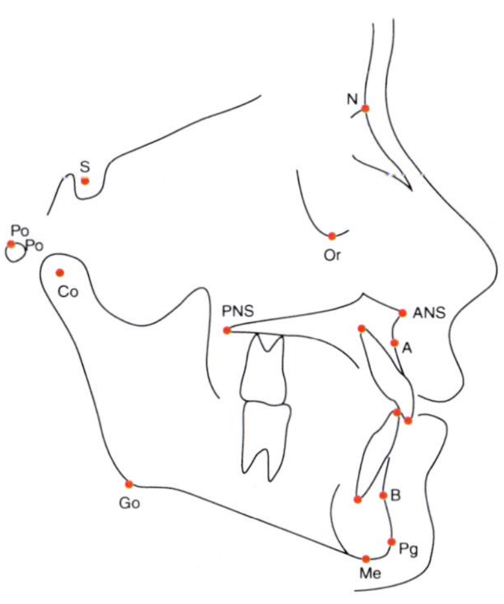

Step 7. Identify the soft-tissue landmarks.

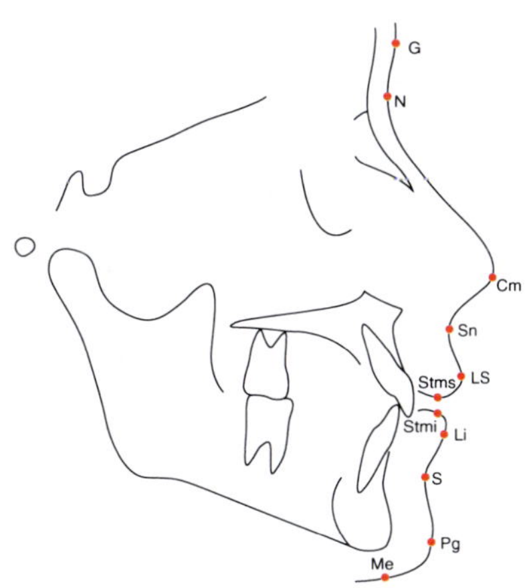

Identify Skeletal Reference Planes

Horizontal Planes (lines)

1. Sella–nasion (S-N)—a line connecting S to Na (cranial base as reference plane)
2. Frankfort Horizontal (FH) plane—a line connecting Po to Or (standard reference plane)
3. Palatal plane (PP)—a line connecting the ANS to PNS
4. Occlusal plane (OP)—a line that bisects the occlusal plane of the maxilla and the mandible
5. Mandibular plane (MP)—a line connecting Go to Me

Vertical Planes (lines)

6. Facial plane (N–Pg)—a line connecting N to Pg
7. Nasion–A point (Na–A)—a line connecting Na to A
8. Nasion–B point (Na–B)—a line connecting Na to B

Incisor Axis

9. Upper incisor (U1)—a line connecting the incisal edge and the root apex of the most prominent maxillary incisor
10. Lower incisor (L1)—a line connecting the incisal edge and the root apex of the most prominent lower incisor

Skeletal Analysis

Maxilla to Cranial Base

SNA

Sella–nasion–A point
82° ± 3°

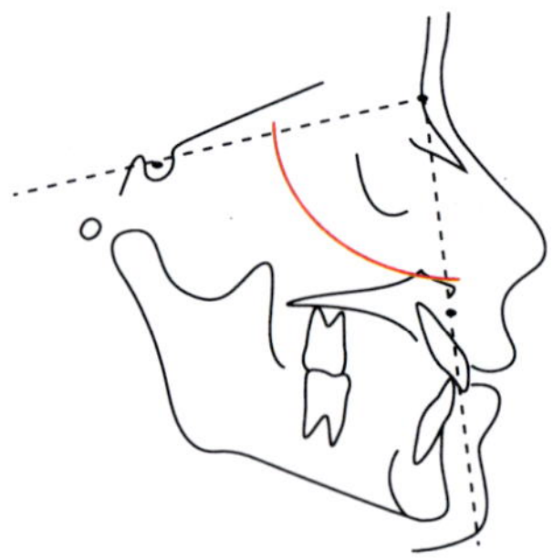

Reference line: sella–nasion

This angle indicates the horizontal position of the maxilla relative to the cranial base

- >85°—protrusive or prognathic maxilla
- <79°—deficient or retrognathic maxilla

NA–FH

Nasion–A point to FH
90° ± 4°

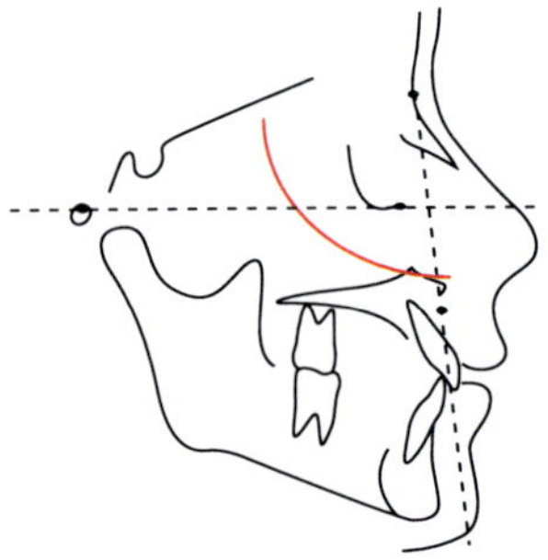

Reference plane: Frankfort Horizontal (orbitale–porion)

This angle (also called maxillary depth, Landes angle) indicates the horizontal position of the maxilla relative to the cranial base

- >94°—protrusive or prognathic maxilla
- <86°—deficient or retrognathic maxilla

Mandible (Body) to Cranial Base

SNB

Sella–Nasion–B point
79° ± 3°

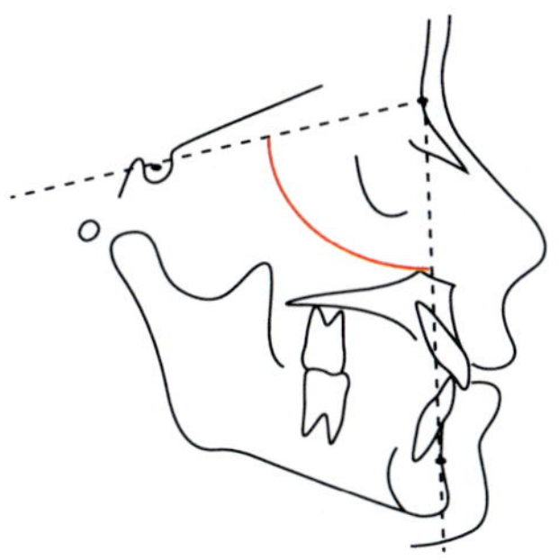

Reference line: sella–Nasion

B point is the most anterior measure point of the mandibular apical base. This angle expresses the horizontal position of the mandible relative to the cranial base using B point as a cephalometric landmark

>82°–prognathic mandible

<76°–retrognathic mandible

Chin

Pg–SN

Sella–nasion–pogonion
80° ± 3°

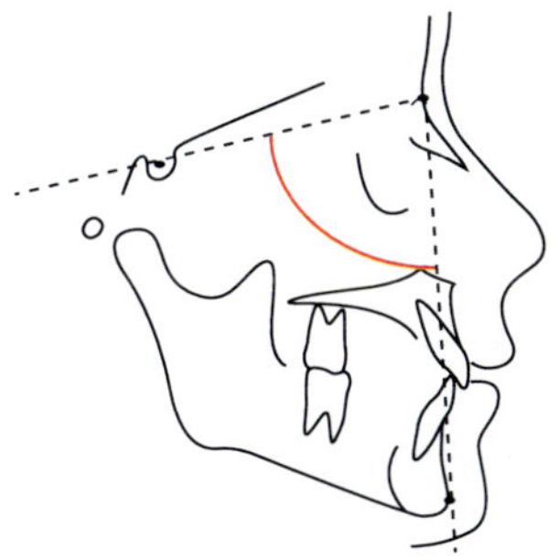

Reference line: sella–nasion

This angle represents the extent of chin prominence relative to the reference plane SN. It also indicates the horizontal position of the mandible relative to the cranial base using pogonion as landmark

>83°—prognathic mandible

<77°—retrognathic mandible

N–Pg–FH

Nasion pogonion to FH
87° ± 4°

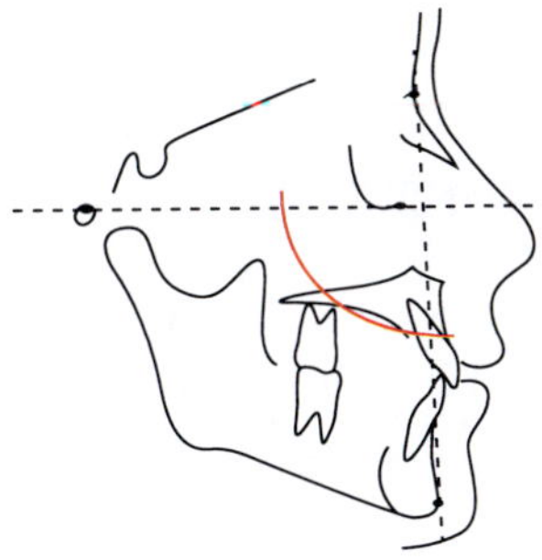

Reference plane: Frankfort Horizontal (orbitale–porion)

N–Pg is the facial plane. Similar to SN–Pg, this angle measures the degree of protrusion and retrusion of the chin but uses Frankfort Horizontal as a reference plane. It also indicates the horizontal position of the mandible relative to the cranial base

>91°—prognathic mandible

<83°—retrognathic mandible

Note: using all three angles and both reference planes, the diagnostician can make a good evaluation of the position of the mandible and determine whether the mandible is normal, protrusive, or retrognathic. In addition, the prominence of the chin may also be determined. It is possible to have a retrognathic mandible but prominent chin

Pg–NB

Pogonion to nasion–B point
3 mm ± 2 mm

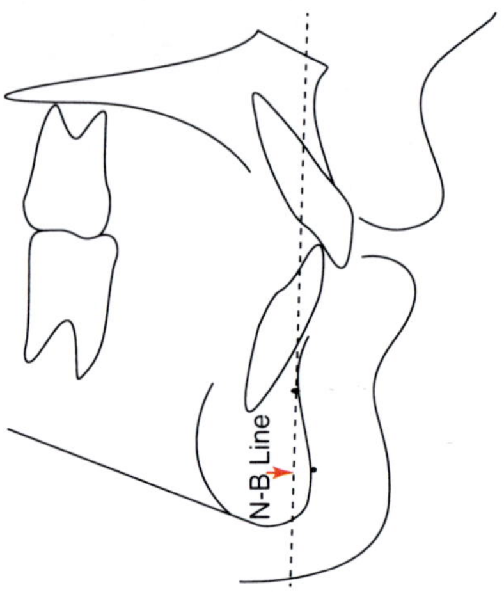

Reference line: nasion–B point

The prominence of the bony chin is measured by the distance of pogonion (the most anterior point of the chin) to the reference NB line

A smaller than average value indicates a recessive chin, while a greater than average indicates a prominent chin

Chin prominence is also affected by autorotation of the mandible (hinge axis rotation at centric relation). Rotation of the mandible in an anterior–superior direction (forward) increases chin prominence relative to NB. Rotation of the mandible in an inferior–posterior direction (backward) decreases chin prominence relative to NB

Pg–SN and N–Pg–FH also measure chin prominence with respect to SN and FH reference planes

Mandible to Maxilla

ANB

A point–nasion–B point
3° ± 2°

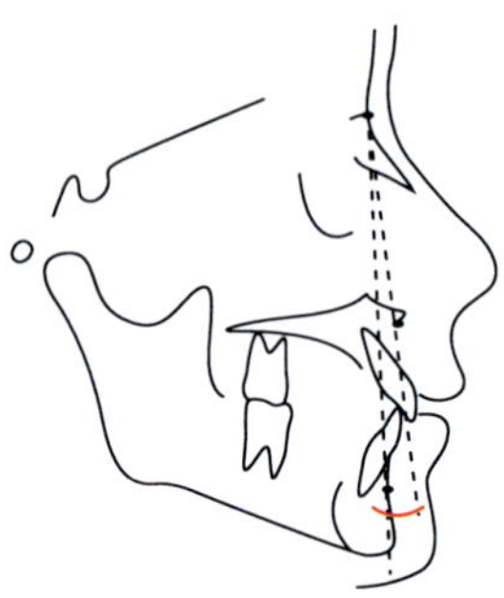

The ANB angle measures the relative position of the maxilla to mandible. The ANB angle can be measured or calculated from the formula: ANB = SNA − SNB

- A positive ANB angle indicates that the maxilla is positioned anteriorly relatively to the mandible (Class I or Class II malocclusion cases)
- A negative ANB angle indicates that the maxilla is positioned posteriorly relative to the mandible (Class III malocclusion cases)

The normal range is 1°–5°

- >5° indicates a Class II skeletal jaw relationship, protrusive maxilla, or retrognathic mandible
- <1° indicates a Class III skeletal jaw relationship, deficient maxilla, or prognathic mandible

Facial convexity at A point

Acute angle between the lines NA and APg

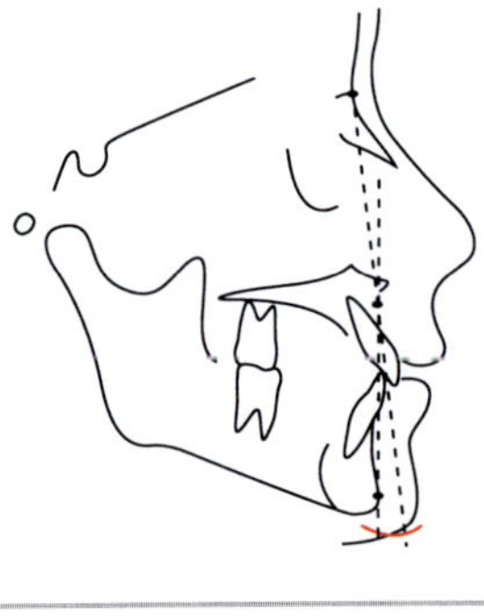

The facial convexity at A point measures the degree of convexity (positive angle) or the concavity (negative angle) of the face. The more convex the face, the greater the positive angle as an indication of Class II skeletal relationship between the maxilla and mandible. The more concave the face, the greater the negative angle as an indication of a Class III skeletal relationship between the maxilla and the mandible. The face should have a slight convexity

The normal range is 0° ± 8°

- > +8° indicates Class II skeletal jaw relationship
- <0° indicates Class III skeletal relationship

Anterior Facial Height

UFH	LFH
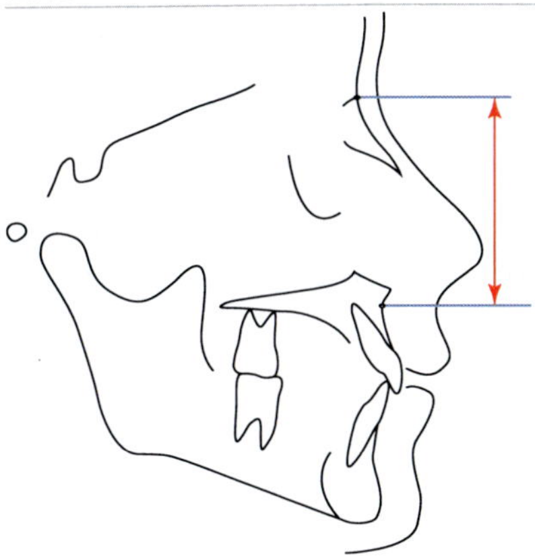	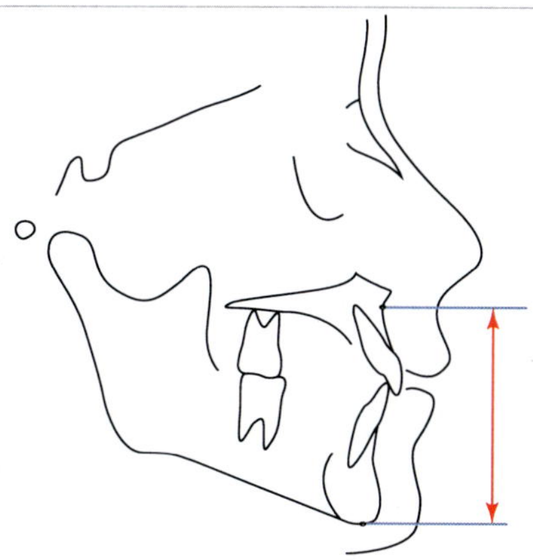
Upper anterior face height	Lower anterior face height
Linear measurement from nasion to anterior nasal spine (N–ANS)	Linear measurement from anterior nasal spine to menton (ANS–Me)

UFH/LFH ratio based at a Point

The ratio of UFH to LFH is more important than the individual linear measurements of UFH and LFH. UFH varies with the superior–inferior dimension of the size of an adult skull, while the ratio of UFH/LFH indicates the balance of facial proportions

- UFH/LFH ratio <0.8 indicates a greater LFH, or longer lower anterior face height
- UFH/LFH ratio >0.8 indicates a smaller LFH, or shorter lower anterior face height

Dental Analysis

Maxillary Incisors

U1 to SN

Max. incisor to SN
103° ± 6°

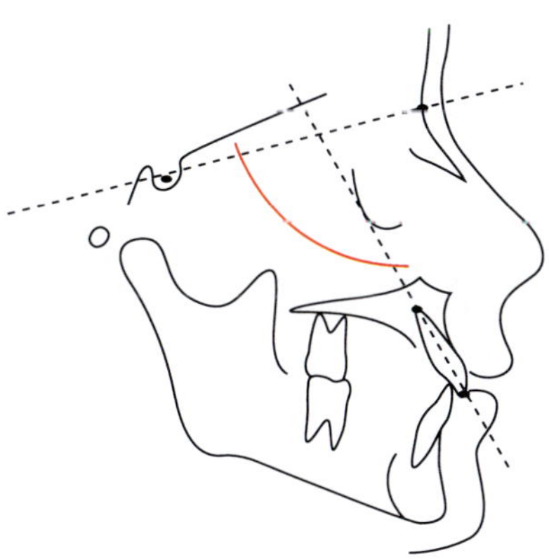

Reference line: sella–nasion

This angular measurement determines the inclination of the central incisor relative to the anterior cranial base

- A greater than average angle indicates proclination (labioversion) of incisors as often seen in Class II division 1 cases
- A smaller than average angle indicates upright or retroclined (lingually inclined) incisors as often seen in Class II division 2 cases

U1 to NA

Max. incisor to NA
Angular: 22° ± 6°

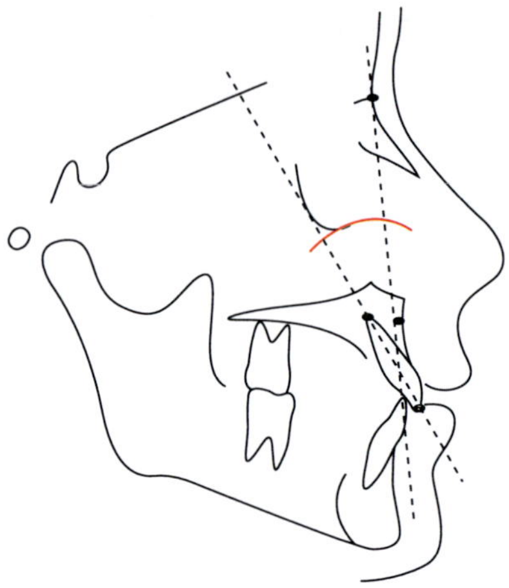

Reference line: nasion–A point

The relationship of the maxillary central incisor to the N–A reference line is used to establish the position of maxillary incisors relative to the maxillary apical base

The angular measurement indicates the amount of maxillary dental protrusion

- Labially proclined incisors will have a greater than average angular measurement (Class II division 1 cases)
- Upright or retroclined (lingually inclined) incisors will have a smaller than average angular measurement (Class II division 2 cases)
- Positive values are recorded if the labial surface of the incisor is anterior to the NA line, negative values if it is posterior

Interincisal Relationship

Overjet

Max. to mand. incisor
Horizontal distance

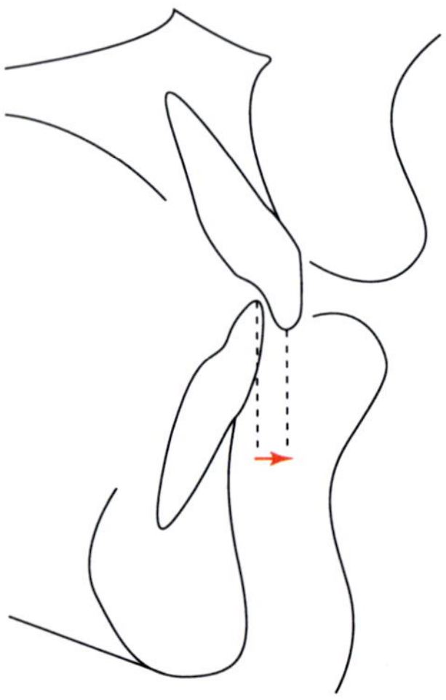

Overjet is the interincisal horizontal linear measurement

Normal 2 mm ± 1 mm

Positive overjet greater than normal range indicates a Class II relationship

Negative overjet indicates a Class III relationship

Overbite

Max. to mand. incisor
Vertical distance

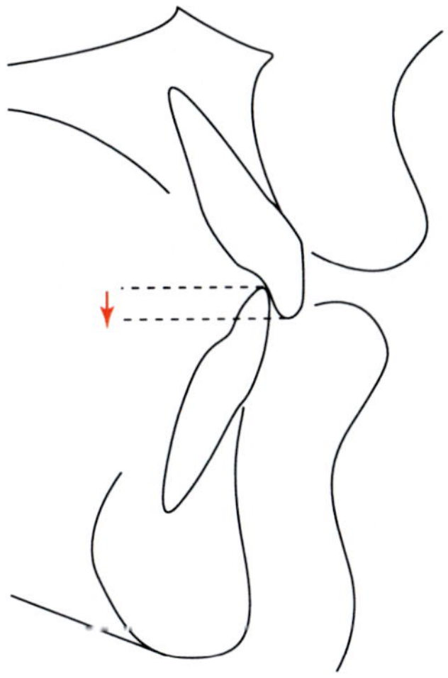

Overbite is the interincisal vertical linear measurement

Normal 2 mm ± 1 mm

Positive overbite greater than normal range indicates a deep bite

Negative overbite indicates an anterior open bite (apertognathia)

Occlusal Plane

OP–FH

FH to mand. lower borders
24° ± 3°

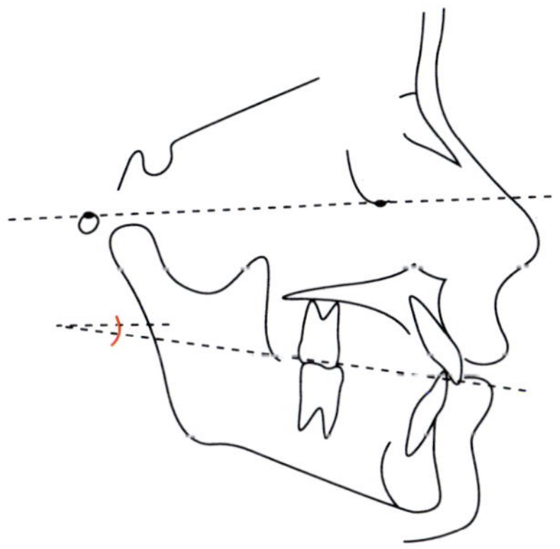

Reference plane: Frankfort Horizontal (orbitale–porion)

The occlusal plane is a line from the maxillary–mandibular molar to the maxillary–mandibular incisor. There may be two occlusal planes one for the maxilla and one for the mandible as in cases of anterior open bite

Soft-Tissue Analysis

Facial convexity at Sn

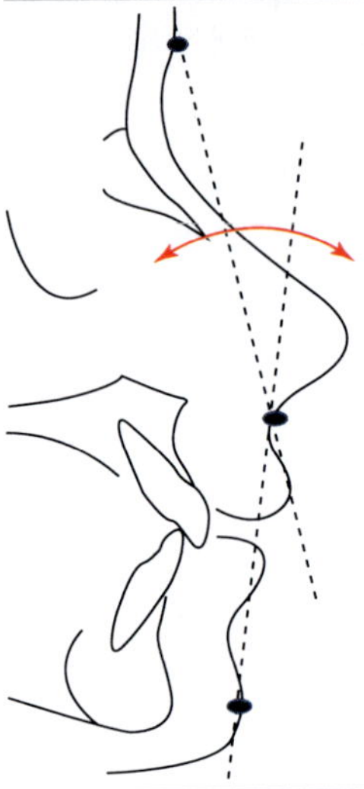

The facial convexity at Sn point measures the degree of convexity (positive angle) or the concavity (negative angle) of the face. This angle is measured between the line glabella (G)–Sn and the line Sn–chin (Pg)

The angle G–Sn–Pg should be 12° ± 4°

The more convex the face, the greater the positive angle as an indication of Class II skeletal relationship between the maxilla and mandible. The more concave the face, the greater the negative angle as an indication of a Class III skeletal relationship between the maxilla and the mandible. The face should have a slight convexity

Zero–meridian

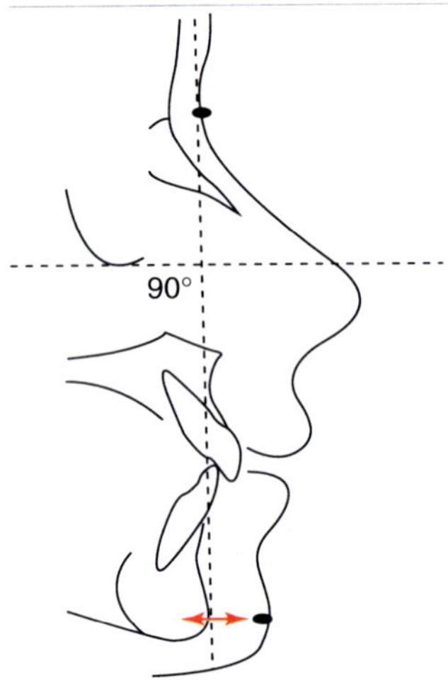

The Gonzalez–Ulloa line (zero–meridian). A perpendicular line relative to the Frankfort Horizontal (FH) is dropped from the nasion (N). The chin point as the soft-tissue pogonion (Pg) is assessed relative to Gonzalez–Ulloa line. The "ideal" chin position in the sagittal plane is at this line and should be adjusted to the personal goals of the patient

Vertical proportion

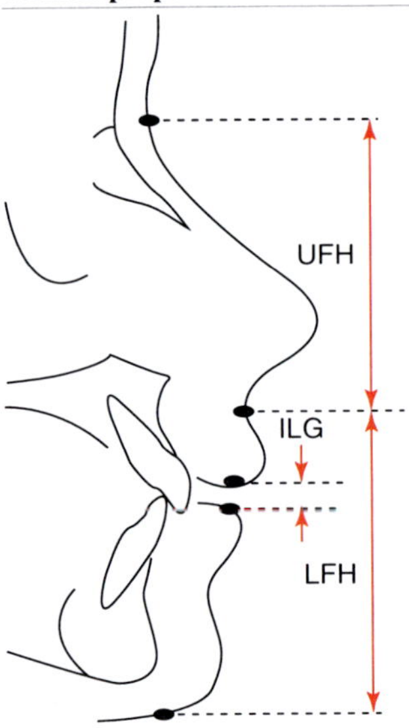

UFH/LFH ratio based at Sn point

The upper facial height (UFH) is measured from glabella (G) to subnasale (Sn)

The lower facial height (LFH) is measured from subnasale (Sn) to menton (Me)

The ratio of UFH to LFH is more important than the individual linear measurements of UFH and LFH. The ratio of UFH/LFH indicates the balance of facial proportions

The interlabial gap

The interlabial gap (ILG) is measured when the lips are at rest (repose). ILG is 0–3 mm. If it is greater than 3 mm, it indicates lip incompetence

Nasal–labial angle

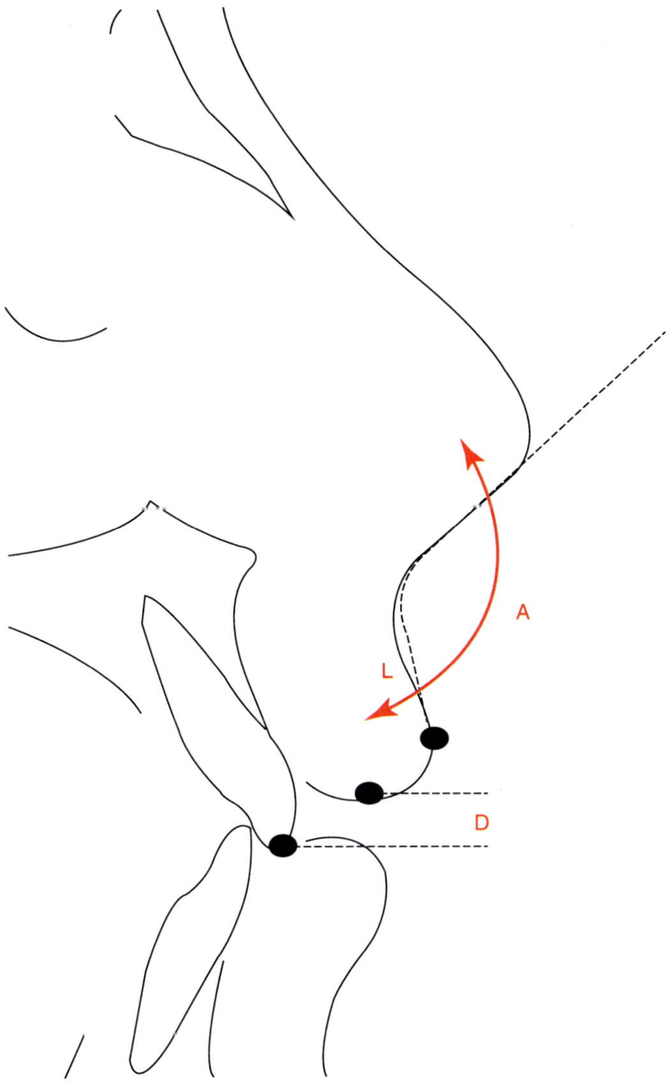

Nasal–labial angle (A) is measured at subnasale (Sn)

Maxillary surgery affects the nasolabial angle with repositioning of the anterior nasal spine. With sagittal maxillary advancement, the nasolabial angle becomes more obtuse. With vertical maxillary impaction, the nasolabial angle becomes more acute

Normal value: 102° ± 8° (In males the angle is more acute than in females)

<94°—the nasolabial angle is overly acute and the upper lip procumbent

>110°—the nasolabial angle is overly obtuse and the upper lip retrusive

Dental display

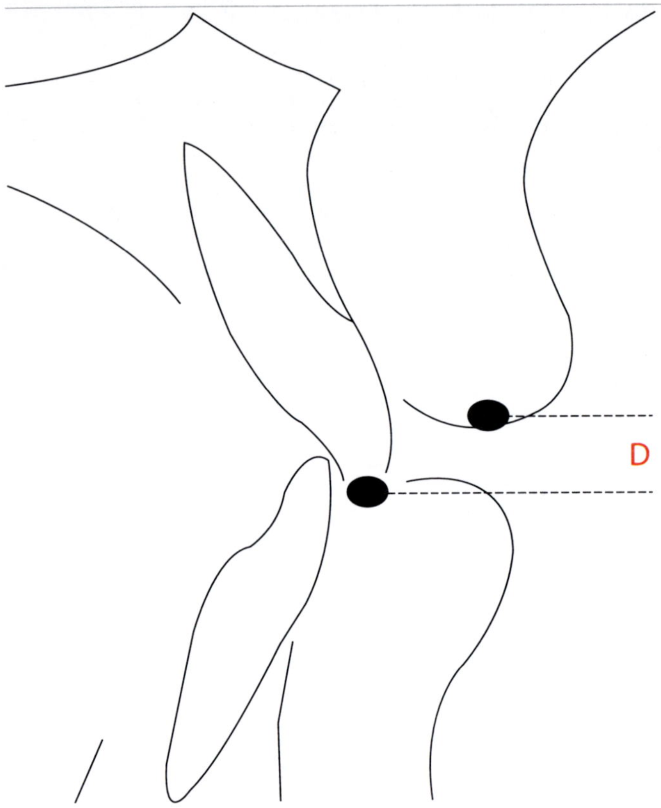

Dental display is measured from the upper lip vermilion border to the maxillary incisor tip when the lips are relaxed (repose) and when the patient is asked to smile

With the lips at rest, the incisor display is:

Males: 2 mm (±2 mm)

Females: 3.5 mm (±2 mm)

With full smile, the incisor display is full crown with less than 2 mm gingival display

Bibliography

Bhatia SN, Leighton BC. A manual of facial growth: a computer analysis of longitudinal cephalometric growth data. USA: Oxford University Press; 1993.

Cevidanes LHS, Styner MA, Proffit WR. Image analysis and superimposition of 3-dimensional cone-beam computed tomography models. Am J Orthod Dentofacial Orthop. 2006;129(5):611–8.

Chirani RA, Jacq JJ, Meriot P, et al. Temporomandibular joint: a methodology of magnetic resonance imaging 3-D reconstruction. Oral Surg Oral Med Oral Pathol Oral Radiol Endod. 2004;97(6):756–61.

Elolf E, Tatagiba M, Samii M. Three dimensional computed tomographic reconstruction: planning tool for surgery of skull base pathologies. Comput Aided Surg. 1998;3(2):89–94.

Harrell Jr WE, Hatcher DC, Bolt RL. In search of anatomic truth: 3-dimensional digital modeling and the future of orthodontics. Am J Orthod Dentofacial Orthop. 2002;122(3):325–30.

Hatcher DC, Aboudara CL. Diagnosis goes digital. Am J Orthod Dentofacial Orthop. 2004;125(4):512–5.

Hajeer MJ, Ayoub AF, Millett DT, et al. Three-dimensional imaging in orthodontic surgery: the clinical application of a new method. Int J Adult Orthodon Orthognath Surg. 2002;17(4):318–30.

Hajeer MY, Ayoub AF, Millett DT. Three-dimensional assessment of facial soft-tissue asymmetry before and after orthognathic surgery. Br J Oral Maxillofac Surg. 2004;42(5):396–404.

Jacobson A, Jacobson RJ. Radiographic cephalometry: from basics to 3-D imaging. Chicago: Quintessence Pub Co; 2006.

Kim N-K, Lee C, Kang S-H, Chang Y-II, et al. A three-dimensional analysis of soft and hard tissue changes after a mandibular setback surgery. Comput Methods Programs Biomed. 2006;83(3):178–87.

Kitaura H, Yonetsu K, Kitamori H, et al. Standardization of 3-D CT measurements for length and angles by matrix transformation in the 3-D coordinate system. Cleft Palate Craniofac J. 2000;37(4):349–56.

Lagravère MO, Major PW. Proposed reference point for 3-dimensional cephalometric analysis with cone-beam computerized tomography. Am J Orthod Dentofacial Orthop. 2005;128(5):657–60.

Lagravère MO, Hansen L, Winfried H, et al. Plane orientation for standardization in 3-dimensional cephalometric analysis with computerized tomography imaging. Am J Orthod Dentofacial Orthop. 2006;129(5):601–4.

Legan HL, Burstone CJ. Soft-tissue cephalometric analysis for orthognathic surgery. J Oral Surg. 1980;38:744–51.

Maki K, Inou N, Takanishi A, et al. Computer assisted simulations in orthodontic diagnosis and the application of a new cone beam x-ray computed tomography. Orthod Craniofac Res. 2003;6 Suppl 1:95–101.

Mah J, Hatcher D. Current status and future needs in craniofacial imaging. Orthod Craniofac Res. 2003;6 Suppl 1:10–6.

Miller AJ, Koutaro M, Hatcher DC. New diagnostic tools in orthodontics. Am J Orthod Dentofacial Orthop. 2004;126(4):395–6.

Moorrees CF, Kean MR. Natural head position; a basic consideration in the interpretation of cephalometric radiographs. Am J Phys Anthropol. 1958;16:213–34.

Ngan DC, Kharbanda OP, Geently JP, et al. Comparison of radiation levels from computed tomography and conventional dental radiographs. Aust Orthod J. 2003;19(2):67–75.

Nkenke EN, Zachow S, Benz M, et al. Fusion of computed tomography data and optical 3D images of the dentition for streak artifact correction in the simulation of orthognathic surgery. Dentomaxillofac Radiol. 2004;33(4):226–32.

Ono I, Gunji H, Suda K, et al. Method of preparing an exact-size model using helical volume scan computed tomography. Plast Reconstr Surg. 1994;93(7):1363–71.

Swennen GRJ, Schutyser F, Hausamen JE. Three dimensional cephalometry. A color atlas and manual. Berlin: Springer; 2006. p. 364.

Walker L, Enciso R, Mah J. Three-dimensional localization of maxillary canines with cone-beam computed tomography. Am J Orthod Dentofacial Orthop. 2005;128(4):418–23.

Wolford LM, Karras SC, Mehra P. Considerations for orthognathic surgery during growth. Part 1: mandibular deformities. Am J Orthod Dentofacial Orthop. 2001;119(2):95–101.

Xia J, Samman N, Yeung RWK, et al. Three-dimensional virtual reality surgical planning and simulation workbench for orthognathic surgery. Int J Adult Orthodon Orthognath Surg. 2000;15(4):265–82.

Xia JJ, Gateno J, Teichgraeber JF. Three-dimensional computer-aided surgical simulation for maxillofacial surgery. Atlas Oral Maxillofac Surg Clin North Am. 2005;13:25–39.

Ziegler CM, Woertche R, Brief J, et al. Clinical indications for digital volume tomography in oral and maxillofacial surgery. Dentomaxillofac Radiol. 2002;31(2):126–30.

28 Orthodontics

Neil Warshawsky, Henry Schupert, and Howard Aduss

Introduction

In correcting dentofacial skeletal deformities, the role of the orthodontist and surgeon are equally important. The responsibility of the orthodontist is to diagnose and treatment plan the case, decompensate the dentition, and provide the surgeon a stable intra-arch dental framework. The surgeon must then place the skeletal components into the most pleasing and functional position possible to achieve the pretreatment goals established for the patient. Clear communication is essential as the goals of presurgical orthodontic treatment generally are opposite that of the routine orthodontic regimen used to camouflage the skeletal discrepancies in patients who choose not to pursue surgery. Successful occlusal relationships can be achieved with orthodontic treatment alone in minor skeletal discrepancies and at times even in more significant deficiencies; however, it is frequently at the expense of a pleasing facial appearance or a precarious position of a tooth that can risk its vitality relative to its position within the cortical and cancellous bone alveolus. These same patients who have had orthodontic treatment without consideration for combined surgical-orthodontic management may seek plastic surgical procedures later in life to address this residual skeletal deformity. Skeletal correction, once the occlusion is achieved, is compromised and frequently requires the use of prosthetic implants and soft tissue procedures to camouflage the deformity: the results of which are less than ideal.

When is the problem too severe for orthodontic treatment alone? It depends on the severity and the age of patient. Given the same degree of severity, orthodontic treatment in a growing child is likely to have a favorable influence and may avoid the necessity for orthognathic surgery with the exception of extreme growth and congenital birth defects such as clefting of the jaw, alveolus, or palate and craniofacial conditions. In the adult (i.e., an individual who has reached facial skeletal maturity) with the same degree of severity, since growth is not an option, surgery is the only option to mimic or imitate growth. However, when the malocclusion persists in the growing child despite orthodontic treatment used to modify growth, surgical consideration should be considered either during active growth or at the time of skeletal maturity. A successful outcome occurs when both the occlusal goals and the aesthetic goals are achieved. In the opinion of many orthodontists, the limits of orthodontic treatment lie within an envelope of a positive overjet of +8 mm, a negative overjet of −4 mm, and a transverse width discrepancy of 3 mm. Proffit and White's well-known discrepancy diagram illustrates the envelopes of achievable outcomes based on orthodontic treatment alone (inner envelope), orthodontic treatment in a growing child (middle envelope), and with orthognathic surgery (outer envelope) (See Fig. 28.1). The envelopes are asymmetrical and differ for the maxilla and the mandible. The precise dimensions of the envelopes are less important than the philosophical concepts that must be applied to each case.

Dental development plays an important element in the maxillary-mandibular alveolar development. There are two aspects. One is dental eruption itself and the other is the "drifting" of the tooth as a whole within the alveolar process. Orthodontic movement of the tooth itself involves a tension/pressure gradient causing a boney remodeling of the associated alveolus aided by the periodontal ligament. While growth is present, the orthodontist can guide the individual teeth into position taking advantage of the active phase of development with "braces." In contrast other orthodontic interventions such as headgear, face masks, and restraining chin cups can alter the vector of the displacements of the maxilla and mandible including the dental unit as a whole by affecting the sutures and sites of regional growth. These orthodontic maneuvers can only have significant and stable impact on future facial skeletal development while growth is active and can be modulated (orthodontic growth modification).

N. Warshawsky, DDS (✉) • H. Schupert, DDS • H. Aduss, DDS
The Craniofacial Center, Division of Plastic Reconstructive and Cosmetic Surgery, University of Illinois, Chicago, IL 60612, USA
e-mail: neilwars@UIC.EDU

P.J. Taub et al. (eds.), *Ferraro's Fundamentals of Maxillofacial Surgery*,
DOI 10.1007/978-1-4614-8341-0_28, © Springer Science+Business Media New York 2015

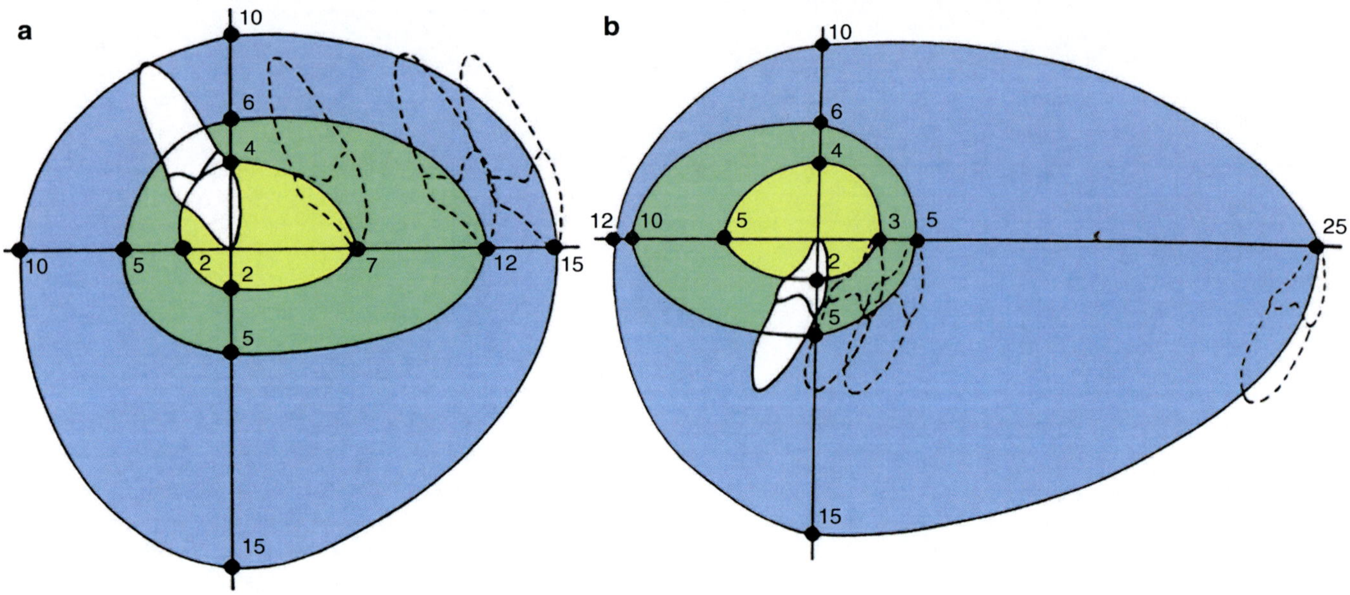

Fig. 28.1 Profitt and White's discrepancy diagram for the maxillary dentition (**a**) and mandibular dentition (**b**). The envelopes represent the amount of dental repositioning possible by orthodontic movement alone (*yellow*), orthodontic movement with growth modification (*green*), and with orthognathic surgery (*blue*). Note that the envelopes are not symmetrical and that for example orthodontic movement in the growing child is more effective with mandibular deficiency than with mandibular excess

Surgical intervention at an early age is often not questioned in the child with a severe deformity as a result of either a congenital or acquired condition. However, the child with a moderate deformity and a dental malocclusion is the one that poses the problems in timing and sequencing of treatment. A fundamentally correct treatment plan instituted at the wrong time in the child's development can yield a poor result. Thus, timing of the "ortho/surgical" intervention becomes the more critical question.

If the skeletal malalignment is minimal to moderate, then it is possible to achieve correction by influencing the pattern of jaw growth with interceptive facial orthopedic treatment. This interceptive treatment must be initiated during the periods of active growth in early to late childhood, but before the completion of the adolescent growth spurt. By the time the child has reached sexual maturity, it is usually too late to attempt such treatment.

It makes sense in most circumstances of moderate deformity to wait until skeletal maturity when planning for orthognathic surgery to avoid reoperation because of recurrence of the deformity with continued disproportionate growth. There is a gender variation with the timing of skeletal maturity. Serial cephalometric x-rays will objectively indicate deceleration of growth and a hand-wrist film or cervical vertebrae maturity can be used to determine skeletal age. However, there are circumstances when relying solely on ensuring stability of correction to determine the timing of surgery may be inappropriate. Adolescents who have poor self-image, socially introverted, or are victims of ridicule can greatly benefit from early intervention. Similarly functional indications—speech, airway difficulties, and malocclusion—may dictate earlier intervention.

An Overview of Orthodontic-Surgical Management

Treatment planning begins by reviewing the various orthodontic and surgical options available that would address the problem list. The primary decision that needs to be made is whether the deformity is significant enough to require surgical repositioning or can growth modification and orthodontic alignment of the dentition alone achieve a satisfactory result without significantly compromising the facial aesthetics. If surgical intervention is contemplated, then the question arises whether to intervene prior to completion of skeletal growth or to await skeletal maturity to eliminate the variability of subsequent growth and need for further surgical intervention. Once the decision is made for combined dental-surgical correction, the overall treatment must be carefully planned. Formulation of a treatment plan thus requires close cooperation of the surgeon working with the orthodontist. Unlike many of the surgical procedures, outcome depends not only on the surgical procedure itself but also on a multitude of factors that begin long before the actual surgery and control of the variables long after the surgery. The management (see Fig. 28.2) is divided into five phases: (1) pre-orthodontic preparatory phase,

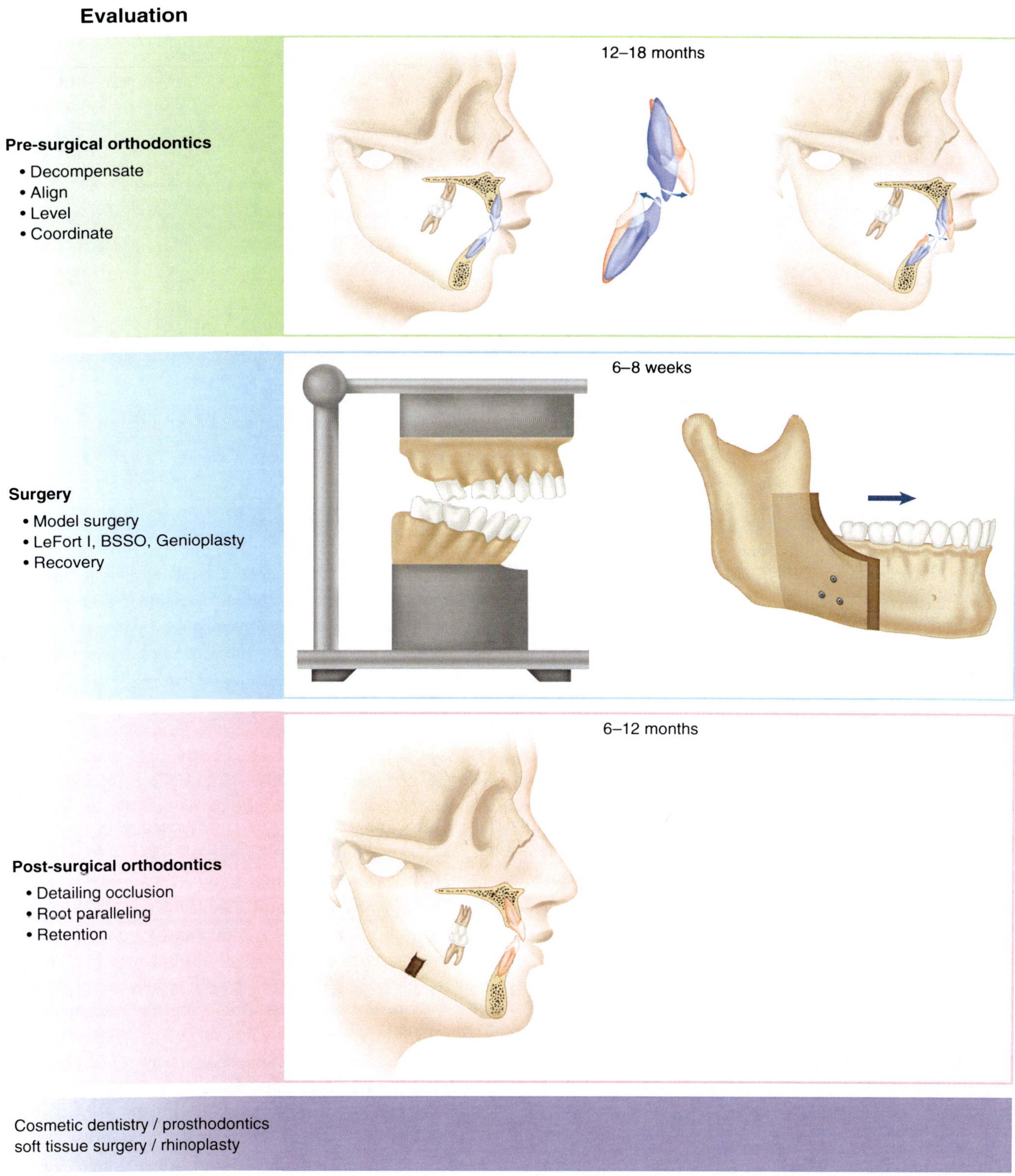

Fig. 28.2 An overview of orthodontic-surgical treatment in patients with dentofacial skeletal deformities that represents in most cases 18–24 months of treatment time. The majority of that time is under orthodontic management with the surgical team involved at the initial treatment planning stage and typically 6–8-week period at the time of surgery

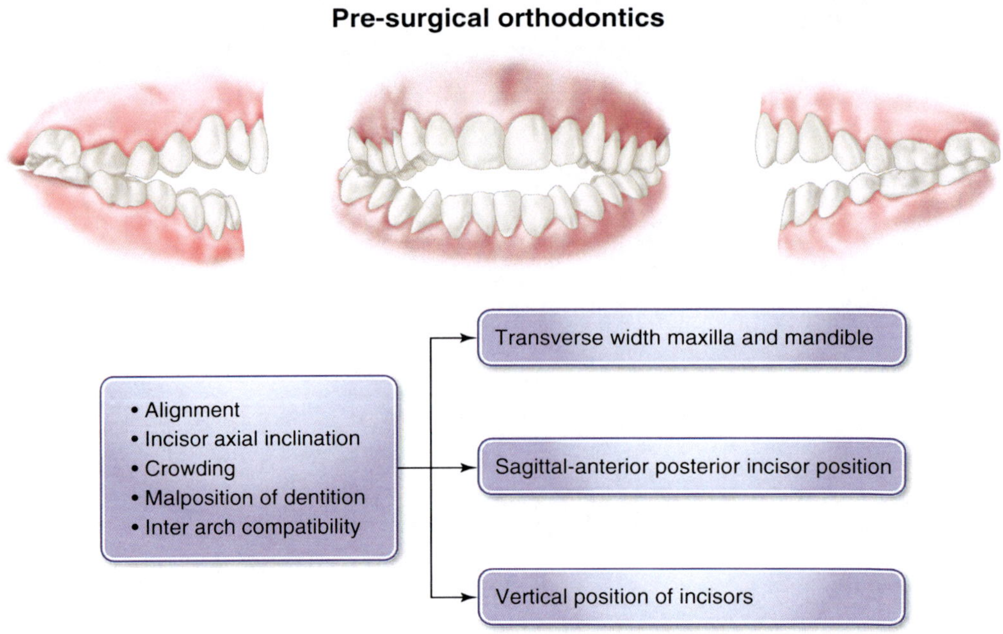

Fig. 28.3 An overview of presurgical orthodontic management decompensation in all three planes. The dental arches are assessed for alignment, incisor axial inclination, crowding, and interarch compatibility

(2) presurgical orthodontic treatment phase, (3) surgical phase, (4) postsurgical orthodontic phase, and (5) prosthodontic and/or restorative treatment phase.

Pre-orthodontic Preparatory Phase

Prior to the initiation of the presurgical orthodontic treatment, creation of good oral health and the elimination of caries must be managed as part of this initial phase. Patients with periodontal disease or gingivitis will have an increased risk with the long-term application of orthodontic appliances, tooth movement and during the postoperative surgical period. A lack of sufficient attached gingiva must also be managed prior to orthodontic tooth movement. Interim temporary restorative or prosthetic restorations must be used to stabilize a mutilated dentition prior to the initiation of orthodontic and surgical treatment.

Pre-surgical Orthodontic Management

Once oral health is achieved, the presurgical orthodontic treatment phase can begin. In skeletal discrepancies, the teeth naturally compensate to establish as functional an occlusion as possible within the limitations of the deformity. The goal of the presurgical orthodontic preparation is to remove the dental compensations to reveal the true extent of the skeletal deformity. The teeth are orthodontically returned to their ideal position (axial inclination and alignment) within their respective maxillary and mandibular dental arches. This may require the extraction premolar teeth. The occlusion and facial appearance is often made worse until surgical correction occurs. Without appropriate dental decompensation, the surgeon is limited by the tooth position to fully correct the skeletal deformity. The decompensation must be accomplished in all three dimensions: the transverse plane (width), the sagittal plane (anterior-posterior), and the coronal plane (vertical) (see Fig. 28.3).

In the transverse plane, the maxillary and mandibular dental arches need to be coordinated with the postsurgical occlusion (see Fig. 28.4). Because of the relative transverse arch width discrepancy with Class II and Class III malocclusions, the dentoalveolar compensations need to be removed. As with removing the sagittal compensations, the arch width discrepancy is worsened. Depending on the discrepancy the options are transpalatal orthodontic expansion with or without surgical assistance versus segmental maxillary osteotomies at the time of the orthognathic surgical procedure. Expansion may be accomplished orthodontically alone with a palatal expansion device if the mid-palatal suture is open, otherwise this may require surgical assistance with an osteotomy. When interdental osteotomies are needed, orthodontic root divergence must be created. Minor width discrepancies may be acceptable with some degree of orthodontic compensation and can be corrected postsurgically.

The anterior-posterior decompensation involves the correction of the maxillary and mandibular incisors (see Fig. 28.5). In an adaptive Class II malocclusion, the maxillary incisors are often retroclined and the mandibular incisors proclined to allow a functional bite as a natural compensation to the skeletal deformity. Thus, the decompensation involves orthodontically uprighting the proclined mandibular incisors and advancing the maxillary incisors in the proper position to create adequate lip support. To develop

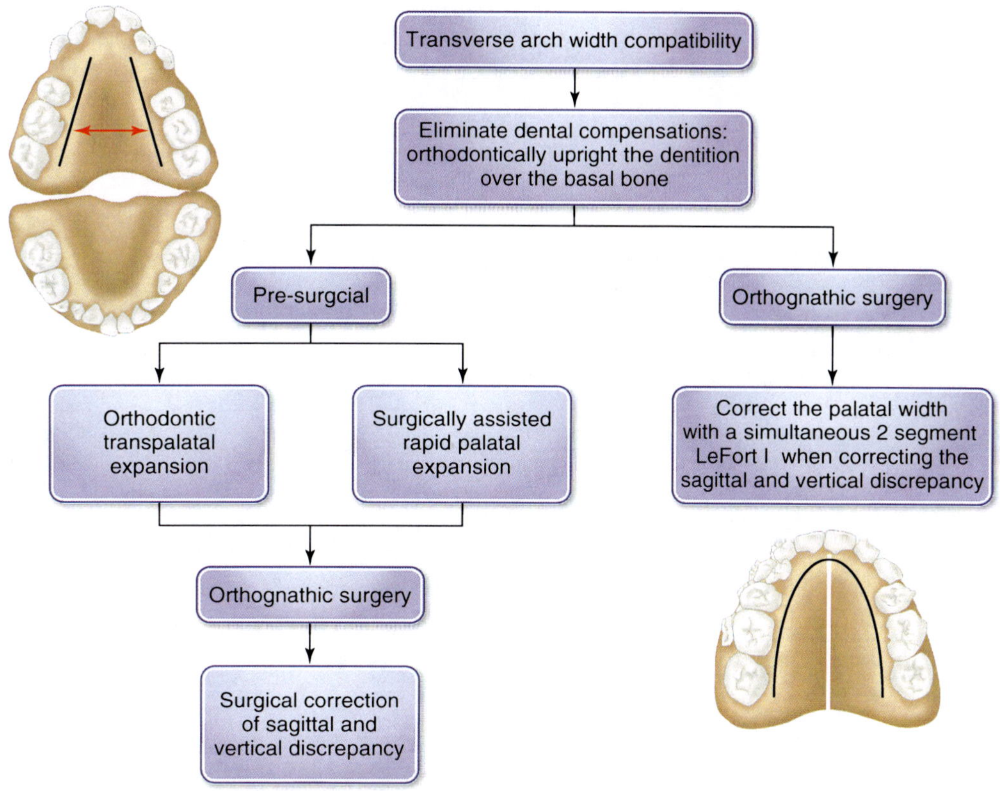

Fig. 28.4 Orthodontic management of transverse component of dentofacial skeletal deformities

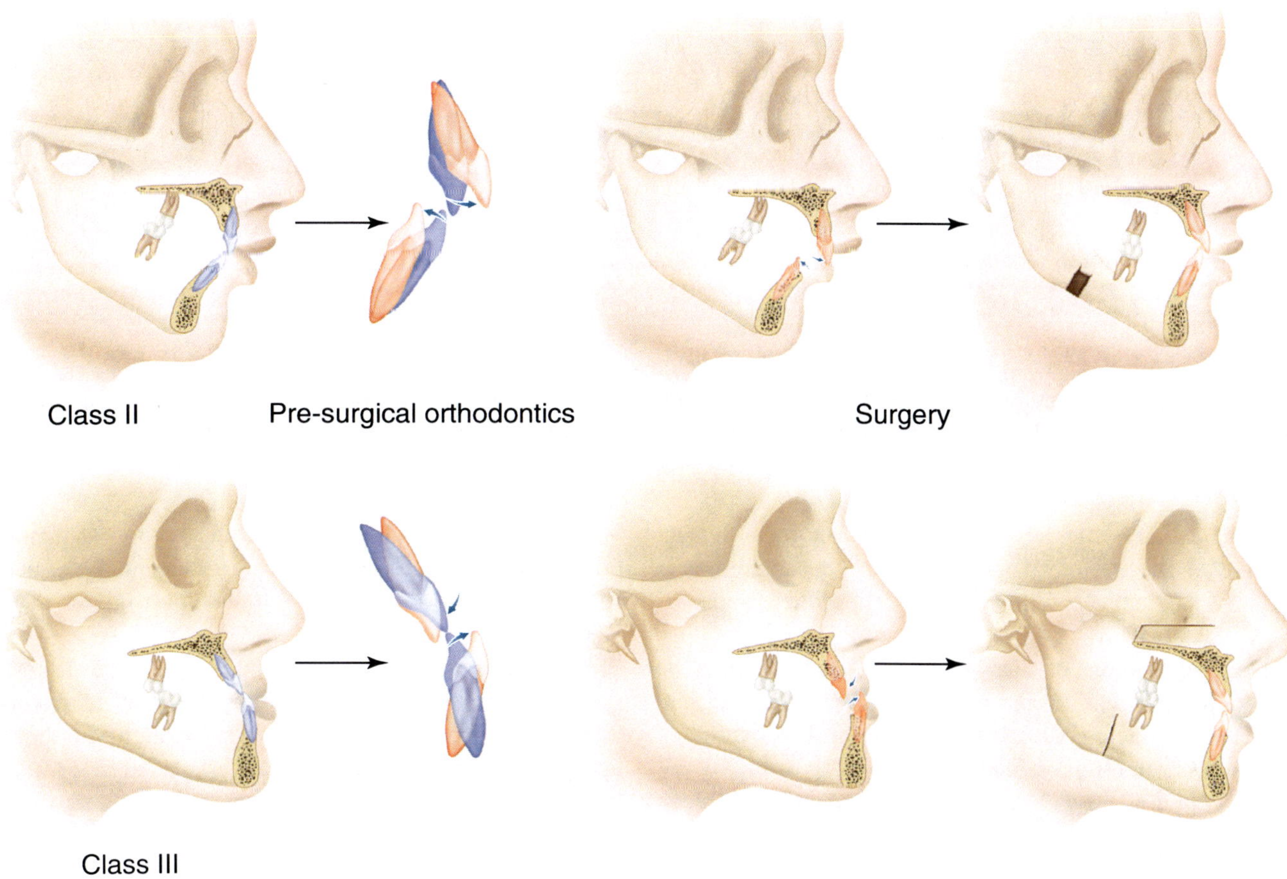

Fig. 28.5 (**a**) Orthodontic management of the sagittal (anterior-posterior) component of dentofacial skeletal deformities. (**b**) Class II decompensation followed by mandibular advancement. Class III decompensation to allow maxillary advancement and mandibular setback

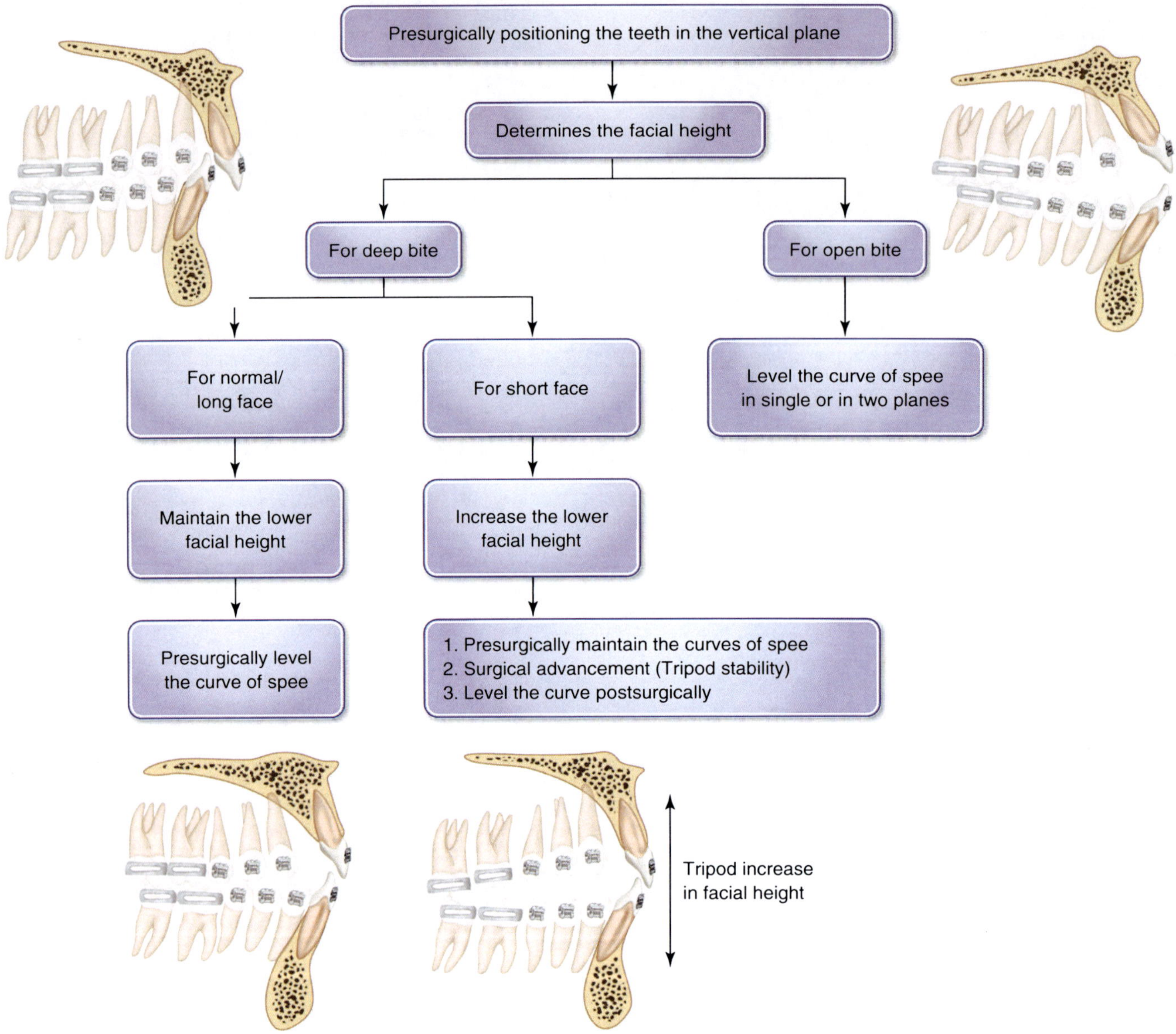

Fig. 28.6 Represents orthodontic management of the vertical component of dentofacial skeletal deformities. Whether or not to level the Curve of Spee prior to surgery depends on the lower facial height. By advancing the mandible first with a tripod stability, the lower facial height increases. The lateral open bite is closed after the surgery. With an open bite deformity, the decision is whether leveling the curve in one plane will result in stability versus in two planes and a segmental maxillary procedure

a Class I dental occlusion with proper tooth-to-tooth contact often requires the removal of the maxillary second premolars and the mandibular first premolars to relieve the compensations and dental crowding.

Decompensations of Class III malocclusion occur in the reverse pattern with advancement of the lower incisors and retraction of the maxillary anterior teeth. The extraction sequence is often represented by the removal of the maxillary first premolars and the mandibular second premolars, thereby attaining a functioning Class I posterior presurgical occlusion.

In the vertical plane, dental decompensation of the anterior dentition depends on three factors: the amount of dental display of the maxillary incisors to the upper lip, the interlabial gap, and the lower anterior facial height (See Fig. 28.6). When there is excessive dental display with gingival show in skeletal anterior open bite deformities, the extruded maxillary teeth that compensate the open bite can be intruded orthodontically only to a limited extent in an effort to develop a level occlusal plane that permits a single piece maxillary LeFort impaction surgical procedure. Orthodontic correction alone will be unstable. Frequently, the posterior teeth may be in a significantly different occlusal plane than the anterior dentition. In such cases, if segmental maxillary repositioning is needed, the presurgical orthodontic treatment correspondingly involves segmental leveling in two or more different planes. In such cases root diversion is needed to allow for interdental osteotomies for a multi-segmented LeFort I procedures.

In patients with a deep anterior incisor overbite, the decision to whether to level the occlusal plane orthodontically depends on the lower facial height. When the lower facial height is normal, the deep bite is corrected by both intruding the incisors and extruding the first molars and premolars. In contrast when the lower facial height is reduced as in deep Class II skeletal conditions, the arches are not leveled until after mandible has been advanced. By maintaining the Curve of Spee, the mandibular advancement will result in a "tripod" occlusion: the incisors anteriorly and the molars and premolars posteriorly on either side. This will allow a natural increase in the lower facial height. The resulting lateral open bite will then be closed by extruding the mandibular first molars and premolars and leveling the Curve of Spee. If the occlusal plane was instead leveled presurgically, a more anterior than vertical projection of B Point will be produced.

When a mandibular osteotomy such as sagittal split is contemplated, it is generally wise to have the mandibular third molars extracted well in advance, typically 8–12 months, to allow for new bone formation. This minimizes the risk of unfavorable fractures and allows for successful internal fixation. During this phase, the dentition is coordinated, the Curve of Spee may/may not be leveled, and the anterior dentition decompensated. The resultant malocclusion is frequently made worse and the patient must be made aware of this prior to the initiation of treatment. The maxillary and mandibular dentition is coordinated. Handheld dental casts are obtained throughout the orthodontic treatment, and when they can be manually coordinated or tripoded, then planning for surgery can begin (see Fig. 28.7). If segmental osteotomies are planned, then the dentition must be accordingly prepared. If osteotomies are not approached through planned extraction sites, then interdental space must be orthodontically prepared with the roots widely divergent to prevent injury with the space favorably closed at the time of surgery or by orthodontics following surgery. Periapical or CBCT films should be used to evaluate the space for osteotomies. Segmental dental casts will then confirm the readiness for surgery.

At the time of surgery, the orthodontic arch wires should be fully engaged in the bracket slots, the arch wires should be completely passive, and surgical hooks should be soldered or crimped in place to facilitate intermaxillary elastic traction for the surgeon. If segmental osteotomies are planned, the arch wires can be segmented prior to surgery. This presurgical phase typically varies from 12 to 18 months depending on what needs to be accomplished to maximize the final surgical stability.

The Postsurgical Orthodontic Phase

The postsurgical orthodontic phase begins typically 6 weeks after the surgery. The patient is then returned to the orthodontist for finishing dental alignment with the relative position of the skeletal bases in their final position. Any remaining interdental spaces are closed and the dentition is brought into maximal intercuspal relationship. This phase typically lasts for about 8–12 months and ends with the removal of the orthodontic appliances and instructing the patient on the use of a retainer to maintain long-term stability. Photographs, radiographic studies, and dental models are obtained on debanding and at 1 year from completion of treatment. Ideally when possible the patient should be followed annually for an extended period of time to assess for long-term results.

Retention Phase

Management of orthognathic surgical patients following combined orthognathic surgery usually presents similar problems posed by the traditional orthodontic patient—failure to cooperate in wearing the retainers, breaking the retainers, or loosing the retainers. The unique problem presented by the Class III patient is the potential for residual mandibular growth and this fact must be carefully outlined to the family and the patient. It would not be uncommon to have some orthodontic posttreatment regimen necessary to address the minor mandibular positional changes occasionally seen when a small amount of residual growth occurs following active care.

Management of Specific Dentofacial Deformities

Mandibular Deficiency

Patients with mandibular deficiency clinically present with a convex facial profile (see Fig. 28.8). The aesthetic soft tissue analysis of the upper and middle thirds of the face is within an acceptable norm, and the lower third of the face is retruded. The lower lip is everted with a deep labial mental crease and as there is lip incompetence and mentalis muscle strain is seen with lip closure. The neck length may be short with an obtuse cervical mental angle and redundancy of the soft tissue may be present. Dental examination will show a Class II Angle malocclusion that is further subdivided into Angle Division 1 or Angle Division 2 based on the incisor relationship. In Angle Class II Division 1, the maxillary incisor angulation is within an acceptable range, there is significant overjet, but the lower facial height is usually normal. In Angle Class I Division 2, the maxillary incisors are

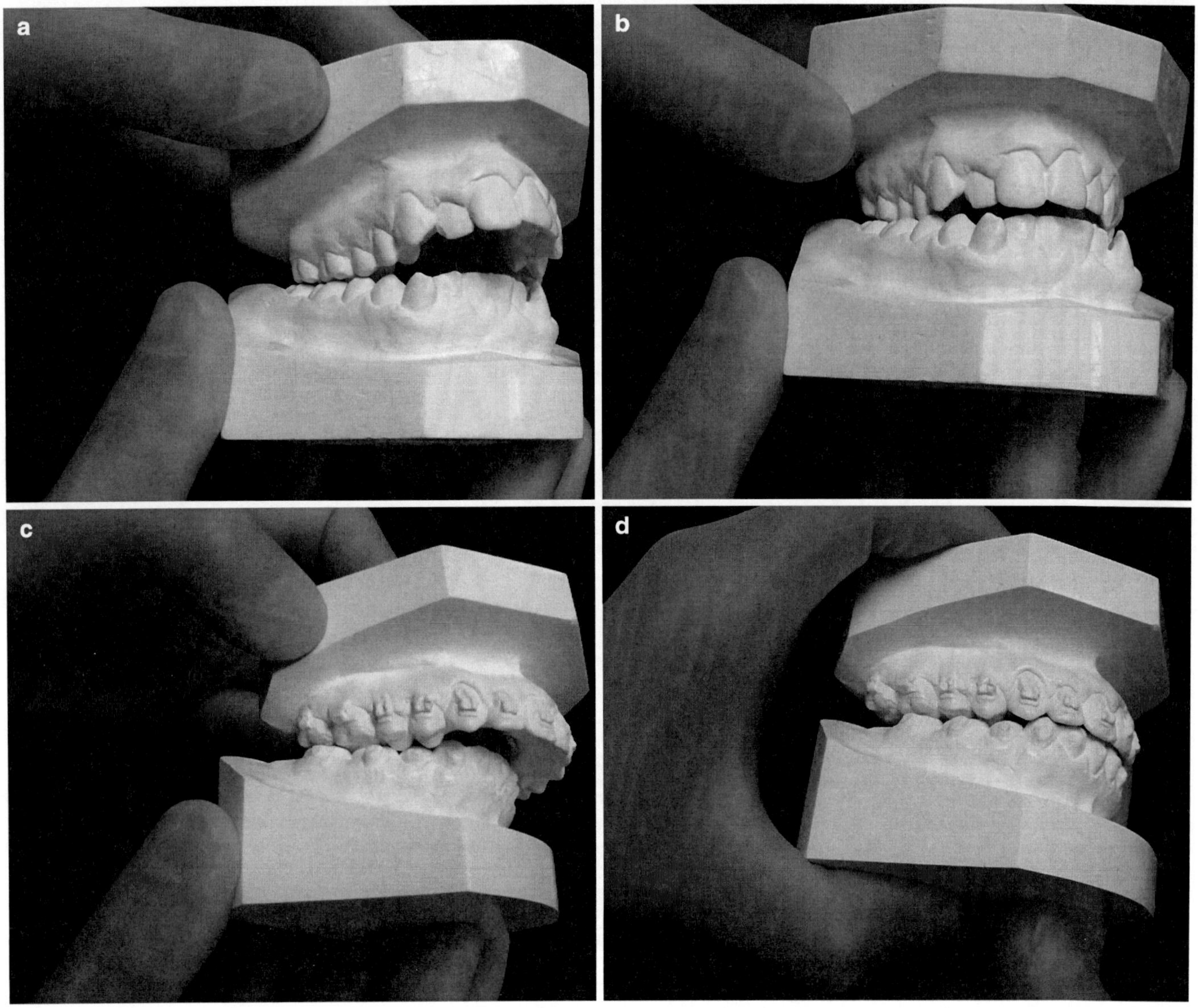

Fig. 28.7 Hand articulating the models to simulate the occlusion with surgery. (**a**) Pretreatment occlusion (**b**) Hand articulating the models without orthodontic treatment. There is no occlusal stability to support the surgical plan. (**c**) Presurgical occlusion after orthodontic treatment. (**d**) Hand articulating the models will show that with surgery, there is good occlusal stability and the patient can now be scheduled for surgery

retroclined giving the appearance of less overjet, and in addition there is an associated deep bite and an over accentuated Curve of Spee resulting in a decreased lower facial height.

As the location of the incisors often dictates the degree of surgical movement, the orthodontist positions the maxillary and mandibular incisors in the "ideal" position in both the anterior-posterior and vertical planes. Failure to adequately decompensate limits the surgical correction and aesthetic outcome. When there is crowding of the mandibular dental arch, it is frequently necessary to extract the lower first premolars and retract the anterior dentition. This allows for maximal mandibular advancement. In comparison, maxillary crowding in many circumstances can be managed by transpalatal expansion or when severe extraction of the upper second premolars to minimize retraction of the maxillary incisors and allow for maximum mandibular advancement. Routine leveling of the occlusal plane to obtain arch compatibility needs to be individualized depending on the severity of the Curve of Spee. If the Curve of Spee is orthodontically leveled prior to surgery, this is accomplished by intrusion of the mandibular incisors and will further adversely decrease the lower facial height in Class II Division 2 patients. It is instead preferable to skeletally advance the mandible to incisor Class I prior to leveling to maximally increase the lower facial height. The resultant lateral open bite is then closed orthodontically in the postsurgical phase by extrusion of the first molars and premolars. With only three-point contact (anterior and the two posterior molar regions), a surgical

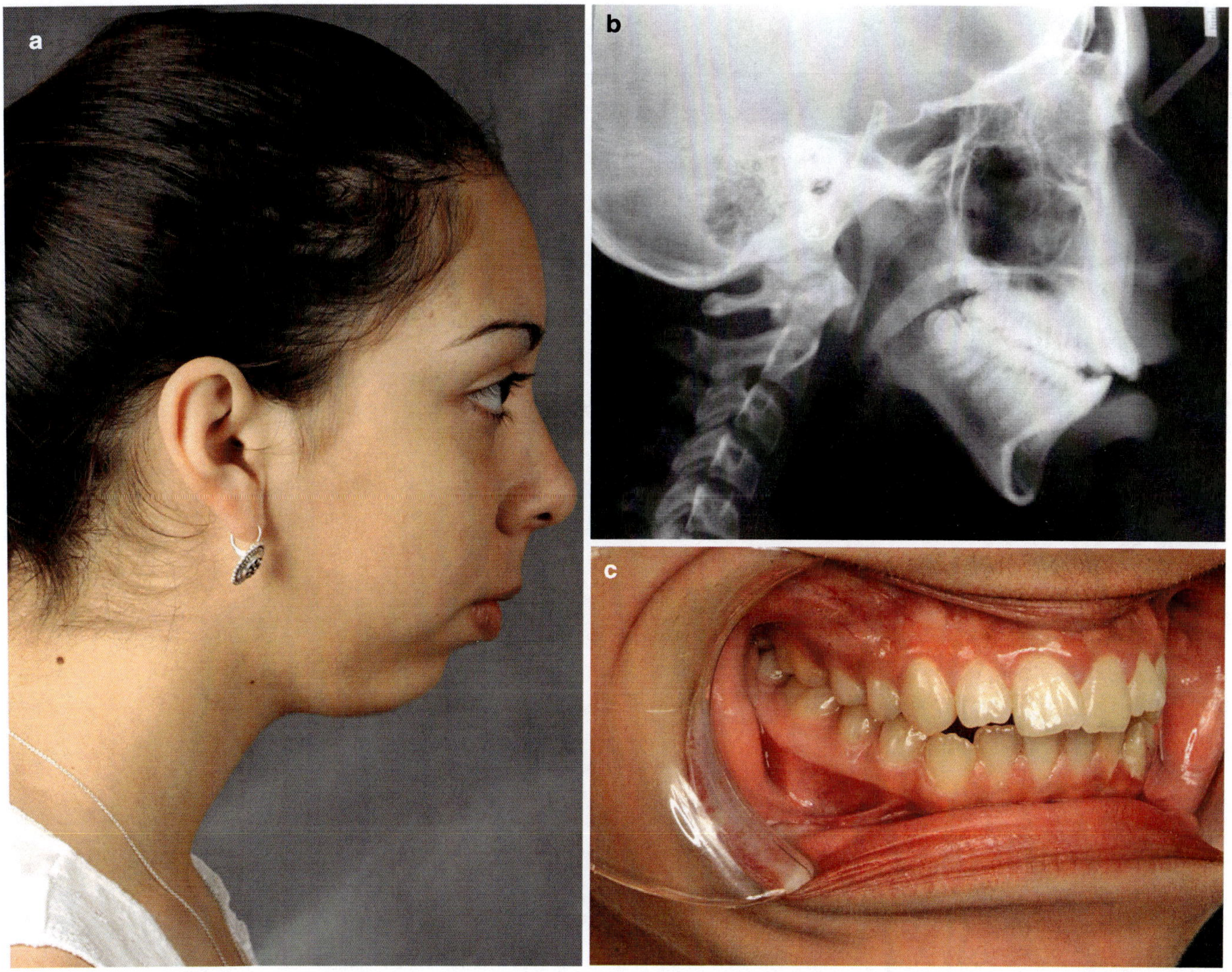

Fig. 28.8 Mandibular deficiency. Lateral photograph and cephalogram demonstrate recession of the lower face (**a**, **b**). Note that in the treatment planning lower first bicuspids are extracted to increase the overjet that will allow sufficient mandibular advancement (**c**) (Courtesy of Dr. Pravin K. Patel, MD, Chicago, IL)

splint is needed to ensure stability. The greater the lower facial height, the more likely the leveling should be done by incisor intrusion prior to surgery. With the exception of the patient with severe Curve of Spee and decreased lower facial height discussed above, establishing maximal arch compatibility and occlusal interdigitation prior to surgery is important to ensure immediate postoperative stability.

The skeletal advancement is achieved by the bilateral sagittal split osteotomy of the mandible using well-described techniques in the literature. The postsurgical management includes using "light" Class II elastics to override proprioception and guide the new occlusion in the immediate postoperative period. Orthodontic management then finalizes the coordination of the dental arches by definitive leveling of the Curve of Spee, closure of any spaces, and correction of any minor occlusal interferences.

Mandibular Excess (Prognathism)

Patients presenting with mandibular excess (prognathism) will present with a concave facial profile where the deformity is primarily isolated to the lower third (see Fig. 28.9). However, the vast majority of the patients will also show to some extent mid-facial skeletal deficiency, and the patient should be made aware of this. A number of patients will also have overclosure of the mandible further accentuating the prognathism and mid-facial deficiency. Dental examination will show a Class III malocclusion with lingually inclined mandibular incisors and often procumbent maxillary anterior teeth.

Presurgical orthodontic preparation includes decompensating the maxillary and mandibular incisors to an "ideal" position; however, in many patients, this presents

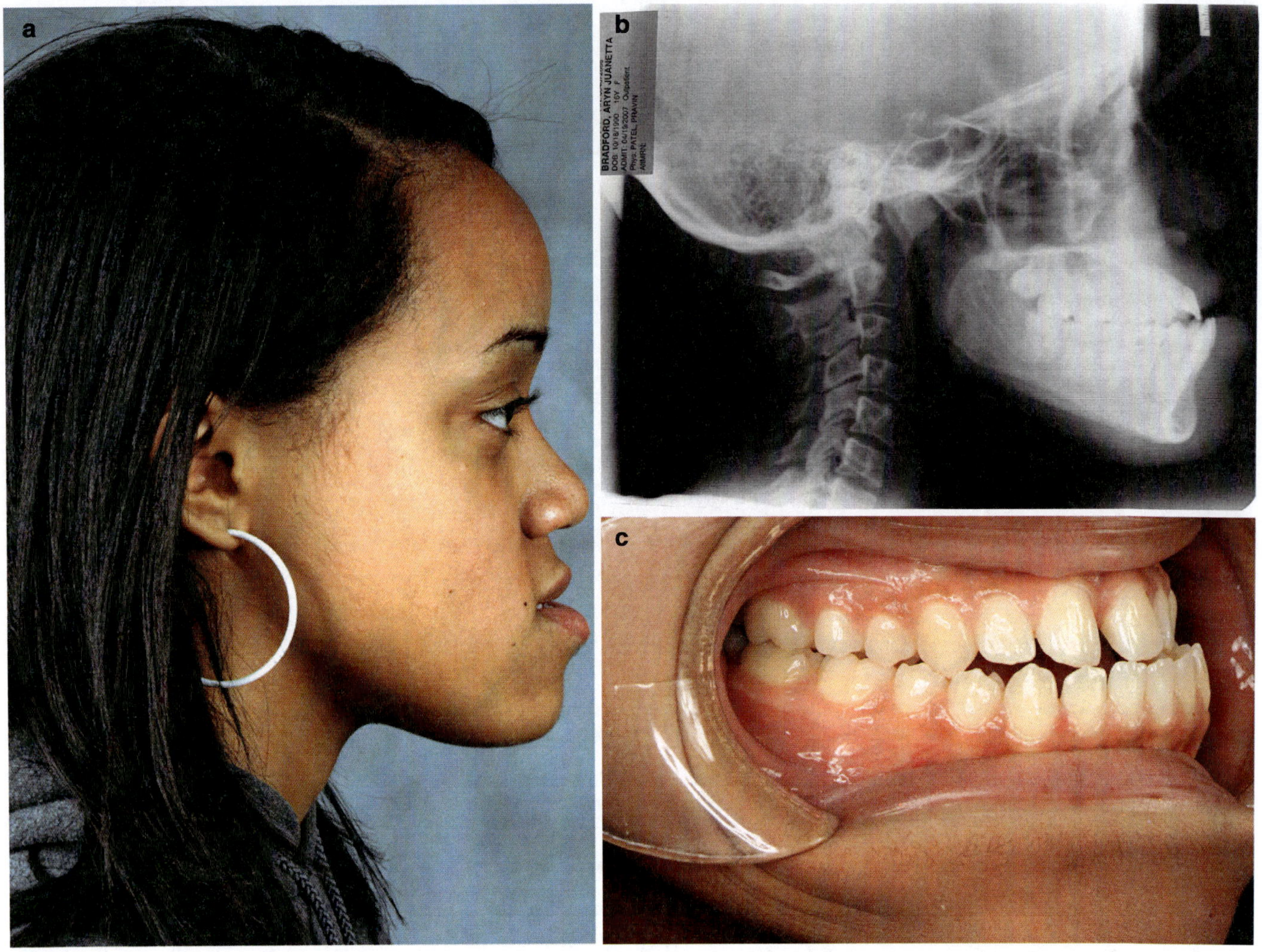

Fig. 28.9 Mandibular prognathism with maxillary deficiency. Lateral photograph and cephalogram demonstrate long mandibular body length, acute nasolabial angle, and piriform deficiency (**a**, **b**). Intraoral photograph demonstrates compensatory flaring of the incisors (**c**). (Courtesy of Dr. Pravin K. Patel, MD, Chicago, IL)

some clinical challenges as often these types of patients present with a thin alveolar process in the symphyseal region accompanied by thinly attached gingiva. Any transverse maxillary width discrepancy needs to be addressed by either orthodontic expansion of the maxillary dentition or if needed surgically assisted rapid palatal expansion prior to formally correcting the Class III sagittal discrepancy.

The surgeon's options to correct the Class III skeletal relationship are either the intraoral vertical ramus osteotomy (IVO) or the bilateral sagittal split osteotomy (BSSO) of the ramus. For minimal setbacks, it is frequently preferable to correct the Class III malocclusion with a maxillary advancement as the skeletal expansion allows "filling" of the soft tissue envelope and is more favorable over time with aging of the face. For large setbacks, similarly combining mid-facial skeletal advancement will limit the amount of mandibular setback required and a BSSO instead of an IVO can be accomplished. Similarly, with mandibular setback, the surgeon must be cognizant of the tongue confined to a smaller intraoral volume and the potential for sleep apnea.

Sagittal Maxillary Deficiency

Because of the similarity in clinical presentation, maxillary anterior-posterior sagittal deficiency has often been diagnosed solely as mandibular excess (prognathism) and a mandibular setback procedure is planned. However, in many circumstances, the deformity also includes the mid-face, and instead of a mandibular setback alone, the patient is better served with a mid-facial skeletal advancement either solely or combination with mandibular surgery. Both present with a Class III skeletal pattern. Clinically, the patient presents with concave facial profile, deficiency of the maxilla that may extend to involve the zygoma, paranasal deficiency with a narrow alar base, an acute nasolabial angle, short upper lip length, and a retrusive upper lip with a thin vermilion and in many circumstances an accompanying lack of dental display (vertical deficiency). Dental characteristics include a class III molar and canine relationship, maxillary dental crowding with canines blocked out of the dental arches, and in many circumstances deficient transverse palatal arch width (posterior lingual crossbite), proclined maxillary incisors, and mandibular incisors either in a normal or retroclined inclination.

The orthodontist eliminates the dental compensations prior to surgery. This is termed "surgical decompensation" where an ideal incisor position is established and coordinates the maxillary and mandibular dental arches. If there is an absolute transverse width discrepancy, this may require increasing the transverse palatal dimension as a two-segment LeFort I osteotomy with simultaneous correction of the sagittal discrepancy. The roots of the central incisors then need to be deviated to safely perform the interdental osteotomy. In many circumstances, it is preferable to stage the orthognathic surgery by first correcting the transverse width discrepancy by orthodontic expansion that may require surgically assistance rapid palatal expansion (SARPE) and then subsequently correcting the sagittal discrepancy as a single piece LeFort I osteotomy to postoperative skeletal stability. With maxillary crowding and the need for incisor retraction, the decision to extract the first or second premolars is based on the extent of crowding and degree of incisor decompensation needed. When the advancement of the mandibular incisors is limited by lack of attached gingiva and/or minimal alveolar bony support, then mandibular second premolar extraction may be necessary to provide the necessary space. Under most circumstances, the maxillary first premolars are extracted or where needed combined with extraction of mandibular second premolars as a most common extraction pattern.

Vertical Maxillary Excess

Patients with vertical maxillary excess (VME) or long face syndrome will present with increase in the lower facial height with clockwise rotation of the mandible a convex facial profile. The chin may be vertically increased and retrusive (see Fig. 28.10). Lip incompetence (increased interlabial gap) is present and mentalis strain occurs with attempted lip closure. There is excessive dental display on repose and a "gummy" smile. The alar base is frequently narrow in width, the paranasal regions deficient, and there is lack of malar projection in many of the patients. Intraoral examination reveals an anterior open bite deformity in the majority of the patients, a high-arched palate with a "V"-shaped transversely narrow maxilla, and dentition in palatal crossbite. While the occlusal relationship is Class II in the majority of the cases, Class I and Class III, VME can occur. With downward and posterior rotation of the mandible (clockwise rotation of the mandibular plane) as a result of excessive vertical maxillary growth will make associated mandibular deficiency appear worse and mandibular excess not as severe. While anterior open bite is the usual presentation, patients with a deep bite can exhibit VME.

The orthodontic management involves elimination of dental compensations and minor leveling of the mandibular arch. In cases where the open bite is severe and there is an excessive reverse Curve of Spee in the maxillary arch, it is preferable to level the arch in segments with appropriate root divergence to allow interdental osteotomies and surgical leveling with a three-piece LeFort I osteotomy. When the vertical discrepancies are minimal then the arch can be leveled in a single plane and the open bite corrected by differential posterior-anterior impaction single piece LeFort I osteotomy. The open bite should not be closed orthodontically to minimize dental relapse. Relief of dental crowding and transverse palatal expansion (surgically assisted) should be addressed prior to definitive orthognathic surgery.

In many circumstances correction of significant VME requires double jaw surgery: differential LeFort I impaction of the maxilla either as a single segment or multi-segment with mandibular BSSO advancement. However, occasionally LeFort I impaction with or without a genioplasty with reliance on auto-rotation of the mandible will result in a stable occlusion and a satisfactory aesthetic outcome. Prediction cephalometric tracings are beneficial to assess the need for concomitant mandibular surgery.

Summary

The treatment of complex malocclusions with overriding skeletal discrepancies requires an exceptional amount of pretreatment planning. It is necessary before any patient care is delivered that there has been sufficient input from each member of the orthognathic surgical team. As the goals of presurgical orthodontic treatment are more often than not opposite of the routine orthodontic regimen, detailed planning utilizing diagnostic orthodontic set-ups and predictive visual imaging are often needed to affirm the necessary procedures needed to create an aesthetic and functional result. Without this "integrated team approach," successful outcomes of treatment can be problematic.

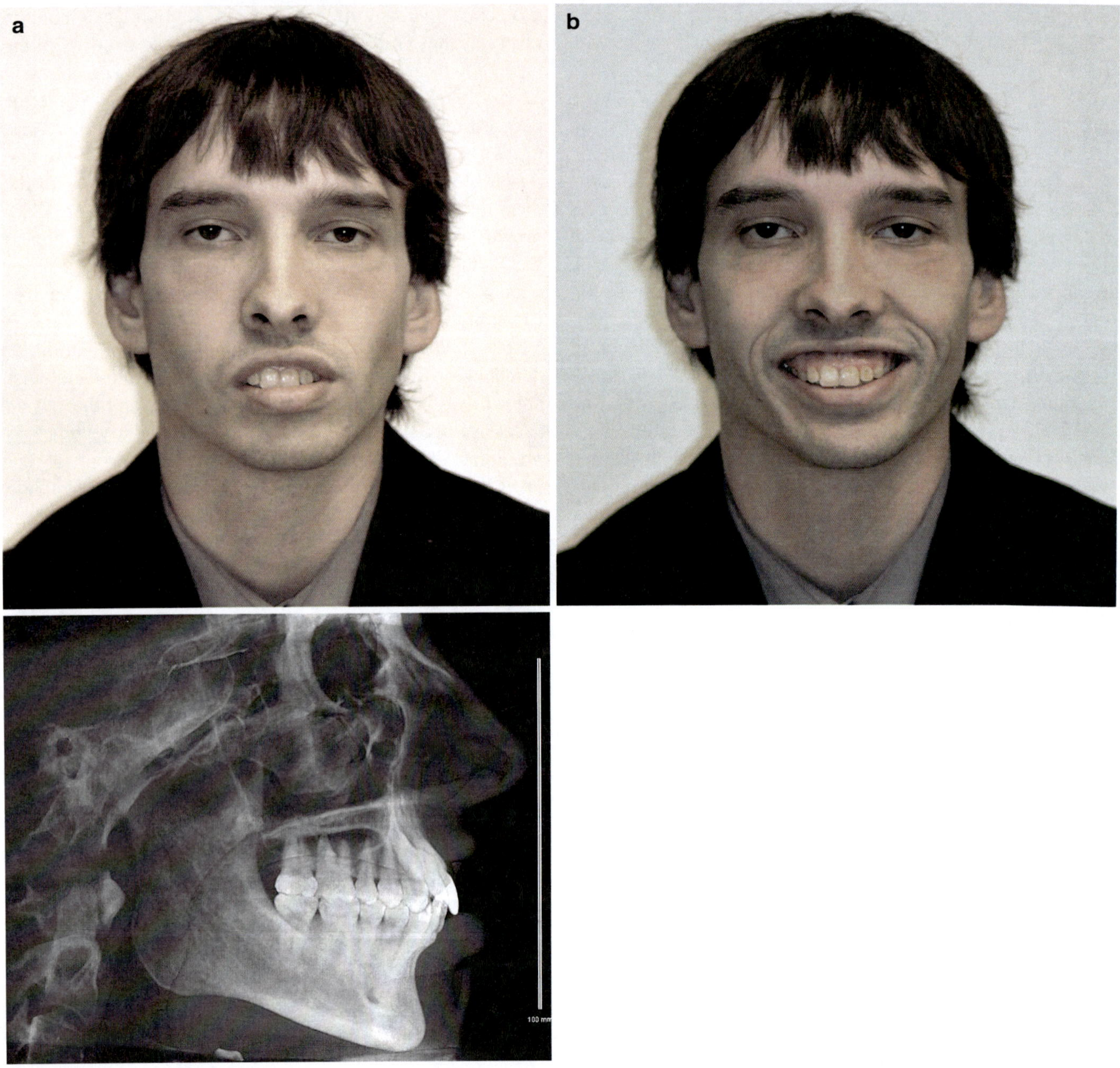

Fig. 28.10 Vertical maxillary excess. Photographs demonstrate abnormal lip posture at rest and the excessive "gummy" smile (**a**, **b**). Lateral cephalogram is demonstrated in image (**c**)

Bibliography

Baccetti T, Franchi L, McNamara JA. An improved version of the cervical vertebral maturation (CVM) method for assessment of mandibular growth. Angle Orthod. 2002;72:316–23.

Carlson DS. Biological rationale for early treatment of dentofacial deformities. Am J Orthod Dentofacial Orthop. 2002;121:554–8.

Fox ME, Stephens WF, Wolford LM, el Dee M. Effects of interdental osteotomies on the periodontal and osseous supporting tissues. Int J Adult Orthodon Orthognath Surg. 1991;6:39–46.

Freihofer HPM. Results of osteotomies of the facial skeleton in adolescence. J Maxillofac Surg. 1977;5:267.

Freihofer HPM. The timing of facial osteotomies in children and adolescents. Clin Plast Surg. 1982;9(4):445.

Grave KC, Brown T. Skeletal ossification of the adolescent growth spurt. Am J Orthod. 1976;69:611–9.

Greulich VVW, Pyle I. Radiographic atlas of skeletal development of the hand and wrist. 2nd ed. Stanford: Stanford UP; 1959.

Haralabakis N, Papadakis G. Relapse after orthodontics and orthognathic surgery. World J Orthod. 2005;6:125–40.

Jacobs JD, Sinclair PM. Principles of orthodontic mechanics in orthognathic surgery cases. Am J Orthod. 1983;84:399.

Lo FM, Shapiro PA. Effect of presurgical incisor extrusion on stability of anterior open bite malocclusion treated with orthognathic surgery. Int J Adult Orthodon Orthognath Surg. 1998;13:23–34.

Mao JJ, Wang X, Kopher RA. Biomechanics of craniofacial sutures: orthopedic implications. Angle Orthod. 2003;73:128–35.

Proffit WR, Ackerman JL. Diagnosis and treatment planning. In: Graber M, Vanarsdall Jr RL, editors. Orthodontics: current principles and treatment. St. Louis: Mosby; 1994.

Proffit WR, White Jr RP. Surgical orthodontic treatment. St. Louis: Mosby; 1990a. p. 96–140.

Proffit WR, White WR. Who needs surgical-orthodontic treatment? Int J Adult Orthodon Orthognath Surg. 1990b;5:81.

Reyneke JP, Tsakiris P, Becker P. Age as a factor in the complication rate after removal of unerupted/impacted third molars at the time of mandibular sagittal split osteotomy. J Oral Maxillofac Surg. 2002; 60:654–9.

Ricketts RM. The influence of orthodontic treatment on facial growth and development. Angle Orthod. 1960;30:103.

Riolo ML, et al. An atlas of craniofacial growth. Ann Arbor: Center for Human Growth and Development; 1974.

Rosen H. When osteotomy should be considered. Clint Plast Surg. 1991;18(1):205.

Sabri R. Orthodontic objectives in orthognathic surgery: state of the art today. World J Orthod. 2006;7(2):177–91.

Schultes G, Gaggl A, Karcher H. Periodontal disease associated with interdental osteotomies after, orthognathic surgery. J Oral Maxillofac Surg. 1998;56:414–7.

Shanker S, Vig K. Orthodontic preparation for orthognathic surgery. In: Fonseca RJ, Betts NJ, Turvey TA, editors. Oral and maxillofacial surgery, vol. 2. Philadelphia: W B Saunders Company; 2000.

Squire D, Best AM, Lindauer SJ, Laskin DM. Determining the limits of orthodontic treatment of overbite, overjet, and transverse width discrepancy: a pilot study. Am J Ortho Dentofacial Orthop. 2006; 129(6):804–8.

Wolford LM. Periodontal disease associated with interdental osteotomies after orthognathic surgery. J Oral Maxillofac Surg. 1998;56:417–9.

Wolford LM, Stevao ELL, Alexander CM, et al. Orthodontics for orthognathic surgery. In: Gahli GE, Larsen PE, Waite PD, editors. Oral and maxillofacial surgery, vol. 2. Hamilton, ON: BC Decker Inc.; 2004.

Genioplasty

29

Stephen Baker and Kevin Han

Introduction

The chin is an important structure in creating an aesthetic facial shape. Not only does it contribute to facial proportion in frontal and lateral views, but it also supports the overlying soft tissues. The chin can be moved three dimensionally with an osteotomy (osseous genioplasty) or can be augmented with an alloplastic implant (implant genioplasty) for more limited changes in chin position. The versatility of an osteotomy provides more precision to move the chin to its ideal position, but it is a more invasive procedure when compared to an implant (Fig. 29.1). Most surgeons consider an alloplastic chin augmentation a simpler procedure with a faster recovery, but in the majority of indications, an implant cannot provide the same result as an osseous genioplasty. When compared to other maxillofacial procedures, either type of genioplasty is a relatively straightforward procedure that produces a predictable result with a fast recovery.

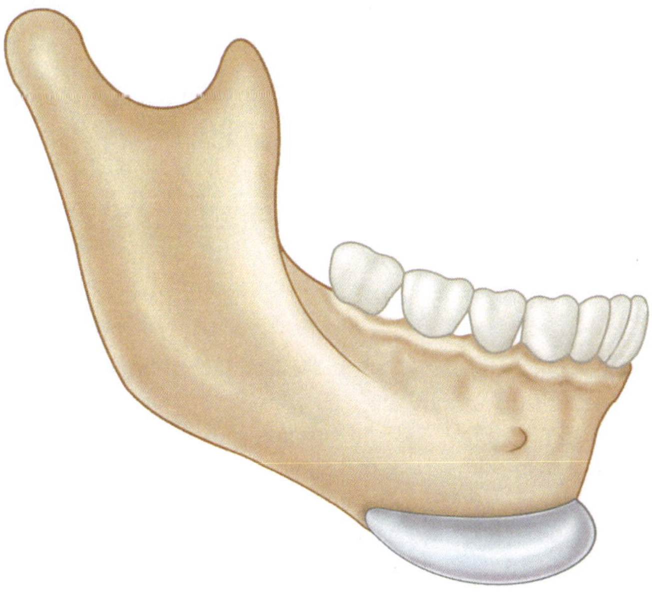

Fig. 29.1 Placement of an implant to augment the chin

Anatomy

The chin is comprised of skin, subcutaneous tissue, fat, muscle, and bone. The *depressor angularis oris*, *depressor labii inferioris*, and *mentalis* muscles attach to the anterior plane of the chin. The *geniohyoid*, *genioglossus*, *mylohyoid*, and anterior belly of the *digastric* attach to the lingual aspect of the chin at the genial tubercle. The blood supply to the mental area is from the inferior alveolar artery and vessels from the geniohyoid, genioglossus, and anterior belly of the digastric muscles. The mental nerve supplies sensation to the anterior mandibular gingival mucosa and lower lip. This nerve is a continuation of the inferior alveolar nerve and becomes the mental nerve after it exits the mental foramen between the first and second premolars. The mental foramen has been shown to be located 14.61 mm superior to the inferior border of the mandible. Because the inferior alveolar canal runs lower than the mental foramen, an osteotomy must be planned at least 6 mm caudal to the foramen.

Diagnosis and Treatment Planning

Frontal View

Because the chin contributes to facial proportion, it is important to have an understanding of normal and aesthetic values prior to treatment planning a genioplasty. When examining the face, it is important that the teeth are in occlusion and the lips are in repose. The vertical height of the face can be divided into thirds. The trichion to the glabella is the upper third, the glabella to subnasale is the middle third, and subnasale to menton is the lower third. The lower facial third can

S. Baker, MD, DDS, FACS (✉) • K. Han, MD
Department of Plastic Surgery,
Georgetown University Hospital, Washington, DC, USA
e-mail: sbb6@gunet.georgetown.edu

P.J. Taub et al. (eds.), *Ferraro's Fundamentals of Maxillofacial Surgery*,
DOI 10.1007/978-1-4614-8341-0_29, © Springer Science+Business Media New York 2015

be further subdivided so that the distance between the stomion and the menton should be twice as long as the distance from subnasale to stomion.

When examining transverse symmetry of the chin, it is useful to mark several points (glabella, nose, dental midlines, vermillion, and chin) to see if all are congruent. Occasionally, these points are not aligned, and the surgeon needs to point this out to the patient preoperatively and explain the limitations of surgery. Ideally, the center of the chin is congruent with the mandibular skeletal and dental midlines. If the chin is not centered, a simple centering genioplasty is indicated. If both the chin and the mandible are not centered, a mandibular osteotomy is necessary to correct the asymmetry. In rare cases, both the chin and the mandible are off the midline, and the patient desires improved symmetry but does not wish to undergo a mandibular osteotomy. In these cases, the chin alone can be moved to improve lower facial symmetry without moving the mandible. When the chin is moved, a 1:1 ratio of bone to soft tissue movement is anticipated when planning the final position.

Lateral View

From a lateral view, the three aspects of the chin that affect aesthetics the most are the sagittal projection of the chin, the labiomental angle, and the submental soft tissue support. The sagittal projection of the chin may be determined by several methods. Byrd has described a method using the mid-dorsum of the nose and dropping a line from this point inferiorly and tangential to the upper lip. Assuming the nose is of normal length, the chin should be about 3 mm posterior to this line. Another method is to drop a line inferior and perpendicular to Frankfurt horizontal that is tangential to the lower lip. The chin should be just posterior to this line in females and at or slightly anterior to it in males. A final analysis is Riedel's line. This line connects the most prominent points of the upper and lower lips. The most prominent point of the chin should be the third point on this line.

The labiomental angle is another important dimension that contributes to the aesthetic appearance of the chin in profile. Vertical reduction or anterior movement will increase the acuity of the labiomental angle, and vertical elongation or posterior positioning will make the angle more obtuse. Farkas described the normal adult female labiomental angle as 121° and the adult male angle as 114°, and Reyneke has stated it to be 130°. However, it is important to remember that in the majority of cases, the patient does not necessarily want to be normal but beautiful. Iglesias-Linares et al. reviewed the labiomental angles of the 40 most beautiful white and black females as voted by a popular beauty magazine, and the average labiomental angle in this group is 108.75° for the 40 white women and 104.75° for the 40 black women. There is no statistical significance between the two groups. The ultimate judgment of the result is the patient, but it is important to note that norms do not always equate the aesthetic ideals.

The submental soft tissue needs to be assessed prior to modification of the chin. In patients who desire to have their chin projection reduced, one must be careful not to compromise submental laxity by posteriorly positioning the chin and therefore reducing skeletal soft tissue support. Occasionally, it is better to leave the patient with a slightly strong chin in order to avoid creating laxity of the submental tissue. If a patient requires posterior chin positioning that will lead to submental laxity, an adjunct neck lift may be necessary to reduce the resulting submental laxity. In contrast, anterior chin movements will stretch and tighten the submental tissue thus improving the cervicomental angle. In older patients, this increased skeletal support will have rejuvenative effects in the lower face.

Influence of Facial Features on the Perception of the Chin

Other factors that affect the perception of chin position but are not intrinsic to the chin itself are nasal projection, vertical maxillary position, and mandibular projection. An overprojected nose may give the illusion of a small chin and vice versa. Vertical maxillary excess will cause the mandible to be rotated in a clockwise position, which will decrease anterior chin projection. A vertically short maxilla will lead to counterclockwise mandibular rotation that will increase chin projection. Problems related to abnormal vertical maxillary position are best treated by maxillary osteotomies.

The labiomental fold and chin-lip relationship will aid in determining whether deficient chin projection is due to the chin, the mandible, or both. A deficient chin with a normal labiomental angle and lower lip relationship is likely due to mandibular retrognathia. If the labiomental crease is obtuse and the chin is well posterior to the lower lip, the deficiency is likely due to the chin. The degree to which the mandible contributes to chin projection may be evaluated by examining the occlusion. If an overbite is noted on physical examination, the degree to which the mandible would need to be advanced to achieve a class I occlusion is typically the degree of mandibular deficiency. This value assumes normal maxillary projection and normal dental alignment. If after advancing the mandible, the chin would remain deficient, the chin can be advanced to achieve an ideal projection based on the criteria discussed previously (see Part III).

Orthognathic Camouflage

A patient may exhibit mandibular retrusion but will present with a class I occlusion. This is typically a patient who originally would have been ideally treated with orthognathic surgery but opted for nonsurgical orthodontic treatment. Achieving a class I occlusion using only orthodontics in a patient whose skeletal discrepancy would ideally be treated with orthognathic surgery is known as dental compensation. These patients will demonstrate a dental class I occlusion but at the expense of facial disharmony. Frequently orthodontists will extract upper premolars to allow room for the upper teeth to be pulled back to meet into a class I occlusion with the lower teeth. As the upper teeth are moved posteriorly, lip support is lost giving the perception of an overly projected nose. This commonly encountered group of patients will have the appearance of a large nose and a small jaw/chin yet possess a class I occlusion. In addition to an advancement genioplasty, these patients also may be candidates for a rhinoplasty.

Facial Rejuvenation

Previous studies have demonstrated that skeletal projection has beneficial effects on the overlying soft tissue envelope. In middle age to elderly patients who present with deficient chin projection and soft tissue complaints of redundant submental skin and an obtuse cervical mental angle, an advancement genioplasty will have beneficial effects on the overlying soft tissue. The muscles attached to the genial tubercle underneath the neck are advanced and tightened analogous to a rubber band as the chin segment is moved forward. Additionally, the increase in the length of the distance from the cervical mental crease to gonion will be elongated giving the illusion of a more well-defined neck. A tightening of skin that occurs in the area of the lower lip, jowls, and marionette lines is also achieved as the underlying skeleton is projected in the area of the chin. Genioplasty is a good procedure in patients who do not desire the scars or stigmata of a facelift yet seek some soft tissue improvement in the lower facial third.

Cephalometric Evaluation

A lateral cephalometric radiograph is a standardized lateral radiograph of the face that shows both the bone and soft tissue and can be easily obtained at any orthodontist's office. This image is useful in determining the degree to which the chin will be advanced or setback. Clear acetate tracing paper is taped over the radiograph, and the soft tissue and skeleton of the chin and mandible are traced in pencil. A second small piece of tracing paper is then used to just trace the bone and overlying soft tissue of the chin. The smaller tracing is then moved over the original tracing so that the soft tissue pogonion (most anterior chin point) is in the optimal location relative to the face. The measured difference between the original and newly positioned skeletal chin is the distance the surgeon will move the osteotomized chin segment to achieve that result. The soft tissue moves with the bone in approximately a 1:1 ratio making this an accurate predictive tool. Software programs are also available to analyze the image and provide similar information.

Digital Imaging

Digital imaging is important for both treatment planning and documentation. Recommended views include a frontal, right and left lateral, right and left oblique, worm's eye, and bird's eye views of the patient's face. From these images, a dimensional analysis of the patient's chin can be made incorporating the previously mentioned normative values. Predictive digital imaging can also be performed giving the patient an idea of the final result. However, it is important to inform the patient that the predicted image is not a guarantee of the result but a prediction to make sure the surgeon and the patient have the same goals in mind. In order to improve accuracy in treatment planning, it is recommended to apply a ruler to the patient's face and enlarge the image to a 1:1 reproduction. This allows movements in the prediction to be accurately quantified in millimeters and produce the most accurate assessment of the patient's goals. The ruler taped to the face can easily be calibrated to actual size using calibration tools found on both Adobe Photoshop and Mirror imaging software. The amount of movement that is desired by the patient in the image will dictate the amount of skeletal movement the surgeon will move the chin. Studies have shown that soft tissue follows skeletal movements in a 1:1 ratio, so the millimeter difference between the preoperative and predicted image can be directly translated to the skeletal movements of the chin. When using an implant, the soft tissue to implant ratio is 0.8:1. Radiographic imaging should be obtained as well to document the absence of osseous pathology prior to performing osseous surgery of the chin.

Basic Genioplasty Technique

- Infiltrate lower lip mucosa and mentalis with 10 cc of 1 % lidocaine 1/100,000 epinephrine. Because the injection is done before prepping and draping the patient, it has redistributed by the time of the procedure so that the volume of infiltration does not compromise accuracy.
- The patient is prepped after the injection allowing the epinephrine to take effect.
- The throat pack is placed and Peridex is poured into the oral cavity and remains for 5 min prior to suction.
- Use non-dominant hand to evert the lip, using the index finger to palpate below intraoral incision.
- Using a guarded blunt tip Bovie, make the initial mucosal incision from canine to canine. Then, redirect the Bovie towards the bone to divide the mentalis muscle. The left

index finger is used to make sure that the Bovie tip does not inadvertently cut through the cutaneous surface.

- A periosteal elevator is then used to dissect from the incision to the inferior border of the mandible in an inferior direction. Once the inferior border has been identified, the periosteal elevator can be used to dissect laterally in the subperiosteal plane along and parallel to the inferior aspect of the mandible. Because the mental foramen is 14 mm superior to the inferior mandibular border and the widest Obwegeser periosteal elevator is 10 mm, this dissection can be done rapidly and blindly without worry of hitting the mental nerve. I refer to this region as a dissection "hot lane" meaning the dissection can be done very quickly without risk of injury to the mental nerve as long as the surgeon keeps the elevator flush with the inferior border of the mandible. Once this dissection has been done bilaterally, careful superior elevation easily identifies the mental nerve.
- A reciprocating saw with a long blade is used to make a vertical line between the midline of the lower central incisors and additional lines 10 mm lateral to midline on both sides. The midline cut is typically made between the lower central incisors; however, if it's slightly off midline, it is of no relevance as it is drawn merely as a reference to make sure that the chin remains midline when the plate is secured.
- Genioplasty retractors are placed to retract the mucosal tissue as well as to identify the mental foramen and to protect the mental nerve. The osteotomy cut should be at least 6 mm inferior to the mental foramen because the nerve runs through the mandible inferior to the mental foramen before exiting and rises superiorly as it exits the mental foramen.
- It is important to use the reciprocating saw to get around the lateral aspect of the chin when making the osteotomy; and it is also important to go far posteriorly so that in addition to the chin button, the wider portion of the inferior mandible is also advanced. Initiating the osteotomy from a more posterior position (around the first molar) reduces an iatrogenic appearance after chin surgery when advancement is being performed. Frequently, if there is an area that does not appear released after the osteotomies are complete, it is usually in the far lateral areas of the osteotomy. The problem usually relates to the fact that the tip of the saw blade has not made it completely around the lateral genial segment during the osteotomy. When making the cut, it is also important to be aware of the angle of the osteotomy. If the cut slopes from low to high as it goes posterior, the chin will be elongated as it is advanced. It is important the surgeon be aware of the three-dimensional nature of the movement to avoid an unanticipated result.
- If the surgeon feels as though the osteotomy should be complete but the genial segment is not mobile, he needs to avoid the temptation of snapping it free with the periosteal elevator. Although this will usually free the segment, it does so leaving a spicule of bone that will likely interfere with the continuous slide of the osteotomized segment and thereby may introduce a degree of err to the final result. Instead, it is recommended that the osteotomy be checked with the saw to see where the incomplete cut is in order to free it where the bone remains intact.
- It is the author's preference not to dissect the soft tissue off of the genial tubercle because as the genial segment is advanced, the musculature under the neck gets stretched which enhances the overall neck chin profile from the lateral view.
- The genioplasty advancement plates come in sizes that differ by 2 mm increments. The desired advancement plate is picked. The inferior mobile genioplasty segment is typically secured to the plate first, with the midline mark being directly under the middle hole of the plate. A Kocher or a small "L" retractor or elevator can be used to pull the segment from below and stabilize the bone segment. This may help orient the mobile segment as well as provide some resistance as screws are being inserted. It is important to ensure that the shaft of the drill does not touch the lip as the screws are inserted. If this occurs, a friction burn may result and be noticeable postoperatively.
- Once the inferior segment is secured, the top screws will be easier to place in the superior or stable mandibular segment. It is important to make sure that the vertical reference lines are congruent if no lateral movement of the chin is desired. If an asymmetry is going to be corrected, the degree of lateral movement can be calculated from the difference between the reference lines.
- Once the chin plate is secured, the incision is loosely approximated, and the patient is evaluated from the side to make sure that both the anterior movement and the acuity of the labiomental fold are acceptable to the surgeon.
- If the anterior movement is sufficient but the labiomental fold is too acute, it is possible to inferiorly position the chin segment to soften the acuity of the labiomental fold while preserving the sagittal projection of the chin segment.
- After the final chin position is established, the lateral edges of the chin are assessed. If an irregular transition is present between the mandible and the newly positioned chin, the lateral bony edges can be smoothed with a burr or a power rasp.
- Once the chin has been plated in the proper position, 2–0 Monocryl sutures on an SH needle are used to approximate the mentalis muscle. It is recommended to put two or three sutures in the muscle to restore to its anatomic position and prevent postoperative chin ptosis. It is important

when passing the needle through the mentalis on the skin side that the skin is not puckered as the suture is tightened. Gentle traction on the suture after it has been placed can check this. If puckering is noted, redo the suture with a bite less superficial to the skin. Also, the bites should correspond to the labiomental fold to minimize soft tissue distortion from the mentalis closure. Finally, the sutures are held on snaps until all have been placed to maintain visualization while placing them. After all the sutures are placed, they are tied to approximate the mentalis. After the mentalis was approximated, the mucosa is closed with interrupted 4–0 chromic sutures on a tapered needle.

- The postoperative dressing consists of either an elastic compression jaw bra or an elastic adhesive dressing to provide soft tissue support over the osteotomized chin.

Types of Osseous Genioplasty

The basic steps outlined above generally apply to the following osteotomies. Any variance or modification specific to a desired osteotomy will be mentioned under each specific type of osteotomy mentioned below.

Sliding Genioplasty (Anterior-Posterior Movements)

The osteotomy is performed as a single cut through the chin at least 6 mm inferior to apices of the mandibular teeth and the mental foramen. It is important to be aware of the angle of the osteotomy because a sloped cut will change the vertical position of the chin as it is advanced or set back (see technique section). Once the osteotomy is complete, the caudal segment can be moved anteriorly or posteriorly while maintaining contact between the two bone segments. Prefabricated genioplasty plates come in 2 mm increments and can be used to secure the segments in the desired position. For a setback genioplasty, the plates are just inverted and bent to fit the contour of the bone. These plates can then be used to set the chin back to the desired number of millimeters. When performing advancement genioplasty, it is important to assess the labiomental crease as well as chin projection. If the desired projection results in an excessively deep labiomental crease, the degree of advancement should be reduced or the chin elongated to reduce the acuity of the crease if the lower facial third will not be excessively elongated (Fig. 29.2).

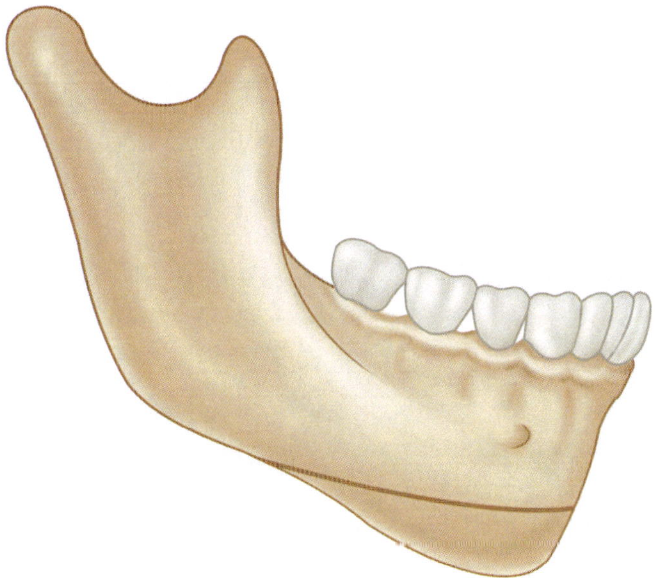

Fig. 29.2 Lateral view of basic sliding advancement genioplasty

Vertical Reduction Genioplasty

When the vertical height of the chin is excessive, two horizontally parallel osteotomies are made with removal of the intervening segment. The amount of bone to be removed is based on the preoperative determination from radiographs and clinical examination. Once the bone is exposed, two horizontal lines are marked and measured using a sterilized pencil. If a cant exists in the inferior chin, the lines may be adjusted to remove more bone from the elongated side of the chin. The inferior osteotomy is performed first followed by the superior cut. This allows the surgeon to make both cuts on stable bone. If the superior osteotomy is done first, the inferior osteotomy will be difficult to perform since the genial segment will be mobile. In large vertical reductions, it may be necessary to remove some bone from the inferior mandible just posterior to the osteotomy to prevent a boxy appearance in the frontal view. It is recommended to evaluate the labiomental fold after mentalis approximation because vertical reduction may cause it to become too acute (Fig. 29.3).

Vertical Elongating Genioplasty

The horizontal osteotomy is marked and performed in the usual manner. If the vertical elongation is less than 5 mm, a genioplasty plate is used to secure the segments apart in desired distance. A caliper is used intraoperatively to confirm the degree of elongation. If the segments are to be spaced greater than 5 mm apart, a bone graft or a piece of hydroxyapatite (HA) is placed between the bone segments to add stability to the lower portion of the chin. It is recommended to evaluate the labiomental fold after mentalis approximation because vertical elongation may cause it to become too obtuse.

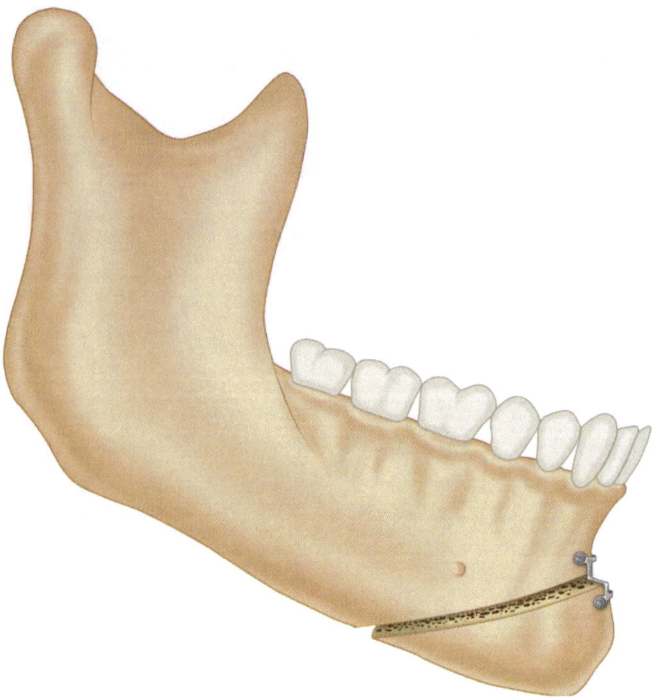

Fig. 29.3 Movements to advance and vertically shorten the chin

Narrowing Genioplasty

To narrow the wide chin (facial feminization, softening lower face), a genioplasty is performed with the removal of a central segment of bone (typically about 1 cm) in the inferior segment to allow the two lateral segments to be medialized and secured to each other as well as the mandible with a plate. The sequence is to first mark the mandibular midline with a reciprocating saw. Second, make two vertical reference lines on the inferior segment that are separated by the degree to which the chin needs to be narrowed. It is important that this distance is split evenly on each side of the upper midline reference mark, so the chin remains symmetric after surgery. The first cuts in bone are the two vertical cuts in the inferior segment. Second, the horizontal osteotomy is made. As you come across horizontally with the saw, the lateral segments and central segment of the inferior chin will become mobile as they are released. The central segment can now be removed and cautery is used to release it from its lingual muscle attachments with minimal bleeding. The two inferior segments are medialized and secured so the line between them lines up with the midline vertical reference in the mandible. If an advancement or setback is planned in addition to the narrowing, a standard chin plate is used with one screw in each of the inferior segments and three screws in the superior segment. It is the author's feeling that one screw in each inferior segment is sufficient to prevent rotation because the segments abut one another and the chin is not under any functional loading (Figs. 29.4).

Widening Genioplasty

Dividing an osteotomized segment in the midline and moving each piece laterally to the desired degree will widen the narrow chin. After the bone is exposed, the horizontal osteotomy is marked with a sterile pencil. A midline vertical mark is also made that extends from the inferior chin to the horizontal mark. The vertical cut is made first, and then the horizontal cut is made. Once each piece is free, it is evaluated to make sure that any irregular edges are smoothed. If the widening of the chin is greater than 5 mm, a bone graft or piece of block hydroxyapatite will be required as a midline spacer for stability. Widening the chin may prevent the prefabricated genioplasty plates from being used because the lateralized segments may be moved beyond the dimension of the plate. In these cases, two plates can be adapted laterally to secure each segment, and a transverse plate can be used to secure the graft or hydroxyapatite.

Centering Genioplasty

A centering genioplasty is performed when the chin midline deviates from the facial midline. It is important to identify the asymmetry prior to performing the genioplasty. Commonly used midline landmarks for the face are the intercanthal midline, nasal tip, Cupid's bow, upper and lower dental midlines, and the center of the chin. If all of these landmarks are on midline except the chin, it is reasonable to assume the chin is accounting for the asymmetry. If, however, the chin midline is centered to the mandible but off the facial midline, the problem may be due to mandibular asymmetry. Asymmetry due to either jaw is best treated with orthognathic surgery. Occasionally, a patient will have an asymmetry of the lower face that would ideally be treated with orthognathic surgery but refuses this treatment. In these cases symmetry may be improved with a genioplasty even though the chin is not the underlying etiology.

Evaluating preoperative photographs of the patient's face and documenting all preexisting facial asymmetries will assist with planning a centering genioplasty. The surgeon then determines how much the center of the chin needs to move to give the best overall appearance of facial symmetry. After exposure, the midline of the chin is scored with a saw. A second vertical mark is made on the inferior genial segment that corresponds to the distance the chin will be moved. The second mark is made on the opposite side of that to which the chin will be moved. Therefore, when the lateral

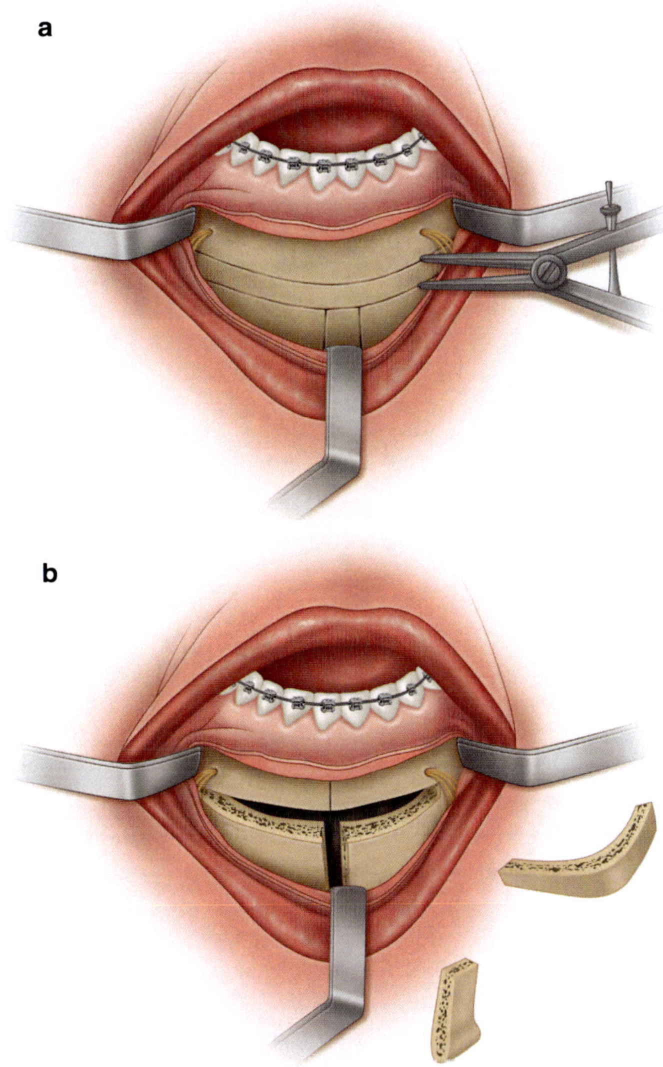

Fig. 29.4 (**a**–**c**) Osteotomies to vertically reduce and narrow the chin

vertical line on the inferior segment is aligned with the midline reference line on the superior segment, the chin will be centered in its desired position.

Leveling Genioplasty

If a cant or vertical asymmetry exists on the chin, it can be corrected with a wedge osteotomy. A posterior-anterior cephalometric radiograph or a frontal image is assessed to determine the degree of cant. Then a decision is made whether to lower the short side, shorten the long side, or perform a combination of both to achieve the desired cant correction and vertical dimension of the chin. A sterile pencil is used to mark the desired dimensions of the wedge osteotomy, and these marks are verified with a caliper. After the osteotomy is performed, the fixation is applied and the chin is assessed for symmetry. If a slight cant persists, bending the plate can achieve minor modifications. Larger discrepancies require replating to get a correct result. For very minor cants, burring may be performed but a caveat of this technique is that it may be hard to reach the inferior border of the chin through an intraoral incision, and a submental approach results in a scar.

Jumping Genioplasty

This is performed usually in the setting syndromic deformities (Treacher Collins). An osteotomy is made through the inferior mandible and then bringing the segment anteriorly and superiorly so the posterior edge of the chin segment rests against the anterior portion of the inferior mandible. This type of genioplasty is used for severe microgenia and because the jumping segment moves superiorly, it will shorten the lower facial third. In many patients who need correction of severe microgenia, they already have a short lower facial third and therefore cannot tolerate further shortening of the facial third. For this reason, the author prefers a double step genioplasty for severe microgenia.

Double Step Genioplasty

This osteotomy is indicated for extreme microgenia (Treacher Collins) and is preferred by some over the jumping genioplasty because it does not vertically shorten the chin. Two horizontal lines are marked on the chin taking care to ensure that each of the segments is of sufficient width to receive a fixation screw. The two osteotomies are then made making sure to do the most inferior cut first. After both cuts are made, the two mobile segments can be aligned for fixation. One technique is to use two separate genioplasty plates. One plate is used to secure the middle segment to the superior, intact mandible. Only the middle screw is placed in the middle segment leaving the lateral holes open to receive screw from the second plate. After the middle segment is attached to the mandible, the inferior segment is plated to the middle segment by overlapping the plate holes so that the lateral holes of the second plate overlap the lateral holes from the first plate on the middle segment. Screws are then inserted that secure the lateral holes from both plates. The inferior segment is secured with using three screws in the three holes.

A second technique is to use two lattice plates that are cut and bent to the desired dimensions and place one on each side of the chin. This type of plate application can be difficult because the plates need to be bent to accommodate all three levels of screw fixation, maintain symmetry, and preserve overlapping bone at each step. Both of these techniques require that some overlap of bone be maintained at each step so that healing can occur between the osteotomized segments and maintain stability. It is also important to note that the fixation be of sufficient strength to maintain the projection of the chin in these severe cases of microgenia. As one approaches advance of 18–20 mm, the soft tissue begins to exert a strong force against the fixation, and if the surgeon does not use adequate fixation, the plates may bend, compromising the result (Fig. 29.5).

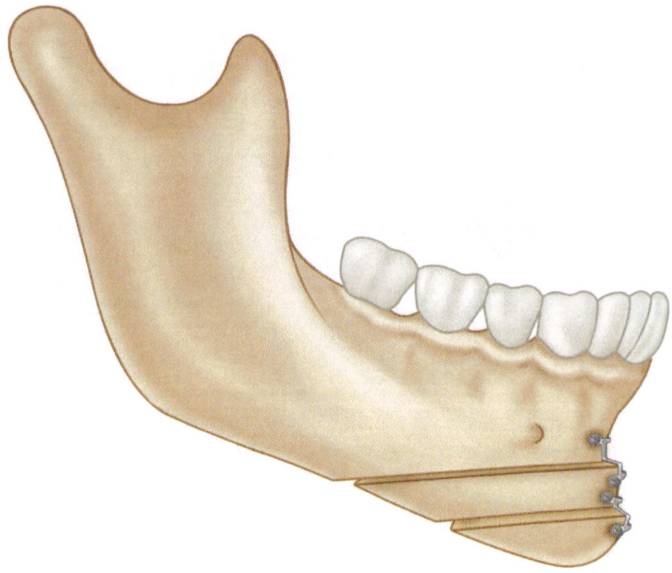

Fig. 29.5 Double-step genioplasty

Management of Soft Tissue

An osseous genioplasty is a powerful tool to improve the appearance of the lower face and neck. Smaller advancements and correction of minor asymmetries are usually well tolerated by the soft tissue envelope and result in a natural look. However, in larger advancements or in correction of asymmetry, overlying soft tissues may be less forgiving. As described previously, a "Pharaoh deformity" occurs when the chin is advanced to the point that it loses a natural transition to the posterior jawline and has the overprojected look of a Pharaoh. This deformity is accentuated from unsupported soft tissue in the parasymphyseal region that results in parasymphyseal hollowing thus exaggerating the prominence of the chin. Additionally, soft tissue irregularities may become apparent when large asymmetric movements are necessary in order to achieve skeletal symmetry of the lower face. Depending on how the soft tissue drapes, noticeable angles or palpable deformities may result and be of significant concern to the patient. Autologous fat grafting has provided a useful tool to ameliorate or correct these persistent soft tissue irregularities that may occur after chin surgery.

Postoperative Care

The patient is sent home with an Elastoplast compressive tape dressing to reduce swelling, decrease hematoma formation, and support the mentalis closure. The dressing can be removed in 5–7 days and patient can resume showering. Peridex mouth rinse is recommended twice a day for 7 days. Occasionally, Peridex may cause a darkening of the teeth; however, discoloration is rare after only 7 days of use and can be treated. Brushing can be done as tolerated but patients are instructed to use a soft brush and stay away from intraoral incisions. The patient can start on a liquid diet on the day of surgery and advance to a regular diet as tolerated within the first 48 h after surgery. Prophylactic antibiotics are given IV in the operating room but are not routinely continued after surgery.

Complications and Side Effects

The surgical risks such as paresthesia, dental injury, infection, and revision must be discussed with patient during the preoperative visits. Wound dehiscence and infections are extremely rare. Infections have been reported to occur in approximately 5–7 % of chin implant procedures and less frequently in osseous genioplasty. If the infection is superficial without any fluctuance or exposed hardware, the standard treatment and follow-up for cellulitis is sufficient. If an abscess is suspected, it is important to avoid a percutaneous drainage if at all possible. The author's recommended approach to an abscess is either repetitive aspirations and oral antibiotics or intraoral incision and drainage. Percutaneous incision and drainage will likely result in skin retraction and a divot that is very difficult to correct without an additional scar.

If dehiscence exposes the hardware, surgical debridement and washout followed by oral antibiotics are recommended. Typically, explant of the hardware is not necessary. Postoperative hematoma should be drained and irrigated adequately to prevent infection. This can be done in an office setting under local anesthesia. Tooth devitalization is uncommon but when it happens, the involved tooth will need root canal treatment. Temporary lip anesthesia or paresthesia is normal in the postoperative period, and a permanent sensory deficit may also occur with an incidence that approximates 10 % in one or both nerves. Traction is generally the etiology and it should resolve in weeks. If there is complete sensory loss with no returning of sensation months after surgery and a true avulsion or transection is suspected, then investigation and repair is required.

When an osseous genioplasty is advanced to more than 5–6 mm, a step off may be palpable at the lateral edge of the osteotomy. This may result in a visible parasymphyseal contour irregularity, and if this persists beyond 6 months, fat grafting can be used to smooth the contour. An over advanced chin also can cause excessive deepening of the labiomental crease therefore creating a prematurely aged appearance. As mentioned previously, the labiomental crease should never be deeper than 4 mm in women and no more than 6 mm in men. Further, excessive vertical elongation can occur as the chin is advanced. The elongated lower third of the face can create a very aesthetically unpleasing appearance known as a Pharaoh deformity.

In contrast, excessive reduction genioplasty (more than 3–4 mm) can create soft tissue redundancy in the submental region. Also, as the symphysis of the chin is posteriorly positioned, a boxy appearance can be created as the facial shape becomes square and loses the ideal oval shape. Narrowing the symphysis and removing some of the inferior mandible posterior to the osteotomy can restore a tapered jawline.

Bibliography

Byrd HS, Burt J. Dimensional approach to rhinoplasty: perfecting the aesthetic balance between the nose and chin. In: Gunter JP, Rohrich RJ, Adams WP, editors. Dallas rhinoplasty: nasal surgery by the masters. St. Louis: Quality Medical Publishing; 2002. p. 117–31.

Farkas L. Appendix A: craniofacial norms in North American Caucasians from birth to young adulthood. In: Anthropometry of the face. 2nd ed. New York: Raven Press; 1994. p. 309.

Iglesias-Linares A, et al. Common standards in facial aesthetics: craniofacial analysis of most attractive Black and White subjects according to People magazine during previous 10 years. J Oral Maxillofac Surg. 2011;69:e216–24.

Oguz O, Bozkir MG. Evaluation of location of mandibular and mental foramina in dry, young, adult human male, dentulous mandibles. West Indian Med J. 2002;51(1):14–6.

Posnick J. Aesthetic alteration of the chin: evaluation and surgery. In: Craniofacial and maxillofacial surgery in children and adults, vol. 2. Philadelphia: WB Saunders; 2000. p. 1122.

Reyneke JP. Systematic patient evaluation. In: Essentials of orthognathic surgery. Chicago: Quintessence Publishing, 2003. p. 29.

Riedel RA. An analysis of dentofacial relationships. Am J Orthod. 1957;43:103.

Rosen HM. Aesthetic guidelines in genioplasty: the role of facial disproportion. Plast Reconstr Surg. 1995;95:463–9.

Rosen HM. Genioplasty. In: Aesthetic perspectives in jaw surgery. New York: Springer; 1997. p. 247–72.

White JB, Dufresne CR. Management and avoidance of complications in chin augmentation. Aesthet Surg J. 2011;31(6):634–42.

Maxillary Osteotomies

30

Pravin K. Patel

Introduction

Among the essential procedures in the surgical armamentarium of a maxillofacial surgeon is the ability to section and reposition the midfacial skeleton. The versatility of the LeFort I and its variations (see Fig. 30.1) allows the surgeon to correct a broad spectrum of midfacial skeletal abnormalities whether of congenital, developmental, or acquired in origin. This chapter will provide an overview of the principles and surgical details used in maxillofacial orthognathic surgery.

History

Historically, the first description of the sectioning of the maxilla was in 1859 when von Langenbeck described removal of nasopharyngeal polyps. In 1867, Cheever performed a hemi-maxillary osteotomy and downfracture to address nasal obstruction and recurrent epistaxis. In 1901, Rene LeFort published his experimentation with midfacial blunt trauma that led to the classic description of natural fracture planes: the LeFort I, the LeFort II, and the LeFort III fracture planes. However, application of LeFort's findings was not until 1927 when correction of the midface deformities was first described by Wassmund using a LeFort I-type osteotomy. However, in Wassmund's description, the pterygomaxillary junction was left intact, and elastic forces were used to gradually bring the midface forward. To improve mobilization of the maxilla, Axhausen in 1934 performed a midpalatal osteotomy. However, Schuchardt in 1942 proposed separating the pterygomaxillary junction, followed by Moore and Ward in 1949 with the horizontal transection of the pterygoid plates. The horizontal osteotomy was abandoned when Wilmar and others reported significant blood loss. Advancement of the midface was fraught with difficulties: limited visualization, significant blood loss, difficulty in downfracture, and inadequate mobilization to achieve a stable long-term outcome. In its infancy, mobilization of the midface could only be achieved by orthopedic traction forces with variable outcomes (today, we would consider it as uncontrolled distraction osteogenesis). Thus many of the deformities were addressed only by anterior maxillary segmental osteotomies as described by Cohn-Stock (1921), Wassmund (1927), and Spanier (1932) and by posterior segmental osteotomies by Schuchardt and Kufner. Total maxillary mobilization as in a "LeFort I" was largely abandoned in favor of limited maxillary segmental osteotomies until Hugo Obwegeser in 1965 in the German literature and in 1969 in the English literature described total mobilization of the maxilla and repositioning in a predicated position with a consistent stable outcome. With Obwegeser's achievement, midfacial skeletal deformities in all three spatial planes could now be addressed. It should be remembered that historically the bilateral sagittal split osteotomy (BSSO) of the mandible was introduced in 1955 by Obwegeser, and many of the deformities that required maxillary advancement were aesthetically and functionally compromised by mandibular setback until the LeFort I became firmly established as viable procedure by the mid- to late 1970s.

Midfacial Skeletal Deformities

Deformities of the midface relative to the cranial base can occur in all three spatial planes and frequently occur simultaneously in multiple planes. Patients with facial clefts will typically present with all three components: palatal transverse width deficiency (collapsed dental arch), midfacial skeletal deficiency in the sagittal plane that may extend to involve the zygoma, and vertical deficiency with clinical lack of dental display. Moreover, there is frequently asymmetry in

P.K. Patel, MD, FACS
Pediatric Plastic and Craniofacial Surgery,
University of Illinois, Division of Plastic, Reconstructive and Cosmetic Surgery, 811 South Paulina Street,
Chicago, IL 60612, USA
e-mail: pkpatel.md@gmail.com

P.J. Taub et al. (eds.), *Ferraro's Fundamentals of Maxillofacial Surgery*,
DOI 10.1007/978-1-4614-8341-0_30, © Springer Science+Business Media New York 2015

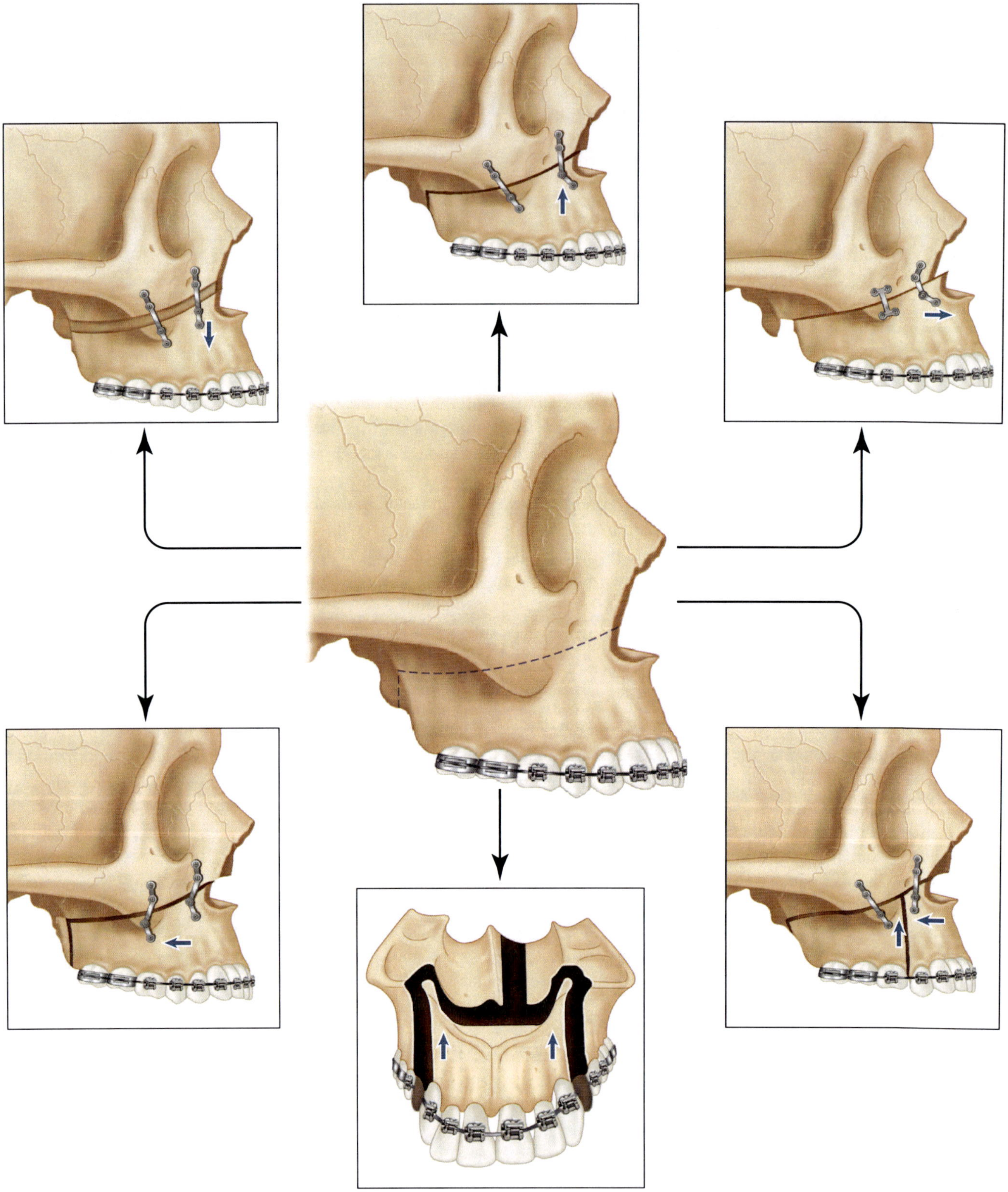

Fig. 30.1 The versatility of the LeFort I osteotomy (clockwise from upper left): vertical lengthening, vertical shortening, horizontal advancement, segmental repositioning, anterior segmental setback, and horizontal setback (Modified from Wolfe SA, Facial Osteotomies. In Georgiade GS, Reifkohl R, Levin LS. Plastic Maxillofacial and reconstructive surgery. Williams and Wilkins, Baltimore, MD 1997)

the three planes resulting in rotational discrepancies that can occur with facial clefts and classically in patients with craniofacial/hemifacial microsomia. Patients with developmental dentofacial skeletal deformities that become evident with adolescence can present with the full range of patterns: from vertical maxillary deficiency to vertical maxillary excess, from sagittal maxillary deficiency to excess, and from transverse width deficiency to excess and in any combination. Even when the primary deformity is in the mandible as in mandibular deficiency/retrognathia, including maxillary repositioning osteotomy in addition to mandibular surgery often improves the postoperative stability and aesthetic outcome. Among the acquired causes, posttraumatic midfacial deformities can present with sagittal and vertical deficiency either because of relapse or inadequate reduction at the initial correction. Patients who present with open-bite deformity as a result of healed bilateral condylar fractures benefit from maxillary surgery to correct the occlusion. Other conditions in which maxillary skeletal osteotomies is a component of surgical management include condylar hyperplasia, hemimandibular elongation, Parry-Romberg disease, fibrous dysplasia, skeletal dysplasias, and obstructive sleep apnea.

Even when the primary skeletal deformity lies with the midface, patients when asked about their appearance will frequently describe their physical concern in terms of their mandible. It is not uncommon for a patient with a Class III facial skeletal pattern to request setting back the mandible. The clinical clues that the surgeon must educate the maxillary deficient patient include acute nasolabial angle, nasal dorsal prominence with depressed nasal tip, lack of dental display, shallow piriform region, and midfacial concavity. When reviewing the photographs with the patient, it is the three-quarter oblique view that best shows the midfacial concavity. Patients may request mandibular advancement, but the excessive overjet may be as a result of maxillary dentoalveolar excess where an anterior maxillary segmental setback would restore the aesthetic facial balance. Good clinical examination without the need for skeletal radiographs will in most circumstances correctly define the maxillary and mandibular components to the deformity. However dental models and 2D/3D radiographs become essential in detailing the surgical-orthodontic plan to optimize skeletal aesthetic goals and occlusal function. This is beyond the scope of this limited overview.

Relevant Anatomy

Osseous Anatomy

The midfacial skeletal anatomy that can be altered with maxillary orthognathic surgery consists of the anterior-lateral surface of the maxilla and the body of the zygoma. The body of the maxilla contains the maxillary sinus, and thus the LeFort I osteotomy invariably must course through the maxillary sinus. The osteotomy through the lateral nasal wall (medial maxillary sinus wall) is limited by the inferior turbinate. Thus the medial limit varies from the piriform base (nasal floor) to the height of the inferior turbinate. The osteotomy through the anterior maxillary wall is limited by the infraorbital foramen superiorly and by the height of the canine root inferiorly medial and by the molar roots posterior laterally. Within this anatomic range, the lateral extent of the osteotomy can course either inferiorly toward the retromolar region or superiorly into the zygoma and the zygomatic arch.

For mobilization of the midface to occur at the various LeFort levels, it must be separated from the sphenoid bone of the skull base. This is the more difficult "osteotomy" as it cannot be directly visualized and is performed by palpation. Thus the surgeon must have a good three-dimensional understanding of the anatomy of the palatine bone and the articulation with the perpendicular plate of the sphenoid bone. The palatine bones are spatially located between the maxilla and the sphenoid forming the posterior portions of the hard palate, the lateral nasal walls, and the orbital floor. The posterior articulation of the palatine bones is with the pterygoid processes of the sphenoid bone. The maxillary tuberosity is located posterior and laterally in maxilla, behind the superior third molar. The pterygomaxillary junction, formed by the palatine bone, superiorly ends in pterygopalatine fissure that communicates with the pterygopalatine fossa. The pterygopalatine fossa is limited anteriorly by the maxilla, posteriorly by the medial plate of pterygoid process and greater wing of sphenoid process, medially by the palatine bone, and superiorly by the body of sphenoid process. Thus repositioning the anterior maxilla can be accomplished by separating at the level of the pterygopalatine junction. Ideally a disarticulation is performed between the palatine and the pterygoid plate of the sphenoid; however, in reality it is technically difficult to accomplish the disarticulation so "cleanly" and more frequently results in various perpendicular sphenoid plate fractures.

Finally mobilization of the midface requires separating the nasal structures from its maxillary base. The lateral nasal walls inferior to the inferior turbinates are sectioned as part of the medial wall of the maxillary sinus. In the midline the maxillary nasal crest articulates with the septal (quadrangular) cartilage anteriorly and the vomer bone posteriorly. The septal cartilage rests in a central groove, which is easily disarticulated from the anterior nasal spine posteriorly; however, the vomer must be sectioned with an osteotome from the maxilla and the palatine bone through the posterior nasal spine.

Vascular

With maxillary osteotomies, an understanding of the vascular blood supply to the mobilized maxilla is crucial. In the 1970s, William Bell's studies in the adult rhesus monkey

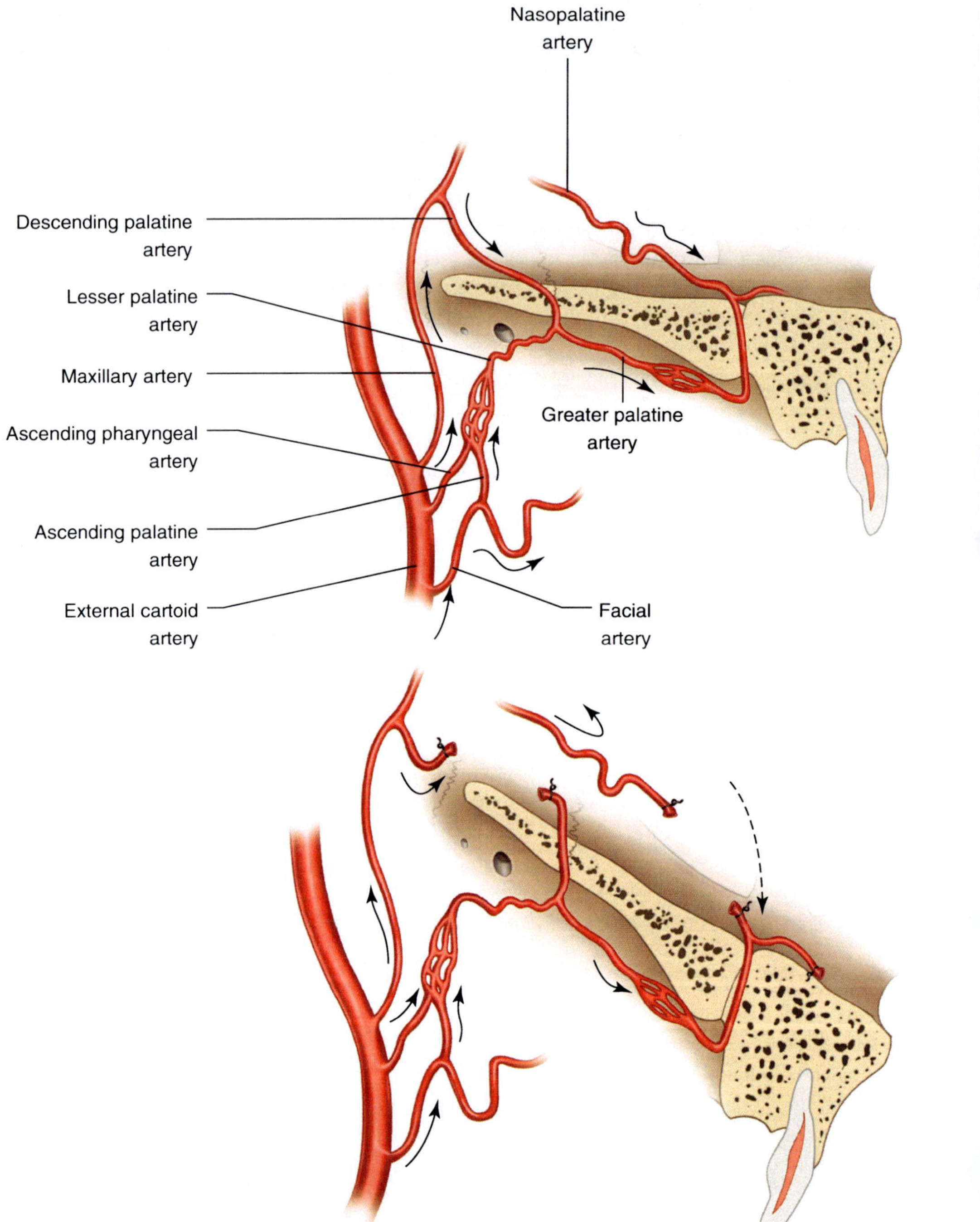

Fig. 30.2 The vascularity of the LeFort segment relies on the ascending pharyngeal artery and the ascending palatine artery branches of the external carotid artery. The descending palatine and nasopalatine arteries are transected with the osteotomy

showed that even when direct blood supply to the maxillary teeth and periodontium was interrupted with a LeFort osteotomy, collateral circulation existed to perfuse the dental pulp and surrounding structures and was responsible for the survival of the rest of the maxilla. Siebert and others confirmed the rich collateral blood supply in human anatomic studies in 1997.

The arterial blood supply to the maxilla is derived from four primary sources (1) the descending palatine branch of the maxillary artery, (2) the ascending palatine branch of the facial artery, (3) the anterior branch of the ascending pharyngeal artery from the external carotid, and (4) the alveolar branches of the maxillary artery. With complete mobilization of the maxilla, the descending palatine vessels frequently are disrupted, and the mobilized maxilla derives its vascularity from the remaining sources, primarily the ascending palatine and pharyngeal vessels (see Fig. 30.2). However, there are times when an intact descending palatine vessels can be well visualized with the downfracture. The author's preference is to isolate and bipolar cauterize to prevent postoperative bleeding rather than preserve the vessels in most circumstances. Moreover, preservation is difficult with the needed mobilization of the maxilla. In patients with palatal clefts who have had conventional palatoplasty reconstruction in infancy, the ascending palatine and pharyngeal vessels is sufficient. It is not uncommon to see some degree of vascular compromise in many patients with advancement in the intraoperative and the immediate postoperative period; however, the vast majority recover uneventfully, and loss of oral mucosa/gingival tissue and segmental maxilla is extremely uncommon. If there is concern, advancement can be delayed as a staged procedure or as an alternative, gradual distraction based on the principles of distraction osteogenesis.

Maxillary Osteotomies: The Technical Details

With its technical ease and dependability of outcome, the LeFort I osteotomy and its variations have become the procedure principally used to solve nearly the full range of anterior-posterior, vertical, transverse, and rotational deformities. Once sectioned, the maxillary dentoalveolar segment can be repositioned in virtually any direction as a single unit and, when needed, subsectioned with interdental osteotomies to differentially move each of the components in all three planes as a multisegmented LeFort I-type procedure. With the LeFort I procedure, the position of the upper lip, the columellar-labial angle, the nasal tip, and the alar base and region can be altered without affecting the orbital-zygomatic region. These standard LeFort-type osteotomies frequently must be modified to address a specific clinical situation. For example, the standard LeFort I osteotomy must be modified to include a portion of the body of the zygoma when the lower maxillary deficiency is accompanied with inadequate zygomatic projection but the orbit itself does not need to be altered, as it would be in a LeFort III when there is exorbitism. In some cases with minor degree of orbital rim deficiency (negative vector), the advancement can be extended to include the orbital rim and body of the zygoma. Thus the osteotomy pattern can be tailored to fit a wide variety of deformity ranging from the LeFort I to the LeFort III requirement.

This section describes the technical details of maxillary orthognathic surgery as follows: (0) surgical preparation, (1) the classic LeFort I osteotomy, (2) the modified LeFort I osteotomy (osteotomy variations), (3) the multisegmented LeFort I, (4) the anterior maxillary osteotomy, (5) the posterior maxillary osteotomy, and (6) the surgically assisted rapid palatal expansion (SARPE). Understanding the technical details of classic LeFort I facilitates the surgeon's ability to understand its variations and to appropriately tailor the osteotomies to the patient's specific deformities.

The Classic LeFort I Osteotomy

Surgical Preparation

Efficiency in executing the surgery involves (1) placing the surgical instruments appropriately in the sequence planned on the Mayo stand and back table, (2) testing the power instrumentation and loading the drill and reciprocating blade, and (3) setting up the plating system with the screwdrivers loaded. The surgical instruments needed (author's preference) to execute the LeFort I are illustrated in Fig. 30.3.

With appropriate monitoring, arterial and venous lines are placed by anesthesia for modified hypotension (systolic pressure of 90–100 mmHg). Prophylactic perioperative antibiotics are started. A single dose of steroids is given. The nasotracheal tube with an accordion extension is secured to the superior aspect of the nasal cartilaginous septum and to the anterior scalp with a protective foam. The nasotracheal tube should be adjusted using the accordion extension to eliminate pressure off of the ala rim. The oropharynx is suctioned, and a throat pack is placed. The eyes should be protected with tarsorrhaphy sutures, clear adhesive eyeshields, or corneal shields.

If interdental surgical hooks that are required for intraoperative intermaxillary fixation have not be placed by the orthodontist prior to the surgery, these should be placed at this time before the start of the formal operative procedure. The occlusal splints should be checked to make certain that they fit to ensure that there have been no occlusal changes since the presurgical models and model surgery.

The mouth is cleansed with using chlorhexidine gluconate 0.12 % (Peridex) oral rinse or alternatively with a dilute povidone-iodine (Betadine) solution.

The operative field is infiltrated with 1 % lidocaine with 1:100,000 epinephrine solution. The solution should be infiltrated into the maxillary labial-buccal vestibule just above the attached gingiva, at the anterior nasal spine and along the base of the nasal septum. Infiltration into the retromolar region is best accomplished through an intraoral approach (palatal) with a Macintosh laryngoscopes used for tracheal intubation. The curvature of the blade helps reflect the tongue, and the light facilitates visualization for infiltrating the local anesthetic with vasoconstriction. For maxillary surgery, further vasoconstriction of the intranasal lining is accomplished with 1 × 3 in. cottonoid sponges soaked in a nasal decongestant.

The medial canthus on both sides is marked with methylene blue. These external marks will be used as a baseline reference to position the maxilla so that the vertical midfacial height is adjusted for the planned final dental display.

The patient is then is prepped with the nasotracheal tube in the field and draped in a standard fashion. The exposure of the operative field should include the entire forehead to the clavicle to allow the surgeon to assess the repositioned facial skeleton fully.

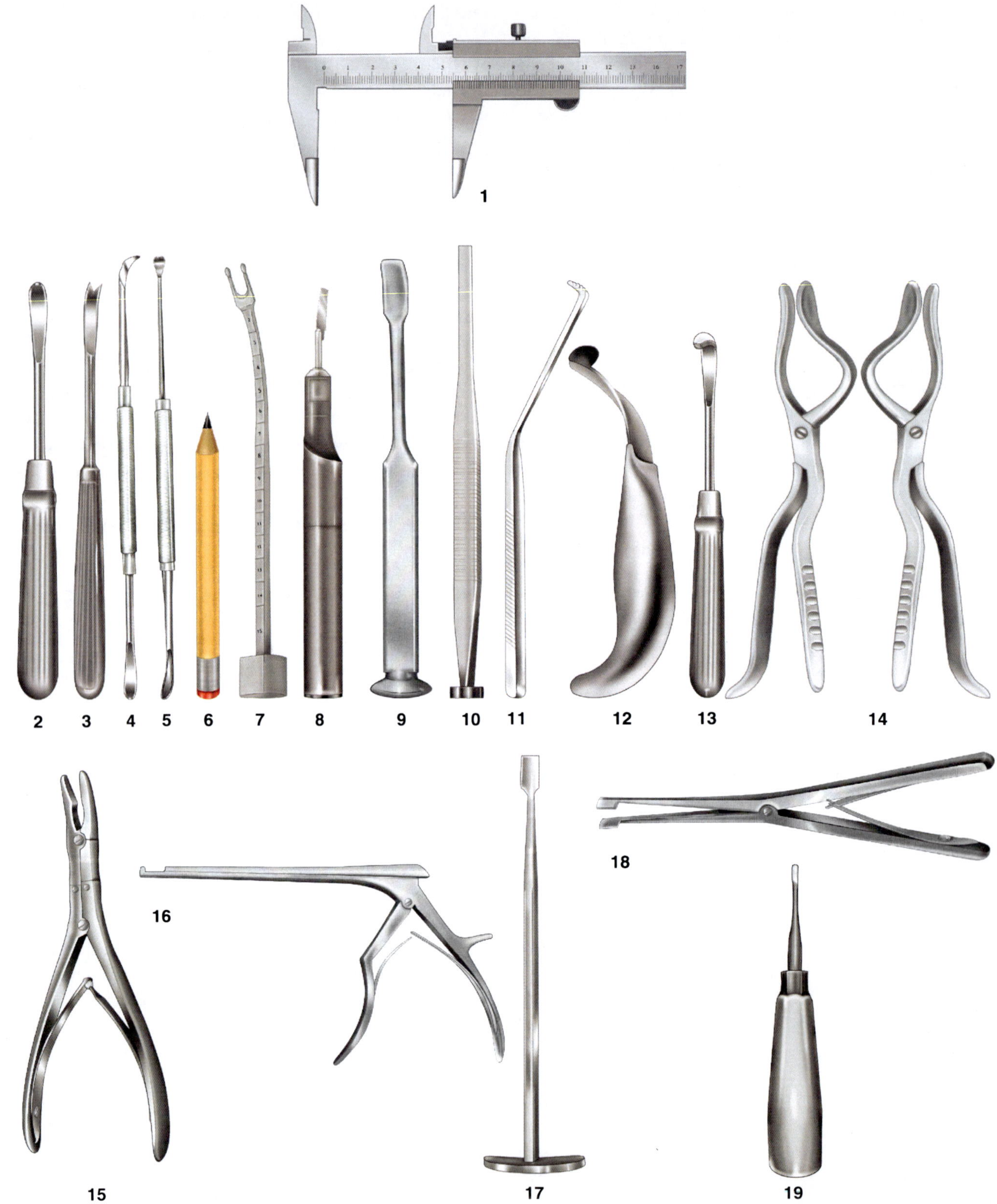

Fig. 30.3 Surgical instruments that are useful for executing maxillary orthognathic surgery in the order of use. (*1*) Caliper used for measuring the vertical height. (*2*) Obwegeser elevators (6 and 9 mm) used for exposure. (*3*) Obwegeser anterior border stripper used to detach anterior masseter from the zygomatic arch. (*4*) Obwegeser long freer elevator for the piriform. (*5*) Cottle elevator for the nasal piriform exposure. (*6*) Pencil to mark the osteotomy. (*7*) Obwegeser septal osteotome. (*8*) Reciprocating saw for the maxillary osteotomy. (*9*) Tessier-Kawamoto pterygopalatine osteotome. (*10*) Marchac osteotome 4 mm for the posterior maxillary wall. (*11*) Tessier bone hook. (*12*) Hargis channel retractor used for mobilization from the retromolar region. (*13*) Obwegeser "J" stripper used for mobilizing the posterior palate. (*14*) Left and right Rowe forceps used for mobilizing. (*15*) Rongeur. (*16*) Kerrison. (*17*) Dunn-Dautrey interdental osteotomes for multisegmental maxilla. (*18*) Turvey palatal spreader for multisegmental maxilla. (*19*) #301 elevator for third molar extraction

Incision and Exposure

1. To facilitate the retraction for the exposure, the author prefers using a clear lip retractor and a combination of wide double-pronged skin hook centrally and Army/Navy retractors laterally. Prior to the incision, the distance from the medial canthus to the maxillary orthodontic arch wire between the lateral incisor and the canine is measured on the right and left side and recorded (Fig. 30.4). Exposure to the midfacial facial skeleton is accomplished through an intraoral labial-buccal mucosal incision well above the attached gingiva from the bicuspid to the bicuspid region, leaving an adequate mucosal edge of a minimum of 5–8 mm from the gingiva to facilitate final closure. The upper lip vestibular frenulum should be spared. The incision is modified centrally as an inverted V so that it peaks above the frenulum when it is retracted by skin hooks (Fig. 30.5). Additionally, by placing this "dart" in the incision, the surgeon will have control of centering the lip at the time of closure and adjusting the lip contour when required. Care must be taken at the lateral extent of the incision to avoid injuring or compromising the papilla of the parotid or Stenson's duct that can be identified typically above the second molar when the lip is retracted superolaterally with the Army/Navy retractor. The incision can be made either with a fine-tip electrocautery or with a knife blade. There is a natural tendency for the surgeon to bevel the incision superiorly as it is deepened. This should be avoided anteriorly in the region between the incisors and the piriform as the incision may enter the nasal cavity.

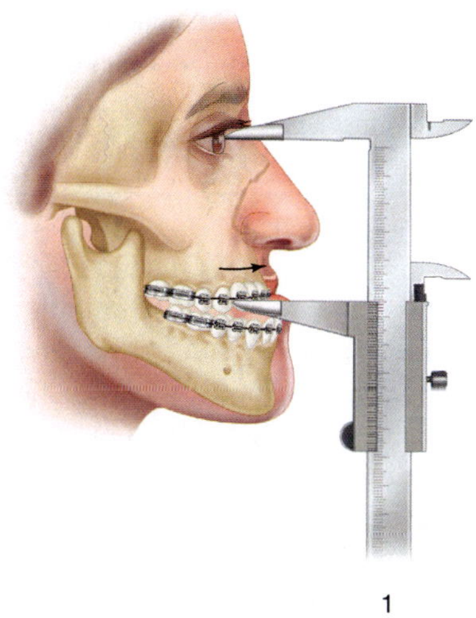

Fig. 30.4 The vertical distance is measured from the medial canthus to the arch wire between the lateral incisor and the caninne. This will be used as a reference for the desired dental display

2. The subperiosteal dissection is directed superiorly, exposing the nasomaxillary buttress and the anterior maxillary wall, identifying the inferior orbital foramen (neurovascular bundle) and exposing the lateral zygomatic-maxillary buttress, the body of the zygoma, and the anterior portion of the zygomatic arch (Fig. 30.6). The anterior maxillary wall is thin, and care must be taken to not fracture it with the exposure. The superior exposure must be sufficient to accommodate the fixation plates. The anterior portion of the origin of the masseter muscle may need to be stripped off by electrocautery and/or by using an anterior V-notched anterior mandibular border stripper. The dissection then is continued posteriorly to the pterygopalatine region, where much of the dissection is accomplished easily and quickly by packing it with 1×3-in. cottonoid sponges soaked in local anesthetic solution. The direction of the periosteal elevator turns sharply medially, and the pterygopalatine junction can be felt easily with the elevator. Care must be taken not to violate the thin overlying periosteum in this region; otherwise the procedure will be plagued with herniation of the buccal fat.
3. While the above exposure can be done quickly, exposure of the anterior nasal spine, nasal piriform aperture, and the intranasal cavity must be done slowly and with care. Although the exposure can be done quickly with the exception of cleft cases, care must be taken in elevating the nasal lining from the bony piriform. The soft tissue is typically more adherent and the surface topography more complex. The piriform lip is thin, and the angle is sharp. Not infrequently tearing of the nasal lining occurs. A Cottle elevator is useful to initially elevate the soft tissue proceeding from the lateral nasal wall to the nasal spine and the mucosa from the rim in this region with the elevator angled sharply against the bone in the premaxillary region (Fig. 30.7).

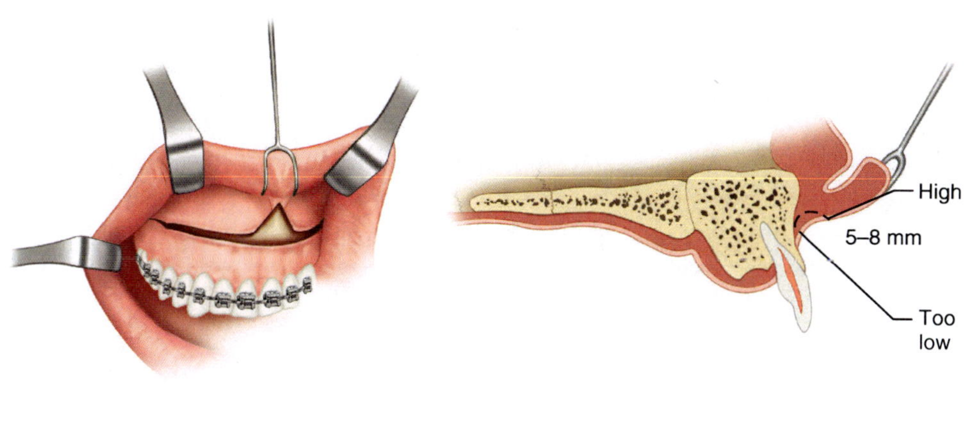

Fig. 30.5 The incision should be made well above the attached gingiva (5–8 mm) with a central inverted V to spare the labial frenulum. This will leave an adequate cuff of attached gingiva for closure, and the central dart will help maintain the midline of the lip to the central incisor

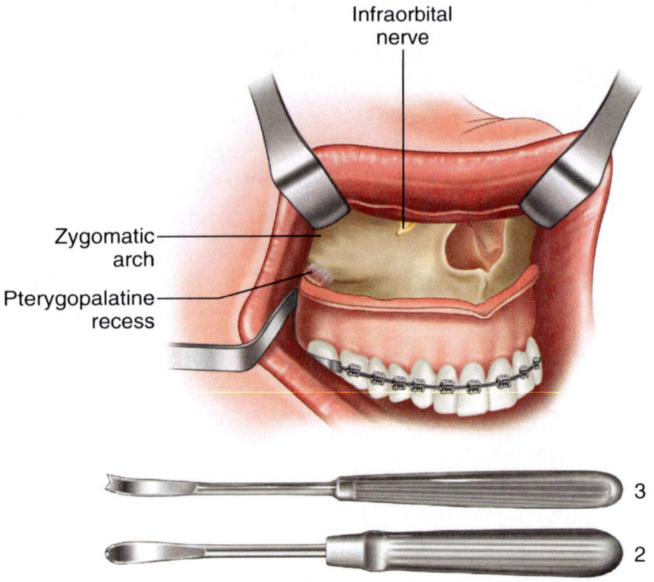

Fig. 30.6 Begin by first exposing the maxilla (*2*) and zygoma to the zygomatic arch followed by the pterygopalatine recess. The infraorbital nerve is visualized and protected. The original of the masseter muscle is retracted with a notched elevator/retractor (*3*) and detached with an electrocautery

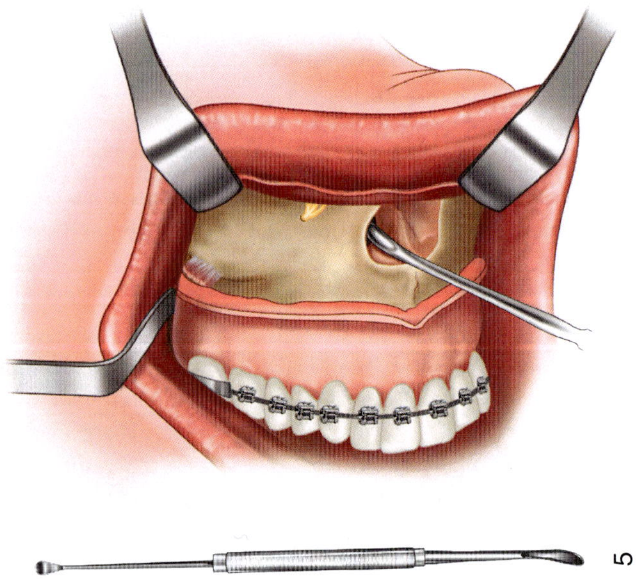

Fig. 30.7 Begin carefully to expose the piriform aperture with a Cottle elevator. It is easiest to begin exposing the lateral nasal mucosa followed by the nasal floor. It will be necessary to expose the anterior nasal spine and the junction of the anterior nasal septum and vomer to elevate the nasal mucosa from the septal-vomer region

As the exposure continues intranasally from anterior to posterior, the intranasal cavity expands, and the elevator must be obliquely angled along the lateral nasal wall with increasing depth. The dissection should continue posteriorly to the junction of the hard and soft palate. Typically the lateral nasal wall and the floor can be elevated with relative ease. However, elevating the nasal lining mucosa intact off of the nasal septum and vomer from the maxillary crest can be difficult. The soft tissue elevation must be complete as possible; completion can be confirmed by placing a finger transorally at the palatal junction while using the Cottle or long Freer elevator in the elevation.

The Osteotomy

4. With skeletal exposure complete, the planned osteotomy is marked noting the tooth root apices and the infraorbital foramen. The osteotomy should be 5 mm above the root apices. The root of the canine is easily located by its prominence and the fossa lateral to it. The osteotomy of the classic LeFort I is marked from the lateral nasal wall and continued laterally toward the molar region. The osteotomy has a downward superior-medial to inferior-lateral slope. There are a number of variations to the classic LeFort osteotomy to tailor to the patient's deformity, and these variations are described in the section on the modified LeFort osteotomy.
5. The osteotomies can be performed in various sequences. The author's preference is as follows. The nasal septum and vomer is separated from the maxillary crest with a septal osteotome that is directed downward and posterior. A finger is placed at the junction of the hard and soft palate to ensure that the separation is complete through the posterior nasal spine by palpating the osteotome (Fig. 30.8). The author prefers to separate the septum first because doing so facilitates placement of the reciprocating saw as far posteriorly as possible by simultaneously deflecting the nasal septum and the nasotracheal tube away from the saw from either side. This technique generally ensures a complete osteotomy of the lateral nasal wall.
6. A reciprocating saw (Fig. 30.9) then is used to complete the horizontal maxillary osteotomies proceeding form the lateral nasal wall across the anterior maxillary wall and through the posterior-lateral maxillary wall. It is important to note that because of the depth of the lateral nasal wall, the serrated portion of the cutting blade cannot be visible when cutting the posterior aspect of the lateral nasal wall; otherwise the posterior osteotomy will not be complete. (The lateral nasal wall measures approximately 50 mm, and the blade is typically only 25 mm in length). As the lateral nasal wall is sectioned from posterior to anterior, the handle of the saw should be angled medially so that the cutting edge becomes visible as it comes through the anterior maxillary wall. The saw is then angled perpendicularly to the anterior surface as the maxilla is cut from medial to lateral. The saw must be controlled tightly, because once the medial buttress is cut, the saw will rapidly section the thin anterior maxillary wall of the sinus until the lateral buttress is reached. The reciprocating saw is then redirected from

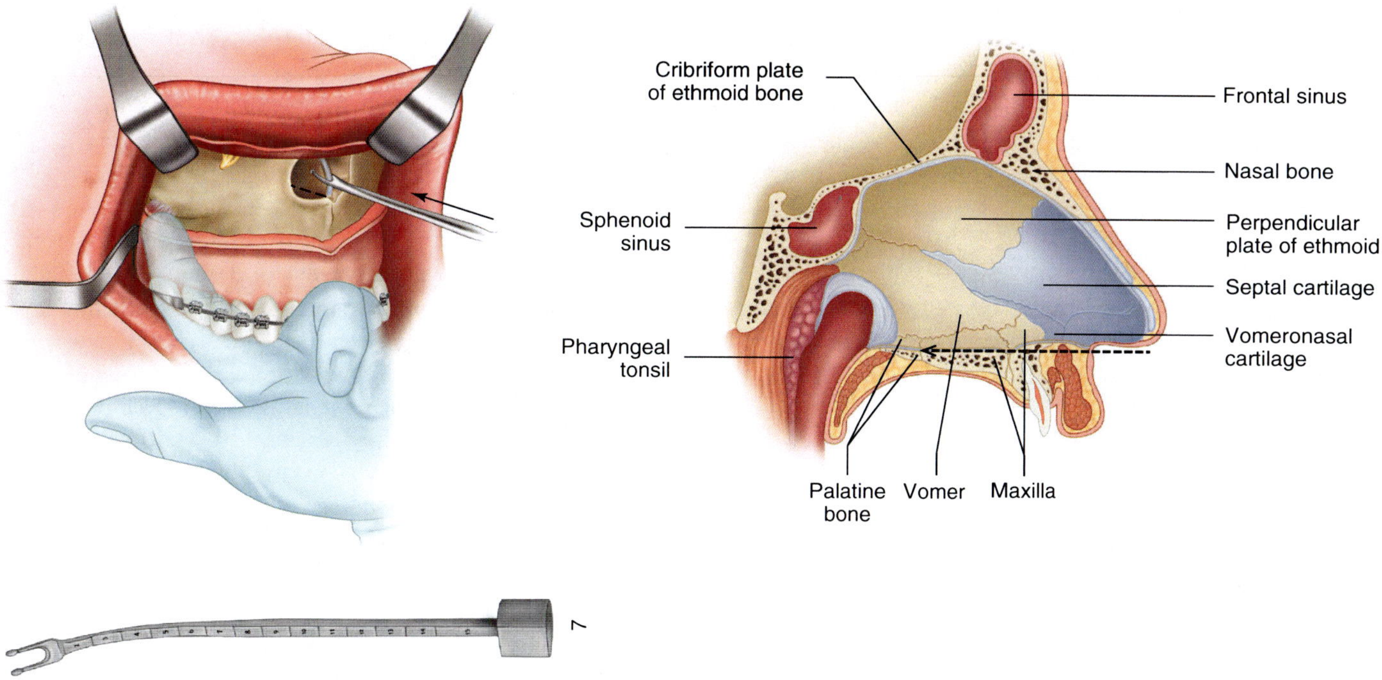

Fig. 30.8 The cartilaginous and bony septum is separated from the maxilla anteriorly and the palatine bone posterior. A finger is placed transorally at the junction of the hard and soft palate to assess the depth of the osteotome as it progresses from the anterior nasal spine to the posterior nasal spine

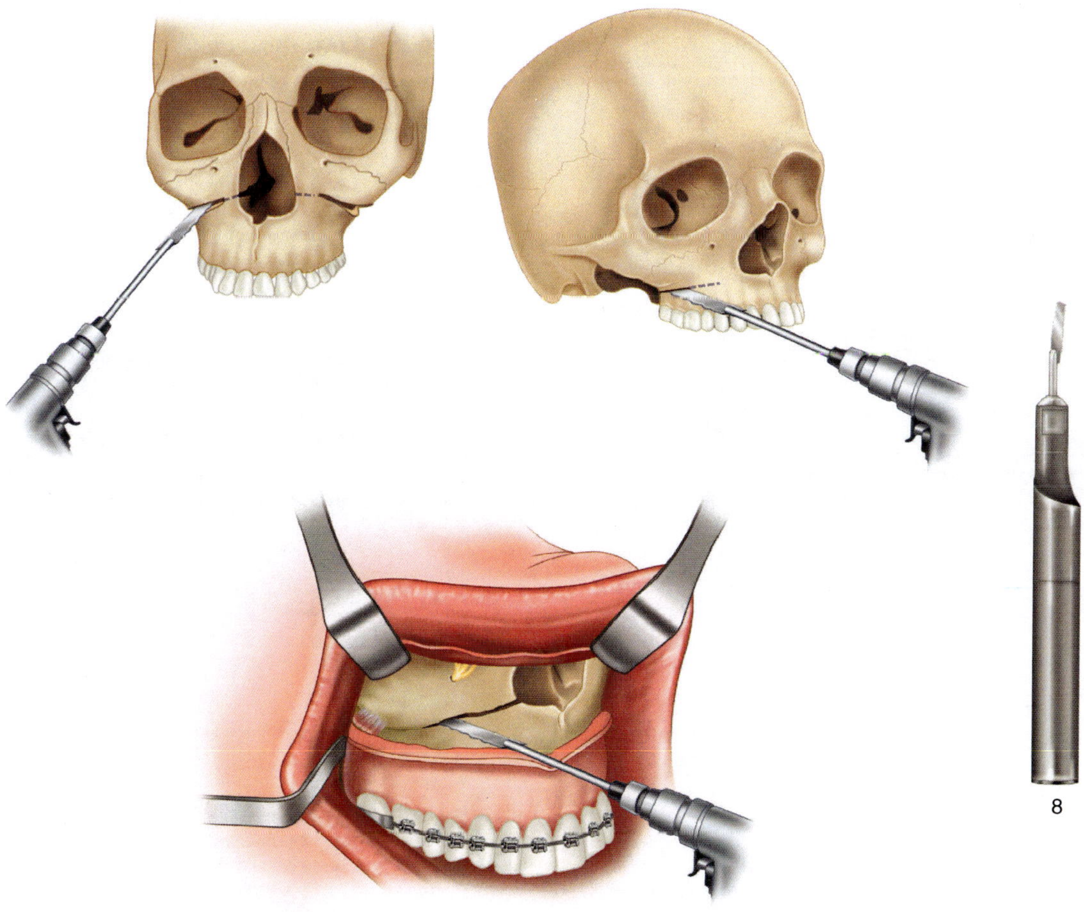

Fig. 30.9 The osteotomy is made with a reciprocating saw from the medial maxillary (lateral nasal) wall from posterior to anterior and then anteriorly across the anterior maxillary wall. The reciprocating saw is then redirected from the lateral to medial completing the osteotomy

lateral to medial sectioning the lateral maxillary-zygomatic buttress to facilitate completion of the osteotomy.

7. Next a curved osteotome is used to separate the pterygoid plate from the maxillary tuberosity (Fig. 30.10). Without direct visualization, typically the pterygopalatine disjunction osteotome can be felt to drops within the junction as it is placed into position. It should be positioned parallel to the occlusal plane and directed inferiorly, anteriorly, and medially. The handle is held as lateral as possible restricted by the buccal soft tissue. A finger placed transorally behind the maxillary tuberosity will facilitate the placement and verify the separation as it is made.

The Downfracture and Mobilization

8. Once the osteotomy is completed, the maxilla is downfractured. When the osteotomy is complete, the downfracture typically can be done with digital pressure alone by placing the thumbs at the base of the pyriform aperture (Fig. 30.11). If there is any significant resistance, it is preferable to revisit the osteotomy sites with the reciprocating saw and a thin osteotome rather than apply more force and use Rowe disimpaction forceps. Using significant force to accomplish the downfracture can lead to unfavorable fractures. The areas that typically are incomplete are the posterior aspect of the lateral nasal walls, the posterior-lateral maxillary wall, and the pterygopalatine disjunction. To facilitate a resistant downfracture, the first assistant can put firm downward pressure on the maxilla, slightly separating the anterior maxillary osteotomy. This then allows placement of a thin osteotome through the distracted osteotomy gap. The intact posterior maxillary wall can be felt with an osteotome and the posterior wall sectioned (fractured) by gently malleting sequentially as each of the areas of resistance is addressed. As the maxilla is mobilized inferiorly, adherent nasal floor mucosal should be elevated simultaneously from anterior to posterior to the junction of the hard and soft palate. Then under direct visualization, areas of bony continuity such as the perpendicular process of the palatine bone and the pterygoid plate can be completely separated from the maxilla using an osteotome. With good visualization, the descending palatine neurovascular bundle is typically isolated, ligated, and divided. Preservation while theoretically ideal may be compromised by the need to reposition the maxilla resulting in either tension or compression of the neurovascular bundle. Additionally, postoperative bleeding has been attributed to descending palatine vessels when not controlled intraoperatively. As described earlier, no deleterious effects have been shown when the descending palatine is not preserved. The surgeon should conscientiously look for bleeding in the posterior region and control it.

9. Once the downfracture is completed, the maxilla is mobilized from side to side (rotational mobilization) and then anteriorly in the sagittal vector with the use of

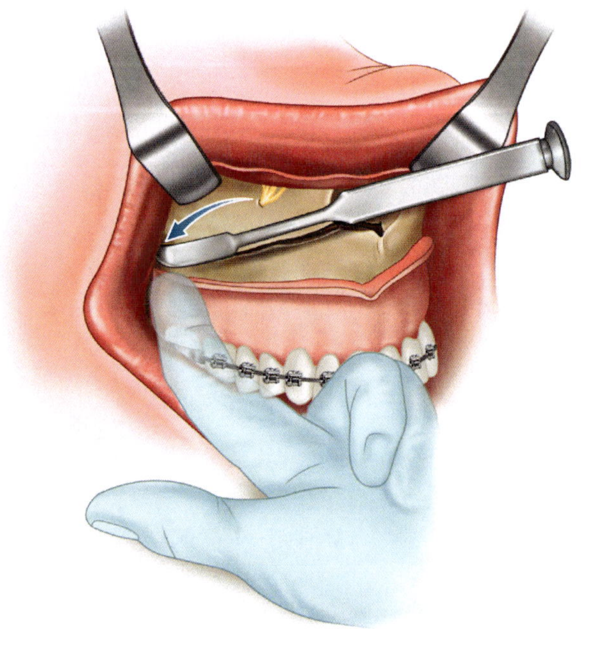

Fig. 30.10 The pterygopalatine disjunction is performed with a curved osteotome. A finger is placed transorally at the retromolar region to help direct the osteotome. The osteotome is positioned inferior to the fossa to minimize the risk to vascular injury

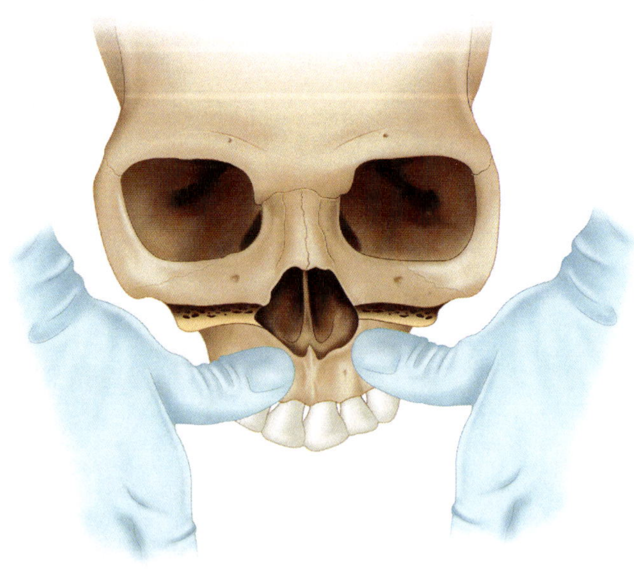

Fig. 30.11 The maxilla is downfractured with digital pressure alone. The surgeon's thumbs are placed at the nasal sill. If there is any resistance, then the osteotomy must be revisited sequentially. Generally the posterior nasal wall and posterior maxillary wall are the sites of resistance. A thin osteotome through the anterior maxillary osteotomy and directed inferiorly may be helpful

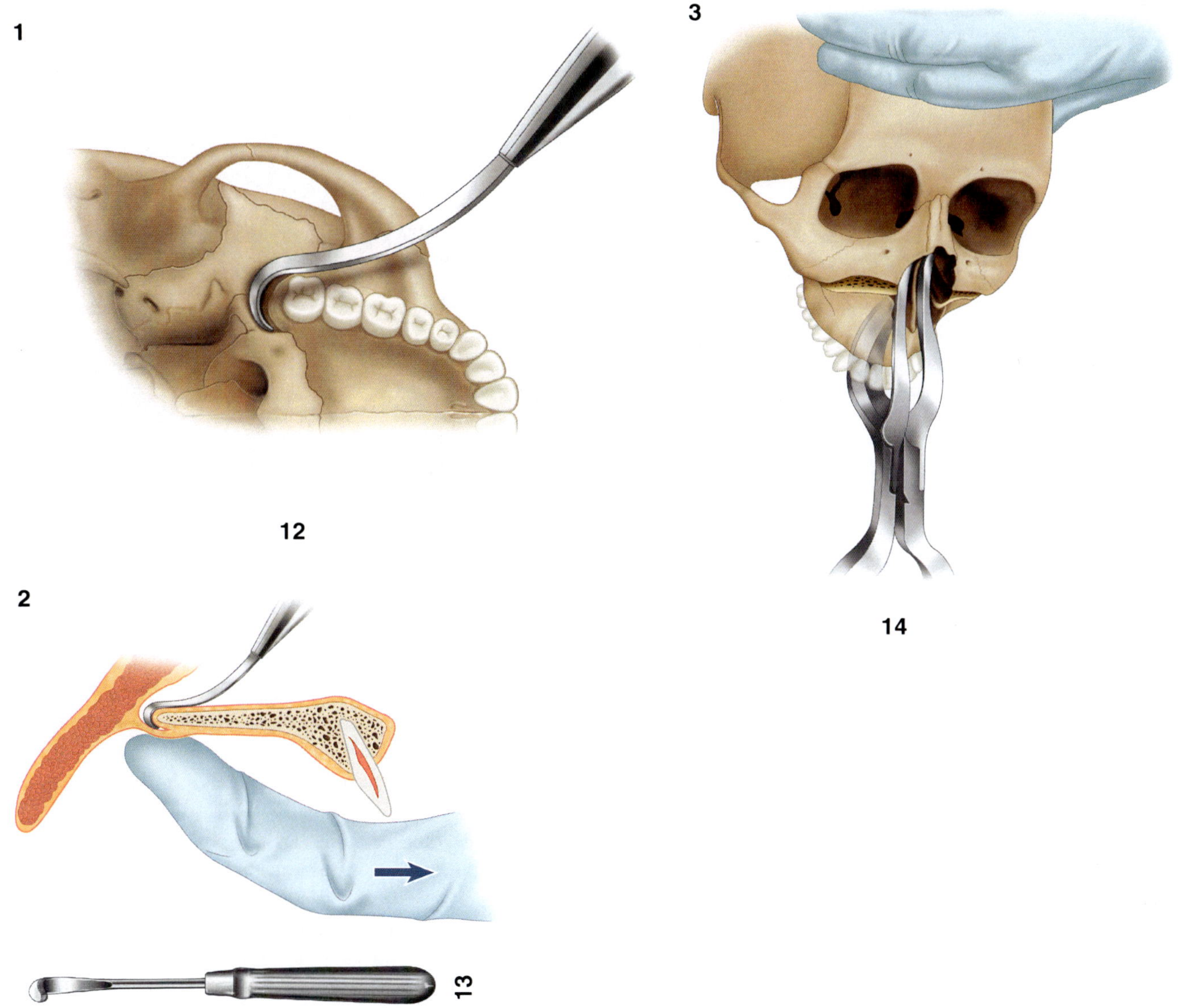

Fig. 30.12 Maneuvers to mobilization of the maxilla. (1) Mandibular inferior border channel retractor is used in the retromolar region for exposure and mobilization laterally. (2) Mandibular "J" stripper can be used at the junction of the hard and soft palate to help mobilize centrally. (3) Rowe disimpaction forceps can be used only after the initial mobilization but should not be used for the downfracture

a mandibular channel retractor positioned behind the tuberosity (Fig. 30.12). The curvature of the channel is ideal for engaging the tuberosity and allows good control of the maxillary mobilization with advancement and torque. Moreover, the shape of the retractor allows reflection of the soft tissue and good visualization in the pterygoid region to remove any restricting adherent soft tissue. Further mobilization can be accomplished by placing a sharply turned (60° or 90°) elevator, or a "J" stripper at the junction of the hard and soft palate helps mobilize the maxilla centrally (Fig. 30.12). Only after the maxilla is fully separated and mobile does the author use Rowe forceps (Fig. 30.12) to accomplish further mobilization (stretching of the soft tissues) should it be necessary; otherwise limit its use. *The maxilla should be mobilized completely so that it can be placed passively in its final position with a pair of forceps.*

10. If the maxillary third molars are present, they can be easily removed through the sinus floor with the maxilla mobilized (Fig. 30.13). A channel retractor is placed at the retromolar region to reflect the soft tissue and simultaneously control the maxilla. The impacted molar is identified through the maxillary sinus. The sinus floor is removed with a sharp end of a #9 Molt elevator, and the tooth is extracted with a straight extraction elevator.

Maxillary Reposition and Fixation

11. Once the maxillary osteotomy is completed, a prefabricated occlusal surgical splint is ligated to the maxillary arch wire with 30-gauge wire. The maxilla and mandible

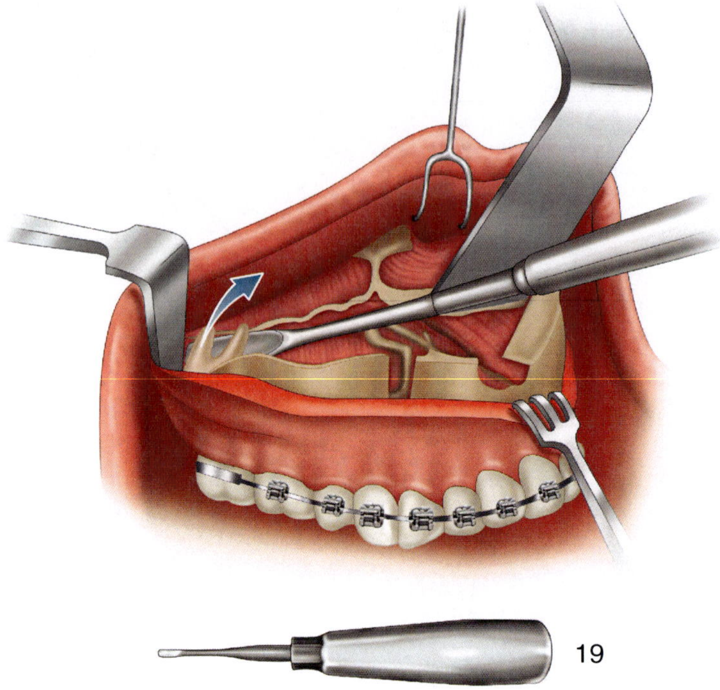

Fig. 30.13 Extraction of impacted maxillary third molars through the maxillary sinus

are placed in maxillary-mandibular fixation with dental elastics. The dental elastic forces will maintain the new occlusal relationship actively, as opposed to a static maxillary-mandibular wire fixation.

12. The newly established maxillary-mandibular complex then is allowed to rotate within its arc of rotation with the mandibular condyle seated in its glenoid fossa (Fig. 30.14). The maxilla then is brought into the desired anterior vertical position based on the amount of dental display desired from the preoperative analysis. The position is confirmed by vertical measurement from the previously marked reference point (either external medial canthus or internal reference drill mark) to the orthodontic arch wire by using a caliper.
13. In superior and posterior maxillary impaction cases, any areas of bony interferences should be removed (Fig. 30.15). The removal of bone should be done selectively to allow maximal bony contact for stability with the use of rongeurs and 5-mm Kerrison. Additionally, the nasal septum may need to be addressed, removing bone along the vomer and resecting the nasal cartilage base to prevent septal buckling. The inferior turbinate may also interfere with the impaction and need to be reduced (Fig. 30.15).
14. With impaction cases, the segments can be stabilized by slotted joints made with either a Kerrison or rongeur (Fig. 30.16). In sagittal and inferior advancement cases, the osteotomy gap after fixation will need to be assessed if it requires bone grafting for stabilization (Fig. 30.17). The author prefers autogenous iliac bone for interpositional buttress grafts over allogenic and alloplastic bone substitutes. A cortical cancellous bone graft is harvested from the medial aspect of the ilium. The cancellous component is removed from the edges allowing the graft to be "wedged" within the osteotomy gap retained by the cortical surface in contact with the maxillary surface.
15. With the maxilla in the desired position, it is stabilized with titanium plates and screws at the medial and posterior-lateral buttresses where the bone is thick and can carry the transmitted occlusal loads (Fig. 30.17). The author prefers to bend the titanium plate to buttress the advancement and not solely rely on the pullout strength of the screw/bone interface. The maxillary-mandibular fixation is released, and the occlusion is verified. The mandible, with the condyle seated within the glenoid fossa, closes passively directly into the splint. If there is any question that the condyle was not seated properly at the time of occlusal check, the osteosynthesis is redone.
16. With the exception of the multisegmented maxilla and unstable occlusal discrepancies, the author's preference is to remove the occlusal splint and reassess the occlusion to match that of the model surgery. If the occlusion is stable, no occlusal splint is required.

Closure

17. Once the maxilla is fixed into position and the occlusion is satisfactory, the anterior nasal spine and the nasal aperture should be assessed in relation to the final nasolabial angle and the alar width as a consequence of the maxillary movement. The anterior nasal spine can be contoured, and in the impaction cases, the piriform

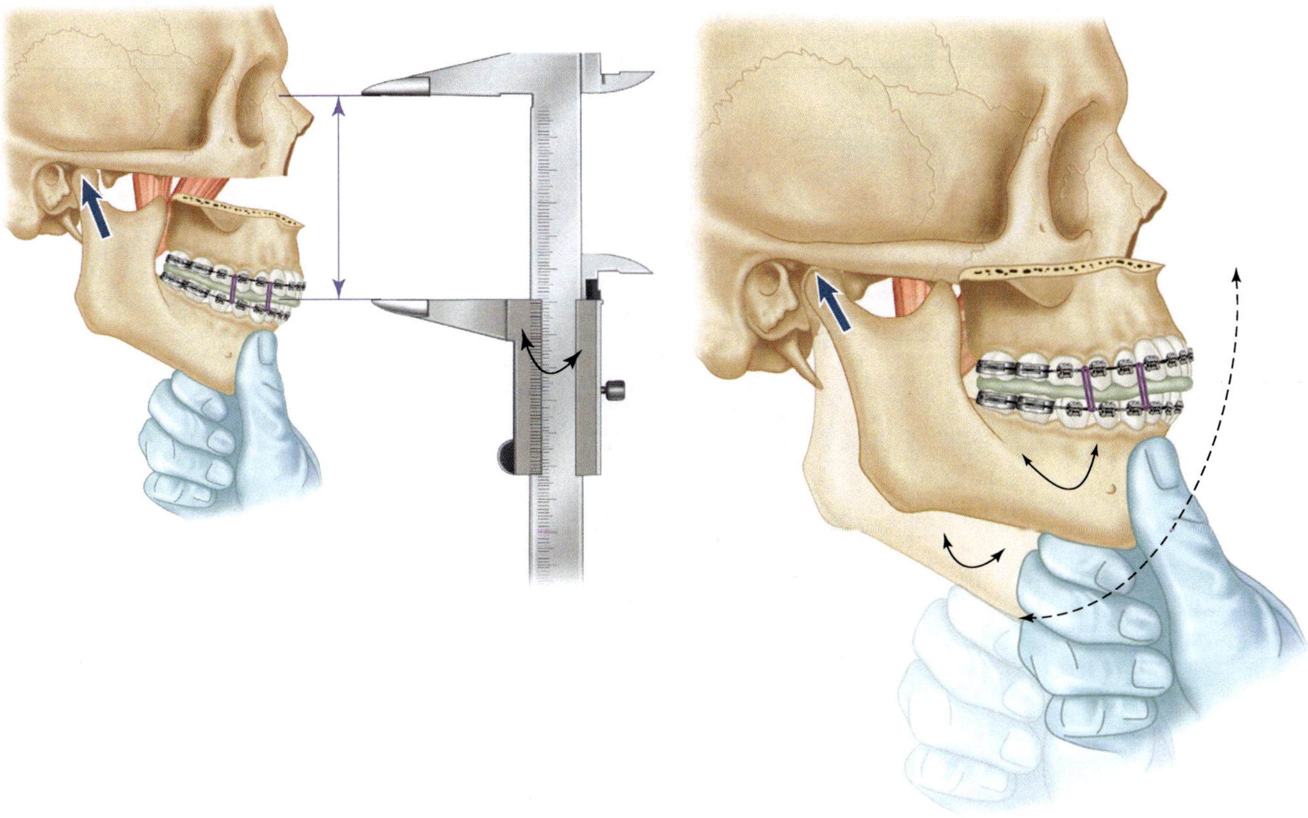

Fig. 30.14 The maxilla is then indexed to the mandible with an occlusal splint and placed in dental elastics. The maxillary-mandibular complex then can rotate clockwise to increase the dental display or counterclockwise to decrease the dental display within the range of the TMJ (condyle seated within the glenoid fossa)

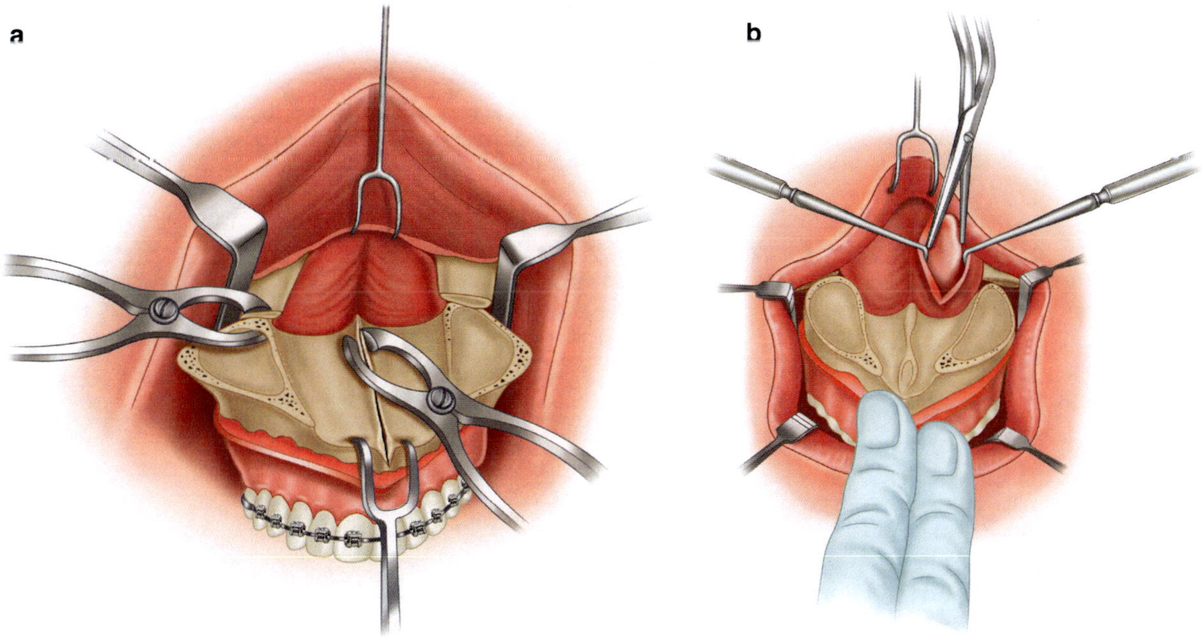

Fig. 30.15 With maxillary impaction, all skeletal interference points must be removed. This may include trimming (**a**) the septum to prevent buckling and if needed (**b**) an inferior turbinectomy

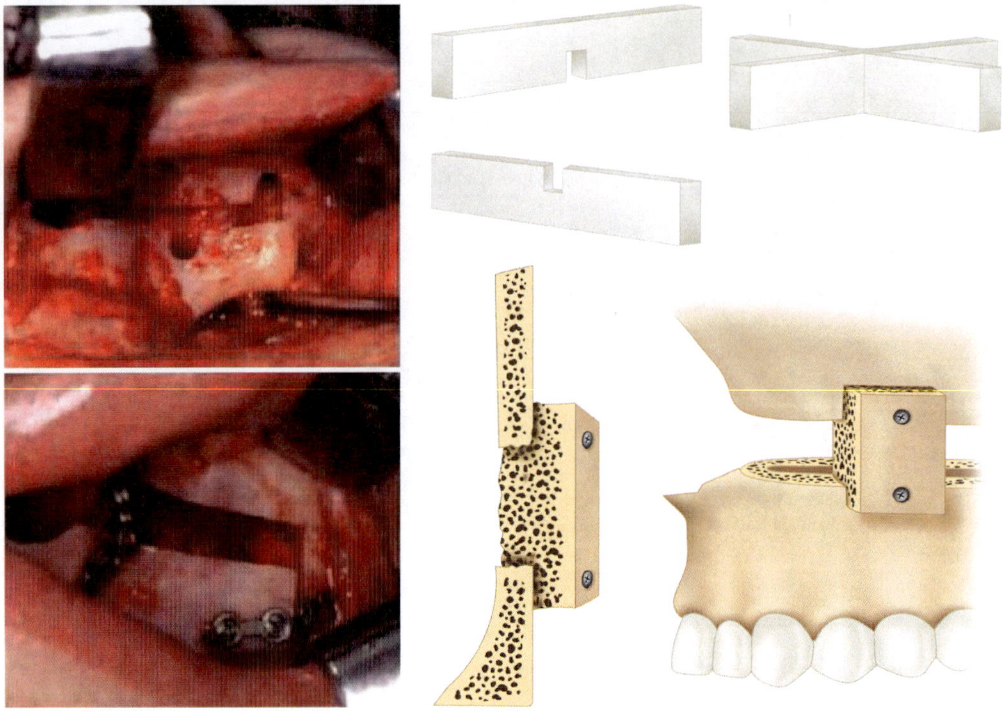

Fig. 30.16 With impaction cases, the segments can be slotted for stability. With vertical advancement cases, bone grafts may be required for stability

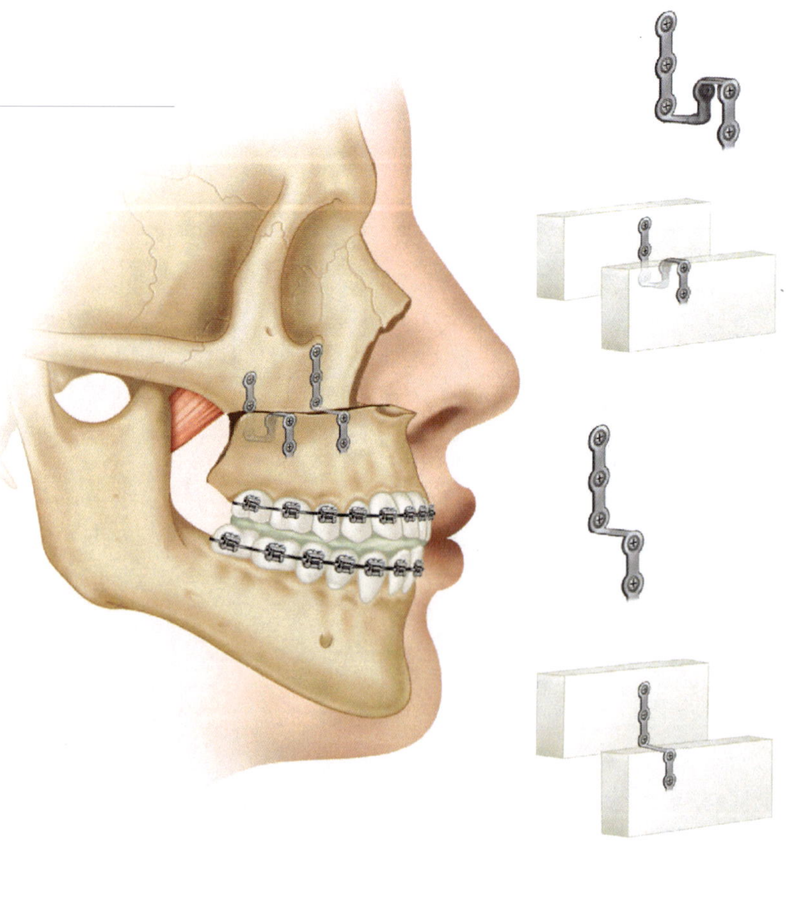

Fig. 30.17 Skeletal fixation plates are placed at the medial and lateral buttresses. With significant sagittal advancement cases, the titanium plates are adapted to provide a posterior buttress for the segment to rest on and not rely solely on the pull out strength of the screw/bone interface with a simple step bend. The occlusal wafer is removed, and the occlusion is then checked

aperture can be deepened if needed. The anterior septum then should be fixed to the midline with a transfixation suture secured through a hole drilled through the anterior nasal spine. When needed, an alar cinch suture is placed to control the width of the alar base.

18. The mucosal incision is then closed with a resorbable suture. At the time of closing the vestibular incision, cheiloplasty with a V-Y advancement or any number of variations can be considered to enhance the lip contour and volume.
19. The throat pack is removed and the orogastric contents are suctioned. The patient is then allowed to emerge from anesthesia. No maxillary-mandibular fixation is utilized in the immediate recovery phase to allow a more comfortable recovery.

The Modified LeFort I

While the classic LeFort I corrects the occlusal discrepancy, it cannot address a broad range of conditions in which patients with dentofacial deformity presents with or aesthetic concerns that they may have. The classic LeFort I osteotomy pattern is "downward" sloping from the piriform aperture to the retromolar region. When among the goals is to increase the dental display by vertically lengthening the anterior maxilla, then the classic LeFort I approach will lead to an opening wedge osteotomy and instability. Bone grafting the skeletal gap is needed. However, if the vector of the osteotomy is changed so that it would be "upward" sloping from the piriform, then as the maxilla is advanced, the skeletal vertical height and the dental display increase, and there is good bony contact. When the osteotomy is well designed, the outcome is stability (Fig. 30.18).

The classic LeFort I addresses only the lower maxilla and dentoalveolar aspects. To address the deformity in patients with deficiencies of the upper maxilla and zygoma, the osteotomy pattern must be tailored to include the component parts of the facial skeleton. From an intraoral approach, the varying portions of the body of the zygoma and zygomatic arch can be approached. In rare instances when the orbital rim needs to be included to correct a negative vector but not to the degree of a LeFort III level, then a transconjunctival approach is also needed to safely and directly visualize the orbital rim and floor (Fig. 30.19).

a

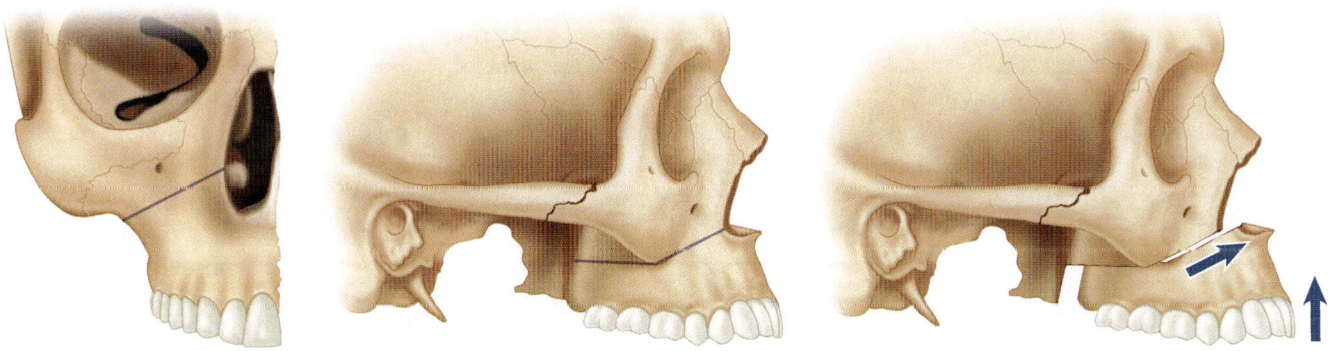

b

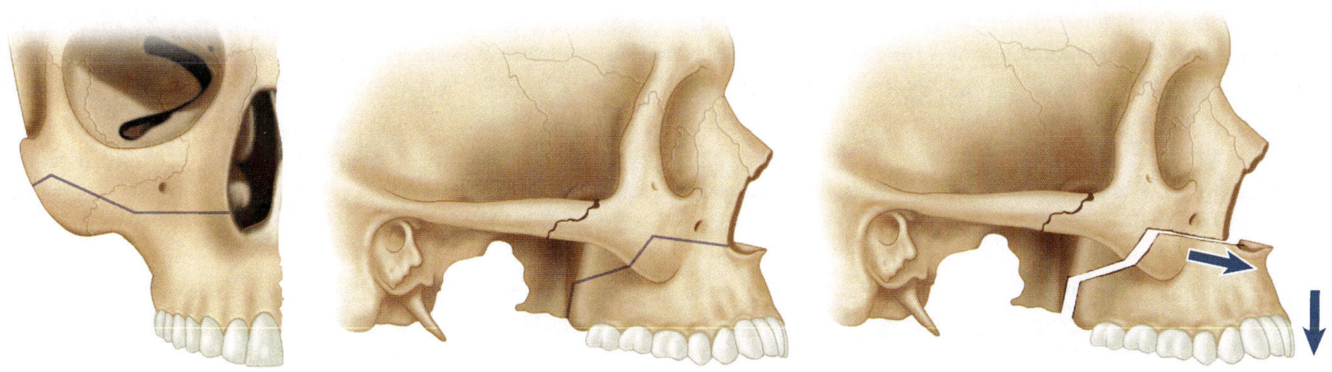

Fig. 30.18 By varying the osteotomy design and angulation, the anterior vertical height and dental display can be controlled. *Top row*: (**a**) With the classic LeFort I osteotomy, increasing the anterior vertical height (dental display) requires increasing the osteotomy gap (opening wedge osteotomy) and bone grafting to ensure stability. *Bottom row*: (**b**) By redirecting the angulation of the osteotomy laterally, the vertical height increases with advancement of the LeFort I segment ensuring a greater degree of stability

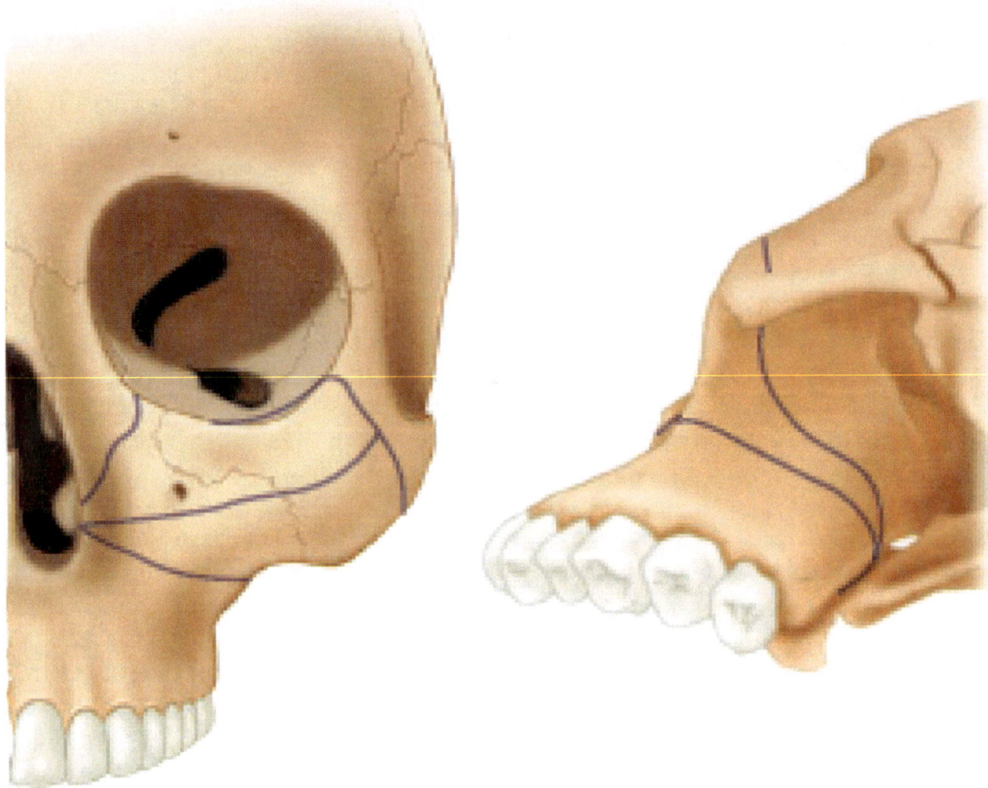

Fig. 30.19 The classic LeFort I and its variations. The classic LeFort I addresses only the maxilla. However, the osteotomy should be tailored to the patient's deformity to address the maxilla, zygoma, and if needed infraorbital rim

In the modified LeFort I with its broad range of variable osteotomy patterns, the details are as described above for the classic LeFort I procedure. The technical detail is different, and the surgeon must have a good understanding of the posterior maxillary wall osteotomy required above the pterygopalatine disjunction. This is an area that cannot be directly visualized. A narrow thin osteotomy must be directed along the lines illustrated in Fig. 30.19. When the osteotomy extends to the zygomatic arch, a right angle oscillating saw may be a useful addition to the reciprocating saw.

Additionally the nasolabial angle will be altered, depending on the position of the anterior nasal spine. With impaction an obtuse angle will become more acute. With advancement, an acute angle will become more obtuse. Thus a decision should be made whether to include the anterior nasal spine with the mobilized segment or to refine it later in the procedure (Fig. 30.20).

Unlike the classic LeFort I that it is primarily driven by an occlusion, skeletal consideration and aesthetic expectations may drive the osteotomy pattern. At times the presurgical orthodontics may be driven by the skeletal goals. There are instances in which the there is a significant midfacial deformity, but the degree of the negative overjet is not nearly as much. By extracting the maxillary first premolars, the occlusal discrepancy can be increased so that the skeletal advancement can be achieved and the occlusion corrected. Thus ideally patients need to be evaluated by both the surgeon and orthodontist prior to treatment to optimize the surgical and orthodontic goals.

The Multisegmented LeFort I

There are instances in which the dentoalveolar arch must be surgically multisegmented to coordinate the dental arches when it cannot be achieved by orthodontic appliances alone. When there is a transverse palatal width deficiency, the interdental osteotomy is typically between the central incisors (8 and 9) resulting in a 2-segment LeFort I. When there are multiple occlusal planes with vertical/torque discrepancies (differential between the anterior and posterior dental arch) and/or transverse width deficiency, then a 3-segment LeFort I may be required with interdental osteotomies either distal or mesial to the canine teeth. In the cleft patients, the maxilla may be multisegmented to close a dental gap such as a canine to lateral incisor substitution to avoid a dental implant or bridge. Thus the need for multisegmentation is coordinated with the orthodontist with model surgery to optimize the occlusion.

In terms of the technical details, the orthodontist diverges the dental roots at the osteotomy sites to minimize root injury with typically 2–3-mm interdental gap. The arch wire is segmented either by the orthodontist or the surgeon at the time of surgery. While others prefer to initiate the interdental osteotomy prior to downfracture, the author's preference is to multisegment the maxilla once it is downfractured and fully mobilized. Interdental osteotomies can be made by tunneling beneath the gingival cuff between the adjacent teeth. A fine side-cutting burr (~1.2 mm) is used to initiate the osteotomy,

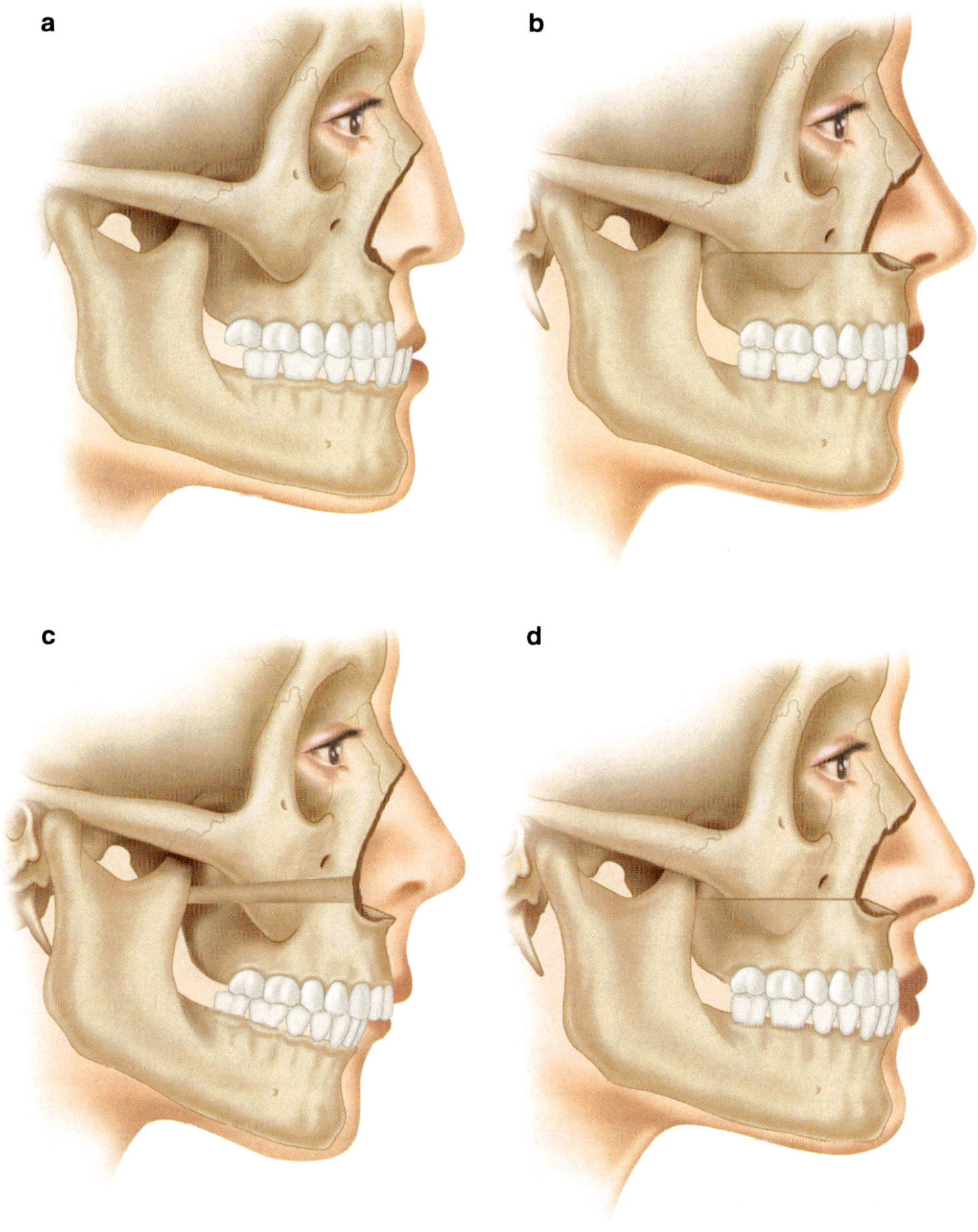

Fig. 30.20 Alteration in the nasolabial angle before (**a**) and after (**b**) maxillary advancement and before (**c**) and after (**d**) maxillary impaction

followed by a thin reciprocating saw superiorly at the level of the horizontal LeFort I osteotomy and a thin flexible interdental or spatula osteotome to complete the osteotomy. With interdental-segmental osteotomies, a finger placed on the palatal surface provides tactile sensation and helps minimize the risk of perforation through the mucosa. In a 2-segment LeFort I, two parasagittal osteotomies are made 6–8 mm lateral to the midline where the bone is thin but the palatal mucosa is thicker. The osteotomies are converged anteriorly in the primary palate to the interdental osteotomy between the central incisors. This is done with either a round-tip burr or a reciprocating saw with a finger placed on the opposite side on the palatal mucosa to minimize injury to the mucosa. Consideration of the anterior nasal spine needs to be taken into account in planning the central osteotomy. In a 3-segment LeFort I procedure, two parasagittal osteotomies are similarly made 6–8 mm lateral to the midline and are joined with the interdental osteotomies along the nasal floor best illustrated in Fig. 30.21.

Once the segmentation is complete, the individual segments are mobilized as vascularized pedicles from the palatal mucosa. Thus care must be taken in the mobilizing with spreader instruments to slowly stretch the gaps without devascularizing the bone. The segments are then placed passively

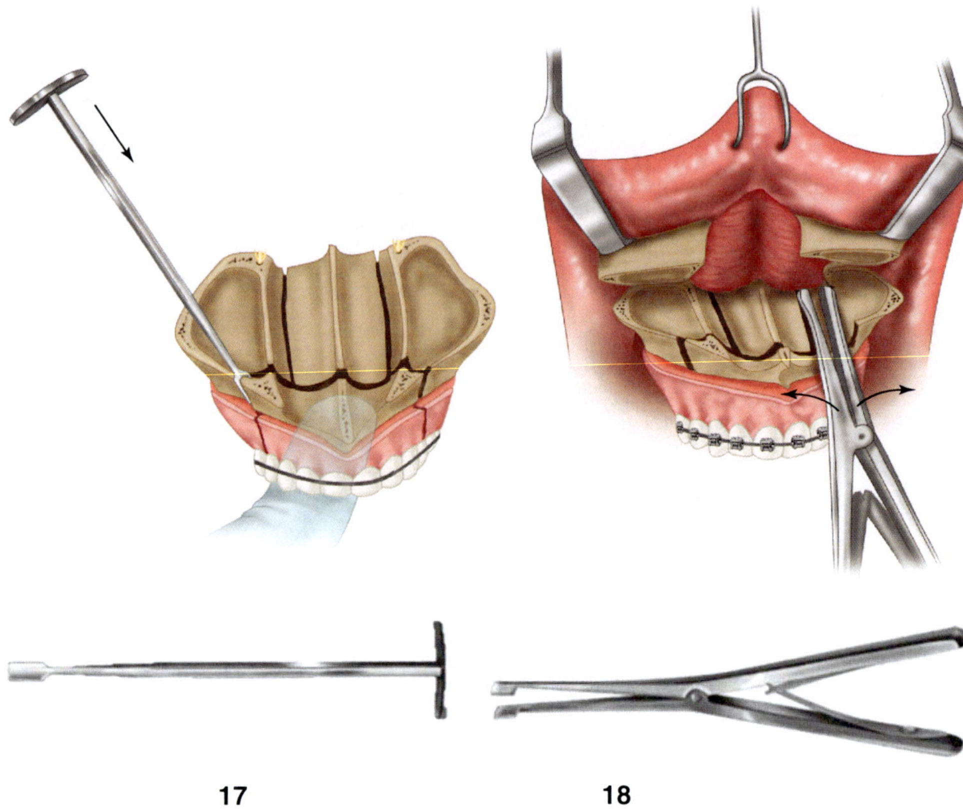

Fig. 30.21 Multisegmenting the maxilla to allow differential movement of the dental arches to accommodate transverse width and vertical leveling. The osteotomy is made with a fine fissure burr, a thin reciprocating saw followed by thin interdental osteotomes. A finger is placed on the palatal surface to guide the procedure

into a prefabricated occlusal splint based on multisegmented dental model surgery and sequentially wire ligated with a 30-gauge wire to the orthodontic arch wire.

In the case of multisegmented maxilla, the author's preference is to leave the splint in place between 2 and 3 weeks. Others will leave the splint in for longer periods of time. The patient is seen with the orthodontist, the splint is removed, and the arch wire is reconstituted. The orthodontist will begin early in the recovery phase (within 2–3 weeks after surgery) to coordinate the dental arches and maintain the stability. As the splint is problematic for patients, orthodontic appliance with transpalatal and lingual support can be made to replace early removal of the occlusal splint to maintain stability.

The Surgically Assisted Rapid Palatal Expansion (SARPE)

In patients who present with transverse palatal width deficiency as a component of multiplanar deformity of sagittal and vertical maxillary discrepancies, surgically assisted rapid palatal expansion (SARPE) should be considered as part of treatment planning. The two options are (1) a single-stage multisegmented LeFort I or (2) two-stage treatment with SARPE as the initial stage to correct the transverse width followed by a single-segment LeFort I to address the vertical and sagittal components of the deformity.

When palatal expansion is needed, the orthodontist will use a transpalatal expander. However, the ability to expand the dentoalveolar arch using dentition for anchorage depends on the patient's age. In children and in early adolescence, the transpalatal expansion works by expansion through the midpalatal suture and the skeletal immaturity of the maxilla. But once the patient has reached skeletal maturity, orthodontic expansion results in buccal-lingual torque instead of widening at the skeletal level. Surgical assistance is then needed by sectioning regions of bony resistance. SARPE is distraction osteogenesis of the maxilla in a transverse plane overcoming the inelastic palatal mucosa (Fig. 30.22). The expander is placed by the orthodontist, the surgeon sections the maxilla, and the palatal expander is activated allowing for gradual expansion at the skeletal level. The results from SARPE are more stable than a segmented LeFort I with immediate surgical expansion. Depending on the need, the SARPE can be bilateral or unilateral with the interdental osteotomy not necessarily between the central incisors. The decision between staged SARPE and immediate multisegmented maxilla depends on the desired arch length, its morphology, the degree of expansion required (small vs. large distance), vertical discrepancies, and need for premolar extractions. This requires careful coordination with the orthodontist.

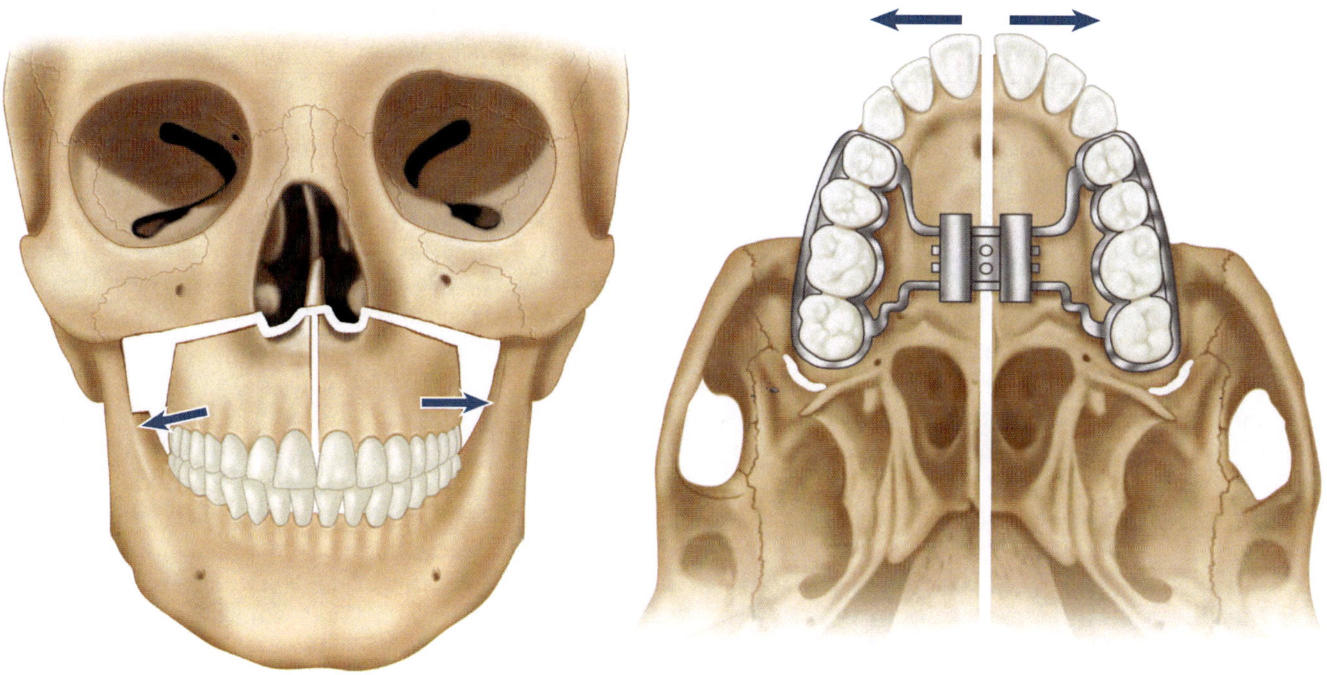

Fig. 30.22 The surgically assisted rapid palatal expansion is a 2-segment LeFort I without the downfracture to correct the transverse width discrepancy by a transpalatal distraction. Note that the osteotomy at the lateral buttress must be well designed so as to interference. A small wedge may be resected to allow expansion

Technical aspects include which skeletal regions need to be sectioned. In the literature there is a wide variety of osteotomies recommended from a 2-segment LeFort I without downfracture to varying degrees of an incomplete LeFort I osteotomy. The author's preference is to section the medial nasomaxillary buttress for a depth of 20 mm where the bone is thickest, to the lateral maxillary-zygomatic buttress as completely as possible, followed by an interdental osteotomy between the central incisors. If significant molar expansion is needed, parasagittal palatal osteotomy and pterygoid separation is made. Consideration should be given to septal deviation with the expansion and whether there is a need for septal-vomer osteotomy. The palatal expander is activated and the above osteotomies are sequentially extended and deepened until there is a 5-mm diastema between the incisors. Both hemi-maxillae must be able to translocate laterally, and areas of bony interference should be addressed. This may occur at the lateral buttress depending on the osteotomy pattern. Once there is no resistance, the expander is contracted until the diastema is 2 mm. There is typically a 5- to 7-day latency period before actively distracting the segments at 0.5 mm/day. The orthodontist will then determine the endpoint.

Subtotal Maxillary Osteotomies

Within this group of procedures are the anterior segmental and posterior segmental osteotomies. While more widely used in the past, these today are indicated only in specific circumstances. Indications for anterior segmental maxillary osteotomy (AMO) include (1) correction of maxillary protrusion to improve the upper lip prominence relative to the nose and face, (2) correction of bimaxillary protrusion with a mandibular subapical osteotomy, (3) correction of an anterior open bite when vertical maxillary excess is not present, and (4) retraction of anterior dentition when it cannot be accomplished by orthodontic means (preexisting condition, e.g., root resorption, ankylosis). There are three basic approaches based on the vascular pedicle: labial (Wunderer), palatal (Cupar), and a combination (Wassmund). Choosing which approach depends on the visualization needed. While the transpalatal approach of the Wunderer provides direct access, the Cupar approach for many is preferred as its approach is that of the classic LeFort I. A labial-buccal mucosal vestibular incision is made that allows access to the anterior segment (canine to canine), the medial anterior maxillary wall, the piriform, and the nasal septum. The sequence is as follows: (1) the nasal septum is first separated from the vomer, (2) the horizontal osteotomy is made, and (3) the vertical osteotomy is then made between the interdental spaces or through the extraction site. The transpalatal osteotomy is made with a finger placed to allow palpation as the osteotomy is made to minimize injury. The author's preference is to hydrostatically elevate the palatal mucosa with saline injection just prior to the osteotomy. Once the anterior segment can be downfractured, the necessary degree of ostectomy can be completed under direct visualization from above to allow mobilization in three planes. The occlusal splint is then placed and the segment is then stabilized internal fixation. The author's preference is a semirigid plate fixation with early removal of the occlusal splint to allow postsurgical orthodontic correction at approximately 3 weeks after surgery.

The posterior segmental osteotomies (PMO) are done for a variety of reasons including posterior maxillary hyperplasia, posterior maxillary open bite, posterior transverse width excess or deficiency, the need for distal repositioning to allow for space for anterior dentition, and segmental cleft dental arch repositioning (canine substitution).

The indications, planning, and the technical considerations that are involved with anterior and posterior segmental osteotomies are beyond the scope of this overview. This section is included to place this group of procedures within the context of maxillary orthognathic surgery. The reader is referred to texts in the bibliography.

Cleft Maxillary Orthognathic Surgery

There is a significant number of patients with facial clefts who would benefit from orthognathic surgery to optimize aesthetic appearance and occlusal stability. Even small maxillary-zygomatic skeletal advancements in the sagittal plane, vertical plane, or clockwise rotation can significantly improve the facial appearance by addressing the typical "convexity" of the midface, deficiency of the piriform region, lack of lip support, and loss of dental display. Moreover there is typically a left/right bony volumetric asymmetry with deficiency on the left side more than the contralateral side (Fig. 30.23). Without surgical input in early adolescence, many cleft patients will be treated with orthodontic management alone or with orthodontics as the primary focus, and only the ones with the severest discrepancies will eventually be referred for surgical assessment. It is not uncommon to see cleft adolescent and young adults with corrected occlusion or edge-to-edge occlusion (camouflage orthodontics) but with the cleft skeletal stigmata. Improving the aesthetic appearance with camouflage procedures and secondary cleft lip and cleft nasal reconstruction never look as good as when the skeletal foundation is in the appropriate spatial relationship. It is important that the surgeon follow the patients as closely as the orthodontist and actively guide the orthodontic-surgical treatment plan to optimize the facial skeletal relationship and occlusion. Ideally skeletal goals should drive the orthodontic management. For example, in instances where the skeletal deficiency is significant, but the maxillary-mandibular dental discrepancy is not, we would request maximal decompensation and, when needed, first maxillary bicuspid extractions so that we can match the degree of negative overjet to the degree of skeletal deficiency. When both are optimized, then the number of patients with facial cleft would benefit with the combined skills of the surgeon, and orthodontist working closer together is much higher than the 25–30 % of the patients cited in the literature.

In our practice, in early adolescence at age 12–14, both the surgeon and the orthodontist will assess the patient and begin the discussion with the family of the possible need for skeletal correction and occlusion depending on mandibular growth and on the deficiency that may already be evident in the midface. Early discussion with the family, monitoring growth, and early close working relationship will alleviate some of the difficulties that may be encountered in late adolescence if treatment planning is delayed. The considerations that the surgeon and the orthodontist must address in adolescence are as follows:

1. The status of the alveolar cleft. Ideally patients have undergone phase I orthodontics that would involve transpalatal expansion, initial alignment of the dentition, and iliac bone grafting of the primary alveolar cleft in early mixed dentition. If this has not been already addressed, then this should be done prior to initiating phase 2 orthodontics when in permanent dentition. This is needed to support the dentition adjacent to the cleft margin, allow canine eruption and orthodontic movement across the cleft site, and improve gingival-mucosal vascularity.
2. The missing lateral incisor. In many cleft patients, the lateral incisor is congenitally missing, has been extracted because of inadequate bone support, or is lost because of dental caries. A decision needs to be made with the family, the orthodontist, and the restorative prosthodontist whether to maintain the dental space for implant-retained dental prosthesis or a bridge versus segmental maxillary osteotomy and closure of the dental space by moving the canine into the lateral incisor position (Fig. 30.24). If a canine substitution is planned for by advancing the lesser alveolar segment, then the cleft site may not need to be grafted prior to segmentation. However, there may be other indications for grafting even in segmented cases.
3. The transpalatal cross-width. In many cleft patients, there is a transverse width discrepancy even after phase I orthodontics that is significant in adolescent at the time of consideration for phase II final orthodontic management. While transverse width discrepancy can be corrected by a segmental LeFort I, it is this author's long-term experience that immediate surgical expansion at the time of surgery is difficult because of the inelastic palatal mucosa that is further made difficult by the palatal mucosal scar. Even when it can be surgically achieved, the long-term stability has not been satisfactory with significant soft tissue palatal mucosa relapsing forces. Our preference is to correct the transverse width with slow expansion using a transpalatal expander and when needed unilateral maxillary osteotomy before formally correcting the sagittal and vertical discrepancies.

Thus, the author's goals in a cleft patient are to (1) convert a multisegmented cleft alveolus to a non-cleft single dental

Fig. 30.23 Typical skeletal features of a patient with a facial cleft that must be addressed

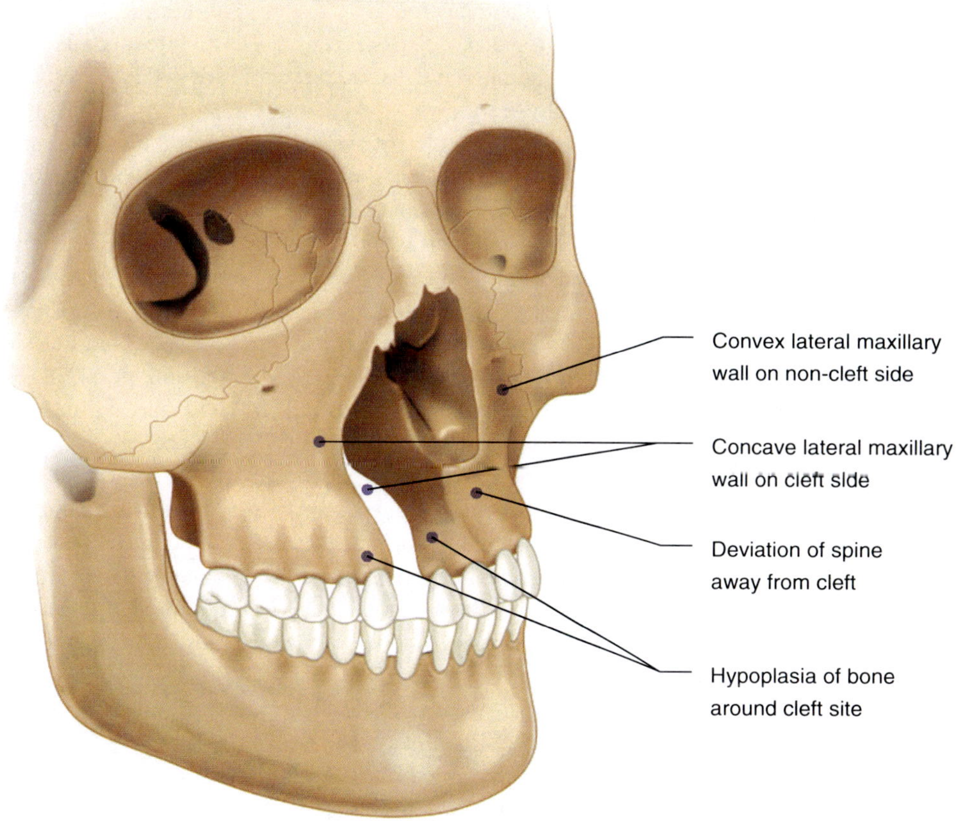

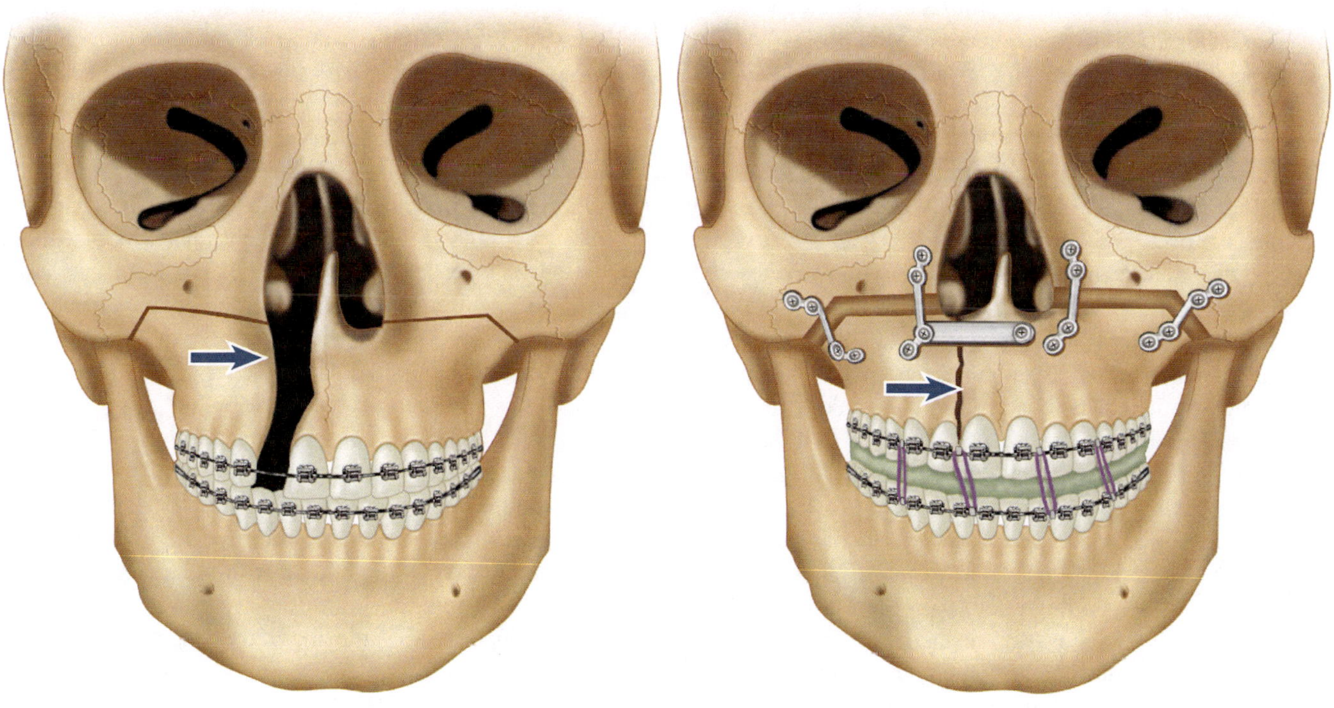

Fig. 30.24 Segmental modified LeFort I to close the dental gap of the typically missing lateral incisor

maxillary alveolar arch, (2) address the missing lateral incisor early in the planning, and (3) correct the transverse width discrepancy prior to sagittal and vertical advancement.

The maxillary osteotomy is as discussed above. However, there are operative details in the cleft patient that the surgeon will need to be familiar with. These are as follows:

1. Nasal intubation may be difficult with the cleft patients because of the typically deviated septum, the small nares with intranasal scar contraction, enlarged turbinates, and previous velopharyngeal surgery. Frequently the surgeon needs to assist the anesthesiologist with the intubation. The challenge is in the patient with the pharyngeal flap requiring fiber-optic placement, introducer guide, and the surgeon assisting intraorally to expose the lateral port of the pharyngeal flap for the passage of the endotracheal tube. In the rare instance when naso-intubation is not possible, the orotracheal tube needs to be positioned in the retromolar region so that the occlusion can be assessed at the time of maxillary-mandibular fixation.
2. In cases where the cleft alveolus has been reconstructed, the incision can be made as described above in which a horizontal incision is made a minimum of 5–8 mm above the attached gingiva. However, in many cleft patients, the labial mucosa is vertically short. The incision is then modified by an inverted "V" at the cleft line so as to lengthen the foreshorten mucosa as a "V" to "Y" at the time of closure. As the incision is deepened, care should be taken at the premaxilla where not infrequently it is significantly vertically short and the incision can be inadvertently carried into the intranasal cavity. In cases where the cleft alveolus is not reconstructed and a segmental osteotomy is planned (2-segment LeFort I) to close the dental gap (canine to lateral incisor), then marginal gingival incisions are made as in alveolar cleft reconstruction.
3. The exposure is more difficult than in non-cleft orthognathic patients. This is especially true in the region of the piriform, the anterior nasal spine, and the septal-vomer junction with the nasal floor. Even when the cleft has been bone grafted, the intranasal exposure is difficult and tedious as the nasal mucosa is in continuity with the palatal mucosa along the reconstructed cleft palate. Typically, there is no bony continuity through the majority of the length of the hard palate distal to the alveolar bone graft (primary palate). The intervening soft tissue has to be sharply divided with scissors from anterior to posterior. The nasal floor mucosa then needs to be approximated after the downfracture. When the cleft alveolus is not bone grafted, then the elevation of the labial gingival mucosa and of the nasal floor mucosa is similarly developed and reconstructed at the time of closure with secondary bone grafting (Fig. 30.25).
4. In cleft patients, the septal-vomer disjunction from the maxillary crest is typically done without difficulty but should be remembered that it will be asymmetric with the typical deflection of the nasal septum and vomer that are deflected toward the left side in unilateral cases.
5. The typical advancement in cleft patients must be in both the sagittal and vertical plane. Thus it is the modified LeFort I in which the upward sloping osteotomy design that may include varying degrees of the upper maxilla and zygoma is ideal. As the maxilla is advanced, the dental display increases, and there is bony contact for stability, limiting the need for bone grafting as with a conventional classic LeFort I osteotomy. Moreover, in the unilateral cleft cases, there is typically asymmetry with the sagittal projection, and the osteotomy pattern can be varied to improve the final outcome with the advancement.
6. The downfracture is typically more difficult than in non-cleft cases. The nasal mucosa is in continuity with the palatal mucosa along the palatal cleft. This may not be completely elevated and divided at the time of the exposure. As the anterior maxilla is downfractured, the intranasal visualization improves and the tissue is divided from anterior to posterior under direct vision. The posterior-lateral nasal wall and the descending palatine vessel are exposed and can be better addressed under direction vision as discussed above.
7. The mobilization is more difficult because of the initial cleft palatal mucosa repair and further limited by previous velopharyngeal surgery. Stripping the soft tissue from the skeletal maxilla may at times be tedious. A channel retractor is helpful to visualize the posterior maxilla and removal of adherent soft tissue. A sharply turned elevator or a mandibular inferior border stripper placed at the posterior hard palatal junction can be useful to distract the maxilla forward in conjunction with the channel retractors. The maxilla must be completely mobile and capable of being repositioned in 3-dimensional space without "relapsing" tension. If the maxilla cannot be placed in the desired position, then either a mandibular sagittal split osteotomy is performed or a placement of either internal or external distraction devices is considered. In our practice this is an intraoperative decision and discussed with the patient and patient's family members prior to surgery. Maxillofacial distraction is discussed in Chap. 34.
8. In this author's practice, consideration is given to turbinectomy in cleft patients to improve the intranasal volume. With the maxilla downfractured, the turbinectomy can be performed easily through the mucosal incision, bone reduction, and tailoring of the mucosal closure.
9. The nasal lining should be repaired, though in many of the cases, complete repair is not possible. In the areas of

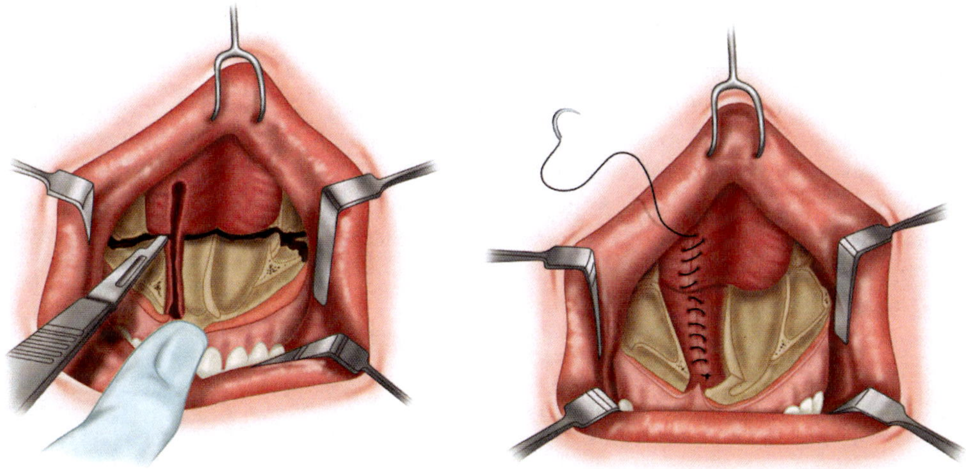

Fig. 30.25 The intranasal exposure is tedious, and the adherent soft tissue along the reconstructed cleft palate must be sharply divided. The nasal lining and palatal lining is repaired when the maxilla is downfractured before the final fixation. Bone is added at the primary palate

incomplete repair, intranasal mucosal lining heals by secondary intention. We have the patients use a saline nasal rinse after surgery for several months. The occurrence of intranasal adhesions and synechiae is extremely low. The lining heals remarkably well.

10. If there are any significant osteotomy gaps, then our preference in cleft patients is to use iliac corticocancellous bone graft. In our experience, the need has been less with well-designed osteotomies.
11. At the time of closure, the nasal ala base position can be set with a fixation suture through the spine. The septum can be centered through the anterior nasal spine with a transfixation suture. In addition any minor lip contour and mucosa can be corrected at this time.

Postoperative Management

Patients who have undergone SARPE or subtotal anterior maxillary osteotomy procedures can be managed as outpatient procedures. Their recovery is within 5–7 days and they present with few concerns. The transpalatal expander is activated between 5 and 7 days after surgery when the patient can comfortably open their mouth and turn the expansion key. This is typically at a rate of 0.5 mm/day to minimize vascular compromise of the gingiva and overcome the palatal mucosa resistance without creating an oral-nasal fistula. With activation of the transpalatal expander, the patients with SARPE will experience pain and discomfort at the points of bony interference (maxillary-zygomatic buttress), at the nasal-glabella region (intact lateral nasal wall and maxillary rotation) and occasionally at the posterior orbital region (intact articulation of the palatine bone). These are managed by nonsteroidal anti-inflammatory agents. The orthodontist will primarily monitor the length of the distraction phase to achieve the arch length needed and the transverse width to correct the lingual crossbite.

The LeFort I maxillary osteotomies are admitted for monitoring of airway and bleeding to an observation unit overnight. With maxillary surgery alone, the author's preference is to not use maxillary-mandibular fixation or place guiding elastics in the immediate postoperative recovery phase because of concerns for airway, bleeding, and postoperative nausea and to more easily allow oral intake and oral care. The vast majority of patients are discharged the following day. Patients are instructed in oral care (frequent mouth rinses with diluted hydrogen peroxide and water), nasal care (intranasal saline spray, humidifier), diet (oral fluids and mechanically soft diet advanced as tolerated), and facial edema (cool compresses to the face). Patients are encouraged to ambulate and to resume non-strenuous daily living activities. Patients are seen at 2 weeks with the orthodontist. Occlusal splint when used in multisegmented and instability cases is removed, and the orthodontic arch wire is reconstituted. It is at 2 weeks postoperative that guiding elastics are placed to begin coordinating the dental arches. The patients are seen at 2-week intervals, more frequently if needed, to assess the occlusion and adjust the vector pattern of the guiding elastics. At 4 weeks patients are instructed in TMJ range of motion exercises, increasing their diet that requires more masticatory force. By 6 weeks patients are on an unrestricted diet though many will have put themselves on an unrestricted diet much earlier.

The first 2 weeks are difficult for many patients having to cope with facial edema, limited TMJ opening, drooling, and adjustment to a new occlusal relationship with oral intake further aggravated with an occlusal splint. Pain and discomfort are typically well controlled with nonsteroidal anti-inflammatory agents that are continued as a baseline and the occasional use of oral narcotics to help with sleeping. However, there is a turning point that occurs physically and psychologically between 2 and 3 weeks when the majority of patients feel that surgery is behind them, resumed noncontact sports/exercise, and have returned to school and work.

Complications

With maxillary orthognathic surgery, the most common surgical complications are related to neurovascular compromise. However, uncommon or rare unpredictable events have been described in the literature. Among these include avascular necrosis, pseudoaneurysm, carotid-cavernous sinus fistula, nasolacrimal duct injury, orbital compartment syndrome, and blindness. These are isolated cases and, because of their rarity of occurrence, cannot be anticipated.

Vascular

Postoperative nasal bleeding after LeFort I osteotomy typically resolves spontaneously but may require packing. Ongoing bleeding requires further treatment and evaluation. Anterior and posterior nasal packing with release of maxillomandibular fixation may be necessary for hemostasis. If bleeding persists, then this should be followed by angiography with possible embolization and surgical exploration. External carotid ligation is the last resort for hemostatic control.

When not ligated, the descending palatine artery is the primary source of postoperative bleeding from the LeFort I osteotomy. It is typically injured during the posterolateral nasal wall osteotomy. While such injuries can be avoided by stopping the osteotomy at the palatine bone and keeping it as low as possible near the tuberosity, it is in reality difficult to avoid. Once downfractured, the surgeon should look for the descending palatine and control it. The internal maxillary arterial branches may be partially or completely transected during posterior maxillary wall osteotomy and the pterygopalatine separation. When this occurs, it is generally best to complete the downfracture and control the bleeding with vascular clip and bipolar electrocautery under direct visualization after temporary packing and the use of various hemostatic agents.

With degloving osteotomy and repositioning of the facial skeletal elements, there is a reduction in blood supply to the osteotomized segment. The vascular compromise affects not only the skeletal component but also the dentition and the associated soft tissue elements (pulp, periodontia, and gingiva). However, in the overwhelming vast majority of cases, this vascular compromise is transient and has no significant clinical impact on outcome.

The vascularity of the LeFort I downfractured segment is derived primarily from the soft palate and from the buccal soft tissue pedicle because the greater palatine vessels are frequently divided in the course of the osteotomy and mobilization. Although the reduction in blood supply is transient, devitalization of the teeth, periodontal gingival defects, and segmental bone loss have been described. These often have been attributed to incisions that may compromise the vascularity, stripping of the periosteum, compromised palatal mucosa (secondary to previous cleft palate surgery), interdental or segmental osteotomies with loss of the attached gingiva, and transverse expansion with excessive stripping of the palatal mucosa. When cyanosis of the gingiva is noted intraoperatively and vascularity does not return with reversal of hypotension, thought should be given to returning the maxilla to the original position and reassessing the surgical approach. In this case, delayed advancement can subsequently be done gradually or using distraction osteogenesis, either surgically controlled with implanted devices or with orthopedic elastic traction forces.

Neural

With the exception of the nasopalatine and superior alveolar nerves that are inevitably transected as an intrinsic part of t the LeFort I osteotomy, sensory loss in the infraorbital nerve distribution is temporary with nearly complete recovery, because the infraorbital nerve is well visualized and the vast majority of osteotomies are inferior to the foramen. The long-term incidence of sensory loss is approximately 1.5–2 % and may occur as a result of extensive traction from soft tissue retraction or from compression at the time of plate fixation. The greater palatine nerve is frequently transected with the posterior osteotomy but without apparent significant sensory disturbance to the patient with collateral innervation. Sensory deficits of the teeth, palatal mucosa, and buccal mucosa tend to gradually resolve over a 12- to 18-month period.

Summary

Since Obwegeser first introduced the LeFort I procedure in 1965, it has become the workhorse to solve a wide range of deformities that the maxillofacial surgeon may encounter in his practice. The LeFort I and its multitude of variations allow the surgeon to tailor the midfacial skeletal osteotomy to the patient's deformity. With the sagittal split osteotomy of the mandibular ramus and the osseous genioplasty, the surgeon can disassemble the facial skeleton and reconstruct it to reach a desired aesthetic and functional goals.

Bibliography

Bays RA. Complications of orthognathic surgery. In: Kaban LB, Pogrel MA, Perrott DH, editors. Complications in oral and maxillofacial surgery. Philadelphia: WB Saunders Co; 1997.

Bell WH. Le Forte I osteotomy for correction of maxillary deformities. J Oral Surg. 1975;33(6):412–26.

Bell WH, editor. Modern practice in orthognathic and reconstructive surgery. Philadelphia: W. B. Saunders Company; 1992.

Bell WH, Fonseca RJ, Kennedy JW, et al. Bone healing an revascularization after total maxillary osteotomy. J Oral Surg. 1975; 33:253.

Kawamoto Jr HJ. Simplification of the Le Fort I osteotomy. Clin Plast Surg. 1989;16:777.

Obwegeser H. Surgery of the maxilla for the correction of prognathism. SSO Schweiz Monatsschr Zahnheilkd. 1965;75:365–74.

Obwegeser H. Surgical correction of small or retrodisplaced maxillae. The "dish-face" deformity. Plast Reconstr Surg. 1969;43:351–65.

Obwegeser HL. Mandibular growth anomalies. Berlin: Springer; 2001.

Patel PK, Margulis A. Orthognathic surgery in adolescents. In: Bentz ML, Bauer BS, Zuker RM, editors. Principles and practice of pediatric plastic surgery, vol. 1. St. Louis: Quality Medical Publishing, Inc; 2008.

Patel PK, Novia MV. The surgical tools: the LeFort I, bilateral sagittal split osteotomy of the mandible and the osseous genioplasty. Clin Plast Surg. 2007;34:447–75.

Patel PK, Morris DE, Gassman A. Complications of orthognathic surgery. J Craniofac Surg. 2007;18(4):838–43.

Posnick JC. LeFort I, osteotomy, sagittal splitting of the mandible and genioplasty: historical perspective and step-by-step approach. In: Posnick JC, editor. Craniofacial and maxillofacial surgery in children and young adults, vol. 2. Philadelphia: W. B. Saunders; 2000.

Siebert JW, Angrigiani C, McCarthy JG, et al. Blood supply of the LeFort I maxillary segment: an anatomic study. Plast Reconstr Surg. 1997;100:843–51.

Wolfe SA, Berkowitz S. Plastic surgery of the facial skeleton. Boston: Little, Brown and Company; 1989.

Mandibular Osteotomies

31

Mitchell A. Stotland, Jeffrey Y. Wu, and Derrick C. Wan

Orthognathic surgery involves segmental movements of the tooth bearing maxilla and/or mandible for the correction of skeletal deformities. This chapter focuses on the various osteotomy techniques available for mandibular repositioning. As for any surgery, the pathway towards an optimal outcome in orthognathic surgery involves precise diagnosis and planning. This requires careful clinical history-taking and examination, dental/orthodontic consultation, standard photography and cephalometric analysis, an appraisal of patient expectations, and conventional laboratory or computer-assisted model surgery and splint fabrication. These preliminary steps are covered in depth elsewhere in this text.

The clinical indications for mandibular osteotomy include correction of skeletal distortion in the sagittal (AP), coronal (cephalocaudad), and axial (transverse) dimensions. These changes can be manifested in the following clinical patterns:

Sagittal (AP) distortion:

- Mandibular retrognathia
- Mandibular prognathia
- Mandibular alveolar protrusion
- Mandibular alveolar retrusion

Coronal (cephalocaudad) distortion:

- Vertical mandibular hypoplasia
- Vertical mandibular hyperplasia

Axial (transverse plane) distortion:

- Transverse hypoplasia
- Transverse hyperplasia

The skeletal distortions above are most commonly caused by congenital growth disturbance but may also occur secondary to trauma, infection, radiation exposure, remote oncologic surgical intervention, etc. Severe changes in the mandible are associated with aesthetic facial disharmony and with dental malocclusions that can impact an individual's chewing efficiency, bite force, and mandibular excursion. Mandibular skeletal abnormality can also contribute to lip incompetence, as well as breathing and swallowing dysfunction. Over the past 150 years, a variety of orthognathic surgical techniques have been described to address these disorders. The bilateral sagittal split osteotomy (BSSO) is currently the workhorse approach to surgical repositioning of the mandible, while the vertical ramus and inverted-L osteotomies are also important methods that are employed. Far less commonly utilized are the mandibular body and subapical (block) osteotomy.

Mandibular Retrognathia

Mandibular retrognathia, or anteroposterior deficiency, results in a medialized position of the maxillary first molar relative to the mandibular first molar, referred to as an Angle Class II malocclusion. This is further subdivided into Class II, Division 1 (with proclined incisors and an increased overjet) and Class II, Division 2 (with retroclined incisors and an increased (or deep) overbite). Mandibular retrognathia results in a convex facial profile and a weak-appearing chin. There is an obtuse cervicomental angle, reduced chin-throat length, and an acute labiomental fold. The skeletal disharmony of the upper and lower jaws, along with incisor displacement, results in poor lip seal, mentalis strain with attempted oral closure, and a tendency towards lower lip eversion.

Bilateral sagittal split osteotomy is the procedure of choice for surgical advancement of the mandible due to its broad contact area of bone fragments and amenability to rigid fixation. The inverted-L osteotomy may be considered for patients requiring secondary advancement following prior sagittal split or when an abnormal anatomy of the ramus is encountered. Furthermore, for correction of micrognathia-associated upper airway obstruction in children, the inverted-L osteotomy is employed in concert with distraction osteogenesis.

M.A. Stotland, MD, MS (✉) • J.Y. Wu, MD
Section of Plastic Surgery, Dartmouth-Hitchcock Medical Center, Geisel School of Medicine at Dartmouth, Lebanon, NH, USA
e-mail: mitchell.a.stotland@hitchcock.org

D.C. Wan, MD
Division of Plastic and Reconstructive Surgery, Stanford University Medical Center, Palo Alto, CA, USA

P.J. Taub et al. (eds.), *Ferraro's Fundamentals of Maxillofacial Surgery*,
DOI 10.1007/978-1-4614-8341-0_31,

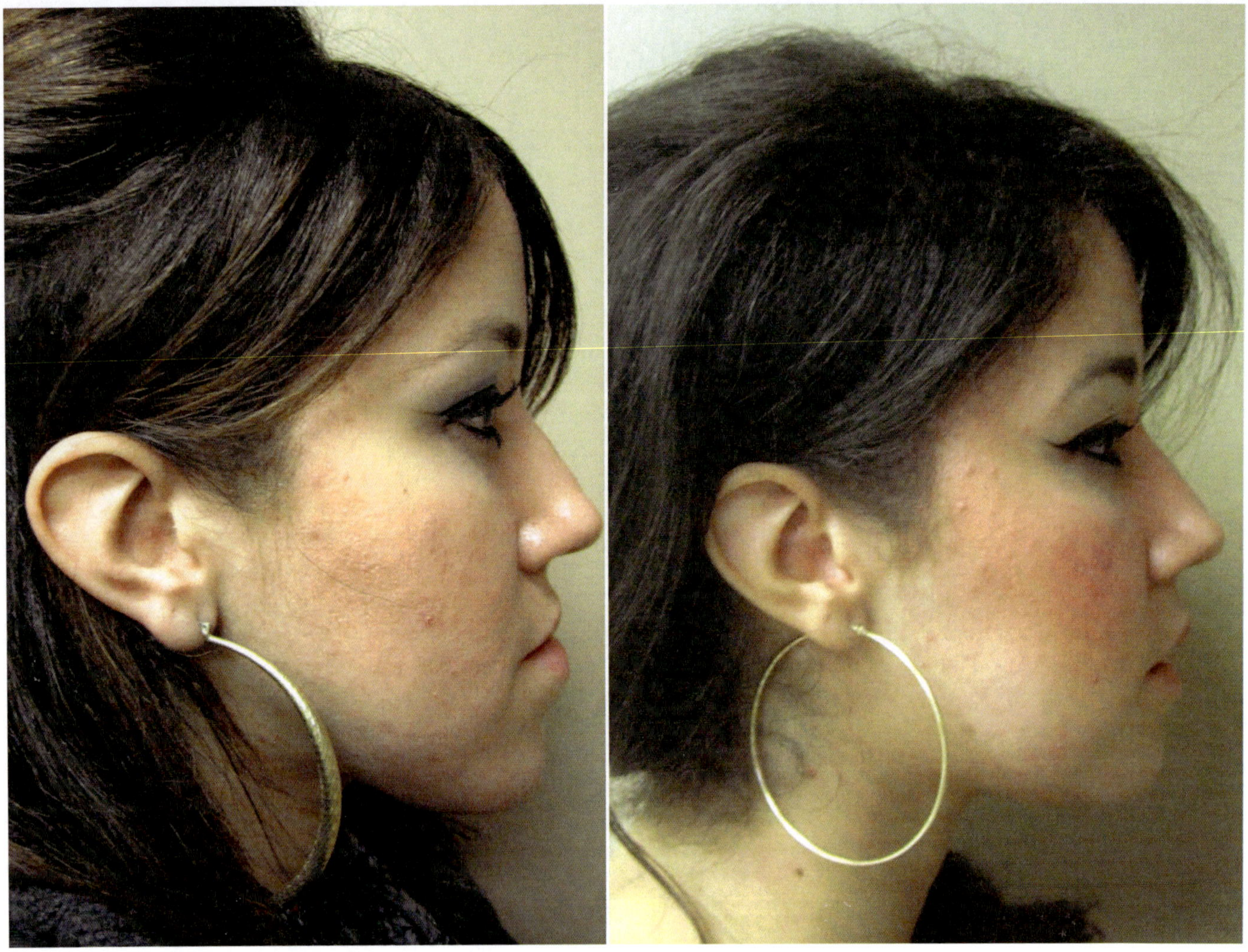

Fig. 31.1 Patient with mandibular prognathism preoperatively (*left*) and following setback by bilateral sagittal split of the mandible (*right*)

Mandibular Prognathia

Mandibular prognathia, or anteroposterior excess, results in a distalized position of the maxillary first molar relative to the mandibular first molar, referred to as an Angle Class III malocclusion. The facial contour assumes a concave profile, and the lower third of the face appears prominent with a protrusive chin and well-defined lower border of the mandible (see Fig. 31.1). There is an acute cervicomental angle, increased chin-throat length, and obtuse labiomental fold.

Surgical options for mandibular setback include the bilateral sagittal split osteotomy, vertical ramus osteotomy, and inverted-L osteotomy. The choice between bilateral sagittal split osteotomy and vertical ramus osteotomy remains controversial. Bilateral sagittal split osteotomy allows for better bony contact between the proximal and distal segments, immediate jaw mobilization (although final bite strength is not different between the techniques), better oral hygiene, and earlier initiation of postsurgical orthodontics. However, unfavorable osteotomy is an uncommon but well-documented, technical complication. Proponents of the vertical ramus osteotomy cite the lower incidence of inferior alveolar nerve injury, technical ease (shortened operative time and easier technique), and ability for larger mandibular setback. Vertical ramus osteotomy does require maxillomandibular fixation when performed transorally. This impairs nutrition and can lead to osteoarthritic changes in the temporomandibular joint if immobilization is prolonged.

Mandibular Alveolar Protrusion/Retrusion

Mandibular alveolar protrusion can be a normal finding in some ethnic groups, but it can also represent an anomalous finding. Most commonly, harmful habits such as thumb sucking or tongue thrusting contribute to alveolar protrusion and malocclusion. In growing children, functional appliances can be used to modify these habits in an attempt to eliminate such causative factors. Mandibular alveolar retrusion in otherwise healthy children is usually caused by genetic factors and may be associated with a deep labiomental sulcus. In either situation, alveolar protrusion or retrusion can be corrected in most cases with fixed orthodontic therapy. However, unless the underlying cause is removed or long-term retention is employed, relapse rates are high. In the rare situation where a patient has an appropriately positioned maxillary and mandibular skeletal base and malocclusion is caused by a mandibular dentoalveolar deformity alone, a subapical (block) osteotomy may be performed. This technique may also be indicated in a patient with alveolar protrusion or retrusion not amenable to orthodontic treatment alone.

Surgical Techniques

Bilateral Sagittal Split Ramus Osteotomy

The first large clinical series of mandibular osteotomies were published by Blair and later Kostecka. These involved ramal osteotomies located cephalad to the lingula utilizing an extraoral approach. A high rate of complications was associated with these procedures including relapse, pseudoarthrosis, open bite, irreversible injury to the mandibular or facial nerves, and parotid gland fistula. Schossmann and Kazanjian later performed an oblique osteotomy to increase the bony contact area. Obwegeser described the intraoral sagittal split osteotomy of the horizontal ramus. Dal Pont later modified Obwegeser's technique by transitioning the distal osteotomy to the vertical retromolar osteotomy. In order to reduce the risk for bad splits, Hunsuck proposed that the posterior split only extend past the lingula instead of the posterior border of the mandible.

The Obwegeser-Dal Pont bilateral sagittal split osteotomy is approached through a vestibular incision, made well lateral to the mandibular gingivobuccal sulcus in the molar region in order to allow for an optimal mucosal closure. The incision is extended superiorly approximately 2 cm towards the coronoid process. A periosteal elevator exposes the posterior body, angle, and ascending ramus (see Fig. 31.2), and an inferior border stripper ("J stripper") completes the exposure of the inferior mandibular border (see Fig. 31.3). Care must be taken to leave the masseter attached to the posterolateral ramus in order to preserve the blood supply and stability of the proximal segment (see Fig. 31.4). The anterior ramus is exposed using a notched "V"-shaped elevator and the anterior attachment of temporalis muscle divided with electrocautery. An angled Kocher clamp is placed high on the coronoid process for control (see Fig. 31.5). A medial tunnel is developed superiorly to inferiorly using a curved periosteal elevator, watching for the inferior alveolar nerve. A retractor is placed to protect the inferior alveolar nerve and keep the lingual soft tissue at bay. A Lindemann side-cutting burr or reciprocating saw creates the medial ramus osteotomy along the width of the ramus. The corticotomy is deepened to approximately half the thickness of the ramus and is gradually extended in an oblique fashion towards the external oblique line. Care is taken to maintain a lat-

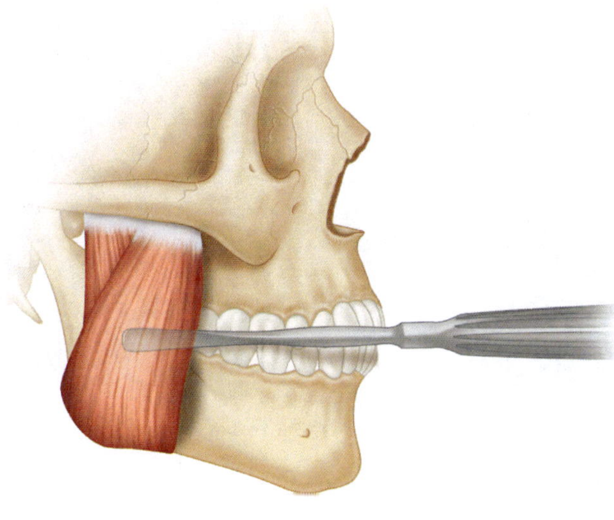

Fig. 31.2 Stripping the masseter off the lateral border of the mandible

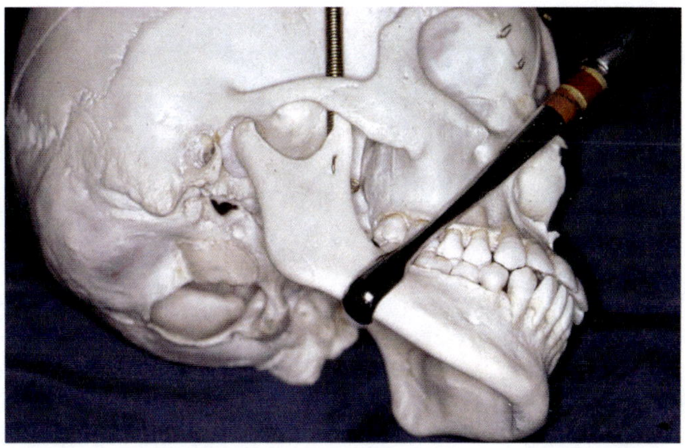

Fig. 31.3 Stripping the pterygomasseteric sling off the inferior border of the mandible

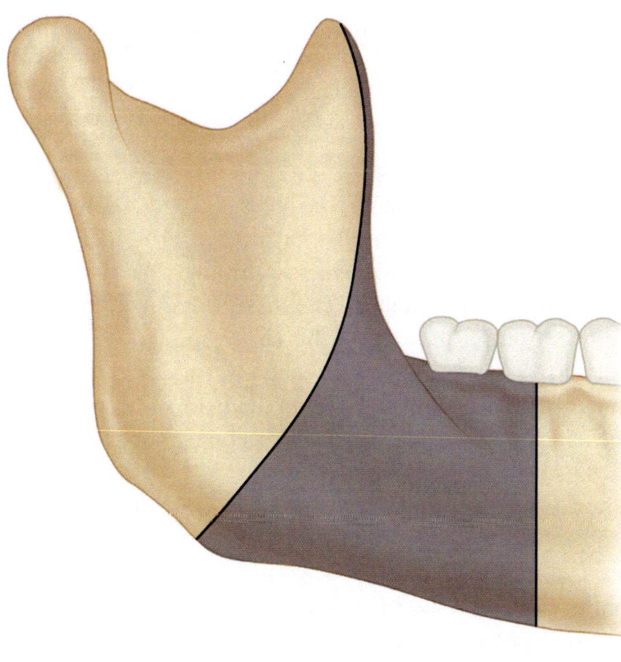

Fig. 31.4 Area of muscle stripping with preservation of the posterior attachments to preserve blood supply to the proximal segment

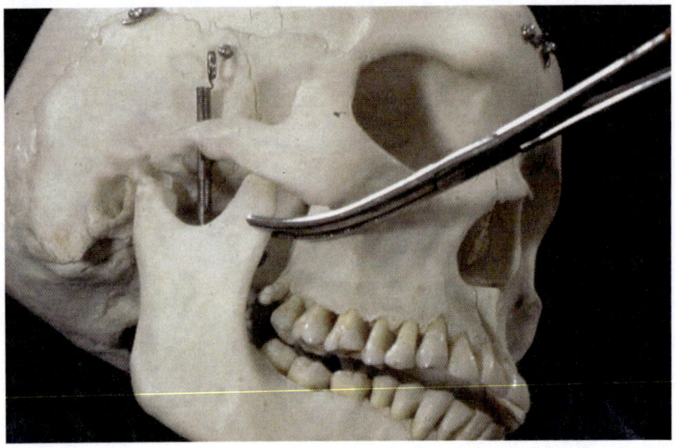

Fig. 31.5 Kocher clamp used to stabilize the coronoid process

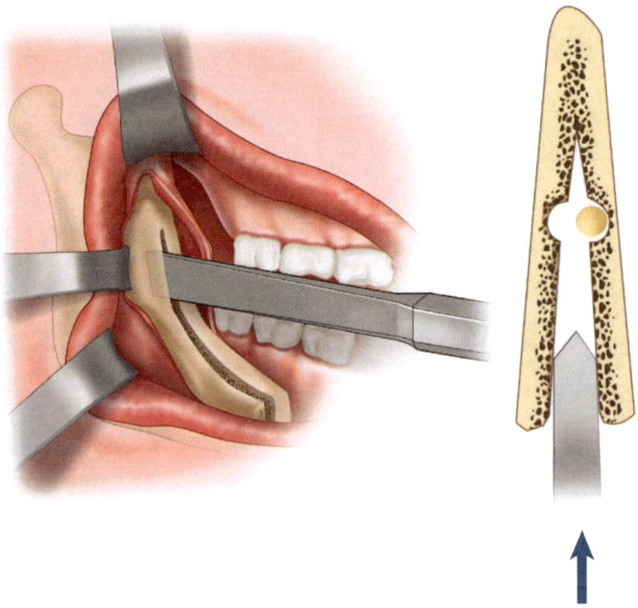

Fig. 31.6 The "sagittal" split of the mandible using thin osteotomes. The orginal description involved a split through the alveolar nerve canal. Modifications attempt to split the bone just inside the buccal plate, leaving the canal of the nerve intact

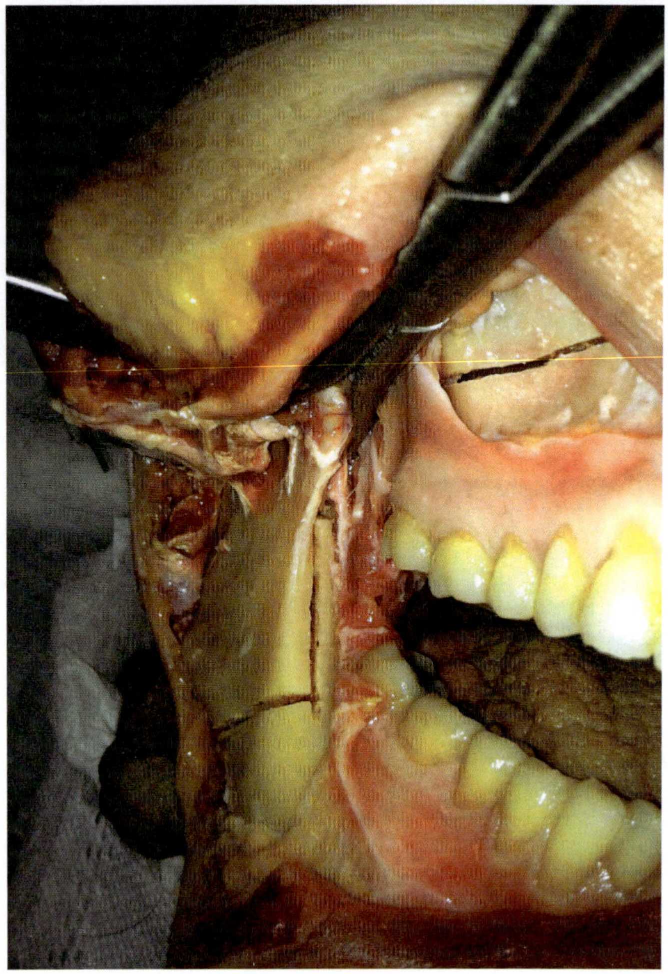

Fig. 31.7 Cadaver dissection showing the osteotomies of the sagittal split

eral path across the region of the anterior oblique ridge. The vertical corticotomy along the buccal border is made with a reciprocating saw extending towards the space between the first and second molars. The vertical corticotomy must continue through the inferior border to the medial lingual cortex in order to allow subsequently for an expeditious and clean split with osteotomes. Finally, a series of osteotomes are used to split the cancellous bone, completing the sagittal split (see Figs. 31.6, 31.7, and 31.8). Newer piezoelectric saws have been recommended to minimize injury to the intraosseous alveolar nerve. The distal segment is advanced or setback into proper occlusion using a prefabricated occlusal splint with care taken to ensure that the condylar segment is seated within the glenoid fossa. Fixation is completed with positional screws or monocortical plates (see Figs. 31.9 and 31.10). The mucosa is then closed with resorbable sutures.

Bad splits during sagittal split osteotomy describe an unfavorable or irregular fracture of the mandible. These include a split on the superior corner of the proximal segment, a split that leaves the inferior border on the distal or proximal segment intact, nerve trapped in the proximal segment, an inadvertent cut through the ramus, a distal segment vertical fracture, and a buccal plate or proximal segment fracture. The incidence of bad splits ranges from 0.21 to 22.72 %, occurring most commonly on the buccal plate of the proximal segment or the posterior aspect of the distal segment. Risk factors associated with bad splits are younger age and presence of third molars. It is recommended that patients younger than 20 with unerupted third molars should have removal 6–9 months before surgery; however, in patients older than 20, the removal of third molars before or concurrently with orthognathic surgery remains controversial.

Relapse after mandibular orthognathic surgery is multifactorial and is related to the amount of advancement/

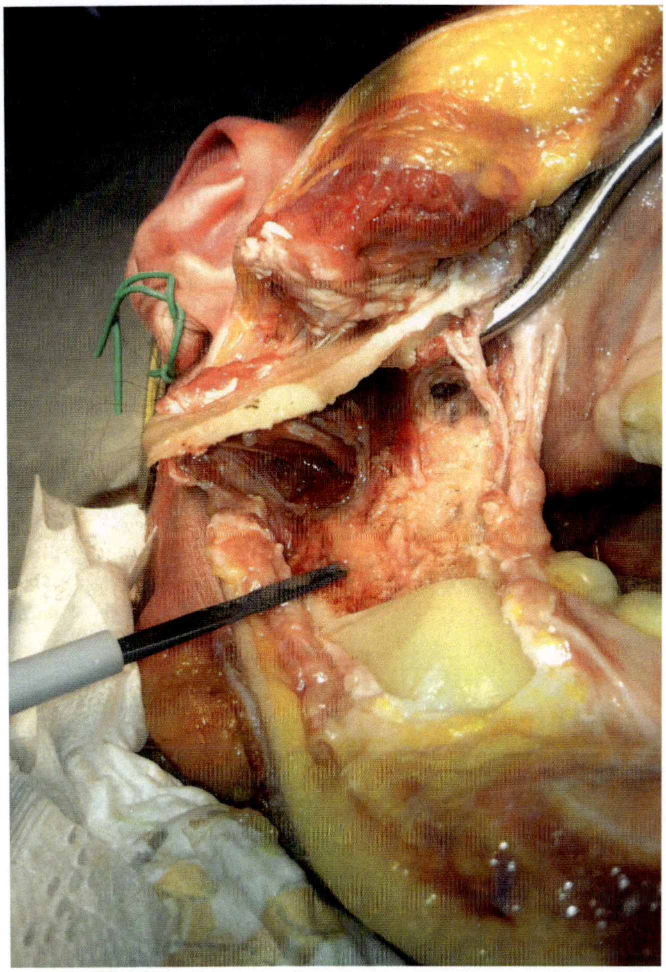

Fig. 31.8 Cadaver dissection with the proximal portion reflected highlighting the canal of the inferior alveolar nerve

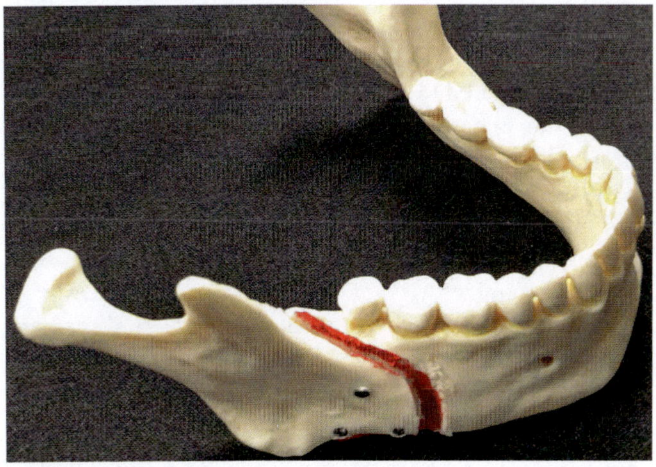

Fig. 31.9 Model demonstrating the sagittal split segments fixed with bicortical screws on either side of the nerve

setback, proper seating of the condyles, disrupted tension of the stomatognathic system, mandibular plane angle, remaining growth and remodeling, age, and gender. After

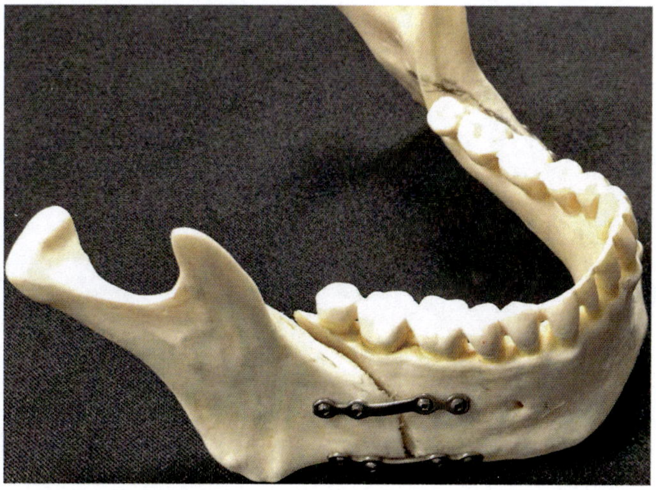

Fig. 31.10 Model demonstrating the sagittal split segments fixed with monocortical plates

bilateral sagittal split advancement surgery, the short-term relapse (within 1.5 years) was 1.5–32.7 % at point B and 2.0–37 % at pogonion using bicortical screw fixation. Long-term relapse (after 1.5 years) was 2.0–50.3 % at point B and 6.4–60.2 % at pogonion. With miniplates, the short-term and long-term relapses were 1.5–80 % at point B and 1.4–18.7 % at pogonion and 1.5–8.9 % at point B and 1.6–16.1 % at pogonion, respectively. After bilateral sagittal split setback surgery, the short-term relapse was 9.9–62.1 % at point B and 15.7 and 91.3 % at pogonion. Long-term relapse was 14.9–18.5 at point B and 11.5–25.4 % at pogonion.

The incidence of inferior alveolar nerve injury with sagittal split osteotomy has considerable variation, depending on subjective versus objective measures of nerve function. Clinical diagnosis of inferior alveolar nerve injury is mostly subjective and consists of perception of light touch, pain, or two-point discrimination along the distribution of the nerve. While nerve injury usually results in transient paresthesia which most patients tolerate well, injuries to the inferior alveolar nerve may also result in hyperesthesia or painful dysesthesia, which is poorly tolerated. The incidence of inferior alveolar nerve injury detected clinically is 73.6 % (range 55.5–88.2 %) at 2 weeks and 36.7 % (range 10.5–53.8 %) at 6 months. Permanent nerve symptoms persisting beyond 1 year were found in 23.8 % (range 5.3–38 %). Objective tests include trigeminal somatosensory evoked potentials, orthodontic sensory nerve action potentials, and blind reflex. At 1-week postoperatively, the incidence of inferior alveolar nerve disturbance was 63.3 % (range 50–73.2 %), diminishing to 33 % (range15.4–80 %) at 6 months. Continued nerve disturbance was detected in 12.8 % (range 5–40 %) of sagittal split osteotomies at 1 year. The reported incidence of complete transection of the nerve is 2–3.5 % for sagittal split osteotomies.

The incidence of facial nerve injury ranges between 0.125 and 0.38 % in the literature. The exact etiology of facial nerve injury is not entirety known and may result from damage to

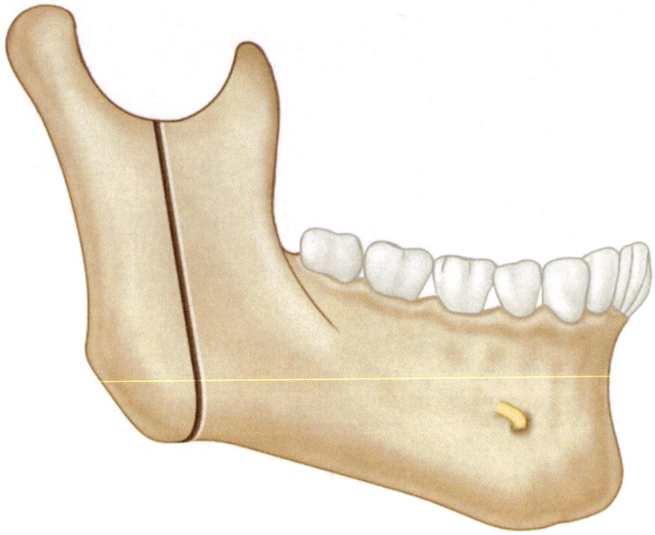

Fig. 31.11 Beveled, vertical osteotomy of the mandibular ramus

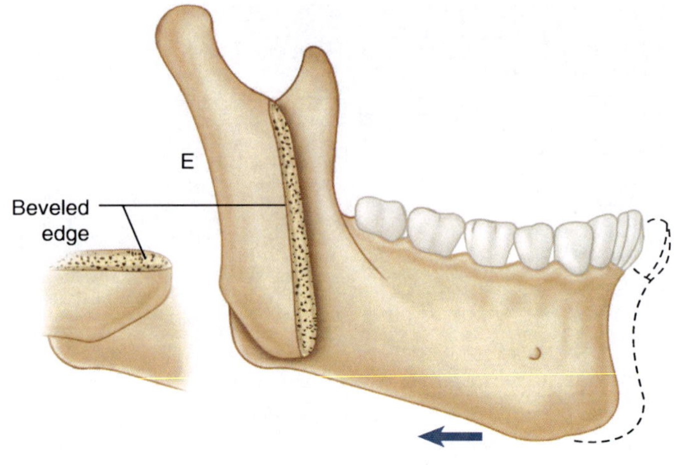

Fig. 31.12 Overlapping segments of the vertical ramus osteotomy

the nerve during placement of medial retractors, compression by postoperative edema, nerve ischemia caused by injection of vasoconstrictor deep into the perimandibular region, and/or compression of the nerve by the distal segment. In the vast majority, there is only transient facial nerve palsy, and recovery may be accelerated by a short course of oral steroids.

Intraoral Vertical Ramus Osteotomy

The intraoral vertical ramus osteotomy is frequently employed for the treatment of mandibular prognathism. Often cited benefits to this approach over that of sagittal split osteotomy include lower incidence of alveolar nerve injury, technical simplicity, and ability to achieve greater mandibular setback and repositioning of the condyle, if necessary. The main disadvantage of this technique, however, is that it is primarily limited to mandibular setback.

A vestibular incision is made well lateral to the mandibular gingivobuccal sulcus in the molar region in order to allow for an optimal mucosal closure. The incision extends superiorly along the anterior border of the ramus. The masseter is stripped off the lateral (but not posterior) ramal surface. Exposure of the lateral ramus is optimized with retractors placed in the sigmoid notch and inferior border of the mandible. The osteotomy is then performed with a 30° oscillating saw from superior to inferior starting at the sigmoid notch, following a course of 5 mm posterior to the antilingular prominence (see Fig. 31.11). The angled saw blade allows the osteotomy to be beveled away from the alveolar canal and also improves bony contact when the tooth-bearing segment is retropositioned. The condylar fragment ends up positioned buccally (lateral) to the tooth-bearing segment (see Fig. 31.12). Maxillomandibular fixation is then implemented after first placing a prefabricated occlusal splint to ensure correct occlusion. Upward pressure is applied to the mandibular angles in order to seat the condylar segments properly into the glenoid fossa bilaterally. Importantly, when encountering patients who cannot tolerate maxillomandibular fixation, an edentulous mandible, or when a large retrusive movement (>1 cm) with higher risk for relapse is being performed, rigid fixation following vertical ramus osteotomy may be necessary. In such instances, an external approach is required.

One of the largest advantages reported for intraoral vertical ramus osteotomy relative to sagittal split osteotomy is the lower incidence of damage to the inferior alveolar nerve. The reported incidence of nerve injury after vertical ramus osteotomy is less than 1 %. Furthermore, studies evaluating the incidence of neurosensory deficit following ramal osteotomies have shown a higher rate of diminished sensation in the lower lip for sagittal split osteotomies (up to 40 %) compared to 9 % for the vertical ramus osteotomy. Reports have described long-term sensory disturbances following vertical ramus osteotomy to range between 2 and 14 %. The main reason for a lower incidence of neurologic injury is the ease in placing the osteotomy posterior to the mandibular foramen. In addition, the lack of rigid fixation minimizes risk of injury secondary to hardware placement. Finally, the potential for inadvertent damage to the nerve caused by compression of bony segments is eliminated.

An additional benefit with intraoral vertical ramus osteotomy is the ability to reposition the condyle, which may be considered in patients with internal derangement of the temporomandibular joint. By detaching the masseter, temporalis, and a portion of the medial pterygoid muscle, this results in anterior movement of the condyle under influence of the lateral pterygoid muscle. For patients with an anteriorly displaced articular disc, this repositioning of the condyle may help to reintroduce proper joint relationship. During healing, the condyle tends to move superiorly and posteriorly, restoring jaw function. Of note, while the incidence of temporomandibular joint derangement after a sagittal split osteotomy is low, a lower incidence following an intraoral vertical ramus osteotomy has been noted.

The relapse rate of the vertical ramus osteotomy is not well described and ranges from 10.2 to 18.5 % with 6–24-month follow-up. Higher rates of relapse have been noted with larger setback of the mandible, particularly when the vertical ramus osteotomy is performed transorally and maxillomandibular fixation is implemented postoperatively. This provides one particular advantage for rigid fixation following sagittal split osteotomy. Early descriptions of the intraoral vertical ramus osteotomy also described stripping of the medial pterygoid muscle which was associated with significant condylar sag and proximal segment necrosis. Modifications have since been described limiting such stripping to reduce this occurrence.

Inverted-L Osteotomy

The inverted-L osteotomy was first described for correction of mandibular prognathism. However, subsequent reports have also shown this technique suitable for correction of mandibular deficiencies. In patients with large mandibular asymmetry, an inverted-L osteotomy may be preferable to the sagittal split osteotomy. Secondary correction of proximal segment malrotation following prior sagittal split osteotomy may also be accomplished using an inverted-L osteotomy. While an inverted-L osteotomy is technically easier to perform through an extraoral approach, this can similarly be accomplished transorally with proper knowledge of ramal anatomy and techniques for transbuccal fixation.

An intraoral incision is made from the second molar to the anterior border of the ramus. Subperiosteal dissection is performed to expose the lingula and sigmoid notch medially and angle laterally. The horizontal osteotomy is made with reciprocating saw above the lingula, visualizing the inferior alveolar nerve at all times. The vertical osteotomy is performed with an oscillating saw. The distal segment is moved into its final position. The proximal segment must be positioned correctly in the condyle. Adequate condylar positioning can be obtained with gentle pressure on the horizontal cut. Alternatively, a Wurzburg plate can be placed on the proximal segment to secure it to the zygomatic buttress of the maxilla. The plate is manipulated to ensure correct seating of the condyle. For mandibular advancements, a bone graft is placed between the proximal and distal segments. Two L-plates on the anterior border and angle secure the distal segment. For mandibular setbacks, the distal segment is retropositioned and secured with transosseous wiring. The incision is sutured with an absorbable stitch. Occlusion may be maintained with maxillomandibular fixation.

For an extraoral approach, an incision is made two fingerbreadths below the angle of the mandible in a curvilinear fashion. The platysma is then divided to expose the pterygomasseteric sling. The marginal mandibular nerve is now identified and retracted out of the operative field. The pterygomasseteric sling is divided, and subperiosteal dissection is performed to expose the ramus to the sigmoid notch laterally and lingula medially. Osteotomy and advancement/setback are performed in a similar fashion to the intraoral technique. The pterygomasseteric sling does not have to be reapproximated at closure as it was initially described. The remainder of the incision is closed in layered fashion, approximating the platysma, dermis, and skin.

Similar to the vertical ramus osteotomy, the incidence of inferior alveolar nerve injury is lower following inverted-L osteotomy compared to the sagittal split osteotomy. By performing horizontal and vertical osteotomies superior and posterior to the mandibular foramen, no exposure of the inferior alveolar nerve is encountered with the inverted-L osteotomy. Subjective postoperative neurosensory deficits have been reported to be less frequent following inverted-L osteotomy than after sagittal split osteotomy. Furthermore, this difference in sensory disturbance was found to be greater on long-term evaluation. While Naples et al. reported a 33 % incidence of moderate hypoesthesia of the lip and 22 % of the chin after sagittal split osteotomy, no patients were found to have moderate hypoesthesia of these areas after inverted-L osteotomy.

Relapse following inverted-L osteotomies is dependent on the mandibular deformity treated and the amount of setback or advancement required. For treatment of significant retrognathia, use of an interpositional bone graft may be necessary to improve postoperative stability. Reported relapse rates have ranged from 4 to 22 % at 1–3 years following correction of mandibular deficiency with an inverted-L osteotomy.

In the pediatric setting of upper airway obstruction secondary to congenital micrognathia, surgical advancement of the mandible can be accomplished using the inverted-L osteotomy and distraction osteogenesis. The inverted-L osteotomy is preferred as it potentially minimizes injury risk to developing tooth buds and allows for sufficient space on both the proximal and distal bone fragments for placement of distractor foot plates. Large reviews of significant long-term mandibular dental injuries following inverted-L osteotomy and distraction have reported rates from 0.002 to 2 %. However, when complications were expanded to perforation of dental buds, root malformations, and shape anomalies of the teeth, the rate of adverse events was reported as high as 76 %.

Anterior Subapical (Block) Osteotomy

The mandibular subapical (block) osteotomy is one of the oldest known procedures to correct jaw deformity and was first described by Hullihen in 1849. Subsequent modifications have been described by Hofer and Koele who popularized this technique. Today, the mandibular subapical osteotomy is less commonly performed, as it designed to reposition only portions of the dental alveolus. Such a need may be encountered to level the occlusal plane or to correct asymmetries and change the anteroposterior angulation of the teeth when orthodontic treatment alone is insufficient. As the mandibular skeletal base is not altered with this technique, occlusal discrepancies can be corrected without unsatisfactory changes to aesthetic facial relationships.

A circumvestibular incision is made from the retromolar region one side of the mandible to the opposite side. The mental nerve is identified by blunt dissection and subperiosteal exposure of the anterior mandible is performed. Anterior to the mental foramen, a vertical corticotomy is marked between tooth roots and the buccal cortex is cut with a fissure bur or oscillating saw. The horizontal component is similarly cut 0.5 cm below the apices of the tooth roots to preserve pulpal circulation. A fine osteotome is used to complete the osteotomy with care taken to preserve the lingual mucoperiosteum which serves as the vascular pedicle. The mobilized anterior alveolar segment is then positioned into a prefabricated occlusal splint to ensure correct occlusion and internal fixation is achieved with monocortical plates. Once again, care should be taken to preserve dental roots when placing screws. Finally, any gap in the alveolus can be filled with autogenous bone graft. Postoperatively, the splint may be left in place to reinforce proper occlusion during healing.

While the subapical osteotomy avoids detrimental forces placed on the mandible by suprahyoid musculature, relapse rates are still high, particularly when underlying causative factors such as thumb sucking or tongue thrusting have not been addressed. Cephalometric studies following dentoalveolar advancement have also shown posterior drift of the mandibular incisors after 1 year. Long-term retention is thus frequently employed to reduce risk of relapse.

Another frequent complication following subapical osteotomy is tooth loss or damage. Collectively, injury to teeth following this technique has been reported to range between 7 and 50 %. These complications are more common with mandibular subapical osteotomies than when similar osteotomies are performed in the maxilla. This has been attributed to differences in neurovascular supply and tooth length. Perfusion studies of dental pulp have shown blood supply to the pulp chamber of the teeth in the osteotomized segment is maintained by vascular anastomoses. Therefore, the horizontal component of the subapical osteotomy must be completed 0.5 cm or more from the apices of the teeth.

Conclusion

Multiple techniques have been described for segmental movement of the mandibular tooth-bearing region. Selection of the appropriate strategy for correction of skeletal malocclusion is dependent on the type and complexity of the individual deformity. Clinical assessment of skeletal distortion thus begins with evaluation in the sagittal, coronal, and axial dimensions. For most patients, the sagittal split osteotomy is preferred, as it is a versatile technique that can address both mandibular prognathism and retrognathism. In certain situations, however, the vertical ramus osteotomy, inverted-L osteotomy, or subapical osteotomy may be more appropriate. The orthognathic surgeon should therefore be experienced with all of these techniques.

Bibliography

Banks P. Pulp changes after anterior mandibular subapical osteotomy in a primate model. J Maxillofac Surg. 1977;5(1):39–48.

Bell WH. Mandibular prognathism. In: Modern practice in orthognathic and reconstructive surgery. Philadelphia: Saunders; 1992. p. 2111–37.

Chen C-M, Lee H-E, Yang C-F, Shen Y-S, Huang I-Y, Tseng Y-C, Lai S-T. Intraoral vertical ramus osteotomy for correction of mandibular prognathism. Ann Plast Surg. 2008;61:52–5.

Chrcanovic BR, Freire-Maia B. Risk factors and prevention of bad splits during sagittal split osteotomy. Oral Maxillofac Surg. 2012;16:19–27.

Colella G, Cannavale R, Vicidomini A, Lanza A. Neurosensory disturbance of the inferior alveolar nerve after bilateral sagittal split osteotomy: a systematic review. J Oral Maxillofac Surg. 2007;65: 1707–15.

De Santana Santos T, Albuquerque KM, Santos MESM, Filho JRL. Survey on complications of orthognathic surgery among oral and maxillofacial surgeons. J Craniofac Surg. 2012;23(5):e423–30.

Datillo DJ, Braun TW, Sotereanos GC. The inverted L osteotomy for treatment of skeletal open-bite deformities. J Oral Maxillofac Surg. 1985;43:440–3.

Farrell CD, Kent JN. Evaluation of the surgical stability of 20 cases of inverted-L and C osteotomies. J Oral Surg. 1977;35(3):239–45.

Ferraro JW. Mandibular excess and deficiency. In: Fundamentals of maxillofacial surgery. New York: Springer; 1997. Print.

Ghali GE, Sikes JW. Intraoral vertical ramus osteotomy as the preferred treatment for mandibular prognathism. J Oral Maxillofac Surg. 2000;58:313–5.

Grubb J, Evans C. Orthodontic management of dentofacial skeletal deformities. Clin Plast Surg. 2007;34(3):403–15.

Hall HD, Chase DC, Payor LG. Evaluation and refinement of the intraoral vertical subcondylar osteotomy. J Oral Surg. 1975;33(5):333–41.

Hall HD, McKenna SJ. Further refinement and evaluation of intraoral vertical ramus osteotomy. J Oral Maxillofac Surg. 1987;45(8):684–8.

Hay AD, Ayoub AF, Moos KF, Singh GD. Euclidean distance matrix analysis of surgical changes in prepubertal craniofacial microsomia patients treated with an inverted L osteotomy. Cleft Palate Craniofac J. 2000;37(5):497–502.

Hong P, Graham E, Belyea J, Taylor SM, Kearns DB, Bezuhly M. The long-term effects of mandibular distraction osteogenesis on developing deciduous molar teeth. Plast Surg Int. 2012. Available from http://www.ncbi.nlm.nih.gov/pmc/articles/PMC3483672/pdf/PSI2012-913807.pdf.

Joss CU, Vassalli IM. Stability after bilateral sagittal split osteotomy setback surgery with rigid internal fixation: a systematic review. J Oral Maxillofac Surg. 2008;66:1634–43.

Joss CU, Vassalli IM. Stability after bilateral sagittal split osteotomy advancement surgery with rigid internal fixation: a systematic review. J Oral Maxillofac Surg. 2009;67:301–13.

Kleine-Hakala M, Hukki J, Hurmerinta K. Effect of mandibular distraction osteogenesis on developing molars. Orthod Craniofac Res. 2007;10(4):196–202.

Levine B, Topazian DS. The intraoral inverted-L double-oblique osteotomy of the mandibular ramus: a new technique for correction of mandibular prognathism. J Oral Surg. 1976;34(6):522–5.

McMillan B, Jones R, Ward-Booth B, Goss A. Intraoral technique for intraoral inverted 'L' osteotomy. Br J Oral Maxillofac Surg. 1999;37:324–6.

Mofid MM, Manson PN, Robertson BC, Tufaro AP, Elias JJ, Vander Kolk CA. Craniofacial distraction osteogenesis: a review of 3278 cases. Plast Reconstr Surg. 2001;108(5):1103–14.

Obwegeser HL. Orthognathic surgery and a tale of how three procedures came to be: a letter to the next generations of surgeons. Clin Plast Surg. 2007;34(3):331–55.

Patel PK, Novia MV. The surgical tools: the LeFort I, bilateral sagittal split osteotomy of the mandible, and the osseous genioplasty. Clin Plast Surg. 2007;34(3):447–75.

Petersson A, Willmar-Hogeman K. Radiographic changes of the temporomandibular joint after oblique sliding osteotomy of the mandibular rami. Int J Oral Maxillofac Surg. 1998;18(1):27–31.

Rai KK, Shivakumar HR, Sonar MD. Transient facial nerve palsy following bilateral sagittal split ramus osteotomy for setback of the mandible: a review of the incidence and management. J Oral Maxillofac Surg. 2008;66:373–8.

Reyneke JP. Basic guidelines for the surgical correction of mandibular anteroposterior deficiency and excess. Clin Plast Surg. 2007;34(3):501–17.

Sandler NA, Buckley MJ. Total mandibular subapical osteotomy. In: Oral and maxillofacial surgery. 2nd ed. Philadelphia: Saunders; 2008. p. 343–6.

Schneideman GB, Kawamura H, Finn RA, Bell WH. Wound healing after anterior and posterior subapical osteotomy. J Oral Maxillofac Surg. 1985;43(6):408–16.

Swennen G, Schliephake H, Dempf R, Schierle H, Malevez C. Craniofacial distraction osteogenesis: a review of the literature. Part 1: clinical studies. Int J Oral Maxillofac Surg. 2001;30(2):89–103.

Tornes K. Osteotomy length and postoperative stability in vertical subcondylar ramus osteotomy. Acta Odontol Scand. 1989;47(2):81–8.

Tuinzing DB, Greebe RB. Complications related to the intraoral vertical ramus osteotomy. Int J Oral Surg. 1985;14(4):319–24.

van Merkesteyn JP, Groot RH, van Leeuwaarden R, Kroon FH. Intraoperative complications in sagittal and vertical ramus osteotomies. Int J Oral Maxillofac Surg. 1987;16(6):665–70.

Westermark A, Bystedt L, von Konow L. Inferior alveolar nerve function after mandibular osteotomies. Br J Oral Maxillofac Surg. 1998;36:425–8.

Wolford LM. The sagittal split ramus osteotomy as the preferred treatment for mandibular prognathism. J Oral Maxillofac Surg. 2000;58:310–2.

Dental Extractions

32

Thaddeus S. Boucree II and Jose I. Garri

Introduction

The extraction of teeth is a common therapeutic procedure performed for a variety reasons, including dental caries, odontogenic pathosis, trauma, or for orthodontic treatment. A detailed clinical examination and proper radiological studies help to determine how the extraction should be approached. Proper technique will optimize outcome and minimize complications. For those practitioners who will perform exodontias as part of their clinical responsibilities, it is paramount to have a sound working knowledge of dental anatomy and the basic principles of oral surgery.

Applied Anatomy

The extraction of teeth is a surgical operation involving bony and soft tissues of the oral cavity. Before any tooth is extracted, a thorough exam of the oral cavity should be performed. Both the tooth morphology and position will dictate the extraction technique. It is important also to ascertain if the tooth is fully erupted (crown fully visible in the oral cavity) or impacted (crown partially or fully covered by gingival and/or bone) as this will have certain implications as to the technique needed for extraction. The clinician must also study the patient's radiographs (orthopantomogram, periapical plain film, CT scan, etc.) in order to evaluate the formation, size, and number of the roots, as well as their relationship to vital structures such as the inferior alveolar neurovascular bundle, adjacent teeth, or the maxillary sinus. It is also extremely important for the clinician to understand dental morphology, as different teeth may have multiple roots and these roots might be oriented differently in the alveolar bone, depending on whether the tooth is positioned in the maxillary versus the mandibular arch.

T.S. Boucree II, MD, DDS
Department of Oral and Maxillofacial Surgery, Larkin Community Hospital, Miami, FL, USA

J.I. Garri, MD, DMD (✉)
Department of Plastic Surgery, University of Miami, Miami, FL, USA
e-mail: drgarri@drgarri.com

Dental Terminology

A working knowledge of dental terminology is important not only for the purpose of understanding this chapter but also is imperative in communicating with other medical and dental colleagues. Some of the relevant terminology includes

"Incisal": refers to the cutting edge of anterior teeth

"Occlusal": refers to the chewing surface of posterior teeth

"Apex": the most extreme end of the root; the root tip

"Mesial": anatomic area of the crown which is the anterior surface of any given tooth or the surface which is oriented towards the midline along the path of the arch

"Distal": anatomic area of the crown which is the posterior surface of any given tooth or the surface which is oriented away from the midline along the path of the arch

"Buccal": area of the tooth oriented towards the cheek (posterior teeth)

"Labial": area of the tooth oriented towards the lip (anterior teeth)

"Lingual": area of the tooth oriented towards the tongue (mandibular teeth)

"Palatal": area of the tooth oriented towards the hard palate (maxillary teeth)

"Alveolus": the tooth-bearing bone of the maxilla or mandible, which supports the tooth roots

"Periodontal ligament": collagen fibers that attach the teeth into its surrounding bone in the socket

Tooth Nomenclature

In the USA, the most commonly used dental notation is the Universal Numbering System. In the pediatric population, the primary teeth are counted using letters A through T,

P.J. Taub et al. (eds.), *Ferraro's Fundamentals of Maxillofacial Surgery*,
DOI 10.1007/978-1-4614-8341-0_32, © Springer Science+Business Media New York 2015

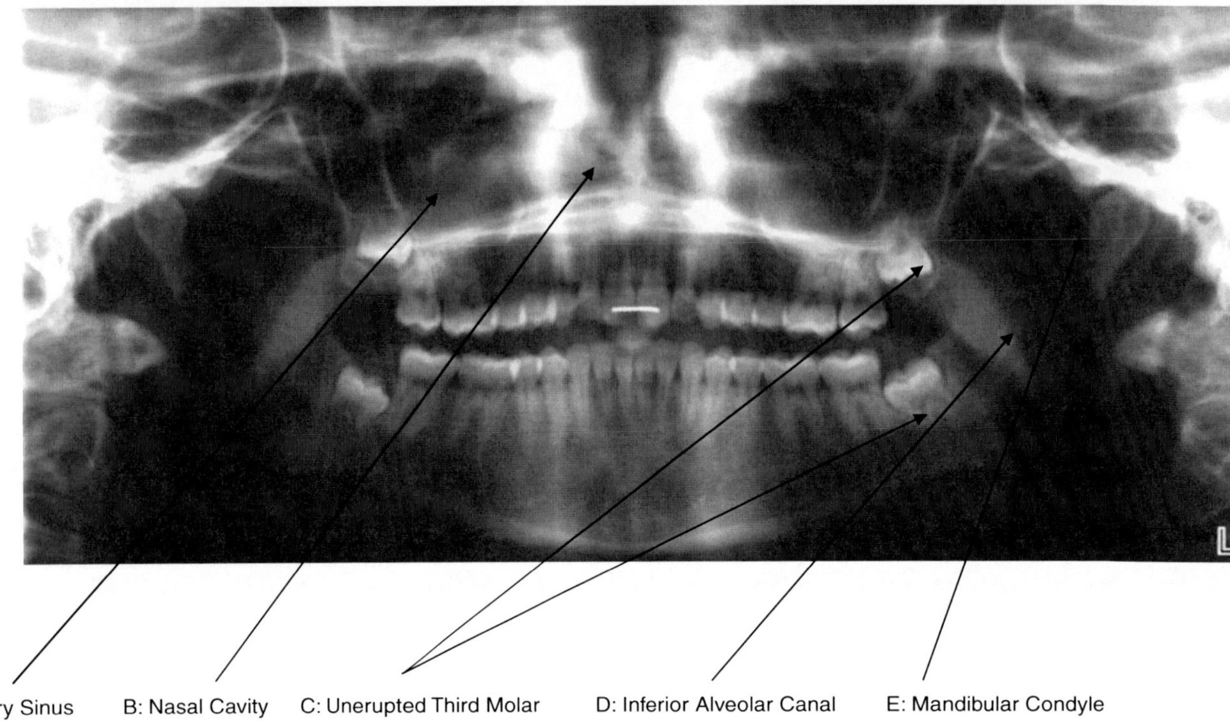

Fig. 32.1 Panoramic radiograph showing pertinent anatomical landmarks: *A* maxillary sinuses, *B* nasal cavity, *C* unerupted third molars, *D* inferior alveolar canal, and *E* mandibular condyle

starting at the maxillary right with the letter A and proceeding towards the last tooth on the left maxilla with the letter J. The sequence then moves to the last tooth on the mandibular left with the letter K and then moves sequentially towards the last tooth on the mandibular right with the letter T. The primary dentition, also referred to as deciduous, consists of 20 teeth. The permanent dentition is delineated by numbers and uses the same sequence as the deciduous dentition. The numbering starts with the right maxillary third molar #1 and continues from right to left. The last tooth in the maxilla is #16, the maxillary third molar. The next tooth counted is the left mandibular third molar, #17. The count then continues along the mandible from left to right. The last tooth is #32, the mandibular right third molar.

Dental Radiographs

Good radiographic studies of the dentition are not only a great adjunct to diagnosing disease of the teeth, periodontium, and surrounding bony structures, but it is also paramount in the planning of odontectomies. With the proper studies, not only can roots be examined but the density of the labial and buccal cortices can be evaluated. Anatomic boundaries like the maxillary sinus, mental foramen, inferior alveolar canal, and the thickness of the mandible can be further surveyed. The orthopantogram is the gold standard for radiological evaluation prior to exodontias. While a hospital-based CT scan can give invaluable information as it relates to odontogenic pathosis, it is rarely needed in routine dental extractions. A cone beam CT scan (CBCT), not to be confused with a hospital-based CT scan, is a 3-dimensional orthopantomogram that can be performed in the dental office. A CBCT can give beneficial information as it relates to nerve, cysts, or the maxillary sinus. While a CBCT has proved to be a great asset in the surgical placement of dental implants, it is not routinely indicated in routine dental extractions, where an orthopantomogram suffices. A periapical x-ray shows usually one or two teeth only and can give useful information as it correlates to a particular tooth, as when evaluating the tooth for a possible root fracture. The reliance on a periapical radiographs alone during exodontias makes it difficult to evaluate adjacent structures to the tooth in question and makes it difficult to assess adjacent and potentially relevant bony pathosis (see Fig. 32.1).

Local Anesthesia

Ensuring local anesthesia is paramount in order to be able to perform painless exodontia on the awake patient. It is important to block not only the nerve supply to a particular tooth but also the soft tissues surrounding the tooth. Thus, for dental extractions, multiple nerve blocks are usually necessary, even when extracting a single tooth. Local anesthesia not only helps with pain control but also helps to reduced bleeding due to the epinephrine content of some local anesthetics. Whether extractions are performed while the patient is awake or sedated, the surgeon should consider local nerve blocks to help with hemostasis during the procedure and postoperative pain.

Nerve Blocks Used in Exodontia

Posterior Superior, Middle Superior, and Anterior Superior Nerve Blocks

Nerves arise from the second division and maxillary branch of the trigeminal nerve and provide innervation to the unilateral maxillary dentition, gingiva, and upper lip. The needle is inserted 3 cm superior to the maxillary tooth or teeth to be excised within the vestibule and advanced to the alveolar bone.

Greater Palatine Nerve Block

The nerve is also a maxillary branch of the trigeminal nerve and provides innervation to the unilateral palatal mucosa from the molar region to the first premolar. The needle is inserted in the palatal depression located 3 cm from the second maxillary molar. The greater palatine canal is located at the junction of the horizontal and vertical components of the hard palate.

Infraorbital Nerve Block

The nerve is a division of the maxillary branch of the trigeminal nerve. It exits the infraorbital foramen and provides innervation to the maxillary dentition, gingiva, upper lip, and cheek. The infraorbital rim is palpated at the level of the mid-pupillary line and the needle is inserted 1 cm inferior to this point. This block can be given intraorally by injecting the needle 2 cm in a superior orientation in the vestibule at the interproximal area between the maxillary first and second premolars.

Incisive Canal Nerve Block

The nerve is the terminal division of the maxillary branch of the trigeminal nerve. It exits the incisive foramen and provides innervation to the canine, lateral incisors, and central incisor on its respective side. The nerve is blocked by injecting right at the incisive papillae to provide anesthesia to the palatal mucosa of the anterior teeth from canine to canine.

Inferior Alveolar Nerve Block

The nerve is the third division and mandibular branch of the trigeminal nerve. It enters the mandible at the inferior alveolar foramen (adjacent to the lingula in the medial aspect of the ramus) and provides innervation to the mandibular dentition (from the third molar to the incisors), gingiva, and lower lip. A division of the nerve exits through the mental foramen, located on the buccal aspect of the mandible in the area of the second premolar, and provides innervations to the mucosa of the anterior teeth, the ipsilateral half of the lower lip, and skin of the menton. The anterior aspect of the ramus is palpated and the needle is inserted at a 45° angle to the contralateral side of the jaw (opposite maxillary canine) until contact is made with the bone. The insertion of the needle should be approximately 1 cm superior to the level of the occlusal plane. The orientation of the needle is then changed to lie more parallel to the medial aspect of the ramus and it is then inserted about two centimeters before injecting.

Lingual Nerve Block

The nerve is also a mandibular branch of the trigeminal nerve. It branches from the mandibular branch before the inferior alveolar nerve enters the lingula and provides innervation to the lingual surface of the tongue on its respective side. This nerve is anesthetized using the inferior alveolar nerve block technique. Local anesthetic is deposited as the needle is about half way (1 cm) from the location of the inferior alveolar foramen.

Long Buccal Nerve Block

The nerve is also a mandibular branch of the trigeminal nerve and provides innervation to the buccal mucosa and dentition from the molar region to the first premolar. The needle is advanced into the mucobuccal fold adjacent to the mandibular second or third molar and deposit anesthesia along the buccal surface of the mandible.

Mental Nerve Block

The nerve is the terminal division of the mandibular branch of the trigeminal nerve. It exits the mental foramen and provides innervation to the mandibular dentition (from the second bicuspid to the incisors), gingiva, and lower lip. The foramen is usually located at the level of the second mandibular premolar about half way along the vertical dimension of the mandible at this point. The needle is inserted in the buccal vestibule at this location about 2 cm into the tissues adjacent to the buccal plate of the mandible.

Periodontal Ligament Nerve Block

The needle is inserted into the periodontal ligament and the anesthetic is deposited into the space between the tooth and alveolar bone. This is done to reinforce any of the other nerve blocks and augment anesthesia to any particular tooth.

Intrapulpal Nerve Block

The needle is inserted into the dental pulp and the anesthetic is deposited into the central chamber inside the tooth. This zone of both nerve and blood vessels, rich in connective tissue, is known as the plexus of Raschkow. In order to perform this block, access to the pulp chamber of the tooth must exist either through carious disease or through tooth sectioning. This technique is used to augment anesthesia to a particular tooth when other blocks are not sufficient. Alone, this block is not adequate for dental extraction, as it does not provide anesthesia to the periodontal ligament and adjacent soft tissue structures.

Surgical Armamentarium

The proper knowledge of the indications and use of the specialized instruments used in exodontias will lead to better technique with less risk of complications. Some of the instruments used in the extraction of teeth are:

1. Molt retractor: mouth prop covered with rubber ends used to hold mouth open
2. Minnesota cheek retractor: retracts the cheek and retracts a third molar flap
3. Weider ("sweetheart") retractor: tongue and cheek retractor
4. Periosteal elevator: frees attached gingiva and elevation of a mucoperiosteal flap
5. Small straight (301) dental elevator: loosens alveolar ligaments
6. Large straight (46) dental elevator: used interproximally to further loosen alveolar ligaments
7. 31 Large Cryer (East) dental elevator: removes roots using a wedge technique
8. 32 Large Cryer (West) dental elevator: removes roots using a wedge technique
9. #33 Ash mandibular forceps: removes lower anterior teeth and roots
10. #150 maxillary universal forceps: removes maxillary anterior teeth and bicuspids
11. #151 mandibular universal forceps: removes maxillary anterior teeth and bicuspid
12. #88 maxillary forceps: removes maxillary first and second molars
13. #85A mandibular forceps: removes lower cuspids, bicuspids, and molars
14. #24 maxillary forceps: removes maxillary molars
15. #23 Cowhorn mandibular forceps: removes lower first and second molars
16. #17 mandibular forceps: removes lower molars
17. #210 maxillary forceps: removes maxillary third molars
18. Miller elevator: removes soft tissue impacted maxillary third molars
19. Apical elevator ("root pick:): removes small root tips
20. Bone rongeurs: used for post-extraction trimming of alveolar bone
21. Curette: exploratory instrument to remove granulation tissue and apical cysts from extraction socket
22. Bone file: smoothes down rough margins of the alveolus following an extraction
23. Surgical drill and burr: removes bone, splits tooth crown. #557 surgical burr or #2 or #4 round burr
24. Surgical mallet: used with bone chisel to remove bone for treatment of tori (see Figs. 32.2, 32.3, 32.4, and 32.5).

Surgical Technique

The essence of exodontia involves loosening (luxating) the tooth within its socket and then retrieving or removing the tooth. Luxation is done by severing the periodontal attachments between the tooth and the surrounding bone. This is usually done with the aid of dental elevators, which there is a variety of different shapes and sizes, specially designed for a particular situation or set of teeth. The removal of the tooth is performed with extraction forceps. Like elevators, extraction forceps are customized for each individual tooth or for a group of teeth with similar morphology.

Positioning of the patient and surgeon during an extraction is very important for both visualization of the surgical site and access by the surgeon. For maxillary extractions, the patient should be slightly reclined or supine with the chin slightly elevated as in a "sniffing position." The mandible should be slightly open and in a relaxed position, as maximum mandibular opening is usually not required to access the maxillary teeth. For mandibular extractions, the patient should be in a more upright position and a bite block should be used. A bite block has two benefits. First, it maximizes mouth opening, and second, it stabilizes the mandible to forces applied during the extraction process. This will help with patient comfort and also helps the surgeon by keeping the position of the tooth fixed and steady. A throat pack should be used during all extractions in order to prevent the patient from aspirating or swallowing foreign bodies or tooth fragments. Care should be taken to note the presence of a throat pack and remember to remove it at the end of the procedure. Right-handed surgeons usually approach the patient from the right side.

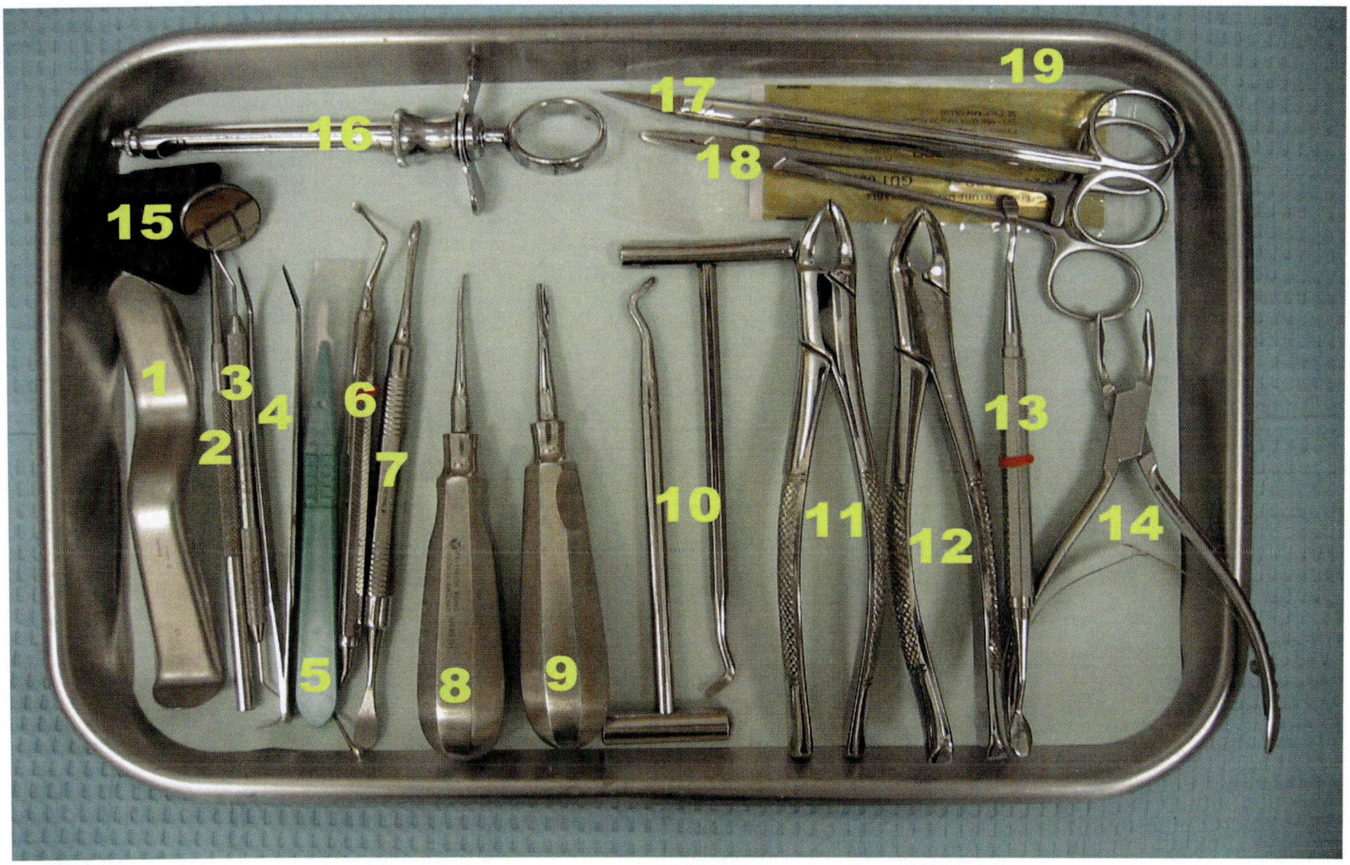

1. Minnesota Retractor
2. Mirror
3. Explorer
4. Forceps
5. #15 Scalpel
6. Curette
7. Periosteal Elevator
8. Small Straight Elevator
9. Large Straight Elevator
10. Potts Elevators
11. Upper Universal
12. Lower Universal
13. Bone File
14. Rongeurs
15. Bite Block
16. Syringe
17. Scissors
18. Needle Holder
19. 3-0 Chromic Sutures

Fig. 32.2 Typical exodontia tray set-up. *1* Minnesota Retractor, *2* mirror, *3* explorer, *4* forceps, *5* #15 scalpel, *6* curette, *7* periosteal elevator, *8* small straight elevator, *9* large straight elevator, *10* potts elevators, *11* upper universal, *12* lower universal, *13* bone file, *14* rongeurs, *15* bite block, *16* syringe, *17* scissors, *18* needle holder, *19* 3-0 chromic sutures

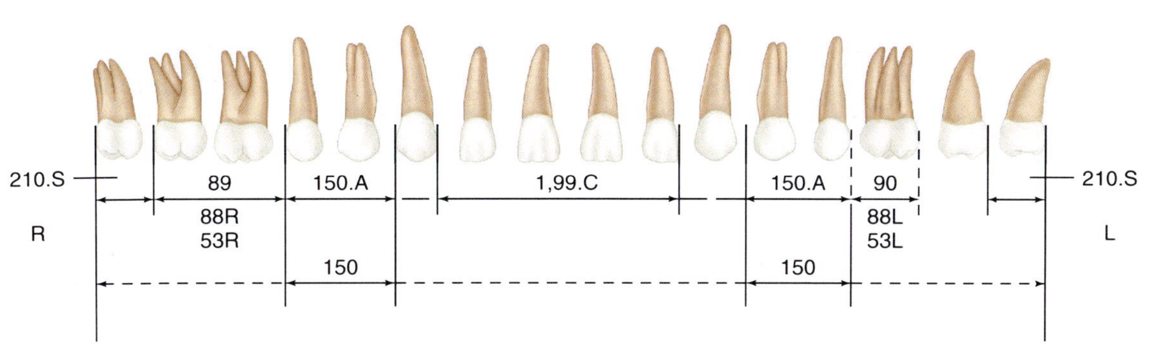

Fig. 32.3 Forceps recommendations for extraction of maxillary teeth

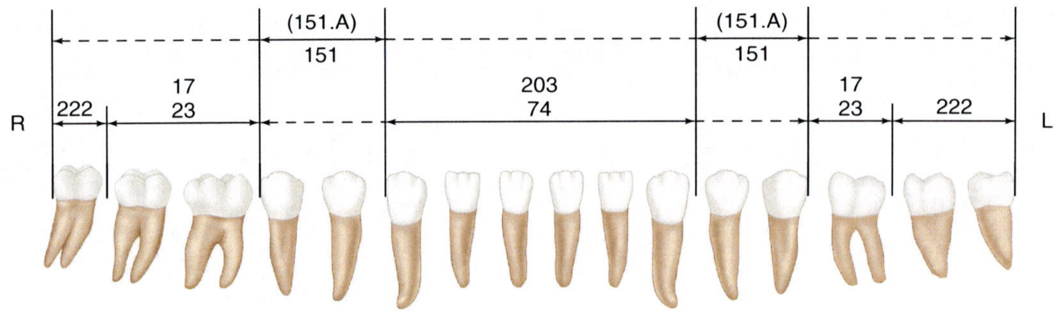

Fig. 32.4 Forceps recommendations for the extraction of mandibular teeth

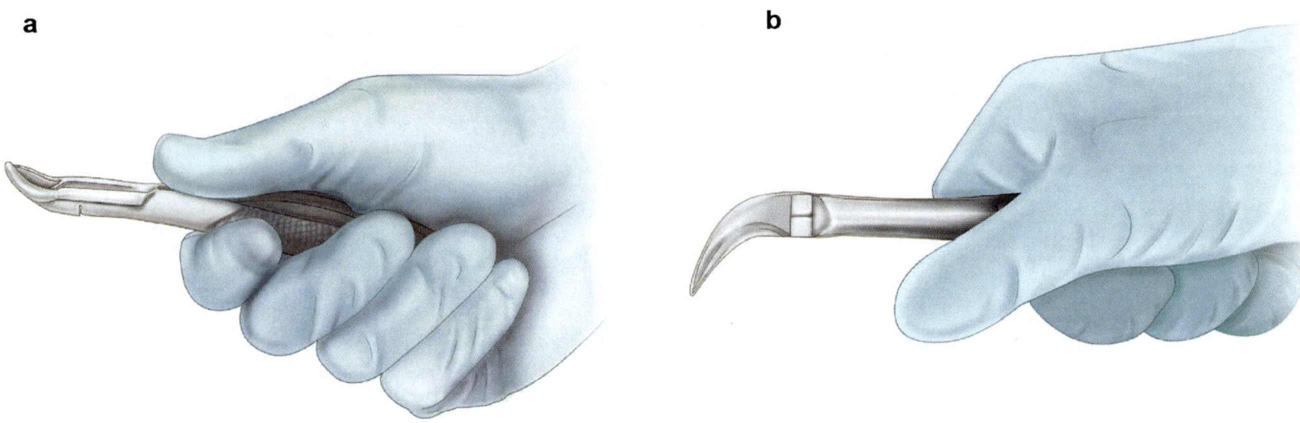

Fig. 32.5 Proper way to hold (**a**) maxillary extraction forceps. (**b**) mandibular extraction forceps

Extractions have been traditionally classified as simple (nonsurgical) and surgical. An extraction is classified as simple when the tooth is removed solely with the use of dental elevators and forceps. Surgical extractions by definition involve raising a soft tissue flap in order to expose the tooth to be extracted as well as the surrounding bone. This is usually done when the crown of the tooth is not visible, present, or is fractured off during the process of extraction. This technique allows easier access to the remaining tooth structures in order to facilitate its removal.

Simple Extractions

The periodontal ligaments can resist masticatory forces as great 590 N. Therefore, extracting a mandibular molar in a healthy young adult using pure strength would be difficult at best. Thus, the cornerstone of dental extractions is the use of the lever. This is why the very first instrument used in a dental extraction is the curette or the periosteal elevator to free the attached gingiva and interdental papillae from the tooth crown in order to minimize damage to these structures during the utilization of the dental elevators. Next follows the insertion of a small dental elevator (#301), followed by a larger one (#46) in order to disrupt the periodontal fibers attaching the tooth to the adjacent bone. The elevator is held in the palm of the hand with the index finger positioned at the shank of the elevator approximately 1–2 cm from its end (to prevent damage in case the elevator slips from its contact point) and it is placed in the mesiobuccal aspect of the tooth to be excised. Using the bone as a fulcrum, rotate the handle. The initial rotation should direct pressure towards the crown of the tooth, as this is the easiest way to begin to luxate the tooth. As the tooth loosens, rotate the elevator to place the force towards the root of the tooth, as this will allow for more mobility of the tooth within its socket, due to increased leverage. This simple action transmits elevating forces to the roots and mobilizes the tooth by severing its collagen attachments to the surrounding bone (periodontal membrane).

Once the tooth is loosened in its socket (luxated), use the appropriate forceps and movement to extract the tooth.

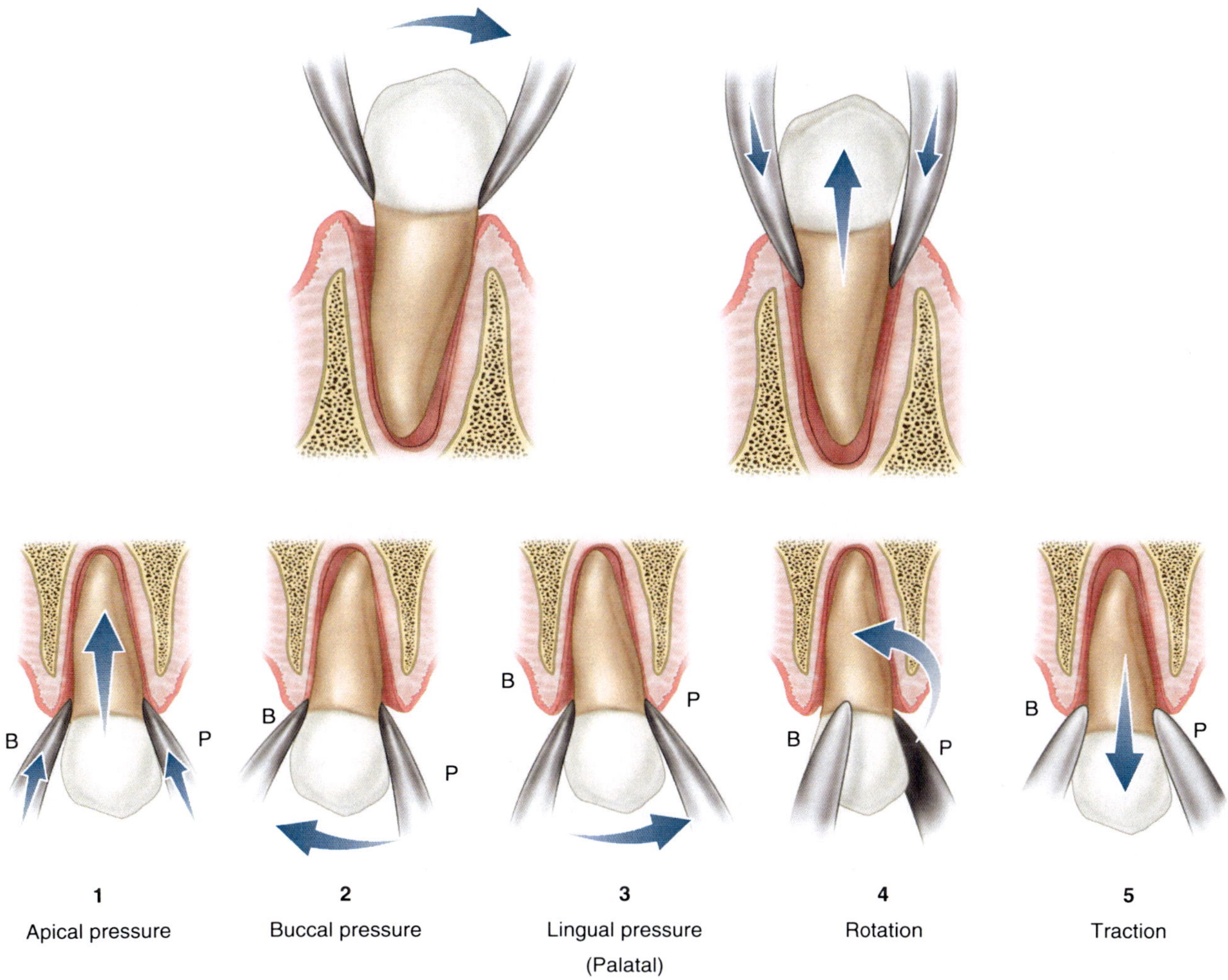

Fig. 32.6 Different movements used in exodontia

There are different forceps designed for specific grouping of teeth depending on crown and root morphology and also on which arch the tooth is positioned. Maxillary forceps in general tend to have a straight or a slightly curved design, whereas mandibular forceps usually have a 90° bend close to the grasping part of the forceps. This is to improve ergonomics as the surgeon approaches the patient usually from front right. With the patient slightly reclined or supine and head in a sniffing position, the orientation of the longitudinal axis of the maxillary teeth will best be reached by a straight force on the surgeon's hand, whereas the orientation of the mandibular teeth will require the forceps to have a 90° angle for better ergonomics.

Once the proper forceps is engaged on the tooth to be extracted, there is an array of movements that can be done in order to further loosen and eventually deliver the tooth (see Fig. 32.6). The movement to use depends on a tooth's morphology as well as the thickness of the surrounding buccal and lingual/palatal bone. Universally, there is usually a combination of rotational and buccolingual forceps movements (often simultaneously) applied in order to complete the extraction. Once the tooth is delivered, the tooth is inspected to make sure it was excised in total or to make sure all tooth and root fragments have been retrieved. Once this is done, the socket is then curetted to remove all granulation tissue and bone fragments that might have been dislodged during the extraction. At this point, the surgeon needs to decide whether the patient might benefit from suturing the soft tissues to ensure better tissue approximation. If suturing is required, this is usually done via a figure of eight suture engaging the interdental papillae on the proximal and distal aspects of the remaining sockets. Pressure with moist gauze packs is recommended over the extraction socket in order to help with hemostasis.

Extraction Techniques for Specific Teeth

#1 and #16: The maxillary third molars, if erupted, may have two roots. During the extraction process of #1 and #16, forceps forces are first applied buccally and then extracted distally. The impacted maxillary third molar will often have one root. When extracting impacted #1 and #16, rotational forces which are applied distally with a Miller elevator. Care must be taken not to place direct apical forces because of the location of the maxillary sinus.

#2, #3, #14, and #15: The maxillary first and second molars have three roots, and thus, rotation forces are useless because of the tripod vector of three roots. During the extraction process of these teeth, forceps forces are first applied buccally, palatally, and then extracted buccally. These teeth are more likely to be removed buccally because buccal bone is more likely to expand. Palatal bone has no direction to expand and has a greater density compared to buccal bone.

#4 and #13: The maxillary second premolar has a single root, and when extracting these teeth, forceps forces are first applied labially, followed by palatal forces, and finally rotational forces. The tooth is usually delivered labially.

#5 and #12: The maxillary first premolars usually have two roots, and when extracting these teeth, forceps forces are applied labially, then palatally, and then slight rotational forces. It is recommended that these teeth be delivered by applying direct traction forces along the long axis of the tooth. This is an attempt to prevent root fractures, as the first maxillary premolars usually have two roots, which are thin and long in configuration.

#6 and #11: The longest tooth in the oral cavity is the maxillary canine, which measures between 25 and 33 mm. When extracting #6 and #11, forceps forces are first applied labially, followed with a mesial (clockwise) rotation for #6 and mesial (counter clockwise) rotation for #11. Due to the long roots that canines have, it is recommended that rotational forces be the main movements applied with the forces, along with a small amount of bucco-palatal movement.

#7, #8, #9, and #10: Maxillary incisors also have one root. Because incisors often have distally positioned root apices, forceps forces are applied labially, then palatally, and then slight clockwise and counterclockwise rotational forces.

#17 and #32: The mandibular third molars, if erupted, have two roots. When extracting an erupted #17 or #32, forceps forces are applied first buccally, followed by lingual forces. The impacted #17 and #32 tend to have two fused roots. When extracting impacted #17 and #32, care must be taken not to apply continuous apical pressure because of the inferior alveolar neurovascular bundle and an iatrogenic fractured mandible. Full bony impacted mandibular third molars tend to be the most clinically challenging extraction procedure for the surgeon. These extractions usually require a soft tissue flap, removal of bone, and sectioning of either the crown of the tooth or its roots.

#18, #19, #30, and #31: The mandibular first and second molars have two roots. During the extraction process of the mandibular first and second molars, forceps forces are applied first buccally, followed by lingual forces. Sometimes rotation forces can also be helpful. The Cowhorn forceps (#23) are very helpful in the extractions of these teeth, as the forceps engage the tooth right at the furcation and between the two roots. The forceps movement should be buccolingual.

#20, #21, #28, and #29: Mandibular premolars have one root and when extracting these teeth, forceps forces are first applied labially, followed by a rotational forces.

#22 and #27: Mandibular canines have one root and when extracting these teeth, forceps forces are first applied labially, followed by rotational forces.

#23, #24, #25, and #26: Mandibular incisors have one root, and when extracting these teeth, forceps forces are first applied labially, followed by rotational forces (see Table 32.1).

Invariably, no matter how well your execution, teeth will break, leaving root tips behind. Decay makes teeth brittle, and trauma can leave the crown absent. In cases like these, better access to the remaining roots is necessary. If the roots are large, the Cryer (East/West) is an excellent choice of instruments. The tip of the Cryer is engaged into the tooth fragment. As the clinician rotates the handle, the opposite side of the tip, the base, will fulcrum off the alveolar bone. This unique fulcrum raises the root out of the socket. For smaller root fragments, the clinician uses root tip picks. When using these thin, long elevators, place the tip adjacent to the cementum, fulcrum off buccal bone, rotate the handle, and roll the root out. If the above techniques do not allow for the extraction of the roots, other techniques will need to be employed in order to gain more access to the remaining tooth structures. When these techniques are used, the procedure is called a surgical extraction (see Figs. 32.7 and 32.8).

Surgical Extractions

This type of extraction requires manipulation of the soft and hard tissue around a tooth or teeth in order to gain better access. This is needed when the tooth is not exposed in the mouth (impacted) or when the tooth is missing parts of the crown, which occurs in cases of decay or trauma. It is necessary to have at least partial access to the roots, in order to extract it.

The first step in gaining access to the inaccessible tooth structures is to elevate a soft tissue flap. The most common flap used for this purpose is called the envelope flap, where

Table 32.1 Summary of teeth, roots, and nerve blocks

Tooth	Tooth numbers	Usual number of roots	Location of roots	Nerve blocks required
Maxillary incisors	#7, #8, #9, #10	1		Anterior superior alveolar and incisive nerve blocks
Maxillary canines	#6, #11	1		Anterior superior alveolar or infraorbital and incisive nerve blocks
Maxillary first premolar	#5, #12	1 or 2 (most common)	1 buccal 1 palatal	Middle superior alveolar and greater palatine nerve blocks
Maxillary second premolar	#4, #13	1		Middle superior alveolar and greater palatine nerve blocks
Maxillary first and second molar	#2, #3, #14, #15	3	2 buccal 1 palatal	Posterior superior alveolar and greater palatine nerve blocks
Maxillary third molar	#1, #16	3 or one fused root	2 buccal 1 palatal Or fused	Posterior superior alveolar and greater palatine nerve blocks
Mandibular incisors and canine	#22, #23, #24 #25, #25, #27	1		Inferior alveolar, lingual, and mental nerve blocks
Mandibular premolars	#20, #21 #28, #29	1		Inferior alveolar, lingual, long buccal, and mental nerve blocks
Mandibular first and second molar	#18, #19 #30, #31	2	1 mesial 1 distal	Inferior alveolar, lingual, and long buccal nerve blocks
Mandibular third molar	#17, #32	2 or 1 fused	1 mesial 1 distal Or fused	Inferior alveolar, lingual, and long buccal nerve blocks

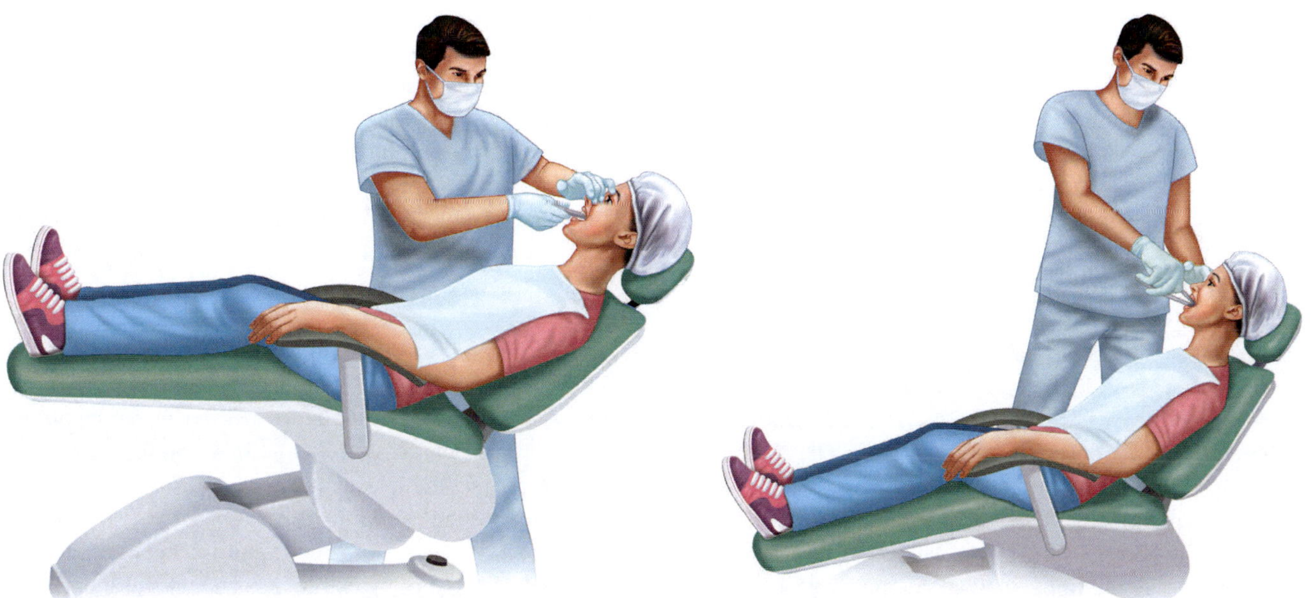

Figs. 32.7 and 32.8 Proper positioning of doctor and patient for extraction of maxillary and mandibular teeth

an incision is made with a surgical blade (usually #15 or #15C) within the gingival sulcus on the buccal aspect of the tooth to be extracted. The incision should encompass the mesial and distal interdental papillae. If further exposure is anticipated, a mesial releasing incision is made from the outer edge of the reflected mesial interdental papillae and extending apically towards the buccal vestibule. The incision should be made down to the bone and the flap should always be wider at the base to insure appropriate blood supply. Elevation of the mucoperiosteal flap is

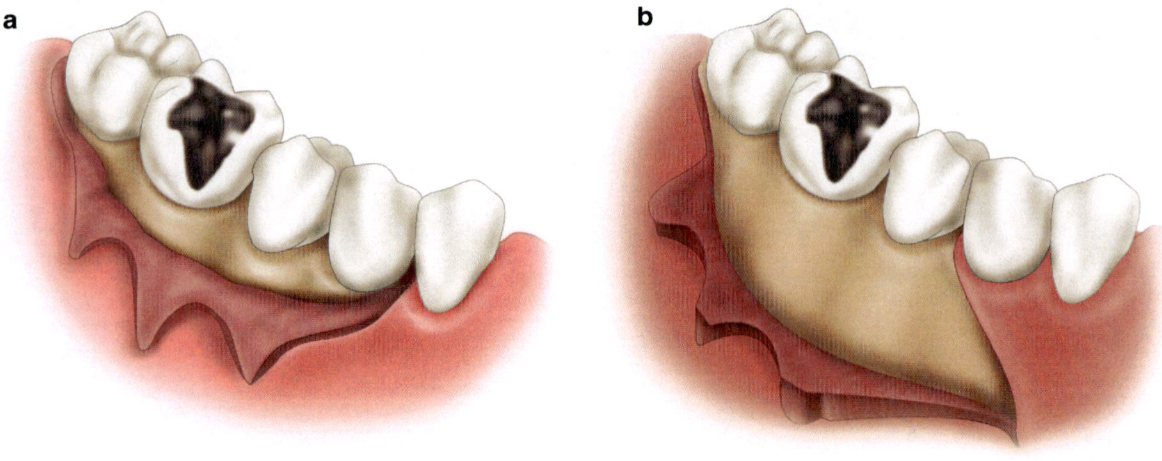

Fig. 32.9 Flap designs for surgical extractions (**a**) envelope flap. (**b**) Envelope flap with anterior release

accomplished using the spear point of a periosteal elevator, exposing the alveolar bone. Careful elevation is essential to avoid tearing the flap. This reflection is continued along the buccal surfaces of the tooth or teeth included in the flap design. Tissue is minimally elevated on the lingual surface of the targeted tooth on the mandible because of the proximity of the lingual nerve, which could potentially result in iatrogenic injury.

Once the soft tissue is reflected, the surgeon will have increased visibility of the remaining tooth structures and the adjacent bone. In order to optimize access, a decision is then made on how to approach the surrounding bone. At this point, a surgical burr can be used to perform maneuvers such as splitting the roots, lowering the level of alveolar bone, or making a trough around the remaining roots. These maneuvers allow easier access to the roots so that dental elevators or forceps can then be used in order to complete the extraction.

If the tooth is impacted in bone, then removal of bone is required for access. A high-speed handpiece and either a fissure (#557) or round burr (#4, #6, #8) is the instrument of choice to remove bone from around the tooth. The motion of the handpiece should be consistent with the motion of an artist holding a paintbrush. Each stroke should gently sweep across alveolar bone, similar to painting on a canvass. Avoiding forceful plunging of the handpiece will prevent destruction of adjacent structures. In some surgical extractions, tooth sectioning is required. The tooth can be sectioned removing the crown with a # 557 fissured burr, followed by sectioning the roots at the bifurcation or trifurcation. Large Cryer (East or West) are used to wedge between the bone and roots. Using the wedge technique, a fulcrum is used for occlusal displacement of the remaining root. Root tip picks are used for smaller root fragments as previously described (see Figs. 32.9 and 32.10).

Complications

Exodontia is a fairly common procedure performed by dentists and oral surgeons. Other specialists such as otolaryngologists, plastic surgeons, and general surgeons might also be called upon to perform exodontias in the treatment of patients with infections, neoplasms, and trauma of the facial region. Although the rate of complication from this procedure is relatively low, it is imperative for the practitioner of exodontia to be aware of the potential complications and their management. One of the first tenets of dealing with complications is to avoid them in the first place. A thorough physical and radiographic evaluation is warranted on all patients who are to undergo extractions. Potential risk factors such as advanced age, history of smoking, oral hygiene, existence of bony pathosis, and anatomical relationships of important structures to the teeth to be extracted should be reviewed.

1. Aspiration of Root Fragments and Foreign Bodies During the Procedure: Complications like the aspiration of root fragments and foreign bodies during dental procedures are associated with poor extraction technique and should be preventable in most cases. Throat packs are routinely used in exodontia to prevent aspiration of surgical debris, ingestion of blood, and tracheal contamination. When performing extractions under local anesthesia, throat packs are placed in the region posterior to the tongue, the pharynx. In the general anesthesia patient, throat packs are placed in the hypopharynx. To minimize complications, the clinician needs to have a systematic algorithm, which reminds him or her to remove the throat packs. Numerous studies have examined the risk versus the benefits of throat packs. Despite conflicting data regarding the use of throat packs, it is our recommendation that they should be used during exodontia.

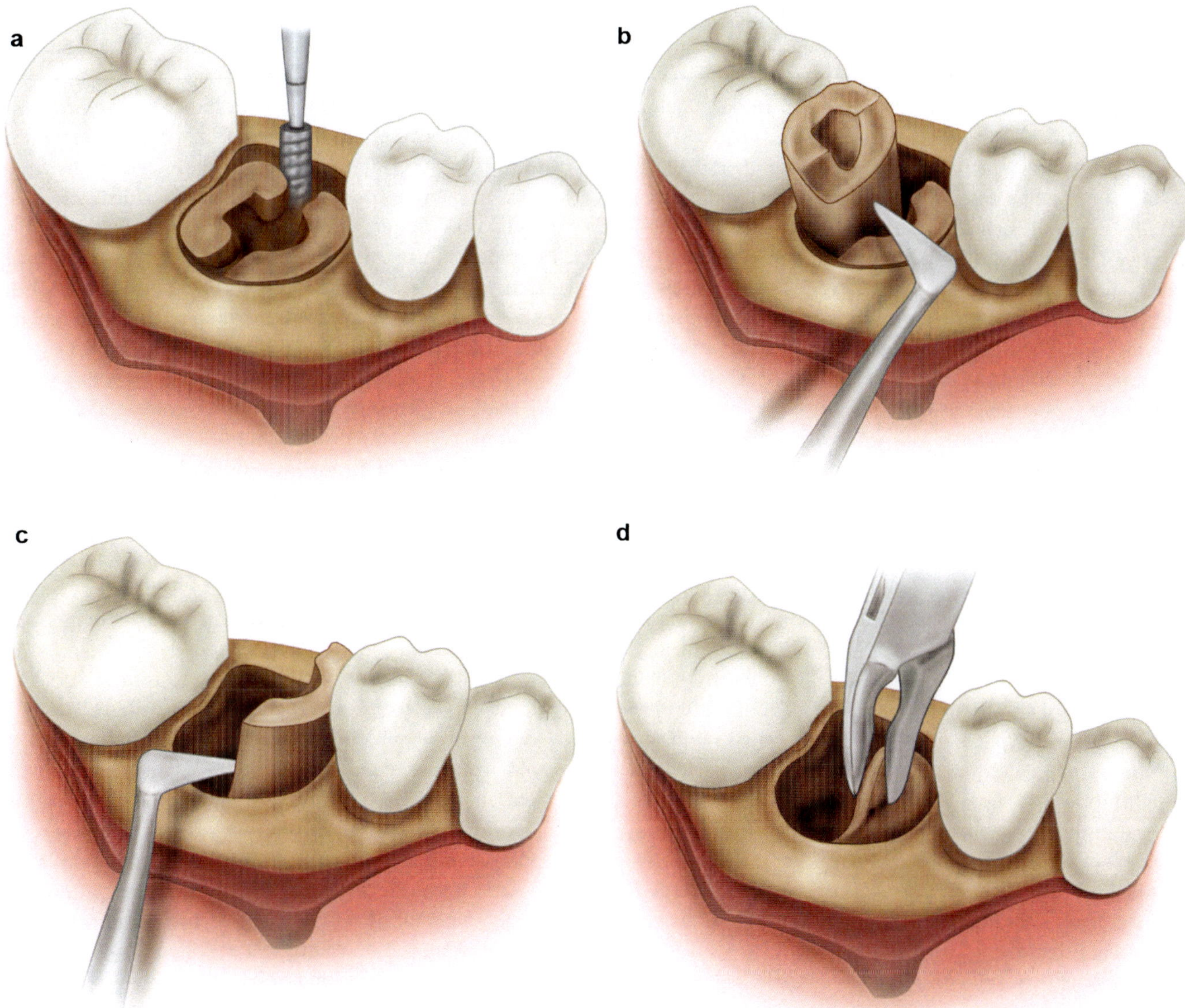

Fig. 32.10 Steps in the surgical removal of a tooth: burring of the surrounding alveolar bone (**a**), retrieval of the tooth root (**b**, **c**, and **d**), and coverage with soft tissue flap

2. Bleeding: A postoperative bleed can be a seemingly minor event that can lead to catastrophic consequences. A detailed medical history is very important in ruling out the potential of a coagulopathy in any surgical patient. Menorrhagia may identify a coagulopathy in young women. While it may be rare in young men, it is not unusual for a tooth extraction to be the first operative procedure that leads to a diagnosis of a bleeding disorder. A family history may be helpful in some coagulopathies, but as many as one-third of all hemophilias are new mutations and, thus, not inherited. Other cases that can cause prolonged bleeding include Von Willebrand disease, aspirin or NSAID use, thrombocytopenia, liver failure, uremia, Glanzmann's thrombasthenia, and Bernard-Soulier syndrome. Sometimes patients may experience dislodgment of a clot, which results in bleeding hours after extraction. Most of these episodes can be controlled by the patient by applying direct pressure with gauze (by placing it over the extraction site and biting on it) for 20 min. If this fails, this same technique can be tried with a tea bag because of the thrombogenic properties of tannic acid. In the perioperative period, bleeding should be subdued by applying direct pressure. The next step is to identify the source of the bleed. If it is determined that the hemorrhage is venous in nature, then try to control bleeding by local measures. Injecting directly into the extraction socket with lidocaine with epinephrine will give you both better vision and may help to gain hemostasis. Cautery can be used once the bleeding is visualized. Other hemostatic modalities

include the application of Gelfoam (absorbable gelatin sponge), Surgicel (oxidized cellulose polymer), sponges soaked with topical thrombin, fibrin glue, and bone wax (sparingly). If the source of bleeding is arterial in nature, cauterization and ligation might be necessary.

3. Infection: Postoperative infection after dental extraction is another rare event. The rate of postoperative infection varies, and in a study of 1,500 teeth, all taking postoperative antibiotics, the reported incidence was 1.5 %. In another study evaluating 550 surgical extractions and no antibiotics administered, the infection rate was 2.2 %. The use of prophylactic postoperative antibiotics is a controversial subject. Most surgeons advocate the use of systemic antibiotics for infection prevention in patients with gingivitis, pericoronitis, or general debilitating diseases. Like many other dental complications, postoperative infection was the highest among the patients with deep impactions and surgical removal of teeth. The incidence of Ludwig's angina is the most feared odontogenic infection but does not usually occur in the postoperative period. This is a rapidly progressive cellulitis of the floor of the mouth and a carious tooth is usually the cause. Symptoms include elevation of the floor of the mouth. The tongue elevation causes dyspnea, which can lead to airway obstruction and death. Treatment includes intravenous antibiotics, surgical extraction, incision and drainage, oral intubation, and sometimes a tracheostomy. The use of aseptic technique, hemostasis, meticulous tissue management, and complete and thorough lavage of extraction sites can decrease the likelihood of postoperative infection.
4. Alveolitis (dry socket): Alveolar osteitis (dry socket) is failure of an extraction socket to form a clot. In normal wound healing, from the time of extraction to day three, platelets will aggregate and thromboplastin will form a clot. Between day 3 and 3 weeks, a careful balance is reached between fibrinolysis and fibroblasts laying down collagen. Patients, who develop a dry socket, have a loss of this homeostasis and have an increase in the fibrinolytic activity. At day 3, instead of granulation tissue formation, healing does not occur. This stagnant wound bed becomes painful by the fifth day, postoperatively. Birn considered that the trauma resulting from extraction, as well as aggressive curettage, might harm the alveolar bone cells, causing inflammation of the osseous medulla and release of cell mediators to the alveolus, where they cause fibrinolytic activity, causing dry socket. Smoking, poor hygiene, gender, and oral contraceptives increase the risk of developing a dry socket. It has been postulated that estrogen indirectly activates the fibrinolytic system. The treatment of dry socket has not changed in a number of years. The use of dry socket paste (composed of acetylsalicylic acid, peru, balsam, eugenol, sodium benzoate, and lanolin) for intra-alveolar application, with the use of gauze, was indicated by Pell in 1934. As in most disease processes, prevention is the best cure. First, instruct the patient not to smoke. Second, curette and irrigate with 1:4 hydrogen peroxide to normal saline mixture. Third, close the extraction sockets, as much as possible, to prevent contamination from the outside and to allow for clot formation. Fourth, tell your patient not to spit or drink through a straw, as these activities may lead to the breakdown of the in mature blood clot.
5. Inferior Alveolar or Mental Nerve Paresthesia: The overall incidence of the inferior alveolar nerve and lingual nerve injury during mandibular extractions ranges between 0.6 and 5 % with the incidence being highest during the extraction of impacted third molars. Nerve damage has been divided into three subtypes, known as the Seddon classification. Type 1, is neurapraxia, causes altered sensation or paresthesia and is the mildest of the three conditions. This condition involves damage to the myelin sheath and can be caused by direct pressure, edema, or ischemia. Once the cause is reversed, conduction is restored, and recovery is complete. Type 2, is axonotmesis, which literally means damage to the axon and myelin sheath. The dysesthesia may be transient and in the young patient, prognosis is encouraging. Nerve regeneration has been well documented at a rate of 1–2 mm/day. Type 3 is known as neurapraxia and occurs once the nerve is transected. The patient will experience anesthesia because of the disruption of the epineurium, perineurium, and endoneurium. This is the worse of the three conditions and at best, recovery is partial. If you lacerate the nerve, it should be reapproximated with interrupted suture placed through the epineurium. The patient should be made aware of the complication and the degree of postoperative proprioception, and serial clinic appointments should be documented. Most nerve injuries resolve spontaneously over time without intervention; however, this resolution may take months.
6. Root Displacement into Maxillary Sinus, Infratemporal Fossa: Extraction of maxillary molars can lead to these complications due to the close proximity of the roots of these teeth to the maxillary sinus. The weakness of the maxilla predisposes it to fractures of the tuberosity. Because of the close proximity of the maxillary sinus, and the thin membrane separating the tooth and the sinus, root tips can easily be displaced into the sinus. If this occurs, the removal of the root can be accomplished through direct exploration through the tooth socket, but can sometimes even require a Caldwell-Luc approach to the maxillary sinus. If a tooth or fragment is displaced

into the infratemporal fossa, an attempt should be made to visualize or palpate the displaced tooth. If the tooth is palpable, an incision can be made intraorally, in the buccal sulcus, and dissection should be made along the buccinator muscle in a superior direction until the tooth is found and retrieved. If the tooth is not palpable, the procedure should be terminated and the location of the tooth should be obtained with the use of a CT scan. In this case, most likely a coronal approach will be necessary to locate and retrieve the tooth.

7. Creation of Oroantral Fistula: It is common during the extraction of maxillary posterior teeth to make an iatrogenic communication between the oral and sinus cavity. This happens because of the close proximity of maxillary posterior root tips to the sinus floor. The intervening bone is extremely thin in some cases and easily fractures during the manipulations required during the process of exodontias. In most cases, these communications close spontaneously after several days to a couple of weeks with no intervention whatsoever. When the communications are large however (over 1 cm), it might be prudent to pack an absorbable collagen sponge into the socket and attempt to attain primary closure of the soft tissues. If an oroantral fistula develops, delayed closure might become necessary utilizing local tissue rearrangement, such as an advancement buccal flap or a pedicled palatal flap.
8. Root Displacement into the Floor of the Mouth: When extracting mandibular teeth, it is important for the clinician not to overestimate the strength of the cortical bone. In the oral surgery literature, posterior mandibular molar roots have been displaced into soft tissue, particularly through the thin lingual plate. Once perforating the lingual plate, root tips can be dislodged directly into the submandibular space. Normally, the mylohyoid muscle acts as a natural barrier of the oral cavity and prevents the migration of these tooth particles. Tooth particles have also been documented, dislodged from the socket, and into the mandibular canals. If a mandibular root tip becomes displaced, an attempt should be made to palpate the soft tissue. In the fortunate situation, external pressure from below can express the foreign tooth debris out of the soft tissue and into the oral cavity. If a tooth particle is in the submandibular space, stop and reassess with radiographs (periapical, occlusal x-ray, or cone beam CT scan). If the root tip continues to be illusive, then a viable option is to use general anesthesia and localize with a needle and C-arm or fluoroscopy. It is important to remember the promise of first doing no harm. Weigh the benefits of continue exploration with the possible complication of injury to the lingual nerve, submandibular duct, postoperative ranula formation, damage to the inferior alveolar neurovascular bundle, and, less likely, damage to the lingual artery.
9. Jaw Fracture: Iatrogenic mandibular fracture associated with the removal of teeth is rare and has been reported incidences ranging from 0.0034 to 0.0075 %. Factors affecting the incidence and etiology of iatrogenic mandibular fractures include the magnitude of tooth impaction, type of tooth angulation, length of roots, patient's age, and experience of the surgeon. Preoperative risk and benefit evaluation, conservative bone removal during extraction, tooth sectioning, and attention to cracking noises are important to avoid fractures. In addition, proper radiographic studies that evaluate bony pathosis around an impacted third molar will aid the clinician to avoid this complication. With a thoughtful and proper extraction technique, an iatrogenic mandibular fracture should not occur. If it does occur, the fracture should be treated utilizing standard techniques.
10. Bisphosphonate-Related Osteonecrosis of the Jaw (BRONJ): First published in 2003, this condition is an osteonecrosis of the bone on patients taking oral or intravenous forms of bisphosphonates. The intravenous formulations are much more likely to lead to this complication, and the risk has been estimated at 0.1 % on these patients after having any type of exodontia. Routine dental extractions and optimal oral hygiene are strongly advocated before starting intravenous bisphosphonates. When a cancer patient is receiving intravenous bisphosphonates, dental extraction should be avoided. A single tooth extraction is responsible for as many as 86 % of cases of BRONJ. At this point, this condition is not preventable but current protocols recommend stopping bisphosphonates if possible prior to elective dental extractions and when BRONJ develops. Treatment recommendations lean towards conservative management (antibiotics, oral antimicrobial rinses, pain control) and extensive debridement and resection are suggested only for longer term palliation of infection and pain (see Figs. 32.9 and 32.10).

Bibliography

Basha SI, et al. The efficacy of pharyngeal packing during routine nasal surgery – a prospective randomized controlled study. Anesthesia. 2006;61:1161–5.

Birn H. Etiology and pathogenesis of fibrinolytic alveolitis ("dry socket"). Int J Oral Surg. 1973;2:211.

Blondeau F. Extraction of impacted mandibular third molars: postoperative complications and their risk factors. J Can Dent Assoc. 2007;73(4):325a–e.

Cankaya AB, Erdem MA. Iatrogenic mandibular fracture associated with third molar removal. Int J Med Sci. 2011;8(7):547–53.

Cardodo C, Rodrigues M. Clinical concepts of dry socket. J Oral Maxillofac Surg. 2010;68:1922–32.

Chiapasco M. Germectomy or delayed removal of mandibular impacted third molars: the relationship between age and incidence of complications. J Oral Maxillofac Surg. 1995;53(4):341–3.

Libersa P, Roze D, Cacart T, Libersa JC. Immediate and late mandibular fractures after third molar removal. J Oral Maxillofac Surg. 2002;60:163–6.

Nelson S. Wheeler's dental anatomy, physiology, and occlusion. 9th ed. St. Louis: Saunders/Elsevier; 2010. p. 1–4.

Nyul L. Kieferfrakturen bei zahnextrationen. Zahnarztl Welt. 1959;60: 1–5.

Pell GJ. So-called dry socket. J Am Dent Assoc. 1934;21:1062.

Pogrel P. The relationship of the lingual nerve to the mandibular third molar region. J Oral Maxillofac Surg. 1995;53:1178.

Ruggiero SL, Mehrotra B, Rosenberg TJ, et al. Osteonecrosis of the jaws associated with the use of bisphosphonates: a review of 63 cases. J Oral Maxillofac Surg. 2004;62:527.

Ruggiero SL, Dodson TB, Assael LA, Landesberg R, Marx RE, Mehrotra B. American Association of Oral and Maxillofacial Surgeons Position Paper on Bisphosphonate-Related Osteonecrosis of the Jaw—2009 Update.

Sakr K, Farag IA, Zeitoun IM. Review of 509 mandibular fractures treated at the University Hospital, Alexandria, Egypt. Br J Oral Maxillofac Surg. 2009;44:107–11.

Tanaka M, Tomitsuka K, Shionoya K, et al. Aetiology of maxillofacial fractures. Br J Oral Maxillofac Surg. 1994;32:19–23.

Thorn JJ, Mogeltoft M, Hansen PK. Incidence and aetiological pattern of jaw fractures in Greenland. Int J Oral Maxillofac Surg. 1986;15: 372–9.

Maxillofacial Augmentation and Reduction

33

David E. Morris and Lun-Jou Lo

Patient Selection

The facial soft tissues largely reflect underlying skeletal structure. Patients may seek consultation in hopes to change facial appearance for a number of reasons: feeling that their features are too angular, not angular enough, that portions of that face project too widely, or are too narrow. There are well-established differences in facial skeletal structure between the sexes. As such, some patients seek treatment in an effort to affect a change in masculinity or femininity. In the transgender patient, facial skeletal contouring may be one component in gender reassignment or transformation.

A number of studies cite measured anthropometric differences across race. In various parts of the world, there are clearly societal differences in how beauty is perceived and what facial features characterize beauty. The popularity of zygoma reduction and mandibular angle reduction in Southeast Asian countries attests to this, as commonly young female patients seek such procedures with the goal of achieving a more oval-shaped facial appearance with soft, gentle contours. Conversely malar and mandibular augmentation with implants has become increasingly popular in many Western countries, where many patients often desire the opposite—more angular cheeks, mandibular angles, and chin.

All humans have some degree of asymmetry between the two halves of the face. While most skeletal asymmetries are below the threshold for even noting at the casual level, there are cases that are clearly noticeable and for which patients seek consultation. Facial skeletal asymmetry may be from a number of origins: developmental, congenital (cleft related, craniofacial microsomia, Romberg's disease, other syndromes), or acquired (posttraumatic, following tumor treatment).

Treatment Planning

There are several essential points to consider in evaluating the patient for facial skeletal contouring.

Age. Most patients seeking such procedures have reached facial skeletal maturity. The authors recommend that facial growth is complete before proceeding with skeletal contouring. With increasing age however, soft tissues become more lax and lose some contractility, making the soft tissue response to skeletal procedures less pronounced than in younger patients, in whom the soft tissues are more likely to conform to underlying skeletal changes. Thus, in patients beyond their 30s, one should consider that subsequent soft tissue procedures (e.g., facelift, necklift) may become indicated secondarily after the skeletal procedure. This should be included in the initial discussion.

Etiology of the Deformity. The patient's anatomic areas of concern must be clearly understood by the surgeon so as to discern if the appearance is indeed due to a skeletal etiology and whether it can be affected by a skeletal change. An example is the patient with a square- or moon-faced appearance seeking mandibular angle reduction; in some such patients, masseter hypertrophy and excess buccal fat significantly contribute to facial contour. This must be recognized preoperatively, the limitations of skeletal contouring recognized, and consideration given to concomitant procedures such as buccal fat resection and masseter muscle resection.

Facial Proportions and Dentofacial Exam

The patient is examined from frontal, lateral, and oblique views. Note is taken as to whether the profile is relatively straight, convex, or concave and frontally whether the face is

D.E. Morris, MD (✉)
Division of Plastic, Reconstructive and Cosmetic Surgery, University of Illinois, Chicago, IL, USA
e-mail: demorrismd@sbcglobal.net

L.-J. Lo, MD
Department of Plastic and Reconstructive Surgery, Chang Gung Memorial Hospital and Chang Gung University, Taoyuan, Taiwan

P.J. Taub et al. (eds.), *Ferraro's Fundamentals of Maxillofacial Surgery*,
DOI 10.1007/978-1-4614-8341-0_33, © Springer Science+Business Media New York 2015

more oval than square. From the frontal view, symmetry is assessed, envisioning a facial midline that descends from the soft tissue nasion and intercanthal midline, as these will remain relatively constant. The dorsum of nose, philtral column, and lip and chin positions are evaluated, taking note of deviations from this midline. The relative proportions of upper, middle, and lower third of face are compared as are deviations from the usual thirds proportions within the lower third of the face. Soft tissue reflections of the bizygomatic width and bigonial width are assessed, as these are largely determined by underlying zygomatic arch and mandibular angle projection, respectively.

Thorough dentofacial exam should include assessment as to whether the upper and lower dental midlines coincide with each other and with other facial midlines and whether there is acceptable occlusion. This is important, as a significant malocclusion should suggest to the surgeon that an orthognathic procedure may be indicated as part of the treatment plan and offered to the patient. In cases where a contour deformity coexists with a skeletal malocclusion, for example, in some craniofacial microsomia cases, the authors' preference is to do any indicated orthognathic procedure first, in order to establish a level occlusal plane, ensure that the upper dental midline is in line with other facial midlines, and that the occlusion is corrected from a skeletal perspective. The patient is counseled that she may later benefit from staged, nonorthognathic contouring procedure (e.g., malar augmentation of the deficient side) or soft tissue augmentation such as fat injection.

Radiographic Planning

For the symmetric patient seeking zygomatic and/or malar augmentation or reduction, radiographic studies are not routinely obtained. Three-dimensional CT and virtual surgical planning software is helpful, however, for asymmetric cases. Here a skeletal midline plane is determined and mirror image function is used to determine areas and degree of asymmetry. This is correlated with clinical exam, as to which side is clinically most acceptable to the patient. This radiographic data can be used in different ways. For example, if the decision is made to augment the zygoma unilaterally with an implant, the shape difference between the two sides is determined. The overall shape, its dimensions, and specific measurements in thickness at various points can be used to help select an appropriate prefabricated implant. Alternatively patient-specific customized implants of a number of materials, including porous polyethylene, can be fabricated based on CT-based virtual planning (see Fig. 33.1).

For patients requiring osteotomies to asymmetrically reduce a portion of the facial skeleton, the same type of planning can be used to either obtain measurements that would guide osteotomy placement or to fabricate a patient-specific custom cutting guide that is fixed to the facial skeleton and guides the osteotomy (see Fig. 33.2).

Facial Skeletal Reduction Through Osteotomies: Technique (See Figs. 33.3, 33.4, and 33.5)

While mandibular angle reduction and zygoma reduction are more commonly sought in parts of Southeast Asia to soften angular facial features, there certainly are patients outside of Asia who seek consultation desiring such procedures, and the same techniques are used for other indications. While a number of approaches/modifications to malar and zygomatic reduction have been described, the authors preferred approach is described here. These procedures are performed under general anesthesia with nasotracheal intubation.

Zygoma Reduction (See Fig. 33.6)

Bilateral upper gingivobuccal incisions are made, and the zygoma is exposed in the subperiosteal plane to the level of the infraorbital nerve. An inverted-L osteotomy is marked which includes a rectangular wedge of bone parallel to the medial limb of the L that is to be removed. These are completed with a reciprocating saw, always taking care to note angle and where the tip of the saw is, so as not to damage adjacent structures such as the orbital floor. A 1 cm incision is made vertically in the sideburn overlying the most posterior aspect of the zygomatic arch, just anterior to where it turns medially. This is cut with a reciprocating saw. Minimal dissection is done here, and the soft tissues are carefully retracted so as to avoid injury to facial nerve branches. Removing the anterior rectangular wedge allows the zygoma to be repositioned medially. The repositioned zygoma is fixed with three two-hole plates and 5–7 mm screws anteriorly. The identical procedure is performed on the contralateral side. The direction and extent of zygoma movement can be adjusted on both sides to achieve symmetry.

Mandibular Angle Reduction (See Fig. 33.7)

The ramus, angle, and mandibular body are exposed subperiosteally through a lower gingivobuccal sulcus incision. An angle stripper is used to take down the muscular attachments. The outer cortex is burred down to enable surgeon to see over the convexity of the body to accurately mark the planned osteotomy. The posterior portion is completed with a reciprocating saw, the hub of which is passed backwards through

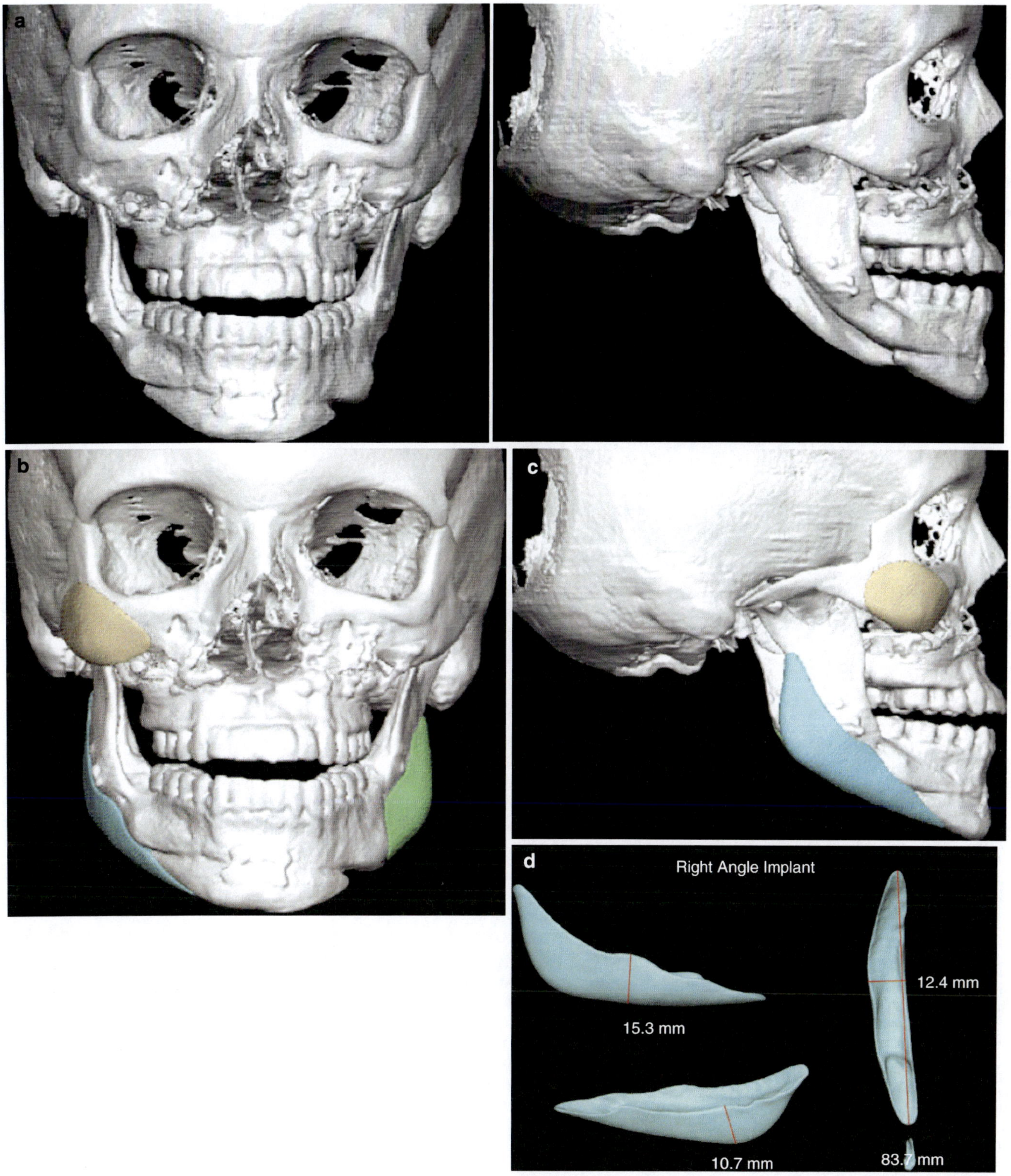

Fig. 33.1 CT demonstrates postoperative change following orthognathic surgery (LeFort 1, BSSO, osseous genioplasty) in an 18-year-old female with craniofacial microsomia. (**a**) Note expected residual complex asymmetries despite achieving the planned orthognathic result. (**b**, **c**) Virtual planning based on mirror imaging demonstrates spatial forms required to optimize skeletal symmetry. (**d**) Dimensions of the planned right mandibular angle implant can be used to select a prefabricated implant, or CT data is used to obtain a patient-specific implant through rapid prototyping

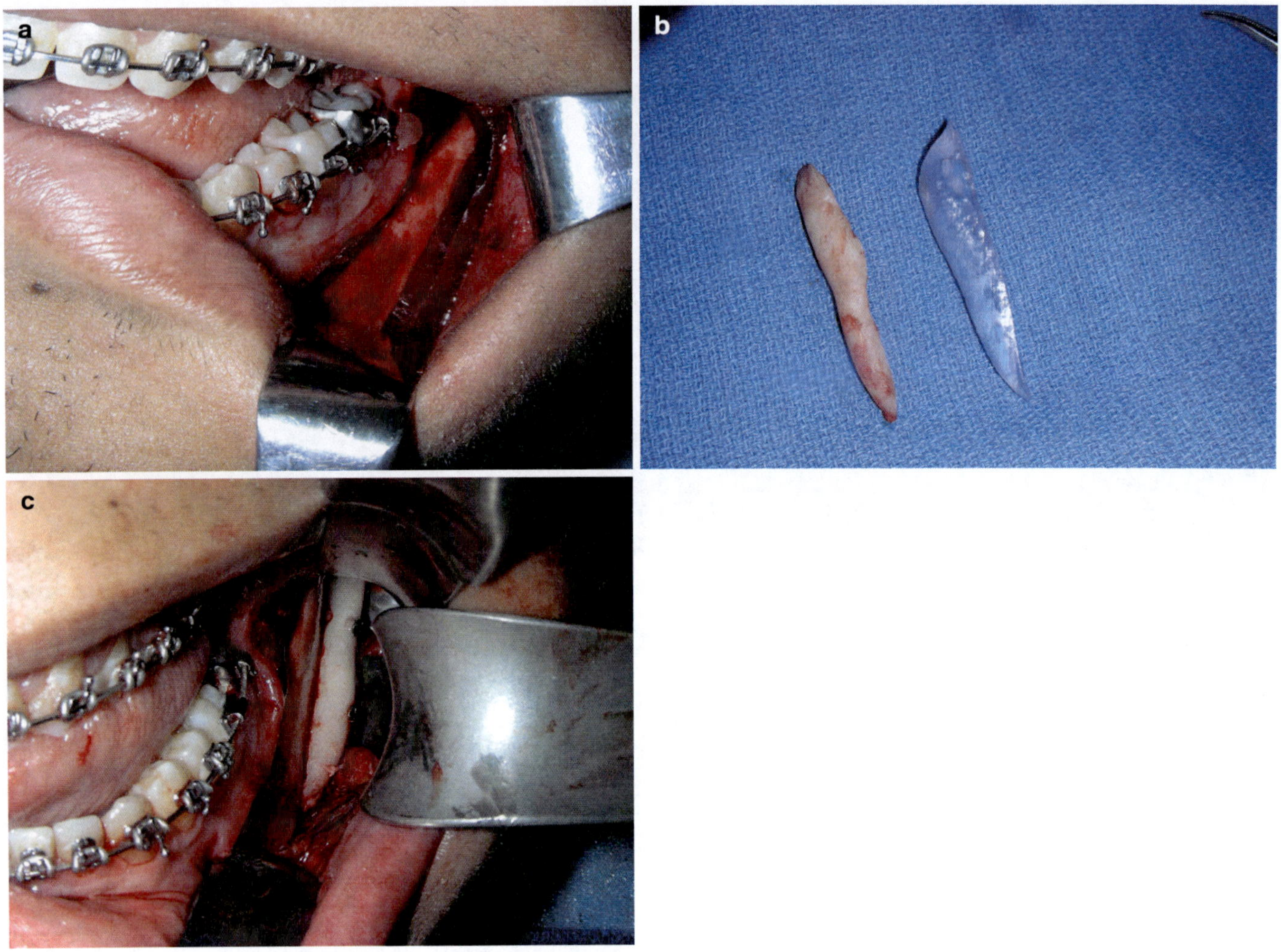

Fig. 33.2 Virtual planning use in designing mandibular angle and body resection for asymmetry case. (**a**) Materialise software was used to plan the amount of mandible to be resected to reduce vertical height; a patient-specific cutting guide is placed along mandibular body to guide osteotomy line. (**b**) Actual resected specimen next to model of what was to be resected based on virtual planning. (**c**) The resected specimen was used as an onlay in order to increase lateral projection

a separate stab incision made just inferior to the lower border of the angle anterior to the osteotomy. A collar around the saw shaft protects the skin from friction. The anterior portion of the osteotomy is competed through the intraoral incision with an oscillating saw and 90° blade. While the entire osteotomy can be completed with the 90° oscillating saw, using the reciprocating saw may allow for a more accurate osteotomy posteriorly in some surgeons' hands. Typically the oblique height of the osteotomized segment measures 15–18 mm. Previous anatomic study based on CT data in a Taiwanese population has demonstrated that the inferior alveolar nerve typically courses at least 20 mm from the inferior border of the mandibular angle (Lo et al.).

Facial Skeletal Augmentation

While there are many implant materials available, there is probably not a single ideal one. Taking available data on advantages/disadvantages of each into consideration, the

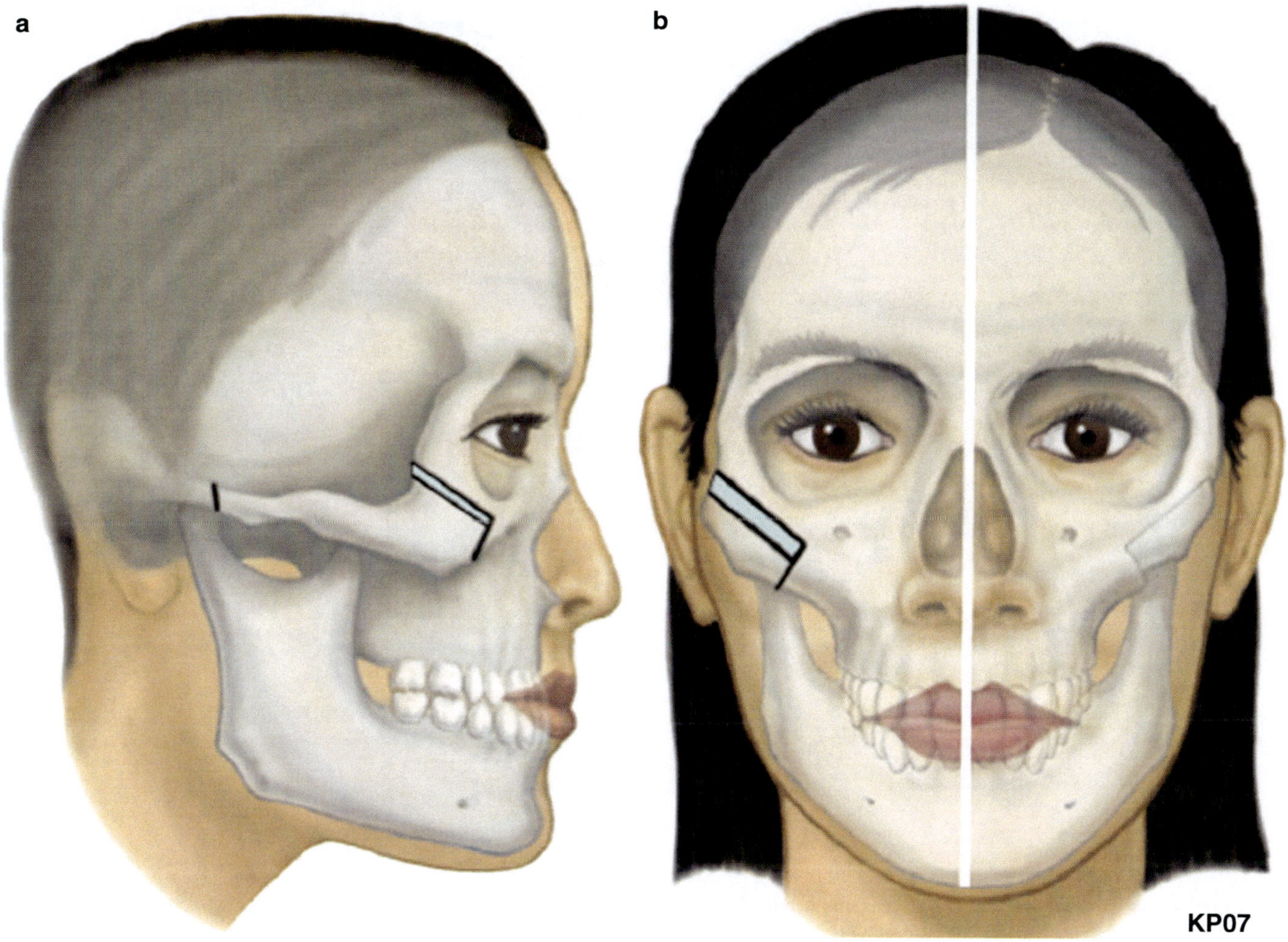

Fig. 33.3 Configuration of osteotomies used in zygoma reduction. The *light blue* rectangular wedge of bone is removed. (**a**) Frontal view, (**b**) lateral view

authors prefer the use of porous polyethylene for facial augmentation in cases where autogenous material is not feasible. As genioplasty is discussed in another chapter, here we focus on malar, mandibular angle, and paranasal augmentation. Such implants may be placed symmetrically for purely cosmetic reasons or for bilateral or unilateral reconstruction for congenital, posttraumatic, or postoncologic defects (see Fig. 33.8).

The authors prefer to place implants under general anesthesia and through the same approaches discussed above for reduction procedures. Reusable silicone sizers are helpful intraoperatively in verifying the appropriate size of implant. A sufficient pocket size is dissected to accommodate the implant and allow for a tension-free closure over the implant. When possible, a several-layer closure is performed. The deep surface of the implant is burred as needed to maximize the area of contact between implant surface and bone, thus minimizing dead space between the implant and bone surface. Implants are secured with at least two screws so as to prevent implant migration (see Fig. 33.9).

Avoiding Complications

To ensure a safe and effective procedure, the surgeon must strive to prevent complications at both the planning and technical levels. With regard to planning, it is imperative to understand the patient's concern and pair this with the procedure that will affect anatomy. Both the soft tissues and

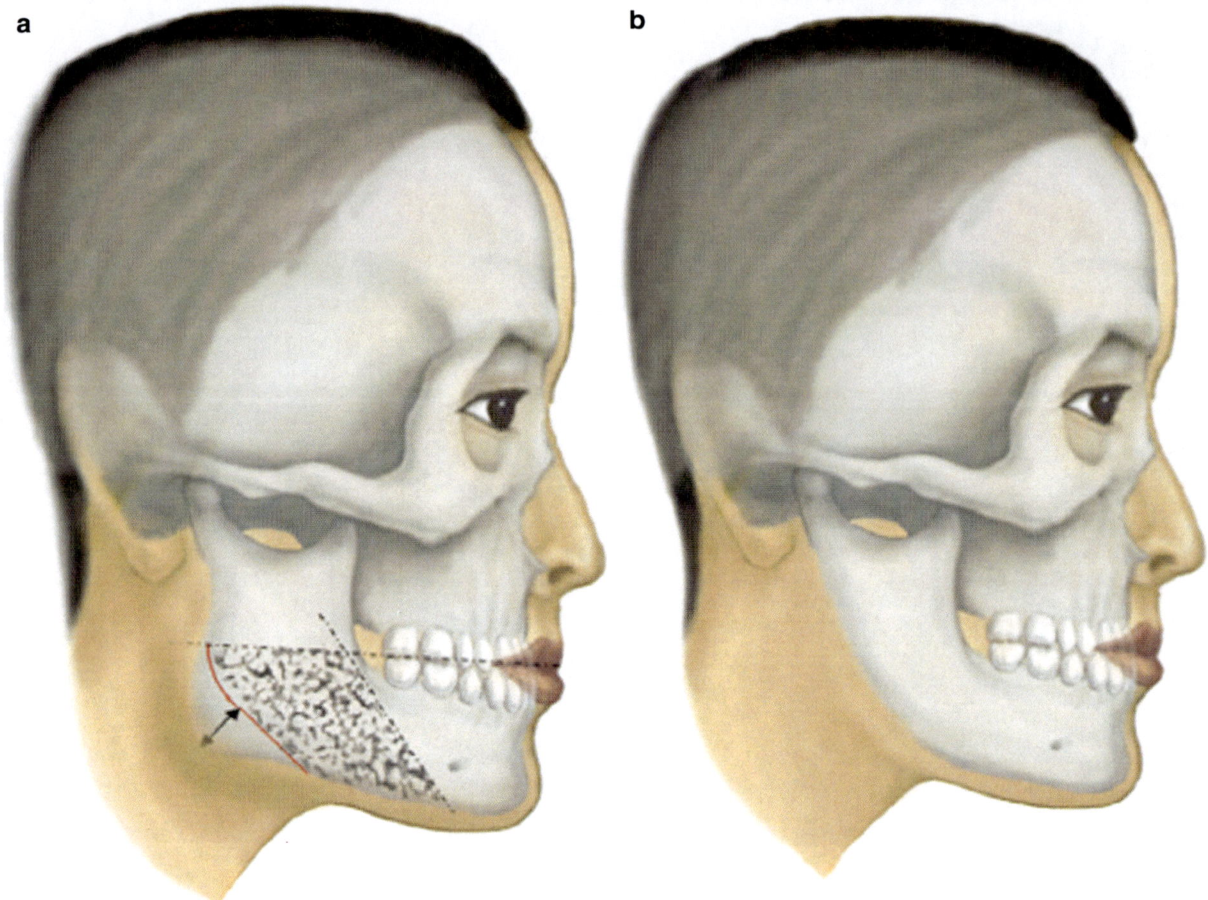

Fig. 33.4 Configuration of osteotomies used in mandibular angle reduction. (**a**) The *shaded region* is the portion of the mandibular body in which the outer cortex is burred prior to osteotomy. The superior level of the osteotomy is at the occlusal plane. (**b**) Note the *softening* of the mandibular angle after the procedure

skeletal components should be considered. Always discuss with the patient the possible need for staged or revisional procedures.

Intraoperatively, the structures vulnerable to injury during osteotomy are dental roots and inferior alveolar nerve (mandibular angle resection), orbital floor, and facial nerve branches (zygoma resection). Care must be taken in safe exposure, adequate visualization, and awareness of where the tip of the saw lies at all times. Postoperative asymmetries following resectional procedures may require revisional resection or placement of an implant. Such deformities are best avoided through careful intraoperative assessment both at the skeletal level and in assessing for visual and palpable asymmetry prior to closure.

With regard to augmentation with implants, key points are matching the appropriate size implant to the pocket and

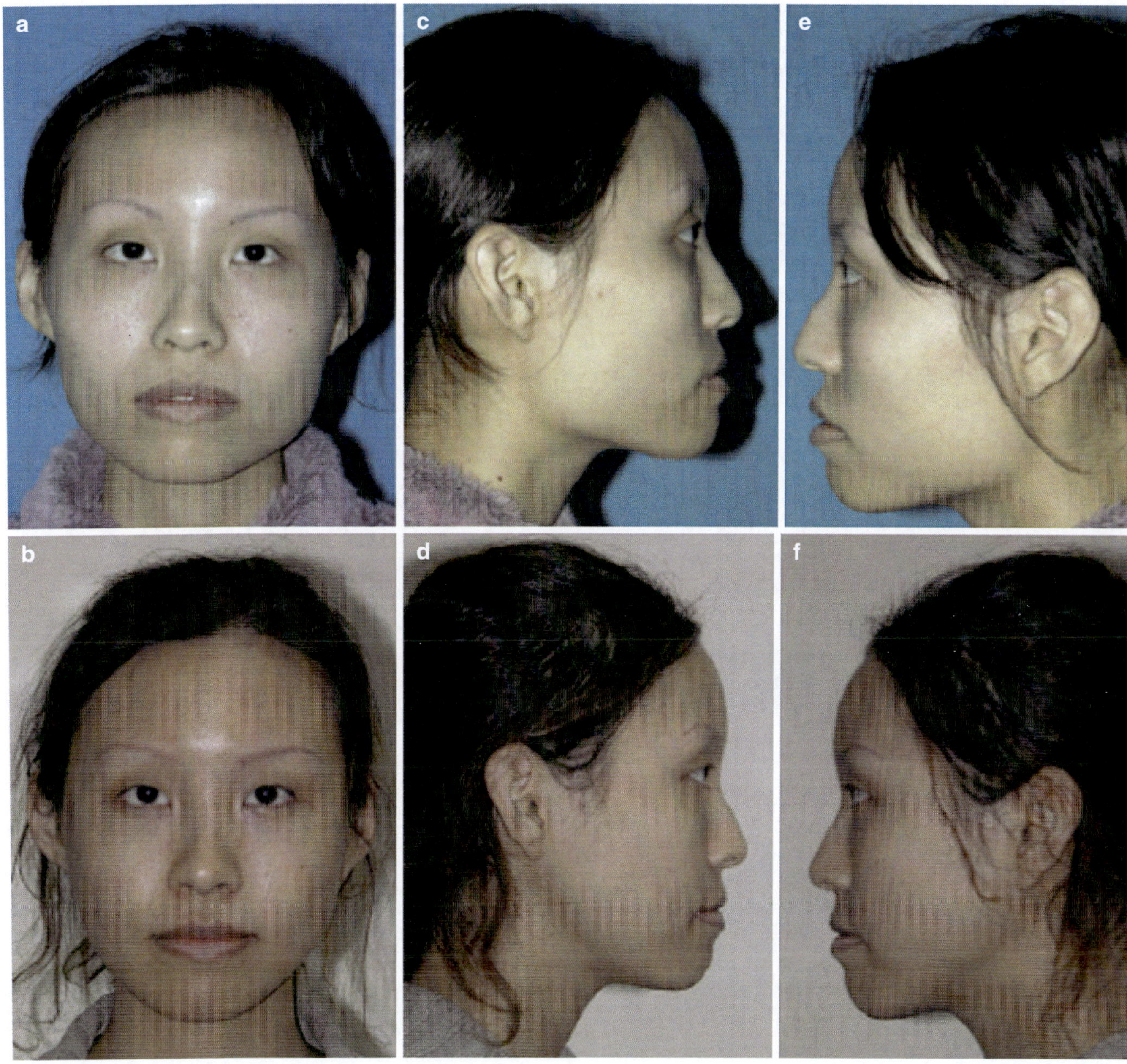

Fig. 33.5 Preoperative (**a**, **c**, **e**) and 9-month postoperative (**b**, **d**, **f**) view of a 26-year-old woman who underwent 6-mm zygoma reduction and mandible angle reduction (18 mm on the right and 20 mm on the left)

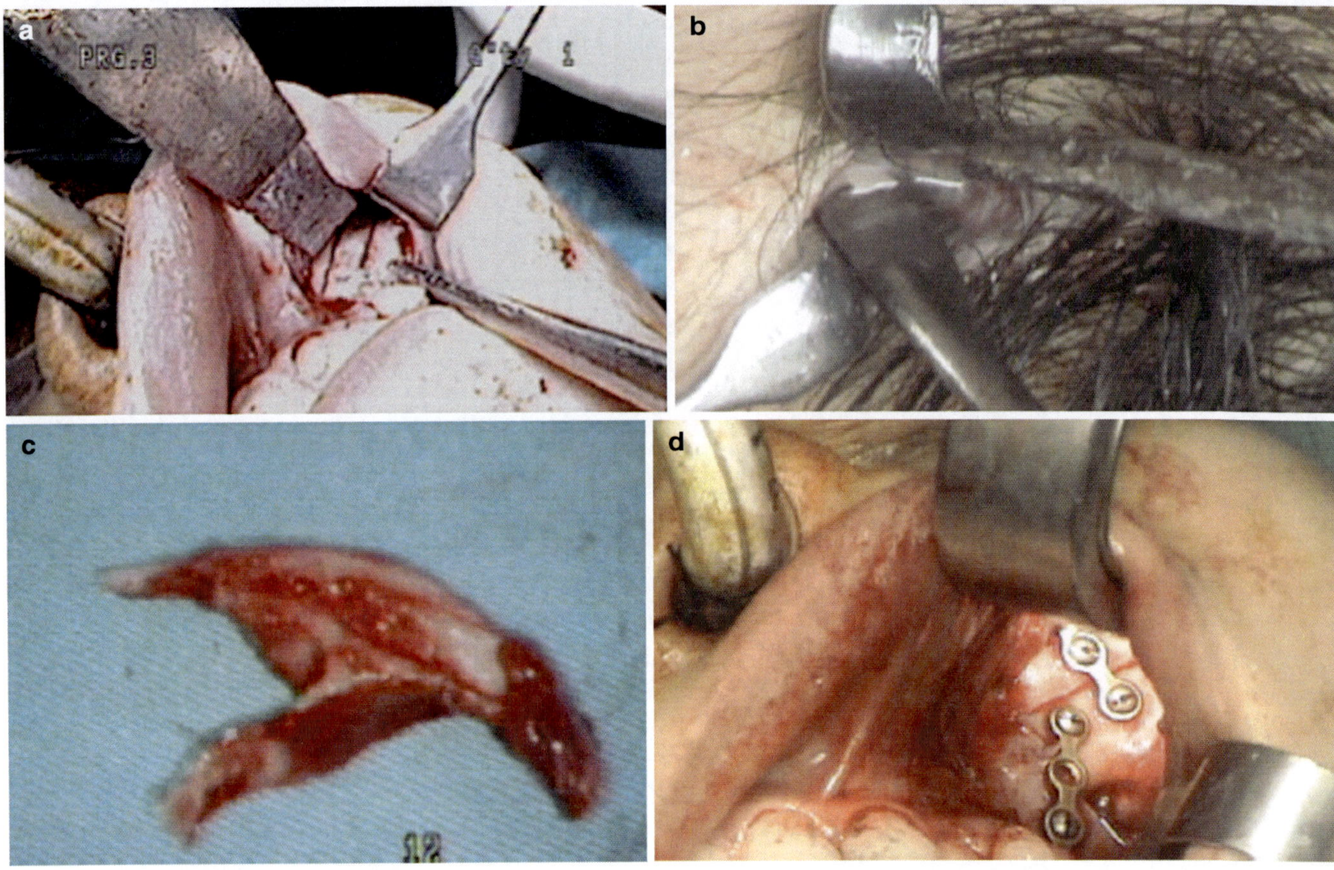

Fig. 33.6 Zygoma reduction, intraoperative. (**a**) The inverted-L osteotomies are demonstrated through upper gingivobuccal sulcus approach. (**b**) The posterior arch is osteotomized using a reciprocating saw through a vertical sideburn incision. (**c**) The wedge of bone removed from the superior aspect of the L osteotomy. (**d**) The anterior aspect of the osteotomized segment is fixated with two two-hole plates

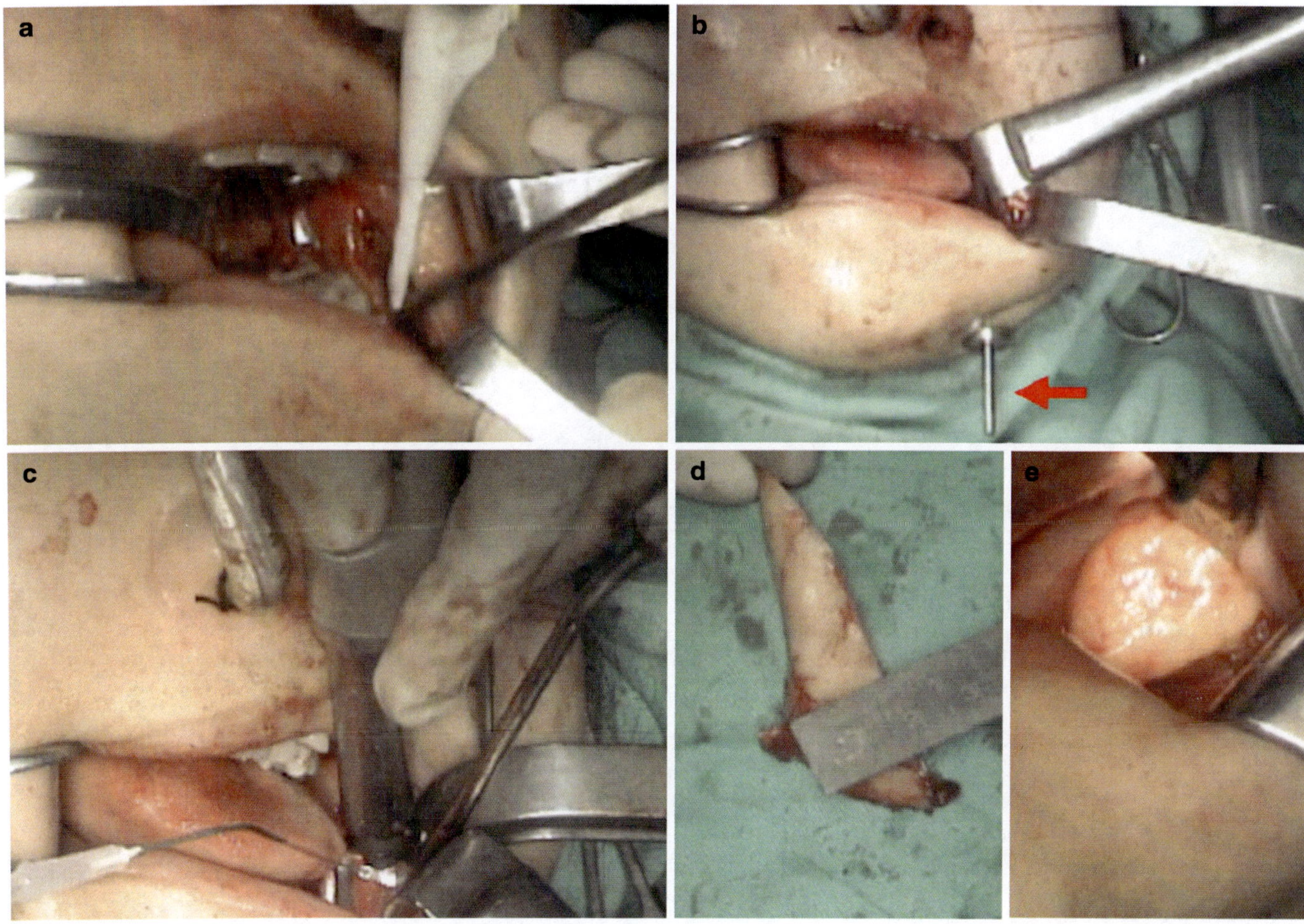

Fig. 33.7 Mandibular angle reduction, intraoperative. (**a**) The lateral aspect of the mandibular body is exposed through a lower gingivobuccal sulcus incision. (**b**) *Red arrow* demonstrates shaft of reciprocating saw used to complete posterior portion of the osteotomy. (**c**) Oscillating saw is used to complete anteroinferior aspect of osteotomy. (**d**) The removed segment. (**e**) Buccal fat is easily removed simultaneously when clinically indicated through opening the buccinator muscle

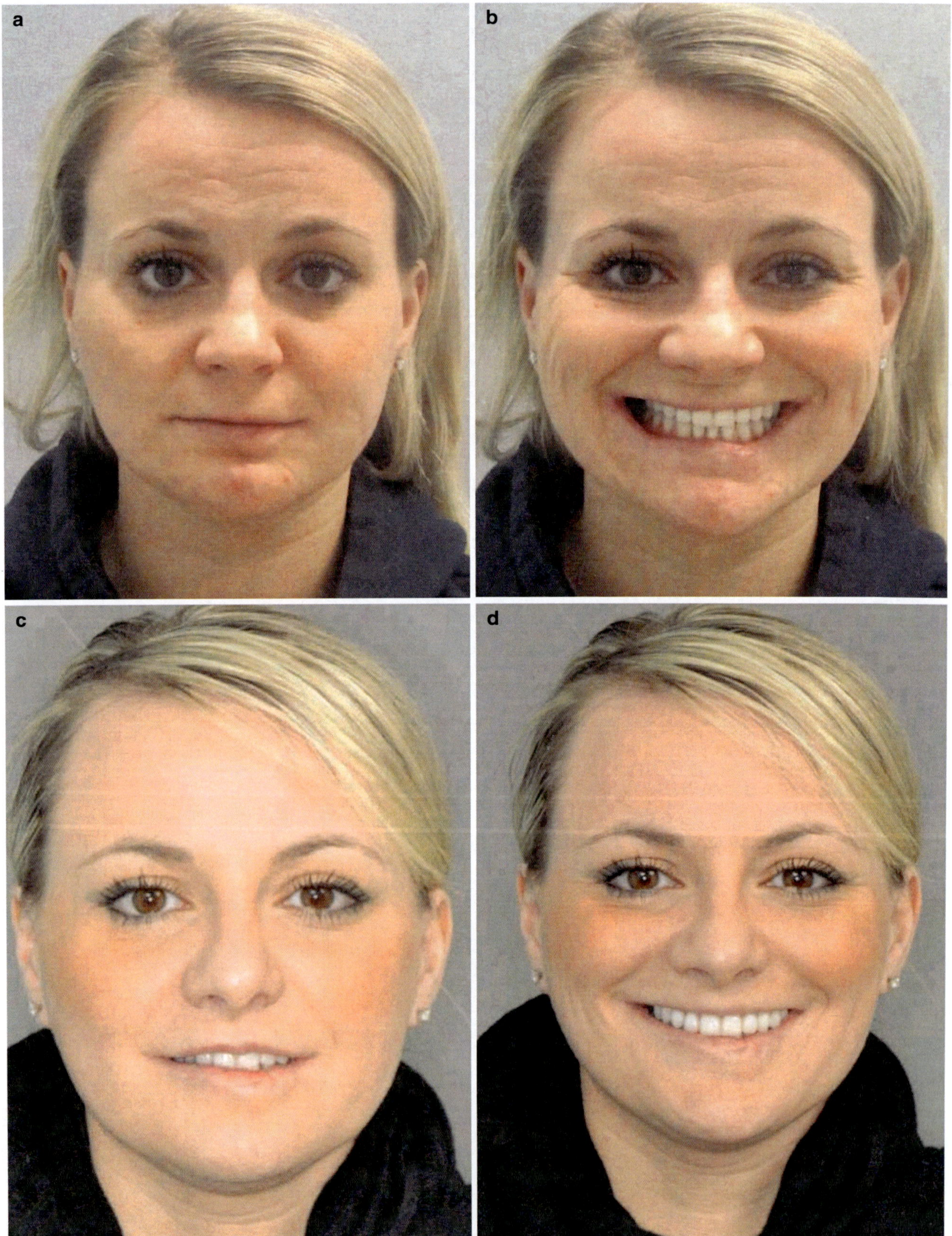

Fig. 33.8 A 26-year-old female who previously suffered multiple facial fractures including anterior maxilla, where she has lost bone and was edentulous. After multiple reconstructive procedures including prosthodontic rehabilitation, she has significant perioral soft tissue laxity with deep nasolabial folds. (**a**, **b**) Preoperative (**c**, **d**) 2 years following placement of bilateral paranasal porous polyethylene implants

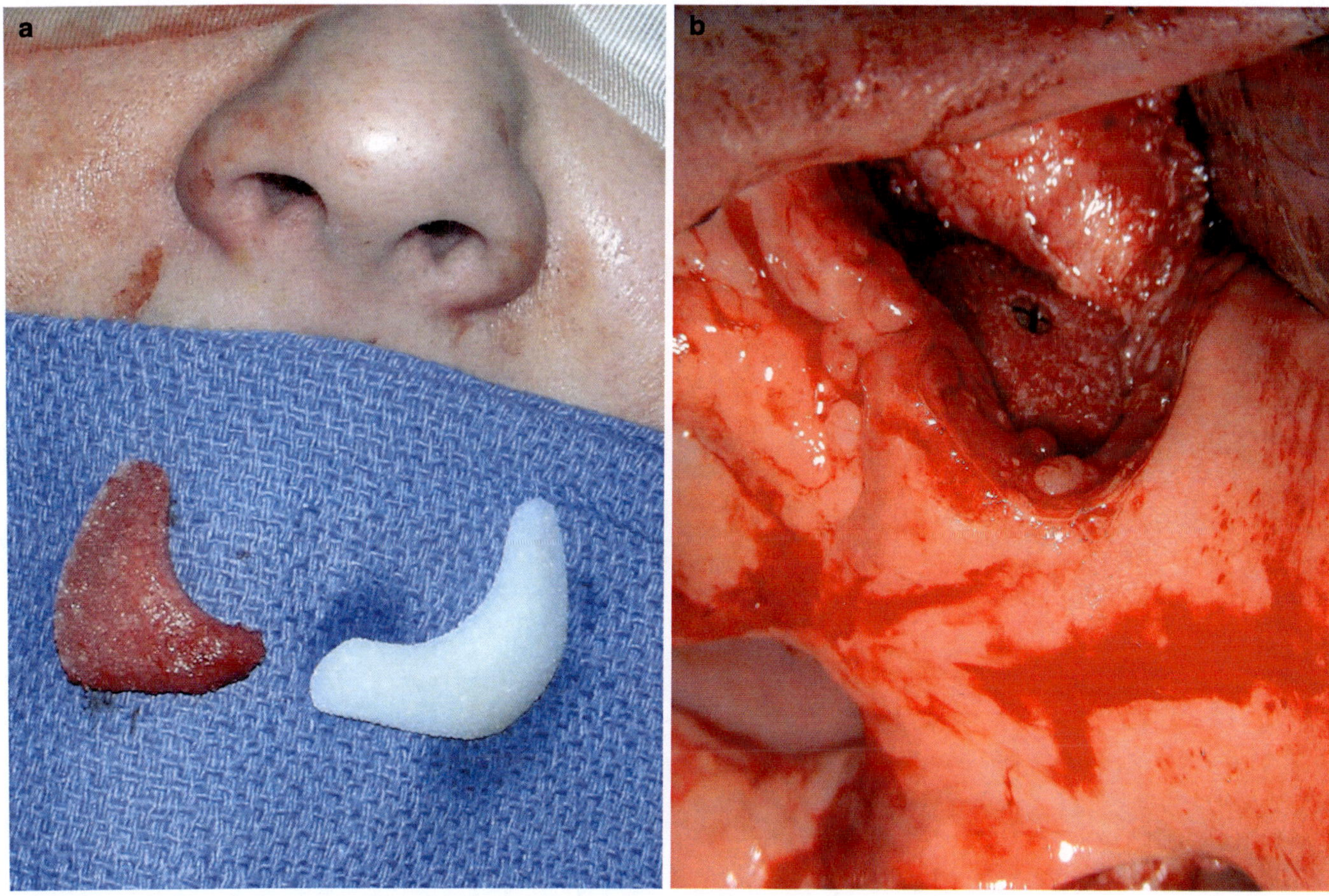

Fig. 33.9 Placement of paranasal implants (intraoperative views of case in 36.7). (**a**) Once implants are selected, size and shape are modified as needed with a burr. (**b**) They are secured to underlying bone with two screws

ensuring ample soft tissue coverage and fixating the implant. The authors have operated on patients who have experienced migration of the implant in cases where surgeons have not adequately fixated the implant. For implants that have started to extrude, our experience has been that these usually require removal.

Bibliography

Lo LJ, Wong FH, Chen YR. The position of the inferior alveolar nerve at the mandibular angle: an anatomic consideration for aesthetic mandibular angle reduction. Ann Plast Surg. 2004;53(1):50–5.

Morris DE, Moaveni Z, Lo LJ. Aesthetic facial skeletal contouring in the Asian patient. Clin Plast Surg. 2007;34:547–56.

Distraction Osteogenesis

34

Raymond Harshbarger and Patrick Kelley

Distraction osteogenesis (DO) of the craniomaxillofacial skeleton has been an adaptation of the original studies on lengthening posttraumatic long bone injuries. Using the principles elucidated by Ilizarov, and building on the work of McCarthy, the scope of DO in the head and neck region has expanded dramatically. Capitalizing on the extensive body of work by orthopedic surgeons in fracture repair, those interested in the congenital and acquired conditions of the head and neck have been able to adapt the technique for bone lengthening throughout the craniofacial skeleton. Using the concepts of tension, stress, and blood supply, the process of distraction osteogenesis is now well anchored in the armamentarium of craniofacial surgeons. Deficiencies of soft tissue, scarring, and limited bone stock can now be overcome by gradual lengthening of the soft callus, along a vector with semirigid fixation; scarless bone formation can lend to the improvement of airway/breathing, masticatory function, eye protection, brain function, and finally craniofacial form.

History

The first recorded attempts at manipulating bone segments for the purpose of elongation dates back to the time of Hippocrates. External traction devices were used in the posttraumatic axial skeleton. In the early 1800s, continuous traction was used in posttraumatic extremities with the introduction of a formal osteotomy. Codivilla, in 1905, further refined these earlier processes reporting femur elongation at the site of former trauma through a process of external traction, using an osteotomy. Russian orthopedic surgeon, Gavril Ilizarov, in the 1950s developed techniques for treating posttraumatic tibial defects which form the scientific basis for modern-day process of distraction osteogenesis. Ilizarov's observations included use of "mechanical tension," a key signal during natural bone growth, and the relationship of blood supply and loading on maintenance of bone. Through Ilizarov's work, the basic principles of distraction osteogenesis were formalized, including osteotomy, latency, and rate/rhythm of distraction. Distraction has since been adapted for use in other regions of the body including the craniofacial skeleton. During the nineteenth and twentieth centuries, early attempts at bone lengthening in the craniofacial skeleton centered on mandibular lengthening. Various osteotomies, combined with acute advancements, and limited ability for skeletal fixation tended to result in variable bone formation, partial relapse, and overall instability (see Fig. 34.1). From 1970 to 1991 investigators began to apply Ilizarov's techniques to the canine mandible. Following this, McCarthy reported the first use of distraction osteogenesis in the human craniofacial skeleton, by successfully lengthening the mandible in a child with craniofacial microsomia (see Fig. 34.2). Since that time, use of DO in the bones of the face and skull has increased dramatically. Currently, DO has been described in the cranium, orbits, midface, and mandible for use in a variety of conditions both congenital and acquired.

Biology and Biomechanics

The principles of bone formation in distraction osteogenesis mirror that of basic fracture repair. Steps to heal a fracture include (1) traumatic impact to bone, (2) induction/inflammation, (3) callus formation, and (4) remodeling (see Table 34.1). After fracture, a hematoma consolidates and is replaced with vascular proliferation, inflammatory cells, and fibroblasts, with recruitment of osteoprogenitor cells from the periosteum. Over time extensive capillary ingrowth occurs with formation of a soft callus made of fibrous tissue,

R. Harshbarger, MD, FACS, FAAP (✉)
Craniofacial and Pediatric Plastic Surgery, Dell Children's Medical Center, University Medical Center Brackenridge, UT Austin, Austin, TX, USA
e-mail: raymond.harshbarger@gmail.com

P. Kelley, MD
Department of Plastic Surgery, Dell Children's Medical Center, Austin, TX, USA

P.J. Taub et al. (eds.), *Ferraro's Fundamentals of Maxillofacial Surgery*,
DOI 10.1007/978-1-4614-8341-0_34, © Springer Science+Business Media New York 2015

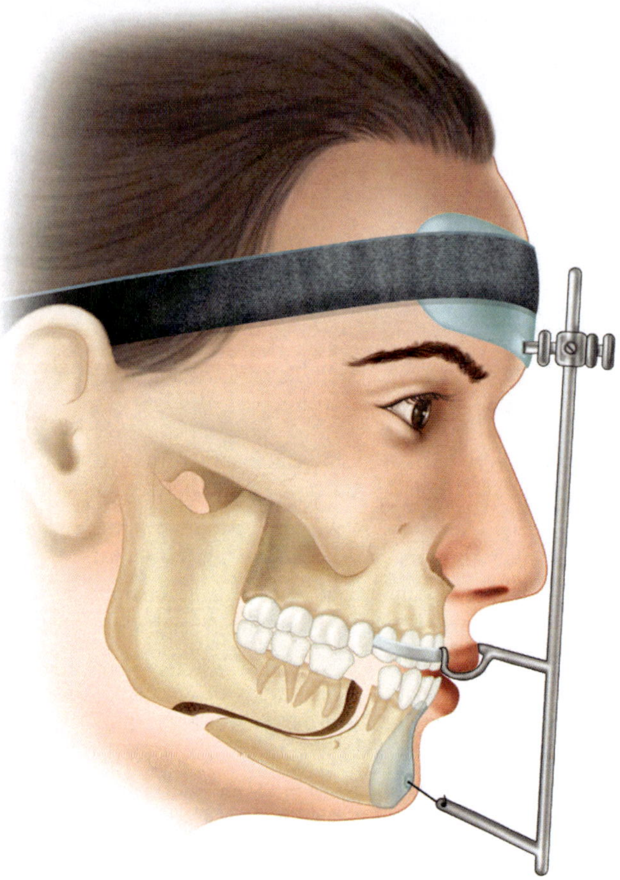

Fig. 34.1 Kasanjian's external "over the face" mandible traction device

the result of the presence of osteoprogenitor cells signaled by factors released at the time of the fracture. Eventually, the soft callus is replaced by hard callus as osteoblasts induce mineralization of bone. Following this, remodeling occurs. The formal stages of DO include (1) osteotomy with application of distraction device, (2) latency, (3) distraction, (4) consolidation, and (5) remodeling (see Fig. 34.3). After osteotomy (instead of traumatic fracture), a latency period ensues, essentially to allow the formation of a soft callus. Through the work of Ilizarov, latency was established at about 1 week after osteotomy. This principle, however, was founded on long bones, with endochondral bone formation, in a posttraumatic state. Through experiments on the canine mandible, and McCarthy's early work in children, the concept of latency of 7 days was transferred for use in the craniofacial skeleton. Formal studies regarding the latency period of various regions of the craniofacial skeleton have not been reported. Alterations in the latency period may be done based on the age of the patient, i.e., less time in younger patients (neonatal) and longer in older patients (adults). Latency must be gauged properly, given that too short a waiting period before active distraction would result in a fibrous distraction versus too long a latency with premature bony consolidation.

A successful active distraction phase relies on the presence of a soft callus, which can be slowly elongated with traction forces to achieve bone lengthening. Within the distraction phase, rate and rhythm of distraction must be established. By convention, with Ilizarov's pioneering work as a foundation, a standard rate of 1 mm/day was determined

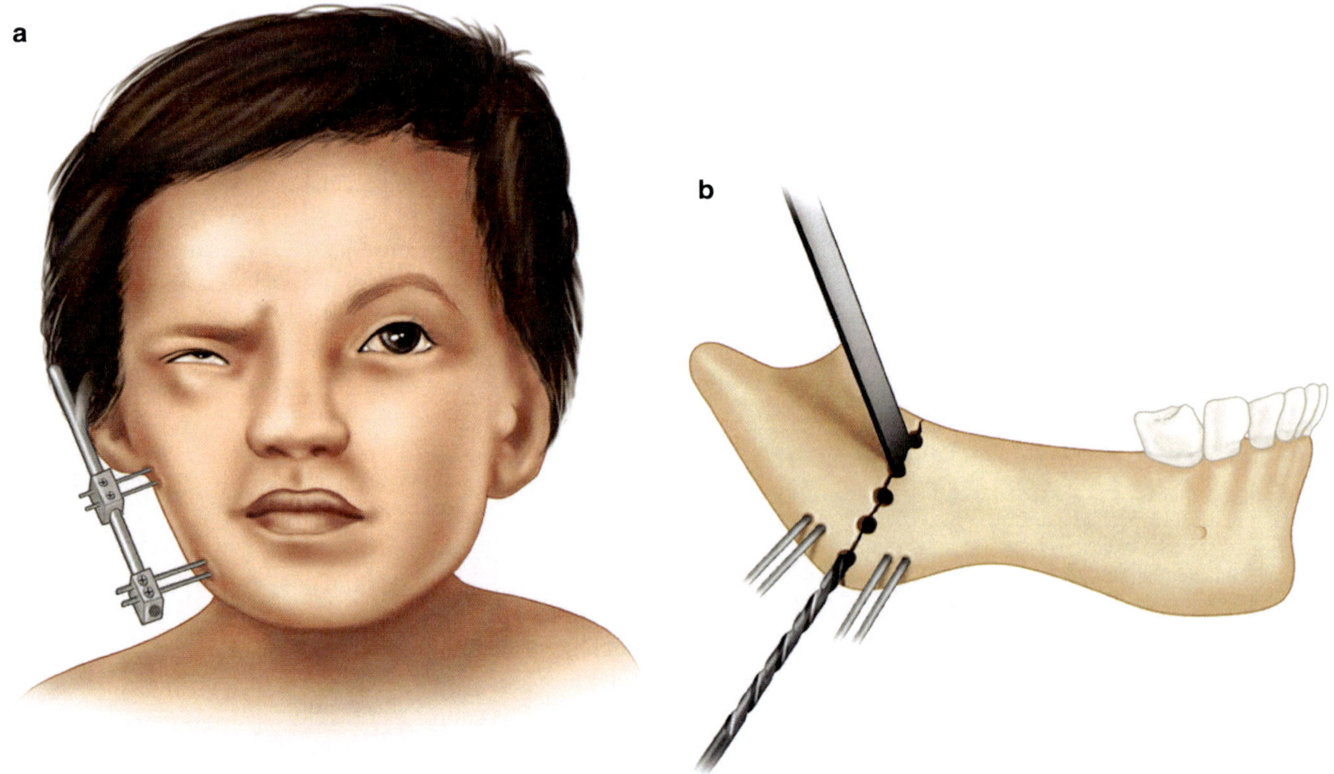

Fig. 34.2 (**a**) McCarthy's patient with hemifacial microsomia undergoing external mandibular distraction with a Hoffman device (Stryker Leibinger, Kalamazoo, MI). (**b**) Schematic showing placement of osteotomy and external traction pins

Table 34.1 Distraction osteogenesis impacts the soft callus phase of typical fracture healing

Fracture healing
Impact
Induction
Inflammation
Soft callus
Gradual traction (distraction)
Hard callus
Remodeling

to produce bone in the distracted gap. Rhythm refers to the frequency of activation (turning) of the device. Many protocols include a rhythm of twice daily activation. Both the rate and rhythm of distraction may vary depending on the age and region to be distracted. Neonatal mandibular distraction may succeed using 2 mm/day, with twice daily device activation, while cranial distraction in the adult may require 0.5 mm/day with once daily activation. After the active distraction phase is completed, consolidation begins. The hallmark of this phase, in which the devices remain for stability, is a transition

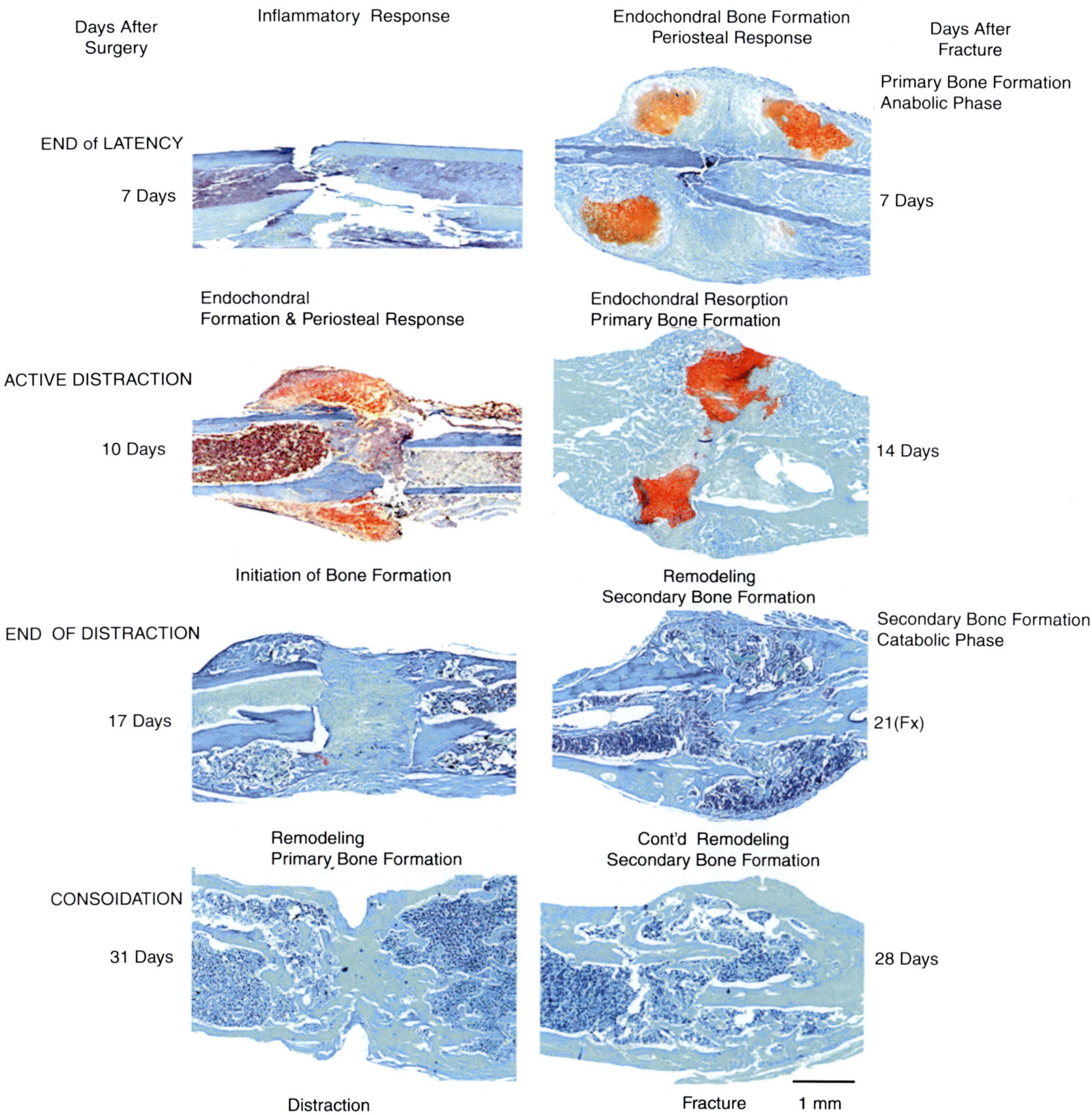

Fig. 34.3 Histologic comparison of healing by distraction osteogenesis (*left*) and healing after fracture (*Right*)

of the fibrous interzone into mineralized bone. Ossification occurs in parallel to the distraction vector. Experimental studies in a rat model have shown the presence of both intramembranous and endochondral bone formation in a distracted mandible. In craniofacial DO cases which involve occlusion, devices may be removed prior to complete ossification to allow for molding of the generate and a more ideal bite relationship. The time to ossification and device removal is not precise, but generally 8 weeks after cessation of active distraction, stable bone has formed, range 6–12 weeks. Again, neonates form mandibular bone faster perhaps in the 4–6-week range, while adults may require longer periods of consolidation. Long-term remodeling of the ossified generate may occur with strengthening of the initial bony scaffold by addition of parallel-fibered lamellar bone.

For most of the indications of DO in the craniofacial skeleton, simple DO would be performed with a single osteotomy between two vascularized regions of bone and lengthening occurring as the segments are moved apart. Occasionally, transport DO is required. Here, an osteotomized segment of bone is transported across a bone gap. For example, transport of a mandibular segment for reconstruction of the ramus/condyle, or across an acquired gap from trauma or cancer resection. Also important to successful outcomes in DO are the vectors of distraction which are vertical, horizontal, and oblique.

Distraction Osteogenesis of the Mandible

The proof of concept of craniofacial DO began experimental animal models and was first shown in humans clinically in a patient with craniofacial microsomia. After McCarthy showed success in lengthening the human mandible through DO, this concept has been applied to a variety of both congenital and acquired conditions involving mandibular deficiencies.

Neonate

The indications for DO of the mandible are numerous and relate to both the age of the patient and particular condition being treated. In the neonatal population, micrognathia with tongue-based airway obstruction may prompt bilateral mandibular DO to prevent tracheostomy in an acutely unstable airway or to reverse severe obstructive sleep apnea, often accompanied by feeding difficulties, gastroesophageal reflux, and general failure to thrive (see Table 34.2). Most frequently, this would be encountered in the patient with Pierre Robin sequence but can be seen in a variety of conditions including Treacher Collins syndrome, Nager syndrome, and craniofacial microsomia. If micrognathia with an unstable airway (unable to undergo polysomnography) is detected in the neonate, operative airway evaluation is indicated to confirm the tongue-based airway obstruction and rule out any other airway anomalies. Bilateral mandibular osteotomies with distractor placement are then performed to prevent a tracheostomy. Neonates, who are stable enough to undergo polysomnography, should do so, and if severe obstructive sleep apnea is detected, they may benefit from mandibular DO to prevent the long-term effects of sleep apnea on the developing brain and to avoid failure to thrive.

Table 34.2 Evaluation of neonate with micrognathia

Neonatal evaluation
Failure of proper respiratory function
Neonatal sleep study (polysomnography)
Feeding evaluation
Genetics
MRI (for central apnea)
Muscular tone
Airway evaluation (direct laryngo-bronchial exam)
3D CT scan

The technique for neonatal DO involves exposure of the lateral mandibular border through a small submandibular incision. In the neonate, the marginal mandibular nerve is typically located along the mandibular border, so an incision 1.5–2 cm below the border should help to avoid this singular structure. Dissection is carried through the investing fascia of the submandibular gland, and then cranially, to the mandibular border. Subperiosteal exposure is undertaken, visualization of the border, angle, ramus, sigmoid notch, coronoid process, and condylar process is important to correctly position the osteotomy. Our preference is for the inverted L osteotomy, beginning on the anterior border of the ramus above the lingula extending horizontally and turning vertically posterior to the nerve and parallel to the posterior ramus down to the border. Sufficient space should be left on the proximal segment of the bone for placement of the footplate. This will avoid injury to tooth buds and to the inferior alveolar nerve. A sagittal saw is used (smaller kerf) to complete 90 % of the osteotomy. A microdistractor with ratchet mechanism (to prevent turning the wrong way) is placed across the osteotomy (see Fig. 34.4). The device is planned so that the turning handle is brought out anteriorly through the incision or posteriorly behind the ear through a separate stab incision. High profile 5 mm screws are placed in each footplate on either side of the osteotomy. The vector of distraction is typically horizontal to slightly inferior in the Pierre Robin patient (see Fig. 34.5a, b) but may be much more vertical in patients without much ramus, i.e., Treacher Collins syndrome. And in those cases, the osteotomy may be modified to a stairstep to allow the device to orient vertically across the posterior aspect of the osteotomy. After device fixation, the remaining 10 % of the anterior osteotomy on the ramus is completed with a micro-osteotome. The turning arm is attached to the device, and it is tested, and then returned to zero position.

Neonates will heal much faster than children or adults, so their overall course of DO is shorter. Latency is typically one night, with an accelerated rate/rhythm of 0.9 mm twice daily.

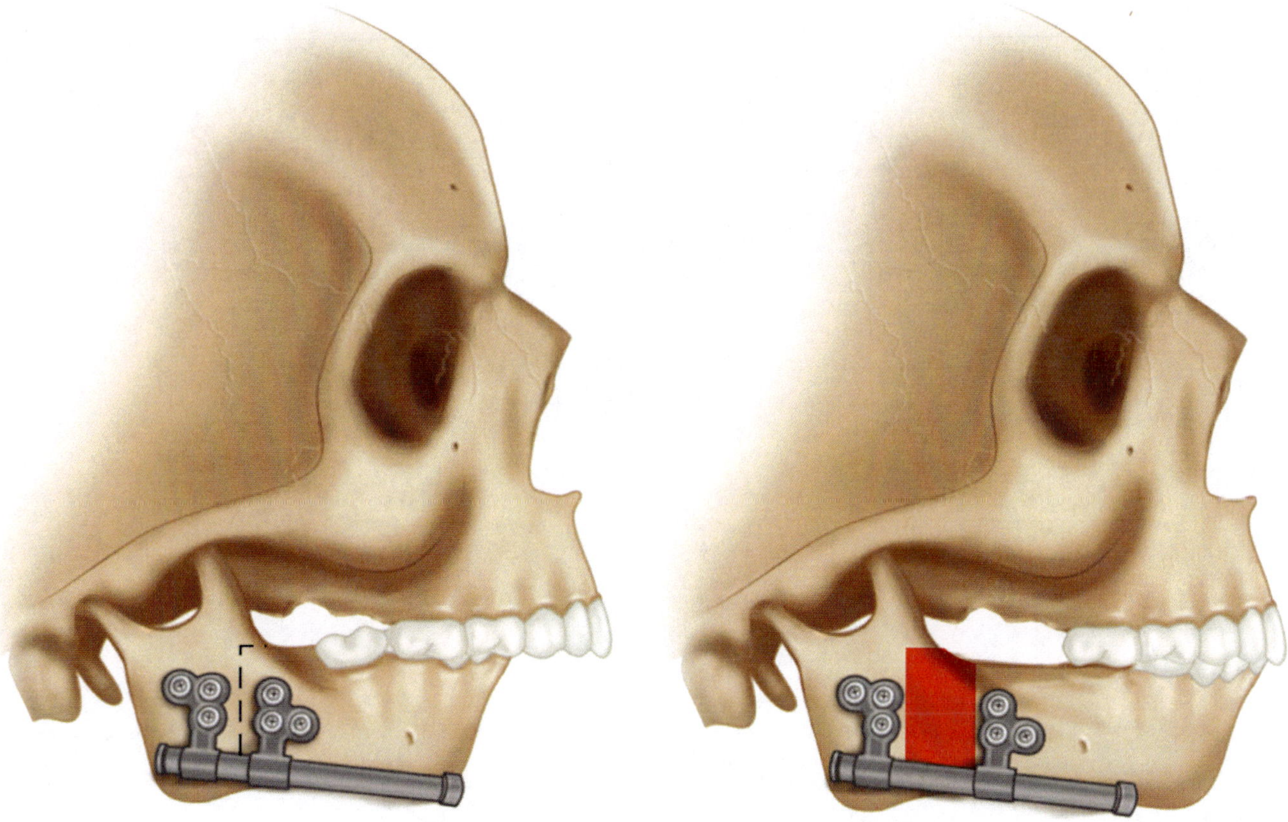

Fig. 34.4 Schematic showing placement of inverted L osteotomy and internal distractor. *Red* represents distractate

In 7–14 days, distraction is completed. Overcorrection is sought with the patient in a class III skeletal relationship at the end of distraction (mainly for airway improvement). Patients may be kept intubated for the first few days after device placement to allow for diminished swelling and increased airway dimension through distraction. Extubation occurs in the OR with nasopharyngoscopy to judge improved airway space. Oral feeding can begin within a day or two after extubation. Consolidation is typically 6 weeks. Postdistraction polysomnography is conducted 2 months after distraction. Limited evidence exists as to the long-term growth of distracted neonatal mandibles.

Childhood

Older children may also benefit from mandibular DO. Some are tracheostomy dependent patients from infancy with micrognathia. Others include micrognathic patients without a tracheostomy but with evidence of severe obstructive sleep apnea on polysomnography (see Fig. 34.6) not tolerating CPAP, or craniofacial microsomia patients with severe mandibular occlusal cants. In evaluating these patients, CT scans are helpful for surgical planning. With all mandibular distraction candidates, the surgeon must ensure that there is sufficient bone stock to place a distraction device. A severity level beyond the Pruzansky 2b category is typically not a distraction candidate. Using a 3D CT scan, the planned osteotomy, distraction vector, and result can be simulated with modern software techniques (see Figs. 34.7 and 34.8).

As with the neonate, mandibular osteotomies in a child must avoid tooth buds and the inferior alveolar nerve. A similar surgical approach is undertaken to access the mandible, except that the submandibular incision should be made lower on the neck. With growth the marginal mandibular nerve migrates inferior to the mandibular border. In children, we also prefer the inverted L osteotomy. Given the greater distance between the Risdon incision and the anterior ramus, an intraoral incision can be used to access the anterior ramus and to visualize the lingua (entrance of the inferior alveolar nerve). When using VSP, footplate and osteotomy guides can be used to precisely execute the bone cuts and position the internal distractors to achieve the desired vector. Internal devices are preferred by many but external devices using pins on either side of the osteotomy can also be used, as was favored early on. The latter offer the theoretical advantages of less dissection, which has not been shown that this would lead to better ossification of the generate. They can be used in a multiplanar fashion and in complex anomalies, although controlling multiple vectors can be difficult. Less desirable aspects of the external devices would include pin loosening and pin track scars on the face (see Fig. 34.9).

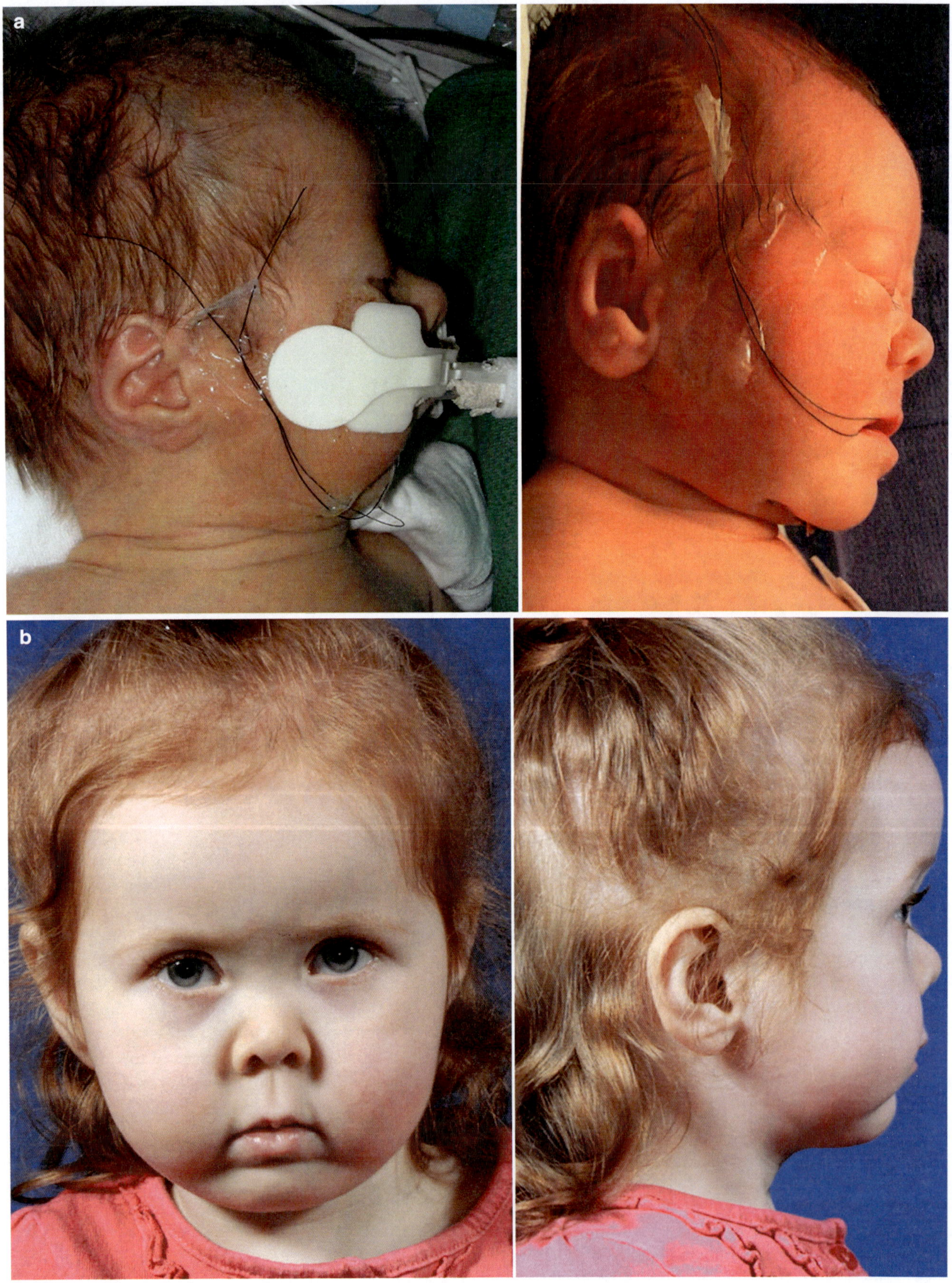

Fig. 34.5 (**a**) Six day old infant with Pierre Robin Sequence prior to mandibular osteotomies and device placement (*Left*), and 1 week later, immediately after extubation upon completion of 14 mm of horizontal mandibular distraction. (*Right*). (**b**) 22 months after bilateral mandibular distraction osteogenesis

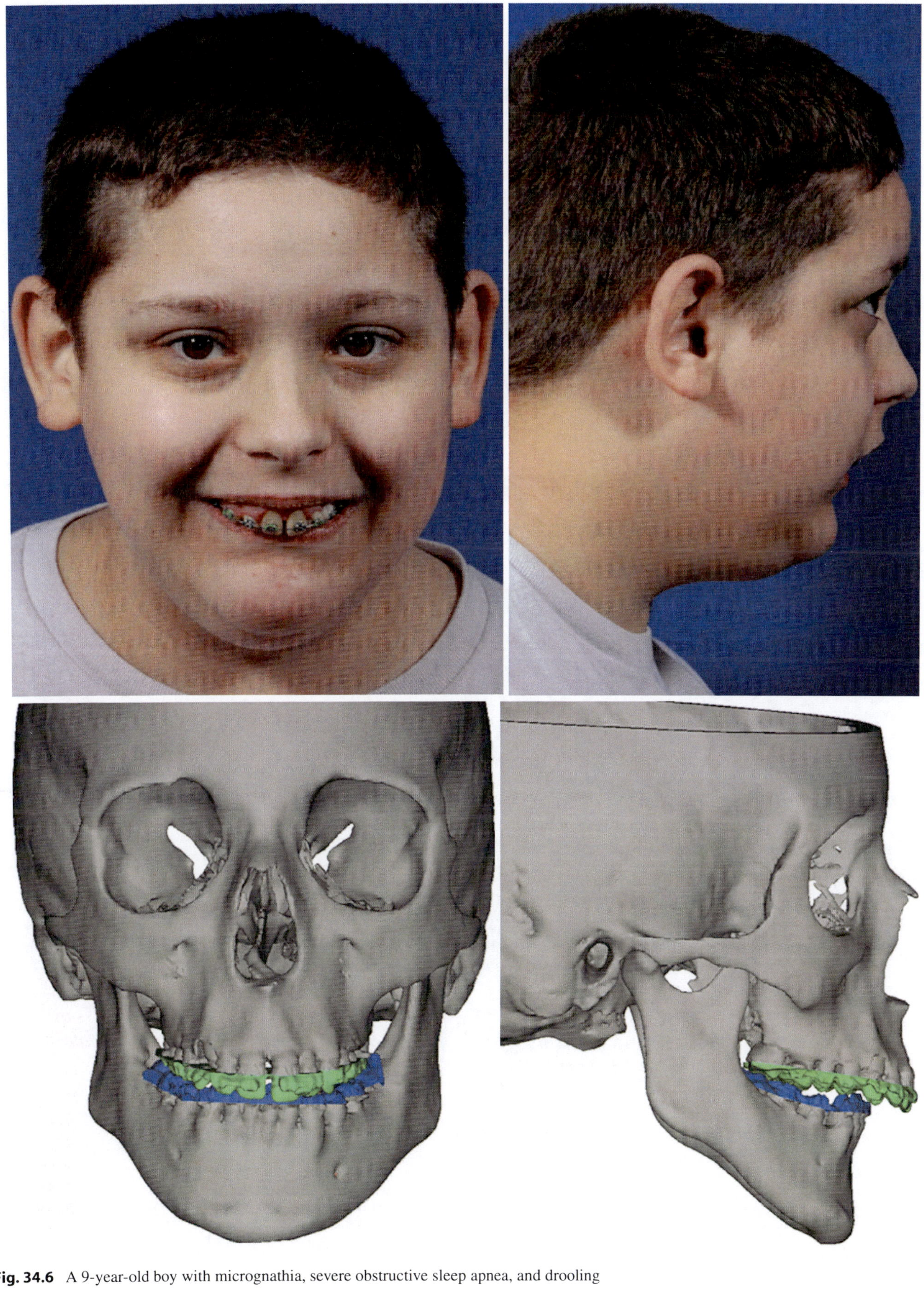

Fig. 34.6 A 9-year-old boy with micrognathia, severe obstructive sleep apnea, and drooling

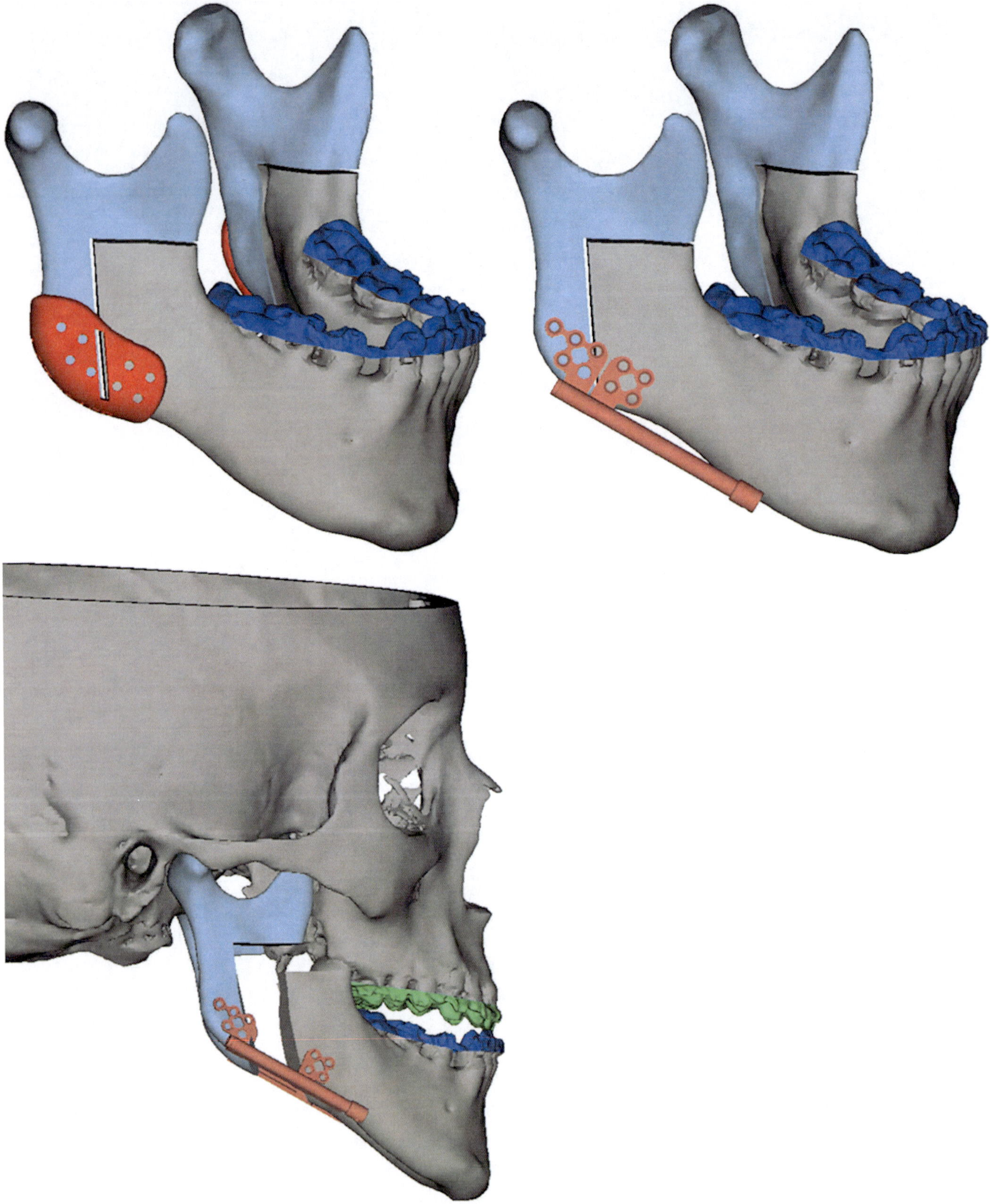

Fig. 34.7 Preoperative CT showing plan for inverted L osteotomy, device footplate guides, device positioning with vector planning, and below, computer simulation of completed distraction (expected mm of distraction) (Medical Modeling, Golden, CO)

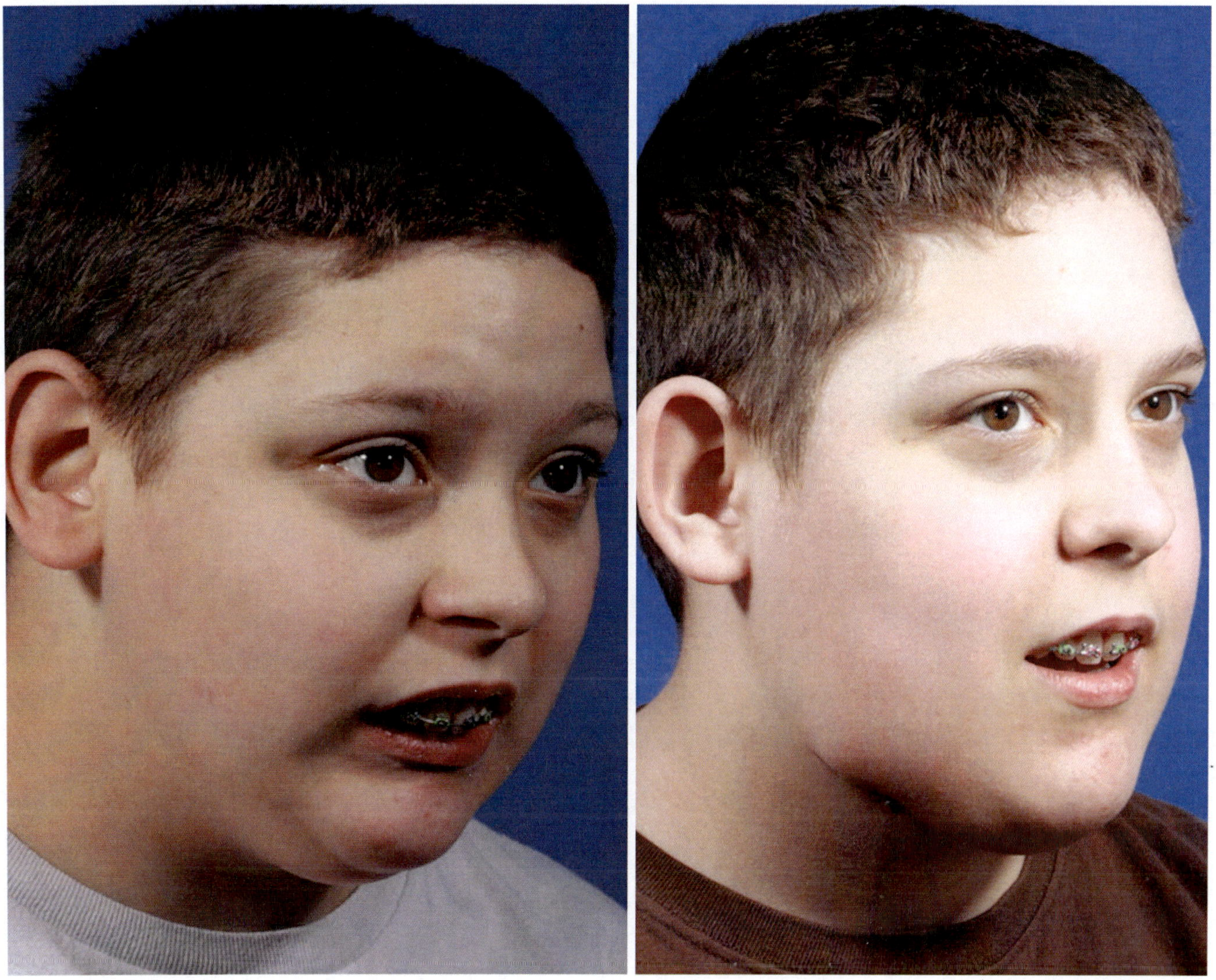

Fig. 34.8 Same patient preoperative oblique view (*left*) and (*right*) early consolidation phase with device present

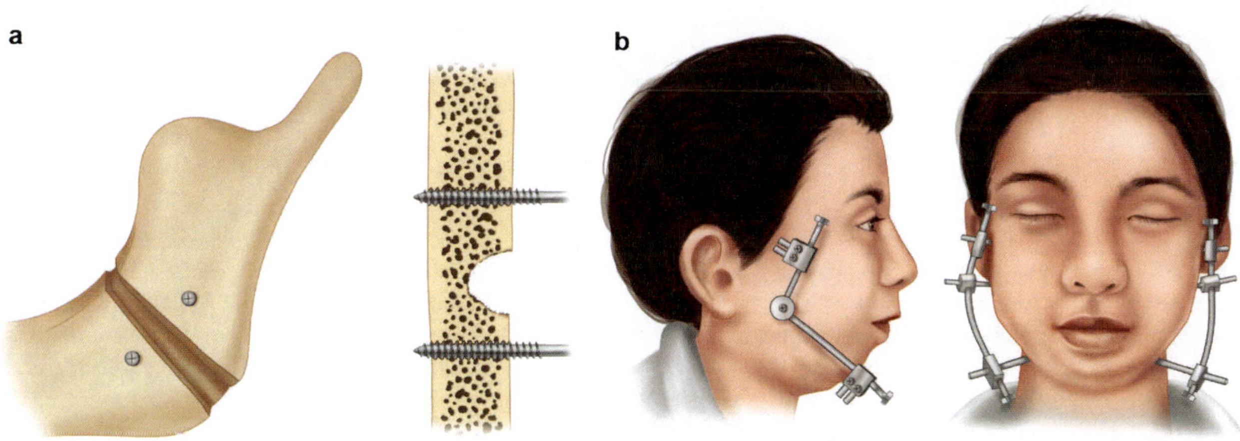

Fig. 34.9 Molina's patient with corticotomy technique (**a**) and (**b**) external distractors in place

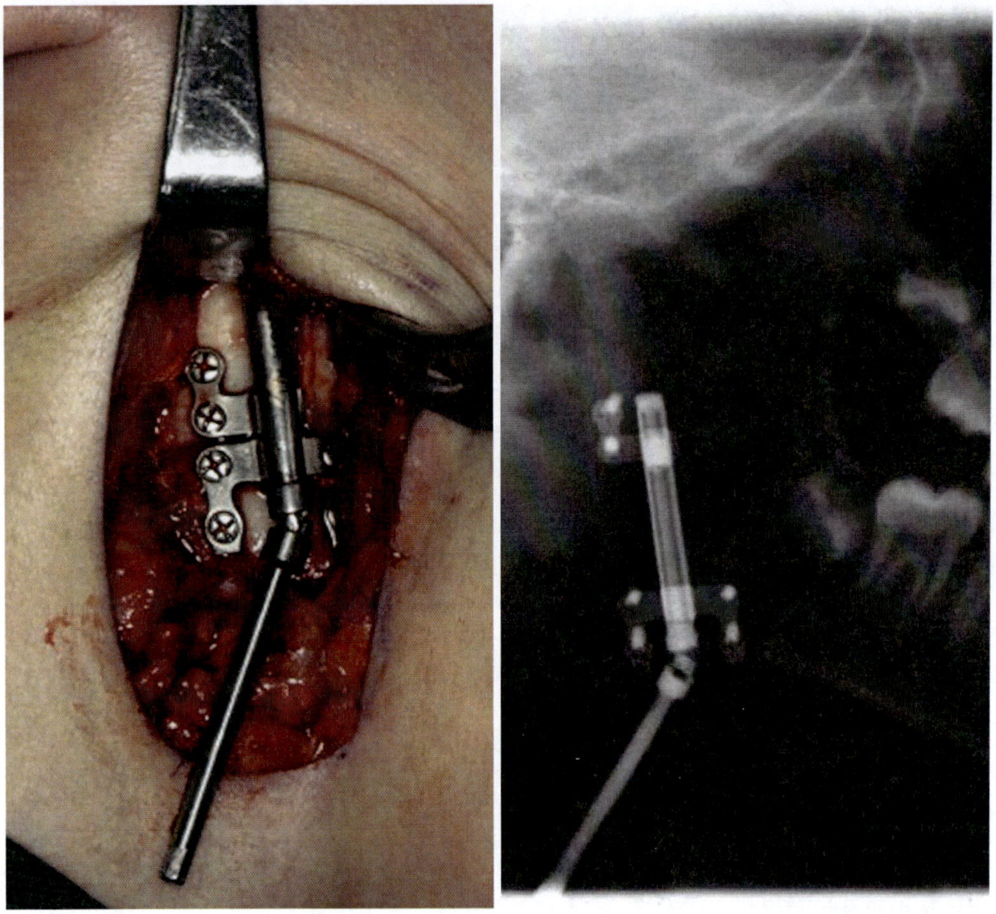

Fig. 34.10 Example of treatment of condylar hypoplasia with transport distraction. Schematic on *left*, with cephalogram on *right* illustrating movement of transport disk

Once the osteotomies are made and the devices placed, the total distraction course is longer than the neonate. Typically a 5–7-day latency is observed prior to device activation. Depending on the patient and indication for mandibular lengthening, a portion of the distraction may be able to be completed at home by the parents. Active distraction is 1 mm/day. Consolidation lasts 8 weeks but may be shortened slightly to allow for molding of the generate through use of orthodontic appliances and elastics. The end point of DO is skeletal class I or slightly class III.

Skeletally Mature Patient

Once growth has completed, certain patients have a significant class II malocclusion with or without the presence of severe obstructive sleep apnea. If patients with severe OSA present prior to completed skeletal growth, DO of the mandible may be an option to treat the OSA, knowing that a completion orthognathic procedure may be needed after growth completion. With skeletal maturity, traditional orthognathic techniques are preferred to correct mandibular hypoplasia with class II malocclusion. However, if there is a significant positive overjet (10 mm or more) and or deficient mandibular ramus to allow a traditional sagittal split osteotomy, or a significantly tight soft tissue envelope, DO would be preferred to achieve lengthening without a risk of relapse. Virtual planning can be used to plan precise osteotomies, vectors, and device placement. Typically, as in childhood mandibular DO, a combined intra/extraoral approach to osteotomy and internal device placement is used. Latency in this population is between 7 and 10 days, with a 1 mm/day rate of distraction and a 2-month consolidation period. Devices can be removed prior to complete consolidation for molding of the generate to achieve a better bite relationship. End point of DO is skeletal class I.

Transport Distraction of the Mandible

There are circumstances when a bone gap is present in the mandible. Congenitally, this may occur with severe hemifacial microsomia, with a Pruzansky 2b or 3 configuration (see Fig. 34.10). Posttraumatic or postresection bone gaps may also exist. Transport DO can successfully bridge segmental gaps, or help to create a neo-functioning TMJ in the case of severe hemifacial microsomia. An internal or external device can be used to achieve transport DO. The concept of transport DO is to liberate a small moveable segment of bone called the transport disk (see Fig. 34.11). This segment will move along a prescribed vector to bridge to another area of

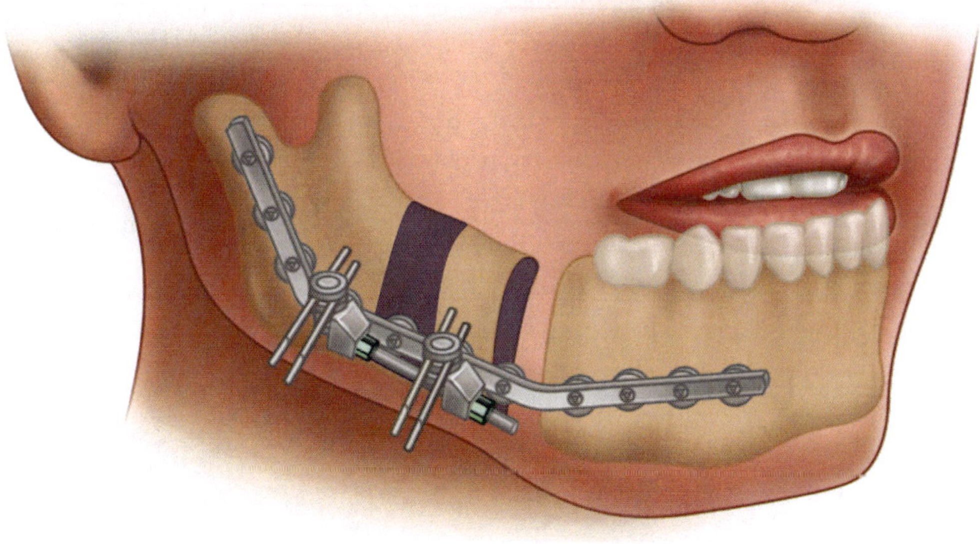

Fig. 34.11 Schematic of posttrauma/resection segmental mandibular defect treated with transport distraction. Transport disk is moving distally along the device, with new bone forming in the pink region

Table 34.3 Advantages of Le Fort I DO

Overcome soft tissue tightness (scar, hypoplasia)
Stable advancement
Preservation of speech
No bone graft

bone, or in the case of a congenital absence of the condyle, up the neo-TMJ. Complications include failure to align the transporting segment with the opposite stable bone and non-union at either the starting or ending points of transport.

Distraction Osteogenesis of the Maxilla

Patients with maxillary deficiency may also benefit from DO. Common diagnoses treated include clefts of the lip and palate, congenital maxillary hypoplasia, and Binder syndrome. Most of these patients require osteotomy at the Le Fort I level; however, patients with Binder syndrome require osteotomy at a higher Le Fort II level. When maxillary growth is complete, around age 12, the deficiency can be treated. When the patient's class III malocclusion (negative overjet) is less than 10 mm, a standard Le Fort I osteotomy with one step correction can be performed. However, with more severe conditions, such as those with a negative overjet of greater than 10 mm, overcoming soft tissue and scar limitations and creation of a stable advancement without relapse can be difficult. In these instances, Le Fort I by DO is preferred. In addition, bone grafting is not necessary when distraction is used. Past reports have shown that large negative overjets can be overcome with Le Fort I DO without degrading speech (see Table 34.3). Of importance when selecting a candidate for Le Fort I DO is that the maxilla is unified. Cleft lip/palate patients who have not undergone alveolar bone grafting to unite the segments are not candidates for DO.

There are several methods to achieve advancement by distraction. An external device fixed to the skull can be used (see Fig. 34.12a) that pulls the maxillary segment anterior via attachments to the bone or to an intraoral splint. The external distraction method moves the Le Fort I segment well and has the advantage of vector control, but the child must wear a large external rig during the consolidation period. Advocates of this technique typically remove the halo prior to complete consolidation (approximately one month after active distraction) and guide the generate with class III elastics. A completely internal device can also be used to achieve Le Fort I DO (see Fig. 34.12b). This device spans the osteotomy and pushes the inferior, mobile segment anteriorly. It is well tolerated by the patients but is more challenging to use in patients with asymmetric hypoplasia and limited bone inferior to the osteotomy above the tooth roots for footplate positioning. A third method involves a partial bone-borne, partial orthodontic-borne device.

Planning for patients undergoing Le Fort I DO with a partially orthodontic and partially bone anchored device involves virtually planning and possibly fabrication of a model. Presurgical planning includes the anticipated amount of distraction, the vector of distraction, and guides for precise placement of preoperatively constructed partial orthodontic, partially bone born distraction devices. The surgical plan may include overcorrection of the existing deformity into a slight class II relationship (see Fig. 34.13a–c).

Intraoperatively, with the patient under anesthesia via nasotracheal intubation, standard subperiosteal exposure of the maxilla is obtained. Positioning guides for the zygoma-borne footplates of the distractors are placed. After predictive footplate holes are drilled, a standard Le Fort I osteotomy is completed. Downfracture at the Le Fort I level is performed with Rowe disimpaction forceps. Any posterior bony interferences are taken down with rongeurs. The Le Fort I segment is reduced. Zygomatic footplates of the devices are mounted using the predrilled predictive footplate holes. The lower device footplates rest along the orthodontic appliances and are secured to the orthodontics with multiple 28-gauge wires. Turning arms are attached to the devices and the distractors are tested and returned to the zero position.

The distraction course for Le Fort I DO is as follows. Standard latency period is 7 days. Devices are activated at 1 mm/day until the desired correction is achieved. Consolidation is typically 6–8 weeks. Molding of the generate can be performed if need be with earlier device removal. Using the partially orthodontic bone device with presurgical virtual planning lends itself to the need for less generate molding, however.

Combined Maxilla/Mandible

In patients with both maxillary and mandibular deficiency, simultaneous DO of both jaws has been described. Skeletally

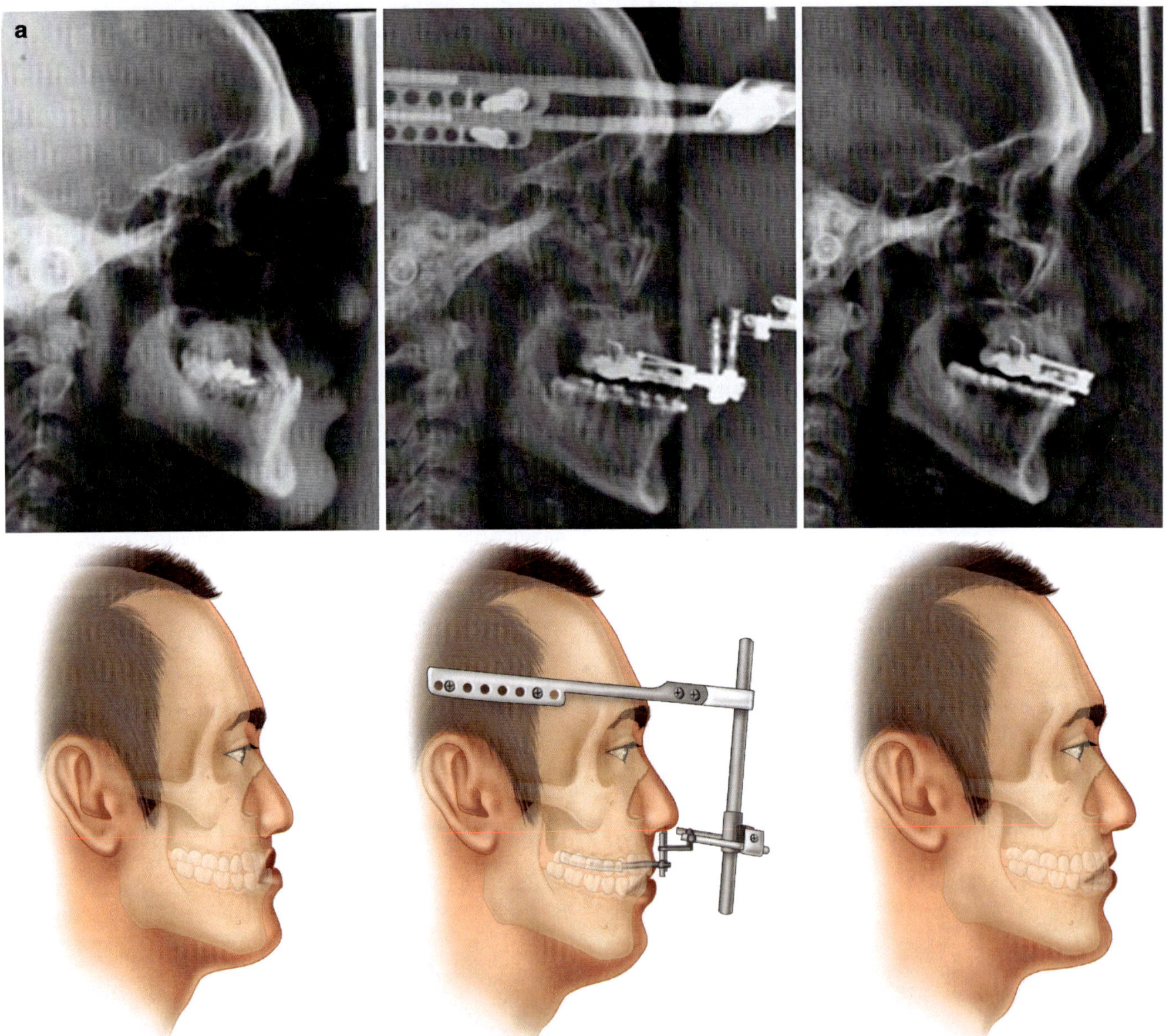

Fig. 34.12 (**a**) Patient with cleft lip/palate and maxillary hypoplasia treated with RED (rigid external device) (KLS Martin Group, Jacksonville, FL). (**b**) Drawing of internal maxillary distraction device

Fig. 34.12 (continued)

b

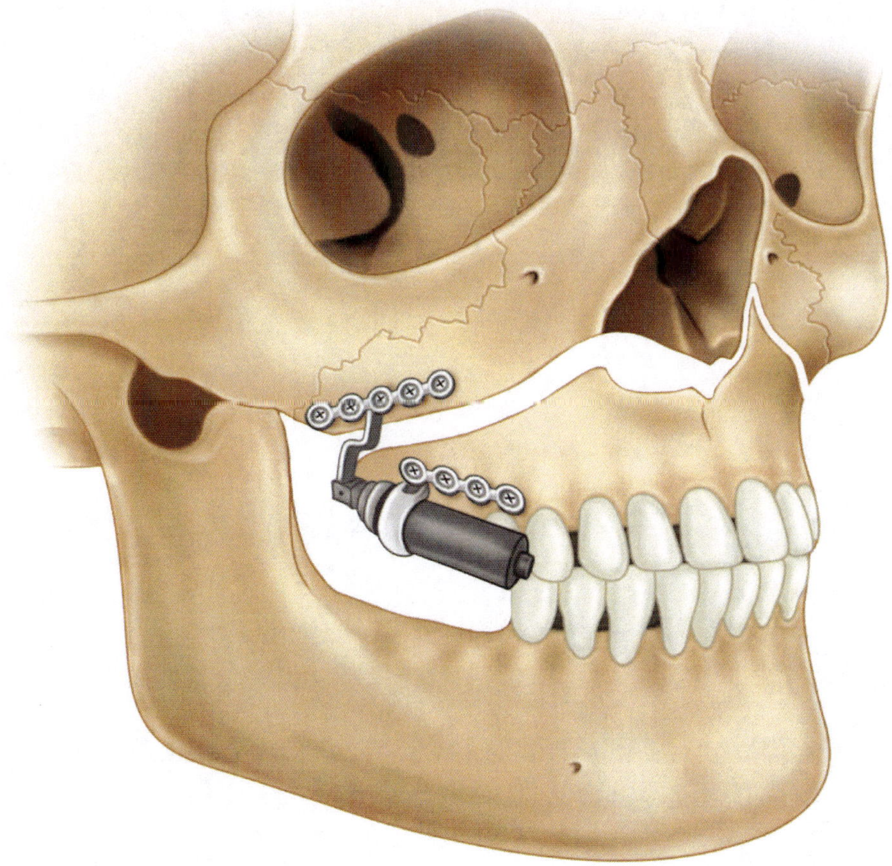

mature patients with severe hemifacial microsomia have roll deformities of both the maxilla and mandible. With limited vertical growth of the mandibular ramus in a patient with severe hemifacial microsomia, who has not undergone mandibular DO in childhood, the maxillary growth on the affected side is limited. These occlusal cant deformities can present challenges when attempting to achieve skeletal correction with traditional orthognathic surgical movements. In addition to the skeletal deformity, soft tissue is limited on the affected side. Monasterio and Molina have addressed this two jaw and soft tissue deformities with bimaxillary DO in patients with Pruzansky 1 or 2 hemifacial microsomia (see Fig. 34.14). After osteotomy of the mandibular ramus on the affected side and Le Fort I osteotomy, the patient is placed in maxillomandibular fixation (MMF). External distraction of the affected mandibular ramus is conducted with the Le Fort segment moving passively in the MMF.

Cranium

Distraction is used in the cranium less frequently than other areas and no real clear indications have developed. Lauritzen performed much of the pioneering work on this concept using springs. It appears that distraction is mostly being used to solve unique and less commonly encountered diagnoses and clinical circumstances. The cranium is different than many other bones in which distraction has developed as a predominant treatment modality. The bones are relatively thin in youth and intimately related to the CSF space presenting the challenge of achieving stable fixation without injuring the meninges and increasing the risk of life-threatening meningitis. Additionally, the cranium does not incur a great deal of stress forces that stimulate bone hypertrophy in healing, yet the cranium has demonstrated remarkable ability to regenerate in gaps in ages below 18 months.

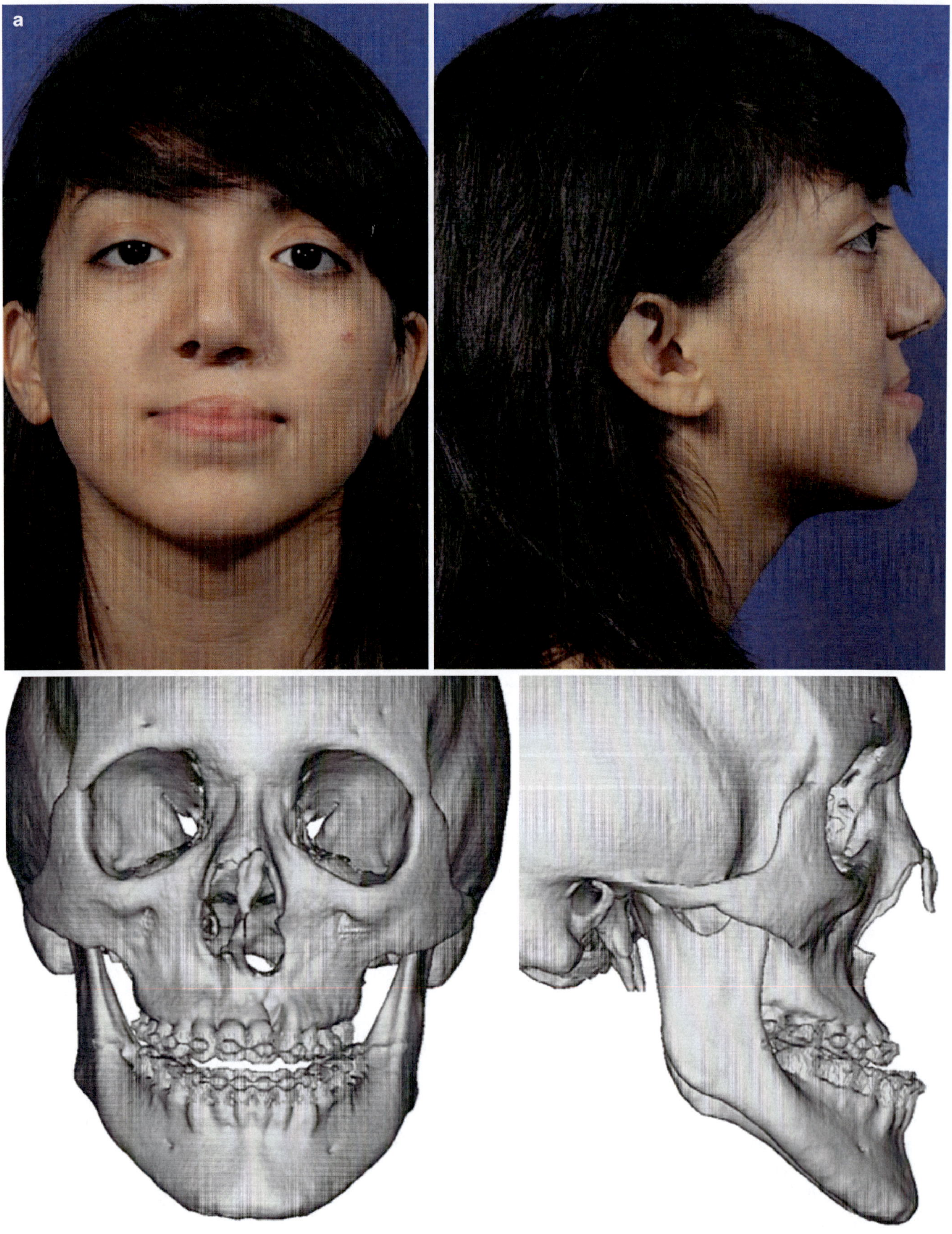

Fig. 34.13 (**a**) Patient with cleft-related maxillary hypoplasia and class III malocclusion. (**b**) *Upper* – Computer-simulated Le Fort I osteotomy with maxillary distractor (Medical Modeling, Golden, CO) (partial bone, partial orthodontic-borne device, KLS Martin Group, Jacksonville, FL). (**c**) Predistraction and 1-year postdistraction cephalograms

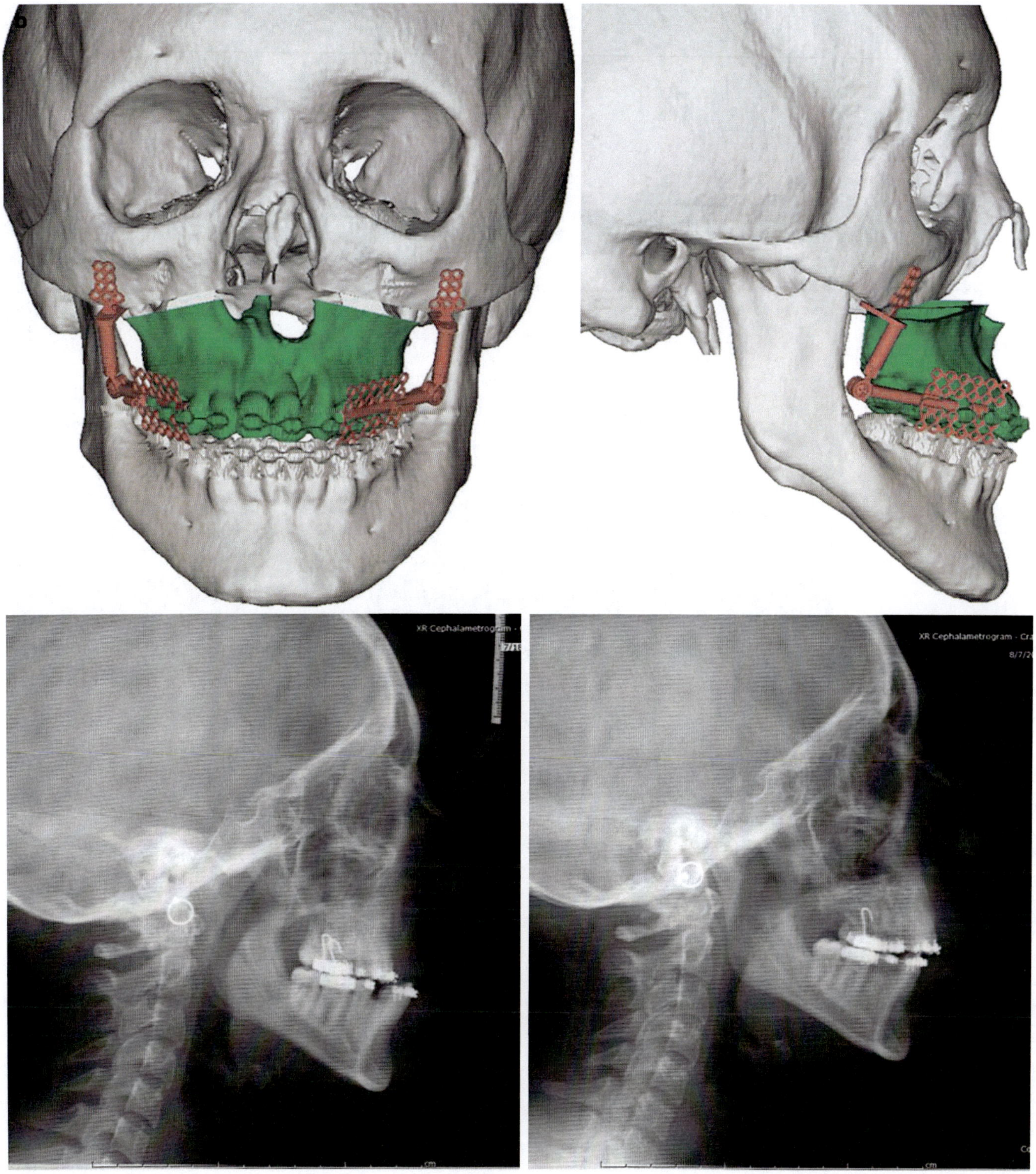

Fig. 34.13 (continued)

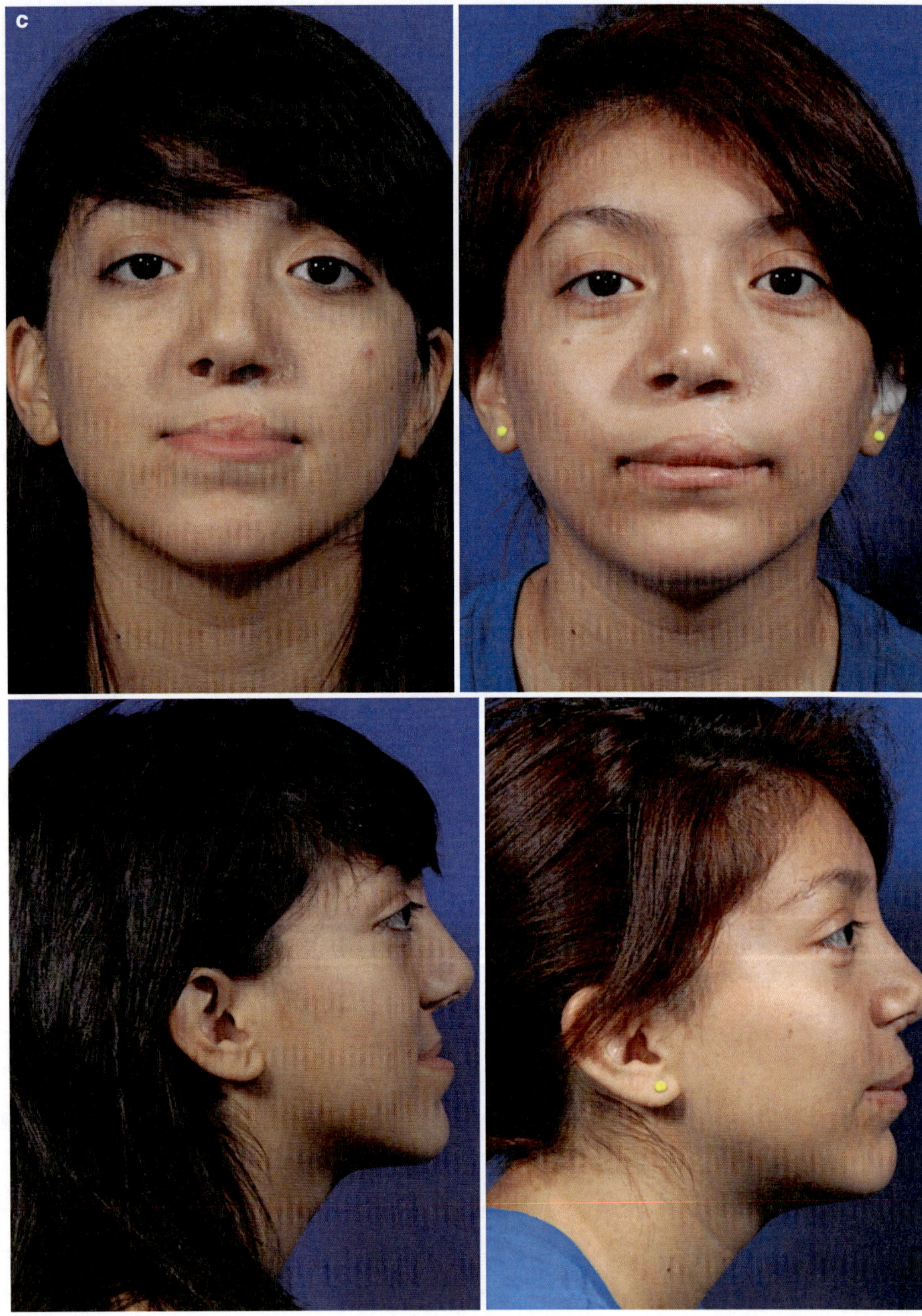

Fig. 34.13 (continued)

Distraction employed as a method to expand the cranium has several advantages over traditional expansion procedures theoretically. Distraction allows for a slower, gradual expansion, which avoids the epidural dead space with its inherent risks created in procedures that acutely expand the cranial volume (see Fig. 34.15). Slower expansion also allows the scalp to more slowly accommodate expansion and therefore great degrees of scalp expansion can be achieved akin to the degrees of expansion afforded by a tissue expander in the scalp versus a large rotation flap of the scalp. This is an

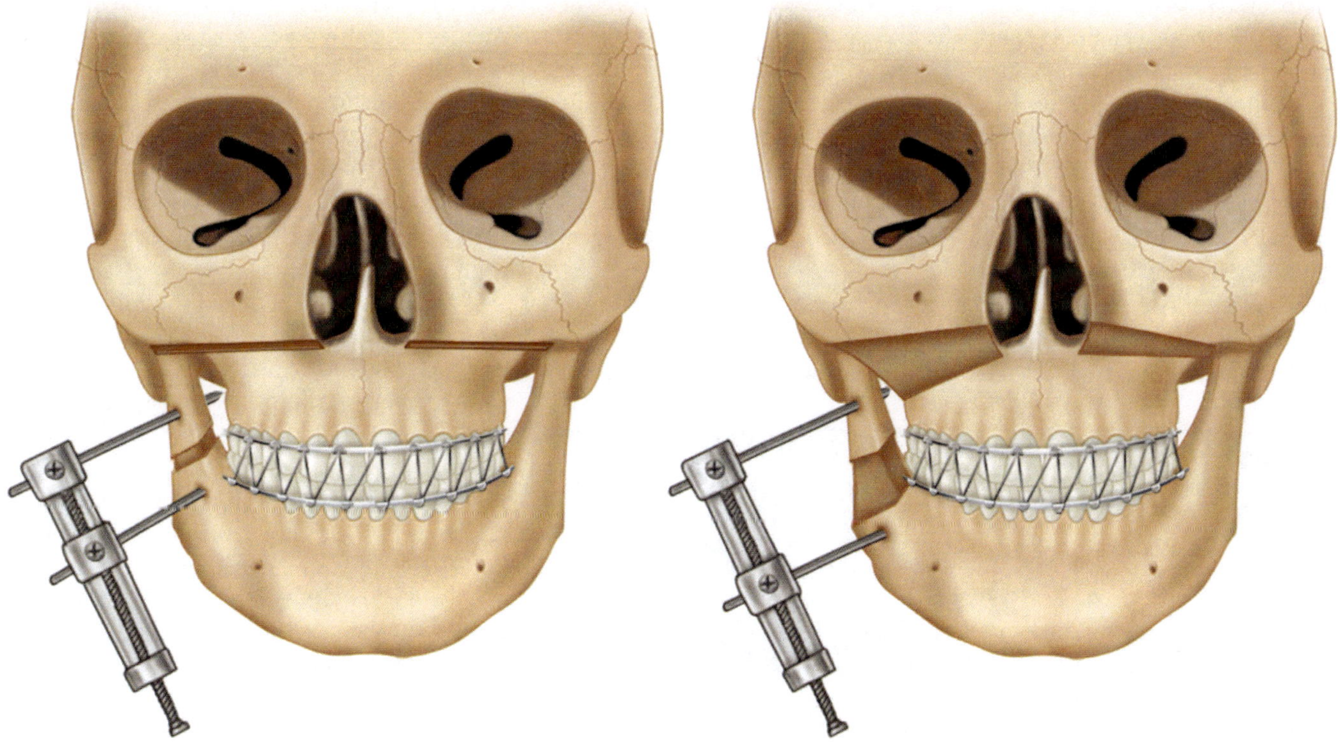

Fig. 34.14 Schematic of Monasterio/Molina simultaneous maxillary and mandibular distraction, treating R-sided hemifacial microsomia. Le Fort I osteotomy and R mandibular osteotomy, placement of maxillomandibular fixation, and mandibular distractor application. Distraction of the mandibular device corrects the roll deformity of both jaws

important factor since it is often the scalp that limits the volume expansion achieved in traditional single-staged expansion procedures. Additionally, there are more opportunities to maintain vascularity of the cranial bone segments using a distraction method, whereas traditional procedures turn the cranial bone into bone grafts. Distraction procedures are designed to create bone, therefore theoretically reducing reliance on donor bone grafts and minimizing long-term bone defects.

On the other hand there are several disadvantages to cranial distraction. The greatest limitation is that the cranium is a complex three-dimensional structure reconstruction which often requires complex three-dimensional movements which is not easily achieved by bulky uniplanar distractors available on the market today (see Fig. 34.16). The cranium is thin in youth, which challenges adequate fixation of distractors, which need to bear the force of expansion. Lastly, secondary procedures are now required to remove the device, the inconvenience of which may be overcome by enhanced bone formation and minimizing secondary cranial defects themselves requiring additional procedures and donor sites.

Patients with multiple-suture synostosis including syndromic patients often experience elevated intracranial pressure and its sequelae early and ideally benefit from total cranial vault expansion. These patients are often remarkable for a progressive turricephaly. There is questionable utility to repeated expansions of the anterior cranial fossa when an

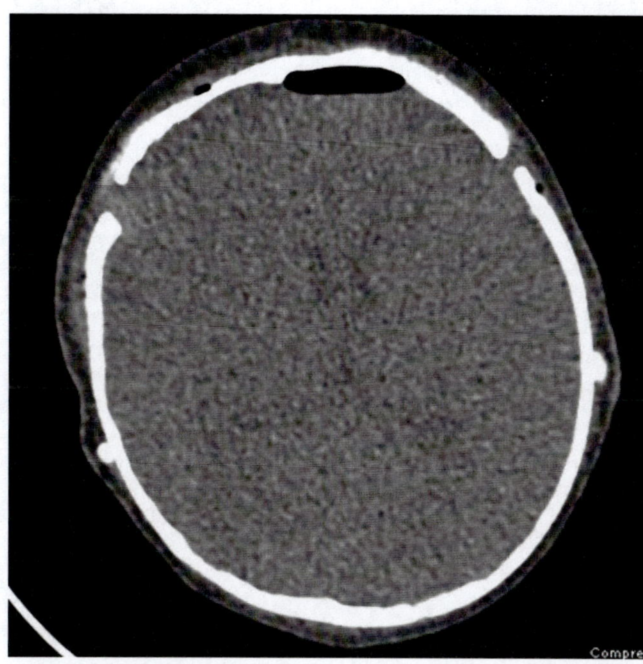

Fig. 34.15 Epidural dead space created by traditional cranial expansion procedures that increases risk of infection and compromises blood flow to cranial bone secondary to lack of contact

underdeveloped cranium restricts other regions. This is the reason that Chiari malformations are treated with a posterior vault expansion and not an anterior vault expansion. Our protocol has been to expand the posterior cranial vault as an initial procedure beginning when the patient first starts to demonstrate signs and symptoms of elevated pressure (usually before 6 months of age) (see Fig. 34.17). Traditional expansions are challenged in this early age group by the fact that the bone is thin and soft and does not lend itself to rigid fixation. The posterior vault often relapses under the pressure of the expanded scalp and with recumbent positioning of the child during sleep, which is difficult to avoid in this age group. Also pertinent here is the fact that these patients have an extreme undersupply of cranial bone (reason for their symptoms) and bone graft donor material. Often the patient has a large number of defects and a fairly weak posterior and mid-vault to base the second-stage anterior cranial vault expansion.

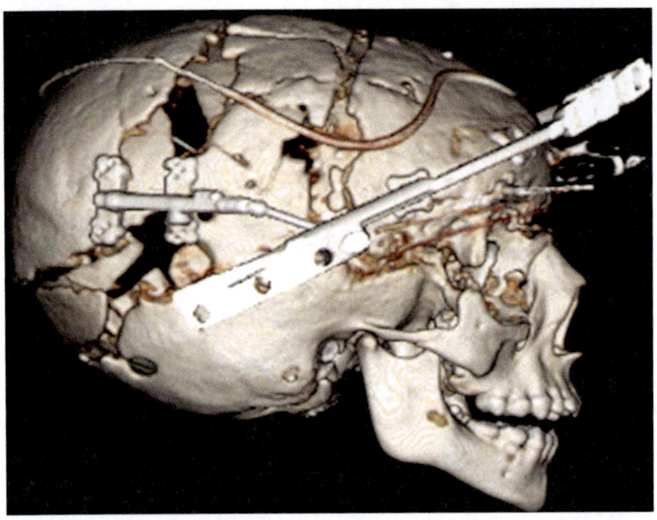

Fig. 34.16 Scaphocephaly induced by distraction secondary to the limited vector of expansion afforded by today's devices

Posterior vault distraction can be used to overcome the limitations of thin immature cranial bone and the late sequelae of cranial defects and its impact on the stability of anterior cranial vault expansion. Expanding the posterior vault at a reasonably early age will also limit the degree of turricephaly that develops in these patients. A traditional zigzag, coronal scalp incision is employed to expose the posterior two-thirds of the cranium. Cranial cuts are made with a side-cutting craniotome leaving the bone attached to the dura in all areas. The posterior cut is made inferior to the transverse sinus at the torcula but traverses it in the region of the asterion. Greenstick out-fracture of the base of the occiput prevents any step-off from developing as the posterior vault is expanded by the distractors. We employ two cranial distractors (KLS Martin), which have ball joints strategically incorporated to relieve stress on the distractors which inevitably occurs as a result of the inability to achieve a single harmonious vector between the distractors due to the asymmetry inevitably present. Distractor arms emerge through the incision anteriorly.

Standard latency protocol for this procedure is 7 days. Once initiated, the devices are turned 0.5 mm twice daily for a rate of 1 mm/day. Consolidation period is limited to 2 months. Some modification of these time frames and rates can be made based on the age and bone regenerating capacity of the patient.

Another group of patients for which cranial distraction has been used are those with a history of multiple cranial expansion procedures yet still need more expansion in context of a heavily scarred and tight scalp. The slow and gradual expansion of the

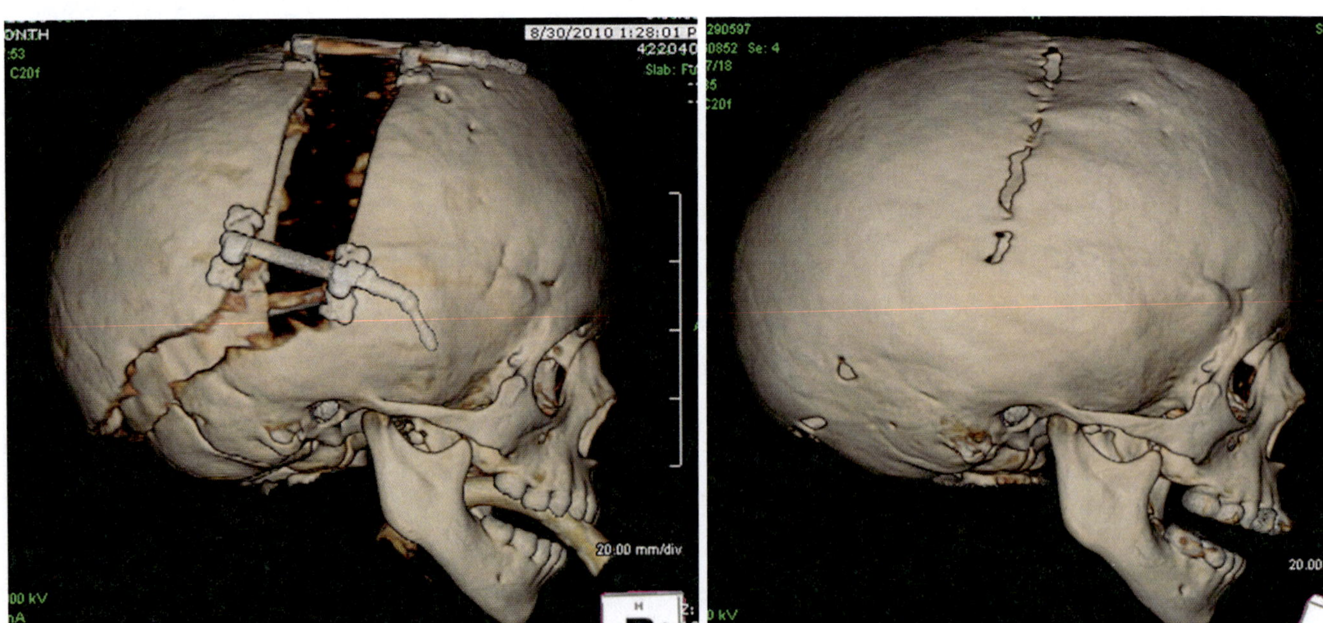

Fig. 34.17 Posterior cranial vault distraction in a patient with multisuture synostosis as an initial stage to prevent progressive turricephaly. Note the amount of generate bone in this early consolidation image

cranium prevents any further deterioration of the scalp. This strategy should only be applied to patients that need expansion in a single plane. The last group of patients where distraction has offered a benefit is patients with late-onset single- or multiple-suture synostosis who present with a normal cranial morphology but inadequate volume and elevated pressure. These patients can usually be treated by a single vector movement, and by using distraction, donor sites are not required and the generate bone can result in a bilaminar skull with excellent quality avoiding long-term activity restriction.

Orbit/Upper Midface

The application of distraction to the orbital and upper midface region has significantly improved outcomes of the procedures used to address exorbitism and midface hypoplasia, when severe presents as obstructive nasal breathing and sleep apnea. Distraction applied to the Le Fort I segment was discussed earlier but will be addressed here as well, as it applies to the movement of the maxillary dentition along with the orbits. The two primary procedures are the Le Fort III and Monobloc. These procedures are usually not attempted until the patient has at least completed growth in the orbital region, which is around 7 years of age in boys and girls.

The major functional purpose of the Le Fort III procedure is to advance the lower half of the orbital rim to achieve greater depth to the orbit to accommodate the globe and position the lower eyelid such that it can reach the upper lid for closure and protection of the cornea. There is a strong tendency for function to follow form in this region so reestablishing a normal appearance is often accompanied by a return to functional globe protection. It must be remembered that these operations are first and foremost orbital in nature. Attempts to prioritize the occlusion over the orbit can lead to disastrous results with either under-correction and persistent exorbitism or more commonly enophthalmos which is very difficult to correct once established. The Monobloc procedure additionally aims to increase the intracranial volume in the anterior cranial fossa. Usually an adequate expansion is associated with a precise correction of the orbital position so positioning the lateral orbital rim at the mid-axis of the globe is a good technique for judging the end point of advancement.

The great number of bony interferences and mass of soft tissue that has to move with these procedures generates a great deal of resistance. This is especially true with movements beyond 3–5 mm; distraction with its slow and steady movements is much more effective with much less relapse potential than a single-staged advancement. Additionally, a pulling force on the central face with the lateral components "riding along" is much more reliable and effective for overcoming the resistance than any technique that pushes from the outside margins. This observation comes from the high rate of failures generated by internal distractors pushing from the temporal fossa region relative to the very reliable RED distractor (KLS Martin), which pulls from an anterior and more central vector. Our preference is to use the RED almost exclusively. Although this is an external distractor, the transcutaneous anchoring points are in line with the vector of distraction so pin track scars are not an issue with the use of this device. The patient is left with very little permanent hardware and the device can be removed without making any surgical incisions other than minor pin site suturing. The most important advantage of the RED is that the surgeon maintains complete three-dimensional control of movement. This device does require sturdy bone in the supra-auricular region for securing the device and is almost impossible to use when not present.

Le Fort III

The Le Fort III procedure is completed in the same fashion as the traditional procedure and with the same degree of mobilization of the mobile segment. Failure to mobilize the segment adequately is the most common reason for failure to advance sufficiently. Our most common approach to the orbital and upper midface is via a coronal scalp incision although a subcranial approach using a series of palpebral incisions has been described. It is best to avoid lower eyelid incisions and complete the orbital osteotomies via the coronal and a complete degloving of the orbit. Care is taken to avoid the detachment of the medial canthal tendon. The nasoglabellar osteotomy must be completed in such a manner that it avoids entrance into the anterior cranial fossa and CSF violation and leak. The point of osteotomy of the lateral orbit depends on where the orbit becomes hypoplastic. If the entire lateral orbit is underdeveloped, then the superior-lateral orbit can be included with a greenstick in the mid-lateral orbit so that a gradual movement occurs superiorly and a greater advancement occurs inferiorly. Every attempt should be made to avoid any stairstepping at the mid-lateral orbit where the soft tissue envelope is thin and the step-off will look odd. If the lateral orbit is in reasonable position, then a lower osteotomy can be performed in the region of the upper edge of the inferior orbital rim and the superior edge of the arch. The soft tissues are thicker there so any stairstep is easily concealed. Osteotomy of the arch is best made as posterior and possible to avoid and mid-lateral cheek depression. The temporalis muscles should be completely mobilized if the osteotomy is anywhere above the mid-lateral orbital rim to avoid any soft tissue contour depression. While mobilizing the temporalis the surgeon should pay careful attention to avoid injuring the deep temporal motor nerve on its deep surface to avoid any atrophy. The muscle and canthal tendon are reattached to their respective places on the transport segment to maintain the normal soft tissue-bone relationships.

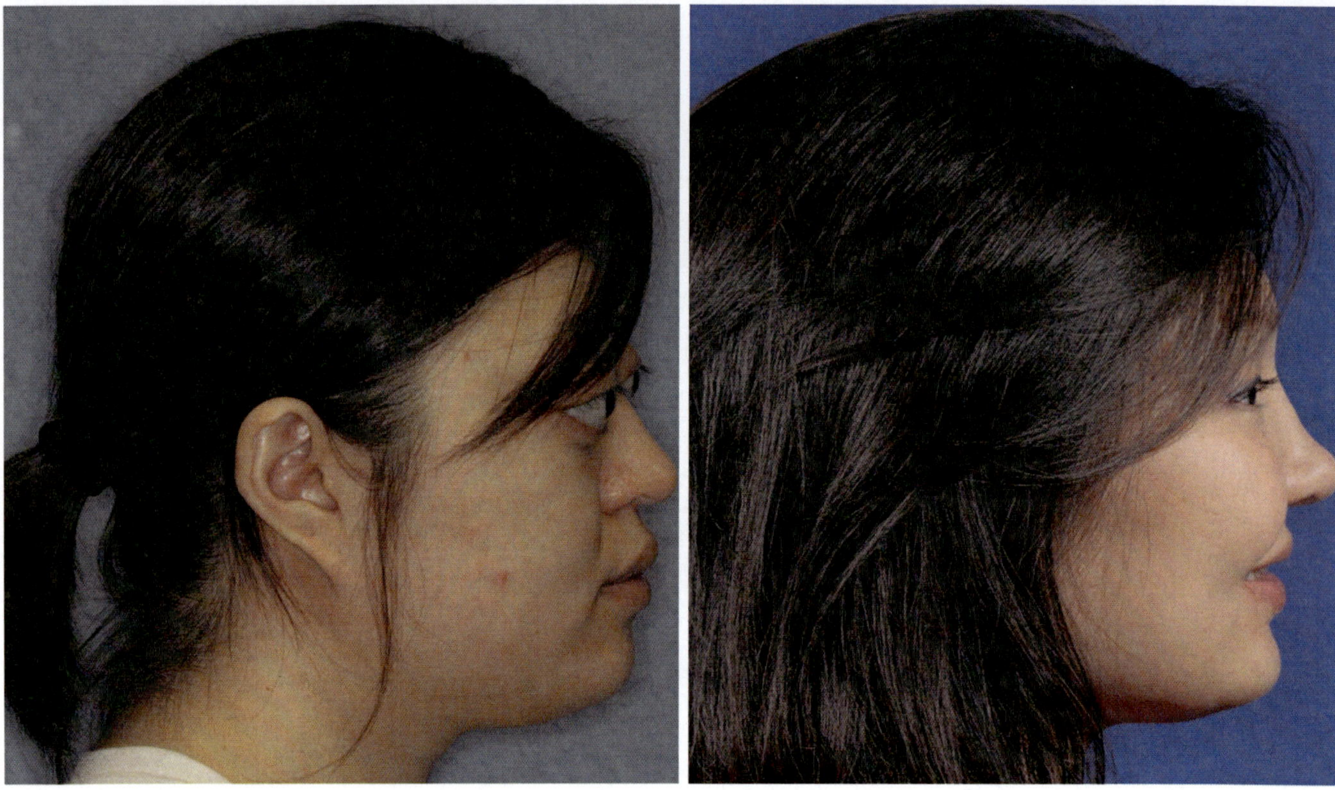

Fig. 34.18 Preoperative and postoperative lateral photos of a patient who underwent a distraction Monobloc procedure to treat exorbitism and elevated intracranial pressure. Note the natural appearance around the orbit because the orbit is kept as a single unit

Inclusion of the Le Fort I segment requires a pterygoid dysjunction; exclusion requires a septal osteotomy at the maxillary crest. It cannot be stressed enough that the Le Fort III segment must be mobilized very well as if the segment was going to be advanced without distraction; it should then be allowed to settle back into its native location to initiate callus formation during the latency period.

After the segment is mobilized and settled back into position, a decision is made about the location of the wire attachment. A minimum of four wires with two on the upper portion and two on the lower portion of the transport segment ensures true three-dimensional control of the movement. Areas with thick bone where pin-retaining plates can be located include the mid-inferior orbital rim, the body of the zygoma, and the inferior pyriform margin. If the Le Fort I segment is transported, then wire attachment to a dental splint or firm arch wire is arranged to avoid any contact or displacement of the lip, which can easily be ulcerated over time.

Latency for Le Fort III procedure is 7–10 days with transport of 1 mm/day divided twice daily. Of course alterations need to be made as discussed previously. Consolidation for these patients is usually as short as possible since the cranial halo is so uncomfortable and makes it difficult to function and sleep. The advancement can be considered stable when the transport wires become loose. This usually occurs three to six weeks into consolidation. Early in consolidation, the segment is still very easily moved especially by any occlusal forces at play. Therefore, care must be taken to avoid the influence of these forces on the final position especially if the advancement results in a malocclusion which will try to work itself out while the generate bone is still moldable. Either longer consolidation or the strategic use of bite splints can be employed to prevent this effect. Strategic use of non-chew diets is also very effective and awareness of grinding preoperatively is very important in this situation. If circumstances allow the bite to become a priority, then early removal and strategically applied elastics will mold the generate bone into a favorable occlusal relationship if these forces are applied very early in consolidation.

Monobloc

The Monobloc advances the entire orbit so it is a particularly effective and stable way of treating a patient whose orbits are hypoplastic in all dimensions (see Fig. 34.18). Our center uses the Monobloc primarily in syndromic diagnoses who suffer from multiple sutures fusing. We attempt to expand the posterior fossa as much as possible early in life in an attempt to preserve the integrity of the orbits, essentially buying time until a single Monobloc procedure can be performed to address the anterior cranial fossa and the orbits in one operation. The bones must be sufficiently mature and calcified to accept rigid fixation for a Monobloc to be successful.

Distraction of the Monobloc segment is very similar to the Le Fort III with the exception that it requires an intracranial and extracranial approach to mobilize the segment. The addition of the entire circumferential orbit and a variable portion of the forehead to the Le Fort III segment constitutes the Monobloc. In addition, the forehead is turned into a bone graft by the bifrontal craniotomy so it is subject to all issues of a graft especially resorption. By expanding the anterior cranial fossa gradually, there really is very little issue with epidural dead space. This issue is the primary reason why distracting the Monobloc reduced the complications associated with the procedure which were unacceptably high and morbid including a reasonably high risk of death. The primary risk surrounding the Monobloc procedure is the osteotomy in the anterior portion of the floor of the anterior cranial fossa which creates a communication between the nasal cavity and the anterior cranial fossa. This osteotomy violates the integrity of this separating barrier, and distraction seems to prevent both acute and long-term risk of meningeal infections originating in the nose.

The surgical access to the Monobloc procedure is the same as the Le Fort III with the addition of a bifrontal craniotomy. Again, the inferior eyelid access can and should be avoided to prevent degloving if possible. If required, soft tissue suspension should be performed (ala Gruss). Just like the Le Fort III procedure, the Monobloc is primarily an orbital and cranial volume procedure and not an occlusal procedure, so if the Le Fort I segment is included, some degree of malocclusion should be anticipated, understanding that a Le Fort I (and possible a mandible procedure) will be required closer to the time of skeletal maturity to resolve malocclusion. As with the Le Fort III, care should be taken to avoid detaching the medial canthal tendon. The temporalis muscle and the lateral canthal tendon are handled in the same fashion.

Special attention must be focused on the osteotomy through the cribriform plate. We use cortical bone grafts from the inner table of the frontal bone which are fixated to the Monobloc segment with intracranial plates and designed to override the cribriform posteriorly so that as the Monobloc segment advances the bone gradually slides in to fill the void created. Additionally, a large pericranial flap is raised at the time of the coronal exposure. It is used to interpose between the thin dura of the cranial base and the bone to create an additional layer of protection from the nasal cavity. The Monobloc especially requires very aggressive mobilization. Because it is such a large transport segment, it is very susceptible to interferences and resistance. Once allowed to settle back into its native position, a decision about the location of wire attachment is made. Ideally, six wires (two on superior orbit, two on inferior orbit/zygoma, two on maxillary dentition) are employed which will give perfect control over the segment.

Reducing the risk of cerebral and meningeal infection is paramount. While distraction has reduced complication by eliminating the acute creation of a large epidural dead space, complication still can occur and be very severe. Several points on this issue will be discussed. If the patient has a frontal sinus and it is violated during the surgery, cultures should be taken as documentation of resident flora. Strong consideration should be given to cranializing the sinus especially if the drainage of the sinus is damage or compromised. In addition to the bone grafts and pericranial flap, we manage patients with broad-spectrum antibiotics for 72 h postoperatively and maintain intubation for at least 72–96 h to prevent coughing and other causes of elevated positive airway pressure from causing material in the nose from being forced into the anterior cranial fossa, allowing a strong fibrin seal to form. Additionally, this is a very important aspect of safe airway management since nasal swelling and tongue swelling often put the airway at risk for obstruction and reintubation is very difficult in these patients postoperatively especially with a RED device interfering. Temporary tarsorrhaphy should also be considered especially if exorbitism is severe to protect the corneas during the acute swelling phase.

Latency is usually 7–10 days with a rate of 1 mm/day divided twice daily. Position of the lateral orbit again is a good measure for the end point of distraction. Loosening of wires again can be used to determine when to remove the device. The same occlusal concerns as the Le Fort III exist with the Monobloc. The Monobloc is a very big endeavor with significant risks and perioperative changes that the patient and family should be prepared for. The craniofacial team should be ready for supporting the family during the recovery process. Most patients are happy that they had the procedure but would not be willing to experience it again if required so care must be taken to make sure the initial procedure is successful.

Complications

Complications during the distraction process can be broken down into those related to adequate bone generation and those related to effects on the surrounding soft tissue envelope. Inadequate generation of bone is caused by either device failure, errors in technique, inappropriate distraction protocol, or poor environment for bone healing. Choosing the correct device for the forces at play is critical to preventing device failure and providing adequate stability to prevent disruption of the generate bone during distraction and consolidation. While it is often true that greater movements can be achieved with distraction over traditional osteotomies, there are limits. Failure to realize the limits of a particular region or device can lead to treatment failure.

To maximize transport and bone generation, the osteotomy must be performed in such a way that it is complete yet performed using strategies that preserve bone viability at the margins of the osteotomy and minimize any gapping. Overheating the bone using drills and saws or allowing a gap to persist will lead to delays in bone healing (secondary bone healing vs. primary healing) and affect the quality of generate bone that can be produced.

The distraction protocol employed must be adjusted to accommodate the bone healing capacity of the patient and the particular region and condition of the region being distracted. Factors that affect bone healing affect distraction in much the same way. For example, prolonged latency in very young, naïve patients can often lead to premature consolidation, while failure to prolong the latency and slow distraction timelines in a wound that is heavily scarred, or in an older patient, for example, will likely lead to poor bone formation. Age, previous trauma or surgery, radiation, and poor bone stock affect bone healing and therefore require adjustments in the distraction protocol. Use of BMP with proper patient consent in the case of off-label use or import of healthy soft tissues can help overcome some of the negative effects of a poor healing bed.

Distraction procedures have a significant impact on the surrounding soft tissues. The negative effects can often obscure the perceived outcome by the patient despite a successful bone generation. Devices that rely on external pins that are perpendicular to the axis of distraction can cause particularly poor scarring because they drag through the tissues creating a scar track. Preoperative planning should be attentive to placement of any portion of the distractor that traverses the skin to the most concealed area possible so as to minimize the impact of scarring.

Bone is the only tissue capable of significant regeneration capacity. The response of soft tissues in the region of distraction can best be described as an accommodation. As the distraction lengths increase, the ability of the soft tissue envelope to accommodate can be a limiting factor and one can expect neuropractic injuries and pain to be experienced. Most nerve injuries recover, but pain should be perceived as an indication that the soft tissue envelope is reaching its limits.

Bibliography

Aronson J. Experimental assessment of bone regenerate quality during distraction osteogenesis. In: Brighton CT, Friedlaender GE, Lane JM, editors. Bone formation and repair. Rosemont: American Academy of Orthopaedic Surgeons; 1994.

Asonova SN. Morphogenesis mechanisms of limb connective tissue structure in the condition of gradual distraction. Genij Orthopedii. 1996;2–3:124.

Barton FR. On the treatment of anchylosis by the formation of artificial joints. North Am Med Surg J. 1827;3:279.

Beebe DW, Gozal D. Obstructive sleep apnea and the prefrontal cortex: towards a comprehensive model linking nocturnal upper airway obstruction to daytime cognitive and behavioral deficits. J Sleep Res. 2002;11(1):1–16.

Bradley J. Craniofacial distraction osteogenesis. In: Thaller S, Bradley J, Garri J, editors. Craniofacial surgery. New York: Informa; 2008.

Bradley JP, Gabbay JS, Taub PJ, Heller JB, O'Hara CM, Benhaim P, Kawamoto Jr HK. Monobloc advancement by distraction osteogenesis decreases morbidity and relapse. Plast Reconstr Surg. 2006; 118(7):1585–97.

Brighton CT. Principles of fracture healing. In: Instructional course lectures. Rosemont: American Academy of Orthopaedic Surgeons; 1984.

Codivilla A. On the means of lengthening in the lower limbs, the muscles, the tissues, which are shortened through deformity. Am J Orthop Surg. 1905;2:353.

Derderian CA, Bastidas N, Bartlett SP. Posterior cranial vault expansion using distraction osteogenesis. Childs Nerv Syst. 2012;28(9): 1551–6.

Farkas LG, Katic MJ, Forrest CR, Alt KW, Bagic I, Baltadjiev G, Cunha E, Cvicelová M, Davies S, Erasmus I, Gillett-Netting R, Hajnis K, Kemkes-Grottenthaler A, Khomyakova I, Kumi A, Kgamphe JS, Kayo-daigo N, Le T, Malinowski A, Negasheva M, Manolis S, Ogetürk M, Parvizrad R, Rösing F, Sahu P, Sforza C, Sivkov S, Sultanova N, Tomazo-Ravnik T, Tóth G, Uzun A, Yahia E. International anthropometric study of facial morphology in various ethnic groups/races. J Craniofac Surg. 2005;16(4):615–46.

Figueroa AA, et al. Long-term skeletal stability after maxillary advancement with distraction osteogenesis using a rigid external distraction device in cleft maxillary deformities. Plast Reconstr Surg. 2004;114(6):1382–92.

Frost HM. The biology of fracture healing: an overview for clinicians, Par I. Clin Orthop. 1989;248:283.

Gruss JS, Whelan MF, Rand RP, Ellenbogen RG. Lessons learnt from the management of 1500 complex facial fractures. Ann Acad Med Singapore. 1999;28(5):677–86. Review.

Halbower AC, et al. "Childhood obstructive sleep apnea associates with neuropsychological deficits and neuronal brain injury". PLoS Med. 2006;3(8):e301.

Herford AS. Use of a plate-guided distraction device for transport distraction osteogenesis of the mandible. J Oral Maxillofac Surg. 2004;62(4):412–20.

Hibi H, Ueda M. New internal transport distraction device for reconstructing segmental defects of the mandible. Br J Oral Maxillofac Surg. 2006;44(5):382–5.

Hollier L, Kelly P, Babigumira E, Potochny J, Taylor T. Minimally invasive Le Fort III distraction. J Craniofac Surg. 2002;13(1): 44–8.

Hopper RA. New trends in cranio-orbital and midface distraction for craniofacial dysostosis. Curr Opin Otolaryngol Head Neck Surg. 2012;20(4):298–303.

Ilizarov GA. The principles of the Ilizarov method. Bull Hosp Jt Dis Orthop Inst. 1988;48:1.

Ilizarov GA. The tension-stress effect on the genesis and growth of tissues: part I: the influence of stability of fixation and soft-tissue preservation. Clin Orthop. 1989;238:249.

Ilizarov GA. The tension-stress effect on the genesis and growth of tissues: part II: the influence of the rate and frequency of distraction. Clin Orthop. 1990;250:8.

Izadi K, Yellon R, Mandell DL, et al. Correction of upper airway obstruction in the newborn with internal mandibular distraction osteogenesis. J Craniofac Surg. 2003;14:493.

Kasanjian VH. The interrelationship of dentistry and surgery in the treatment of deformities of the face and jaws. Am J Orthop Oral Surg. 1941;27:10.

Kumar A, Gabbay JS, Nikjoo R, et al. Improved outcomes in cleft patients with severe maxillary deficiency after Le Fort I internal distraction. Plast Reconstr Surg. 2006;117(5):1499.

Lauritzen CG, Davis C, Ivarsson A, Sanger C, Hewitt TD. The evolving role of springs in craniofacial surgery: the first 100 clinical cases. Plast Reconstr Surg. 2008;121(2):545–54.

Limberg A. A new method of plastic lengthening of the mandible in unilateral microgenia and asymmetry of the face. J Am Dent Assoc. 1928;15:851.

McCarthy JG, Schreiber JS, Karp NS, et al. Lengthening the human mandible by gradual distraction. Plast Reconstr Surg. 1992;89:1.

McCarthy JG, Stelnicki EJ, Mehrara BJ, et al. Distraction osteogenesis of the craniofacial skeleton. Plast Reconstr Surg. 2001;107:1812.

McCormick SU, et al. Effect of mandibular distraction on the temporomandibular joint: part 1, canine study. J Craniofac Surg. 1995;6(5):358–63.

Michieli S, Miotti B. Lengthening of mandibular by gradual surgical-orthodontic distraction. J Oral Surg. 1977;35(3):187–92.

Monasterio FO, et al. Simultaneous mandibular and maxillary distraction in hemifacial microsomia in adults: avoiding occlusal disasters. Plast Reconstr Surg. 1997;100(4):852–61.

Peltier FL. External skeletal fixation for the treatment of fractures. In: Fractures a history and iconography of their treatment. San Francisco: Norman Publishing; 1990.

Polley JW, Figueroa AA. Management of severe maxillary deficiency in childhood and adolescence through distraction osteogenesis with an external, adjustable, rigid distraction device. J Craniofac Surg. 1997;8(3):181–5.

Schenk RK, Hunziker EB. Histologic and ultrastructural features of fracture healing. In: Brighton CT, Friedlaender GE, Lane JM, editors. Bone formation and repair. Rosemont: American Academy of Orthopaedic Surgeons; 1994.

Stucki-McCormick SU. Reconstruction of the mandibular condyle using transport distraction osteogenesis. J Craniofac Surg. 1997; 8(1):48–52.

Ueda M, Matsuno M, Sakai K, Hata K. Mechanisms of new bone formation during distraction osteogenesis: a preliminary report. In: Samchukov ML, Cope JB, Cherkashin AM, editors. Craniofacial distraction osteogenesis. St. Louis: Mosby; 2001.

Yasui N, Kojimoto H, Sasaki K, et al. Factors affecting callus distraction in limb lengthening. Clin Orthop. 1993;293:55.

Yu JC, Fearon J, Havlik RJ, et al. Distraction osteogenesis of the craniofacial skeleton. Plast Reconstr Surg. 2004;114:1e.

Part IV

Laboratory

Impressions, Models, and Splints: The Basic Maxillofacial Laboratory

35

Stephen A. Chidyllo and Peter J. Taub

The treatment of maxillofacial fractures has evolved over the years from simple stabilization using external bandages and prolonged immobilization to early mandibular function using craniofacial surgical techniques and rigid fixation. The use of splints in the treatment of maxillofacial fractures has been part of the plastic surgeons armamentarium since first reported by Bunon (1743). He used a block of ivory, which he attached by wiring it to two holes into the jaw. During the 1800s, Gunning and Bean devised several types of dental splints, which were secured with an external device. Dental splints have been fabricated in many forms and from different materials. They can be as simple as the patient's existing acrylic dentures or as complex as custom fabricated casted crowns. The most commonly applied are fabricated using quick cure acrylic resin (methyl methacrylate) as either lingual, palatal, or intermaxillary splints.

Today, with advances in rigid fixation, there may be fewer indications for their use. The need for dental splints in the treatment of facial fractures has decreased, and their indications limited. They are rarely indicated in the treatment of simple fractures of one arch when separate dentoalveolar components are not present. However, there are several situations in which a splint will provide assistance in the management of maxillofacial fractures.

Several authors have presented the indications for the use of dental splints in the treatment of maxillofacial fractures. Dental splints should be used in conjunction with the accepted techniques of rigid fixation to assist in establishing and securing the patient's pretraumatic skeletal anatomy and occlusion prior to and during the application of plate and screw fixation. In cases in which the patient is edentulous or missing a significant number of teeth, a splint should be applied to provide interim stabilization of the fractured segments. This is done to accurately reestablish their occlusion and vertical dimension. Similarly, when there are multiple fracture lines or fractures that extend to both sides of the arch, the tendency is toward instability because of differential forces being applied on the bony segments by the muscles of mastication. In patients with severely displaced and comminuted fractures of the mandible, it is difficult to obtain and maintain a bony reduction due to the muscular forces on these segments. A dental splint will assist in reducing the fracture(s) and maintain alignment opposing these forces, preventing rotation or displacement of the segments. In this manner rigid fixation may be passively adapted to the boney segments, while the reduction is secured by the splint.

There are several types of fractures in which conventional mandibular plate and screw fixation cannot be applied because of the risk of injury to tooth roots or developing follicles. Since it is often difficult for mandibular rigid fixation to be adapted to a fractured alveolar segment, dental splints may provide a successful means of stabilizing both the fracture and the involved teeth. Mandibular fractures in children can be effectively managed with the assistance of dental splints. During the period of deciduous or mixed dentition, fractures may occur along the lines of unerupted teeth. This may result in a fracture line that is irregular, long, and oblique. Again, the use of a mandibular plate and screws may cause injury to the developing unerupted teeth. The use of dental splints in these patients can reduce and stabilize the fracture segments without concern for damaging the developing tooth follicles.

In the management of combined fractures of both the maxilla and mandible, it is recommended that the fracture of the least comminuted arch be reduced first. Subsequently, the opposing arch may be reconstructed using this skeletal and occlusal relationship as a foundation. An alternative acceptable technique is with staged operative procedures in which

S.A. Chidyllo, MD, DDS (✉)
Division of Plastic and Reconstructive Surgery,
Department of Surgery, Jersey Shore University Medical Center,
West Long Branch, NJ, USA
e-mail: plasticsurgery1@optonline.net

P.J. Taub, MD
Division of Plastic and Reconstructive Surgery, Mount Sinai
Medical Center, 5 East 98th Street, 15th Floor, New York,
NY 10029, USA
e-mail: peter.taub@mountsinai.org

P.J. Taub et al. (eds.), *Ferraro's Fundamentals of Maxillofacial Surgery*,
DOI 10.1007/978-1-4614-8341-0_35, © Springer Science+Business Media New York 2015

the less comminuted fracture is reconstructed first, a new impression and dental model of this arch performed, and the opposing more comminuted arch is subsequently reconstructed to this new arch form with splints in a delayed operative procedure.

Interocclusal splints are contraindicated in the treatment of comminuted maxillofacial fractures. The use of such a splint alone may not prevent distraction, labial-lingual tilting, or rotation of the fractured segments. Its use may complicate the treatment of mandibular fractures by causing distraction of the fragments at the inferior border. These splints are effective in elective cases in which a specific predicted occlusal relationship between the maxillary and mandibular arches is to be created during surgery.

There are few contraindications to the use of dental splints. They should not be used: If simple wiring or maxillomandibular fixation will suffice, if time is a prime consideration, or if the bulk of the splint will interfere with the patients occlusion. The type of dental splint that is utilized will be determined by the clinical state of the patient's dentition, the radiological evaluation, available laboratory facilities, and experience of the surgeon.

Applied Dental Anatomy and Occlusion

Angle defined occlusion as "the normal relations of the occlusal inclined planes of the teeth when the jaws are closed." He classified occlusion on the basis of what he considered to be optimal morphological relations between the maxillary and mandibular teeth. Occlusion can be simply thought of as the contact between the maxillary and mandibular teeth in all mandibular positions and movements. Occlusion has a physiological and functional component, interrelating the dentition, muscles of mastication, temporomandibular joint, and complete masticatory system into a balanced pain-free state. A physiological occlusion is one in which the components function efficiently without pain and remain in a stable state of health. Few people have an ideal occlusion as described by Angle; however, most have a physiological or functional occlusion.

Various terms are applied to the physiological, nonpathologic position of the condyle within the glenoid FOSSA when the teeth are in occlusion. These include centric occlusion (CO) and centric relation (CR). CO is usually described as the bite when the teeth are in their maximal interdigitated position. CO gives no indication of condylar position. CR, on the other hand, is a term used in conjunction with a description of the condyle position. It is the most posterior unstrained position of the condyle in the glenoid FOSSA, which should occur simultaneous to maximal dental interdigitation. CR is a mandibular condylar position that is consistently reproducible on the patient. CO and CR are not necessarily the same mandibular position, but we must attempt to have the condyle in the unstrained position at the same time as the occlusion of the dentition is in maximum bilateral contact.

The constancy of the dental cusps to FOSSA relationships is important to understand to determine the patient's centric occlusion (maximal intercuspal position). In closure, the buccal cusps of the mandibular posterior teeth distal to the canine are normally seated in the central FOSSA of the maxillary teeth, and the lingual cusps of the posterior maxillary teeth are seated in the central FOSSA of the mandibular teeth. These cusps are called the supporting cusps (maxillary lingual and mandibular buccal). The actual contact points of the cusp-fossa are called the centric stops or holding contacts, because they hold the teeth in a stable position. Their contact relations change with wear of the dentition. With advancing attrition, the supporting cusps seat closer to the depth of the opposing FOSSA. In reassembling models, their pretraumatic anatomical relationship may be determined by a careful evaluation of the occlusal surfaces of the teeth, in particular the facets worn on the teeth by attrition. One should match the wear facets of the cusps with those of the corresponding opposing FOSSA. Angle's classification of the patient's occlusion should be clinically determined and used as a guide in mounting of the casts.

Basic Maxillofacial Laboratory Techniques

The maxillofacial surgeon should be knowledgeable in the techniques available to take impressions of the teeth, transform those impressions into plaster models, and then fabricate acrylic splints to be used either alone or in conjunction with surgical intervention (Fig. 35.1). Fractures involving the maxilla and mandible often occur in edentulous patients where involved teeth have been previously extracted or were lost as part of the injury. To anatomically reduce these fractures and then maintain adequate immobilization with maxillomandibular fixation, or MMF (assuming plate and screw fixation is not preferred), it may be necessary to construct an acrylic splint against which the opposing teeth will occlude. Arch bars are fixed to the existing dentition, secured to the alveolar bone directly, or placed directly on the splint prior to inset in the mouth. Despite the development of computer-aided design and computer-aided manufacturing (CAD-CAM) of splints for orthognathic surgery, the basic laboratory skills remain important. Once the basic techniques are mastered, the learned splinting techniques can be modified to manage the specific clinical problem at hand. Practice may be performed on a typodont, on which impressions can be taken in alginate and then stone models constructed from the alginate impressions. The teeth of the typodont can be selectively removed to simulate edentulous or partially edentulous jaws. Using this technique, various clinical situations can be simulated and splinting techniques demonstrated.

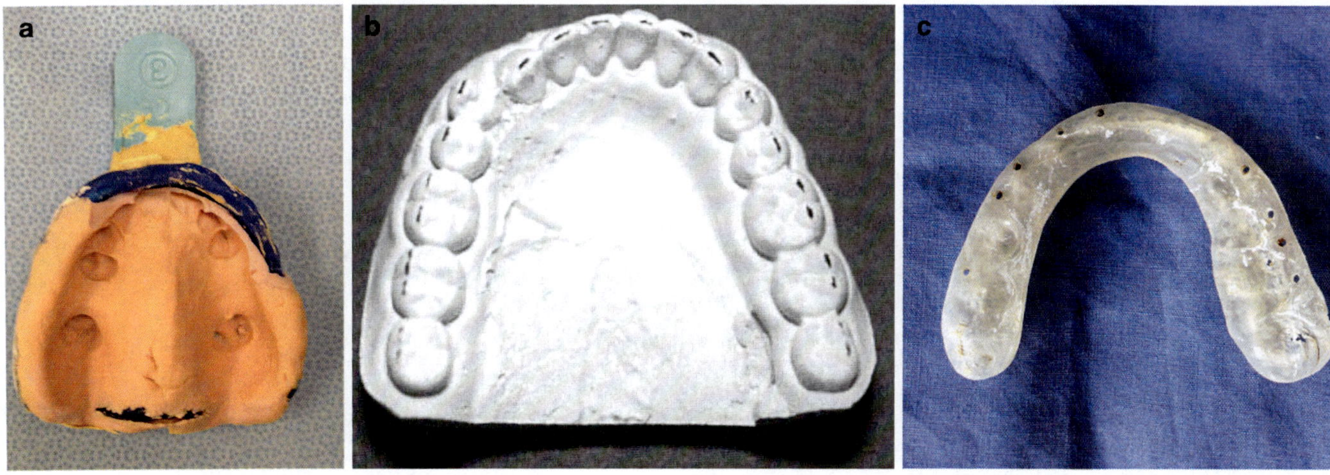

Fig. 35.1 (a–c) The basics of the dental preparation: alginate impression, plaster model, and acrylic splint

A familiarity with the materials, supplies, and equipment needed to take dental impressions is important not only for maxillofacial fracture management but also for orthognathic surgical diagnosis and planning. Dental splints can be useful to provide stability for the reduction of maxillary or mandibular fractures and are critical for orthognathic surgical procedures. Only clinical judgment can help the surgeon decide whether splinting is a preferred option when immobilization of a particular fracture is required. There are certain clinical situations where a constructed acrylic splint may provide a useful role. A patient whose dentition has poor interdigitation may grossly appear to be satisfactory but the cusps of the teeth may be tilted too far lingually. If MMF is selected as a close reduction technique without the use of the splint, then lingual tipping with malunion might result.

The materials used in a basic maxillofacial laboratory include the following:

- Alginate impression material (provided in powder form)
- Plaster of Paris (powder)
- Dental stone (powder)
- Dental utility wax
- Multipurpose (cold-cure) acrylic
- Sticky wax
- Vaseline (for coating models)
- Soft bite wax
- Plasticine

The equipment and supplies used in a basic maxillofacial laboratory include the following:

- Plastic perforated impression trays (small, medium, large for the maxilla and mandible. The latter has a cut out for the base of the tongue)
- Soft rubber mixing bowl and spatula
- Arch bars for application of MMF
- Small electric hand drill with bits, stones, etc.
- Dental wax spatula
- Sharp utility knife
- Dental plaster knife
- Dental articulator on which to mount models
- Facebow transfer device
- Vibrator for pouring stone/plaster
- Electric grinder wheel

Taking Impressions with Alginate

The initial requirement in the fabrication of a dental splint is obtaining an accurate impression of the patient's mandibular and maxillary arches. Care must be taken in securing the impressions accurately, because they provide the foundation for the construction of the dental splints. An impression of the opposing arch is always required to assist in reassembling the fracture segments of the models in occlusion.

When taking alginate impressions, the impression tray size and shape is important. The tray should be wide enough to match the width of the jaw, either maxilla or mandible, and the posterior aspect of the tray should reach the molar teeth. After confirming the correct size of the tray, a strip of utility wax can be placed around the edge of the tray to help confine the impression material and give more comfort to the patient.

Alginate is used to take dental impressions (Fig. 35.2). Sodium alginate is the sodium salt of alginic acid extracted from the cell walls of brown algae, while potassium alginate is the potassium salt extracted from seaweed. Binding of alginate with water forms a viscous gum, which is able to mold the surfaces of the teeth. The higher the temperature of the water, within reasonable limits, the shorter the gelation time of the alginate impression material, and conversely. The alginate scoop and special plastic water vial (Fig. 35.3) are marked so that one *level scoop* full of alginate powder requires one half of a vial of water (i.e., filled to 1/2 mark on vial). For an average intraoral impression of a patient, two scoops are necessary for the mandible and three for the

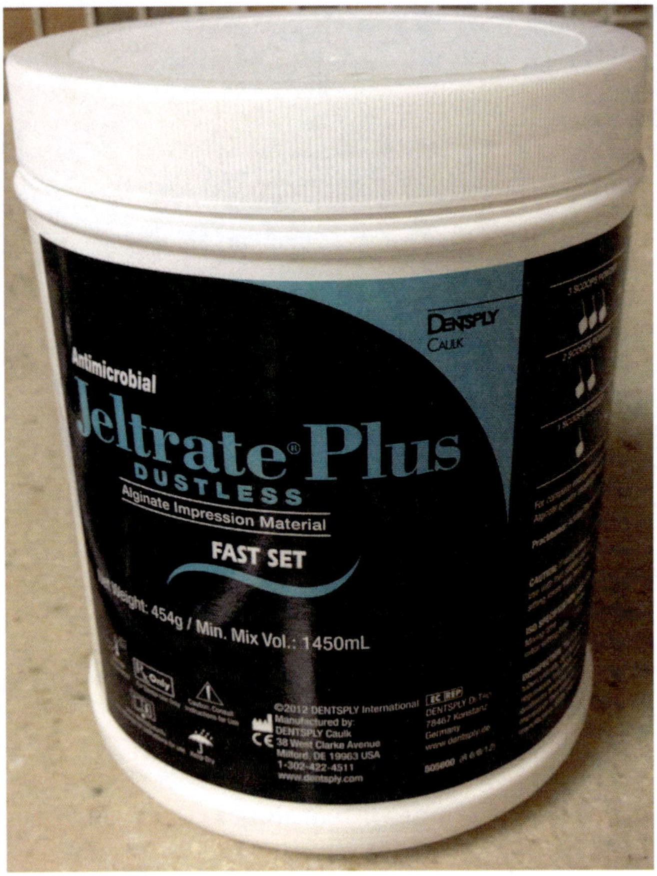

Fig. 35.2 Alginate used to make dental impressions

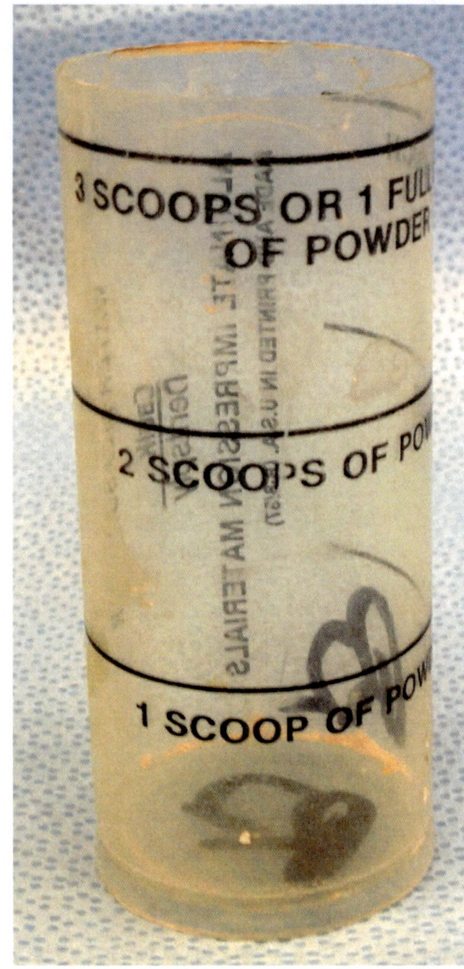

Fig. 35.3 Graduated plastic scoop to accurately measure the amount of water to add to the alginate (usually 3 scoops for the maxillary impression and 2 scoops for the mandibular impression)

maxilla (for the laboratory dentiform, one scoop may be used). By placing the powder into the liquid, there is less chance of air bubbles forming. The contents are mixed with spatula into the consistency of soft butter and placed into one of the trays (Fig. 35.4).

The patient should be seated in a chair in a relaxed forward position and instructed to breath slowly through his or her mouth after the tray is inserted (Fig. 35.5). The setting time for the impression material is approximately 3 min, or when it becomes firm and rubbery. The tray may be easily removed after the impression material has set by pushing down posteriorly on one side with a finger to break the suction seal. Once removed, the tray is wrapped in a moist towel (and possibly placed in a plastic bag) until it is ready to be used. The impression of the other jaw is done next and placed with the first impression.

Pouring the Impressions in Stone

Dental stone or plaster is poured into the impressions to create models of the dental arches. Pouring dental stone (Hydrocal) or plaster of Paris into the alginate trays creates the plaster models. When calcinated, gypsum produces plaster of Paris and kindred products. To obtain plaster of Paris, the gypsum is calcined in open kettles at a temperature of 113–120 °C (235–250 °F), whereas Hydrocal is obtained by calcining the gypsum in a closed kettle under a steam pressure of 17 lb per square inch gage pressure and a temperature of 123 °C (253 °F).

When mixed with water, the plaster first goes into a solution then becomes saturated and finally precipitates. The reaction is exothermic. There are several factors that influence the setting time of the plaster of Paris. The manufacturing process may alter the temperature of calcining (the higher the calcining temperature, the slower the set), the amount of gypsum left in the plaster (the more gypsum left, the faster the set), and the addition of adulterants. Within limits, the longer the spatulation time, the quicker the set. The more water that is added to the mix, the slower is the setting time. The higher the temperature of the water, provided the temperature does not exceed 86 °F (30 °C), the faster is the setting time. When the temperature exceeds approximately

120 °F (50 °C), the setting time is decreased. The effect is not pronounced, however, at any normal room temperature. Finally, the addition of accelerators decreases the setting time, while the addition of retarders causes it to increase.

Hydrocal has smooth and nonporous particles in contrast to the particles of plaster of Paris, which are rough and porous. The result is that Hydrocal can be mixed with much less gaging water than is necessary for the mixing of plaster; consequently the hardened cast will be much stronger. It produces a lower chance of tooth breakage on the model when the hardened cast is removed from the alginate impression.

The plaster (or stone) is mixed in a rubber bowl until it is slightly runny. To avoid or minimize trapping air between the stone and alginate interface, small amounts of the plaster are poured onto the occlusal surface of the impression while the tray is held on a vibrating table (Fig. 35.6). The air bubbles will rise to the surface. Additional plaster is poured from one side and allowed to run around to the opposite side until sufficient plaster has been poured. A continuous stream is maintained so that it rolls around the entire impression by the *force of its own viscosity* to prevent trapping of air bubbles and thus obtain a solid, uniform model. If plaster is introduced from two sides, air may similarly be trapped.

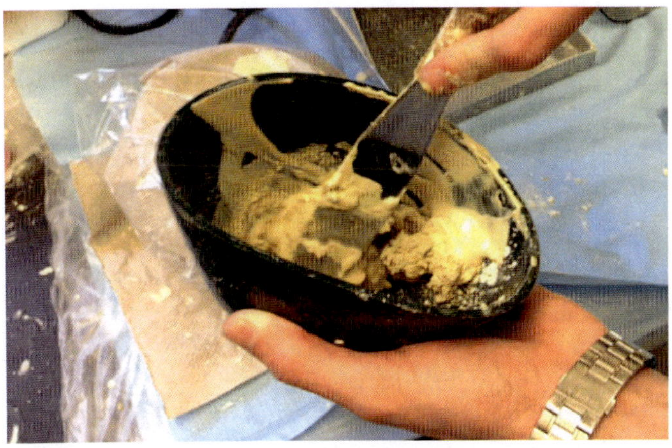

Fig. 35.4 Mixing alginate in a rubber bowl

An additional thicker "cake" of plaster is placed on a paper towel labeled with the patient's and doctor's name to avoid being thrown away. The impression tray with plaster is turned over onto the cake and smoothed around the edges with the spatula (Fig. 35.7). The models are allowed to "set" or harden for a few hours, or preferably overnight. The harder the models are at the time of separation of the models from the alginate impression, the less likely the chance of fracturing the teeth.

Once sufficiently hardened, the plaster impressions are carefully taken out of the impression trays. Every attempt should be made to keep the impression intact since it may be re-wrapped in moist paper towel and be reused if necessary. A grinding wheel is used to trim and smooth out the sides and top of the models (Fig. 35.8).

When the fractures have caused derangement of the arch form, cuts may be made in the model if there is a corresponding fracture line (Fig. 35.9). The sections of the cast are assembled to the opposing nonfractured arch. The fragments are reconstructed and attached together with wax, and a new plaster base is applied to the cast (Fig. 35.10a, b). A duplication of this reconstructed cast is created on which the dental splint is fabricated after articulation of the model to the newly fractured arch. Knowledge of dental anatomy and

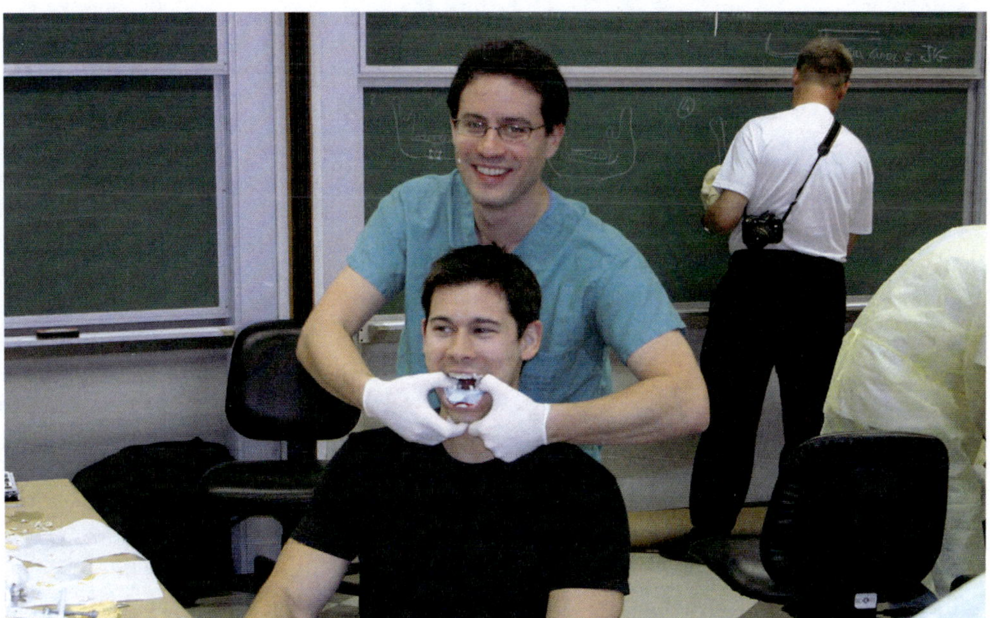

Fig. 35.5 Taking a dental impression

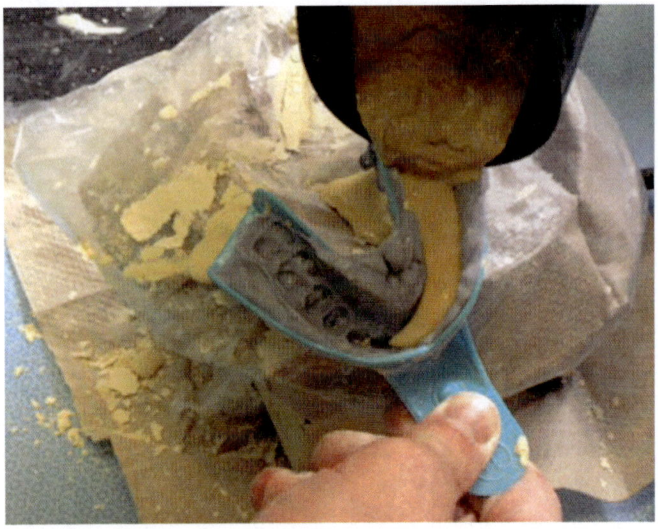

Fig. 35.6 Pouring plaster into an impression tray to avoid air bubbles on the occlusal surface

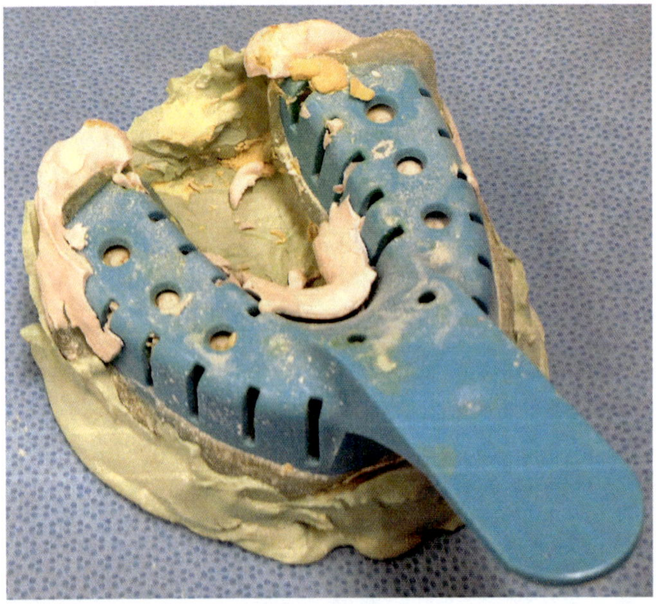

Fig. 35.7 Setting the plaster in the impression tray

occlusion is necessary. The position of the occlusion at the canine and mesiobuccal cusp of the first molar teeth is most pertinent.

Taking a Bite Registration

A bite registration is a record of the way the patient's teeth naturally come together. It is used to mount the dental models on an articulator to recreate the patient's actual centric relation. A single layer of thin, pink baseplate wax is cut to fit the patient's dental arch, extending just beyond the occlusal bite plane. The wax is warmed in hot water (or over a Bunsen burner) and the patient is then instructed to bite down firmly into the soft wax (Fig. 35.11). It is important for the surgeon to guide the patient's condyles (to seat them) in the glenoid FOSSA at the time of biting so that the jaws are in centric relation. This allows for a consistent relationship of the upper and lower teeth as they occlude. The wax may be cooled under cool water and placed on the occlusal surfaces of the poured models. The cusps of the teeth should occlude into the impressions in the wax bite. With the models occluded by the bite registration, the models are mounted into an articulator.

Mounting Dental Casts on the Articulator

One type of articulator is used when only a single jaw is moved, while a different type is used when both jaws are being moved. This is because in the former instance, the stationary jaw is used as a reference for the manipulated one. In the latter instance, an articulator that attaches a facebow is used. The facebow is used to relate the maxilla, which is to be moved to the stable cranial base and then to the mandible. When mounting the models on a handheld articulator, the base of the models may be scored (or scratched) to provide better surface adhesion with the plaster used to hold them on the articulator. The models are mounted to a simple handheld articulator by pouring plaster between the models and limbs of the articulator (Fig. 35.12). They may be mounted to a Galetti-type handheld articulator by simply screwing the models to each half of the articulator (Fig. 35.13). Finally, if a facebow articulator is used, the models must again be affixed with plaster between the tops of the models and the footplates that screw to each side of the articulator (Fig. 35.14). The mounted models are now ready to have an acrylic splint constructed on them.

Constructing Acrylic Splints

Splints are created for use in the operating room to judge how far or how much an individual jaw should be moved. Cold-cure (room temperature setting) acrylic is most frequently used to construct a splint. The models are lubricated with petroleum jelly to prevent adherence of the acrylic to the models. The models may be prepared by blocking out any undercuts with Plasticine to prevent locking of the acrylic into undercuts on the model, as this would prevent removal after the acrylic is hardened. The acrylic powder and liquid are mixed in a small mixing cup as per directions on the container. The acrylic will pass through three phases as it is mixed with a tongue depressor: smooth liquid, "stringy" gel (Fig. 35.15), and then a semisolid. Once in this last phase,

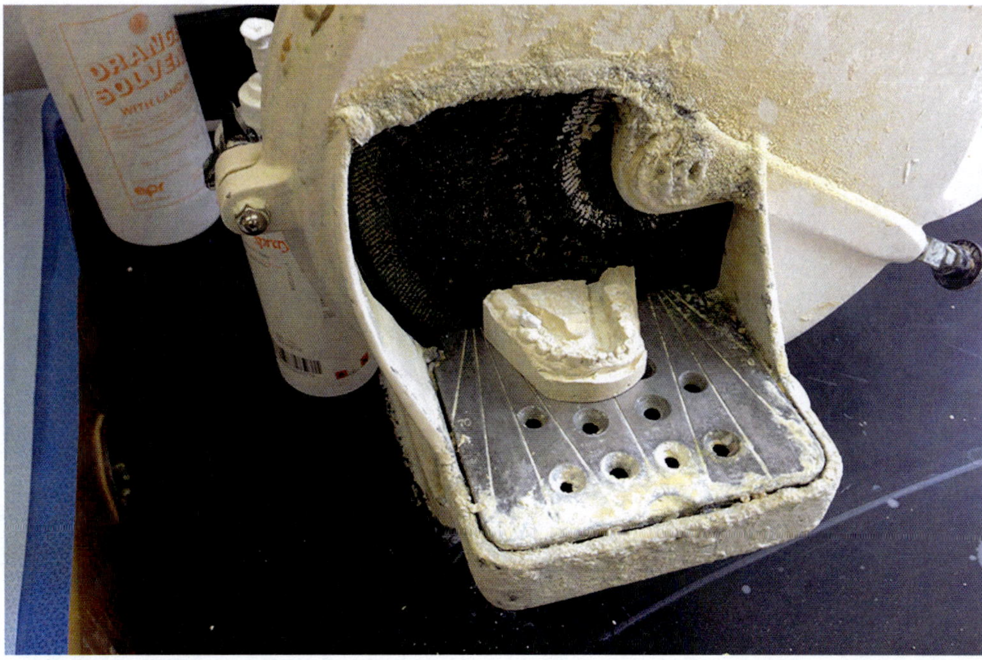

Fig. 35.8 Grinding wheel used to smoothen the edges of the plaster model

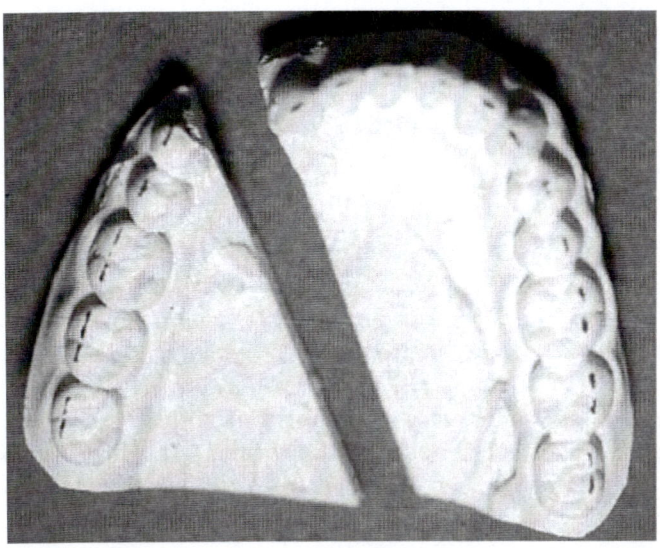

Fig. 35.9 Cutting a plaster model to recreate the line of the fracture

it may be rolled into a thin cigar. To avoiding sticking to the hands, a small amount of petroleum jelly may be spread onto the fingers. The rolled acrylic is placed on the occlusal surface (Fig. 35.16) of the mandibular model and the two models occluded firmly into the soft acrylic to reproduce the desired bite. When still soft, excess acrylic was trimmed away with either a scissors or scalpel before it hardens. The more trimming that is done at this stage, the less grinding of the hardened acrylic will be necessary later.

The splint should remain in place until it has set since its shape will tend to change as it cools. Once set, the splint is removed from the model and trimmed to the desired size and shape using dental burrs and stones. The splint should be thin enough so that the edge should be approximately 1–2 mm above the occlusal surface (Fig. 35.17). The splint should be polished with pumice on a large, electrically driven pumice wheel. Burrs should not be used on the occlusal surfaces of the splint since this will change fit to the patient's teeth.

If a "gunning" type of splint is needed, segments of arch bars can be "welded" to the splint by adding acrylic powder and liquid using a "dusting" technique to gain adherence of the arch bar segment to the underlying acrylic splint. If the splint is being constructed for an edentulous patient, a baseplate of acrylic may be initially made (Fig. 35.18). This is done by greasing (with petroleum jelly) the edentulous model and placing a "pancake" of acrylic "dough" over the edentulous region. The acrylic baseplate is formed over the edentulous dental model with finger pressure; the excess acrylic is cut away with a scalpel. The acrylic is allowed to harden and referred to as the "baseplate." Additional acrylic is mixed, and a cigar-shaped piece is formed. This is spread out over the baseplate in the shape of a bite-block. The bite-block substitutes for the missing teeth. The colorless liquid (from the acrylic set) is added to the hardened baseplate before applying the acrylic "dough" to obtain a good "weld." This bite-block-shaped acrylic is made approximately 1.5 cm in height and, in effect, takes the shape of a full denture without teeth. Once hardened, it is shaped and polished as described. Using similar techniques, a splint is constructed on the mandibular edentulous model. Grease the already constructed acrylic "bite-block" portion of the maxillary splint with petroleum gauze. Another cigar-shaped batch of acrylic dough is made and placed on the lower baseplate after adding acrylic liq-

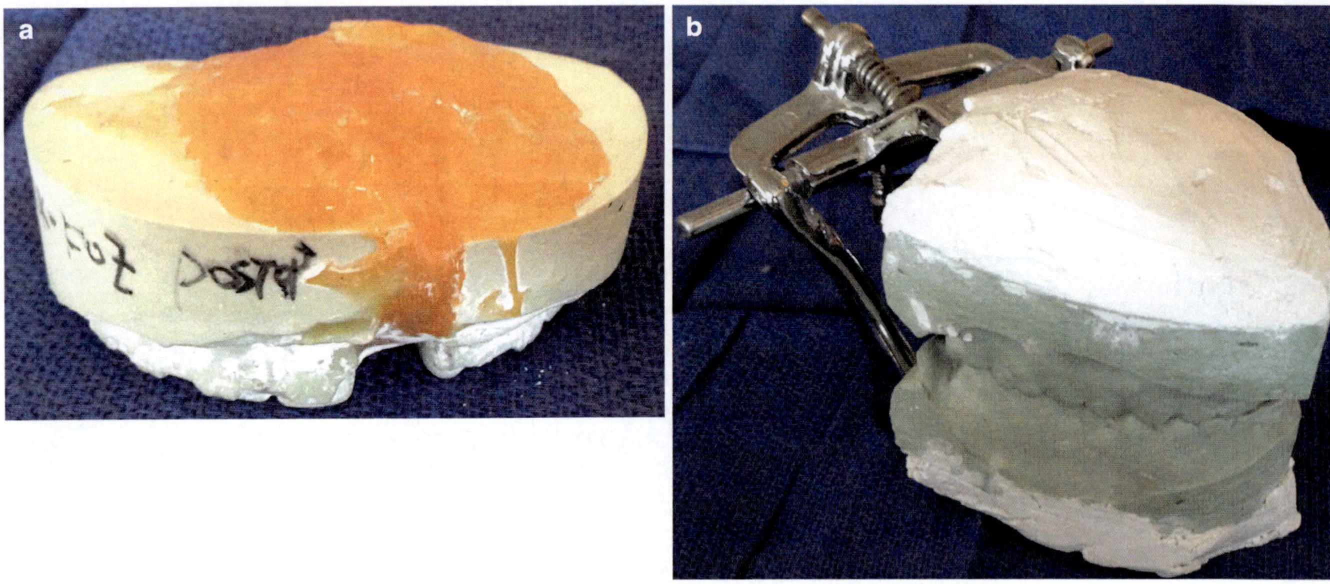

Fig. 35.10 (**a**, **b**) Adding wax and new plaster to the base of the realigned model

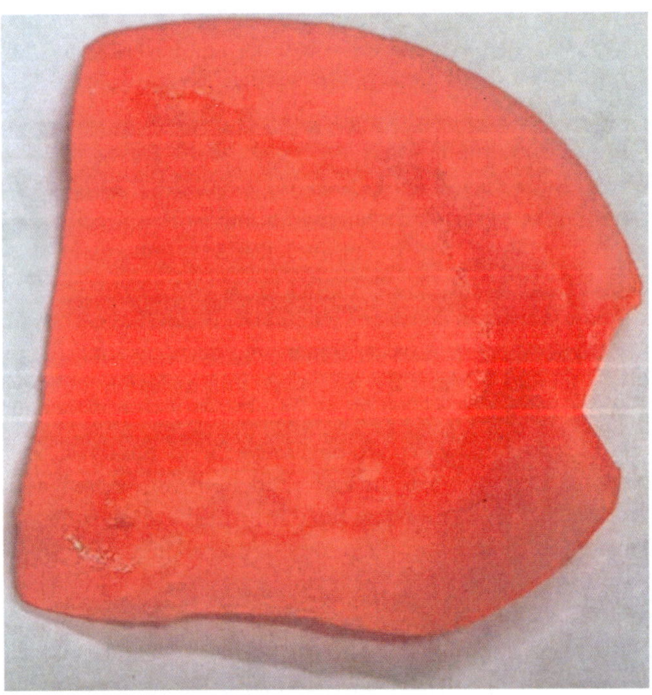

Fig. 35.11 Pink wax bite registration

uid to the surface of the baseplate. The maxillary edentulous bite-block splint (sitting on the articulated dental models) closed onto the mandibular one. After molding the acrylic to the desired shape while it is still soft, excess dough is trimmed off. It is allowed to harden and then finally shaped with a rotary burr and stone, and then polished. Arch bars may be welded to the "full denture" (gunning) splints. It is a good idea to cut an opening in the front to facilitate air intake in feeding. Partial edentulous splints can be made using a similar technique.

When confronted with multiple fractures in the maxilla or mandible, segmentalization of the arches can result. A partial impression tray can be effectively used to take segmental impressions of each of the fractured and dislocated pieces. These alginate (segmental) impressions are then poured in dental stone as independent segments. After each stone cast has hardened, they are trimmed and placed into occlusion with the dental cast of the intact opposing jaw. Hopefully, there will be one-jaw intact. The fragments are applied one by one to the intact opposing dental arch using "sticky" wax to help hold the pieces together. After the fragments have been waxed into occlusion against the opposing intact dental cast, a new base of dental stone is poured to hold the pieces together. This recreates the patient's preinjured arch form from the badly fractured dental arch segments.

Design of Dental Splints

Lingual Splints

Lingual splints are recommended for use in the mandible for treatment of complex, unstable, bilateral fractures or fractures of the symphysis or alveolar ridge. The lingual splint can help prevent inward tilting of the bony segments and counteract the tendency of the inferior border to become distracted (Fig. 35.19). Stabilization of the splint is achieved by either circummandibular or circumdental fixation. It is important that the splint is ligated below the height of the contour of the teeth. If not, circumdental wires may become unstable and

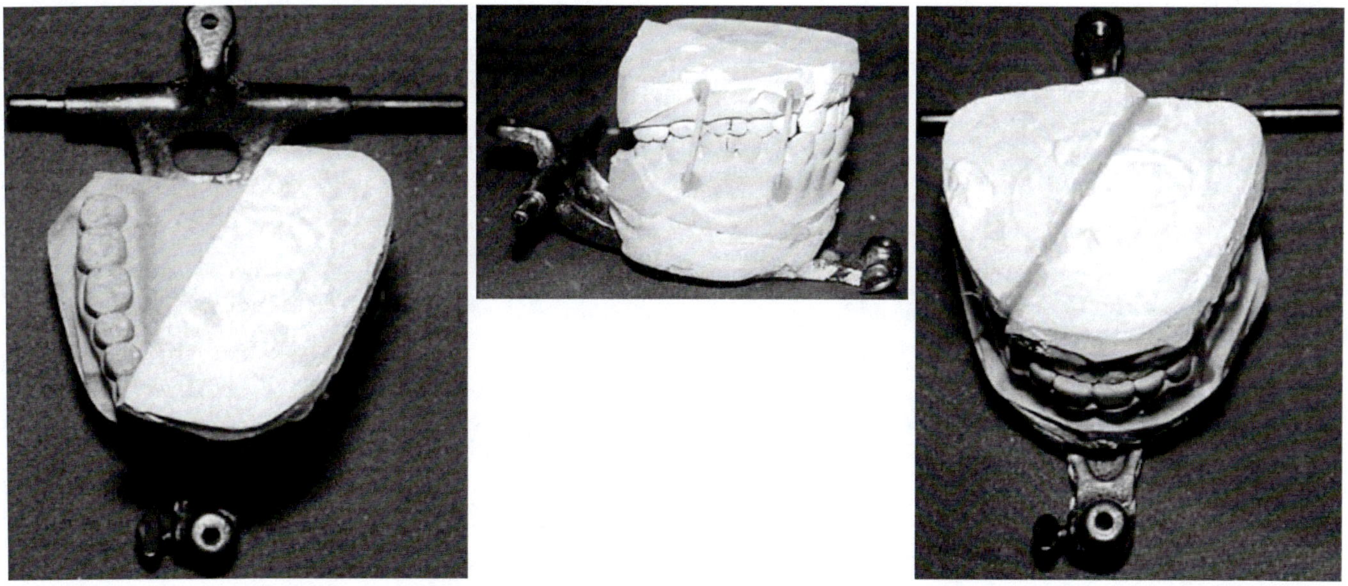

Fig. 35.12 Mounting impressions in a simple articulator for one-jaw surgery

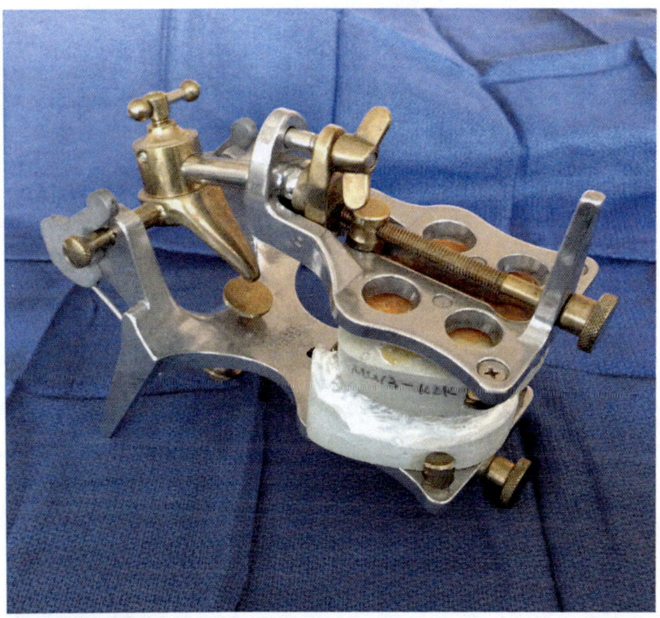

Fig. 35.13 Mounting impressions in a Galetti-type articulator for one-jaw surgery

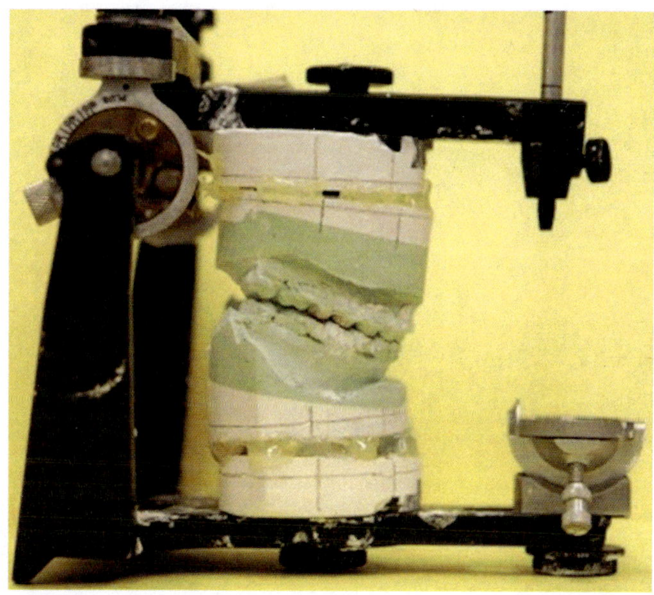

Fig. 35.14 Plaster models mounted on a facebow articulator for two-jaw surgery

the splint displaces occlusally (Fig. 35.20). If there are long edentulous regions within the affected dentalarch, a block of acrylic may be fabricated into the lingual splint in this edentulous segment, between the teeth. This will add stability to the splint and prevent displacement. If must be remembered that if there are teeth in the opposing arch which occlude with this added "acrylicblock" the added acrylic must be reduced to prevent premature occlusion with the opposing dentition.

If the splint interferes with occlusion, it may open the vertical dimension and may affect the reduction. A natural curve exists in the shape of the dental arch (curve of Spee), which should be reproduced with the aid of the splint. If added strength is desired, a metal bar may be inserted into the lingual splint during fabrication. The splint should be used in conjunction with a buccolabial arch bar. This will provide additional support to the fixation. If the application of rigid fixation is indicated, it can be easily applied after all of the bony fragments are anatomically reduced with the aid of the splint. The final fixation of the splint should not be completed until after the anatomic reduction of the bony segments has been performed. The lingual splint allows some leeway in order to accomplish this.

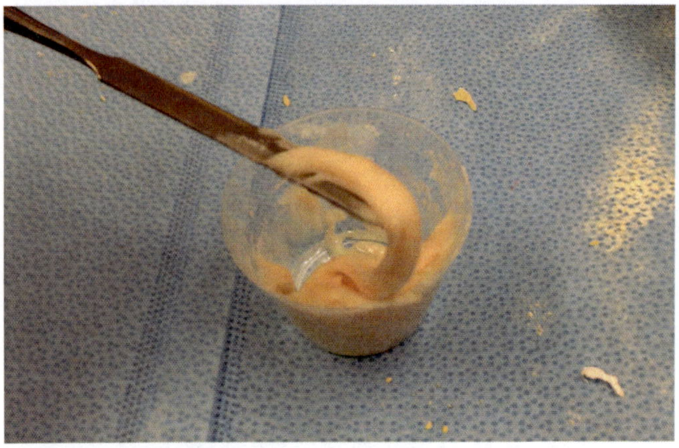

Fig. 35.15 Mixing acrylic into a sticky paste

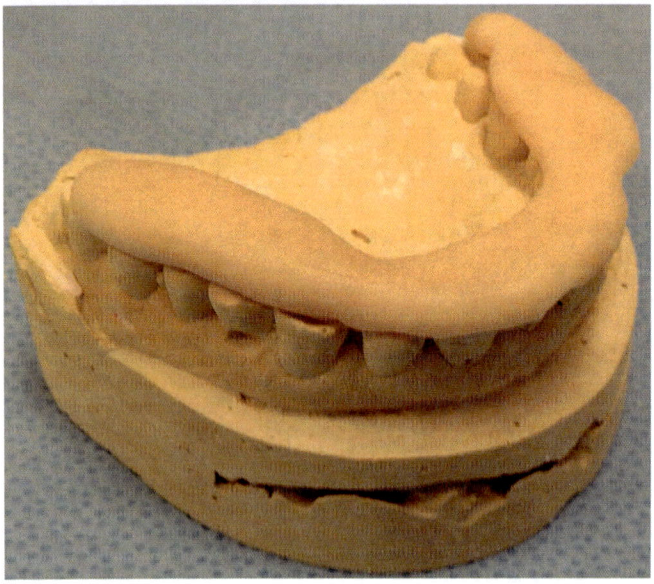

Fig. 35.16 Placing rolled acrylic onto the occlusal surface prior to occluding the maxillary and mandibular models

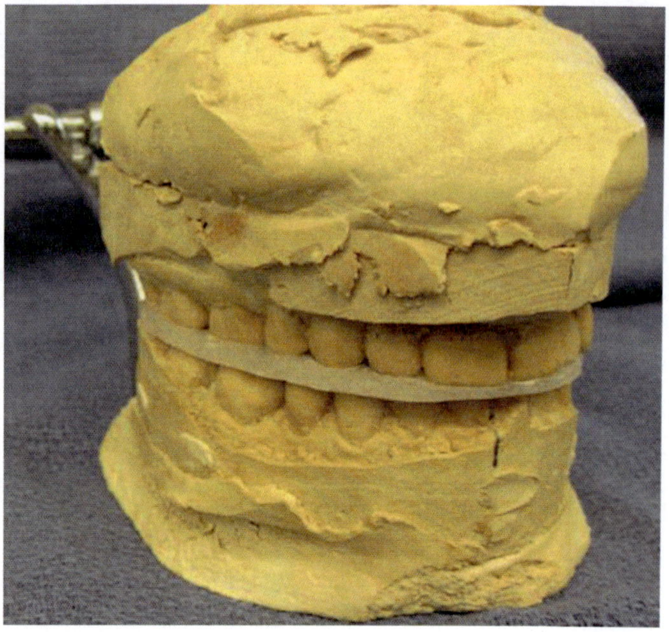

Fig. 35.17 Thin acrylic splint in place

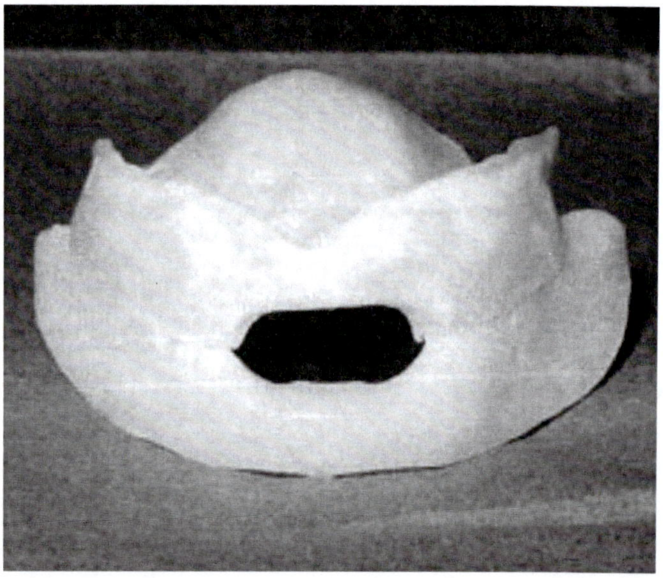

Fig. 35.18 Gunning splint used to maintain space between the occlusal surfaces in an edentulous patient

Maxillomandibular Splints

Maxillomandibular splints are stabilized to both the maxilla and the mandible and are subsequently secured to one another. If the patient wears dentures—either partial or complete—they may be utilized as maxillomandibular splints in the treatment of the patient's fractures. Dentures may assist in reestablishing the pretraumatic centric occlusion of the dental arches (Figs. 35.21 and 35.22). Arch bars are secured to the dentures prior to stabilization. Skeletal fixation of the mandibular denture is obtained by circummandibular or circumdental wires. The maxillary denture is secured by circumdental, piriform aperture, orbital rim, circumzygomatic, or anterior nasal spine suspension wires. A favored method is by transalveolar fixattion utilizing Steinman pins, Kirschner wire or lag screws, directly through the buccal flange of the denture into the alvolar bone.

Steinman pins or Kirschner wire or lag screw fixation. After the skeletal fixation is established, the arches are brought into occlusion and the dentures are secured together with wire ligatures about the attached arch bars.

In the case of an edentulous patient for whom there are no dentures available to utilize as splints, partial lower full upper splints and modified Gunning splints can be fabricated to assist in the reduction and stabilization of the fractures.

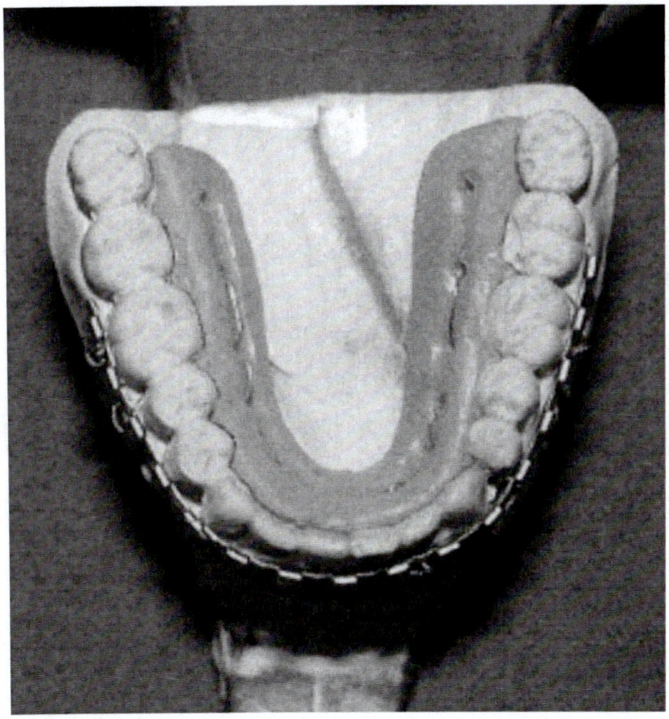

Fig. 35.19 Lingual splint used to hold the mandibular arch held in place with circummandibular wires

These splints are fabricated off an acrylic baseplate that fits intimately over the edentulous arch. Acrylic rims are placed as occlusal stops to maintain the patient's vertical dimension. An anterior opening can be placed in the splint, allowing the patient to ingest a blenderized or liquid diet. The splints are secured by skeletal fixation and subsequently wired together.

These splints may be used in conjunction with rigid fixation or as an interim stabilization prior to the placement of plate and screw fixation. The splints may be immediately removed if the fractured segments are stable, or they may be used to provide additional temporary support. In general, placement of splints over fresh incisions or lacerations should be avoided.

Palatal Splints

Sagittal fractures of the maxilla with dentoalveolar components may be reduced with the assistance of a palatal splint. The splint is inserted off the occlusal surfaces, and the individual bony fragments reduced. Skeleton fixation is achieved as previously described. The splint stabilizes the fractured bony segments either during the application of maxillomandibular or rigid fixation.

It is important that these splints be constructed with palatal relief, contacting only the palatal surfaces of the maxillary teeth. This is ensured by placing a thin spacer of dental wax or foil on the cast in the areas of desired relief prior to the fabrication of the splint. If excessive gingival or palatal contact is allowed, pressure necrosis may result.

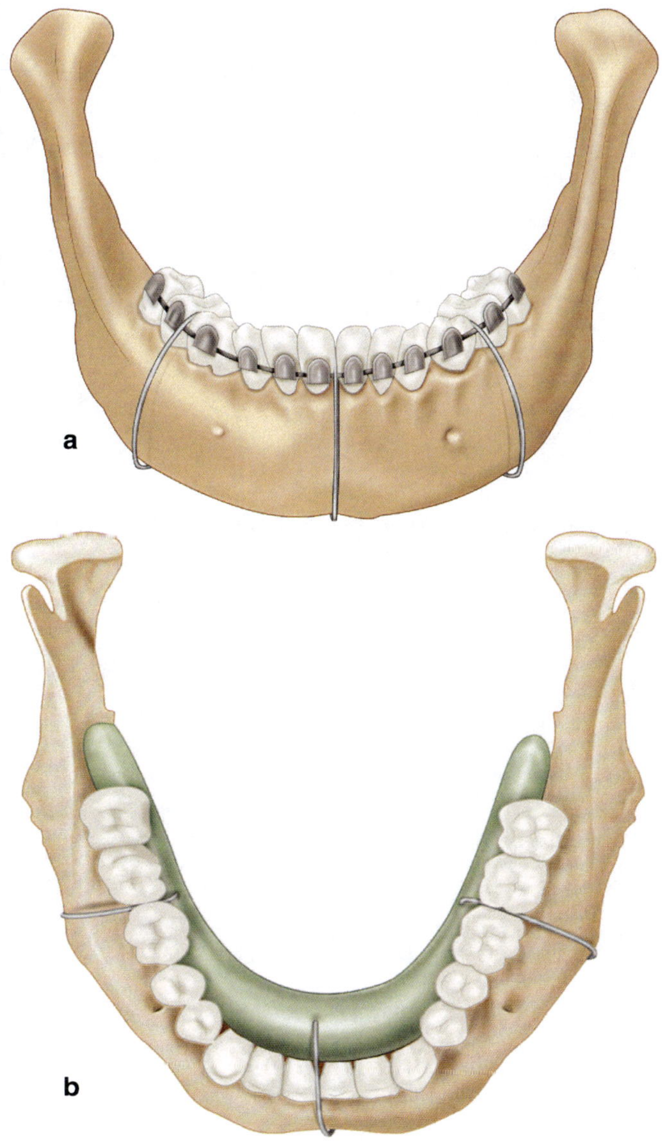

Fig. 35.20 Lingual splint held in place with circummandibular wires. (**a**) Anterior view of lingual splint secured with circummandibular wires. (**b**) Occlusal view of lingual splint secured with circummandibular wires

Cast Crown Splints

These splints consist of casted crowns that are attached together and intimately fit over the existing dentition. The splint is cemented in place over the crowns of the teeth. Their use has been reported in the treatment of mandibular fractures in patients with short crowns, dentoalveolar fractures, periodontitis, and in children with a deciduous or mixed dentition.

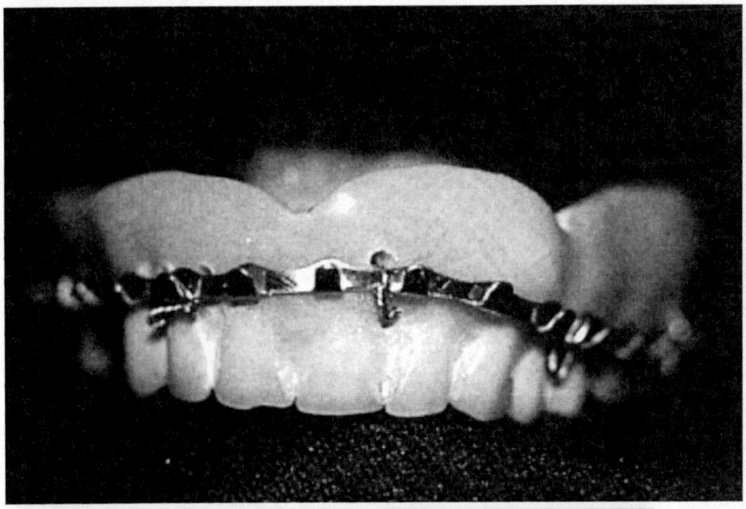

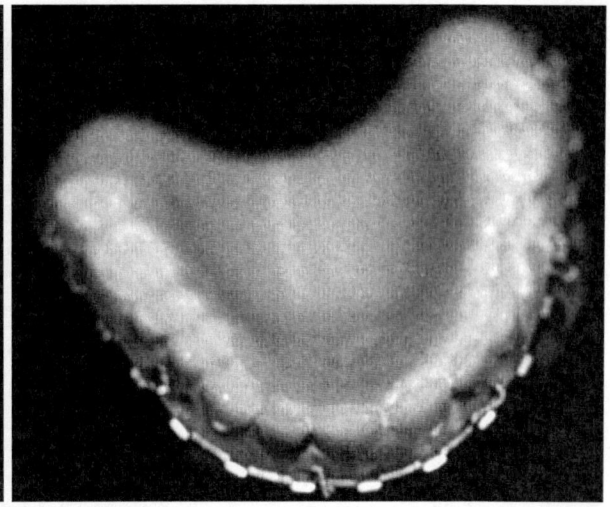

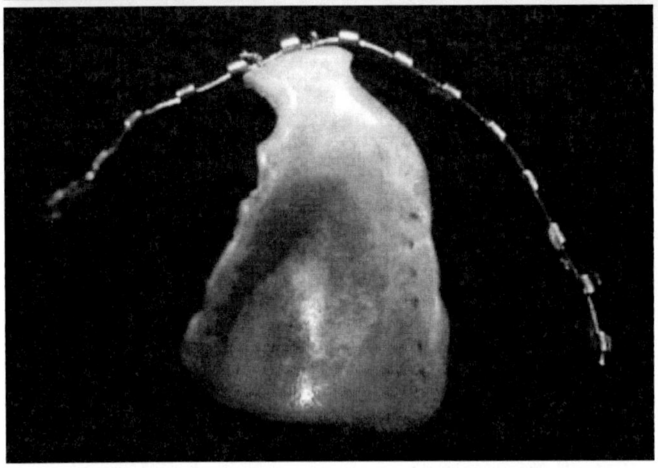

Figs. 35.21 and 35.22 Dentures used to reestablish the pretraumatic centric occlusion of the dental arches

Index

P.J. Taub et al. (eds.), *Ferraro's Fundamentals of Maxillofacial Surgery*,
DOI 10.1007/978-1-4614-8341-0, © Springer Science+Business Media New York 2015

N

R

MIX
Papier aus verantwortungsvollen Quellen
Paper from responsible sources
FSC® C105338

Printed by Books on Demand, Germany